# Ham's Primary Care Geriatrics

# Ham's Primary Care Geriatrics

## A Case-Based Approach

7TH EDITION

**Gregg A. Warshaw, MD**

Professor of Family Medicine
Professor of Internal Medicine (Geriatrics Division)
School of Medicine
The University of North Carolina
Chapel Hill, North Carolina

Professor Emeritus of Family and Community Medicine
Professor Emeritus of Geriatric Medicine
College of Medicine
University of Cincinnati
Cincinnati, Ohio

**Jane F. Potter, MD**

Professor of Geriatric Medicine
Division of Geriatrics, Gerontology and Palliative Care
Department of Internal Medicine
University of Nebraska Medical Center
Home Instead Center for Successful Aging
Omaha, Nebraska

**Ellen Flaherty, PhD, APRN, AGSF**

Director, Dartmouth Centers for Health and Aging
Geisel School of Medicine at Dartmouth
Section of General Internal Medicine-Geriatrics
Lebanon, New Hampshire

**Mitchell T. Heflin, MD, MHS**

Professor of Medicine
Division of Geriatrics
Department of Medicine
Associate Dean and Director
Duke Health Center for Interprofessional Education and Care
Duke University Schools of Medicine and Nursing
Durham, North Carolina

**Matthew K. McNabney, MD**

Associate Professor of Medicine
Division of Geriatric Medicine and Gerontology
Johns Hopkins University School of Medicine
Baltimore, Maryland

**Richard J. Ham, MD, MRCGP**

Director, WVU Center on Aging (Retired)
Professor of Geriatric Medicine and Psychiatry (Retired)
Robert C. Byrd Health Sciences Center
West Virginia University
Morgantown, West Virginia

ELSEVIER

Elsevier
1600 John F. Kennedy Blvd.
Ste 1800
Philadelphia, PA 19103-2899

HAM'S PRIMARY CARE GERIATRICS, SEVENTH EDITION

ISBN: 978-0-323-721684

Previous editions copyrighted © 2014 by Saunders, an imprint of Elsevier Inc.
Copyright © 2007, 2002, 1997, 1992 by Mosby, an imprint of Elsevier Inc.
First Edition, 1983, published simultaneously by John Wright & PSG, Inc.

**Library of Congress Control Number 2020941969**

*Content Strategist:* Charlotta Kryhl
*Content Development Specialist:* Deborah Poulson
*Publishing Services Manager:* Shereen Jameel
*Project Manager:* Rukmani Krishnan
*Design Direction:* Brian Salisbury

Printed in India

Last digit is the print number:  9  8  7  6  5  4  3

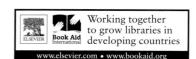

*For Elise, Laura, August, and Alice.*

**GAW**


*To the patients who are my best teachers, to colleagues at the American Geriatrics Society whose energy around patient-centered care inspires me, and my family for their love and support.*

**JFP**


*To my amazing Mom, Ellen Antell, who exemplifies dynamic, graceful aging. Her legacy of nursing, through her daughters and granddaughters, inspires me every day.*

**EF**


*To my wife, Deanna Kay Branscom, MD, the* real *doctor in the family, whose patience and love make all things possible.*

**MH**


*To older adults around the world who have taught me so much over the years, and to my incredible family who are my inspiration for all things.*

**MM**


*In honor of my son Gabriel Ham from whom, as I write this in the late Spring 2020, I have been quarantined for 2 months because he has been nursing COVID-19 victims at a University Hospital. He and all his fellow nurses and therapists are often closer, for longer intervals, to those suffering from this modern plague than their physician colleagues. We hope and pray that they all stayed safe and were reunited with their families and friends.*

**RJH**

**My thoughts on old age . . .**

*A gift for old age is to be able to delight in comfort.*
*Bed, bath, food, drink. To enjoy the simple and immediate.*

*Acknowledge one's disabilities—then try to forget them.*
**Eileen M. Ham (1920-2001)**


*"I feel like my brain is full of tiny drawers, and this little man is running around opening*
*drawers trying to find the thing that I'm trying to remember."*

*"Everybody's in a hurry these days, except old folks."*

*"Getting old sounds like an accomplishment. But it's not, because the last few years all you do*
*is sit around."*

*"I'm not like I used to be, but then again, who is?"*
**Quotes from Grace Heddesheimer (1911-2009) on aging**

# List of Contributors

**Peter Abadir, MD**
Associate Professor of Medicine
Division of Geriatric Medicine and Gerontology
John Hopkins University School of Medicine
Baltimore, Maryland

**Omair H. Abbasi, MD**
Director of Medical Student Education in Behavioral
Health
Assistant Professor, Clinical Sciences
Dr. Kiran C. Patel College of Allopathic Medicine
Nova Southeastern University
Fort Lauderdale, Florida

**Kathleen M. Akgün, MD, MS**
Associate Professor
Department of Internal Medicine
Yale University School of Medicine
New Haven, CT and VA-Connecticut Healthcare System
West Haven, Connecticut

**Robert S. Anderson Jr., MD**
Assistant Professor
Tufts University School of Medicine
Departments of Emergency Medicine and
Internal Medicine
Maine Medical Center
Portland, Maine

**Andrew Artz, MD, MS**
Associate Clinical Professor in Hematology
Director of the Program for Aging and Blood Cancer
City of Hope National Medical Center
Comprehensive Cancer Center
Duarte, California

**Judith L. Beizer, PharmD, BCGP**
Clinical Professor
Department of Clinical Health Professions
St. John's University College of Pharmacy and Health
Sciences
Queens, New York

**Johanna L. Beliveau, BSN, MBA, RN**
President and Chief Executive Officer
Visiting Nurse and Hospice for Vermont and New Hampshire
White River Junction, Vermont

**Christopher R. Bernheisel, MD**
Interim Chair
Fred Lazarus Jr Professor of Family Medicine
Department of Family & Community Medicine
University of Cincinnati
Cincinnati, Ohio

**Karina I. Bishop, MD, CMD**
Assistant Professor, Geriatric Medicine
Division of Geriatrics, Gerontology and Palliative Care
University of Nebraska Medical Center
Omaha, Nebraska

**Stephen J. Bonasera, MD, PhD**
Associate Professor of Medicine
Division of Geriatrics, Gerontology, and Palliative Medicine
University of Nebraska Medical Center
Omaha, Nebraska
and
Director, Home-Based Primary Care
Nebraska/Western Iowa Veteran's Affairs Medical Center
Omaha, Nebraska

**Suzanne F. Bradley, MD**
Professor
Internal Medicine, Infectious Disease
Department of Internal Medicine
University of Michigan Medical School
Research Scientist
VA Ann Arbor GRECC Program
VA Ann Arbor Healthcare System
Ann Arbor, Michigan

**Mallory McClester Brown, MD**
Assistant Professor
Department of Family Medicine
University of North Carolina
Chapel Hill, North Carolina

**Gwendolen T. Buhr, MD, MHS, MEd, CMD**
Duke University Medical Center
Duke Center for the Study of Aging and Human Development
Durham, North Carolina

**Christina Bungo, DO**
Director of Geriatrics
VA Outpatient Clinic
Jacksonville, Florida

**William J. Burke, MD**
Director
Stead Family Memory Center
Banner Alzheimer's Institute
Research Professor
Department of Psychiatry
University of Arizona College of Medicine
Phoenix, Arizona

**Carl Burton, MD**
Clinical Instructor of Medicine
UCLA Geriatric Medicine
David Geffen School of Medicine
Los Angeles, California

**Julie P.W. Bynum, MD, MPH**
Margaret Terpenning Collegiate Professor of Internal Medicine
Professor, Geriatric and Palliative Medicine
University of Michigan Medical School
Ann Arbor, Michigan

**Marco A. Gonzalez Castellon, MD**
Assistant Professor
Department of Neurological Sciences
Medical Director, Nebraska Medicine Telestroke Network
Program Director, UNMC Vascular Neurology Fellowship
University of Nebraska Medical Center
Omaha, Nebraska

**E-Shien Chang, PhD**
Department of Social and Behavioral Sciences
Yale School of Public Health
Yale University
New Haven, Connecticut

**Martha C. Coates, MSN, CRNP, AGPCNP-BC**
Doctoral Nursing Research Fellow
College of Nursing and Health Professions
Drexel University
Philadelphia, Pennsylvania

**Benjamin S. Cooley, MD**
Assistant Professor of Clinical Psychiatry
Indiana University School of Medicine
Indianapolis, Indiana

**Rebecca S. Crow, DO**
Assistant Professor of Medicine
Geisel School of Medicine
U.S. Department of Veterans Affairs Medical Center
Department of Geriatrics and Extended Care
White River Junction, Vermont

**Amelia Cullinan, MD**
Director, Outpatient Palliative Care Services
Assistant Professor
Geisel School of Medicine
Dartmouth-Hitchcock Medical Center
Lebanon, New Hampshire

**Rose Ann DiMaria-Ghalili, PhD, RN, CNSC, FASPEN, FAAN, FGSA**
Professor and Assistant Dean
College of Nursing and Health Professions
Drexel University
Philadelphia, Pennsylvania

**Peter R. DiMilia, MPH**
Research Project Manager
Department of Community and Family Medicine
Dartmouth-Hitchcock Medical Center
Lebanon, New Hampshire

**Brittany M. Dixon, MD**
Cardiology Fellow
Cardiovascular Division, Department of Medicine
Washington University School of Medicine
St. Louis, Missouri

**XinQi Dong, MD, MPH**
Henry Rutgers Professor
Director, Institute for Health Care Policy and Aging Research
Rutgers, The State University of New Jersey
New Brunswick, New Jersey

**Georgia Dounis, DDS, MS**
Professor, Clinical Sciences
School of Dental Medicine
University of Nevada
Las Vegas, Nevada

**Kiki Dounis, DDS, MS**
Adjunct Professor
School of Medicine
University of Nevada, Las Vegas
Las Vegas, Nevada

**Catherine E. DuBeau, MD**
Professor of Medicine
Section of General Internal Medicine—Geriatrics
Department of Medicine
Dartmouth-Hitchcock Medical Center
Lebanon, New Hampshire

**Justin Endo, MD, MHPE, FAAD**
Associate Professor
Department of Dermatology
University of Wisconsin-Madison
Madison, Wisconsin

**Manuel A. Eskildsen, MD, MPH, CMD**
Associate Clinical Professor
UCLA Geriatric Medicine
David Geffen School of Medicine
Los Angeles, California

**Gina S. Fernandez, MD**
Assistant Professor of Medicine
Department of Medicine Dartmouth-Hitchcock Medical
Center
Lebanon, New Hampshire

**Michael Fingerhood, MD**
Associate Professor of Medicine
Director, Division of Addiction Medicine
The Johns Hopkins University
Baltimore, Maryland

**Alfred L. Fisher, MD, PhD**
Neumann M. and Mildred E. Harris Professor of Geriatrics
Chief, Division of Geriatrics, Gerontology and Palliative
Medicine
University of Nebraska Medical Center
Omaha, Nebraska

**Ellen Flaherty, PhD, APRN, AGSF**
Director, Dartmouth Centers for Health and Aging
Geisel School of Medicine at Dartmouth
Section of General Internal Medicine-Geriatrics
Lebanon, New Hampshire

**Aimée D. Garcia, MD**
Associate Professor of Medicine
Baylor College of Medicine
Houston, Texas

**S. Michael Gharacholou, MD, MSc**
Associate Professor of Medicine
Division of Cardiology
Mayo Clinic
Jacksonville, Florida

**Deepta A. Ghate, MD**
Associate Professor
Department of Ophthalmology
University of Nebraska Medical Center
Stanley M. Truhlsen Eye Institute
Omaha, Nebraska

**Danielle Goldfarb, MD**
Neurologist/Psychiatrist, Banner Sun Health Research Institute
Suncity, Arizona
Assistant Professor of Neurology and Psychiatry
University of Arizona College of Medicine
Phoenix, Arizona

**Lisa J. Granville, MD**
Professor and Associate Chair
Department of Geriatrics
The Florida State University College of Medicine
Tallahassee, Florida

**Karen Halpert, MD**
Assistant Professor
Department of Family Medicine
University of North Carolina
Chapel Hill, North Carolina

**Richard J. Ham, MD, MRCGP**
Director, WVU Center on Aging (Retired)
Professor of Geriatric Medicine and
Psychiatry (Retired)
Robert C. Byrd Health Sciences Center
West Virginia University
Morgantown, West Virginia

**Dong-Hun Han, DDS, PhD**
Vice Chair, Institute for Global Social Responsibility
Professor, School of Dentistry
Chairperson, Department of Preventive & Public Health Dentistry
Seoul National University
Seoul, Korea

**Elizabeth N. Harlow, MD**
Associate Professor, Geriatric Medicine
Division of Geriatrics, Gerontology and Palliative Care
University of Nebraska Medical Center
Omaha, Nebraska

**Mitchell T. Heflin, MD, MHS**
Professor of Medicine
Division of Geriatrics, Department of Medicine
Associate Dean and Director, Duke Health Center for
Interprofessional Education and Care
Duke University Schools of Medicine and Nursing
Durham, North Carolina

**Joseph Hejkal, MD**
Assistant Professor, Internal Medicine
University of Nebraska Medical Center
Omaha, Nebraska

**Arthur E. Helfand, DPM**
Professor Emeritus, Temple University School of Podiatric Medicine
Retired Chair, Department of Community Health and Aging,
Temple University, School of Podiatric Medicine
Narberth, Pennsylvania

**Margaret R. Helton, MD**
Professor
Department of Family Medicine
University of North Carolina
Chapel Hill, North Carolina

**Geoffrey J. Hoffman, PhD, MPH**
Assistant Professor
Department of Systems, Populations and Leadership
University of Michigan School of Nursing
Ann Arbor, Michigan

**Peter A. Hollmann, MD**
Chief Medial Officer
Brown Medicine
Providence, Rhode Island

**Gregory J. Hughes, PharmD, BCPS, BCGP**
Associate Clinical Professor
Department of Clinical Health Professions
St. John's University College of Pharmacy and Health Sciences
Queens, New York
and
Assistant Professor
Department of Medicine
Donald and Barbara Zucker School of Medicine at Hofstra/Northwell
Hempstead, New York

**Jessie Jenkins, MD**
Assistant Professor
Division of Geriatrics, Gerontology and Palliative Care and
Section of Hospital Medicine
Department of Internal Medicine
University of Nebraska Medical Center
Omaha, Nebraska

**Jason M. Johanning, MD**
Professor
Department of Surgery
Division of Vascular Surgery
University of Nebraska Medical Center
Omaha, Nebraska

**Philip O. Katz, MD**
Professor of Medicine
Director of Motility Laboratories
Jay Monahan Center for Gastrointestinal Health
Weill Cornell Medical College
New York, New York

**Babar A. Khan, MD, MS**
Associate Director and Research Scientist
Indiana University Center for Aging Research at Regenstrief
Institute
Associate Professor of Medicine
Indiana University School of Medicine
Indianapolis, Indiana

**Soo Kim, PhD**
Assistant Professor
Journalism and Media Studies
University of Nevada, Las Vegas
Las Vegas, Nevada

**Wanda Cook Lakey, MD, MHS**
Division of Endocrinology
Metabolism, and Nutrition
Department of Medicine
Duke University School of Medicine
Durham, North Carolina

**Richard Hsang-Young Lee, MD**
Assistant Professor
Division of Endocrinology, Metabolism, and Nutrition
Department of Medicine, Duke University School of Medicine
Durham, North Carolina

**Susan W. Lehmann, MD**
Director, Geriatric Psychiatry Day Hospital Program
Associate Professor of Psychiatry
Johns Hopkins University
Baltimore, Maryland

**Mengting Li, PhD**
Assistant Professor
School of Nursing and Institute for Health
Health Care Policy and Aging Research, Rutgers
The State University of New Jersey
New Brunswick, New Jersey

**William Lyons, MD**
Professor
Division of Geriatrics, Gerontology and Palliative Care
Department of Internal Medicine
University of Nebraska Medical Center
Omaha, Nebraska

**Phillip D. Magidson, MD, MPH**
Assistant Professor
Department of Emergency Medicine
Division of Geriatric Medicine and Gerontology
Johns Hopkins University School of Medicine
Baltimore, Maryland

**Una E. Makris, MD, Msc**
Associate Professor of Medicine
UT Southwestern Medical Center Department of Internal Medicine
Division of Rheumatic Diseases
Dallas, Texas

**Natalie A. Manley, MD, MPH**
Assistant Professor
Department of Internal Medicine
Division of Geriatrics, Gerontology, and Palliative Medicine
University of Nebraska Medical Center
Nebraska Medical Center
Omaha, Nebraska

**Alayne D. Markland, DO, MSc**
Associate Professor
Department of Medicine
Division of Gerontology, Geriatrics, and Palliative Care
University of Alabama at Birmingham
Birmingham, Alabama
and
Department of Veterans Affairs
Birmingham/Atlanta Geriatric Research, Education, and Clinical
Center
Birmingham, Alabama

**J. Marvin McBride, MD, MBA**
Assistant Professor
Division of Geriatric Medicine
University of North Carolina
Chapel Hill, North Carolina

**Eleanor McConnell, PhD, RN**
Duke University School of Nursing
Durham, North Carolina
and
Geriatric Research, Education and Clinical Center
Durham Veterans Affairs Health Care System
Durham, North Carolina

**Matthew K. McNabney, MD**
Associate Professor of Medicine
Division of Geriatric Medicine and Gerontology
Johns Hopkins University School of Medicine
Baltimore, Maryland

**Devyani Misra, MD, MS**
Instructor in Medicine
Beth Israel Deaconess Medical Center
Divisions of Geriatrics and Rheumatology
Boston, Massachusetts

**Erik Monson, DPM**
Chief, Division of Podiatry
Director, Podiatric Medicine and Surgery Residency Program
Assistant Professor, Department of Orthopaedics
Ohio State University Wexner Medical Center
Gahanna, Ohio

**Hillary R. Mount, MD**
Associate Professor of Family Medicine
University of Cincinnati College of Medicine
Cincinnati, Ohio

**Thomas Mulligan, MD**
Medical Director, Senior Services, St. Bernards
Health Care
Jonesboro, Arkansas

**Aurelio Muyot, MD**
Assistant Professor
College of Osteopathic Medicine
Touro University Nevada
Henderson, Nevada

**Lauren J. Parker, PhD, MPH**
Assistant Scientist
Department of Health, Behavior, and Society
Johns Hopkins Bloomberg School of Public Health
Baltimore, Maryland

**Margaret A. Pisani, MD, MPH**
Associate Professor
Department of Internal Medicine
Yale University School of Medicine
New Haven, Connecticut

**Alice K. Pomidor, MD, MPH**
Professor
Department of Geriatrics
Florida State University College of Medicine
Tallahassee, Florida

**Jane F. Potter, MD**
Professor of Geriatric Medicine
Division of Geriatrics, Gerontology and Palliative Care
Department of Internal Medicine
University of Nebraska Medical Center
Home Instead Center for Successful Aging
Omaha, Nebraska

**Michaela Preiss, LPN, BS**
Project Coordinator
Dartmouth Centers for Health and Aging
Dartmouth-Hitchcock Health
Lebanon, New Hampshire

**Micah T. Prochaska, MD, MSc, FHM**
Assistant Professor
Department of Medicine, The University of Chicago
Chicago, Illinois

**Michael W. Rich, MD**
Professor of Medicine
Cardiovascular Division, Department of Medicine
Washington University School of Medicine
St. Louis, Missouri

**Carly B. Robbins, DPM**
Fellow
American College of Foot and Ankle Surgeons
Marysville, Ohio

**Jeffrey M. Robbins, DPM**
Fellow American College of Podiatric Medicine
Director Podiatry Service VACO
Director, Preservation of Amputations in Veterans Everywhere
Clinical Assistant Professors, Case Western Reserve University
School of Medicine
Louis Stokes Cleveland VAMC
Cleveland, Ohio

**Miriam B. Rodin, MD, PhD**
Professor of Medicine
Division of Geriatric Medicine
St. Louis University School of Medicine
St. Louis, Missouri

**Jeffrey D. Schlaudecker, MD, MEd, FHM**
Associate Professor of Family & Community Medicine
Kautz Family Foundation Endowed Chair of Geriatric Medical
Education
University of Cincinnati
Cincinnati, Ohio

**Gabrielle Scronce, PT, DPT**
Department of Health Professions
Medical University of South Carolina
Charleston, South Carolina

**Melissa A. Simon, MD, MPH**
George H. Gardner Professor
Department of Obstetrics and Gynecology
Feinberg School of Medicine
Northwestern University
Chicago, Illinois

**Julie Zacharias Simpson, DO**
Assistant Professor
Specialty Medicine Department
Touro University Nevada
Henderson, Nevada

**Amir E. Soumekh, MD**
Assistant Professor of Clinical Medicine
Jay Monahan Center for Gastrointestinal Health
Weill Cornell Medical College
New York, New York

**Daniel Stadler, MD**
Director, Geriatrics
Assistant Professor, Geisel School of Medicine
Dartmouth-Hitchcock Medical Center
Lebanon, New Hampshire

**Monica Stallworth, MD, MPH, MM**
Associate Professor
Department of Family Medicine
Georgetown University School of Medicine
Washington, District of Columbia
and
Faculty
Department of Family and Community Medicine
Penn State College of Medicine
Hershey, Pennsylvania

**Lorraine S. Sease, MD, MSPH**
Assistant Professor
Duke Department of Family Medicine and Community Health
Durham, North Carolina

**Philip D. Sloane, MD, MPH**
Professor
Department of Family Medicine
University of North Carolina
Chapel Hill, North Carolina

**Monica A. Stout, MD**
Advanced Geriatrics Fellow in Wound Care
Baylor College of Medicine
Houston, Texas

**Niharika Suchak, MBBS, MHS**
Associate Professor
Department of Geriatrics
Florida State University College of Medicine
Tallahassee, Florida

**Paul Thananopavarn, MD**
Associate Professor
Department of Physical Medicine and Rehabilitation
University of North Carolina
Chapel Hill, North Carolina

**Jonathan R. Thompson, MD**
Assistant Professor
Department of Surgery
Division of Vascular Surgery
University of Nebraska Medical Center
Omaha, Nebraska

**Roland J. Thorpe Jr, PhD**
Professor
Department of Health, Behavior and Society
Johns Hopkins Bloomberg School of Public Health
Baltimore, Maryland

**Victoria S.T. Tilley, PT, GCS**
Project Facilitator
Center for Aging and Health
University of North Carolina
Chapel Hill, North Carolina
and
ElderFit In Home Rehab-NC
Hillsborough, North Carolina

**Sophia Wang, MD**
Assistant Professor of Clinical Psychiatry
Department of Psychiatry
Indiana University School of Medicine
Indianapolis, Indiana

**Gregg A. Warshaw, MD**
Professor of Family Medicine
Professor of Internal Medicine (Geriatrics Division)
School of Medicine
The University of North Carolina
Chapel Hill, North Carolina
Professor Emeritus of Family and Community Medicine
Professor Emeritus of Geriatric Medicine
College of Medicine
University of Cincinnati
Cincinnati, Ohio

**Heidi K. White, MD, MHS, MEd, CMD**
Duke University Medical Center
Duke Center for the Study of Aging and Human Development
Durham, North Carolina

**E. Foy White-Chu, MD**
Geriatric Fellowship Program Director
Portland VA Medical Center
Oregon Health and Science University (OHSU)
Portland, Oregon

**Sandra M. Winter, PhD, OTR/L**
Research Assistant Scientist
Department of Occupational Therapy
College of Public Health and Health Professions
University of Florida
Gainesville, Florida

**Sara Wolfson, DNP APRN GNP-BC**
Division of Geriatrics, Gerontology and Palliative Care
Home Instead Center for Successful Aging
Nebraska Medical Center
Omaha, Nebraska

**Kahli Zietlow, MD**
Division of Geriatric and Palliative Medicine
Department of Medicine
Michigan Medicine
Ann Arbor, Michigan

**Robert A. Zorowitz, MD, MBA, FACP, AGSF**
Regional Vice President
Health Affairs, for the Northeast Humana, Inc.
New York, New York

# Preface

It is my pleasure to write the preface to the seventh edition of *Ham's Primary Care Geriatrics: A Case-Based Approach*, a book first published in 1983 as a pioneering, case-based textbook on geriatric medicine. Geriatric medicine was not thought of, nor defined, as an American medical specialty at that time.

Conceived from the outset to use the case-based model, this textbook was a project of the American Geriatrics Society (AGS) led by Richard Ham, MD and an AGS advisory group. Dr. Ham, a pioneering academic geriatrician, has been actively involved in each edition of this textbook since that first edition. The sixth edition was dedicated to him for his long-standing commitment to the specialty. The textbook is now known as *Ham's Primary Care Geriatrics*.

The first edition aimed to appeal to and inform any clinician tackling the problems of older adult patients. The intent was to help readers categorize the complex and often ambiguous clinical problems these patients present. The editors and contributors know that the book has been appreciated and that it has a loyal following. Every clinician likes a "good" case, and the book's text is driven by the progress of each case. This method is, after all, the way we learned the art and science of medicine when we were young trainees.

Two additional returning editors have joined Dr. Ham and me to prepare this edition. Jane Potter, MD, Professor of Geriatric Medicine, University of Nebraska, Omaha, and Ellen Flaherty, PhD, APRN, co-director for the Dartmouth Centers for Health and Aging. All four of us are proud to have served as presidents of the AGS. Two outstanding educators have joined us as first-time editors: Mitchell Heflin, MD, and Matthew McNabney, MD. Mitch Heflin is a Professor of Medicine at Duke University and he directs the Duke Geriatric Medicine Fellowship program. Matt McNabney is an Associate Professor of Medicine at The Johns Hopkins University, and he directs the Geriatric Medicine Fellowship program there. Drs. Heflin and McNabney bring exceptional expertise and new perspectives to this edition of our textbook.

Missing from the editorial team for this edition is Philip Sloane, MD, the Goodwin Distinguished Professor in the Department of Family Medicine at the University of North Carolina, Chapel Hill. Phil Sloan retired from his role as an editor for the seventh edition to focus on his wide-ranging research activities. His longstanding contributions to this textbook are, nevertheless, clearly evident in this new edition. Drs. Sloane and Ham together ensured that a second edition of *Primary Care Geriatrics* was published nearly 30 years ago, and they have worked on each subsequent edition. They are the two most important links in the chain of authors and editors who have contributed to this book's success.

Although originally designed with the primary care physician in mind, this book is useful to any health professional who provides primary care services to older patients. In addition, all clinicians with adult patients, even clinicians in the subspecialties, regularly care for older patients and must be able to recognize and refer problems, such as early dementia, increased fall risk, and polypharmacy.

All the chapters in this edition have been updated to current evidenced-based practice. There are many new cases, and more than one-third of the chapters have been written by new authors. Topics included in the expanded content are integrative medicine, opioid management, gastroenterology, and—for the first time—a chapter on the care of older lesbian, gay, bisexual, and transgender adults.

Chapter questions, and all the references for each chapter, are now included on Expert Consult. (See the inside cover for details on how to access this content online.) Each chapter in the book cites the references numerically, but only Key References are listed at the end of chapters in the printed version. In many chapters, Web resources with suggested readings or Web guidelines are included at the end of the chapter. A dermatology quiz and a dizziness assessment video guide are included only on Expert Consult.

An outline of the basic format of the book follows:

- Three units: Principles and Practice; Geriatric Syndromes and Common Special Problems; and Selected Clinical Problems of the Organ Systems.
- Each clinical chapter has core text with the following subheadings to assist readers when using the text for reference: Prevalence and Impact; Risk Factors and Pathophysiology; Differential Diagnosis and Assessment; Management; and Summary.
- In all but a few chapters, cases and case discussions (generally in several numbered parts and set in a font that differs from that used in the core text) are interspersed within the text at appropriate points. Although the case and its discussion illustrate the text and show the text "in action," the text itself stands alone. With few exceptions, all the core information—as in a conventional textbook—is in the text itself.

The editors wish to thank the excellent Elsevier team for their investment in this textbook. Once again, they have provided superb editorial support and a pleasing layout for our rather complicated format.

It is a privilege to practice medicine. For many, practicing primary care geriatrics is especially rewarding. Our patients trust us to look after their health and to hear their stories, to learn how they came to be the people they are now. I hope this book will assist you as you care for your older patients.

*Gregg Warshaw, MD*
*Chapel Hill, North Carolina*

# Acknowledgments

I wish to acknowledge my colleagues at the University of Cincinnati and the University of North Carolina — Chapel Hill for their inspiring dedication to improving the health care of older adults.

—*Gregg A. Warshaw*

Thanks to all the contributing authors who made this an enjoyable learning opportunity for me and who made the whole process a joy. Also to the faculty at the University of Nebraska Medical Center who agreed to contribute updated chapters and those who joined the project for this edition.

—*Jane F. Potter*

In gratitude to all the patients and families who inspire me to humbly practice nursing. None of my work would be possible without the love and support of my husband Mel Aaron, our children, and the entire team at the Dartmouth Centers for Health & Aging.

—*Ellen Flaherty*

I wish to acknowledge all those who inspired me to pursue a career in geriatrics and who, along the way, have taught me the right blend of patience, persistence, and creativity that makes this work so uniquely rewarding. This includes my many teachers, mentors, and colleagues at Duke University and the Durham VA; my students, residents, fellows, and mentees; and generations of older adults, families, and other devoted caregivers.

—*Mitchell T. Heflin*

I would like to thank the older adults and their caregivers who have taught me so much about medicine, as well as the meaning and value of life. I also thank the many incredible mentors and teachers I have had over the years, especially my colleagues at Johns Hopkins University.

—*Matthew K. McNabney*

My heartfelt thanks to Gregg Warshaw who, as I expected, has been a splendid, efficient, patient, and considerate leader of the editorial team. He has remained a good friend over the years in which we have seen many medical advances that have been especially useful in the care of older adults: noninvasive investigations, safer surgery (if well planned!), more specific pharmaceuticals—the list is long. I am truly delighted that Ellen Flaherty and Jane Potter returned to work on this edition. I am thrilled to have had two such committed new editors as Mitch Heflin and Matt McNabney. I can see how much work they have done! It is vital to rewrite and refresh a book for a new edition and they have helped to do just that. I am also very glad that Phil Sloane helped us, too—without him there would not have been a second edition and certainly no seventh! This textbook has been such a large part of my professional life! And thank you so much to everyone at Elsevier, especially Deborah Poulson, Lotta Kryhl, Brooke Kannady, Sarah Barth, and Rukmani Krishnan for their patience, understanding, and skill.

—*Richard J. Ham*

# A Note on Level of Evidence Ratings

Where A through D ratings are used, they correspond (as appropriate) to:

A, Evidence from well-designed metaanalysis, or well-done synthesis reports, such as those for the Agency for Healthcare Policy and Research or the American Geriatrics Society; B, evidence from well-designed controlled trials, both randomized and nonrandomized, with results that consistently support a specific action; C, evidence from observational studies of controlled trials with inconsistent results; D, evidence from expert opinion or multiple case reports.

A, Supported by one or more high-quality randomized trials (RCTs) in an appropriate population, without contradictory evidence from other clinical trials; B, supported by one or more high-quality nonrandomized cohort studies or low-quality RCTs; C, supported by one or more case series and/or poor-quality cohort and/or case-control studies; D, supported by expert opinion and/or extrapolation from studies in other populations and/or settings; X, the preponderance of evidence supports the treatment being ineffective or harmful.

# Contents

## Unit 3: Selected Clinical Problems of the Organ Systems

# Principles and Practice

*An archeologist is the best husband any woman can have; the older she gets, the more interested he is in her.*

**AGATHA CHRISTIE, 1890–1976**

*You know, by the time you reach my age, you've made plenty of mistakes if you've lived your life properly.*

**RONALD REAGAN, 1911–2004, at 86, in The Observer, March 8, 1997**

*I haven't felt this well since I was 70!!*

**A 93-year-old patient (of RH), to her daughter, after she had inflicted extra fluids on her mother for 2 complaining weeks.**

*Oh, to be seventy again!*

**GEORGES CLEMENCEAU,
French statesman, on seeing a pretty young girl
on the Champs-Elysées on his 80th birthday.**

*Being over seventy is like being engaged in a war. All our friends are going or gone and we survive among the dead and dying as on a battlefield.*

**DAME MURIEL SPARK, 1918–2006, in Memento Mori**

*It's not that I'm afraid to die. It's just that I don't want to be there when it happens...*

**WOODY ALLEN, b.1935, in Without Feathers, "Death (A Play)"**

*It is not by muscle, speed or physical dexterity that great things are achieved, but by reflection, force of character, and judgement; in these qualities, old age is not only not poorer, but is even richer.*

**CICERO, 106–43 BC, Roman statesman and orator, in On Old Age, V1**

*A medical revolution has extended the life of our elder citizens without providing the dignity and security those later years deserve.*

**JOHN F KENNEDY,
1917–1963, in his Democratic Party nomination acceptance speech, 1960**

*Optimistic lies have such immense therapeutic value that a doctor who cannot tell them convincingly has mistaken his profession.*

**GEORGE BERNARD SHAW, 1856–1950, in Misalliance, Preface**

*Old men are dangerous; it doesn't matter to them what is going to happen to the world.*

**GEORGE BERNARD SHAW, 1856–1950, in Heartbreak House**

*The key to a long friendship or marriage is a great sense of humour—and a weak memory!*

**JEH, married to RJH for 46 years**

*Old age is not a disease—it is strength and survivorship, triumph over all kinds of vicissitudes and disappointments, trials and illnesses.*

**MAGGIE KUHN, 1905–1995, U.S. activist, founder of the Grey Panthers**

*It is as natural to die as to be born; and to a little infant, perhaps, the one is as painful as the other.*

**FRANCIS BACON, 1561–1626, in Essays, "Of Death"**

*Now more than ever seems it rich to die,*

*To cease upon the midnight with no pain. . ..*

**JOHN KEATS, 1795–1821, in Ode to a Nightingale**

# 1

# Principles of Primary Care of Older Adults

GREGG A. WARSHAW, JANE F. POTTER, ELLEN FLAHERTY, MITCHELL T. HEFLIN, MATTHEW K. MCNABNEY, RICHARD J. HAM, AND PHILIP D. SLOANE

## OUTLINE

*Additional online-only material indicated by icon.*

## OBJECTIVES

*Upon completion of this chapter, the reader will be able to:*

- Describe and identify at least one clinical implication of each of the following key aspects of physiologic aging: the rule of fourths, normal physiologic changes, functional reserve, reduced stamina and fatigue, increased physiologic diversity, the relationship between environment and function, and immobility in older persons.
- Describe and identify at least one clinical implication of each of the following key aspects of psychological aging: looking old but not feeling or thinking old, ageism, life review and adjustment to changes, the activity and disengagement theories of healthy aging, cognitive impairment, and the importance of relationships in older age.
- Describe and identify at least one clinical implication of each of the following key aspects of healthcare provision involving older persons: multiple morbidity, function-oriented care, underreporting of symptoms, iatrogenic disease, deliberate medicine, polypharmacy, the US healthcare system, transitions in care, interprofessional care, and the value of a generalist in primary care geriatrics.

When is a person old? Most people would say 65 years—the age adopted by Germany under landmark legislation introduced by Otto von Bismarck to implement its new social welfare model in the 1880s. The United States later followed this precedent with the Social Security Act of 1935 which established the age of 65 years as appropriate retirement age and was thus considered the "beginning of old age." Ironically, Germany had initially adopted 70 years as the retirement age, lowering it to 65 years in 1916. Now, with increases in life expectancy, many countries are making efforts to raise the retirement age, and we may eventually come full circle.

Of course, the question of how to define *old* often depends on the age of the person you ask. A recent poll of 1000 adults aged ≥ 50 years found that the majority thought middle age began at 55 years and older age at 70 years.[1] In fact, for many persons throughout life, *old* is defined as "somewhat older than I am." Indeed, the feeling that "I'm not old yet" can persist long beyond age 65 years, as many older adults equate "old age" with disability.

Regardless of one's perspective on aging, it is clear the body, mind, and social circumstances change over time, such that people who are older are different from young adults in many ways. These changes affect health risks, health behavior, and healthcare decisions. Therefore health professionals who care for older persons need to understand how older persons differ from younger adults. This chapter provides an overview of the most important principles of aging, beginning with physiologic principles, followed by psychological factors, and then discussion on aging and the healthcare system.

## Aging and the Body

Aging brings about physical and physiologic changes, some of which are universal and many more of which are unique to the individual person. This section highlights some of the key principles of physiologic aging that have therapeutic implications.

## The Rule of Fourths

"Is this a normal part of aging?" Clinicians are frequently asked to answer this question about a new symptom or sign in an older patient. Perhaps the presenting complaint is a problem with memory, possibly an accidental fall. Maybe it is a sore joint, declining vision, or falling asleep during the day.

In the past, medical providers were much more likely to write off symptoms such as these as normal (Box 1.1). In fact, research during recent decades has taught us that much of the disability that we used to attribute to "normal aging" is not normal at all.

One way to think about changes in aging is the *rule of fourths* (Fig. 1.1). This rule clarifies that changes often attributed to normal aging by the general public (and sometimes by medical professionals) are caused by disease, disuse, misuse, and physiology—about one-fourth of the time for each.

*Disease-related disability*, for example, could manifest as decreased exercise tolerance in a chronic smoker with chronic lung disease; *disuse-related disability* as shortness of breath on minimal exertion in a sedentary older person; *misuse-related disability* as knee arthritis in a former football player; and *disability related to physiologic aging* as trouble reading fine print in a 50-year-old.

The job of healthcare providers is to determine whether and to what extent a new symptom is caused by each of these etiologic categories and then develop an appropriate treatment plan.

THE RULE OF FOURTHS

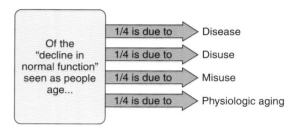

• **Figure 1.1** The rule of fourths. In the past, all of the decline in function that occurs between young adulthood and old age was called normal aging. We now know that approximately one-fourth can be attributed to disease, one-fourth to disuse (e.g., sedentary lifestyle, lack of mental stimulation), and one-fourth to misuse (e.g., smoking, injuries from contact sports, and adverse effects of prescription and/or recreational drugs). Only about one-fourth can be attributed to physiologic aging.

- If the problem is disease, then medical treatment is indicated.
- If the problem is disuse, it can often be cured with an activity regimen.
- If the problem is misuse, prior damage cannot be reversed but steps can be taken to prevent deterioration and to preserve function.
- If the problem is physiologic aging, then steps should be taken to adapt and compensate for the disability.

## Normal Physiologic Changes

Whereas much of the change seen with aging results from causes other than physiologic aging, some changes are inevitable. Table 1.1 lists and describes many common physiologic changes noted with aging. Among the many notable changes are the following:
- The age at which reading glasses are needed because of reduced lens elasticity is between 42 and 50 years.
- Vestibular sensitivity gradually increases until about age 60 years, which is one of the reasons why adults have increasing trouble on amusement park rides as they age.
- Fertility in women peaks between 15 and 25 years and declines thereafter, with menopause typically occurring about age 50 years.
- Reaction time tends to increase with age (which explains why teenagers are usually far better at games of speed—including many video games—than older persons).
- The amount of sway a person will experience if asked to stand still with eyes closed is high in early childhood, is minimized between about ages 15 and 16 years, and then gradually increases beyond age 60 years.

**TABLE 1.1  Some Common Anatomic and Physiologic Changes With Aging (in the Absence of Identified Disease)**

| System or Function Affected | Change Noted |
|---|---|
| **Body composition:** | |
| Percent body water | Decreased |
| Percent body fat | Increased |
| **Brain:** | |
| Weight | Decreases by 7% |
| Anatomy | "Atrophy" commonly noted |
| Sleep patterns | Markedly reduced stage 3 and 4 sleep |
| | More frequent awakenings; reduced sleep efficiency |
| **Vision:** | |
| Lens accommodation | Markedly reduced after age 40–50 years |
| Amount of light reaching the retina | Diminished by up to 70% |
| Color perception | Reduced intensity (especially of blues and greens) |
| Hearing | Acuity declines beginning about age 12 years, with decline steepest in high frequencies (> 5000 Hertz [cycles/second]) |
| **Taste/smell:** | |
| Number of taste buds | Reduced by 70% |
| Changes in preferences | Increased tolerance for very sweet and very salty foods (as a result of reduced perception) |
| **Cardiac function:** | |
| Maximum heart rate | Reduced from about 195 to about 155 beats per minute |
| Reduced cardiac output during stress | Predisposes to heart failure during sepsis, pneumonia, surgery |
| Renal perfusion | Decreased by 50% |
| Bone mineral content | Diminished by 10%–30% |
| Prostate gland anatomy | Size increases by 100% |
| **Sexual function:** | |
| Men | Reduced intensity and persistence of erections; decreased ejaculate and ejaculatory flow |
| Women | Menopause; reduced lubrication; vaginal atrophy |

(Modified from Sloane PD. Normal aging. In: Ham RJ, Sloane PD, Warshaw GA, eds. *Primary Care Geriatrics: A Case-Based Approach.* 4th ed. St. Louis: Mosby-Yearbook; 2002:15–28.)

- Ankle jerk reflexes are increasingly diminished or absent with older age, in the absence of detectable musculoskeletal pathology.
- Bone density plateaus between ages 20 and 50 years, then gradually declines, with the slope of decline being more rapid in women than in men.

The list of physiologic changes with age is long, and the clinical implications vary from merely interesting to very important. Also, the line between "normal physiology" and changes caused by other factors is frequently blurry.

What is important for the clinician to recognize is that aging does result in real, profound changes. Many of these changes cannot be reversed, and the older person will need to make adjustments. An important role of primary care clinicians is therefore to help provide access to the variety of mechanisms that can help compensate for bodily change and preserve function. In addition, the clinician may need to help the patient successfully make changes in goals and lifestyle that will help him or her successfully adjust to aging.

## Functional Reserve

All body systems tend to have functional ability over and above what is used during everyday activities; this is called *functional reserve.* For example, the average adult's cardiac output is around

5 L/min when sedentary, whereas the heart of a trained athlete is capable of generating 40 to 50 L/min.[2] All other key body systems, such as the kidney, the lungs, the liver, and the brain, have reserve capabilities as well, so fairly significant impairment from disease, disuse, misuse, or physiologic aging is needed to result in impaired function during normal activity.

Clinically significant impairment in function occurs when demands exceed functional reserve. As people age, patterns of disease, disuse, misuse, and physiologic aging combine to decrease functional reserve. Among the losses in functional reserve that have particularly common implications in geriatric care include the following clinical situations:

- Delirium is common in postoperative older persons, because brain functional reserve capacity is overwhelmed by the stress of the surgery and the persistence of anesthetic agents in the central nervous system and the bloodstream.
- Nocturia is almost ubiquitous in older persons, largely because of changes in bladder physiology (decreased capacity and increased residual volume) combined with altered control of fluid excretion (related to low nighttime antidiuretic hormone levels and increased nighttime natriuretic polypeptide levels).
- An older person will often fall when a younger person would not, because neuromuscular mechanisms to reestablish

equilibrium from a minor perturbation (e.g., tripping on the edge of a rug) are impaired, often by a combination of disuse and normal aging changes in nerve conduction and vibratory sensation in the feet

When functional reserve is impaired, the clinician should work with the patient to explore ways to improve this capacity and thereby to improve function. For a patient with chronic obstructive pulmonary disease, for example, solutions include continuous low-flow oxygen and pulmonary rehabilitation exercises. For a patient with impaired brain reserve, minimizing sedating and anticholinergic medications is often the best approach.

## Reduced Stamina and Fatigue

One of the inescapable physiologic declines with aging is reduced stamina. Beginning in one's 20s and terminating in advanced age, an insidious reduction in stamina occurs (Fig. 1.2). Of course, this gradual decline in stamina and increased fatigue can be accelerated by disease, disuse, and misuse; however, gradual decrease in stamina and need for more frequent rest is a universal phenomenon as one ages. Therefore medical interns in their 20s can pull an all-night shift much more easily than they would be able to if asked to follow the same schedule when in their 50s.

When reduced stamina and fatigue are so great that they become the defining feature of one's physiologic status, we refer to this as *frailty*. Fried et al. developed an evidence-based definition of frailty, which aids in the assessment of older adults defining *frailty* as the occurrence of three or more of the following: unintentional weight loss (10 lbs. in past year), self-reported exhaustion, weakness (reduced grip strength), slow walking speed, and low physical

activity.[3] One can see that all but the first of these criteria are manifestations of reduced stamina and fatigue. Frailty is a common and important geriatric syndrome (see Ch. 29).

## Increased Physiologic Diversity

Another characteristic of aging is physiologic diversity increases. Indeed, the range of "normal" (i.e., the range that encompasses the performance of 95% of people) becomes increasingly wide as populations age. When we say, for example, "Jason is a normal 5-year-old child," we have a pretty good idea what Jason can and cannot do. The same is also generally true at age 20 years. However, with each advancing decade the range of normality becomes wider (Fig. 1.3), to the point that saying, "George is a normal 75-year-old man," tells you practically nothing about George other than how long ago he was born.

This increased diversity with age has many clinical implications. For example, it is easy to develop age-related guidelines for children, because, except in rare cases of chronic or developmental illness, age predicts performance in children. In older adults, however, age is not very helpful in determining healthcare norms or needs, and age-related protocols and guidelines are less helpful. The clinician must individualize most aspects of assessment, goal setting, and care planning.

❖ **Because of increasing diversity with age, protocols and guidelines are less useful in geriatric care than for younger ages, and care must be individualized.**

## Environment and Function

An often-unappreciated aspect of aging is the importance of the environment in which an older person is asked to live and function. Indeed, the environment within which one lives and functions can make the difference between being independent and being unable to carry out basic everyday activities.

In healthcare, it is useful to think about three distinctive types of environments: the physical, the social, and the organizational environment.[4] The physical environment refers to the physical setting in which a patient lives; it includes such things as size and decor of spaces, lighting, temperature, acoustic properties, and access to outdoors. The social (caregiving) environment refers to the people who

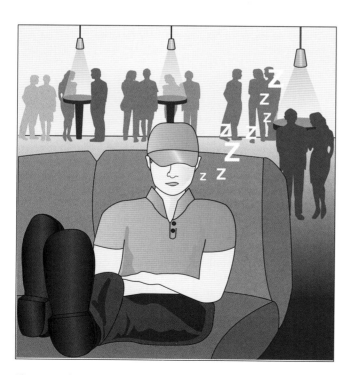

• **Figure 1.2** Inability to party all night is one of the earliest signs of aging. With increasing age and disability, diminished stamina can progress to the point where the older person no longer has enough energy to complete the necessary activities of daily living. This severe fatigue is the cardinal symptom of the frailty syndrome.

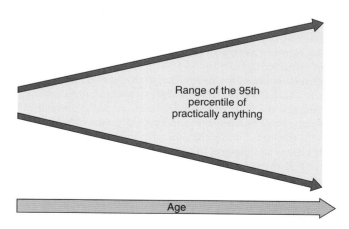

• **Figure 1.3** As people age they become more diverse. This explains why individualized care rather than protocol-based care is especially important in the geriatric population.

interact directly with the patient—how they approach the person and what they do. The organizational environment refers to rules and regulations that affect a patient's life (especially in licensed facilities such as nursing homes), such as when they can eat, whether and how they can go outdoors, and what type and amount of services they receive. Needless to say, these environmental characteristics can have a huge impact not only on function but also on quality of life for a dependent older person.

The design of living units can greatly influence an older adult's independence. Fortunately, with the aging of the population has come increased interest in housing design features that make it easier for persons who have a variety of disabilities to function. For example:

- Doorknobs that are levers can markedly improve ease of door use for persons with arthritis.
- Widened doorways can permit entry for persons in wheelchairs.
- Motion sensors that turn on lighting can help prevent falls at night among cognitively or physically impaired older persons.

Universal design is an approach to designing products and environments to be appropriate for all people, including those with physiologic, cognitive, or sensory impairments. A movement to improve the usability of housing for older adults and persons with disabilities is called *visitable housing*. The goal of the visitable housing movement is to have all housing units built in such a way as they can be visited by people with disabilities, which includes many older adults. Visitable housing includes these three basic features: at least one no-step entrance, doors and hallways that are wide enough to navigate through in a wheelchair or walker, and a bathroom on the first floor big enough to get into in a wheelchair and close the door.[5]

## Immobility

A common case scenario: An 80-year-old woman has an episode of dizziness, for unclear reasons, and her daughter encourages her to go to bed. The family mobilizes to help her; a bedside commode is brought in, and she is encouraged to "relax and get better." Nearly a week passes with family attending to her every need. She feels better and decides to join the family for dinner and falls on the way to the table.

Her postural reflexes have been blunted by a week in bed, and her blood pressure drops when she stands up. "Don't hurt yourself," the daughter says. "We'll bring your dinner, and you can eat in bed." As a result of these good intentions to "help" her during this time, the woman never walks again.

This scenario happens all too frequently. Older persons need to move it or lose it, but well-meaning caregivers may overcompensate in providing total care and the result is permanent disability.

Numerous studies have verified that immobility is bad for older persons. Among younger adults, a week in bed in the hospital is like adding 10 years to your age. Among older persons, extended immobility is often the end of ambulation.

Wheelchairs present a particular problem. They are useful for transportation, making it easier for disabled persons to get around, but they increase the risk for many medical complications and adverse events, which they share with overall sedentary existence. Among these complications are muscle atrophy, constipation, pressure sores, urinary tract infections (caused in part by bladder outlet obstruction from constipation), decreased involvement in activities, and increased risk of radial nerve palsy.[6,7]

In summary, the physiologic changes of normal aging mean that older persons are at a heightened risk for a permanent loss of function if they are kept immobilized in bed or in a wheelchair for as little as a few days. So as soon as older persons can get up, they should be encouraged to get up and if older persons can still walk independently, or with some assistance, they should walk. For older persons, the well-known statement, "Use it or lose it," could be extended to, "Use it or lose everything."

## Aging and the Mind

Health professionals, especially younger persons who have little firsthand experience with the emotional aspects of aging, often underappreciate psychological aspects of aging. Yet identifying and addressing these factors is often the most important aspect of an encounter with an older person. This section introduces a few key neurologic and psychological issues that are common in geriatric medicine, many of which are discussed in greater detail in subsequent chapters.

### Looking Old but Not Feeling or Thinking Old

It is common for older persons to say, "I don't feel old." In doing so, they are reflecting a very prevalent feeling among persons of "geriatric" age—that they have energy and interests that are not different from those of many younger adults.

In fact, the characteristics that health professionals most associate with older adults—aging, disease, and disability—are rarely foremost in the minds of older persons. Instead, they are more often concerned with personal finances, family problems, national politics, world events, issues in the community, the health of a pet, or other areas of personal interest. Furthermore, the common belief that older persons are interested only in themselves is just not true. Older persons are often among the most active and vocal supporters of such issues as environmental preservation, quality education, and help for disadvantaged persons.

### Ageism

One reality that confronts older persons repeatedly is the ubiquity of ageism in society. *Ageism* can be defined as the systematic stereotyping of and discrimination against people because they are old. The reasons for societal ageism are numerous and have their origins in older persons as well as younger ones. Studies have verified that older persons often have negative attitudes toward people in their own age group, particularly if they have an aging-related condition or disability, such as slow walking speed (or driving speed), impaired hearing, or cognitive impairment.[8] Ageism is not only pervasive; it can also lower self-esteem, reduce opportunities, and lead to isolation, loneliness, and depression.

The following are a few of the many examples of how ageism is perpetuated in society:

- Older persons who are out of work have greater difficulty reentering the workforce than younger persons, and opportunities for meaningful engagement in part-time work for older persons are limited in today's society.
- Images of older adults in popular media, including print publications and television, often depict them as infirm and objects of pity or ridicule.
- The language used to describe the population growth among older adults often has negative connotations, including terms such as "graying of America" or "silver tsunami." In addition, broad descriptors such as "the elderly" or "seniors" imply that older adults are a homogeneously frail sector of the population.

Ideas for counteracting ageism include adopting language and images to more regularly include depictions of most older adults who are, in fact, highly engaged and capable of continuing contributions to society. More information about "reframing" aging is available online.[9]

In medical practice, ageism is also a major concern. A study revealed that one in five older adults reported some form of age-based discrimination in a healthcare setting.[10] For example, health professionals may assume that their older patients are incapable of accurately or effectively communicating their needs and may be more likely to ignore or dismiss complaints such as memory concerns, gait instability, or chronic pain. Although decisions to withhold care based on age have been increasingly challenged in recent years, rates of application of lifesaving interventions, such as cardiovascular procedures and organ transplantation, continue to decline with increasing age; when resources are limited, youth is prioritized.[11] Through a shared decision-making process using an individualized assessment of risk and benefit that accounts for factors other than age, such as comorbidity and function, primary care providers can discern which of their older patients actually stand to benefit from more aggressive care and advocate for them. It is true that behind many ageist notions is more than a grain of truth. As people age, they do change, often insidiously losing capability to optimally perform. A surgeon described his experience with this process in an essay published in *The Journal of the American Medical Association*, in 1983. At 67 years, he thought that he was performing as well as ever, but a couple of small lapses, both easily correctable without any adverse impact on patient care, raised his concerns about his own ability to operate. "I began to inspect the anesthesiologists' charts," he wrote. "I noticed that my operating times had moved from 50 to 60 minutes, and then over a period of 1 year to about 70 to 80 minutes—always for the same procedure." Because longer operating times are associated with increased risk of adverse outcomes, he decided that it was time for him to retire.[12]

◆◆ **Ageism can lower self-esteem, reduce opportunities, and lead to isolation, loneliness, and depression.**

## Life Review and Adjustment to One's Changing Life Status

The story of the surgeon who decided to retire provides an excellent example of our next principle of aging—that the aging process involves active reflection on one's life (life review) and that the changing nature of one's physical state necessitates psychological adjustment. The surgeon we discussed in the previous section had to, as he put it, "kneel at the grave of memories," reflecting on what he had accomplished and what he wished he had accomplished. "All of a sudden you are in an unfamiliar, ill-defined world," he wrote.

Adjusting to losses is a key element of successful aging—loss of one's role as a worker through elective or forced retirement; diminished physical strength and stamina; reductions in vision and hearing; impaired or lost sexual capability; loss of a sense of physical attractiveness; death or disability of a spouse, of siblings, and/or of close friends; the sadness of saying good-bye to the home that houses memories of children; and the loss of vigorous independence. In addition, as one progresses through the decades, the horizon of one's future becomes increasingly limited; hopes and dreams become increasingly replaced by memories.

All this requires continual psychological adjustment, and a key part of this process is life review. This process of adjustment to one's changing life status is gradual; it begins in middle age, with the "midlife crisis" often representing initial awareness of the finiteness of life. During older age, key elements of successful psychological adjustment include developing a sense of satisfaction with one's accomplishments; enjoying the advantages that come with being older, such as time with grandchildren, a slower pace to life, and more ability to choose how one spends time; and developing a new sense of both serenity with and ability to enjoy each day as it comes. This process usually is successful and explains why happiness increases with age and persists throughout most of the geriatric years, only fading when chronic illness, disability, and pain take over.[13]

## Activity Versus Disengagement

In the 1950s and early 1960s, gerontologists disagreed as to which psychological approach to aging was healthier. Many endorsed the *disengagement theory*, who posited that letting go of the trappings of earlier life was the key to successful aging. The icon of this theory was an old man in a rocking chair on the front porch. Other gerontologists were advocates of the *activity theory*, who believed that staying active and engaged was the key to healthy aging. Their icons were people who some referred to as representatives of *exceptional aging*, people like Pablo Casals, who in his 90s was still actively performing as a musician.

As the data came in, it became clear that activity and engagement are healthier for most older persons than disengagement. That is, of course, provided the individual is realistic and makes the needed adjustments to losses and changing life circumstances discussed in the previous section.

Unfortunately, the retirement industry was founded based on the disengagement theory and has been slow to adjust. The developers of Sun City, Arizona—the prototypical retirement community on which thousands of others were subsequently modeled—hired gerontologists who were proponents of disengagement.[14] This led to creation of communities prohibiting adult residents younger than 55 years (and children), focused on leisure activities, such as golf and shuffleboard, and encouraged the attitude, "You've worked hard; you deserve to relax."

Attitudes are, however, beginning to change, but they still have a long way to go. To promote healthy engagement in late life, more work opportunities need to be created for older adults that are interesting, part time, flexible, and adapted to promote continued productive engagement. More older persons need to be engaged as volunteers and entrepreneurs; and older adults need more opportunities to be integrated into the rest of society. Such developments are consistent with current theories of "successful aging" and may well keep older adults in the workforce and volunteer service longer, providing a clear benefit to broader society.[15]

## Cognitive Impairment and Worry

Cognitive impairment is a central concern of healthcare providers and older persons. Indeed, dementia or worry about memory is the reason for nearly 50% of consultations to geriatric assessment clinics, and dementia is the most common reason for nursing home placement. Because the prevalence of dementia is strongly correlated with age, the increasing life expectancy of today and tomorrow's older adults means that increasingly more persons are likely to have dementia.

Worry about memory is ubiquitous among older persons. BF Skinner, in an address to the American Psychological Association when he was 78 years old, described some of his experiences:

*Forgetting is a classical problem. It is most conspicuous in forgetting names because names have so little going for them by way of context. . . . When I have time—and I mean something on the order of half an hour—I can almost always recall a name. . . . But that will not work in introducing your wife to someone whose name you have forgotten. My wife and I use the following strategy: if there is any conceivable chance that she could have met the person, I simply say to her, "of course, you remember . . .?" and she grasps the outstretched hand and says, "Yes, of course. How are you?" The acquaintance may not remember meeting my wife but is not sure of his or her memory either.[16]*

At the time that Dr. Skinner delivered his address, what he was describing would have been termed "benign senescent forgetfulness" and unequivocally distinguished from "dementia." Over the past couple of decades, however, the lines between normal and abnormal cognition have become increasingly blurred. For one thing, it has become clear that good social skills (as in Dr. Skinner's example) can cover up considerable cognitive impairment (Fig. 1.4). More importantly, recent discoveries have made it clear that measurable reductions in neuronal anatomy and function occur years—often decades—before the onset of dementia. The terms *mild cognitive impairment* and *executive function impairment* have emerged as clinically important entities to define and screen for—the former primarily because it increases the risk of Alzheimer disease; the latter, because it identifies persons at risk for poor decision making (including susceptibility to scams). As a result, the medical profession is increasingly concerned about early cognitive impairment, and perhaps as a result there is an increasing fear among the older population that they may be "starting to get Alzheimer's."

Although a significant investment in research to delay the onset of or slow the process of Alzheimer disease and other dementias is ongoing, progress is slow. In the United States, a comparable investment has not been made in the long-term care support that older adults with cognitive decline require. As a result, a large amount of this care is provided by families, at a considerable economic, psychological, and physical cost.[17]

## Relationships and Family Are Crucial to Health and Survival

Medical students are taught to obtain a family history of illness (e.g., Who had what? Who died of what?). However, in geriatric medicine, a family history is often more useful if it is reframed to include the social and relational context of a person's living situation and care network (e.g., Who lives with the patient? Who provides support? Who should be consulted if a surrogate decision maker is needed? What are the dynamics within the family unit?). This information is critical because it can be a harsh world for people who are old and limited by disability, and they need help. Things they may need help with can include maintaining a household, managing medications, doing personal care activities (such as bathing), navigating the healthcare system, and deciding what to do when new symptoms develop. Not surprisingly then, the availability of family and/or an established circle of friends has a tremendous impact on health outcomes and overall quality of life. Without such bonds, older persons are at high risk for isolation, depression, and institutionalization (Fig. 1.5).

Approaching one's later years in an established long-term relationship, with the intimate knowledge and actual obligations such a relationship implies, provides a built-in caregiving dyad. Ideally each can help the other as problems develop, "in sickness and in health," thereby reducing the actual dangers and limitations of

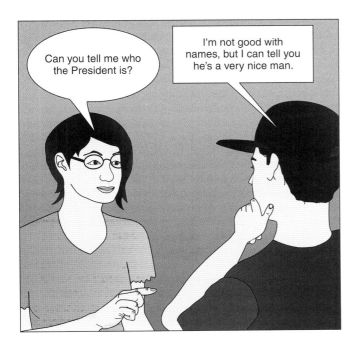

• **Figure 1.4** Good social skills can cover up a considerable amount of cognitive impairment, as in this example involving a patient with moderate dementia. Therefore formal screening and evaluation of cognitive status is a key element of geriatric practice.

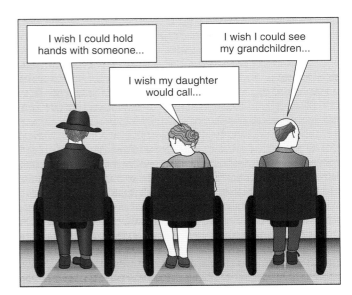

• **Figure 1.5** Loneliness is profound for many older persons, not just in long-term care (as pictured here) but for many living alone in community settings.

living alone. However, not everyone can be so blessed, and in most partnerships one dies or becomes disabled before the other, so couplehood is only a partial answer. If there is a younger generation, the loyalty of good family bonds can immeasurably enhance the security and quality of the life of an older person. Often, based on traditional gender roles, a daughter or daughter-in-law is compelled to step forward to fulfill this role, although men are increasingly caregivers as well. The caregiver role often subjects the caregiver to stress and an increased likelihood of illnesses, such as acute infections and depression (see Chs. 3 and 19). However, if done well, caregiving, which may continue for years, can be experienced as a profound responsibility that enhances life for both members of the dyad. Box 1.2 lists some of the areas in which a well-informed, well-supported family caregiver can enhance the health and life of a care recipient. Here the primary care clinician can be invaluable by caring directly or indirectly for the caregiver's own health and by assisting the caregiver in obtaining access to available resources.

## Delivery of Primary Healthcare to Older Persons

Providing excellent primary care for older persons requires an in-depth knowledge of general clinical medicine. In addition, older persons practically never have one disease, so the approach needs to be functionally oriented and to consider multiple morbidities. It requires the primary care provider to look for hidden functional problems; to be aware of the potential to interfere with homeostasis, causing unanticipated complications; to treat the patient in the context of his or her values and family; and to understand the many options and pitfalls in today's healthcare system.

## Multiple Morbidity and the Geriatric Syndromes

One way that care of older persons tends to differ from that of younger persons is that multiple problems are the norm rather

than the exception. Decline has typically occurred in multiple systems, leading to an insidious increase in the burden of dysfunction and disability with aging. When looked at in isolation, the deficits may seem modest, but in aggregate the results can be devastating.

Take, for example, an 82-year-old woman named Hazel. She has developing cataracts, so her vision in one eye is 20/40 and in the other is 20/50 (see Ch. 26). She had an episode of labyrinthitis 20 years ago, which left her with a clinically undetectable but measurable reduction in vestibular function. She has type 2 diabetes, which is well controlled, with a glycosylated hemoglobin ($HbA_{1c}$) of 7.1, but after 25 years of living with diabetes she now has proprioceptive deficits in both lower extremities. Taken individually, none of these sensory deficits would cause functional disability. However, together they make Hazel at very high risk for falls. Furthermore, she exercises little and is a bit overweight at 180 lbs and 5 foot 2 inches.

This accumulation of multisystem deficits is responsible for the existence of geriatric syndromes—problems that are typically multifactorial in etiology and that therefore are rare in younger persons and common in the elderly. Among the most important geriatric syndromes are falls, frailty, dizziness, gait problems, weakness, incontinence, and confusion (see Unit 2).

## Function, Not Diagnosis, Is What Counts

Another implication of the multiple morbidities in geriatric medicine is that the most important issue is what the patient can and cannot do, not what medical diagnoses the physician can identify. In geriatric medicine, the role of the primary care physician (PCP) should be to identify functional deficits that adversely affect the patient's prognosis and quality of life, to identify potential evidence-based medical interventions for the patient, and to identify what cannot be improved with medical treatment but can be helped with rehabilitation, social support, and empathy.

Activities of daily living (ADLs) and instrumental activities of daily living (IADLs) are useful approaches to defining the function of geriatric patients. ADLs are tasks that people need to do every day, often multiple times each day, such as dressing, bathing, eating, changing position, and going to the toilet. People who are dependent in two or more ADLs generally will qualify for nursing home care; if they remain at home, they will require daily assistance to continue to live in the community. IADLs are tasks that are required to maintain a household but do not need to be done every day; examples include talking on the telephone, shopping, and making the bed. People who are dependent in two or more IADLs generally need someone to help them several times a week; with adequate support, these people will be able to continue to live in the community (see Ch. 3).

The most effective provider (or team) is not the one who makes the most diagnoses or prescribes the most medications, but the one who identifies and addresses the functional problems of greatest importance to the patient and caregiver.

## Advance Care Planning and Shared Decision Making

*Advance care planning* is an activity that allows patients and their clinicians to discuss the patient's goals of care and preferences for care during a serious illness. This may include the completion of a living will, durable power of attorney for healthcare, and/or a physician order for life-sustaining treatment (e.g., POLST, MOLST, or MOST) (see Ch. 8).

The process of *shared decision making* is an attempt to move away from one-way conversations where the clinician presents the patient with a plan of care without exploring options with the patient. Shared decision making builds upon the tradition of informed consent. Shared decision making is a conversation between the patient and clinician to develop a plan for medical care. Clinicians share their knowledge of the clinical problem and possible treatments; patients share their goals of care, values, and preferences.[18]

Advance care planning and shared decision making require that the patient still retains decision making capacity. In older adults, with the increased risk for cognitive impairment, the assessment of decision-making capacity is an essential, and prerequisite activity to ensure that the patient has the capacity to understand the facts and can weigh the options for care (see Ch. 8).

## Underreporting of Symptoms

Some key symptoms and functional impairments in older persons are often not reported during routine office visits. Sometimes this is because the older person thinks the problem is part of normal aging; this is especially true about musculoskeletal complaints, such as bilateral weakness or joint pain. At other times, it is because the older person is embarrassed to report the problem; this is especially true when the issue involves urinary or fecal incontinence, sexual problems, and depressive symptoms (particularly in men). Also, the problem may be unreported because the older person is not aware that a problem exists; this is particularly common when the problem is dementia. In some circumstances, the patient may deliberately withhold information because of a fear of losing independence. For example, in a recent study of patients who experienced a recent fall, nearly three-fourths failed to report the fall when asked. Failure to report a fall occurred more often in younger individuals, men, non-White individuals, and individuals with better function and health.[19]

For the primary care clinician to avoid missing important problems such as these, primary care office visits must be organized to conduct systematic case-finding for common unreported symptoms in older adults. Symptom checklists help some. In addition, specific screening for cognitive function, depressive symptoms, and physical function (e.g., falls risk) should be routine for all persons age >75 years. The Medicare Annual Wellness Visit addresses all of these recommended screens, plus the Advance Care Plan can be completed by a team nurse with supervision of a provider and is well reimbursed relative to other evaluation and management services.

## Iatrogenic Disease

Illness caused by medical interventions, known as iatrogenic illness, is one of the most common medical problems of older persons. Healthcare is not as safe as it should be. A substantial body of evidence points to medical errors as a leading cause of death and injury. Even when using conservative estimates, deaths in hospitals caused by preventable adverse events accounts for one-sixth of all deaths in the United States each year.[20] Increasing age is a risk factor for virtually any medical complication. Older people have more diseases and therefore have more tests and treatments despite their increased risk. Hospitals are particularly hazardous, but no medical venue is safe. The list of possible iatrogenic complications is long and includes many of the geriatric syndromes, such as falls, delirium, dizziness, and urinary incontinence.

Three especially common iatrogenic problems in geriatrics are adverse drug effects, acute kidney injury, and adverse surgical outcomes.

- Adverse drug events (ADEs). This is an expensive problem for the healthcare system and all too frequently a morbid (and occasionally fatal) problem for patients. So ubiquitous are ADEs that one expert suggested, "any symptom in an elderly patient should be considered a drug side effect until proven otherwise."[21] The majority of persons aged ≥65 years take five or more medications, and more than one in three will experience an ADE during a year.[22] Because taking five or more medicines is a potent predictor of ADEs, regular review and discontinuation of unnecessary prescription and over-the-counter drugs is a critical preventive measure (see Ch. 7).

- Acute kidney injury (AKI). At least two-thirds of persons age >65 years have a significant decline in renal function, making them vulnerable to AKI. On top of baseline decline in renal function in all older adults, risk factors for AKI are multifactorial and include nephrotoxic drugs, sepsis, hypotension, and radiologic contrast media. By some estimates 7% to 10% of hospitalized older people experience AKI.[23] Therefore nephrotoxic drugs and contrast agents should be avoided when possible in hospitalized older patients, and hydration should always be maintained. Also, when considering a study using radiologic contrast, we need to ask whether the test results will lead to an important change in care that would be consistent with the patient's care goals.

- Adverse surgical outcomes. Surgery has the potential to provide tremendous benefits for many older adults but with substantial increases in risk of postoperative complications. Replacing a painful hip that limits mobility, for example, can improve function and help maintain independence—if the patient is not too frail or unmotivated to do the necessary rehabilitation exercises. It would be appropriate to assess for frailty status (see Frailty chapter) and share this information with the surgery team. The challenge is that older people are more prone to poor outcomes after surgery; thus many operations leave the patient worse off than before. Frail patients are at especially high risk; therefore surgeons increasingly are interested in frailty measures to assess risk and benefits of surgical interventions.[24] When patients ask if they are "too old" for surgery, the question we should pose is whether they are "too frail," and if they are, whether the potential benefits justify the risks. These are hard decisions, because the patient and/or family members will often grasp at any possibility of improvement, no matter how remote. Therefore it is essential to promote shared decision making (older adult, family/caregivers, medical providers) throughout the entire process to ensure that the goals of any intervention are established.

❖❖ **Iatrogenic illnesses are among the most common preventable problems experienced by older people.**

## Deliberate Medicine

"Don't just do something, stand there." This is useful advice not only for doctors in training but for the healthcare system. The reason is that aggressive treatment, when applied to older persons, often leads to adverse consequences rather than to improvement. If, for example, an older person has florid pulmonary edema, the best treatment is often to give oxygen and a little intravenous furosemide, see what happens, and then decide about the second drug. If a more aggressive regimen were used instead, the patient might experience a drop in blood pressure and possibly even suffer a stroke.

"Start low, go slow." This is another mantra of geriatrics; it refers to the best way to approach pharmacotherapy in older persons. Once again, the issue is that adverse effects are more common in the elderly than in younger persons and treatments will react differently for each older adult. In addition, beneficial effects are often more uncertain in older persons. Organ dysfunction, comorbidities, and overall prognosis, among other factors, can impact this. An example is the use of antidepressants. They do sometimes work in older persons but less reliably than in younger populations and with a greater risk of adverse effects. Concomitantly one should not so underdose older patients that they have no chance of responding to a drug; instead, starting at a low dosage and gradually increasing is the way to proceed.

*"Deliberate" medicine* describes a philosophy and approach that applies the principle of beneficence (i.e., "first do no harm") to the general care of geriatric patients. The idea is to pace care decisions so that both patients and healthcare providers have a chance to evaluate care options before proceeding, because acting hastily is more likely to do harm than not acting at all. Dennis McCullough elegantly advocates for slow medicine in the book *My Mother, Your Mother*:

*The practice of Slow Medicine has taught me that it is wise to slow down and moderate the urgent pressures of decision-making that are often pushed prematurely on elders by society, the medical profession, worried friends and family. Well-intentioned, we want to make good and humane choices for ourselves and for those we love.[25]*

❖❖ **In caring for older patients, we should not act hastily as it is likely to cause harm and a more deliberate approach is often ideal.**

## Polypharmacy

Older persons take a lot of medicine. As of 2011, persons age >65 years comprised only 13% of the US population but consumed one-third of all prescription drugs. In 1 year, the average older adult with five or more chronic illnesses will see 14 different physicians, make 37 physician office visits, and fill 50 prescriptions (see Ch. 7).[26]

Taking so much medicine has its drawbacks. The risk of adverse drug-drug interactions or drug-disease interactions rises with the number of medications. Considering the number of medications taken by older persons, it should be no surprise that ADEs are the primary cause of more than 10% of hospital admissions by older adults.[27]

The term *polypharmacy* was coined to describe persons (most of whom are older) who take a lot of medications. During the past 15 years, the level of polypharmacy among older persons has risen markedly, despite admonitions that it is dangerous.

The challenge is that, although too many drugs can be bad, so can too few. In fact, much of the rise in prescription drug use over the past 10 to 20 years has been because of appropriate use of preventive medications, such as beta-blockers after myocardial infarction, anticoagulants for persons with atrial fibrillation, plus more aggressive treatment of hypertension and congestive heart failure, all of which are supported by evidence-based disease-specific guidelines from professional organizations and expert panels.

However, such disease management guidelines must be applied selectively when the patient is an older adult with multiple chronic illnesses.[28] Disease management guidelines are usually developed from research on patients age <65 years without comorbidities, not on patients with multiple and complex problems.

The challenge of applying disease management guidelines in older adults is illustrated by the following example:

*A physician's 92-year-old mother was hospitalized with a mild heart attack. Following standard guidelines, her cardiologist prescribed atenolol. Not long after, the woman complained of considerable fatigue and a "fuzzy" head. The physician daughter had heard these complaints from her mother 6 years earlier when she had been prescribed the same medication for her hypertension. At that time, stopping the atenolol had alleviated the symptoms, so the daughter called the cardiologist on behalf of her mother to request that the atenolol be discontinued. The cardiologist's response was that this was impossible, because not using a beta-blocker after a heart attack was tantamount to malpractice! The daughter debated with the cardiologist the potential benefits of this protective medication versus its adverse effect on her mother's quality of life. The daughter won the debate, the medication was discontinued, and her mother felt much better. So far there has been no recurrent heart attack.*

## Fragmented Components of US Healthcare: Implications for Older Adults

The US healthcare system for older adults has traditionally had an acute care focus, with access to services largely driven by illness episodes. Thus the major insurers—Medicare, Medicaid, and Veterans Health Administration benefits—tend to provide coverage primarily for active medical treatment. Older adults and the clinicians who care for them experience significant gaps in coverage for primary, preventive care, and proactive interventions. Integration of services is limited between care settings: the hospital, assisted living and the nursing home, home- and community-based services, and the PCP's office. This is a problem for older adults who require more time to recover from acute illness and frequently have multiple chronic illnesses. The result is a fragmented system that funds the most intensive and expensive settings, while requiring individuals and their families to privately fund less expensive alternatives.

Health spending per capita in the United States was $10,586 in 2018. This amount was 30% higher than in the next highest spending country (Switzerland), and almost twice the average of other wealthy developed countries.[29] The cost of providing medical care services to older adults is substantial. Medicare spending was 15% of total federal spending in 2018 and is projected to rise to 18% by 2029. In 2018 Medicare benefit payments totaled $731 billion, up from $462 billion in 2008.[30]

To contain the rising costs of care, Medicare has created numerous complex rules to control costs. These rules are confusing for providers and for patients and their families. Although the majority of healthcare funding for older Americans is public, many older adults also have high out-of-pocket expenses. More than one-third of Medicare beneficiaries spend at least 20% of their household budget on healthcare costs. By 2030, this percentage is projected to rise to more than 40%[31] (see Ch. 9).

The most significant coverage gaps for older adults involves long-term care. Many older adults believe their Medicare benefits under Part A and B will cover long-term care services; however, Medicare offers only limited skilled nursing benefits at home or in a nursing home and no coverage for assisted living. Furthermore, Medicare benefits are designed to be intermittent and are triggered by hospitalization. As a result, more than 90% of bed days in nursing homes and virtually all assisted-living bed days are paid for either privately or (once private funds are depleted) by Medicaid.

Putting all this together, it is probably most accurate to describe US healthcare as a nonsystem (Fig. 1.6). *System* usually implies not just a series of parts but the concept of working together in harmony. US healthcare consists of a variety of separate providers and service types, each of which tends to have its own access requirements, structure, record system, and billing. Having many providers and services leads to duplication, high cost, fragmentation, access barriers, and problems when patients transition from one setting or provider to another.

A recent project to improve care for older patients is the effort to encourage health systems to become "Age Friendly." Age-Friendly Health Systems is an initiative of The John A. Hartford Foundation and the Institute for Healthcare Improvement in partnership with the American Hospital Association and the Catholic Health Association of the United States. The goal of the initiative is to rapidly spread the 4Ms Framework to 20% of US hospitals and medical practices by 2020.[32] The four essential elements of an Age-Friendly Health System are known as the 4Ms Framework for Age-Friendly Care:

- **What Matters**: Know and align care with each older adult's specific health outcome goals and care preferences including, but not limited to, end-of-life care, and across settings of care.
- **Medication**: If medication is necessary, use Age-Friendly medications that do not interfere with What Matters to the older adult, Mobility, or Mentation across settings of care.
- **Mentation**: Prevent, identify, treat, and manage dementia, depression, and delirium across care settings.
- **Mobility**: Ensure that older adults move safely every day to maintain function and do What Matters.

## Transitions in Care Are Dangerous

Care transitions occur whenever a patient changes level or location of care, and a new set of care providers must get to know a patient. In today's healthcare, these transitions occur with dizzying frequency. They are especially problematic around hospitalizations, because patient information must be passed at least twice—and three times if, as usually happens, an emergency room visit is part of the admission. In addition, hospital stays are increasingly short, with patients often being discharged before they are ready to return home. This leads to an additional transition involving a posthospitalization nursing home stay. All these handoffs can lead to misunderstandings of diagnoses and plans, to medication discrepancies, and to confusion on the part of patients and families.

In years past, a primary care provider who knew the patient would oversee hospital care and arrange follow-up, so transitions were more seamless. The advent of hospitalists and other aspects of healthcare specialization changed all that. Nowadays, provider continuity rarely occurs; thus special effort must be undertaken to ensure that accurate information on a patient's history, capabilities, disabilities, care preferences, medications, allergies, and family/social support are communicated across transitions. Failure to address these issues will lead to complications, hospital readmissions, and patient dissatisfaction.

Fortunately, essential elements of safe transitions have been identified and studied. A widely acknowledged program is the Care Transitions Program[33,34]. Among its key elements are the following indicators of high-quality transitional care (and reduced hospital readmissions):

- Accurate and timely information transfer to the next set of providers
- Patient and family education about the disease process, self-management recommendations, and expectations for the next level of care
- Empowerment of patients to assert their preferences for the type, intensity, and location of services received

Hospital readmissions have been a focus of Medicare healthcare reform,[25] largely because of cost concerns. Under the Affordable Care Act considerable funding has been allocated to foster strategies that will improve care transitions for Medicare beneficiaries. In addition, the Centers for Medicare and Medicaid Services has approved two transitional care management service codes that provide a modest reimbursement for a Medicare patient's primary provider for non−face-to-face, as well as face-to-face transitional care

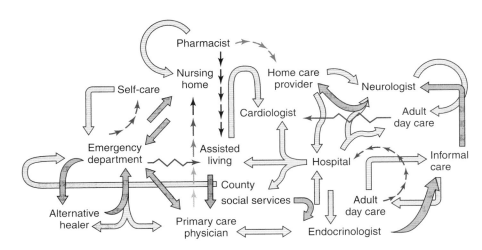

• **Figure 1.6** The US healthcare system for older persons is a confusing array of largely independent providers. Anyone with significant cognitive, physical, or sensory impairment—and many persons who are quite intact but are not good at understanding and navigating complex systems—requires assistance to understand and appropriately use the resources that are available.

management services provided within 30 days of discharge. This change will help to place primary care providers back in the center of care coordination during transitions out of the hospital and postacute care (see Ch. 11).

❖ **Transitions from one provider or care setting to another can lead to misunderstanding of diagnoses and plans, medication discrepancies, and confusion on the part of patients and families.**

## Interprofessional Nature of Geriatric Care

Evidence from numerous studies supports the use of interprofessional teams in the care of older adults. Managing patients as a team leads to better continuity, enhanced care coordination, improved patient safety, better chronic illness care, enhanced medication adherence, fewer adverse drug reactions, preserved function, and decreased hospital readmissions.[35-38]

Several publications, federal legislation, and new care models, including the following, have led to an increased emphasis on geriatric care teams in primary care:

- The 2008 Institute of Medicine report, *Retooling for an Aging America: Building the Health Care Workforce*, emphasized the importance of training all healthcare professionals in the skills needed to work effectively in teams and calls for the implementation of new geriatric care models that use interprofessional teams.[39]
- The Affordable Care Act, with its encouragement of Accountable Care Organizations, holds clinicians and hospitals accountable not only for treating patients once they get sick but also for helping to keep them out of the hospital and emergency rooms.
- The Patient Centered Medical Home (PCMH) model of primary care, which focuses on use of interprofessional teams to provide improved continuity, comprehensiveness, and coordination of care. Implementation of the PCMH model requires additional resources that have not been provided through traditional payment mechanisms; thus payment models that encourage and reward primary care practices for achieving improved outcomes are an essential component necessary to drive this interprofessional team model.

Whereas the importance of teamwork is evident, it can be challenging to implement in an effective yet cost-efficient manner. For years, academic medical centers had "geriatric assessment and management clinics" in which interprofessional teams took several hours or longer to evaluate a patient; however, this model was never feasible in primary care. Instead, primary care geriatricians tend to use virtual, ad hoc interprofessional teams consisting of an office-based core (usually a physician and a nurse) supplemented as needed by consultations or referrals to other professionals who may work for different organizations (e.g., medical offices, home care agencies, hospitals). For less complex patients, the team is often small, whereas for very frail elders managed at home, the care team can be large. In addition to a variety of health professionals, interprofessional teams usually include an identified care manager and must always explicitly include the older person and family at the center of the team.

The essential elements of teamwork include coordination of services, shared responsibility, and communication. Because each profession has its own approach to care, differences in values, expectations, and/or language can occur within a team. Therefore a good team requires its members to not only have excellent clinical skills but also be knowledgeable and skillful at working as a team. Good teamwork does not happen by accident but is a function of a

well-developed structure that includes mutual respect and shared goals; clarity about each member's roles and responsibilities; frequent, clear communication; and mechanisms for working together and managing team conflict. Fulfilling these requirements can lead to care goals and care planning that emphasize the needs of the older adult (see Ch. 2).

❖ **Interprofessional care is important but challenging to implement in an effective yet cost-efficient manner.**

## A Generalist Is Often the Best Clinician for a Geriatric Patient

Because older persons so often have impairments in multiple organ systems, a generalist clinician (family physician, general internist, geriatrician, or advance practice nurse or physician assistant) is often better able to set priorities and identify the remediable problem than a multitude of specialists. Therefore specialist clinicians should generally be viewed as *consultants*, and patient *referrals* should only be made once the primary care provider has weighed the evidence and decided on the best course of action. Often this process of decision making involves not only obtaining specialist opinions but also meeting with the patient and family to identify goals and priorities and putting all available information in the context of the patient's overall health status and prognosis.

The view of specialists as very useful but secondary adjuncts to the primary care process can best be illustrated by the story of the blind men and the elephant (Fig. 1.7). As the case study illustrates,

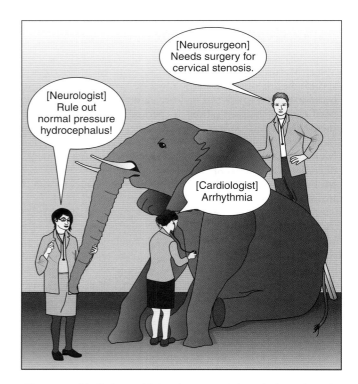

• **Figure 1.7** Medical specialists often approach geriatric patients in a manner reminiscent of the blind man and the elephant. In this case of a patient with a gait disorder and multiple falls, three specialists viewed the situation through the lens of their own subspecialty and recommended invasive procedures that could have harmed the patient. The actual diagnosis was failure to adhere to a medication regimen because of mild cognitive impairment. See text for details.

specialists may view patients through a narrow lens and at times can fail to see the forest because they are accustomed to looking at trees. For these reasons, a good generalist is often the best clinician for an older person.

---

**CASE 1**

**Frieda (Part 1)**

Frieda is a 79-year-old woman who was hospitalized after falling and bruising her face and shoulder. Once a significant orthopedic injury had been ruled out, several subspecialists were consulted to evaluate the patient's recurrent falls (see Fig. 1.6). A neurologist ordered a head computed tomography (CT) scan, thought the cerebral ventricles were unusually large for a person with her degree of cerebral atrophy, and wanted further evaluation and possibly shunting for normal pressure hydrocephalus. A neurosurgeon ordered a CT scan of the neck, which was interpreted as showing spinal stenosis, and wanted to operate. A cardiologist noted that the patient had a right bundle branch block and three to five premature ventricular contractions per minute and, when the echocardiogram showed an ejection fraction of 30%, recommended evaluation for possible implantable cardioverter defibrillator (ICD).

Frieda, a stubborn woman, refused all of these.

1. What other next steps might be possible in Frieda's care?
2. Which of the proposed interventions if carried out would be most likely to help Frieda?

---

**CASE 1**

**Frieda (Part 2)**

Frieda's primary care physician reassessed her status considering the conflicting specialist recommendations and her own frame of mind. He noted that she had mild short-term memory loss and admitted to not always knowing whether she had taken her medications; thus he recommended that a family member place Frieda's daily medication in a pill dispenser. She took a sleeping pill each night, which he discontinued, advising her to read in bed and consider taking melatonin. He also noted that Frieda was highly deconditioned, with weak leg and hip muscles but intact peripheral nerve function, so he arranged for her to have physical therapy at home three times a week. The frequent falls stopped and, 3 years later, Frieda continued to do well.

---

**CASE 1**

**Discussion**

Frieda's case history illustrates that, although subspecialists can often be invaluable in clarifying a diagnosis or providing needed therapy, they can at times make recommendations that are not the best course of action for a particular patient. Because conducting multiple tests on complex older persons always reveals a host of abnormal or questionable findings, it often takes a generalist to identify what is most important and what will be most helpful to the individual patient.

## Summary

The clinical characteristics and physiologic changes of older adults and the principles of delivering good care for older adults, as described in this chapter, should serve as the foundation for providing optimal primary care for older patients. Our approach to the older patient starts with a careful clinical assessment to identify correctable or manageable acute or chronic medical problems and geriatric syndromes. Next, the management of chronic problems is conducted in the context of the patient's goals of care, always assessing the risk versus benefit of therapy. Finally, we maintain an emphasis toward restoring and maintaining the older adult's function and independence.

### Web Resources

Website of the Care Transitions Program, which aims to support patients and families and increase skills among healthcare providers around care transitions: www.caretransitions.org.

https://www.choosingwisely.org/societies/american-geriatrics-society/.

Kaiser Family Foundation's website provides a trustworthy resource about health policy, including up-to-date information on Medicare and Medicaid programs: www.kff.org.

A nonprofit information resource devoted to helping people in need find assistance programs to help them afford their medications and costs related to healthcare: www.needymeds.org.

Hartford Institute for Geriatric Nursing's *Practice* website with resources on geriatric assessment and other key topics, including "Try This" evidence-based assessment tools: http://hartfordign.org/practice.

Official website of the American Geriatrics Society provides access to a variety of guidelines and clinical tools and free public education tools at the foundation site https://www.healthinaging.org/tools-and-tips?type = Tip: www.americangeriatrics.org.

## Key References

18. Fried TR. Shared decision making—finding the sweet spot. *N Engl J Med.* 2016;374(2):104—106.
28. Tinetti ME, Bogardus ST, Agostini JV. Potential pitfalls of disease-specific guidelines for patients with multiple conditions. *N Engl J Med.* 2004;351:2870—2873.
34. Naylor MD, Aiken LH, Kurtzman ET, Olds DM, Hirschman KB. The importance of transitional care in achieving health reform. *Health Affair (Millwood).* 2011;30:746—754.

*References available online at expertconsult.com.* ▶

# 2

# Interprofessional Team Care

KAREN HALPERT AND GABRIELLE SCRONCE

## OBJECTIVES

*Upon completion of this chapter, the reader will be able to:*

- Describe three traits of effective geriatric care teams.
- Describe four components of an effective geriatric care team.
- Describe the role of the patient and the family in the team.
- Describe the importance of the team in new models of care.

## Introduction

A team-based approach plays a critical role in the care of the older patient. Older patients tend to have multiple chronic conditions, geriatric syndromes, polypharmacy, functional deficits, and social needs. Older adults benefit when their primary care providers (PCPs) think beyond the patients' medical conditions and consider other contributors to health and wellness. The most comprehensive and patient-centered approach requires the skills of an interprofessional team. It is valuable and productive for the PCP to engage with a team of professionals from other disciplines to provide comprehensive assessment and management of complicated patients. It is necessary that all the members of the team understand the importance of team-based care and how everyone adds to the health of the patient.

Clinician training to work effectively in teams is now emphasized by most health profession societies. For example, the Accreditation Council of Graduate Medical Education (ACGME), as part of the competency "interpersonal and communication skills" requires residents to "demonstrate interpersonal and communication skills that result in effective information exchange and teaming with patients...and professional associates."[1] Medical residents should be trained to "work effectively with others as a member or leader of a healthcare team." Training

in teamwork is also recommended under the ACGME "systems-based practice" competency. The core competencies in collaborative practice have also been agreed upon by the major organizations in health professional training[2] (Box 2.1).

There are a number of terms used to describe team-based approaches to healthcare, such as *interprofessional, multiprofessional, interdisciplinary,* and *multidisciplinary.*[3] In this chapter we will use the term *interprofessional,* defined as a cohesive, patient-centered practice among professionals from different disciplines who work interdependently to optimize patient outcomes.[3–5]

### CASE

#### Emily Jones (Part 1)

Mrs. Jones is a 76-year-old who was living independently in an apartment. During the night, she tripped while going to the bathroom and landed on her right hip. She immediately felt pain in her hip and was unable to get up. She stayed on the floor of her apartment until her daughter found her the following morning. You now see her in the emergency room where she was diagnosed with a femoral neck fracture.

## BOX 2.1 Core Competency Domains for Interprofessional Collaborative Practice

- *Values/ethics for interprofessional practice*: Work with individuals of other professions to maintain a climate of mutual respect and shared values.
- *Roles/responsibilities*: Use the knowledge of one's own role and those of other professions to appropriately assess and address the healthcare needs of the patients and populations served.
- *Interprofessional communication*: Communicate with patients, families, communities, and other health professionals in a responsive and responsible manner that supports a team approach to the maintenance of health and the treatment of disease.
- *Teams and teamwork*: Apply relationship-building values and the principles of team dynamics to perform effectively in different team roles to plan and deliver patient-centered/population-centered care that is safe, timely, efficient, effective, and equitable.

◆◆ **During Mrs. Jones's treatment and rehabilitation for her femur fracture what are the likely health disciplines she will encounter?**

## Evidence Supporting Team-Based Care

The patient experience in healthcare is rapidly changing. As the US population ages and individuals are living longer with a greater number of complex medical problems, the field of medicine has responded with an increase in specialist providers who focus on each individual pathology, body part, or impairment.[6] In fact, because of the increasing complexity of medical conditions and their impact on older adults' health and function, comprehensive care from only one provider is often simply not possible. However, when patients receive care by a number of specialized providers who operate independently to address distinct medical issues, there is an increased risk for medical errors affecting patient safety.[7] For these patients who require multiple providers, quality of care is optimized when providers work together as a team.[7–9]

Lemieux-Charles and McGuire (2006) reviewed studies of interdisciplinary teams working in a variety of healthcare settings. They found that older adult patients receiving care from teams in the Veterans Administration (VA) compared with usual care in that setting experienced higher functional status, improved mental health, decreased dependence, and decreased mortality. For patients in the VA and elsewhere, receiving interdisciplinary team care was associated with higher quality of life, decreased depression symptomatology, and greater patient satisfaction with care.[10] In a review of studies describing interprofessional teams in hospitals, Epstein[8] summarized that effective communication and collaboration within interprofessional teams can reduce adverse events such as hospital-acquired pressure ulcers and surgical errors, decrease patients' length of hospital stay, and increase patient and family satisfaction with care.

Ritchie et al.[11] evaluated the role interdisciplinary team-based care has to play in the care of patients with healthcare needs that are complicated by significant medical and psychosocial factors. Through implementation of the Geriatric Resources for the Assessment and Care of Elders (GRACE) program, a healthcare delivery model intended to improve care and control costs for geriatric patients with complex needs, it was shown that interdisciplinary care could be realistically performed at an urban teaching hospital. The GRACE team model led to a significant reduction in emergency department (ED) visits, reduction in frequency of hospitalization, and increase in patient self-rated health, as compared with usual care. As a result, those who participated in GRACE realized a reduction in healthcare costs associated with hospital and ED visits.[11]

Research also demonstrates that the benefits of team-based care occur not only for patients and their families but also for members of the teams. Providers involved in interprofessional teams report increased job satisfaction and less burnout than providers who do not provide team-based care.[8,12] This evidence speaks to the inherent challenges associated with working as a solo provider in primary care. Older adult patients often have multiple chronic conditions requiring several medications. Mental health issues, functional limitations, financial challenges, and family and social stresses may also be present and can require additional time and resources from the provider. For providers who work in a team of colleagues with diverse skills and viewpoints, the multifaceted issues brought by a patient can be more easily digested and addressed than by a provider working alone.

Public health authorities and organizations have recognized the benefits of team-based care and support the use of teams to address the challenges of caring for an aging population with chronic conditions. The World Health Organization,[13] American Geriatrics Society,[14] and US Department of Health and Human Services[15] indicate that interprofessional teams are the solution to growing demands on clinicians. However, the benefits from interprofessional teams do not occur effortlessly. Instead, proactive steps must be taken to facilitate successful teamwork.[16]

◆◆ **Team-based care improves the health of the patient and increases patient and team satisfaction.**

## CASE

### Emily Jones (Part 2)

Mrs. Jones undergoes a hip replacement without complication. Her pain is well controlled although she feels unsteady on her feet. She also finds during her hospital stay that she is weaker and has difficulty bathing herself. When Mrs. Jones returns to her home, she will need to walk up 12 steps to get to her bedroom.

Who are the key members of the team that would enable Mrs. Jones to successfully transition from the hospital back to her home environment?

**Specific Roles of the Care Team.** Working as a team is imperative to meeting the patient's complex needs. Although it may be easier to meet as a team while the patient is in the hospital, communication is required across all settings to help patients meet their goals. Brief descriptions of the overall roles or scope of practice of team members are provided in Table 2.1.

## CASE

### Emily Jones (Part 3)

Mrs. Jones is transferred to a rehabilitation floor. While there, she is found to have orthostatic blood pressure that is limiting her working with physical therapy. Multiple medications for pain control and management of constipation have been added since her initial admission to the hospital.

What is the role of the PCP in managing Mrs. Jones and ensuring that she can participate in rehabilitation?

**TABLE 2.1   Geriatrics Team-Selected Discipline Participants**

| | |
|---|---|
| Primary care provider | Responsible for managing the team, certifying the need for rehabilitation, and treating medical comorbidities. Orders medical tests, reviews associated findings to make medical diagnoses, prescribes medications, and facilitates referral to other providers. |
| Physical therapist (PT)<br>PT assistants (work under the supervision of a PT) | Provides education and assistance to patients managing the development of disease processes affecting movement, such as chronic pain, arthritis, diabetes, pelvic floor dysfunction, tendonitis, peripheral joint pain, weakness, and instability. Assesses joint range of motion, muscle strength, gait, and mobility; instructs appropriate use of assistive devices; and provides exercise training to increase range of motion, strength, endurance, balance, coordination, and gait to address the underlying causes of movement dysfunction. |
| Dietician | Assesses nutritional status and recommends changes to diet to promote informed dietary choices to take advantage of the benefits of a healthy diet when managing disease or simply when trying to achieve a health-related goal. |
| Nurse (registered nurse [RN])<br>Licensed practical nurse (LPN)<br>Certified nursing assistants (work under the supervision of a nurse) | Performs physical examinations, takes vital signs, assists with medication administration, assists with wound care, and takes patients' health history. Provides continuous patient observation identifying various signs of patient health deterioration in addition to providing for the patient's basic needs such as feeding and hydration. Assists in coordination of care by informing other providers concerning medication administration, patient status. Provides health promotion, counseling, and education in the clinic and community at large. |
| Social worker | Evaluates family, support, and home care factors; assesses psychosocial factors. Aids family and patient concerning transitioning from hospital to home or other care facility assisting in discharge planning. Assists the patient and family understanding a particular illness and works through emotional stress of dealing with an illness. Provides counseling and guidance about what personal and medical decisions the patient and family need to make and how that will affect them personally. Reports to care providers concerning the social and emotional state of the patient and the family. Addresses social, financial, and psychological problems related to patient's health condition. Performs psychosocial assessments, provides patient education of treatment options and associated consequences, helps patient adjust to being in the hospital and social role changes of the patient and family, and coordinates patient discharge and continuity of care planning. |
| Recreation therapist | Assists in developing skills, knowledge, and behaviors for daily living and community involvement. Provides patient treatments and recreational activities, including techniques such as arts and crafts, animals, sports, board games, video games, music, dance, and social outings. Promotes physical, mental, and emotional well-being by reducing depression, stress, and anxiety. Activities focus on addressing recovery of motor function, coordination, critical thinking, and reasoning. Therapy sessions will incorporate specific tasks: reaching or weight shifting in the format of a game or other recreational activity to promote patient participation and to assist in generalization of motor skill. |
| Speech therapist | Assesses all aspects of communication, treats communication deficits, assesses swallowing disorders, and can recommend changes in diet or positioning to treat dysphagia. Provides skilled interventions to improve patient communication and address oral-motor dysfunction. Performs aural rehabilitation for those who are deaf or hard of hearing. Facilitates use of augmentative and communication (AAC) systems to help patients communicate more effectively. |
| Occupational therapist (OT)<br>OT assistant (works under the supervision of an OT) | Evaluates self-care skills and other activities of living (ADLs), provides self-care skills training, makes recommendations and trains in use of assistive technology, fabricates splints, and treats upper extremity deficits. Focuses therapeutic interventions on maximizing the patient's ability to perform everyday ADLs. Provides a holistic perspective that focuses on adapting a patient's environment to fit the person. |
| Audiologist | Evaluates, diagnoses, and treats hearing loss and balance disorders. Appropriately applies technologies, such as hearing aids and cochlear implants, and provides fitting, programming, and audiologic rehabilitation. Other responsibilities include treatment of central auditory disorders; screening of factors affecting communication, including patient's speech, use of sign language, and cognitive deficits; and patient education on the psychosocial adjustments of hearing loss. |
| Pharmacist | Prepares medications, identifies therapeutic incompatibilities, monitors drug therapy, and proposes alternative medications. Advises patients on recommended diet and activities that they should avoid while taking a medication. Provides guidance to patients concerning dosage and consequences of missing a dosage, side effects, financial cost, and therapeutic effect of name brand versus generic forms of a medication. Also identifies harmful drug reactions and makes recommendations accordingly. |
| Behavioral health support | A psychologist, psychiatrist, or clinical social worker who assesses, treats, or manages mental health disorders. Provides counseling and guidance for patient and family psychosocial function. |

## Roles of Core Team Members

**Primary Care Provider (Physician, Nurse Practitioner, Physician Assistant).** The PCP on the geriatric team has the responsibility of assessing and managing the patient's medical problems. In addition to the pharmacist, the PCP must be mindful of medication side effects and the polypharmacy cascade that can occur in older patients. In a team-based approach, the PCP elicits insight and recommendation from other team members' assessment to develop a comprehensive care plan. For example, in a patient with balance problems, a physical therapist may identify a neuropathy that requires further evaluation by the PCP. Furthermore, the PCP is crucial in bringing the patient and family into the discussion to ensure the patients' goals and wishes are clarified. This model of shared decision making is crucial in caring for older adults, as the plan for care is dependent on the patient's wishes and goals. Because of the potential for complexity of their patients, PCPs must prioritize and determine which problems to address first.

PCPs are also responsible for balancing the benefits and risks of treating multiple conditions. For example, while targeting blood pressure to a goal of less than 130/80 mmHg may be important for a patient with chronic kidney disease, being mindful of orthostatic blood pressure and the risk of falls with low blood pressure will be equally important. It is important for PCPs to be mindful of different treatment goals for older patients. For example, blood sugars in diabetics may not need to be as tightly controlled as in younger patients.[17] Similarly, decisions on the appropriate approach to preventive screening will be important. The PCP is also responsible for monitoring the patient's medication regimen, assessing the use of over-the-counter medications and when it may be appropriate to continue or discontinue medications.

PCPs also play a key role in advance care planning. Although this discussion may originate with the social worker, it is imperative the PCP explores the patient's goals and wishes for care. It is important the provider discusses the medical implications of the patient's wishes and updates the medical record. It is essential all PCPs understand their role in filling out Do Not Resuscitate Orders or Physician Orders for Life Sustaining Treatment forms.

The PCP also provides a crucial role as patient advocate within the medical system. Given the diversity of older patients along with opinions of family members and other members of the care team, the PCP will have to advocate for patients and ensure patients feels their goals and wishes are being met. Older adults may see multiple other medical specialists and the PCP may have to interpret what other providers say and help navigate the patient through the desired treatment course. The PCP has a role in helping patients choose among treatment options and understand the risks and benefits of their choices. When a patient is unable to provide consent, the PCP works with a healthcare proxy or surrogate decision maker to ensure the decisions being made reflect the choice that would have been made by the patient. Furthermore, as a patient moves from the outpatient setting to the hospital to a nursing facility, the PCP plays a crucial role in ensuring that the patient's goals of care are acknowledged during care transitions.

Although the PCP has many responsibilities, this person is not always the leader of the care team. It may be assumed the PCP is the team leader, but this may not always be the case. Leadership varies by the type of team and by the situation. For example, in the nursing home, nurses are often the team leaders because they have the most face-to-face interactions with patients. In a well-functioning team, the leadership role may shift depending on the primary problem being addressed. For example, if a move from independent living to an assisted living facility is being made, the social worker may assume the leadership role. Clinicians working in care teams must be comfortable at changing roles and supporting the team as needed to achieve the best patient outcome.

**◆◆ The PCP has the responsibility to inform other team members of the patient's conditions and learn from other team members about what else the patient may need.**

---

### CASE

#### Emily Jones (Part 4)

During her stay in short-term rehab, the nursing staff notes that Mrs. Jones is having increased difficulty with urinary incontinence, which is contributing to skin breakdown. They also find she has difficulty swallowing, which limits her nutritional status. Mrs. Jones reports these issues have been ongoing but a bit worse than usual.

What is the role of nursing when alerting the team to changes in the patient's status?

---

**Nurse.** Nurses often have the most direct contact with patients and ensure that the patient receives accessible, high-quality care. From the primary care office, hospital wards, inpatient rehabilitation, to home health, nurses have a key role in assessing and evaluating the patient. Because nurses are often providing the day-to-day care of patients, they are best positioned to advocate when they identify problems and to ensure that the team follows up. Beyond the patients and their families, nurses are frequently required to act as an advocate for patients.

Finally, nurses have a distinct role communicating with patients and their families. The nurse tends to be the eyes and ears for the team; therefore clear, succinct communication is necessary to ensure proper triage and patient care. Nurses also must be able to communicate with social work and care managers to ensure transfers are occurring safely, especially as patients move between care facilities (see the section later on team communication). Nurses may be the primary communicator of treatment plans from the PCP or other healthcare team member. Nurses ensure all information is understood and well presented. If the patient or family member does not understand the information, the nurse needs to inform the care team so that there will be appropriate follow-up. In the outpatient clinic, nurses play key roles in triaging patient complaints, scheduling appointments and referrals, and helping fill out forms.

**◆◆ Nurses play a key role in communicating the plan between the patient and family, as well as being the eyes and ears for the rest of the care team.**

---

### CASE

#### Emily Jones (Part 5)

Mrs. Jones completes rehabilitation and feels safe to go back to living independently. Mrs. Jones's daughter raises concerns for lack of equipment and safety at her mother's current apartment. The social worker on the team is called to assist the daughter and Mrs. Jones with helping with this transition and ensuring appropriate support at home is available.

Given their broad training, what other role is the social worker on the team able to provide?

**Social Worker.** Social workers are essential members of the care team for older adults. Social workers can provide important information to the providers and nurses regarding the social and psychological impacts of disease upon the patient and family. Given shorter hospitalizations and the multiple transitions patients may make after a hospitalization, more health-related social work services are needed in the community.[18]

A social work assessment is multifactorial and brings a wealth of information to the care team. The social work assessment includes crucial information concerning the patient's past, as well as current social, psychological, spiritual, and financial issues. This collateral information can help the healthcare team understand the patient's reasons for making decisions and encourages the team to incorporate that information into the care planning process. Furthermore, social workers have training in some formal psychological assessments, such as depression or cognitive screening that may help the care team.

The care manager is a role that may be filled by a social worker or a nurse depending on the healthcare system. This role is essential in linking the patient or families of patients with resources. The care manager may assist with filling out paperwork, facilitate meetings with Medicare or Medicaid professionals, and help to set up home health or hospice care. The care manager is key in helping patients transition between various care settings and ensuring the patient has the appropriate support.

◆ **Psychosocial assessments are the basis of social work practice in the geriatric population.**

# Defining Effective Teams and Interprofessional Team Care

Successfully expanding patient care from an individual PCP to a team of multiple health professionals requires intentional, organized collaboration, communication, and understanding.[19,20]

## Components of Effective Geriatrics Team Care

Various models have been proposed to facilitate these characteristics within interprofessional teams in healthcare. The Agency for Healthcare Research and Quality developed Team Strategies and Tools to Enhance Performance and Patient Safety (TeamSTEPPS), an evidence-based training program to optimize performance of healthcare teams.[15] TeamSTEPPS promotes five key characteristics

of effective teams: team structure, communication, leadership, situation monitoring, and mutual support.

### Team Structure

Effective team structure is patient centered and includes a diversity of professions. Individuals on effective interprofessional healthcare teams understand and respect the roles of other professionals on the team.[15,19,20] A practical understanding of the other professionals' patient care skills is essential for appropriate referrals and efficient management of the patient's healthcare.

### Mutual Support

In addition to simply knowing what services are provided by other professionals, members of effective healthcare teams respect and appreciate the contributions of their collaborators. Mutual respect for team members' skills and knowledge is necessary for provider relationships and for patient wellbeing. When interprofessional team members display mutual support, they protect each other from work overload by offering to help other team members when appropriate and by actively asking for help when they need it.

### Communication

Effective communication among healthcare teams is essential for patient safety.[21] Effective communication occurs in both formal and informal meetings, includes all team members, and involves sharing information, asking questions, and listening.[19] TeamSTEPPS recommends the SBAR technique to facilitate effective communication within healthcare teams.[15] SBAR, an acronym for Situation, Background, Assessment, and Recommendation/Request, was adopted from the US military to provide clear and accurate information regarding a patient's condition. Table 2.2 defines the components of SBAR and provides an example.

For improved communication during transitions in care, TeamSTEPPS recommends using a strategy with the acronym I PASS the BATON, which is described in Table 2.3.

### Team Leadership

Leaders on interprofessional healthcare teams may be designated or may step into the role as the situation demands. Effective team leaders help to organize the team, ensure participation and input from all team members, and both model and facilitate effective communication. It is not the leader's role to make decisions for the team; instead, an effective leader fosters collaboration and shared responsibility. TeamSTEPPS suggests that leaders coordinate team members through briefs, huddles, and debriefs. Briefs are short

| TABLE 2.2 | Situation, Background, Assessment, and Recommendation/Request: A Tool for Team Communication | |
|---|---|
| **SBAR Component** | **Example** |
| Brief statement describing the patient and **Situation** | "I am calling about Ms. Costa in room 251. Chief complaint is shortness of breath of new onset." |
| **Background** information relevant to this situation | "Patient is a 62-year-old female postoperative day 1 from abdominal surgery. No prior history of cardiac or lung disease." |
| **Assessment**: What do you think is happening? | "Breath sounds are decreased on the right side with acknowledgment of pain. Would like to rule out pneumothorax." |
| Your **Recommendation** and **Request** | "I feel strongly the patient should be assessed now. Can you come to room 251 now?" |

**TABLE 2.3** Introduction, Patient, Assessment, Situation, Safety Concerns, Background, Actions, Timing, Ownership, Next: A Tool for Team-Based Communication for Hand-Off of Care

| I PASS the BATON | Meaning |
| --- | --- |
| Introduction | Introduce yourself and your role |
| Patient | Patient's name and pertinent identifiers |
| Assessment | Patient's overall assessment, including chief complaint, diagnosis |
| Situation | Patient's current status and situation as well as recent changes and response to treatment |
| Safety concerns | Precautions, critical lab values, allergies |
| the | |
| Background | Comorbidities, pertinent medical history, medications, pertinent family/social history |
| Actions | Actions recently taken or soon needed |
| Timing | Level of urgency and priority of necessary actions |
| Ownership | Clear identification of who is responsible for upcoming actions |
| Next | Plan for next step as well as contingencies |

sessions that occur to clarify team roles, share goals, and establish or share plans. Huddles occur as needed to discuss the current plan or adjust, as well as to ensure that all team members are still aware of the situation and their roles. Debriefs occur after plans are completed to highlight things that went well and consider ways to improve team effectiveness. These short meetings help with situation monitoring, which is described in the next section.

### Situation Monitoring

Situation monitoring occurs when all members of the team are on the same page regarding the patient's status and plan in the present environment. Situation monitoring occurs with open and ongoing communication among team members. Effective situation monitoring requires team members to be aware not only of the situation with the patient but also within themselves. This is the place for team members to examine their own fatigue, workload, skill, and stress and to consider whether these may be affecting their performance. Situation monitoring also occurs when team members look beyond the patient, as well as the team at the environment to assess how healthcare system administration and resources may affect team performance. By creating an awareness of the multiple challenges affecting the interprofessional team and the patient, situation monitoring builds a safe space for problem solving and positive change.

◆◆ **Clear, concise communication is key to providing high-quality patient care.**

## Barriers to Effective Teams

Team performance suffers when these characteristics of effective teams are lacking. Specific barriers that can occur include absenteeism, disorganization, inadequate time for team building, and physical barriers to communication, such as working in separate spaces. When barriers occur that restrict the ability of interprofessional teams to provide high value care for patients, healthcare providers and health system administrators must provide the foundation for teams to have effective team structure, mutual support, communication, leadership, and situation monitoring.[22–24]

**CASE**

### Discussion

During recovery from her hip fracture, Mrs. Jones encounters and interacts with many members of the healthcare team. It is imperative to remember that the patient's needs are the top priority. Patient-centered care involves placing the patient and the family at the core of the team and using their input throughout the process. By maximizing the patient's and family's voice, it ensures the team aligns the goals of therapy and rehabilitation with the patient. This helps everyone achieve the desired outcome and reduces errors and iatrogenic disease.

Mrs. Jones completes her rehabilitation and with occupational and physical therapy feels strong enough to transition home and conquer those steps! The provider in rehabilitation has adjusted her medication so she is no longer lightheaded, her pain is well controlled, and she is moving her bowels. She is more mobile now so there are less concerns from nursing concerning incontinence and skin breakdown. Mrs. Jones's daughter has worked with the social worker to set up support at home with assistance with meals and appropriate equipment for Mrs. Jones. The discharge summary from the rehabilitation center has been sent to the PCP, and an appointment within 1 week has been set up for Mrs. Jones to follow up with her outpatient care team.

## Transitions of Care

For ill, older patients, an episode of illness may require care in multiple settings. Transitions of care are crucial times for the patient, and team-based care is imperative in ensuring patient safety. Transitions of care can negatively affect a patient's health and increase healthcare costs by contributing to preventable hospital admissions.[25] One in five (20%) Medicare patients is readmitted within 30 days (2.6 million patients annually), and lack of coordination, poor communication, and unidentified psychosocial stressors are often significant contributors to these readmissions.[26–29] During acute hospitalizations, early discharge planning has been associated with fewer hospital readmissions and lower readmission lengths of hospital stay.[30] It is imperative to recognize that the roles of the team may change depending on where

• **BOX 2.2** **Successful Transition of Care**

Begin planning at the time of admission with early assessment of needs and barriers.
Encourage a multidisciplinary input.
Involve patients and families.
Provide clear communication between team members.
Provide patient and family with medication list.
Ensure a thorough information transfer between hospital and receiving facility.
Use a multifaceted and holistic approach.

---

the patient is receiving care. While in the outpatient setting, a patient may be using more of the PCPs' and nurses' time; in a long-term care facility, however, the nursing staff and rehabilitation team may be the team members delivering most of the patient's care.

Team-based care is integral for ensuring smooth transitions and avoiding readmissions or errors. Inadequate communication with facilities, including postacute care rehab facilities or home health agencies, can lead to increased rates of hospital readmissions. Teams can be successful by identifying a clear plan for close follow-up care. Communication of the plan via discharge summaries is crucial especially when discharging to subacute rehabilitation or back to home.[31] There is no one solution to ensure a successful transition of care especially with increasing patient complexity. Some suggestions for successful transition are listed in Box 2.2.[32]

❖ **Transitions of care can be successful with early discharge planning and clear communication between the team and the family.**

## Role of Patient and the Family

One of the most important, although challenging, aspects of effective team care is including the patient and the family. Although the rest of the healthcare team may speak a common language, this is not always understood by laypersons. It is crucial to incorporate the patient and the family to provide patient-centered care. Shared decision making is essential because the goals of the team are developed based on the patient's goals and wishes. It is imperative to incorporate a multidisciplinary evaluation as patients may tend to overestimate or underestimate problems, especially functional deficits. For example, patients with cognitive impairment may be able to mask their deficits in the outpatient setting, but in the hospital their functional impairment may become clearer. Incorporating information from multiple sources and comparing notes between the team is a helpful way to build a complete picture of the individual.

The best approach to any patient is to assess early on the patient's goals and wishes. The team can offer a variety of interventions or management pathways, but the patient or the decision maker must be the one to choose among them. Treatment plans may vary based on the patient's goals, or unnecessary care may be provided when we do not understand what the patient's wishes are. For example, if a patient's goal is symptom control and desire to be at home for as long as possible, a rehabilitation stay after an acute hospital stay or a prolonged hospital stay may be unnecessary. Clear documentation of patient wishes in the chart or electronic medical record is crucial as patients move between home, hospital, or different specialists. During times of transition, it is

important the patient and the family understand the plan and how it aligns with patient goals. Given the complexity of health problems and the potential for continued decline, high-quality care for an older adult involves helping the patient and the family anticipate future problems. Although a patient after a hip fracture may recover and continue to live independently, there is the potential for decline that will require a higher level of care. Clear communication between the team and the patient is crucial in anticipating future problems.

❖ **Keep the patient's goals and wishes at the heart of the team.**

## Team-Based Care in New Models of Care

As healthcare systems move toward value-based reimbursement, team-based care becomes even more important. These new care models emphasize the importance of team-based care but expand the care from the usual settings to virtual visits and enhanced home-based services. These models are rapidly changing with healthcare systems continuing to adjust to taking the best care of patients. Some of these new models of care are briefly described in this section. All PCPs and health team members need to be aware of this evolution in healthcare and adapt the team to best serve the patient.

*Accountable care organizations* seek to improve the quality of care while using improved care coordination to reduce overall cost.[33] Frail elderly patients are one subset of high-need patients that have been found to account for higher costs. Although frail elderly account for less than 10% of the Medicare population, they account for more than half of potentially preventable spending for admissions related to ambulatory care, such as dehydration and urinary tract infections.[34] Inpatient and postacute care are high-cost settings for providing medical care for older adults.[35] Developing and using team-based interprofessional care is crucial to managing these costly services. A team-based approach may include care management by a care coordinator, who helps the patient via phone or in person to manage transitions of care. One benefit of moving toward value-based care would be the ability to financially support team-based care that was not possible with the fee-for-service payment model (see Ch. 9).

*Population health management* refers to an organization that accepts responsibility for all three aspects of the Triple Aim (improving the patient experience of care; improving the health of populations, and reducing per capita costs), with the goal of using available resources to address the areas of need within a defined population.[36] Population health management takes a systemwide approach to managing the health of the population it serves. Interprofessional teams play a key role as projects tend to go beyond the scope of the clinic. Successful examples include nurse discharge advocates who call to arrange follow-up appointments, confirm medication reconciliation, and conduct patient education along with a clinical pharmacist who called the patient 2 to 4 days after discharge to review medications. Pharmacist telephone calls were found to reduce the rate of unplanned hospital use.[37] As healthcare systems become responsible for the costs of patients outside the hospital, team-based care will need to adapt and become more creative.

*Home-based primary care (HBPC)* is another value-based program that focuses on providing care to patients in their own home. HBPC is a multidisciplinary, ongoing care strategy to provide cost-effective, in-home treatment to the approximately 4 million homebound, medically complex older adults in the United States.[38] Currently there is no single model of HBPC that can be adopted across all types of health organizations or geographic regions. Recent studies have demonstrated that HBPC can be a cost-effective strategy for delivering care to frail patients while maintaining or improving quality of care and patient satisfaction.[39] One example of HBPC is Independence at Home (IAH). IAH provides mobile interdisciplinary care to frail Medicare beneficiaries with multiple chronic conditions who need assistance with two or more basic ADLs, have had a recent nonelective hospitalization, and received acute or subacute rehabilitation services within the past year.[40] Home-based care provided by IAH must include availability by telephone at all hours, use of an electronic health record, and access to mobile diagnostic technology. During the first 2 years of this new model, IAH has been shown to provide cost savings.[40] HBPC works best with an interprofessional team that is supported by a healthcare system that supports value over volume of care.

## Summary

Older patients tend to have multiple, interacting chronic conditions along with functional limitations and family or social stresses. It is crucial that a team-based approach is adopted given the benefit of different disciplines with additional skills and knowledge to assist the PCP. The team must use clear communication with efforts to include the patients and the families in decision-making activities. As we move toward new, innovative models of care, incorporating and maximizing team care will improve the health and wellbeing not just of the patient but of all the clinicians involved.

### Web Resource

World Health Organization. Framework for action on interprofessional education and collaborative practice. WHO. http://www.who.int/hrh/nursing_midwifery/en/. Published 2010. Accessed April 16, 2014.

## Key References

14. Farrell TW, Luptak MK, Supiano KP, Pacala JT, De Lisser R. State of the science: interprofessional approaches to aging, dementia, and mental health. *J Am Geriatr Soc.* 2018;66(suppl 1):S40−S47.
15. Pocket Guide: TeamSTEPPS. Content last reviewed January 2020. Rockville, MD: Agency for Healthcare Research and Quality; https://www.ahrq.gov/teamstepps/instructor/essentials/pocketguide.html. Accessed 01.08.2020.
20. Sargeant J, Loney E, Murphy G. Effective interprofessional teams: "contact is not enough" to build a team. *J Contin Educ Health Prof.* 2008;28(4):228−234.

***References available online at expertconsult.com.***

# 3

# Geriatric Assessment

KARINA I. BISHOP AND ELIZABETH N. HARLOW

## OUTLINE

## OBJECTIVES

*Upon completion of this chapter, the reader will be able to:*

- Recognize that a detailed history is the first component of initial geriatric assessment.
- Understand how functional assessment provides a window into a patient's overall wellbeing and helps prioritize treatment plans.
- Describe how the geriatric physical examination should focus on systems that affect function.

- Maintain realistic expectations when planning for the visit; complete geriatric assessment will often take several clinic visits to accomplish.

## Introduction

Geriatric assessment is a challenging process that integrates patient-centered medical care and broad medical knowledge. A special approach is needed to care for older adults given the complexity in this patient population. Older adults often have subtle manifestations of disease and an increased prevalence of chronic illness, which make caring for them a challenge. In addition, many older adults will evolve in their healthcare priorities, which require an adjustment in the provider's clinical approach. Priorities often change from prolongation of life to prolongation of independence and quality of life. These attributes of older adults necessitate individualized care. Caring for older adults does not tend to follow an algorithm, nor is it "cookie cutter" medicine; rather, it requires attention to specific patient needs. Successful care plans align with patients' individual preferences and values.

❖ **Geriatric assessments encompass four main domains of patient care: mental, physical, functional, and social/economic.**

Adequate evaluation of this challenging, yet very rewarding, cohort requires both an organized approach and flexibility. Geriatric assessments encompass four main domains of patient care: mental, physical, functional, and social/economic. Not all elements need to be addressed during the initial assessment for every patient; however, each element should be considered eventually because each significantly contributes to overall patient wellbeing. Complete geriatric assessment will take planning and organization to accomplish over a series of visits. Time is often a limiting factor in assessment of the geriatric patient.

Geriatrics by nature is interprofessional. Nursing staff play an essential role in data collection and patient assessment. Other professionals, such as pharmacists, social workers, home healthcare providers, physical, occupational, and speech therapists, provide services that will greatly enhance patient care. Communication with these team members will provide insights that otherwise would go unnoticed.

One practice model through which geriatric interprofessional care works well is the patient-centered medical home. This model of patient care emphasizes the team approach, with the primary provider (physician and/or advanced practice provider) as the team leader of professionals focused on providing care that follows the patient's individual priorities. That primary provider coordinates and facilitates care provided by different participants in the healthcare team. Disciplines within the patient-centered medical home typically include nursing, pharmacy, and social work, and sometimes physical and occupational therapy. This care model focuses on shared decision making with patients.

---

**CASE**

**Ms. M (Part 1)**

Ms. M is a 68-year-old female here today to establish care. She currently resides in her own home with her husband and is here with her daughter today. Her prior primary care provider is retiring. Today she tells you that her biggest concern is dizziness for which an otolaryngologist evaluated her recently. The nurse begins the encounter by obtaining vital signs and reviewing the medications that she brought with her. You review notes from her past medical records. On medical record review, you learn that Ms. M has a history significant for diabetes mellitus that is diet controlled, hypothyroidism, and osteoarthritis. Her healthcare maintenance is up to date for the annual flu shot and pneumococcal immunization, but is due for tetanus and zoster immunization. She had a bone density scan 3 years ago showing osteopenia. Her last colonoscopy was 5 years ago, with recommended 10-year follow-up. Her last pelvic examination was at age 65 years at which time her last Papanicolaou smear was done with cotesting. She visits her dentist twice a year and just saw him last month.

What elements in the history would be helpful to understand her complaint?

What preparation is helpful before the clinic visit with this new patient?

---

## When To Do an Assessment

In general, geriatric assessments should be done on stable patients and not in those acutely ill or hospitalized because you may encounter patients who are delirious or unable to do their activities of daily living (ADLs) because of intravenous (IV) lines, monitors, and so on. A common time for a geriatric assessment is at the time of the initial visit with a patient in clinic when the patient is establishing care. These can then be repeated at annual visits. Many times, serial assessments collected over time provide more information than that collected at one point in time.

The direction of these assessments will depend on the patient's goals of care and current state of health, the level of disability, the place where the visit is taking place, time, and the availability of a care team. In addition, if the patient is cognitively impaired, the assessment should be done with the presence of the caregiver to provide collateral history.

To efficiently perform a geriatric assessment, one should take advantage of tools available in electronic medical record. This allows more time to focus on areas of specific concern. Many screening tools (e.g., questionnaires) can be filled out by the patient ahead of time or in the waiting room or applied by trained office staff once the patient is in the room.

## Previsit Planning

When preparing for a new patient visit, it is prudent to review the patient's medical record ahead of time for an overall understanding of the patient's past medical history. This preview of the available medical information guides the visit, allowing the provider to prioritize the pertinent medical issues. It will also aid in efficiency because there is often much to cover in little time at the initial visit. A medical record review identifies gaps in history that need attention and gaps in healthcare maintenance, including vaccinations and screenings. Ideally records will include eye and dental exams, areas often neglected with older patients. Medical record review also starts to compile a list of specialists involved in the patient's care with whom coordination will be needed. Previsit instructions for patients should include a request to bring their medications (including over-the-counter preparations, and preferably all medications in their original containers), assistive devices (canes, walkers), glasses, dentures, and hearing aids with them to the first visit. If needed, involve family members and caregivers in the visit. Caregivers will be needed for collateral history if there is a question of cognitive impairment, and their presence allows assessment of available caregiver support.

Ideally, the office design and patient flow keep older patients in mind. The needs of older individuals vary, but it is often necessary to ensure wheelchair accessibility and close parking. It is also helpful to use rooms large enough to accommodate the patient and family members who may accompany the patient. When possible, scheduling should allow adequate time for a new patient encounter (about 50—60 minutes) (Box 3.1).

---

**• BOX 3.1   Appropriate Environment for a Geriatric Assessment**

- Quiet room with good lighting
- Comfortable seating for the patient and caregivers
- Hearing amplifiers for hearing impaired, and reminder to wear glasses
- Staff available to help fill out forms if necessary

## Communicating With the Patient

Low health literacy and sensory impairment is common in older patients. Rates of low health literacy approach 30% by age 65 years[1] and only increase with age. By age 75 years, visual impairment affects 20% to 30% and hearing impairment 25%. Older patients often pretend/attempt to understand even when they do not. A well-lit room and written large-print instructions should be the norm; similarly, with a patient who is hard of hearing, ensure that the room is quiet, face the patient, speak slowly and clearly, and check understanding. A pocket talker or auditory amplifier will facilitate communication; these are inexpensive, so consider purchasing one for the clinic. These simple maneuvers ensure that the patient has the best chance of retaining the information. Undiagnosed sensory deficits can lead to inadequate understanding of care plans.

Beyond sensory impairments, low health literacy decreases a patient's ability to process information in either a verbal or a written format. To assess a patient's health literacy, consider using an assessment tool, such as the Rapid Estimate of Adult Literacy in Medicine—Short Form (REALM-SF)[2], a word-recognition tool with scoring based on the pronunciation of 66 common health-related terms. It is crucial that a provider use a "teach-back" or "ask-me-3" method to ensure appropriate understanding of the treatment plan. The teach-back method asks the patient to explain the medical plan back to you. The "ask-me-3" program, developed by the Institute for Healthcare Improvement,[3] motivates patients and family members to ask: (1) What is the main problem? (2) What do they need to do? (3) Why it is important? Chances are improved that patients will be able to carry through with plans if they are able to perform either of these methods.

◆ **To improve communication with older patients, assess vision, hearing, and health literacy.**

Cognitive impairment is a common impediment to executing a plan of care. Screening for cognitive impairment should be routine (see later). It is more difficult to collaborate with a patient on a treatment plan if that patient is unable to articulate symptoms or concerns and follow instructions. A caregiver or family member's corroborative history in such circumstances is invaluable. However, it is important not to ignore the patient; always keep eye contact when asking questions. Involve patients with cognitive impairment in decision making to the greatest extent possible. This builds rapport with and reasserts the patient's position as central in the healthcare team. Building a treatment plan based on a patient's preferences and priorities facilitates adherence to the treatment plan regardless of cognitive abilities. Providing written instructions for later reference is especially important for those with cognitive impairment. Written instructions should be in layman's terms or at the patient's health literacy level.

Another barrier to care is the predisposition of some older adults to attribute symptoms to normal aging and pass over important complaints as "no different than anyone else my age." They may not want to be seen as complainers or burdensome to their caregivers. In addition, some older patients will be embarrassed by symptoms, such as urinary incontinence, constipation, or falls. Patients may not bring up such symptoms unless asked directly. For this reason, it is important to conduct a complete review of systems, focused on geriatric syndromes (Box 3.2).

---

**• BOX 3.2 How to Communicate With an Older Adult[23]**

- Use a proper form of address (Mr. Mrs., Ms.), unless you are told by the patient not to do so.
- Avoid using familiar terms such as Granny, Dear, or Sweetie.
- Greet everyone as you enter the room and apologize if late.
- If you know the patient, try asking about family or a hobby to help relieve stress.
- Speak slowly and allow time to reply.
- Face the patient and make eye contact and use brief responses, such as "okay," "go on," to let the patient know you are following.
- Demonstrate empathy.
- Avoid medical jargon and explain particular procedures or studies that will be done.
- Be aware of cultural or ethnic background where words can have a different connotation.

---

**CASE**

**Ms. M (Part 2)**

Ms. M feels more tired, in part because her dizziness is preventing her from doing her routine exercises. She has also been taking meclizine for her symptoms, but this has not really helped. Her dizziness is worse when standing quickly, and she has noticed it has been worse the past couple of days that have seen record-breaking hot days in her town.

---

## History

A detailed history is often the majority of the initial assessment and remains a crucial part of follow-up visits. Although it is unnecessary (and often not feasible) to discuss all of the following with every visit, it is important to maintain a complete understanding of the full patient history and problem list. Consider allowing the patient to remain dressed for this portion of your patient encounter. This allows patients to remain comfortable (many older adults do not tolerate temperature extremes) and maintain their dignity. It is wise to ensure that enough chairs are available for all parties to be seated. Sitting down while eliciting the history gives reassurance that you are interested in what the patient has to say. It also minimizes dominance in a provider's body language. Finally, it gives the appearance of being unrushed. At some point during the encounter, it is appropriate to ask any accompanying family members to step out of the room. This allows for privacy for the patient to speak about any sensitive issues, including but certainly not limited to elder abuse or sexual dysfunction. It also presents an opportunity for a member of the clinic staff to obtain a collaborative history from the patient's family member(s).

## Chief Complaint

The history begins with addressing the patient's chief concern. This may be a bothersome symptom, or it may be why the patient is transferring care to a new healthcare provider. Asking an open-ended question such as, "What can I help you with today?" allows the patient to set the agenda, feel more in control, engender trust, and increase your chances of addressing the most pressing problem. After understanding what is most important to the patient, you should proceed with other concerns that are pressing from either previous visits or review of the medical record. When evaluating new patients, important insight can be gained into patients' understanding of their own health by eliciting their understanding of their medical diagnoses.

◆◆ **Family history for an older person may reveal the number and health and location of children who might become future caregivers**.

## Past Medical History, Past Surgical History, and Family History

Recapping the prior medical history and determining which medical problems have resolved is useful in creating a succinct and current problem list. Inquiring about prior surgical procedures is also helpful and prevents further imaging studies from being performed and discards possible etiologies from problems that may arise.

Family history in the traditional sense is relatively less important in an older adult, because hereditary conditions have usually declared themselves before old age. A family history of dementia can be informative, especially if it was of early onset. A particular benefit of taking a family history is in learning a patient's perspective on the illnesses and treatments received by his or her family members. Both positive and negative experiences with the healthcare system bring to light what the patient's preferences may be. Inquiring about the health of children can provide information regarding potential future caregivers for the patient.

### CASE

#### Ms. M (Part 3)

Ms. M was born and raised in this area and has a college education. She has been married for 33 years and has three children. She still works as a teacher, teaching language arts to junior high students. She denies smoking and has minimal alcohol use, a beer rarely. She denies any drug use. She is not currently sexually active because of vaginal dryness. She was offered topical estrogen but is using an herbal supplement instead. She does not have an advance directive. Ms. M notes that she feels safe in her place of residence. When asked to talk a little more about herself, her interests, and her values she mentions that her family has always been the most important thing in her life. She attends church and finds a great deal of comfort in her faith. She has always been active in her community, volunteering and participating in civic organizations. She also mentions that she enjoys playing cards, although she does not get much time to play anymore.

1. Beyond health-related habits, how can obtaining a social history be useful?
2. How can the social history be used to obtain information regarding a patient's healthcare goals?

## Social History

Social history can be enlightening. Habits, such as tobacco use, alcohol consumption, and exercise, and recreational drug use, should be discussed. Alcohol use disorders can masquerade as other conditions common in the older population. Alcohol misuse can present as gait instability, falls, or confusion. A long-time consumer of two drinks/day can get into trouble when the volume of distribution of alcohol declines with age. Similarly, alcohol use slows cognitive function or makes underlying cognitive dysfunction worse. Being aware of a person's alcohol habits can be helpful if the patient is ever admitted to the hospital, where withdrawal can be an occult cause of delirium.

Beyond a patient's health-related habits, it is important to inquire about a patient's support system. Who lives at home? Are there adult children who live in the area? Is the spouse still living? What is the health status of each? Does the patient serve in a caregiving role? The overarching goal of this discussion is to determine the strengths and limitations of an elder's support system. The majority of older adults will experience a period of dependency in later life. Inquiring about who would help, in the case of illness or emergency, can help identify people at risk, the so-called unbefriended elderly. It might also identify the patient's preferred surrogate decision maker. This might be an opportunity to have the patient designate a durable power of attorney for healthcare and document that individual in the medical record. Knowledge of family resources in such cases is helpful in providing optimal care. In addition, it is important to evaluate home safety. Does the person feel safe in his or her own home? Is the patient able to navigate stairs in case of emergency? Are there any firearms in the home? When there are concerns, have a visiting nurse or an occupational therapist (OT) go into the home to assess home safety, level of risk, and modifications to improve safety. Are there concerns for elder abuse (financial abuse, caregiver, or self-neglect)?

◆◆ **An important goal in taking the social history is to determine the strengths and limitations of an older person's support system**.

Consider beginning new patient encounters by expressing a desire to get to know the patients and asking them to tell their story. For example, "Can you tell me a little about yourself?", followed by, "What are some of the things that I need to know to help me take the best care of you?" In a way it is possible to begin to understand in detail what the patient values and what some of his or her priorities are. In this discussion attempt to determine what it is that the patient expects from the healthcare provider. Discuss what the patient's goals are with regard to healthcare. For example, does the patient desire a primary emphasis on life prolongation? Or an emphasis on preserving independence and self-care function? Or a focus on comfort and symptom control? If the patient is open to it, this may be an opportunity to discuss goals of care and code status. Many providers prefer to wait to start this more difficult conversation until they know the patient better and have a deeper understanding of the patient's medical conditions. Regardless, it is important to pursue this topic early in the relationship because it sets the framework for many future healthcare decisions. It also establishes rapport and ensures the patient that his or her opinions and values are important in how you direct their care. This process of listening to patients tell their story enables the provider to practice medicine with empathy and understanding.

Asking, "What do you like to do for fun?" may help elicit gambling or drinking issues or, on the contrary, elicit serious thought from patients and realization that they do very little and/or are depressed.

Bringing up sexual history is often forgotten as well. Patients may be sexually active or may want to be, and not be able to, secondary to a medical condition (see Ch. 32). Past history of violence, abuse, or high-risk behaviors could be contributing to problems as well. Lastly, asking about prior incarceration or time in prison for them or a close family member can shed light into the social support system.

◆◆ **Ask patients to bring all prescribed and over-the-counter medications to each clinic visit.**

## Medication Review

During each encounter, it is necessary to document an updated, reconciled medication list. Accurate knowledge of a patient's medications is crucial to appropriate prescribing and for quality medical care. Similar to discerning a patient's understanding of medical diagnoses, checking for a patient's understanding of medications can give important information about adherence and cognitive abilities. Discuss with patients their method of medication administration (e.g., pillboxes) to see if education or simplification of the regimen might improve adherence.

Medication changes and generic medication names are often not recalled accurately, so asking patients to bring all medications (prescribed and over the counter) to each clinic visit is very helpful. Having access to the actual medication bottles also provides insight into the number of pharmacies and prescribers involved, and refill dates may also be useful in assessing adherence. This helps to reduce redundant prescribing and polypharmacy. On review of a patient's medication list, one should scrutinize for problem medications (medications that may be inappropriate for older adults, medications requiring lab follow-up, etc.) (see Ch. 7). It is also important to ensure that the list of patient allergies is up to date.

## Review of Systems

The goal of the review of systems is to ensure that all systems are adequately covered using a method of direct questioning. This is of particular importance in the older population because of their many "hidden symptoms." Patients will often not bring up symptoms owing to embarrassment, normalization, or skepticism that anything can be done (see Ch. 1). Review of systems typically focuses around geriatric syndromes, many of which patients attribute to normal aging and will not be mentioned unless asked.

### Sensory

Hearing and vision impairment is common in older age. Cataracts, macular degeneration, and glaucoma may be advanced when diagnosed because older adults may not notice their visual deficits. Ask about driving or difficulty reading the newspaper to elicit patient's comments.

Hearing loss is most common in the high-frequency range and is usually bilateral. Acknowledgment of hearing loss by the patient or failing a whisper test[5] should prompt a referral to audiology. Hearing loss can lead to isolation, depression, and avoidance of social events. Changes in vision or hearing can exacerbate, or be mistaken for, other common geriatric problems.

### Nutrition

Asking about difficulty with chewing and swallowing food (ill-fitting dentures, dry mouth) or something as simple as who the patient is eating with provides clues to why a patient is losing weight. Asking who does the cooking and grocery shopping at home (and who has traditionally done these tasks if it has changed) may provide insight into a patient's worrisome nutritional status. Also, ask about use of community services, such as Meals on Wheels or church-delivered food. Weight and height should be assessed and compared over the past year. Unintentional weight loss of more than 5% in 6 months or a low body mass index should trigger a nutritional assessment.

### Sleep

Asking about bedtime routines and latency time before falling asleep, as well as nocturia and presence of naps, will most likely give clues to underlying causes of sleep problems. Screening for and evaluating for appropriate treatment for sleep apnea should also be addressed at this time.

## Continence

Ask about changes in bladder habits, specifically problems with urinary incontinence, frequency, or urgency. Similarly, bowel habits, such as constipation or diarrhea, can be difficult problems for an elder to bring up but extremely important to their perception of health. A complaint (or admission) of diarrhea should prompt a question about fecal incontinence. Use of tools like the International Prostate Symptoms Score[4] can quickly help with diagnosing prostatic obstruction problems, which are often present in older men.

## Mobility

Ask about falls (if yes, how many), fear of falling, and feelings of unsteadiness. Has the patient experienced any associated dizziness or presyncope? Does musculoskeletal pain impair mobility? Ask about joint mobility because limited range of motion can restrict function. Asking about the use of assistive devices, canes, walkers, and wheelchairs is also important for the assessment.

## Mood

Screen all patients for depression with the Patient Health Questionnaire−2.[6] It includes the following two questions:
- In the past 2 weeks have you had little interest or pleasure in doing things?
- In the past 2 weeks, have you often been bothered by being down, depressed, or hopeless?

A positive screen is appropriately followed up with a more in-depth assessment, usually a Patient Health Questionnaire−9 or the 15-item Geriatric Depression Scale.[7]

Depression can often go unrecognized. It can be a primary condition or associated with comorbid illnesses, such as dementia. In many cases, older adults do not meet criteria for depression, but endorse many, often somatic, symptoms like poor sleep, gastrointestinal complaints, and fatigue. Keeping a close eye on patients with subsyndromal depression, those with symptoms that do not meet full criteria for depression, should be a priority as the disease can present itself at any time and then require treatment.

## Cognition

Many patients recognize early cognitive deficits, such as recall of names or item placement. In such cases, it is important to screen for dementia. Other older adults may not be aware, and family members more often bring up their concerns about the older persons cognition. People with cognitive impairment have a higher risk of delirium and accidents. Later on in the chapter we further discuss screening for cognitive problems (see also Ch. 18).

## Social Support

Caregivers may accompany an older adult to clinic visits. They can be invaluable sources of collateral history or provide clues as to subtle changes or problems that the patient may be unaware of or unconcerned about. The more dependent a patient is, the more demands are placed on the caregiver. In such situations it becomes important to recognize the importance of the caregiver in the overall wellbeing of the patient. Although the health of the caregiver of your patient is not your primary concern, caregiver health does indirectly affect the health of your patient. Take a few moments to acknowledge the hard work that is being done by the caregiver on behalf of the patient. Emphasize to the caregiver the importance of looking after his or her own health and wellbeing. Stressed caregivers have been shown to suffer increased mortality.[8] The caregiving role can have negative psychological effects resulting in anger, depression, and anxiety. Maintaining the health of the caregiver therefore can be vital in maintaining the stability of an elder's health and preventing institutionalization. It can be helpful to have a list of resources available in the community that may be helpful should a need arise (Alzheimer associations [www.alz.org], Area Agencies on Aging [www.n4a.org], www.caregiver.org, driver evaluation programs, etc.).

---

**CASE**

### Ms. M (Part 6)

Ms. M continues to care for herself. She tells you that she performs all of her own ADLs without difficulty. She has had someone come in to help with her cleaning for many years because it was "never something I was good at." She does make all of her own meals, and states that she eats three meals a day. Ms. M manages her own finances, with her husband. She states proudly, "For years I have been perfect in balancing my checkbook to the penny," but later admits to a few mistakes more recently. She has not missed paying bills or had overdrafts on her account.
1. What can the patient's functional status tell you about her overall health?
2. What is the most efficient way to determine functional status in an office setting?

---

## Functional Screen

⁍ **Functional assessment is a crucial piece of the initial assessment because it reflects a patient's overall health status and quality of life.**

Assessment of functional ability is critical to caring for older patients. Functional status refers to the ability to perform the tasks necessary to participate in daily life. Function gives the provider a picture of the interaction between medical conditions, physical aging, cognition, and overall health in the setting of the patient's environment. Function is a predictor of mortality and a reflection of a patient's level of independence and, by extension, quality of life.[9] A patient's functional abilities are a window through which to view and prioritize medical conditions. Knowing a person's baseline functional abilities will allow you to appreciate when a change in function signals emerging or worsening illness. Functional loss is often the common pathway for progression of multiple chronic conditions. Despite this fact, healthcare providers often do not recognize the importance of functional disabilities in their patients. Care of diseases is just a portion of the care of an older adult. At times, disease management is less important than maximizing a patient's function. In addition, knowing a patient's functional status is the only means by which to assess the patient's resource needs and appropriate level of care. Loss of independence is often a sign of the need for involvement of other members of the care team, such as physical or occupational therapist.

It is important to assess both basic ADLs and more complex instrumental ADLs (IADLs). Basic ADLs, listed in Table 3.1, are skills necessary to get ready for the day. IADLs require more

## TABLE 3.1  Activities and Instrumental Activities of Daily Living

| Activities of Daily Living | Instrumental Activities of Daily Living |
| --- | --- |
| Bathing | Managing finances |
| Dressing | Driving |
| Toileting/continence | Shopping |
| Transferring | Preparing meals |
| Feeding | Medication management |
| Grooming | Technology use/ability to text or use internet |
|  | Housekeeping/laundry |

complex mental processes, such as executive function and judgment. Difficulty in IADLs may precede a decline in cognitive screening tests in persons with a developing dementia. Such a decline should prompt more thorough cognitive testing. Bathing is the ADL with most prevalence of disability and the reason for bath aides through home healthcare.

There are two methods by which to gain information regarding the functional status of a patient: self-report and performance. Self-report is significantly more practical (because it is quicker) but less reliable. Self-report methods of determining functional status are limited by patients' tendencies to overestimate their true abilities. Confirmation of function by family members is often helpful especially in patients with cognitive impairment. Several tools are available for use as an aid in assessing ADLs and IADLs, such as the Katz index for ADLs[10] and the Lawton scale for IADLs.[11]

Driving is often an important but sensitive issue to address with older people. If a patient is driving, it is important to ask not only if he or she has had any driving-related problems, but also specific questions, such as recent accidents, moving violations, passenger complaints, or problems with getting lost in familiar areas. Any of these are red flags and may indicate a need for further examination and formal driving evaluation. Safety concerns should be discussed honestly with the patient and family, particularly if the patient lacks insight into the deficits. Suggesting a driving evaluation by an OT is a good next step for those where it is not clear if they should be completely off the road. Although an initial OT consultation is generally a Medicare covered service, on-road testing is not and costs at least $300 to $500 depending on location. However, remember that recommending that a patient stop driving can lead to decreased activity and increased depressive symptoms (level of evidence = B).

The American Geriatrics Society in collaboration with the National Highway Traffic Safety Administration has developed the Clinician's Guide to Assessing and Counseling Older Drivers[12] where more information can be obtained.

### CASE

#### Ms. M (Part 7)

After you have finished your history, you politely ask the daughter to step out as one of your nurse helps Ms. M get dressed in a gown. You take this opportunity to verify the history you have just obtained. Ms. M's daughter agrees with much of what has been said, but further expresses a concern for her mother's memory. She explains that her mother has always been very bright, but that she has been making more mistakes in her financial management, and has difficulty putting together classes for her students. She also expresses concern that her mother is not, in fact, eating or drinking well. She confides that they have recently had to go shopping for smaller-sized clothes and that she thinks that her mom has lost more than 20 pounds in the last year. You then direct her to the waiting room for the examination portion of the visit, reassuring her that someone will come and get her to wrap up this initial visit.

When is it important to take a collateral source history?

## Collateral History

A collateral history provides an opportunity for those who care about the patient to express their concerns about the patient's health. It is especially important when there is a change in cognition. Determining if the changes have been gradual or sudden "step downs" can help identify the cause of the impairment. The AD-8[13] is a brief tool in which informants describe changes in behavior from baseline that may indicate a cognitive problems. Asking about prior personality traits can also help understand patient behavior. Recognizing their temperament, mood, and outlook on life, as seen by those who are close to them, may bring further insights. The Neuropsychiatric Inventory Questionnaire (NPI-Q) is a self-administered questionnaire completed by informants about patients. It contains questions about 12 domains related to cognition and provides a brief assessment of neuropsychiatric symptomatology.[14]

Also asking the informants about who assists the patient with ADLs and IADLs and how many hours per week, provides a look into their life, and helps assess caregiver stress.

### CASE

#### Ms. M (Part 8)

On physical examination, Ms. M's vital signs are temperature 97.7° F, heart rate 68 beats per minute, respiratory rate 16 breaths per minute, and blood pressure lying down 132/86 mmHg. Standing blood pressure after 3 minutes is 116/67 mmHg. Her weight is 142 lb (which from your review of the medical records is about 20 lb less than a year ago, but stable since her visit with her previous provider 6 weeks ago). Before she leaves the chair, you ask her to cross her arms and rise without using her arms. She is able to do so without difficulty, but quickly grabs on to the wall next to her to adjust her balance. As she ambulates to the examination table, you observe that she has a narrow-based gait with normal strides and a mildly forward-flexed posture. The head, ears, eyes, nose, and throat examination reveals intact vision (acuity of 20/30 in each eye tested individually, with correction). She fails the whisper test bilaterally, but is found to have cerumen blocking her ear canals bilaterally. You make a note to proceed with cerumen removal, and to recheck before a referral to audiology. Her oropharynx is mildly dry but otherwise clear. Her dentition and oral hygiene are good. Chest examination reveals regular cardiac rhythm with occasional premature beats and an S4 gallop. No murmurs were heard. Lungs are clear to auscultation bilaterally. Her abdomen is benign. On pelvic examination she has atrophic vaginal mucosa but no other abnormalities. On musculoskeletal exam, she has full range of motion in both hips and shoulders. Her strength is minimally decreased bilaterally. Her cranial nerves, with the exception of olfactory, are intact. She demonstrates positive palmomental and glabellar reflexes. Her neurologic examination is otherwise intact. On cognitive evaluation, she recalls two of three on the 3-item recall. She draws a clock that is the right shape with accurate numbering; however, the hands are placed incorrectly. You move on to perform a Montreal Cognitive Assessment (MoCA), in which she scores 23/30 (she loses 2 points in the visuospatial part, 1 point in naming, 1 point in abstraction, 3 points in delayed recall, and orientation is intact). Before bringing her daughter back into the room, you confirm that Ms. M feels safe in her home. Finally, you step out as Ms. M redresses to gather all of the information you have collected and to formulate orders for further workup.

1. What should be the focus of the geriatric physical examination?
2. How does a geriatric physical examination vary from that of a younger patient?

## Geriatric-Specific Physical Examination

A geriatric-specific physical examination embraces an increased focus on systems that affect function. Many of the components remain the same as those for a younger individual, but the examination typically includes a more in-depth musculoskeletal and neurologic assessment. A general survey of the patient can provide a wealth of information during the history portion of the exam. It is helpful to take note of the patient's level of alertness and ability to answer questions appropriately. Note also the use of language, in particular, any slurring of speech, word-finding difficulties, or repetitiveness. Evaluate the patient's thought content (is it logical, requiring redirection, or delusional?) and listen for tangential thought patterns. Observe the way the patient is dressed, including grooming and hygiene, as well as the appropriateness of dress for the current weather conditions. This may provide insight into underlying cognitive and functional status. Observe the fit of a patient's clothing, and examine for temporal wasting to determine nutritional status.

Vital signs deserve careful review. Abnormalities, such as weight loss, irregular pulse, or tachypnea, have important implications. Elevated blood pressure is not unusual with new patients, given an expected level of anxiety, so this should be rechecked, preferably at home. Home blood pressure monitoring is an accurate and useful measure of blood pressure.[15] It is helpful to check orthostatic blood pressure and heart rate as part of routine vital signs taken with older adults. Blood pressure should be taken in the sitting or supine position, then at 1 and 3 minutes after standing. The prevalence of orthostatic hypotension (a drop in systolic blood pressure >20 mmHg, or a drop in diastolic blood pressure >10 mmHg with standing) significantly increases with age, and the finding is common in patients over the age of 85 years.[16] This reflects altered baroreceptor sensitivity and provides information about why a patient may be dizzy or unsteady (two common geriatric complaints). A pain scale should be included as part of the vital sign intake because pain, similar to other parts of the review of systems, may be viewed as normal by an older patient. In addition, this provides a way in which to objectify and trend chronic pain.

During the head, ears, eyes, nose, and throat examination, visual acuity and visual fields should be checked for deficits. Visual assessment becomes particularly important if the patient has a problem with falls or if there are questions regarding driving abilities. When examining visual acuity, make sure to use corrective lenses. Using a Snellen chart or Rosenbaum card and scoring worse than 20/40 is the cutoff for visual impairment.[17] There are several methods by which to quickly screen for hearing deficits. The whisper test is an accurate screen for hearing loss, as it detects inability

to hear speech. If the patient fails the whisper test screening, the next step is evaluation for occluding cerumen. If present, one should retest after removal. If the screen is again failed, the provider should offer referral to audiology for definitive diagnosis and treatment. The oral examination is a useful portion of the geriatric exam because it can give clues to unexplained weight loss (e.g., if dentition is poor) or give a potential explanation for falls (if mucous membranes are dry, may indicate dehydration and a cause for orthostasis).

Examination of the chest may reveal dry crackles at the lung bases that do not necessarily imply pathology. Similarly, atrial or ventricular ectopy is also typically benign. A fourth heart sound is common among older adults, even among those without hypertension or heart disease. However, a third heart sound is always pathologic and suggests heart failure. Systolic heart murmurs are common in many older adults. Many are benign, for example, representing turbulence over a sclerotic aortic valve. If unsure, further evaluation with an echocardiogram is helpful.

A genitourinary exam is helpful based on patient presentation. With patients who complain of urinary incontinence, it is an important part of the evaluation for etiology. Examine for stress incontinence by locating the urethral meatus and asking a patient to cough. Leakage of urine with cough is positive for stress incontinence. In addition, one should evaluate for signs of cystocele as possible contributors to urinary incontinence. In addition, vulvar malignancies are not uncommon, and palpable ovaries in an older woman are always pathologic. A rectal exam is helpful if there is concern for bowel incontinence (assessment of sphincter tone, for stool impaction, and perirectal hygiene). In addition, checking for occult blood may explain anemia. Abdominal palpation may detect a fullness in the colon as a sign of impaction that points to the etiology of fecal soiling. In a male with urinary symptoms consistent with benign prostatic hyperplasia (urgency, frequency, nocturia, etc.), a rectal examination can give clues to prostate size and more worrisome symptoms of malignancy, such as nodules. Because hyperplasia limited to the vicinity of the urethra (median lobe hypertrophy) can impair urine flow significantly, a gland that feels normal on palpation does not rule out benign prostatic hyperplasia as the cause (see also Ch. 23 and Ch. 24).

The musculoskeletal and neurologic examinations provide direct information regarding functional ability. Performance-based measurements are more objective assessments of functional status and can be used to confirm a patient's self-report. Several tests that can be performed quickly provide useful information. The Timed Up and Go (TUG) test[18] is an assessment of gait and lower leg function. This is done by observing a patient rise from a chair without use of the arms, walk 3 meters or 10 feet, turn around, and return. A wealth of knowledge can be gained by watching this simple maneuver. Gait speed, for example, is a predictor of mortality, and an older adult who takes more than 12 seconds to complete the TUG test is at risk for falling. The ability to rise from a chair gives information regarding lower extremity strength and the ability to transfer. Inability to rise from a chair suggests hip flexor weakness and is a predictor of future disability (level of evidence = A). Examine the gait for step length, arm swing, and base width. Be sure to note unsteadiness, favoring of one side versus the other, or staggering during a turn. Shoulder function can be assessed by having a patient touch the back of the head and then placing hands together behind the back to test range of motion. Hand function can be easily tested by having the patient pick up a pencil. Balance can be assessed using a modified Romberg test, during which the

**Eyes**
Cataracts
Decreased visual acuity

**Ears**
Decreased hearing
Excess cerumen blocking ear canals

**Mouth**
Poor dentition
Dry mucous membranes

**Neck**
Elevated jugular venous pressure
Carotid bruits
Limited range of motion in the cervical spine

**Chest**
Kyphosis/scoliosis

**Cardiovascular**
Irregular heart rhythm
Systolic murmurs and S4 are common

**Abdomen**
Palpable aorta
Abdominal bruit

**Genitourinary**
Male: prostatic enlargement/nodules
Female: cystocele, rectocele, adnexal masses

**Musculoskeletal**
Gait abnormalities
Asymmetry in strength

**Neurologic**
Apraxia
Loss of coordination

patient stands with the feet together and eyes open. Simple observation of patients' ability to dress and undress themselves and put on socks and shoes provides information regarding independence. Occupational therapy can be usefully consulted for more extensive performance-based functional testing.

Examine any assistive devices needed for ambulation. Check the height of the device to ensure proper fit. With the patient in a standing position, and with the arms fully extended, the top of the cane or walker should be at the break of the wrist. Once the patient is on the examination table, test range of motion, particularly in the hips, shoulders, and hands, because these are most closely related to functional activities. Assess for strength, muscle tone, and bulk. Assess for manual dexterity or clumsiness with rapid alternating movements. In addition, observe for tremor that may inhibit the ability to perform tasks requiring fine coordination. Finally, with regard to the musculoskeletal system, observe for signs of osteoporosis (e.g., kyphosis) and examine specific joints of complaint. When testing cranial nerves, observe for signs of facial droop or tongue deviation that may be indicative of prior stroke. Loss of sense of smell (cranial nerve 1) may occur early in

Alzheimer disease, although this is nonspecific. Primitive reflexes, such as the glabellar, snout, or rooting reflex, indicate evidence of brain dysfunction, although they are not specific to location. Stereognosis and graphesthesia test cortical integration (the ability to integrate multiple areas of input), as well as sensation. Some neurologic changes are commonly seen in older adults, and there is debate about the extent to which these changes are pathologic or simply part of normal aging.

◆◆ **Examine the height of canes and walkers to ensure proper fit. Devices are often inherited or borrowed and not fit for the patient**.

Skin examination in older adults is often overlooked; however, skin is an important source of pathology. Evaluate closely for skin tears and early signs of pressure ulceration in at-risk patients (e.g., patients with poor mobility). In particular, examine areas of increased pressure (sacrum and heels) for signs of ulceration. Also, evaluate for bruising patterns as possible indicators of falls or elder abuse. Monitor lesions for growth, color change, and border irregularity as signs of malignancy (Box 3.3).

## Cognitive Testing

Cognitive assessment should be done with corrected vision and hearing aids (if appropriate) and in the patient's native language. Proven screening tools include the mini-cog (3-item recall and clock drawing[19]) or 3-item recall alone.[20] When positive, examining with the MoCA, Mini Mental State Exam (MMSE), or St. Louis University Mental Status Examination should be performed. The MMSE is proprietary and the MoCA has required training and certification before its use. With this brief testing, it might be unclear how much impairment a person has and it becomes important to know to whom to refer for further cognitive evaluation of persons who are difficult to diagnose. A full evaluation by neuropsychology is very useful in individuals whose cognitive deficits are difficult to tease out during brief testing. Although geriatricians do these evaluations routinely, the US Preventive Services Task Force currently concludes that the current evidence is insufficient to assess the balance of benefits and harms of screening for cognitive impairment; this recommendation is being updated.

**CASE**

**Ms. M (Part 9)**

For further laboratory workup, you are interested in Ms. M's kidney function, given her ibuprofen usage. You are also interested in further workup for her cognitive impairment. At this time, it seems that she is experiencing orthostatic drops in her blood pressure that are making her dizzy.

## Routine Laboratories and Imaging

The primary purpose of laboratory and imaging investigations is to inform clinical decision making in a way that is beneficial for the patient. There is no global evidence-based approach for deciding appropriate laboratory and imaging studies for older adults. To conserve resources and avoid false-positive findings, testing should be based on a patient's presentation and complaints. Overly aggressive testing also runs the risk of finding "incidentalomas," unexpected lesions, or results with uncertain significance. Workup of incidentalomas can be costly, risky, and provide ambiguous results. Testing should only be pursued if the result will change the patient's treatment plan and if likely benefits outweigh risks. It is important to think about what would be done with the knowledge gained by the results. Is the patient an operative candidate, and does surgery fit with the patient's stated goals of care? Is the patient's life expectancy (which reflects age, gender, disease burden, and functional status) long enough that treatment of discovered colonic polyps or cancer would make a difference in his or her life expectancy? Using tools such as e-prognosis,[21] available at eprognosis.ucsf.edu, can help with graphs and information to better perform shared decision making. Overall, diagnostic and screening investigations for older patients should be ordered after careful deliberation, with consideration given to procedural risk, "incidentaloma" findings, and patient preferences.

---

### CASE

#### Ms. M (Part 10)

You now feel that you have gotten to know Ms. M fairly well, and you are getting familiar with many of her medical issues. At this point, you feel that a strong enough connection has been made for you to broach the topic of goals of care. You start the conversation by saying to Ms. M, "I would like to talk with you about your healthcare goals. I have patients who tell me that they want me to do everything I can to keep them alive. On the other side, I have patients who request that I make their comfort and quality of life the top priority. Other patients are somewhere in between. What is your thinking on these things?" After much thought, Ms. M comes down somewhere in the middle. She states, "I understand I am getting old, but I still think I have a lot in me. I feel if we can fix my dizziness I will be able to get back to my usual routine." She determines that at this time she would like to remain "full code" (meaning that she wants everything done to prolong her life).

1. What is one way to ask a patient about his or her goals of care?
2. What is the patient's role in decision making regarding the treatment plan?

---

## Advance Directives, Quality of Life, and Goals of Care

The geriatric assessment is a great opportunity to discuss advance directives. Taking into consideration cultural, ethnic, and spiritual background is of utmost importance when carrying out these discussions. It is important to have conversations about who the designated decision maker would be in the event the assessed patient was unable to make decisions and what aggressive behaviors, if any, would be preferred by the patient in the event of him or her being found unresponsive.

Discussion regarding goals of care is an important, and ongoing, part of geriatric care. This tends to be a combination of advice and directed decision making based on the information gathered during the social history (the patient's values and treatment preferences). It is helpful to ask the patient, "What is most important to you at this stage in your life?" This question can be followed up by determining what the patient would want if doing whatever was most important to him or her was no longer possible. Consider subsequent questions to understand the patient's priorities (e.g., is life prolongation the priority? remaining independent? symptom control?). It is helpful to understand how the patient wants major

healthcare decisions to be made (e.g., if the patient wants to involve family). Finally, given the patient's current quality of life and healthcare goals, consider discussion regarding resuscitation efforts in the event of cardiac or respiratory arrest. This portion of the discussion may need to be tailored based on a patient's culturally based beliefs and preferences as well.

The most widely used instrument to measure quality of life is the Short Form-36 Health Survey[22] (SF-36), which includes 36 items organized into eight domains. It has been tested among older adults, but may lose sensitivity with those who are frail. Another option is to ask, "How would you rate your quality of life today: excellent, very good, good, fair, or poor?"

Discussion of goals of care may include screening and prevention. The importance of screening and prevention in a patient's care is a balance of the patient's preferences and overall prognosis. In addition, the feasibility of the test to be performed given the functional status of the patient must play a role in decision making. Health promotion, or health and wellness education, should be an important part of this discussion regardless of goals of care. This involves encouragement toward smoking cessation and reduction of alcohol use. In addition, education should be provided on the benefits of exercise in aging, including reduced mortality and better balance, cognition, and function. This is also an opportunity to encourage patients to be socially active. These topics may be more aptly covered in a "Welcome to Medicare" or the Medicare Annual Wellness Visit, which is also an excellent time to ensure vaccinations are up to date.

---

### CASE

#### Discussion

With Ms. M's daughter back in the room, you now begin to wrap things up. It is unclear at this time, given her cognitive screening results, how well Ms. M is able to self-manage her health, although she has not shown much difficulty in the past. For this reason, you write down all of your instructions for Ms. M to take home with her and to discuss with her husband. You have arranged for further cognitive evaluation because of her cognitive screen. You recommend increased oral hydration and reducing her blood pressure medication in an attempt to reduce orthostatic drops that make her symptomatic. You also recommend stopping the sleep aid and the meclizine, which can be contributing to her dizziness or worsening her cognition. You additionally have encouraged her to change from ibuprofen to acetaminophen because it has a more favorable side effect profile. You will also proceed with cerumen removal between now and her next visit. As they are leaving, you reiterate to both Ms. M and her daughter the importance of follow-up. Much was accomplished in this first visit, but you still feel like there is much to do. You then sit down to construct your to-do list for their next visit in 1 month: (1) follow up results of cognitive testing and discuss implications in her job; (2) arrange meeting with social worker for additional support for Ms. M and her daughter; (3) rescreen hearing in the absence of cerumen, and refer to audiology as needed; and (4) query regarding gait and balance after these changes have been made, and send to physical therapy if needed for balance training and strengthening.

1. How can you avoid becoming overwhelmed by complicated older patients?
2. What can you realistically expect to accomplish on the initial clinic visit?

---

## Patient Education and Self-Management

Patient education is a crucial step toward successful patient management outside of the office setting. Assess the ability and willingness of your patient to self-manage his or her medical issues. This can be done by demonstration of understanding of medical problems and the treatments proposed. Self-management can be difficult in older patients given the complexity of medical illness, cognitive deficits, complex drug regimens, and other factors. It may be necessary to involve family members or other supportive individuals in this discussion because they can be helpful in promotion of self-management at home. In discussion with the patient, it is important to set reasonable healthcare goals. Appropriate goals can include increasing exercise or socialization or setting up a pillbox for medication management. As the clinical encounter ends, it is important to reiterate many of the main points established during the visit and check for understanding (teach back). As electronic health records are nearly universal, meaningful use of those records includes a written after-visit summary that includes any medication changes or important points for the patient to take home for future reference or sharing with caregivers. It is a good idea to ensure that any information provided to the patient is at an appropriate level of health literacy and appropriate font size; we suggest bold font, size 14 to 16.

## Summary

Geriatric assessment is a comprehensive review of a patient's mental, physical, functional, and socioeconomic status. It includes a complete history focused on function and quality of life with enough room to allow flexibility in the conversation. Assessing for geriatric syndromes and evaluating ADLs and IADLs can help elicit the problems that should be addressed first. Establishing good rapport and understanding what the patient values will make for a more efficient visit and for better communication. Making

## Follow-Up Visits

Commonly, new geriatric patients will require follow-up shortly after their initial visit (typically 4–6 weeks) for continued evaluation. It is very likely that much evaluation work has been left undone after the initial visit. It is nearly impossible to cover every medical problem a person age > 65 years has had throughout life, so planning for a future visit and keeping a to-do list is helpful for you as well as the patient. This is also a good opportunity to determine if prior records are needed, or pharmacies need to be called to verify medications. Follow-up visits certainly do not need to readdress all aspects of the initial history and physical. Focus your encounter first on things that have changed since the last visit. In addition, spend time tying up loose ends from previous visits and any aspects that are most important to patient function (cognition, mobility, hearing, and vision in particular). Review medications and functional status with every visit. With complex geriatric patients, it can be helpful to cultivate a habit of creating a next-visit to-do list at the end of your clinic notes. This helps provide focus and structure for an otherwise challenging patient population.

to-do lists of things left undone is useful. In addition, making sure to discuss goals of care, and having the patient relay his or her goals to those who are close, is also important and encouraged to be discussed ahead of time. Taking advantage of available resources, whether they be nursing, social work, pharmacy, or other professions, will help because good geriatric care necessitates a team-based approach.

## Key References

9. Lee PG, Cigolle C, Blaum C. The co-occurrence of chronic diseases and geriatric syndromes: the health and retirement study. *J Am Geriatr Soc*. 2009;57(3):511–516.
19. Borson S, Scanlan J, Brush M, Vitaliano P, Dokmak A. The mini-cog: a cognitive 'vital signs' measure for dementia screening in multi-lingual elderly. *Int J Geriatr Psychiatry*. 2000;15:1021–1027.
20. Lin JS, O'Connor E, Rossom R, et al. *Screening for Cognitive Impairment in Older Adults: An Evidence Update for the U.S.* *Preventive Services Task Force*. Evidence Report No. 107. AHRQ Publication No. 14-05198-EF-1. Rockville, MD: Agency for Healthcare Research and Quality; 2013.
23. National Institute on Aging. *Understanding Older Patients*. May 17, 2017. Available at: https://www.nia.nih.gov/health/understanding-older-patients. Accessed 25.07.19.

**References available online at expertconsult.com**.

# 4

# Lesbian, Gay, Bisexual, Transgender Medicine in Older Adults

CARL BURTON AND MANUEL A. ESKILDSEN

## OUTLINE

*Additional online-only material indicated by icon.*

## OBJECTIVES

- To create a welcoming practice environment for the lesbian, gay, bisexual, and transgender (LGBT) community.
- To expertly assess a sexual history in older LGBT adults and offer age-appropriate screening and counseling.
- To understand community structures that contribute to older LGBT adults' health.
- To provide age-appropriate primary care screening to all LGBT patients.

---

### CASE 1

#### Hector Ramirez (Part 1)

Hector Ramirez is a physically active 76-year-old male with history of hypertension, type II diabetes mellitus, hyperlipidemia, and history of myocardial infarction 2 years prior, now presenting to establish care with you. He comes into your clinic with a man he introduces as his roommate. Hector has no acute complaints. He reports his health is robust and he is independent in his activities of daily living (ADLs) and instrumental ADLs (IADLs). He walks independently without an assistive device and denies any recent falls. He still does some part-time work as a lawyer. For leisure, he enjoys swimming in the morning and walking his dog throughout the day.

He denies hearing or vision issues and reports he is up to date on routine vaccinations.

He continues answering your questions, denying any substance use, and reporting that he is currently sexually active with men only. He then pauses, grasping the hand of his roommate. He endorses that he has never told any health provider about his sexuality before because no one had ever cared to ask if he had sex with men. He reports he has been with his roommate for 35 years and self-identifies as gay.

1) What additional information would be helpful for determining his care needs and appropriate laboratory testing?
2) What may be additional healthcare considerations in care for this older gay male?

# Introduction

Providers care for a group of patients with diverse sexual and gender identities (Box 4.1). As a social term of identity, *gay* can refer to men who identify as MSM (men who have sex with men), although not all MSM will identify as gay. Indeed, some adults will not use any categorical term to identify themselves. Other adults may use the term *bisexual* to identify themselves as being sexually attracted to both sexes, for instance. Gay men are part of the larger lesbian, gay, bisexual, transgender (LGBT) community (see Box 4.1). Women who have sex with women (WSW) may also identify as gay or lesbian. The groups within the LGBT community share societal stigmatization for their status as a gender or sexual minority.

A manifestation of this stigmatization is the presumption of people, as a society and on an individual level, to be heterosexual, a phenomenon called heterosexism. Older adults are diverse. It is important to ask open-ended, nonjudgmental questions that prompt patients to share information they are comfortable with, such as their sexual identity. Gathering information regarding a patient's sexual and gender identity is helpful in the setting of a diverse community and affects the care geriatric healthcare practitioners provide. Beyond sexual orientation or sexual identity, our patients have various gender identities (see Box 4.1). A patient may identify as a cisgender man, congruent with the natal gender, or may identify as a transgender woman, for example. There is also variability in how individuals express their gender, independent of their identity. Many individuals will pursue gender affirming

therapies, for example, but this is a diverse group where not all individuals will pursue these treatments (Box 4.2).

To best serve patients, it is important to understand their sexual and gender identity and therapies related to their care. Within the LGBT community, disclosure of one's sexual or gender identity to another person, including a provider, is considered "coming out" or "coming out of the closet." There are degrees of coming out, meaning that people will disclose their identity along a spectrum, from the invisible to completely transparent individual. With the geriatric LGBT community, there is a variety of societal and cultural experiences that intersect across a lifetime affecting identity disclosure, making them more prone to withholding information on their sexual identity.

## Asking About Sexual Orientation and Gender Identity

A helpful starting point in a busy primary care practice to facilitate sexual and gender identity disclosure is intake paperwork. For example, including standardized questions with open-ended responses to prompt patients for their identity encourages disclosure. One example would be asking patients their preferred pronouns (e.g., if they refer to themselves as "he/him/him," "she/her/hers," "they/their/theirs," or other pronouns in their social history). Other important social history questions to explore include if persons are having sex with men, women, or both, and then asking if they identify as gay, lesbian, or bisexual. Both with gender and sexual identity, it is important to ask for this information and to not make assumptions. Using a standard, open, nonjudgmental manner helps LGBT older adults feel they are in a safe space, despite historical experience to the contrary.

## Minority Stress

LGBT older adults have lived through times when being LGBT was illegal, when acquired immunodeficiency syndrome (AIDS) was an epidemic ravaging the community, and when being gay or transgender was considered a mental illness. These

---

**• BOX 4.1** **Lesbian, Gay, Bisexual, Transgender Terminology**

- **LGBT**: An umbrella term to describe the lesbian, gay, bisexual, and transgender community. Now also appended with terms, such as queer. There is no consensus on sole acronym because there may be others (e.g., LGBTQI) to describe the community.
- **Sexual orientation:** An enduring, inherent emotional, sexual, or romantic attraction on a fluid spectrum.
- **MSM:** Men who have sex with men.
- **WSW**: Women who have sex with women.
- **Gay**: A term of identity for sexual orientation to refer to people who have sex with the same gender. Traditionally used to describe men, it can also be applied to WSW.
- **Lesbian**: A term of identity for a woman whose sexual orientation is toward women.
- **Bisexual:** A person whose primary sexual and emotional orientation is to both genders. Their orientation toward other people may also be regardless of gender.
- **Transgender**: a person whose gender identity does not fit the natal gender assigned at birth. This person may be genderqueer and not identify within the gender binary.
- **Queer**: a term of inclusion for younger LGBT community members, for people who do not clearly identify with other gender or sexual identities. In geriatric medicine, older adults may see it as a slur because of the implications the term has historically carried. When in geriatrics practice, queer can then be perceived as a pejorative term and should be avoided.

(Modified from LGBT Resource Center. *General Definitions*. 2019. Available at: https://lgbt.ucsf.edu/glossary-terms.)

---

**• BOX 4.2** **Gender Identity Terminology**

- **Gender dysphoria:** Distress that is caused by a discrepancy between a person's gender identity and that person's sex assigned at birth. This distress may also be from the associated gender role or attributed sex characteristics.
- **Gender identity:** A person's intrinsic sense of being male, female, or an alternative gender.
- **Sex:** Sex is assigned at birth as male or female, usually based on the appearance of the external genitalia. Natal gender.
- **Gender expression:** The way an individual socially expresses gender, such as style of clothing, speech, and mannerisms. Gender identity and gender expression may differ. There may also be people who do not present in the binary or masculine or feminine roles, presenting as an alternate gender, such as genderqueer.

(Modified from Coleman E, Bockting W, Botzer M, et al. Standards of care for the health of transsexual, transgender, and gender-nonconforming people, Version 7. *Int J Transgend*. 2012;13 (4):165–232; LGBT Resource Center. *General Definitions*. 2019. Available at: https://lgbt.ucsf.edu/glossary-terms.)

past experiences represent important intersections with the medical system and society that have deeply affected older LGBT adults and how comfortable they are coming out to providers about their gender and sexual identities. For patients, being out with their gender or sexual identity is a complex, multifaceted issue that includes personal safety at times, predisposing LGBT people to stress.

The treatment of LGBT people across a lifetime as a minority not only affects identity and expression, but also health. In a situation called minority stress, LGBT older adults have experienced a hostile social environment filled with discrimination and stigma that creates stress within the person.[1,2] For example, persons may be increasingly vigilant of their actions, expecting rejection regardless of the situation or even hide their identity for fear of harm. With this expectation of harm, they may be less likely to come out. Someone may even experience societal stigma that has become internalized, a phenomenon called internalized homophobia. Together these factors contribute to stress, which leads to higher rates of mental disorders in LGBT individuals and may be connected to physical illness. This is an area of continuing study.[1]

## Preventative Screening in Lesbian, Gay, Bisexual Populations

In primary care for lesbian, gay, bisexual (LGB) populations, there is little population-level data to guide practice. Instead, expert opinion and small case studies inform our practice. For example, translating minority stress into primary care practice, routine screening for depression would be recommended in LGBT older adults, in addition to assessing for suicide risk. These practices augment typical age-appropriate screening in older adults, such as cancer screening. However, there are certain considerations that are more specific to LGB patients.

In gay men, there is consideration of the risk of anal cancer and screening. An HPV (human papillomavirus)—related cancer, anal cancer is more common in MSM because of lifetime exposure to HPV through receptive anal intercourse. This translates to being 20 times as likely as a heterosexual man to develop anal cancer.[3] Besides receptive anal intercourse, human immunodeficiency virus (HIV) infection is an important risk factor for anal cancer, even with highly active antiretroviral therapy (HAART), potentially because of increased activity of HPV in an immunocompromised host.[4] (HAART is a customized combination of different classes of medications that can control viral load, delaying or preventing the onset of symptoms or progression to AIDS, therby prolonging survival in people infected with HIV.) Despite known risk factors and higher prevalence of cancer, guidance for screening is unclear.

For better screening guidelines, there is still a need for quality prospective studies to guide care, despite known risks in this population and increased prevalence of cancer.[5] No current consensus exists to formally recommend screening at-risk populations for anal dysplasia. However, experts in infectious disease advocate for anal dysplasia screening in high-risk individuals. In HIV-positive MSM populations, annual anal Pap smears are suggested and can also be considered in HIV-positive women with history of receptive anal intercourse, abnormal cervical Pap smears, or history of genital warts (grade C).[6] The reasoning behind screening is largely extrapolated from the screening used for cervical cancer cytology, another HPV-related cancer, and attempting to detect lesions,

such as anal intraepithelial neoplasia and anal cancer, before significant complications develop. There are no guidelines for HIV-negative MSM and use of anal cytology, although biannual screening can be considered as a cost-effective option (grade D).[7]

There are additional considerations for anal cytology in MSM. For older adults, there is no consensus on an age at which to stop screening for anal cancer, unlike guidelines for cervical Pap smears. Healthcare providers also must consider steps after positive screening tests. If a screen returns positive, the next step would be diagnostic high-resolution anoscopy, comparable with cervical cancer screening followed by colposcopy. However, not all healthcare systems have access to high-resolution anoscopy. If the healthcare system cannot provide high-resolution anoscopy or further evaluation after positive anal Pap smear, the system is unable to effectively triage and treat these patients. In this situation, referral to a center with resources and the capability of anal colposcopy would be preferable, particularly in patients with multiple risk factors.

For other cancers, such as prostate cancer, there are no specific changes in screening guidelines in the LGBT population. For example, the US Preventative Services Task Force (USPSTF) recommended against screening for prostate cancer with prostate-specific antigen in all men age $> 70$ years (grade D).[8] With respect to colon cancer, there are no published studies to examine difference in risk across different gender or sexual orientations.

In WSW, cancer screening follows guidelines established for older adults at large with differences in risk factors. With respect to breast cancer, for example, there may be more prevalent risk factors, such as nulliparity, alcohol use, smoking, and obesity in lesbian women when compared with heterosexual women.[9] In addition to increased prevalence of risk factors in lesbian women for breast cancer, there are inconsistent data on participation in mammogram screening in WSW.[6] With increased risks and unclear uptake of mammography, a study using the National Health Interview Survey estimated the age-adjusted relative risk (RR) for disease-specific mortality attributed to breast cancer was greater in WSW (RR, 3.20; 95% confidence interval [CI], 1.01–10.21).[10] Despite disease-specific differences in WSW, mammogram screening in WSW follows current society guidelines for the general population. Similarly, Pap smear recommendations for cervical cancer screening follow population-wide society guidelines, with no further recommendations specific to LGBT women.

LGBT people have higher rates of smoking compared with heterosexual peers across all age groups, which also has implications for primary care of LGBT older adults.[6] This higher smoking prevalence underscores the importance of screening for smoking and smoking cessation counseling in this population. Given this prevalence of smoking, it is also important to appropriately offer lung cancer and abdominal aorta aneurysm screening based on latest society guidelines for the general population.

A final consideration for LGBT preventative health is vaccination guidelines. The Centers for Disease Control and Prevention (CDC) as of 2019 recommends offering MSM patients hepatitis A and hepatitis B vaccinations, but does not clarify age cutoffs. In certain areas, such as urban settings, meningitis vaccination is also recommended to MSM patients. When questions arise regarding vaccination schedule, the CDC website and local resources can help guide vaccination management.[11]

## Sexual History

Older adults often still engage in sexual intercourse, which includes older adults in the LGBT community. Besides remaining sexually active, there is also potentially lower barrier condom use for all older adults, which carries increased risk of sexually transmitted infections (STIs). In one study, 17% of older adults used condoms between ages 60 and 69 years compared with 24% aged 50 to 59 years.[12] For older MSM, despite risks associated with unprotected anal sex, they may not perceive themselves at risk of HIV or other STIs. To complicate this situation further, older MSM may be reluctant to take preventative measures after diagnosis of HIV. These attitudes may place MSM at higher risk of STIs as older adults.[13]

Given older LGBT community members may remain sexually active, we recommend obtaining a sexual history, similar to care for heterosexual older adults. A sexual history should consist of sexual activity, the number of partners a patient has, use of barrier protection, and gender of sexual partners. These items help clarify risk and inform screening strategies in a LGBT population (Box 4.2). It is also important to ask about the type of sexual intercourse that individuals are having (e.g., whether it be receptive oral, receptive anal, receptive vaginal, or insertive sex) (see Box 4.2). Depending on the type of sexual intercourse, throat swab, rectal swab, vaginal swab, or urine testing can be pursued for STIs. These tests can be obtained in addition to HIV testing and syphilis testing for those engaging in unprotected sexual intercourse. For those with multiple sexual partners, more frequent testing every 3 to 6 months is recommended by the CDC, versus annual testing or less frequent testing for those with a single partner or a monogamous sexual relationship. Finally, the fastest growing group of HIV-positive individuals is those aged over 50 years, so continued screening for HIV is another cornerstone of STI screening.[13]

Given this increased risk of HIV in MSM, there are preventative measures to take to reduce risk of HIV transmission. Barrier condom use should be part of a strategy to prevent HIV transmission, but if sexual risk factors are present, preexposure prophylaxis (PrEP) is a potential additional consideration. PrEP is a combination medicine (tenofovir disoproxil fumarate/emtricitabine) taken on a daily basis to prevent HIV. Taking PrEP daily is a strategy that, alongside condoms, has been proven to mitigate HIV transmission risk. Although not studied specifically in older adults, PrEP has been studied in sexually active adults. Given these recommendations and although there is no age cutoff for PrEP use, PrEP would be a consideration in higher risk older adults. A shared decision-making discussion about the risks and benefits of PrEP would be warranted in patients with multiple sexual partners and those who are engaging in unprotected sex or those with diagnosis of an STI in the last 6 months. If taken every day, PrEP has efficacy in preventing transmission of HIV, with few reported breakthrough cases of transmission. However, there are side effects to PrEP, including renal injury and decreased bone mineral density. Regular monitoring of kidney function is recommended, and this side effect profile may limit use in an older population.[14]

For WSW, there are additional sexual health considerations. Despite disclosing their current sexual activity with women, many WSW have had sexual experiences with men, which can predispose them to STIs, such as HIV. Obtaining a thorough sexual history is important to understand these risks. In general, WSW have higher risks of bacterial vaginosis but not necessarily STIs.[15] More research is needed to understand the risks for other STIs among WSW, including chlamydial infection.[16] For those WSW with multiple partners or partners of both sexes, it would be prudent to offer STI testing, again taking into account the type of sexual intercourse the patient is having and the STI testing offered. We recommend evaluating if a patient is having anal, vaginal, or oral intercourse and the number of partners to determine appropriate STI testing.

---

## CASE 1

### Hector Ramirez (Part 2)

With an open discussion, you screen Hector for depression, which he currently denies, although he states he has been treated for depression in the past. He reflects that he is well supported by his roommate, Roy. At this time, your patient seems a bit worried and asks you what would be appropriate preventative healthcare screening for him today.

He states that he has heard of anal Pap smears from friends and would be open to scheduling an appointment for testing. He understands that if he has positive results, he may need to undergo further testing.

You ask him about his sexual habits, and he states he has had multiple sexual partners in the last year and is versatile, both bottoming (or receptive anal intercourse) and topping (insertive anal intercourse) with multiple men. He rarely uses barrier protection and has at least three sexual partners.

You offer him rectal, oral, and urine testing for gonorrhea and chlamydia, in addition to syphilis testing and HIV testing. You counsel him on using protection as well, given he has multiple sexual partners. Finally, you have some time left in your visit today. You ask open-ended questions about who would make decisions for him in emergencies or care for him if he was unable to care for himself. He reports it would be his roommate, Roy. You ask him if Roy is his partner and if they have any legal documentation showing these are his care preferences. He reports he does not have any legal documentation or license showing Roy is his surrogate decision maker and partner.

1) What are important advanced care planning considerations in the LGBT community?
2) What social structures do LGBT adults rely on?

---

## Social Structures

In primary care, care plans often involve a patient's family of origin and, less commonly, people who have been chosen by the patient to be involved in his or her life and care. For older LGBT adults, it is more common to develop and rely on these families of choice compared with their heterosexual peers. Part of this reliance on families of choice arises from differences in societal discrimination against LGBT people, including issues with familial acceptance of LGBT people. However, despite ostracization across a lifetime, there is resiliency in older LGBT adults. In spite of rejection from families of origin, LGBT people sought out people who they could fully depend on and trust, forming families of choice, which may even be hybridized with families of origin.

Families of choice face serious implications as they age, suffering from vulnerability to diseases of aging. There may be a lack of children in this family structure for LGBT people, which limits the potential caregivers and advocates from a younger generation. Although families of origin may include members of various ages, families of choice can be from friends of similar ages. In geriatrics, this similarity in age in families of choice may mean when one member of the family is becoming older and dependent on others, other members may be suffering from their own age-related issues, including falls, increasing dependence, worsening frailty, or impaired cognition. This effect on potential caregivers from families of choice can limit care options for older LGBT adults. Older LGBT adults may be less likely to have someone care for them, with three-quarters of LGBT people being worried about having adequate social or family support.[17] Some LGBT older adults find themselves living alone as their families of choice dwindle, making social isolation common.

With reduced caregiver access, older LGBT adults may have needs that cannot be met with their own resources, leading to entry into long-term care facilities. LGBT older adults entering nursing homes may fear discrimination similar to that they have met across their lifetime. Unfortunately, state laws protecting their rights in nursing homes vary. With this fear and potential lack of protection, many older adults will return to the closet and keep their identity secret, fearing repercussions if they disclose sexual or gender identity. There may also be issues with same-sex couples requesting to room together. From a care perspective, it is important to be able to support these patients and direct them to appropriate advocacy resources.[18]

There is also legal vulnerability in families of choice because they do not enjoy the same legal recognition as blood relations. For instance, someone recognized and treated as a patient's sister, without blood relation, does not have the ability to act as legal surrogate decision maker unless there is legal documentation present.

Legal status for LGBT adults is changing. In 2015, the US Supreme Court recognized a right to marry for same-sex couples. Having legal marriage allows LGBT adults to have legal recognition of their partners, which protects healthcare decision-making rights as a surrogate, in addition to economic rights. Benefits extended to married couples include inclusion on health insurance, social security benefits and Medicare benefits, and financial incentive sharing, with the ability to share unlimited assets to a spouse without penalty. Moreover, with respect to financial planning, if a person dies without a will or trust, his or her assets will transfer to the spouse without penalty. These are substantial benefits that marriage equality provides LGBT older adults. Previously, to protect these rights, advance care planning was imperative.

Advance care planning remains essential for those with large families of choice and those without legal recognition, such as partners who remain unmarried. It is crucial to discuss this topic with LGBT older adults. Clarify who appropriate surrogate decision makers are before persons reach a situation where their decision-making capacity is impaired. The primary care office is an ideal setting to address a well older adult and document advanced care planning.

A final consideration in families of choice is the presentation of geriatric syndromes, such as dementia. Typically, dementia is a disease process where collateral information proves essential in diagnosis because functional decline is most apparent to close companions or loved ones. Many LGBT people may then present later in their dementia course owing to social isolation. Although there are no formal guidelines on screening for dementia in this population, dementia should be considered in primary care settings. The diagnosis of dementia in older LGBT adults may be delayed further if they are living alone and compensating despite functional impairments, so the primary care office remains the likely setting for detecting dementia.

## CASE 1

### Discussion

After speaking with Hector, you clarify that his primary surrogate decision maker would be his roommate, Roy, with a secondary surrogate his close lifelong friend, Martha. You firmly tell Hector that he will need to file advance directive paperwork to recognize his chosen individuals as surrogate decision makers. You arrange for follow-up in 4 weeks to continue your goals of care discussion. You have given Hector several items to think about, and he is excited to continue his healthcare with you.

## CASE 2

### Margaret Getty (Part 1)

Margaret is a 74-year-old female with a history of hypertension, prior smoking, and high cholesterol who is presenting to establish care with you after she moved into assisted living. You greet Margaret and see she looks noticeably uncomfortable. You go through your routine interview—touching on past medical history and medications—and note that Margaret has been on long-term estrogen therapy and has had a vaginoplasty. Knowing this information, you pause and ask Margaret what pronouns and names she prefers to use. She endorses her pronouns as "she/her/hers" and states her preferred name is in fact Margaret. She breathes a sigh of relief and reveals that she has jumped from provider to provider because of not feeling accepted as a transgender woman and has deferred much of her medical care because of not feeling safe with her last provider. When you ask what her chief concern is today, she reveals that she seeks a refill of her estrogen as she is about to run out.

She specifically asks you if she can continue using her estrogen therapy and if you would provide the refill. She has been using the same dose of estrogen patch for the last 30 years.
1) What are issues specific to the care of transgender women and men and how do we effectively manage these concerns?
2) What risk factors may transgender patients have for osteoporosis?

## Transgender Health

Like diversity in sexual orientation, there is great diversity in gender identity, with some individuals expressing a different gender or having a different gender identity than their natal sex (see Box 4.2). Transgender patients with gender dysphoria may have particular healthcare needs that require a thorough understanding of their past medical and social history. The first step in obtaining that history is the creation of a welcoming environment. Much as for LGB older adults, transgender people have experienced discrimination across a lifetime, including in healthcare. For example, providers may have called a transgender person "it" instead of the preferred pronoun; in 2019, only 20 states had laws that protected LGBT people against discrimination.[19]

A nonjudgmental, accepting environment helps welcome all LGBT older adults. For example, standardized questioning, such as asking about sexuality, sexual activity, and gender identity of everyone, facilitates care for transgender patients. These questions can even be asked on forms, providing patients the option to fill out the form with options outside of the gender binary, or using open-ended questions, such as asking patients' preferred name or how would they like to be addressed. Simply asking can enable patients to be safe, allow the space to share their needs, and empower them to advocate for their own care. Nevertheless, despite our best efforts, missteps can happen during interviews. When missteps happen, apologize succinctly and move on, using it as a learning experience.

Another important step in care for transgender patients is focusing on a gender affirming approach, which refers to when social interactions affirm a person's gender identity. To accomplish this goal, providers should refer to patients by their preferred name and pronoun. Engaging in gender affirming care requires first engaging in how persons prefer to be addressed and enacting this terminology. Although not every visit may center around their sexual or gender identity, nor should every visit, we can still affirm their identity through our interactions. For example, an urgent care visit for influenza evaluation need not review what medications a transgender patient takes for gender affirming therapy, but the patient should be referred to by the preferred name and pronouns.

Once the therapeutic patient provider alliance is established, the provider can explore specific concerns to older transgender patients in primary care. Keep in mind that although typical examinations may be described as well woman examinations, gendering of examinations and preventative testing should be avoided. There may be a gender identity mismatch for transgender patients, where they forego screening when the organ to screen for (i.e., prostate) does not match their gender (female). An important starting point is an organ inventory for these patients to understand what organs they have, and the screening then required. By documenting which organs a patient still has, the provider can offer appropriate preventative screening in a patient-centered approach. For each transgender patient, regardless of gender identity, obtain this inventory and ask about the presence of a penis, testes, prostate, breasts (and residual tissue), vagina, cervix (with cuff), uterus, and ovaries.

For example, in breast cancer screening in transgender men, there is recommended screening if there is residual breast tissue (grade D). For transgender women, breast cancer screening would follow normal guidelines, with evidence suggesting male-to-female persons are not at a higher risk for breast cancer than are biologic women.[20]

In female transgender patients who still have their prostates, prostate cancer screening is per society guidelines for all older adults. However, this screening could be burdensome because it is not synchronous with this woman's gender identity. Similarly, for breast cancer screening for a transgender man with residual tissue, a mammogram would be recommended per society guidelines, but could be distressing because it represents screening for a female, a gender he does not identify with. Shared decision making should take place for the screening examinations, holding a discussion over the risks and benefits and aligning with the patient's needs.

For osteoporosis screening, an approach similar to all older adults can be considered. With continuing hormonal treatment, there would theoretically be mitigated risk of osteoporosis, which has been seen in short-term studies on hormone replacement therapy. However, it would be reasonable to screen those individuals aged over 65 years in transgender individuals regardless of assigned sex at birth (grade D).[21]

## Gender Affirming Therapies

Certain transgender adults pursue gender affirming therapies to affirm gender identity. These therapies can be ongoing. Despite decreasing levels of hormones over time and a natural decrease in hormone levels, many continue therapy. On the other end of the spectrum are individuals who express their gender differently, with some people not pursuing gender affirming therapy. Understanding your patients' goals is important to determine what options would be available to them.

Although many older transgender patients may approach you wishing to continue their current hormone therapy, there may also be patients who are presenting wishing to start gender affirming therapies and consider gender affirming surgery. In these individuals, it is prudent to assure diagnosis of gender dysphoria and refer them to specialist care for full psychosocial assessment. Gender affirming therapies are still options open to older adults.

For transgender women, gender affirming therapy can include a feminizing hormone, with an antiandrogen in addition to this

estrogen. Estrogen in older adults is associated with its own risks. Estrogen is absolutely contraindicated in the presence of an estrogen-sensitive cancer and increases the risk of venous thromboembolic (VTE) events. For older transgender patients on estrogen therapy, other risk factors, such as obesity or smoking, can further increase their VTE risk, making smoking cessation and weight loss counseling important items to review in primary care visits.[22] The form of prescribed estrogen also contributes to risk because patches can help minimize the risk of VTE.[23] Finally, estrogen use can also carry cardiovascular and stroke risk.[24] Although there is no evidence for or against continuing or stopping hormones for older transgender women, there are these associated risks.[25] In the setting of the risks associated with ongoing hormone treatment, a patient-centered discussion about stopping hormones after age 50 years to mirror the hormonal changes of menopause to mitigate VTE and cardiovascular risks can be considered (grade D). There is no expert consensus on next steps for hormone therapy in an aging population. However, stopping feminizing hormones, such as estrogen, in transgender women can lead to virilization.[25,26] Ongoing stable estrogen therapy would require yearly monitoring.

For transgender men, gender affirming therapy can include masculinizing hormone therapy, typically with injectable testosterone, although many formulations are available. Like transgender women, there are no clear guidelines for ongoing hormone use in older adults and for testosterone. Without guidelines, clinicians can consider discontinuing testosterone therapy around age 50 years, when nontransgender women would go through menopause. Again, a risk-benefit discussion would need to be held regarding the risks of ongoing therapy and the risks of withdrawal of testosterone. Risks associated with ongoing testosterone use include male pattern hair loss and polycythemia, with transgender men's hemoglobin following the normal hemoglobin range for males. Cardiovascular risk is unchanged in transgender men receiving testosterone therapy when compared with nontransgender women, an important difference versus general older adults' risk of testosterone therapy.[27] Meanwhile, cessation of testosterone can lead to changes in body hair, loss of muscle mass, and loss of libido. If choosing to continue therapy, ongoing testosterone use also requires monitoring, such as hematocrit and for injections and midcycle testosterone levels. Note that any active hormone sensitive malignancy would also be an absolute contraindication to continuing therapy.[28]

---

**CASE 2**

### Margaret Getty (Part 2)

Talking with Margaret, you learn she is independent in all her ADLs, although for her IADLs she no longer drives or goes grocery shopping on her own. She reports with the loss of some of her night vision and slower reaction speed, she simply did not feel safe behind the wheel anymore. She enjoys assisted living and getting help with cleaning and her meals. Otherwise, she reports no recent falls and denies depression. Asking about her advanced care planning, Margaret does tear up and states her surrogate decision maker is her friend, Anne, after her partner of 10 years had passed away. She provides her advanced directive showing Anne as her primary healthcare surrogate.

You then ask her if she is sexually active with men, women, or both. She notes that she is currently sexually active with both men and women.

## • BOX 4.3    Obtaining a Sexual History

- I am going to ask you a few questions about your sexual health that I ask all of my adult patients, regardless of age, gender, or identity.
- Are you currently sexually active? If no, have you ever been sexually active? With men, women, or both?
- How many sexual partners have you had in the last year?
- What kind of sexual contact do you have or have you had? Genital contact (involving penis or vagina), anal (penis in the anus), or oral (mouth on penis, vagina, or anus)?
- For MSM: Have you engaged in receptive (bottoming) or insertive (topping) intercourse?
- Do you and your partner use any protection against sexually transmitted diseases? If not, could you explain the reason? How often do you use this protection?
- Have you been diagnosed with any sexually transmitted infections in the past? When? How were you treated?

(Modified from US Department of Health and Human Services Center for Disease Control and Prevention. *A Guide to Taking a Sexual History.* 2019. Available at: https://www.cdc.gov/std/treatment/sexualhistory.pdf.)

## Further Considerations

Transgender older adults face similar social issues to LGB older adults. These issues include minority stress and discrimination across a lifetime, which can be associated with its own health issues and mental illness. Transgender people may also be reliant on families of choice, especially if they have faced ostracism from their families of origin.

In transgender individuals of all ages, risk of HIV is higher than the general population. Some 14% of transgender women in general and 44% of transgender Black women are HIV positive.[29] Transgender women are also three times as likely to receive a new diagnosis of HIV.[30] Higher rates of HIV in transgender women underscores the importance of screening for HIV and other STIs in this population.

Throughout this chapter, in the LGB community there is discussion of MSM and WSW, which includes bisexual individuals. Bisexual adults are a diverse group who may not be visible within the LGBT community. For bisexual adults, they can often be assumed to identify as the relationship they are in, for example, being assumed to be gay in a relationship of a man with another man. However, despite a relationship with one sex, their attraction to both sexes does not change. This assumption of their sexuality or sexual identity can contribute to bierasure and diminish the visibility of bisexual adults, in addition to the internal LGBT community discrimination bisexual adults may face.[31] In turn, this means bisexual older adults are less out about their sexuality, which can affect their ability to receive adequate healthcare in clinic. It remains important to ask standardized questions of all patients who enter the clinic to facilitate the sharing of important healthcare related information (Box 4.3).

## CASE 2

### Discussion

You conclude your visit offering her STI testing, offering her mammogram screening, and letting her know you are here to support her. You will refill her estrogen prescription at this time, after discussing the long-term risks of estrogen use, including DVT risk and screening her for smoking. However, you wish to hold an ongoing discussion about her estrogen use and referral to one of your colleagues who specializes in transgender health. She smiles and shakes your hand before you leave the room.

## Summary

Care for our LGBT patients begins with our paperwork, our office design, and how we address our patients. It is important to be inclusive in care for this growing population, making sure prompts regarding their sexuality and gender identity are included in how we interview and gather information about our patients. Without this information, we would not be aware of appropriate screening, diagnostic lab testing, support networks, community issues, and advanced care planning concerns that are necessary to fully care for any of our geriatric patients.[32-35]

- Care for LGBT patients begins with your paperwork and interviews. Without a welcoming space, they may not be empowered to share their full history.
- Collect patient data in a standardized fashion to collect a robust sexual, gender, and social history.
- LGBT people are often part of families of choice, which may be vulnerable to aging. Advocate for advanced care planning in your patients to respect their goals of care.

## Key References

22. Coleman E, Bockting W, Botzer M, et al. Standards of care for the health of transsexual, transgender, and gender-nonconforming people, Version 7. *Int J Transgend.* 2012;13 (4):165–232.
32. Centers for Disease Control and Prevention. *Sexual Orientation and Gender Identity.* 2016. Available at: https://www.cdc.gov/nchhstp/sexual-id-orientation.htm.
33. Deutsch MB. *Guidelines for the Primary and Gender-Affirming Care of Transgender and Gender Nonbinary People.* 2016. Available at: https://transcare.ucsf.edu/guidelines.
34. SAGE - Advocacy & Services for LGBT Elders. 2019. Available at: https://www.sageusa.org/.
35. National LGBT Health Education Center: A Program of the Fenway Institute. 2019. Available at: https://www.lgbthealtheducation.org/.

**References available online at expertconsult.com.**

# 5
# Wellness and Prevention

SARA WOLFSON

*Additional online-only material indicated by icon.*

## OBJECTIVES

*Upon completion of this chapter, the reader will be able to:*

- Define the purpose of health promotion, wellness, and disease prevention in older adults.
- Describe an appropriate immunization schedule for older adults.
- Describe lifestyle modifications that can prevent disease.

- Delineate the use of prophylactic medication on cardiovascular, musculoskeletal, and cancer prevention.
- State appropriate cancer screening guidelines for older adults.
- Engage patients in putting prevention and wellness into practice.

## Essentials of Health Promotion for Aging Adults

Health promotion is the science and art of helping people change their lifestyle to move toward a state of optimal health, defined as a balance of physical, emotional, social, spiritual, and intellectual health.[1] Health promotion and disease prevention can reduce the potential years of life lost to premature mortality, while ensuring better quality of life.

Health promotion activities include immunizations to prevent infectious diseases and their complications, and reduction of risk factors through lifestyle modifications, such as smoking cessation or regular physical activity, and the prophylactic use of medication to reduce risk of cardiovascular disease (CVD).

In addition, health promotion includes screening for malignancies to facilitate the early identification of disease so the proper treatments can be initiated. There are multiple guidelines available for clinicians, as well as patient-specific information to aid patients in selecting among health promotion activities. Guidelines for overall health screening decisions[2] can help direct clinicians and patients, or their proxy, in this process. An individualized approach is critical when working with older individuals in the area of health promotion and should drive decision making.

## CASE 1

### Mrs. W

Mrs. W is an 81-year-old White female new to your outpatient clinic. Her history includes Parkinson disease, hypertension, lactose intolerance, urinary incontinence, hypothyroidism, glaucoma, alcohol abuse (with no alcohol intake for 25 years), and a one half-pack per day smoking habit for 50 years and she continues to smoke. She lives in a senior high-rise and is independent with personal care activities and meal preparation. She gets medication set-up help with her weekly pillbox. Her weight has been stable, with a body mass index (BMI) of 29.2 kg/m².

She is concerned about her health and fears future health impairments. She participates in regular screenings, including routine colonoscopies, annual mammograms, and Pap tests, all of which have been negative. She is unable to tolerate aspirin, calcium, and bisphosphonates because of diarrhea. Attempts to cut back and/or stop smoking have been unsuccessful. She does not exercise regularly. However, she is motivated to learn ways of improving her health and wants to be proactive in preventing future problems. She acknowledges not always following through with health provider recommendations. Her medications include carbidopa-levodopa 25/100 mg orally three times daily for Parkinson disease, amlodipine 10 mg orally daily for blood pressure, loperamide up to 12 mg orally daily as needed for diarrhea, and tolterodine 4 mg orally daily for incontinence.
1. What interventions might improve Mrs. W's health?
2. How would you prioritize your interventions?
3. What motivational strategies might help Mrs. W change her behavior in areas such as smoking cessation and exercise?

## Prevention of Disease

### Immunizations

The aging process increases the risk of developing preventable - diseases. These illnesses confer higher morbidity and mortality in older adults who already have significant chronic conditions. Influenza, for example, accounts for upwards of 36,000 deaths and 200,000 hospitalizations yearly.[3] Despite older adults comprising 15% of the US population, they accounted for 50% of influenza-related hospitalizations and 64% of deaths linked to influenza and pneumonia during the 2015 to 2016 seasonal outbreak. Immunization rates to prevent pneumococcal pneumonia are currently about 61.3% for adults age ≥ 65 years, and 27.9% for herpes zoster immunization of adults age ≥ 60 years. It is essential to screen patients for their immunization history during routine visits and offer the needed vaccinations. Screening should also be done during hospital and long-term care stays. It is also important to pair screening with patient education as to the importance of immunizations in preventing diseases that worsen overall health

**TABLE 5.1  Immunizations Recommended for Older Adults**

| | |
|---|---|
| Influenza inactive (IIV), or recombinant (RIV) | 1 dose annually |
| Tetanus, diphtheria, pertussis (TDAP) | 1 dose after age 65 years then Td every 10 years |
| Varicella recombinant (Shingrix) | 2 doses 2–5 months apart. Give to those who had zoster |
| Pneumococcal | 1 dose of PPSV23 (Polysaccharide, Pneumovax); consider 1 dose PCV 13 in high-risk patients |
| Hepatitis A/hepatitis B | Only if high risk, and at least once |

PCV13, Pneumococcal conjugate vaccine 13; PPSV23, pneumococcal polysaccharide vaccine 23. (From Advisory Committee for Immunization Practices, United States, 2020 Advisory Committee for Immunization Practices.)

while negatively impacting chronic conditions. Keep up to date with yearly vaccination schedules from US Advisory Committee for Immunization Practices (ACIP).[2]

Table 5.1 provides an overview of recommendations for immunizations for older adults. Guidelines come from the Centers for Disease Control and Prevention (CDC) and ACIP. Currently, all adults age ≥ 65 years are advised to get a yearly influenza vaccination because of high risk of serious complications from the flu.[4] The target percentage for 2020, as set in *Healthy People 2020*, is 90% adherence for noninstitutionalized adults aged ≥ 65 years.[5] To promote adherence in long-term care and home health settings, the federal government approved standing orders for annual influenza vaccinations and pneumococcal pneumonia vaccination for all Medicare and Medicaid beneficiaries. Medicare Part B covers vaccines to prevent influenza and pneumonia, as well as hepatitis B if the patient is at medium to high risk for this disease. No copay is associated with these vaccines. All other vaccines are covered under Medicare Part D; this includes the vaccine for zoster.

The second shingles vaccination, Shingri was approved in January 2018. This varicella recombinant vaccine is strongly recommended for all adults over age 65 years, even those who previously received Zostavax. In clinical trials, Shingrix had an effectiveness of 90% in preventing shingles, versus 50% with the zoster vaccine. Protection against shingles and postherpetic neuralgia is greater than 85% for a minimum of 4 years postimmunization. Zostavax can be used when there is a Shingrix allergy, if a patient prefers the Zostavax, or the patient wishes an immediate vaccination and Shingrix is unavailable. The vaccination is recommended even if a patient is unsure about having chickenpox in the past. According to the CDC, approximately 99% of Americans aged ≥ 40 years had contracted chickenpox.[6]

◆◆ **Adults should receive immunizations for influenza, pneumococcal disease, diphtheria/pertussis/tetanus, herpes zoster, and selectively for other infectious diseases**.

Persons age ≥ 65 years also should have pneumococcal vaccination, with the pneumococcal polysaccharide (Pneumovax) vaccine. If a person received the Pneumovax before turning 65 years, it should be repeated once after the age of 65 years. In late 2019, ACIP retracted its previous recommendations on routine use of pneumococcal conjugate vaccine (Prevnar). Prevnar is now only recommended for high-risk persons such as those with asplenia or cochlear implants.

The ACIP Pertussis Vaccines Work Group in 2011 concluded that the burden of disease resulting from pertussis was 100 times higher than previously suspected at an incidence of 66 to 500 cases per 100,000 older adults. Adults over 10 age 65 years should receive the tetanus toxoid, reduced diphtheria toxoid, and acellular pertussis (TDAP) booster once followed by the diphtheria toxoid every 10 years. Trade names are Boostrix (preferred) and Aquacel.[6]

## Lifestyle Behaviors

### Tobacco Use

No matter one's age or smoking history, quitting improves health by promoting better blood circulation, lowering the risk of cancer, stroke, and heart attack, improves breathing, and lowers blood pressure. Smoking increases the likelihood of getting the flu, pneumonia, and other respiratory illness; it weakens bones and can lead to vision loss, development of type 2 diabetes, erectile dysfunction, and delayed wound healing.[7] Smokeless tobacco, pipes, and cigars are unsafe substitutes for cigarette smoking. Nicotine addiction can still occur with these products along with gum disease and precancerous lesions of oral mucosa.

Despite common assumptions, older adults are not more likely than younger individuals to have nicotine addiction (8.9% after 65 years vs. 17.3% aged 18−24 years, 21.6% aged 25−44 years).[8] Studies suggest rates of smoking cessation are lower in older adults than in younger individuals. However, when cessation interventions are tailored to older adults, their rate of smoking cessation equals that of younger persons.[9] Unfortunately, older adults are less often offered smoking cessation interventions and support. This accounts for many missed opportunities in primary care. Smoking cessation is most successful when pharmacotherapy is in combination with counseling[10] (level of evidence [LOE] A). Medicare covers "intermediate cessation counseling" (3−10 minutes per session) and "intensive cessation counseling" (>10 minutes per session), and two quit attempts per year (details available on the Center for Medicare & Medicaid website).[11]

❖❖ **The most effective smoking cessation approach uses a combination of behavioral approaches and pharmacotherapy.**

The Agency for Healthcare Research and Quality recommends the use of the "five As" (assess, advise, agree, assist, and arrange) in patients age ≥ 50 years. Counseling interventions, physician/healthcare provider advice, buddy support programs, age-tailored self-help materials, telephone counseling, and the nicotine patch are effective interventions to facilitate smoking cessation in adults age ≥ 50 years (Box 5.1).

Pharmacologic interventions for smoking cessation include seven first-line medications (five nicotine and two nonnicotine): bupropion SR; nicotine replacement therapy (NRT) with gum, inhaler, lozenge, nasal spray, or patch; and varenicline (Chantix). In a 2015 meta-analysis, behavioral interventions, NRT, bupropion, and varenicline all improved smoking abstinence at ≥ 6 months; varenicline was most effective, while behavioral interventions combined with pharmacotherapy had the best quit rates (LOE A).[9]

Potential side effects of pharmacologic agents include the following: The nicotine patch may cause local skin irritation, gum

---

**• BOX 5.1** **The "Five As": Interventions That Can Be Applied by a Variety of Clinical Staff in Primary Care**

**Assess**
Ask about behavioral health risks and other factors that affect health goal change.

**Advise**
Provide clear, targeted behavior change advice, along with information as to potential harms/benefits.

**Agree**
Work together on selection of appropriate, achievable treatment goals, and methods, based on patient's buy-in and willingness to change.

**Assist**
Guide the patient to achieve the agreed-upon goals by fostering self-confidence, along with providing additional medical treatments when needed. Help the patient with social/environmental supports for behavior change.

**Arrange**
Schedule follow-up visits or phone conversations to provide ongoing support, and adjust treatment plan as needed. Include any referrals for more specialized treatment.

---

may cause mouth soreness or dyspepsia, nasal irritation may occur with nasal spray (or oral irritation if used as an inhaler). Nicotine may also cause insomnia. Likewise, bupropion can cause insomnia and dry mouth, whereas varenicline can cause nausea, and caution is needed for persons with history of depression who are at risk of suicide.

According to a National Academies Press 2018 report, although tests have shown that e-cigarettes are less harmful than tobacco cigarettes, the risks of vaping are still undetermined; a spate of reports of serious lung injuries associated with vaping in 2019 has dimmed interest in this approach. Some products contain harmful substances along with nicotine. The concentration of these varies by product and method of use, and the amount of nicotine inhaled through vaping (among experienced users) may be similar to that in tobacco cigarettes.[12]

### Opioid Use

Although opioids are safe for many older adults with chronic pain, clinicians need to be aware of the national conversation regarding opioid use and misuse. For many older adults, chronic pain is the overriding symptom, and primary care management is a challenge. The National Health and Nutrition Examination Survey from 1999 to 2014 showed that 25.4% of opioid users were adults aged ≥ 65 years.[13] The longer the duration of opioid use, the greater the risk of developing an opioid use disorder. Opioids should never be first-line treatment for chronic pain. According to the CDC, nonpharmacologic interventions, such as exercise, topical analgesics, Tai Chi, physical therapy, acupuncture, and massage, have good evidence for pain management goals along with nonopioid medications (see Ch. 27). It is important to emphasize to the patient that opioids should be taken only as prescribed and with consistent follow-up on the part of the clinician as to effectiveness: (1) Does use of the medication meet the individual's goals? (2) Is it correctly dosed? (3) Are there other interventions that can take the place of this, or work as adjuvant treatment? (4) Does use of the opioid medication promote daily function and independence?[14]

◆◆ **Opioid misuse is to be avoided while maintaining a focus on relief of pain in older adult patients.**

### Prevention of Polypharmacy

Polypharmacy is the use of more medications than are clinically needed or indicated. Older adults are at particular risk for polypharmacy because of multiple comorbidities and because they see multiple healthcare providers. One way to reduce polypharmacy is to try nonpharmacologic therapies first. Interventions may include diet, exercise, stress management, and cognitive-behavioral therapy. Moreover, combining behavioral interventions with medications may reduce the drug dosages needed for effect. Clinicians should also make certain to be very clear about drug use instructions and possible side effects. Always provide both verbal and written instructions on how to use the medication. Drug regimens should be as simple as possible and medications need thorough review and updating at each provider–patient interaction (see Ch. 7).

### Screening for Alcohol Use/Abuse

As the body ages, there is a decrease in total volume of body water; this reduces the volume of distribution of alcohol that produces a higher blood concentration with the same amount of intake. Thus alcohol's effects are greater even when an older individual's alcohol intake remains unchanged.[15]

The current recommendation on alcohol intake, from the National Institute on Alcohol Abuse and Alcoholism, for healthy adults over age 65 years is no more than one drink per day (maximum of seven drinks in 1 week) and never more than three drinks on a given day. Alcohol can worsen certain chronic conditions, such as osteoporosis, memory loss, congestive heart failure, hypertension, impaired balance, and liver disease. It increases hypertension by negatively affecting the mechanisms for blood pressure control, specifically baroreceptors, cortisol levels, and the renin-angiotensin/aldosterone systems. In addition, changes to blood vessels and the heart can be harder to detect as alcohol dulls the pain sensations that can warn of a heart attack.[16]

The interaction of medications with alcohol may change the metabolism of one or the other. Either alcohol intensifies the medication's effect, especially in the central nervous system, or it interferes with metabolism of the medication in the liver (Box 5.2).

It was long believed that small amounts of alcohol were beneficial for heath. Data from a 2019 study suggest that the amount of alcohol intake that is optimal to maximize longevity and minimize years living with disability is zero alcohol intake. The signs and symptoms associated with alcohol abuse in the older adult include the same spectrum of physical, behavioral, and psychological problems as in younger individuals[15,16] (see Ch. 34).

The most commonly used and reliable screening instrument for alcohol use disorders is the CAGE self-report questionnaire (Box 5.3). When used with older adults, it has reported sensitivities ranging from 43% to 94% for detecting alcohol abuse and alcoholism.[17] The CAGE questionnaire is well suited to busy primary care settings because it poses four straightforward yes/no questions. It may fail, however, to detect low but risky levels of drinking and often performs less well among women and minority populations. Other measures include the 25-question Michigan Alcohol

Screening Test (MAST),[18] which was revised to be more relevant for older adults, or the Alcohol Use Disorders Identification Test[19] (see also Ch. 34).

◆◆ **Aging alters the distribution of alcohol in the body, so that a single drink produces higher blood levels.**

## Nutrition

Aging changes dietary needs. Metabolism slows, physical activity declines, and absorption of nutrients becomes problematic because of chronic conditions and medication-nutrient interactions. Requirements can actually increase related to the amount of body mass. This prompted the Institute of Medicine to issue a different set of guidelines for adults aged ≥70 years. In addition, food and nutrients impact overall health to a greater degree. With loss of appetite, poor oral hygiene, decreased gastric motility, and mobility challenges, intake of nutrient-dense foods declines and food choices become limited. Undernutrition becomes more prevalent in older adults.[20]

Evaluating food intake in older adults is important because inadequate intake can result in weight and muscle mass loss, decreased strength and walking speed, impaired balance, and activity/functional decline. Nutritional screening assesses number of daily meals, unintentional weight loss, dental issues, financial circumstances, daily function for shopping, and meal preparation. Nutritional screening using the Mini Nutritional Assessment[21] helps identify individuals who are malnourished or at risk.

◆◆ **Physiologic changes of aging create a greater risk of dehydration.**

## Age-Relevant Requirements

The presence of undernutrition can reflect medical illness, depression, dementia, inability to perform the functional tasks of shopping or cooking, inability to self-feed, financial challenges, or poor oral health, among other problems. In addition, undernutrition contributes to frailty. A low BMI (kg/m$^2$ <20) or an unintentional weight loss of ≥ 10 lb in 6 months suggests poor nutrition and requires evaluation.

Overall, calorie needs decline as we age, from a slowing of metabolism, decline in lean body mass, and a decrease in physical activity. However, general requirements do not change. The US government recommends a daily caloric intake, for women over the age of 65 years, of 1600 calories for a sedentary lifestyle, and 1800 and 2000 calories respectively for moderately active and active lifestyles. For men in the same age group, the recommendation is 2000, 2200, and 2600 calories, respectively, for sedentary, moderately active, and active lifestyles.[22] The MyPlate Table (Box 5.4) shows the recommendations from the US government Dietary Guidelines for Americans 2015 to 2020.[23] Encourage choices of nutrient-dense foods from all food groups.

❖ **Protein intake must be maintained in older patients, and it is important to distribute that intake throughout the day**.

### Protein

In addition, intake of protein paced throughout the day can strengthen muscles and may reverse muscle loss. A recommended daily intake for protein of 1 to 1.5 g/kg promotes rebuilding and retention of muscles. Protein should make up 12% to 20% of total calories.[24] It is common for acutely ill older adults to become protein deficient.

### Fiber

Fiber, an indigestible residue of food, is a natural laxative, adds bulk to stool, absorbs water, and reduces gut transit time. Fiber sources are grains, nuts, seeds, fruits, and vegetables. The recommendation for older adults is 14 g of dietary fiber per 1000 calories consumed. Ideally, fiber intake should include cereal fibers and be consumed with 64 ounces of fluid daily.[24]

### Water

Older adults on average experience physiologic changes that predispose to dehydration. The mechanisms are reduced renal response to antidiuretic hormone and often a relative hyporeninemic hypoaldosteronism (sodium wasting and potassium retention). Thirst sensation is blunted with age. Older adults need to be conscious of hydration especially during periods of illness.

Water is essential for joint lubrication; transport of nutrients and salts; hydration of skin, eyes, nose, and mouth; removal of waste products; regulation of body temperature; and adequate blood volume. Inadequate hydration can result in constipation, fatigue, hypotension, hyperthermia, dizziness, breathing difficulties, and palpitations. Fluids are best as water, juice, or milk; alcohol, caffeinated tea and coffee, and soft drinks have a diuretic effect and raise fluid level more modestly.

### Vitamins and Minerals

Vitamins and minerals are important to overall health with foods preferable as the source over dietary supplements. Five servings of fruits and vegetables daily optimize intake of potassium and vitamins A, C, and E. Absorption of vitamin $B_{12}$ is less efficient in many older people possibly related to gastric atrophy. Vitamin $B_{12}$ intake is generally adequate, although older adults should be encouraged to increase intake of the crystalline vitamin $B_{12}$ found in fortified foods, such as whole-grain breakfast cereals. Water-soluble vitamins (C and eight of the B vitamins) exit the body in urine, while fat-soluble vitamins are stored in body tissue. Exceeding upper level recommendations for fat-soluble vitamins can result in toxicity (Table 5.2).

## Approach to Obesity

On average, weight increases throughout adult life, although that gain slows in later life. A majority of that weight increase is located in the central part of the body increasing waist circumference. The healthier the diet, the less is the weight gain. Central (abdominal) obesity as part of the metabolic syndrome is waist circumference of more than 40 inches for men and more than 35 inches for women. The importance of central obesity is its link to risk of insulin resistance, hypertension, and dyslipidemia leading to diabetes, and CVD.[25]

BMI of 30 to 34.9 kg/m$^2$, 35 to 39.9 kg/m$^2$, and 40 kg/m$^2$ or higher constitutes grades I, II, and III obesity, respectively.[25] However, in diagnosing obesity in older adults, consideration must also be given to body fat composition (lean vs. fat body mass), and retention of fluid. A subgroup of individuals are at risk for sarcopenic obesity, which is low muscle mass and function despite being overweight. Low muscle mass in conjunction with

---

**• BOX 5.4    My Plate for Older Adults**

Fruits and vegetables→rich in fiber and nutrients. Choose those with deeply colored flesh. Choose canned varieties packed in their own juices or low-sodium types.
Healthy oils→Liquid vegetable oils and soft margarines provide important fatty acids and some fat-soluble vitamins.
Herbs & spices→Use a variety of these to enhance food flavor and reduce the need for salt.
Fluids→Drink plenty of fluids. These can come from water, tea, soups, and fruits/vegetables.
Grains→Whole grain and fortified foods provide fiber and B vitamins.
Dairy→Fat-free and low-fat milk, cheeses, and yogurts provide calcium, protein, and other important nutrients.
Protein→Foods rich in proteins provide many nutrients. Choose a variety, including nuts, beans, fish, lean meats, and poultry.

---

**TABLE 5.2    Micronutrient Requirements for Age Over 50 Years**

| Micronutrient | Men | Women |
|---|---|---|
| Riboflavin | 1.3 mg/day | 1.1 mg/day |
| Thiamin | 1.2 mg/day | 1.1 mg/day |
| Vitamin A | 3000 IU/day | 2333 IU/day |
| Vitamin $B_6$ | 1.7 mg/day | 1.5 mg/day |
| Vitamin $B_{12}$ | 100–400 mg/day | 100–400 mg/day |
| Vitamin C | 90 mg/day | 75 mg/day |

low-grade muscle strength or low physical functioning are diagnostic for sarcopenia.

Obesity affects quality of life as well as morbidity. The National Health and Nutrition Examination Survey estimates the prevalence of obesity after age 60 years at about 40%. Obesity is associated with physical deconditioning, functional decline, immobility, and greater risk for acute illness.[25]

Engaging patients in behavioral change to prevent and address obesity is a focus of primary care. Counseling, education, and guidance toward safe weight loss should incorporate other professional providers (dietician, physical therapist, or exercise specialist) to maintain nutrition, strength, and lean body mass during weight loss.

For individuals who have hypertension and are overweight, the Joint National Committee on Prevention, Detection, Evaluation, and Treatment of High Blood Pressure[26] suggests counseling patients on adopting a salt-restricted diet, increasing physical activity, and decreasing alcohol consumption. The Dietary Approaches to Stop Hypertension (DASH) eating plan consists of fruits, vegetables, whole grains, low-fat dairy products, poultry, and fish. In addition, obesity counseling by clinicians is reimbursable under Medicare.

According to Centers for Medicare and Medicaid Services, obesity counseling is for patients with a BMI $\geq 30 \, kg/m^2$, and includes dietary evaluation along with in-depth behavioral therapy and exercise guidance. The goal is successful weight loss with continued nutrition and exercise as part of daily routine. Reimbursement began in 2011 with the billable code G0447 (face-to-face behavioral counseling for obesity, 15 minutes).[27]

## Prophylactic Medication Use

### Aspirin

Aspirin for the prevention of cardiovascular events was called into question in 2019. The ASCEND (A Study of Cardiovascular Events in Diabetes), ARRIVE (Aspirin to Reduce Risk of Initial Vascular Events), ASPREE (Aspirin in Reducing Events in the Elderly) trials showed less benefit from aspirin in preventing first-time cardiovascular events than previously noted and significant bleeding risk from daily aspirin in people over age 75 years. As a result, clinicians are now identifying patients who should no longer take daily aspirin (Box 5.5).

A stepwise approach is recommended, as to whether aspirin is initiated, continued, or stopped for primary prevention. Discussion with the patient on risk versus benefit and patient

---

**• BOX 5.5   Discussing Low-Dose Aspirin for Primary Prevention**

**What does the patient know about the role of aspirin in prevention of heart attack?**
Is the patient confused between current and previous study results?
Any interest in learning more during the current visit?

**Cite the current evidence while educating on potential:**
Benefits→reduced ASCVD risk   Harms→brain bleed; GI bleed; skin bothersome bruising

**What is the patient's concern regarding development of these conditions?**
Would skin bruising be a nuisance?
Would the patient take a daily aspirin for years if indicated?

*ASCVD*, Atherosclerotic cardiovascular disease; *GI*, gastrointestinal.

---

preferences is paramount. The benefit of aspirin exceeds risk when CVD risk is high, and bleeding risk is low, and also when patient preference for avoiding CVD events is a goal. Consider starting therapy when 10-year CVD risk is > 15%.[28] Consider continuing daily aspirin if 10-year CVD risk is > 10% and the patient has already been taking aspirin for ≥ 10 years. Stop aspirin therapy for 10-year CVD risk > 5%, high risk for bleeding, or patient preference to avoid bleeding.[28] Always promote lifestyle interventions to prevent CVD: physical activity, low alcohol intake, heart-healthy diet, smoking cessation, and adequate sleep. Adequate management of chronic conditions can also prevent cardiovascular events.

⧫⧫ **Use of aspirin for prophylaxis against cardiovascular disease must be balanced against bleeding risk. For many patients over age 75 years, this means eliminating aspirin.**

## Physical Activity

### Guidelines for Physical Activity

Physical activity is key to healthy aging. The US Department of Health and Human Services recommends engaging in 150 minutes of activity weekly at moderate intensity, or 75 minutes at a vigorous intensity. Ideally, activity should include muscle strengthening, endurance, flexibility, and balance to reduce risk for falls. Additional benefits include overall fitness, better freedom of movement, and maintenance of day-to-day function and independence.[29] To promote consistency with physical activity, clinicians can help older adults set specific, practical activity goals that are achievable. Then, revisit these goals with patients to check progress. Give patients an "exercise prescription" that also notes any pertinent exercise limitations because of chronic conditions. Medicare Advantage plans may provide coverage of the Silver Sneakers or comparable fitness program for older adults.

Some older individuals require screening before initiating a physical activity program. Screening incorporates current level of activity; presence of renal, cardiovascular, or metabolic disease; and the level of activity sought by the individual.[30]

The National Institute on Aging is an excellent resource for older adults, including workout videos, ways to exercise without leaving home, and tips for staying safe while exercising. In addition, patients should consider the benefits of Tai Chi on balance as a way to reduce fall risk.

For some older adults, with preexisting balance or gait impairment, starting first with physical therapy provides a good segue into regular physical activity.

⧫⧫ **Exercise is key to successful aging and functional independence and to control of many chronic illnesses. Exercise also promotes brain health.**

## Bone Health

### Dual Energy X-Ray Absorptiometry

Bone mineral density (BMD) testing screens for osteoporosis and, when used in conjunction with the Fracture Risk Assessment Tool (FRAX), predicts future fracture risk. Serial BMD also tracks response to bisphosphonate treatment. T-scores reflect bone density in the lumbar spine (L1-L4), radius (one-third), and femoral neck/femur. The US Preventive Services Task Force (USPSTF) recommends BMD testing at least once in women age 65 years and above and postmenopausal women younger than age 65 years who are at increased risk for osteoporotic fractures (e.g., previous minimal trauma fracture, history of hyperparathyroidism, use of medications that reduce bone density). The National Osteoporosis Foundation, International Society for Clinical Densitometry, and the Endocrine Society recommend BMD testing for all men older than age 70 years and in men age 50 to 70 years when risk factors are present.[31]

The standard for site selection is a T-score at the femoral neck. According to Up-to-Date, however, clinical diagnosis also comes from the lowest T-score whether at the lumbar spine, radius, and femur, which carry predictive value in calculating fracture risk.[32]

Presence of a fragility fracture (fracture from a fall from the standing position, or with preexisting low BMD) confers a diagnosis of osteoporosis as a matter of course. Repeat or serial testing is done every 1 to 3 years after initiation of a bisphosphonate to gauge effectiveness of treatment, looking for improvement in bone density. In addition, repeat BMD testing if clinical decision making depends on the results. Testing at the same facility on the same machine provides consistent comparison of scores.[32]

Initiation of bisphosphonate treatment, for the prevention and management of osteoporosis, rests on an individual's comorbidities, lifestyle, cognition, and personal preferences. The FRAX calculates the 10-year risk of an osteoporotic fracture. The FRAX tool uses BMD at the femoral neck to calculate risk. Adherence to the treatment protocol for safe and effective use of bisphosphonates may be challenging for older individuals and should be explicitly included in patient education.

## Calcium and Vitamin D

The nutritional needs for bone health may be met by a diet high in fruits and vegetables, adequate in protein but moderate in animal protein, and that includes dairy or calcium-fortified foods. When calcium from diet is inadequate, calcium supplementation, spread out through the day, for a total intake of 1200 to 1500 mg, is recommended. No more than 500 mg should be consumed at any one meal to optimize absorption. The safe upper limit of total calcium intake is 2500 mg per day. Calcium citrate is better absorbed than calcium carbonate and does not need to be taken with food; this is the correct formulation for individuals taking acid suppressant medications, such as proton-pump inhibitors. Vitamin D intake is generally below recommendations, which range from 400 to 600 IU daily. Supplementation is generally needed; it enhances absorption of both calcium and bisphosphonates (if treatment is indicated) and decreases fracture risk (see Ch. 43).[33]

❖ **Calcium absorption is best when consumed in food sources; for those who do not meet requirements, supplements are necessary to meet a goal of 1200 to 1500 mg of elemental calcium daily.**

## Exercise

To maintain optimum bone health, as well as overall function and mobility, exercise should include strength, resistance training, balance, and aerobics. Bone, as "living tissue," becomes stronger with exercise just as muscle does; consistent exercise improves strength and balance while preventing falls and the fractures that can result.[34]

## Cognitive Health

Convincing evidence attests to the positive benefit of physical activity on brain health. Through exercise, brain cells receive increased blood flow and oxygen. In addition, a good night's rest serves to clear amyloid from the brain. Although evidence also supports social engagement as lowering risk of cognitive decline, the mechanism is not yet clear. Other important lifestyle changes include eating a healthy diet (such as the Mediterranean diet), maintaining heart health, and treatment of any sleep disorder. The Alzheimer's Association promotes "10 Ways to Love Your Brain," an excellent and concise resource that encourages older adults to affect healthy lifestyle change.[21]

Cognitive screening may be necessary if a patient has subjective memory complaints or if clinician observation of a patient raises red flags that may indicate cognitive change (e.g., decrease in daily function/skills of daily living, word finding difficulties, or visualspatial difficulties). The Mini-Cog, a 3-minute assessment tool, contains a clock-drawing test combined with three-item recall. It is public domain and can be downloaded at no charge (see Ch. 18).

❖ **Periodic screening for colon and breast cancer improves survival. Benefits of prostate cancer screening are uncertain and should focus on high-risk patients.**

## Cancer Screening

Medicare reimburses for screening tests that are recommended by the USPSTF. Determining whether an older adult should undergo screening depends on factors such as the risk of the disease, the benefit of screening, implications of not screening, whether treatment is an acceptable option, and life expectancy. Strict adherence to guidelines for all older adults, however, can result in unnecessary stress and burden to the individual. Decisions about screening should be individualized, with both potential benefit and burden assessed by patient, or proxy, and clinician together. According to the American Geriatrics Society, consideration of the patient's life expectancy and the risks of testing, overdiagnosis, and overtreatment should be considered.[35]

### Breast Cancer Screening

Breast cancer screening guidelines from organizations differ on when to stop screening, frequency of screening, and whether to include clinician or breast self-examination. The USPSTF recommendation is for biennial screening mammography for women age 50 to 74 years. In women age ≥ 75 years, there is insufficient evidence to determine the benefits versus harm to continued use of screening mammography. There is also insufficient evidence to assess the additional benefit versus risk of clinical breast examination beyond screening mammography in women age ≥ 40 years. After age 75 years screening is up to the patient and clinician. The American Geriatrics Society recommends continued screening is reasonable as long as the patient has a 10-year life expectancy.

### Colon Cancer Screening

Colon cancer is the third most common cancer and the second leading cause of cancer death among older adults. The incidence of adenomatous polyps increases with age as does the risk of polyps becoming cancerous. The majority of colorectal cancers are found in adults above age 50 years, with a median age at diagnosis of age 68 years for men and age 72 years for women.[36] The natural history of polyps is evolution to cancer over a 5- to 10-year period. The USPSTF recommends screening for colorectal cancer for persons age 50 to 74 years of age with one of the following: yearly fecal occult blood or fecal immunochemical testing (FIT); every 1 to 3 years FIT deoxyribonucleic acid; every 5 years sigmoidoscopy or computed tomography colonography; every 10 years colonoscopy. In adults age 76 to 85 years, this same set of screenings should be done selectively based on professional judgment and patient preference. In addition, colon cancer screening of any type is not recommended until 10 years have elapsed following a high-quality negative colonoscopy for patients without elevated risk for the cancer (positive family history, personal history of polyps, or inflammatory bowel disease).[37]

## Cervical Cancer Screening

The USPSTF recommends against screening for cervical cancer in women older than age 65 years who have had adequate prior screening. Women with precancerous lesions, immunosuppression, or human immunodeficiency virus (HIV)/human papilloma virus (HPV) infection are at high risk for developing cervical cancer and require screening at any age. Women for whom previous screening is unknown may need screening. Screening is unnecessary in women who have undergone hysterectomy with cervix removal, and with no history of precancerous lesion (grade 2 or 3).

## Prostate Cancer Screening

The USPSTF states that screening offers only a small benefit of decreasing the risk of death in men age 55 to 64 years. In this population, the potential harms of false positives that can lead to overdiagnosis and overtreatment, and treatment complications (urinary/fecal incontinence, erectile dysfunction), outweigh the potential benefit. Persons at higher risk are those with a positive family history and Black men.

For men age $\geq 70$ years, prostate-specific antigen (PSA) testing is not recommended because benefit does not outweigh potential harm. Exceptions to the USPSTF recommendations are for Black men and those with family history of prostate cancer. Any discussion between clinician and patient on whether to screen for prostate cancer must consider risk versus benefit while taking into account the patient's chronic conditions, race/ethnicity, preferences, and values.[37]

## Special Populations

### Lesbian, Gay, Bisexual, and Transgender

*Healthy People 2020* identifies the health needs of the lesbian, gay, bisexual, and transgender (LGBT) population for the first time as a national priority. Currently 2.7 million adults age $\geq 50$ years identify as LGBT.

This number is expected to more than double by 2030.[38,39]

Aging as an LGBT individual presents special psychosocial challenges in addition to aging with the same health issues as other older adults. Health disparities in this population limit both access to healthcare and positive health outcomes. Disparities described include greater economic uncertainty, greater risk of disability, poorer physical and mental health, a greater number of chronic conditions, and higher rates of social risk taking, although some subgroups of LGBT older adults seem to fare much better (see Ch. 4).

Risk-taking habits (excessive alcohol intake, smoking, and drug use) begin in young adulthood and catch up to individuals as they age, resulting in poor physical and mental health, disability, and depression.[40] Although many LGBT older adults are in relatively good health, robust evidence exists that social stigma leads to victimization and discrimination, which in turn are factors in poor physical and mental health, and lack of access to care. In fact, approximately 31% of LBGT older adults delay or do not seek preventive care, such as cancer screening, smoking cessation, and immunizations. Studies also emphasize that social support can mitigate some of these disparities, while contributing to resilience and successful aging.

Of note, in a 2019 study of subjective cognitive decline in LGBT older adults, conducted at the University of California and San Francisco, approximately 25% of participants characterized themselves as having subjective cognitive decline. Although a cause could not be identified, researchers believe elevated rates for stress and low mood and lack of access to healthcare may be factors.[41]

## Human Immunodeficiency Virus and Acquired Immunodeficiency Syndrome

Although risk factors for HIV are the same for any adult, older adults are less likely to undergo testing for the virus. HIV appears to speed up the aging process. According to 2015 statistics from the CDC, approximately 47% of HIV-positive individuals were age $\geq 50$ years. Because of the effectiveness of antiretroviral therapy, persons diagnosed when younger are living into old age. As such, many have comorbidities of aging that can affect continued treatment. The CDC recommends testing up to the age of 64 years. If a clinician believes a patient older than age 64 years to be at risk for HIV infection, then testing should be done. If a patient tests positive, medication choice is individualized taking into consideration other chronic infections that may make management more difficult.[26]

## Putting Prevention Into Practice

### The Annual Wellness Visit

This service is designed to address the recommended preventive services described earlier and creates (initial annual welfare visit [AWV]) or updates (subsequent AWV) the individual's prevention plan. It covers current health status, risk factors, immunizations, and needed screenings, along with functional ability, living environment and safety, and health education. The focus is on disease prevention, as well as disease management. The AWV is covered without copay under Medicare Part B so long as the patient has had Part B for 12 months, and has not had a wellness visit in the prior 12 months. Newly enrolled Medicare beneficiaries who have had Medicare Part B receive a comparable, but slightly different, set of services under the onetime "Welcome to Medicare" preventive visit that must be completed within the first 12 months of Part B enrollment (Tables 5.3 and 5.4). In addition to the services listed later, subsequent AWVs include weight and blood pressure check, updating of medical/family history, advance directives, current

TABLE 5.3 **Medicare Coverage for Preventive Services**

| Service | Who Is Covered | Frequency | Cost to Beneficiary |
|---|---|---|---|
| Welcome to Medicare | All beneficiaries with Part B coverage | Once within 12 months of enrollment | None |
| Annual wellness visit | Part B beneficiaries | Annual after 12 months of enrollment | None |
| Ultrasound screening for abdominal aortic aneurysm | Beneficiaries with risk factors | Once in a lifetime | None |
| Cardiovascular screening (lipid panel, cholesterol, lipoprotein, triglycerides) | Beneficiaries without known cardiovascular disease | Every 5 years | None |
| Diabetes screening | Beneficiaries with risk factors | Two/year if "prediabetic"; one/year if never tested | None |
| Diabetes self-management training | Beneficiaries with diabetes | 10 hours of initial training and 2 hours annually | Deductible applies |
| Medical nutrition therapy | Beneficiaries with diabetes, renal disease, or kidney transplant in the last 3 years | 3 hours counseling in the first year and 2 hours each subsequent year by a nutrition specialist | None |
| Pap screening | All female beneficiaries | Annually if at high risk or childbearing age with abnormal Pap within 3 years; or every 24 months Not provided if age >65 years and three negative tests obtained | None |
| Pelvic screening | All female beneficiaries | Annually if high risk for cervical or vaginal cancer; or childbearing age with abnormal Pap within 3 years Not provided if age >65 years and negative test obtained or no risk factors | None |
| Mammography screening | Female beneficiaries aged 35 and older | Annually for those aged 50–74 and then no screening recommendation | None |
| Bone mass measurements | Estrogen-deficient beneficiaries and at risk; vertebral abnormalities; glucocorticoid therapy for >3 months; primary hyperparathyroidism; or on drug therapy for osteoporosis | Biennial, and as medically necessary | None |
| Colorectal cancer screening | Beneficiaries aged 50–85 years | FOBT/FIT annually; flex sigmoidoscopy every 4 years; colonoscopy every 10 years; Cologuard every 3 years | None |
| Prostate cancer screening | Male beneficiaries aged over 50 years | PSA and DRE; but screening not recommended unless risk factors present | None for PSA; copay for DRE |
| Glaucoma | Beneficiaries with diabetes or family history, Black persons after age 50 years or/and Hispanic persons over 65 years | Annually | Copay applies |
| Influenza vaccine | All beneficiaries | Annually | None |
| Pneumococcal conjugate and polysaccharide vaccines | All beneficiaries | Initial vaccine once and the second vaccine 1 year later | None |
| Hepatitis B vaccine | Beneficiaries at risk for hepatitis B are covered under Medicare Part B; average risk individuals are covered under Medicare Part D | Scheduled dosages | None for Part B coverage; part D copay applies |
| Tobacco counseling | Tobacco users | Two cessation attempts/year; up to eight sessions annually | None |

*(Continued)*

**TABLE 5.3**   Medicare Coverage for Preventive Services—cont'd

| Service | Who Is Covered | Frequency | Cost to Beneficiary |
|---|---|---|---|
| Hepatitis C screening | Beneficiaries at risk; and persons born between 1945 and 1965 | Once in lifetime | None |
| HIV screening | Beneficiaries at risk | Annually | None |
| Behavioral therapy for cardiovascular disease | All beneficiaries | Annually | None |
| Alcohol screening and counseling | All beneficiaries for screening and beneficiaries with alcohol misuse for counseling | Annual screening; four counseling sessions/year | None |
| Depression | All beneficiaries | Annual | None |
| Sexually transmitted | Sexually active individuals with high-risk behaviors | Annual | None |
| Behavioral therapy for obesity | Obese (BMI >30) beneficiaries | One visit/week for 1 month; every other week months 2—6; one/month for months 7—12 | None |
| Advance care planning | All beneficiaries | Annually as part of wellness visit; as needed as illness evolves | No copay as part of AWV; other times copay applies |
| Varicella vaccine medications | All beneficiaries under either Part D or Part C (when medications covered) | Twice for Shingrix (2—6 months apart) and once for Zostavax | Plans must cover; copays will apply |
| Diabetes prevention program: expanded model | Beneficiaries meeting prediabetes criteria | Once for up to 24 sessions within 2 years | None |

*BMI*, Body mass index; *DRE*, digital rectal examination; *FIT*, fecal immunochemical test; *FOBT*, fecal occult blood test; *PSA*, prostate-specific antigen.
For most up-to-date preventive coverage information: https://www.cms.gov/Medicare/Prevention/PrevntionGenInfo/medicare-preventive-services/MPS-QuickReferenceChart-1.html#COLO_CAN

providers/suppliers, fall risk, function, safety, cognitive screening, and advice or referral for health education. A written plan, including patient-stated goals and preferences, is provided to the patient at the AWV.[42]

## Engaging Patients in Health Promotion

Working with older adults to have them engage in health promotion activities and, in some cases, to change lifelong behaviors can be challenging. Barriers to health promotion can include a lack of understanding of its benefits, an assumption that with increased age there is no point to good health behaviors and prevention, financial difficulties, lack of access to services, and having never been told by clinicians what health activities are beneficial to engage in.[43] However, older adults can change behavior. The stronger the individual's self-efficacy (the internal self-confidence that one has the ability to succeed with making a behavior change), the more likely he or she will be to initiate and persist with a given health activity.[44] Self-efficacy also encompasses the idea that if a certain behavior takes place, it leads to a certain outcome. Weighing the pros and cons of a health behavior change with the patient increases the patient's knowledge base and can help motivate the patient to pursue a particular health promotion activity.

## Motivating Patients to Engage in Health Promotion

Motivational interviewing (Box 5.6), which incorporates self-efficacy, has been used with older adults and shows some benefits in changing behavior.[45] As a direct, patient-centered counseling approach, motivational interviewing helps patients explore and resolve any doubt or hesitation regarding behavior change. The responsibility for making a behavior change rests with the patient rather than the clinician, but the clinician provides the guidance. Motivational interviewing is goal and outcome focused via dialogue between clinician and patient, also addressing any challenges and/or ambivalence on the part of the patient. If a patient is cognitively impaired, a family member or surrogate decision-maker can participate to help facilitate goal setting. Examples of health promotion activities include smoking cessation, diet control, reduction of alcohol consumption, and aspects of chronic disease management. Use open-ended questions, recognize patient strengths, practice reflective listening, and provide a recap of each patient visit. At each visit, continue to address health promotion behaviors and provide positive reinforcement to the patient.[46]

Older adults vary in their willingness to engage in health promoting activities. With advancing age, there can be less interest in health promotion activities for the purpose of lengthening life, and

| TABLE 5.4 | Tools for Assessment of Required Elements of the Annual Wellness and Health Promotion Visits |
|---|---|

| Elements | Recommended Tools (Web Access) |
|---|---|
| Alcohol use | • The Michigan Alcoholism Screening Test—Geriatric Version (*MAST - G*) (www.ssc.wisc.edu/wlsresearch/pilot/.../Aging_AppB5_MAST-G.pdf) |
| | • The CAGE (http://pubs.niaaa.nih.gov/publications/arh28-2/78-79.htm) |
| Depression | • Centers for Epidemiological Studies Depression Scale (http://patienteducation.stanford.edu/research/cesd.pdf) |
| | • Geriatric Depression Scale (http://www.stanford.edu/~yesavage/GDS.html) |
| | • Beck Depression Scale (http://www.fpnotebook.com/Psych/Exam/BckDprsnInvntry.htm) |
| | • Cornell Scale for Depression in Dementia (http://www.thedoctorwillseeyounow.com/articles/behavior/depressn_12/) |
| | • The Patient Health Questionnaire-9 or 2 (PHQ-9 or PHQ-2) http://www.cqaimh.org/pdf/tool_phq2.pdf |
| | • Hospital Anxiety and Depression Scale (HADS) http://www.scireproject.com/outcome-measures/hospital-anxiety-and-depression-scale-hads |
| Diet | • The Mini Nutritional Assessment for Older Adults (http://www.mna-elderly.com/) |
| Functional ability | • The Barthel Index (www.healthcare.uiowa.edu/igec/tools/function/barthelADLs.pdf) |
| | • The Katz Index (http://www.mainehealth.org/workfiles/mh_PFHA/Katz%20ADL_LawtonIADL.pdf) |
| Smoking | • The Agency for Healthcare Research and Quality recommends the use of the "4 *As*": ask, advise, assist, and arrange follow-up. |
| Safety/falls | • Check for Safety: A Home Fall Prevention Checklist for Older Adults (http://www.cdc.gov/ncipc/preventionpub-res/toolkit/checklistforsafety.htm) |
| End-of-life | • End-of-Life Care. American Family Physician (http://www.aafp.org/afp/topicModules/viewTopiccounselingModule.htm?topicModuleId = 57) and planning |
| | • The Physician Orders for Life-Sustaining Treatment (http://www.ohsu.edu/polst/) |
| Cognition | • Mini-Cog (www.bami.us/Neuro/MiniCog.html) |
| | • The Brief Interview for Mental Status (BIMS) (dhmh.dfmc.org/longTermCare/.../BIMS_Form_Instructions.pdf) |
| Physical | • The Yale Physical Activity Survey (http://dapa-toolkit.mrc.ac.uk/documents/en/Yal/Yale_Physical_activityActivity_Survey.pdf) |
| | • The CHAMPS Physical Activity Questionnaire (http://sbs.ucsf.edu/iha/champs/resources/qxn/) |

| • BOX 5.6 | The Principles of Motivational Interviewing |
|---|---|

1. Express empathy — Look at things through the patient's eyes and experiences. No criticisms.
2. Support self-efficacy — Emphasize patient strengths first: past successes, skills the patient already has.
3. Work through resistance — Avoid argument. Listen and then validate what the patient has told you. Encourage the patient to come up with solutions instead of just providing them.
4. Develop discrepancy — Guide the patient to understand how current behaviors may be in contrast to values, and goals he/she wants to achieve.

greater interest in engaging in activities to improve quality of life. It is important therefore to select health promotion activities with older adults by using an individualized approach. The goal is to provide individuals with information about each health promotion activity, and the risks and benefits associated with each, while assisting them to engage in activities that will optimize health and overall quality of life.

**CASE**

**Discussion**

The health of Mrs. W. would be improved if she quit smoking and became physically active most days of the week. These are the two most important areas for intervention because both together would provide the greatest positive impact to her overall health. Smoking cessation counseling given by her primary provider includes providing praise for previous efforts on her part, discussion as to the benefits of quitting, shared goal setting to help set Mrs. W up for success, and an agreed upon timetable for telephone/clinic follow-up of her progress. Referral to a local smoking cessation clinic or a state-run program provides support in her efforts, along with careful choice of a pharmacologic agent as adjunct treatment. The best way for Mrs. W to begin, and stay engaged in, a physical activity program is through the social atmosphere of a Silver Sneakers or similar Medicare program. These programs provide a degree of "buddy support" encouraging continued participation. For any noted balance or mobility issues, physical therapy is a good segue into physical activity. There may also be a local

Parkinson disease-specific exercise program Mrs. W. could join. You will check on her progress toward a goal of achieving 150 minutes of exercise and the plan for smoking cessation at scheduled follow-up visits. The two of you agree to 3-month follow-up visits to allow you to reinforce her achievements and develop strategies to address the challenges that she will inevitably experience.

## Web Resources

www.cms.gov/MLNProducts/downloads/MPS_QuickReference_Chart_1.pdf. The Center for Medicare Services list of the Medicare-covered preventive services. https://www.cms.gov/Outreach-and-Education/Medicare-Learning-Network-MLN/MLNProducts/downloads/MPS_QRI_IPPE001a.pdf. Medicare ABC Guide for Wellness Visit.

http://lpi.oregonstate.edu/infocenter/olderadultnut.html. Detailed recommendations for micronutrients for older adults.

https://www.medicareinteractive.org/. Details on Medicare coverage for various services, with patient education guide.

https://www.nia.nih.gov/health/quitting-smoking-older-adults. Tobacco cessation strategies.

Patient education and downloadable handouts on exercise. Includes video demonstrations.

https://hnrca.tufts.edu/myplate. Downloadable patient handout on nutrition.

https://www.nof.org. National Osteoporosis Foundation. Patient education, exercises, guidelines on bisphosphonates and screening

National Institute on Aging (NIA), one of the institutes/center of the NIH. Provides research, free publications for patients and providers, health information from A to Z. https://www.nia.nih.gov/

Centers for Medicare and Medicaid Services (CMS). Part of the US Department of Health and Human Services. Services covered, policies, immunization and screening recommendations/schedules, guidance on regulations, research data, education through the Medicare Learning Network (MLN). https://www.cms.gov/.

Health HealthinAging.org, education portal of the Health in Aging Foundation, a nonprofit organization founded by the American Geriatrics Society. Information for older adults and caregivers on aging and chronic conditions, health management, driving safety, medication use, wellness, and prevention. Downloadable handouts. https://www.healthinaging.org/. For patients, https://www.medicare.gov/.

Area Agency on Aging, part of National Association of Area Agencies on Aging. Access to resources at the local level (geographic area) for older adults. Includes screening of companies providing services (ratings information provided), caregiver respite, nutritional services (Meals on Wheels), legal services, referrals for transportation, and insurance expertise. Find the local agency through the national website. https://www.n4a.org/

Alzheimer's Association. Tips on brain health, information, research, and support for all types of dementia. Locate a local chapter through the national website. https://www.alz.org/

## Key References

2. Centers for Disease Control and Prevention. *Vaccine Recommendations and Guidelines of the ACIP.* Available at: http://www.cdc.gov/vaccines/hcp/acip-recs/general-recs/programs.html.

21. Alzheimer's Association. *10 Ways to Love Your Brain.* 2019. Available at: https://www.alz.org/help-support/brain_health/10_ways_to_love_your_brain. Accessed September 14, 2019.

29. National Institute on Aging. *Go 4 Life: 4 Types of Exercise.* 2018. Available at: https://go4life.nia.nih.gov/4-types-of-exercise/.

42. Medicare Interactive. *Annual Wellness Visit.* Available at: https://www.medicareinteractive.org/get-answers/medicare-covered-services/preventive-services/annual-wellness-visit. 2019.

**References available online at expertconsult.com.**

# 6

# Cultural Competency and Cultural Humility in Caring for Older Adults

LAUREN J. PARKER, ROLAND J. THORPE JR., AND MATTHEW K. MCNABNEY

## OUTLINE

*Additional online-only material indicated by icon.*

## OBJECTIVES

*Upon completion of this chapter, the reader will be able to:*

- Define cultural competency and cultural humility, and describe how the two terms compare and complement.
- Recognize the impact of past inequities in healthcare on future healthcare behavior of both patients and providers.

- Describe the concept of "personhood" and how it can vary across cultural groups.

## Cultural Competency Versus Cultural Humility

It is expected that one in five Americans will be older than age 65 years by 2030, and by 2044 more than half of all Americans will belong to a racial/ethnic group other than non-Hispanic White alone. As the demographics in the United States continue to change, it is imperative to be mindful of the importance of culture while providing care to diverse populations.

 **Culture refers to an everchanging set of shared symbols, beliefs, and customs that shapes individual and/or group behavior.**

Traditionally, culture has been used to categorize ethnic, racial, religious, or geographically bound social groups. However, with its everchanging nature, culture now encompasses other social categories to include sexual orientation, class, and gender. Cultural norms and values related to membership in such bounded groups can, in part, shape individual health behavior and perceptions of health and illness.

Cultural competency is "a set of congruent behaviors, attitudes, and policies that come together in a system, organization, or among professionals that enables effective work in cross-cultural situations." It is commonly accepted that training in cultural competency will raise awareness of the sensitivity that culture has on the health experience.[1] Proponents of cultural competency training promote its use in combating health disparities and providing quality care for all.[2] Although the intended goal of training for health professionals to increase knowledge about a culture and to provide culturally sensitive care has efficacy, there are some critiques.

One major critique of cultural competency is the low likelihood that sufficient cultural understanding can be obtained. Given that culture is an everchanging process, categoric approaches to cultural competence training can potentially result in unintended stereotyping and bias. Another critique of cultural competency contends that many of the observed cultural or ethnic differences in health also represent the downstream consequences of larger structural factors (i.e., access to quality healthcare, structural racism). Reliance solely on cultural attributes may not address the biologic, socioeconomic, and racial impacts of upstream structural factors on health disparities. One alternative approach is cultural humility, which places less emphasis on knowledge acquisition and competency and instead encourages personal reflection.

A dynamic and lifelong process, cultural humility places emphasis on addressing power imbalances and promotes interpersonal sensitivity through partnerships with and learning from patients. This process requires an attitude of openness by placing the practitioner in a learning mode as opposed to an authoritative figure. The interpersonal nature of cultural humility allows for meaningful engagement between the practitioner and client, with potential to develop a better understanding of personal and cultural identities.

---

### CASE 1

#### Wanda and Christopher

Wanda is a nurse practitioner in a community nursing home (NH) in Cleveland, Ohio, where she has worked as the "house provider" for the past 3 years. She is 59 years old, Caucasian, and has worked in a variety of care settings and practices over the past 20 years. Christopher is an LPN who works at the same facility. He is a 37-year-old Black man and is thinking about going back to school to get his Bachelor of Science in Nursing. The clients they serve at this NH are primarily low-income (Medicaid) and people of different races. The mandatory, annual workshop on Cultural Competency Training was held last week. Wanda dutifully attends the workshop and endorses the importance of learning about all types of people and different backgrounds. She proudly displays her workshop certificate on the bulletin board over her desk. Christopher is a little more restless about the content and feels it is a bit oversimplified. The following week, he does the admission intake for a new resident who is Afro-Caribbean (Haitian) and realizes that he is having a hard time understanding the woman and her family, both in language and "other ways." He is not sure why it makes him uncomfortable and he is determined to spend more time with her and the family to ask more questions and demonstrate his curiosity about her life in Haiti and how that impacts her views on day-to-day living and approach to healthcare. This dialogue expands on a daily basis, as Christopher does not allow his lack of familiarity with Haitian culture to be a barrier to a caring relationship.

1. What are the differences between cultural competence and cultural humility?
2. How did the reactions to the workshop differ between Wanda and Christopher?
3. How should professional development "messages" be formatted to allow for greater success when translated to the bedside?

---

## Healthcare Disparities

The demographics in this country are changing dramatically. Along with surge in the number of older adults, there has been a simultaneous shift in the racial and ethnic composition in the United States. Although these dramatic changes in the United States will have a huge impact on the healthcare of this segment of the population, it is unclear if the healthcare system is ready to properly address the care needs of diverse older adults.

There is a large body of research demonstrating that racial/ethnic minorities and those who belong to lower socioeconomic status groups receive inadequate care, lower quality care, have less access to care, health services use, and patient adherence to treatment regimens than White persons. These well-known healthcare disparities have been shown to exist even when accounting for patient

level factors, such as trust in physicians' recommendation, and person preference regarding treatment options, and access-related factors including patients' insurance status and income.[3,5] These very concerns were discussed in the 2003 Institute of Medicine report "Unequal Treatment." The authors of this report deemed these disparities to be complex and often rooted in historical and structural inequities between Black persons and White persons. Examples include discriminatory practices in the 1940s and 1950s when fully licensed Black physicians were not allowed to work at White hospitals, as well as unethical research, such as the Tuskegee syphilis study, which placed minorities in direct harm. Although these horrific practices have since been halted and considered illegal, remnants of this past likely persist in many ways.

In addition, there are likely persistent health disparities stemming from biased clinical thinking and decision making that have the potential to influence the judgment of the healthcare professional. In older adults, these persistent biases are likely cumulative over time that compound the effects. For example, differences in blood pressure control as well as adherence to recommended treatments and preventive health guideline recommendations are significant factors in health disparities in late life. Approaches to providing high-quality healthcare to all individuals is a key component for a healthcare system or provider seeking to achieve health equity. One approach that is gaining attention is cultural humility.

## The Relevance of Cultural Humility in Patient Care

### Establishing a Therapeutic Relationship

An essential goal in primary care is the establishment of a healthy and trusting therapeutic relationship between clinician and patient. This is particularly true with older adults as they deal with an array of medical and psychosocial challenges associated with aging. There are several key components to building these relationships, including respect and congruence with values and beliefs. Providers should maintain an awareness for opportunities, and the need to identify the potential for cross-cultural exchanges—realizing that all relationships have "cross-cultural" qualities. Some indicators are more apparent (language, name, appearance/race) whereas others are not (gender identity, religion, income status). Striving to be skillful at making people comfortable at sharing and trusting the provider is the goal.

As previously discussed in this chapter, promoting cultural awareness in the workplace typically occurs in cultural competency training in professional development workshops. Cultural humility, on the other hand, goes a step further and involves an ongoing process of self-exploration and self-critique combined with a willingness to learn from others.[4] These efforts will foster successful therapeutic relationships regardless of the cultural differences that might exist between clinician and patient.

### Allows Providers to Comfortably Adhere to Person-Centered Care

By incorporating cultural awareness and humility into daily practice, clinicians are able to more naturally connect with older patients to ensure a person-centered approach to care. For example, how providers approach and address patients and families can immediately signal a receptiveness to differences. Readiness to accommodate issues with language and communication barriers is important, including resources, such as use of interpreters (regardless of setting). Some patient characteristics might be overlooked when considering "cross-cultural" issues, such as poverty, level of education, and health literacy. There can be significant differences in how certain individuals relate to the medical community, creating mistrust or a sense of not being understood. This can influence things like adherence to care recommendations and proper use of health services (using primary care offices rather than emergency rooms, for example).

When clinicians are aware of cultural issues and accommodate differences, they will be more comfortable placing the patient at the "center" of the decision-making process.

❖ **"Person-centered care" involves considering a person's desires, family situations, social circumstances, and values. To achieve this level of awareness, clinicians must seek and maintain a level of cultural awareness and sensitivity.**

It is even appropriate for clinicians to "check in" with the older adult (and/or family) to assess how well these connections are being made with regard to the cultural aspects of care. For example, a clinician who is providing end-of-life care for an older adult of a different (less familiar) religion can candidly discuss his/her lack of knowledge. This opens the door for the patient and family to share and educate the clinician creating a safe and comforting space for all.

### Ensures That Flexibility in Care Is Maintained

There are an infinite number of care scenarios with older adults. As stated before, every clinician-patient encounter is, to some degree, "cross-cultural." To remain effective, clinicians must listen and interpret signals from older adults and their families with regard to care preferences. Sometimes, the values and preferences of the patient do not align with the "standard of care" or the recommendation of the clinician. It is important for the clinician to identify when such a deviation might be because of personal values and to respectfully (but clearly) discuss that difference. Likewise, patients and families should be encouraged to do the same when uncertain about the motivation of the clinician.

### Healthcare Provider Shortages (or Malalignment)

Several racial and ethnic groups in the United States are "underrepresented" in the medical field. Therefore there is a high likelihood that clinician and patient will differ with regard to race, ethnicity, or other personal characteristics. Although patients might prefer a provider of the same background, it is often not possible because of availability. Therefore it is necessary to optimally prepare all clinicians to be culturally sensitive and aware of differences to improve circumstances of underrepresentation.[2]

### Promote Diversity and Inclusion in Training and Hiring

To have the greatest impact, it is preferred to positively influence the mindset and approach of clinicians during training. In doing so, it is possible to introduce culturally sensitive approaches to patient care when techniques are still being developed. Informational seminars, role-playing, and sensitivity training are some of the ways to impact practice style while these are still malleable. Conveying sincere interest in the background and values of older adults are essential skills to developing expertise in cross-cultural awareness. Providers should be "mindful" of this effort in patient care and should periodically reflect on meaningful experiences. Intentional efforts to promote a diverse workforce (for the benefit of patient care) should be a priority in hiring practices at all levels.

## Interactions With Coworkers

### Promotes Collective Growth of Healthcare Team (Avoids Dominance of Certain Cultural Identities)

Although some healthcare teams are quite diverse, that is frequently not the case. Therefore it is important that diversity and cultural awareness be a continuous priority among healthcare team members. When diversity among coworkers is addressed thoughtfully and dialogue is encouraged, it can empower the team. An empowered team that feels respected will generally perform at a higher level. In turn, a team that feels respected for its diversity and collective success will likely report higher job satisfaction, which leads to lower staff turnover and the associated expenses that go along with lower job satisfaction.

## Dementia and Personhood

❖ **The dominant US cultural definition of personhood in terms of independence and achievement leads to excess disability and suffering among people with conditions like dementia.**

Such conditions challenge this prevailing definition of "full personhood." In contrast, other cultures may place more value in such qualities as interdependence, spiritual connection, embodied activity, or social relationships and role. In Case 2, we see that Ms. Nettie Mae is still valued as a full person because she still is the family matriarch. The role as a surviving elder is honored as an embodiment of the community's history and the community's ability to survive in a fairly hostile environment (e.g., slavery, Jim Crow, civil rights struggles, ongoing structural and institutional racism in the contemporary United States). Finally, her personhood endures because she still is able to participate interpersonally and emotionally with family and community members. Indeed, we increasingly recognize that emotional and relational abilities persist far into the progression of Alzheimer disease and other dementias. Therefore when personhood is defined as the ability to relate to others appropriately, dementia is less of a threat to the patient's personhood. In contrast, by narrowly defining full personhood as independence and cognitive achievement, the dominant US cultural approach to personhood leads to excess disability and suffering.

❖ **When personhood is defined as the ability to relate to others appropriately, dementia is less of a threat to the patient's personhood.**

### CASE 2

#### Nettie Mae

Nettie Mae is 78 years old and widowed. She is Black and raised her family on a farm in Virginia and now lives with her grandson and his wife and their three small children. Her own children live nearby and join for meals on a weekly basis. The family knows that she is forgetful, and they do not like to leave her at home. She started a small fire in the kitchen last year, and her family no longer lets her cook. In a joking but firm way, they took her car keys away and did not allow her to drive. Over the next 3 years, she became increasingly dependent on family for self-care and was less able to have a conversation. However, she remained a vital part of the family and was assisted to church and all family outings. The stories of days gone by that she had told for decades are now told on her behalf by family members. Her daughter reports a back strain associated with providing the heavy care that is now required by Ms. Nettie Mae. You raise the consideration of assisted living or nursing home. The family politely and repeatedly declines the need for any such assistance.

1. If you had a parent or grandparent who needed assistance at the level of Ms. Nettie Mae, what criteria would you use to determine whether you could maintain her in your home? To what extent do you believe that these criteria differ across different cultures?
2. How does the definition of "personhood" impact how the family responds to her change in care needs and family integration?

## End-of-Life Care

Clinicians should be aware of the varied cultural sensitivities to discussing end-of-life care and impending death. Considerations of cultural beliefs of the family and patient should occur before approaching the patient regarding life-threatening diagnoses. In the US healthcare system, discussion of advanced directives and end-of-life decisions with patients were prioritized in the 1990 Patient Self Determination Act. Such conversations require the clinician to have a keen understanding of the cultural beliefs of the patient, which may be uniquely influenced by intersectional identities and other factors like spirituality. Although the advice of medical providers and the wishes of the patient may conflict, it is pertinent that the decisions regarding care should be a shared decision-making process. Many cultures rely on a family-centered approach (collectivism) as a principle for major decision making, which opposes the autonomic/individual approaches of Western medicine. In collective decision making, family members often receive information about the diagnosis and prognosis of the patient, and make treatment choices without consulting the patient. To manage these situations, the clinician should consult with the patient regarding how he or she would like to make treatment decisions and determine the extent to which the patient/family members would like to be involved in the treatment decision. This requires a skillful and artful approach.

Using cultural humility in developing treatment decisions allows the clinician to learn from the patient regarding his or her cultural beliefs and norms regarding end-of-life care and take such beliefs into account while developing the best course of action. For example, pain management and life-sustaining procedures (i.e., do-not-resuscitate orders) are areas where it is important to consider cultural beliefs. Some cultures may have strict practices that forbid them from using certain life-sustaining procedures. It is important to identify a patients' belief or cultural norms regarding such treatment plans. Further, cultures that have experienced historical disenfranchisement or discrimination from the healthcare system may be reluctant to trust clinicians. This distrust may be enhanced if the clinician is of a different race and/or ethnic background. To address this potential concern, the clinician can encourage the patient or family member to inform them if they have quality-of-care concerns and reinforce to the patient/family that decision-making processes will be a collective effort. Developing rapport with patients and their family members to let them know that you are interested in their cultural heritage will help facilitate more open communication when discussing end-of-life treatments.

### CASE 3

#### Rosario

Rosario is a 79-year-old Mexican-American woman with multiple medical problems, including severe ischemic cardiomyopathy, diabetic neuropathy, peripheral vascular disease, and moderate Alzheimer-type dementia. She had a below-the-knee-amputation 4 years ago. Her renal function is declining and has recently approached the level of considering dialysis. A few days after Thanksgiving, she is hospitalized for an exacerbation of heart failure (likely because of dietary indiscretion). She becomes delirious in the hospital, which is distressing to the patient and family. The inpatient team arranges a family meeting to discuss treatment preferences and is surprised that the family is still wanting to be "full code." The conversation revolves around their mom still being a person, someone they love, and cannot abandon. Because you are her primary care geriatrics clinician, you arrange a follow-up meeting with the family. Several of your office team also attend. It is clear from that meeting that this is not a matter of misunderstanding the prognosis. Instead, it is a matter of living all life that is left to live and the obligation to provide all care that is possible, regardless of the likelihood of success.

1. Describe the sense of "personhood" that is attached to Rosario by her family.
2. How is this impacting their reaction to her health changes and perceived needs for proper care?
3. In future care of other patients with dementia or poor overall prognosis, how should the office staff respond to care decisions that do not make sense to them?

## Advice for Primary Care Clinicians

Prioritize diversity and cultural awareness. Given the many benefits to patient care, as well as other positive effects in the workplace, it is highly recommended that clinicians develop cultural awareness and humility. Evidence supports that these efforts positively impact patient, family, and staff communication and care relationship.

Educate yourself on cultural issues and diversity on the local, national, international level as it pertains to healthcare in your community (especially among older adults and end-of-life issues). Clinicians should recognize how cultural awareness will impact the care they provide and should therefore seek to educate themselves through various methods, including mainstream media. The American Geriatrics Society has published a very helpful handbook, entitled *Doorway Thoughts* (reflections at the doorway before engaging the patient). This book offers many good examples about how different cultural subgroups have subtle variability along the lines of different racial/ethnic groups.

## Summary

The population of older adults in the United States is becoming increasingly diverse, in many ways that were not previously considered. These include race, ethnicity, and religion, as well sexual orientation, gender identity, and many others characteristics. When healthcare providers anticipate this and are flexible in the approach to patients, this reality enriches the experience and sets the stage for better outcomes that are person centered. The goals is to be aware and curious, not simply informed or "competent" about diversity of culture. In addition to adopting this mindset of "cultural humility," clinicians can also access resources to improve communication and understanding. There are many clinical scenarios (such as end-of-life care) that are particularly sensitive to cultural beliefs and values.

## Key References

1. Ferdinand KC, Yadav K, Nasser SA, et al. Disparities in hypertension and cardiovascular disease in blacks: the critical role of medication adherence. *J Clin Hypertens (Greenwich)*. 2017;19:1015–1024.
2. Foronda C, Baptiste, DL, Reinholdt, MM, Ousman K. Cultural humility: a concept analysis. *J Transcult Nurs*. 2016;27:210–217.
3. Jongen C, McCalman J, Bainbridge R. Health workforce cultural competency interventions: A systematic scoping review. *BMC Health Serv Res*. 2018;18:232.
4. Manuel JI. Racial/ethnic and gender disparities in health care use and access. *Health Serv Res*. 2018;53:1407–1429.
5. Sklar DP. Cultural competence: glimpsing the world through our patients' eyes as we guide their care. *Acad Med*. 2018; 93:1259–1262.

**References available online at expertconsult.com.**

# 7

# Appropriate Prescribing

GREGORY J. HUGHES AND JUDITH L. BEIZER

## OUTLINE

*Additional online-only material indicated by icon.*

## OBJECTIVES

*Upon completion of this chapter, the reader will be able to:*

- Describe physiologic changes that may impact how medications should be used in older patients.
- Outline a prescribing strategy to maximize benefit and minimize harm.

- Explain how prescription drug coverage impacts use of medication in older patients.
- Explain how pharmacists add value to the geriatric healthcare team.

The older population uses more prescription medication than any other age group.[1] With the initiation of Medicare Part D in 2006, all 43 million Medicare beneficiaries had immediate access to outpatient prescription drug plans with 90% of beneficiaries enrolling in Medicare Part D or a creditable drug coverage plan.[2] As of 2018, the number of Medicare beneficiaries has grown to 60 million people with 43 million enrolling in a Medicare Part D.[3] A report from the Centers for Disease Control and Prevention states that in 2011 to 2014, 90.6% of older people had at least one prescription drug filled in the last 30 days and that 40.7% had five or more prescription drugs filled, numbers dwarfing those of younger populations.[1] A 2018 study looked at the cost of prescription drug-related morbidity and mortality. They point out that prescription cost is not only direct medication cost but also includes costs attributed to treatment failure from nonoptimized regimen costs when medications cause new symptoms or syndromes. These authors estimated the total burden of prescription drugs to have cost the United States $528.4 billion in 2016.[4]

Over the past 2 decades, the cost of prescriptions has increased more rapidly than increases in the gross domestic product. In 2009 it was estimated that total expenditures for prescriptions in noninstitutionalized patients over 65 years was $86.5 billion in the United States.[5] This figure does not include any over-the-counter medications or medications given in a physician's office, in a clinic, or in the inpatient setting.

### CASE

#### LM (Part 1)

LM is a 76-year-old woman with a past medical history of atrial fibrillation, systolic heart failure, hyperlipidemia, and migraines. She visits you, her primary care physician, complaining of intermittent palpitations. She denies chest pain, shortness of breath, pain, unusual bleeding, swollen extremities, weight gain, or headache. Her chronic medications include warfarin 3 mg daily, metoprolol tartrate 100 mg twice daily, digoxin 0.125 mg daily, lisinopril 20 mg daily, and simvastatin 40 mg daily. She is also taking amitriptyline 150 mg at bedtime for migraine prophylaxis. Her vital signs reveal a blood pressure of 120/75 mmHg, which is near baseline, and an irregularly irregular heart rate of 130 to 150 beats per minute. You perform an electrocardiogram that reveals atrial fibrillation with a rapid ventricular rate. A recent serum digoxin concentration was reported to be 0.9 mcg/L (upper limit considering atrial fibrillation with concomitant systolic heart failure). You decide to initiate LM on amiodarone as her metoprolol and digoxin are at the maximum recommended doses.

What pharmacokinetic and pharmacodynamic age-associated changes will affect LM's medications?

## Pharmacokinetic Changes in the Elderly

Clinical pharmacokinetics is the discipline describing drug behavior with regard to absorption, distribution, metabolism, and elimination with the intent to use medications effectively while limiting adverse effects. Aging brings physiologic changes that affect these four characteristics in a clinically meaningful and relevant way. With age, organ function and physiologic reserve both decline, resulting in enhanced susceptibility to adverse effects of medications[6-8] (Table 7.1).

## Absorption

Medications (except those given parenterally) are subject to variations in absorption. Bioavailability of oral medications may fluctuate with changes that are common in older patients, such as reduced acidity of the stomach, gastric motility, and first-pass metabolism. Medications that require an acidic environment for optimal absorption (e.g., calcium carbonate or ketoconazole) have reduced absorption in patients with hypochlorhydria (whether physiologic or acid suppressant—induced). Fortunately, most medications do not require active transport to be absorbed, and

passive diffusion remains relatively unchanged in most older patients. Absorption of topical medications (e.g., creams, ointments, or patches) may fluctuate because of changes in the skin, such as atrophy and reduced blood flow to the dermal layer. Although some medications may have reduced absorption, this is frequently counterbalanced by a decreased first-pass effect. For medications that have a low bioavailability in average adults, such as propranolol or morphine, a small decrease in the initial first-pass effect may drastically impact drug serum concentrations. Although absorption may be the pharmacokinetic factor least impacted by age, alterations in absorption should be considered when the patient response varies from what is expected.

## Distribution

A medication's distribution describes the extent to which a drug passes into different body compartments. Depending on drug characteristics, such as size, solubility, and plasma-binding affinity, a medication may be more likely to achieve higher concentrations in hydrophilic or lipophilic compartments or to pass through the blood-brain barrier. Older patients have lower total body water and higher body fat. Therefore lipophilic medications have a larger volume of distribution. This leads to a longer elimination phase and prolonged therapeutic or toxic effect because drugs are typically not efficiently eliminated from the lipid compartment. Examples of lipophilic medications include phenytoin, valproic acid, diazepam, olanzapine, amiodarone, and lidocaine.

◆◆ **Higher body fat at older ages means lipophilic medications such as phenytoin, valproic acid, diazepam, olanzapine, and amiodarone are stored in body fat longer causing a longer elimination half-life and prolonged therapeutic or toxic effect.**

Medications reach equilibrium between compartments and also between bound and free forms. As patients age, albumin and alpha-1-acid glycoprotein may decrease or increase, resulting in

<br>

**TABLE 7.1    Pharmacokinetic Changes of Aging and Disease**

| Changes of Age and Disease | Pharmacokinetic Effect | Examples of Some Drugs Affected |
|---|---|---|
| ↓ First-pass metabolism | ↑ Drug serum concentration | Oral nitrates, beta-blockers, calcium channel blockers, estrogens |
| ↓ Rate of absorption | ↓ Clinical effect | Furosemide |
| ↓ Lean mass and total body water | ↓ Volume of distribution | Digoxin, lithium |
| ↑ Fat content | ↑ Volume of distribution | Diazepam, chlordiazepoxide, flurazepam, alprazolam |
| ↓ Food intake/catabolic disease states | ↓ Serum protein concentration with ↓ binding | Warfarin, phenytoin |
| ↓ Approximately one half of CYP 450 metabolic pathways (Phase I reactions) | ↓ Reduction, oxidation, hydroxylation, demethylation → ↑ half-life | Diazepam, chlordiazepoxide, flurazepam, alprazolam |
| ↓ Renal elimination | ↓ Clearance → ↑ half-life | Aminoglycosides, vancomycin, digoxin, salicylates |

*CYP450*, Cytochrome P 450.

(From Stratton MA, Gutierres S, Salinas R. Drug therapy in the elderly: tips for avoiding adverse effects and interactions. *Consultant* 2004;44(3):461–467. ©HMP Global.)

higher or lower free fractions of medication. Alterations to concentrations of these proteins are not caused by aging but rather by chronic conditions. For example, serum albumin decreases with prolonged illness, raising the free fraction of highly bound acidic drugs, such as naproxen, phenytoin, and warfarin. With illness, patients may develop adverse events or side effects from a medication that was previously well tolerated. This is particularly true for medications needing a closely maintained therapeutic range, such as warfarin and phenytoin. Total serum drug concentrations (bound and free fractions) should be monitored because the free fraction may be in a toxic range, while the bound level appears therapeutic.

## Metabolism

Metabolism is the body's process of altering a medication in some way. In the liver, the result of metabolism may be a product that is more or less active in the body or one more easily eliminated by the kidneys or biliary tree. Aging decreases liver size and blood perfusion, but quantitative changes in liver function and histology are minimal. Metabolism of medications usually occurs via reactions that are classified into one of two phases. Phase I metabolism occurs via cytochrome P450 isoenzymes, which have a high interpatient variability even in young adults. Studies of changes in specific isoenzymes with age are plagued by small sample sizes, confounders (such as effects of smoking and genetic polymorphism), and the potential to interpret cohort effects as age-related effects. However, studies suggest a decrease in elimination of substrates 1A2 and 2C19, a decrease or no change in elimination of substrates 3A4 and 2C9, and no change in elimination of substrates 2D6.[6,8] These phase I reactions result in an oxidized, reduced, or hydrolyzed form of the parent drug, but not all medications must pass through this step. Interindividual variability and confounders (listed earlier) affect phase I metabolism more than aging does. Because of these uncertainties, reduced doses of those medications with high hepatic extraction ratios, such as lidocaine, morphine, labetalol, propranolol, verapamil, and imipramine, may be warranted.

Many medications, such as lorazepam and oxazepam, are metabolized only through the phase II reactions glucuronidation, acetylation, or sulfation, resulting in larger, more water soluble, more easily eliminated metabolites. Evidence thus far suggests that phase II is unaffected by aging.

## Elimination

Elimination of medications generally occurs via conversion to inactive metabolites in the liver, excretion in bile, or elimination through the kidneys. The rate at which medications are excreted in the urine is determined by a combination of glomerular filtration, tubular secretion, and reabsorption. With age, most patients experience a decline in glomerular filtration rate. Nomograms and algorithms have been developed and validated to estimate glomerular filtration by calculating the estimated creatinine clearance (CrCl). Creatinine is cleared by glomerular filtration and active tubular secretion. These equations were typically determined using healthy adults. With this in mind, validity of these equations in patients at extremes of age and with active disease is less reliable. Given these limitations, the Cockcroft-Gault equation is the recommended equation for most scenarios. In a longitudinal study of community-dwelling older adults, it was found to more closely estimate the measured 24-hour creatinine clearance compared with equations that estimate the glomerular filtration rate.[9] Equations estimating

the glomerular filtration rate, namely the modification of diet in renal disease (MDRD) equation or the Chronic Kidney Disease Epidemiology Collaboration equation, often automatically calculate the estimated glomerular filtration rate in some electronic medical records, and these results tend to overestimate the creatinine clearance.[9] As with any patient encounter, the entire scenario needs to be considered in addition to the CrCl. The Cockcroft-Gault equation uses the following formula to determine CrCl:

Creatinine clearance (CrCl) mL/min = (140 − age) × weight/(72 × serum creatinine concentration), multiply by 0.85 for females

❖❖ **About two-thirds of all older people experience a decline in creatinine clearance (CrCl). Despite limitations, estimated CrCl is a useful tool for estimating appropriate drug doses of renally excreted drugs.**

This equation uses serum creatinine concentration, which decreases in older patients because of their decreased muscle mass. This may result in a higher calculated CrCl, especially in underweight or malnourished older patients. To correct for these possibilities, many clinicians round the serum creatinine concentration up to 1 mg/dL, which may in turn underestimate CrCl. The estimated CrCl may vary drastically with extremes in weight. It has been suggested to use lean body weight when calculating CrCl in patients who are significantly obese. It is also important to appreciate that drug dosages and recommended dose adjustments for patients with renal impairment are generally based on estimated CrCl rather than on the often reported laboratory estimate of glomerular filtration using equations such as the MDRD.

It is important as a clinician to pay particular attention to dosages for medications that are eliminated unchanged in the urine or that have active metabolites that are eliminated in the urine because these drugs will accumulate in older people.

Because of the variables discussed in this section, predicting a medication's serum concentration or clinical effects may be difficult in an older patient. The starting dose for most renally excreted drugs should be based on the estimated CrCl, but patients must be monitored for both overdosing and underdosing. For medications with a narrow therapeutic range or low ceiling for toxic effects, measuring serum drug concentrations is prudent, particularly when a patient is acutely ill.

In summary, the clinical impact of age-related changes in pharmacokinetics is difficult to predict. Vigilance to adverse effects of medications caused by altered drug pharmacokinetics is necessary in elderly patients, and a thorough medication history is warranted in the presence of any new complaints. The adage to "start low and go slow" applies when initiating medications with potentially adverse effects.

❖❖ **In patients with significant renal impairment (creatinine clearance approaching 30 mL/min), refer to medication monographs for appropriate dosages for renally excreted drugs.**

## Pharmacodynamic Changes in the Elderly

Although numerous studies and reviews describe the pharmacokinetic changes in geriatric patients, there are limited data on age-related pharmacodynamic changes.[10–13] Pharmacodynamics refers to the response of the body to a drug. Older patients may have altered pharmacodynamics because of changes in receptor affinity or number, postreceptor alterations, and/or impairment of homeostatic mechanisms. Unfortunately, it is difficult to generalize age-related changes because studies have shown patients to have a higher "sensitivity" to some medications and a lower "sensitivity" to others. One example of higher sensitivity is increased central nervous system (CNS) effects with benzodiazepines. One small study found that geriatric patients had a higher sensitivity index and a more profound CNS depressant effect, even when receiving a lower dose of midazolam.[14] The opposite is found with beta-agonists/antagonists where patients tend to be less responsive to these agents. Some generalizations that can be made are that geriatric patients will frequently have a greater responsiveness to the CNS depressant effects of benzodiazepines, to the analgesic effects of opioids, and to the anticoagulant effects of warfarin and heparin.

## CASE

### LM (Part 2)

LM's presentation is not uncommon and several pharmacokinetic/pharmacodynamic issues should be considered. The addition of amiodarone to the current medication regimen poses numerous issues. Amiodarone is a highly lipophilic medication with a large volume of distribution and a half-life of weeks to months. In LM, who likely has increased body fat because of her age, a steady state concentration will not be reached for several months. Likewise, if she were to experience an adverse event from this medication, it may take months for the medication to be eliminated and the reaction to resolve. Amiodarone is metabolized to an active metabolite in the liver via the cytochrome P450 complexes and also inhibits the activity of these enzymes, including 3A4, 2D6, 2C9, and 1A2. Amiodarone interferes with the metabolism of warfarin, an anticoagulant that older patients are frequently sensitive to. LM will require frequent monitoring of her international normalized ratio (INR), and her warfarin dose should be carefully adjusted over the next few months until a new steady state therapeutic dose of warfarin is reached. Inhibition of multiple cytochrome P450 enzymes and p-glycoprotein by amiodarone also interferes with the clearance of digoxin, simvastatin, and amitriptyline. Because LM's serum digoxin concentration is already at the upper therapeutic limit for heart failure, the addition of amiodarone is likely to increase her digoxin concentration to a potentially harmful level. Digoxin clearance is dependent on renal elimination, and the dose may need to be decreased to every other day to avoid toxicity. Amiodarone itself has some beta-blockade activity and through its inhibition of the metabolism of metoprolol via 2D6, the extent that the heart rate will decrease in LM is difficult to estimate. This interaction could benefit the patient by reducing the rapid ventricular rate, or it could cause bradycardia. Simvastatin use at the current dose may also become problematic with the addition of amiodarone. The US Food and Drug Administration issued a statement in 2011 that warned of muscle injury with HMG-CoA reductase inhibitors and recommended certain dose restrictions when using these drugs with certain medication classes.[15] Geriatric patients are at an increased risk of statin-induced myopathy and increased exercise fatigue even before the inhibition of simvastatin metabolism by amiodarone.[16,17] In this patient, the dose of simvastatin should be reduced to no more than 10 mg daily to minimize the risk of myopathy. Amiodarone also interferes with amitriptyline metabolism, will lead to increased concentrations, and will increase the risk of QTc prolongation. With all of these issues at hand, amiodarone is still an option although adjustment of other medications will be necessary to avoid toxicities.

## General Guidelines for Safe Prescribing

This section describes strategies to avoid side effects and drug interactions, to minimize the prescribing cascade, to promote medication adherence, and to understand benefits and harms of medications. Writing prescriptions is the most common intervention performed by health professionals in many settings. Older patients, with multiple comorbidities, frailty, and use of more medications, are particularly at risk for adverse drug events. Drug-adverse effects and nonadherence may account for 28.2% of hospital admissions of elderly patients.[18] The Institute for Safe Medication Practices reported 19,551 drug-related deaths in the United States in 2009.[19] This is greater than the 17,520 deaths attributed to homicides in the same year. Creating a therapeutic drug regimen that benefits patients while minimizing ill effects is paramount and requires deliberate planning and careful attention. In 2016 a cost-of-illness analysis calculated the number of deaths related to prescription drugs was over 275,000 when including those caused by nonoptimized medication use.[4]

A principle in geriatric care is that the law of parsimony often does not apply. Problems, especially the geriatric syndromes, often have more than one cause. Geriatric patients frequently have atypical signs and symptoms, and new complaints or increasing dysfunction are frequently related to medication adverse events. The problem of mistakenly identifying adverse medication effects as new medical conditions may lead to a drug-related problem known as the prescribing cascade. This effect occurs when a new complaint is assumed to be from a disease state rather than from a drug, which leads to addition of new medications, further increasing the risk of adverse events. Common examples include the use of nonsteroidal antiinflammatory drugs leading to antihypertensive therapy, the use of thiazide diuretics leading to treatment for gout, and the use of metoclopramide leading to treatment for Parkinson disease.[20] Another example would be a patient taking a benzodiazepine for anxiety who experiences CNS depression that leads to a diagnosis of dementia and prescription of an acetylcholinesterase inhibitor. Acetylcholinesterase inhibitors are known to cause (or exacerbate) urinary incontinence, which could spark the initiation of an anticholinergic medication, further causing cognitive dysfunction. This chain of events demonstrates how with any new complaint, an adverse medication reaction should be in the differential diagnosis. The need for continued use of possibly offending agents must be questioned, and a dose reduction or discontinuation should occur. If treatment is needed for a new condition, nonpharmacologic treatment should be considered.

❖ **The differential diagnosis of any geriatric problem should include an adverse drug effect.**

Creating individualized patient care plans in the face of a growing number of treatment guidelines and diminishing time to spend with each patient is a daunting task. Treatment guidelines rarely have recommendations on when to discontinue therapies in later life. Also older patients are susceptible to medication adverse effects (such as anticholinergic burden).

Deprescribing has been described as the process of withdrawal of an inappropriate medication with the aim of reducing polypharmacy and improving health outcomes.[21] The Canadian Deprescribing Network has developed algorithms and tools for deprescribing five classes of medications available on the website www.deprescribing.org. During any patient encounters, such as when new medications are added or during transitions in care, the opportunity should be taken to review all medications and see if any dose reductions or discontinuations are warranted.

Four criteria have been suggested to assist prescribers in deciding when to start or continue medications in their patients.[22]

These criteria are (1) a patient's life expectancy, (2) the time until benefit from medication, (3) goals of care, and (4) treatment targets. Life expectancy can be estimated based on comorbidities, functional status, and disease markers of poor prognosis. Time until benefit of a given medication can vary drastically. For example, the use of HMG-CoA reductase inhibitors for primary prevention of coronary artery disease will take many years to benefit and have a large number needed to treat, whereas opioids for acute pain control will have a short time to benefit and low number needed to treat. Determining goals of care is challenging because the healthcare provider, the patient, and the patient's family all have input on the goals. Setting treatment targets follows the goals of care discussion. For example, a patient may value a more symptom-targeted approach rather than a disease-modifying approach that may have untoward effects. These decisions are on a spectrum that ranges from a curative to a palliative stance. An optimal plan would consider all of these factors. For example, if life expectancy is likely a few months, and goals of therapy are palliative, then targeting symptoms, rather than prescribing a drug with a long time to benefit, would be appropriate.

❖ **In deciding when to start or continue medications, consider (1) a patient's life expectancy, (2) the time until benefit from medication, (3) goals of care, and (4) treatment targets.**

## Explicit Criteria for Prescribing

Tools are available to guide clinicians in the choice of medications for older adults. A review by Levy et al. compared nine sets of explicit criteria developed by various groups around the world.[23] The best-known criteria in the United States are the Beers Criteria for Potentially Inappropriate Medication (PIM) Use in Older Adults, which were originally developed in 1991.[24] There have been five revisions of the Beers Criteria, with the last three and latest (2019) led by the American Geriatrics Society (AGS).[25] This version is evidence-based and intended for use in all care settings. The AGS Beers Criteria are used as quality measures by the Centers for Medicare and Medicaid Services (CMS) and the National Committee for Quality Assurance. Medications included on the AGS Beers Criteria either have limited effectiveness in older adults or have risk of serious adverse events and safer alternatives are available. Medications are organized by pharmacologic class and listed in tables as drugs to avoid, drugs to avoid in older adults with specific disease states, and drugs to use with caution. In the 2015 update, two new tables were included: Potentially Clinically Important Drug-Drug Interactions and Medication That Should Be Avoided or Have Their Dosages Reduced with Varying Levels of Kidney Function. With the 2015 update, two companion articles were published, one on alternatives to medications on the AGS Beers Criteria and another on how to appropriately use the criteria in clinical practice.[26,27]

❖ **Learn more about the AGS Beers Criteria at** https://geriatricscareonline.org/toc/american-geriatrics-society-updated-beers-criteria/CL001.

The other well-known sets of criteria are the STOPP and START (Screening Tool of Older Persons Potentially Inappropriate Prescriptions, and Screening Tool to Alert Doctors to the Right Treatment), which were developed in Ireland.[28,29] Both sets of criteria are organized by pharmacologic class. The START focuses on prescribing omissions and consists of 22 evidence-based criteria

for use of medications in particular disease states (e.g., use of angiotensin-converting enzyme inhibitors following an acute myocardial infarction). The STOPP, similar to the AGS Beers Criteria, consists of 65 medications that are potentially inappropriate for use in the elderly. There is some overlap between the Beers Criteria and STOPP, but both tools are useful in clinical practice.

A metaanalysis of 33 studies using the Beers Criteria or the STOPP list found a significant association between adverse drug reactions and the use of PIMs in patients age >60 years.[30] This study found a similar association between hospitalizations and use of PIMs, but no association with mortality. The risk of adverse outcomes was increased for those on two or more PIMs.

Older adults are more likely to experience anticholinergic side effects from medication (e.g., sedation, confusion, urinary retention, constipation). There are many medications with strong anticholinergic effects, but there are also medications that have subtle anticholinergic effects. The combination of two or more medications with even subtle anticholinergic effects can cause significant adverse effects in older adults. Hilmer et al. described a "drug burden index" that is based on anticholinergics, sedatives, and total medications used.[31] They found that increased exposure to medications with anticholinergic and sedative effects was associated with poorer physical and cognitive performance. There are at least seven anticholinergic rating scales that have been developed, generally ranking medications from no anticholinergic activity (0) to high/strong anticholinergic activity (3).[32] The AGS Beers Criteria includes a list of medications with strong anticholinergic properties.

❖ **Exposure to medications with anticholinergic and sedative effects is associated with poorer physical and cognitive performance.**

## Medication Adherence

Terms used to describe the ability of a patient to use his or her medications as instructed include adherence, compliance, and persistence. Compliance implies a sense of one-sidedness where the patient is dealing with or adapting to a situation. Persistence refers only to the duration that a patient will continue with a medication treatment, not addressing the issue that an estimated 24% of prescriptions are never even filled.[33] Adherence has a broader, more team-based definition of "the extent to which a person's behavior—taking medication, following a diet, and/or executing lifestyle changes, corresponds with agreed recommendations from a healthcare provider."[34] The World Health Organization defines adherence to account for more than just the use of medications. Adherence is a dynamic process that requires individual patient strategies and follow-up and a multidisciplinary approach (Box 7.1).

**• BOX 7.1  Tips for Assessing Medication Adherence**

- Ask about medication/supplement/over-the-counter use in different ways throughout an encounter.
- Have patient demonstrate inhaler/eyedrop/topical medication use.
- Request that patient bring all medications (preferred) or at least a medication list to all appointments.
- Explicitly inquire about missing doses and difficulties with adherence using open-ended questions.

It is not entirely in the hands of a patient to be adherent, and many determining factors for adherence lie with providers and the health system. It is estimated that adherence to long-term therapy for chronic illnesses averages 50%.[34]

❖ **The first step in ensuring appropriate prescribing is obtaining an accurate and complete medication history.**

Decreasing complexity of a medication regimen will improve adherence.
- **When selecting a regimen, choose a medication requiring fewer doses per day.**
- **Use combination tablets to reduce pill burden.**
- **When adding a new medication, consider whether any other medication could be discontinued or the dose reduced.**

## Adherence Aids

Adherence aids are available to help patients organize and remember to take their medications. The simplest method is to design a schedule for medications and the time of day to take them. Medication boxes that hold one day's or one week's worth of medication are commercially available in a variety of styles, with some boxes having two to four boxes for each day of the week to accommodate different dosing times. There are electronic aids that beep or light up when a dose is due, with some devices connected to the phone line to alert a family member or call center if a dose is not taken on time.

There are other products available to assist with the administration of medications. Tablet splitters and crushers may help patients who have difficulty swallowing tablets. Eyedrop guides fit on the eyedrop bottle, help steady the hand, and direct the drop into the eye (Fig. 7.1). For patients using any type of inhaled medication, their ability to use the device correctly should be assessed. For metered-dose inhalers, spacer devices (e.g., Aerochamber, also requiring a prescription) are available and are recommended for all older people. Transdermal patches can be difficult for older patients to apply if they have decreased vision or diminished manual dexterity. Child-resistant caps, which have been required on

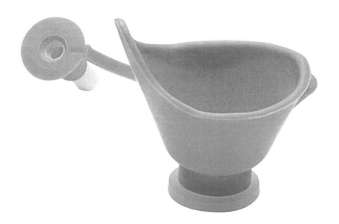

• **Figure 7.1** Eyedrop guide.

prescription medications in the United States since 1970, can be barriers to adherence in older patients. The pharmacist and the prescriber should ask patients if they need a nonchild-resistant cap. The prescriber can note it on the prescription or the patient can tell the pharmacist.

### CASE

#### LM (Part 3)

Because of LM's new complaints, a seventh medication is now being added to her medication list. Adherence should be assessed to ensure that the new findings are not caused by missed doses of her beta-blocker. If uncontrolled heart rate is a result of nonadherence to beta-blocker therapy, adding another agent (amiodarone) may not fix the problem and may only increase the medication burden. Because the complexity of a regimen may affect adherence, efforts should be made to simplify the regimen if possible. LM is currently taking metoprolol tartrate twice daily for heart failure. This could easily be switched to the long-acting once daily metoprolol succinate at a dose of 200 mg daily. Also, there is better evidence for efficacy with the succinate salt in patients with heart failure. If amiodarone is initiated, its interaction with warfarin will require increased frequency of monitoring the INR for several months. Switching warfarin to a direct oral anticoagulant, such as apixaban or dabigatran, would eliminate the need for more frequent lab work but would increase pill burden because either agent is taken twice daily. Patient preference as to which is more convenient should be considered in making such therapeutic decisions.

## Medicare Part D

The Medicare Prescription Drug, Improvement, and Modernization Act of 2003 included a new outpatient prescription drug benefit, known as Medicare Part D. This benefit began in January 2006 as a voluntary component of the Medicare program. All participants in Medicare A and/or B are eligible to enroll in a Part D Prescription Drug Plan (PDP). Although the guidelines for Part D are developed by the CMS, PDPs are offered by private companies and vary from state to state. Each plan has a distinct formulary and restrictions on prior authorization, quantity limits, and step therapy. Prescribers must be familiar with the program to help patients receive the most cost-effective regimens.

The Part D benefit includes a deductible (maximum of $415 in 2019), and then the beneficiary pays 25% of the cost of medications until a predetermined amount ($3820 in 2019). At this point, there is a coverage gap ("the doughnut hole"). When Part D was implemented in 2006, the coverage gap was a true gap—patients paid 100% of the cost of the medications until they hit catastrophic coverage. With the passage of the Patient Protection and Affordable Care Act in 2010, the coverage gap has been gradually phased out so that by 2020 beneficiaries will only pay 25% of the cost of their medications after the deductible is met. As an alternative to the 25% copayment, many Part D plans have a tiered copayment system. The difference in copayment between a Tier 1 medication (preferred generic) and Tier 4 (nonpreferred brand) can be substantial. This added economic burden on the patient may impact adherence, so it is important that prescribers be familiar with the formularies of commonly used PDPs in their patient population.

The intent of Part D was to make medications more accessible to older adults, and studies evaluating the use of medications by patients with Part D coverage have found an increase in the number of prescriptions filled during the initial coverage period.[35–38] However, during the coverage gap, an increase in nonadherence was seen.[38,39] With the elimination of the coverage gap, hopefully adherence and persistence will be maintained.

Pharmacists can assist patients in reviewing their medications and the various plans available to them during the annual Medicare open enrollment period using the Plan Finder tool on the Medicare website. It is recommended that patients review their plan annually because costs and formularies change with each calendar year.

❖❖ **Prescription of generic medications under Medicare Part D will keep copays low and should maintain or improve adherence.**

An important component of Medicare Part D is medication therapy management (MTM). CMS requires that each PDP have a MTM program for enrollees. Patients who have multiple chronic disease states, are on multiple medications, and are projected to use more than $4000 of medications per year are eligible for MTM services. MTM consists of a comprehensive evaluation of the patient's medication regimen by a pharmacist or other qualified provider; the goals are to decrease adverse drug events and improve patient outcomes by promoting appropriate medication use. Starting in 2013, each patient receiving MTM received a Medication Action Plan and Personal Medication List from their MTM provider. The action plan is a summary of the MTM session reminding patients of what was discussed and what they need to do with their medications. In one study of the influence of an MTM program, there was a 47% acceptance rate of the MTM recommendations, mainly in the areas of guideline adherence, cost savings, and safety concerns.[40] Another study found that MTM resolved significantly more medication and health-related problems as compared with a control group.[41] A study of the effectiveness of an MTM program in a large integrated health system found that MTM provided by a clinical pharmacist was associated with a decrease in medications to avoid in older adults.[42] As MTM programs continue to develop, more studies of their impact on patient outcomes are needed.

❖❖ **Learn more about Medicare Part D at** www.medicare.gov **and** www.Q1medicare.com.

---

**CASE**

**1 Discussion**

Because LM is having problems keeping her INR within the therapeutic range, you decide to switch her to dabigatran 75 mg twice daily. On her next visit, LM reluctantly admits to you that she is having trouble paying the copayment for the medication because it is a Tier 4 medication in her Part D prescription plan. LM likes the fact that she does not have to get her INR monitored, but she worries about the expense. You call LM's pharmacist to ask for suggestions and find out that the open enrollment period is soon and that if LM can stay in the plan for a few more months, she could then switch into a plan that has dabigatran as a Tier 3 and a minimal copayment

for all of her generic drugs. In the meantime, the pharmacist suggests looking into the manufacturer's assistance plan. In reviewing LM's drug regimen, the pharmacist notes that LM is on several Beers Criteria medications and suggests that amitriptyline for migraine prophylaxis be discontinued. This will minimize the risks of anticholinergic effects, orthostatic hypotension, and sedation, all of which can increase her risk of falls. The pharmacist notes that metoprolol may also be effective as migraine prophylaxis.

## Role of the Pharmacist in Geriatric Care

Since 1997, pharmacists have had the opportunity to become board certified in geriatric pharmacy and carry the designation BCGP. For more information about this program or to find a BCGP, see www.bpsweb.com. As of 2019, there were more than 4500 BCGP's worldwide.[43]

The role of the pharmacist in geriatric care has traditionally been in nursing facilities. Since 1974, the federal government has mandated monthly drug regimen reviews in skilled nursing facilities. The drug regimen review is "a thorough evaluation of the medication regimen of a resident with the goal of promoting positive outcomes and minimizing adverse consequences associated with medications."[44] For more information, the reader is referred to the American Society of Consultant Pharmacists (www.ascp.com).

Given the benefits and risks of pharmaceuticals, there is an important and evolving role for the pharmacist in geriatric care. There are pharmacists in private practices assisting patients with adherence and disease management. Others operate anticoagulation and hypertension clinics, serve as consultants in hospitals, with hospice agencies, and in Program of All-Inclusive Care of the Elderly programs. Pharmacists assist in designing appropriate medication regimens, including choice of medication, dose, dosage form, and monitoring parameters. Pharmacists provide information on adverse events and drug interactions, assess adherence, and advise about cost issues. Medication reconciliation is a Joint Commission National Patient Safety Goal and is particularly important in geriatrics because of the number of medications used, multiple prescribers, and multiple sites of care (www.jointcommission.org). Pharmacists are the ideal team member to accurately reconcile patients' medications during transitions in care.

Although specific regulations vary by state, community pharmacists are required to counsel patients on all new prescriptions; patients should be encouraged to ask their pharmacist about over-the-counter medications and other health-related products. Most important, patients should be encouraged to use only one pharmacy so that all of their medications are on one computer profile. This allows the pharmacist to monitor for drug interactions, duplications, and potential adverse effects. The pharmacist can also track adherence through refill records and provide advice on adherence and reminder aids.

## Summary

Because of the complexity of physiological, social, and financial issues that older patients experience, care needs to be taken to ensure a logical, pragmatic, and efficient pharmacotherapeutic plan. Aging per se does not explain all or even most of the complexity of prescribing. The most reliable physiologic change is a decline in renal excretion. However, comorbid disease and drug interactions expand the complexity for this population. More and more powerful medications present advantages and also risks.

Providers for patients with complex needs will find pharmacists their allies in provision of safe, reliable, and cost-effective patient care. The aids and resources outlined in this chapter can provide valuable assistance in caring for older people.

## Web Resources

www.medicare.gov or www.Q1medicare.com: Information on Medicare D plans

www.bpsweb.org: Board of Pharmacy Specialties

www.ascp.com: American Society of Consultant Pharmacists

https://geriatricscareonline.org/ProductAbstract/2019-ags-beers-criteria-pocketcard/PC007

https://geriatricscareonline.org/toc/american-geriatrics-society-updated-beers-criteria/CL001: Beers Criteria

https://geriatricscareonline.org/ProductTypeStore/pocketcards/10/: Beers Criteria, available as printable pocket guide or mobile app

www.epill.com: Examples of medication adherence aids for patients

## Key References

6. Delafuente JC. Pharmacokinetic and pharmacodynamic alterations in the geriatric patient. *Consult Pharm*. 2008;23 (4):324−334.

8. Cusack BJ. Pharmacokinetics in older persons. *Am J Geriatr Pharmacother*. 2004;2(4):274−302.

22. Holmes HM, Hayley DC, Alexander GC, et al. Reconsidering medication appropriateness for patients late in life. *Arch Intern Med*. 2006;166:605−609.

25. The American Geriatrics Society 2019 Beers Criteria Update Expert Panel. American Geriatric Society 2019 updated Beers Criteria for potentially inappropriate medication use in older adults. *J Am Geriatr Soc*. 2019;67:674−694.

*References available online at expertconsult.com.*

# 8

# Ethics

ROBERT A. ZOROWITZ

## OUTLINE

*Additional online-only material indicated by icon.*

## OBJECTIVES

*Upon completion of this chapter, the reader will be able to:*

- Discuss the most commonly cited principles of ethical decision making in medical care.
- Understand how to systematically elucidate and resolve ethical dilemmas.
- Discuss the requirements of informed consent and the criteria for decisional capacity.
- Discuss the role and use of different types of advance directives.

- Understand the use of the term *futility* as it applies to medical decision making.
- Discuss ethical concerns regarding assisted suicide and the "double effect."
- Discuss the unique issues involving provision of food and fluid.
- Recognize emerging ethical issues accompanying technological progress.

The rapid advancements in medical technology, the growing population of the elderly, and the increasing awareness of the legal and moral issues confronting the elderly, their families, and their caregivers have resulted in the need for a methodology to evaluate and resolve moral conflicts that may confront clinicians who care for older patients.

Ethics is the field that systematically studies morality, which is defined as the rightness and wrongness of human acts. Medical ethics is the discipline that studies morality in healthcare, using a process that attempts to seek solutions to moral questions or dilemmas that arise in the care and treatment of patients. Medical ethics is a fusion of theory and practice.[1]

Moral dilemmas arise when the rights and wishes of patients conflict with the obligations of clinicians or when there are competing obligations among clinicians. These rights and obligations may be informed by philosophical, social, cultural, religious, or personal principles, beliefs, and values. In geriatric medicine, rights and obligations are often influenced and complicated by factors such as limited life expectancy, cognitive impairment, impaired decision-making capacity, insufficient social and economic resources, and the complexity of polymorbidity and functional disorders.[2]

Ethics committees and related mechanisms for the resolution of ethical conflicts have become a required and necessary presence in hospitals, nursing homes, and other healthcare organizations. The rise of medical consumerism has resulted in a population of patients and caregivers who are increasingly well informed about their rights and choices in healthcare. It is vital that clinicians develop a shared language of ethical decision making.

This chapter introduces the basic principles of ethical decision making and examines common ethical issues encountered in the care of older patients.

---

### CASE 1

#### Alice Oliver (Part 1)

Mrs. Alice Oliver is an 83-year-old woman, an active swimmer and gardener, who suffered a right-sided stroke with mild left hemiparesis and dysphagia. During hospitalization, her motor deficits were improving but the dysphagia persisted. A swallow evaluation indicated that she was able to tolerate a chopped or pureed diet with nectar-thick liquids, but she experienced asymptomatic aspiration with thin liquids. The speech therapist recommended thickening all liquids, and you enter this order on the chart. Mrs. Oliver, however, refuses thickened liquids, insisting that she would rather take her chances with thin liquids. The nurses and the dietician tell you they do not want to provide her with thin liquids; they believe that by doing so, they will be contributing to the risk they were trying to ameliorate.

You are confronted with an ethical dilemma. On one hand, you think the patient should have the right to take risks and eat what she wants. On the other hand, you can sympathize with the other healthcare professionals' discomfort in abetting risky behavior. Medical ethics provides a means for articulating and analyzing such dilemmas.

1. What ethical principles are in conflict in this case?
2. Is there an ethical principle that takes priority over others?

---

## Principles of Medical Ethics

Traditional principles of medical ethics derived largely from the works of Greek philosophers, such as Hippocrates[3] and Pythagorus.[4] During the second half of the 20th century, increasing pressure on the medical establishment from technological change, cultural upheaval, and the increasing complexity of medical care and the issues it raised resulted in the need to more explicitly frame the principles of medical ethics.

Although there are several alternative theories of medical ethics—such as the virtue-based theories favored by the Greek philosophers, the ethics of caring,[5] and casuistry[6]—there remain four prima facie principles that are most often cited as the bedrock of clinical ethics. These are autonomy, beneficence, nonmaleficence, and justice.[7]

### Autonomy

The principle of autonomy refers to the duty to respect a patient's right to self-determination. This has been legally enshrined in the judicial ruling of *Schloendorff vs. Society of New York Hospital* (NY 1914), in which Justice Cardozo found that, "Every human being of adult years and of sound mind has a right to determine what shall be done with his body."[8]

Historically, clinicians have assumed an authoritarian or paternalistic role in the medical decision-making process. This began to change significantly after the discovery of unethical conduct of research on human participants during the Holocaust and in US experiments, such as the Tuskegee syphilis study.[9] With the increase in consumerism and the availability of medical information, patients have been more likely to assert their autonomy. Healthcare providers have been increasingly recognizing autonomy as a fundamental ethical principle.

Integral to the principle of autonomy is the right to receive sufficient factual information to allow self-determination. This is the basis of informed consent, established in the Nuremberg code, which states, "The voluntary consent of the human subject is absolutely essential."[10] In *Nathanson vs. Kline* (KS 1960), a case that centered on the failure to inform a patient of potential surgical risks, the ruling found that, "It follows that each man is considered to be master of his own body, and he may, if he be of sound mind, prohibit the performance of life-saving surgery or other medical treatment."[11]

In addition to establishing the right of an autonomous patient to refuse treatment, these rulings also introduce the "of sound mind" concept, which is indicative of a patient's capacity to understand what has been explained, appreciate the situation and its consequences, rationally manipulate information, and communicate choices.[12] Decision-making capacity is a critical requirement for providing informed consent and therefore for exercising autonomy.

Effective clinician–patient communication is an integral part of providing informed consent throughout the process of reaching an autonomous decision. The clinician has a duty to tell the truth and provide fact-based, objective information to the patient. Such discussions must be free of personal, subjective biases. The information must be fair and lawful and must not be swayed by any financial or personal gain. The clinician may provide advice as to what would be the clinician's own preference, but should assure the patient of support, regardless of the patient's own decision.

Truth-telling is an essential component of the exercise of autonomy. The recognition that there is an obligation to provide truthful information to patients about potentially life-threatening conditions is a historically recent phenomenon. A 1961 survey of physicians in the United States reported that 90% would not reveal a diagnosis of cancer to their patients.[13] A 1979 survey reported that 97% of physicians would reveal a diagnosis of cancer to their patients.[14] A recent survey of hospitalized patients reported that a large majority would prefer to be told of a diagnosis of cancer or Alzheimer disease. Among those who were unsure or who did not want to be told, a majority would want to be told if it was essential to treatment. Preferences did not differ by age.[15]

Age is not, by itself, an obstacle to the full exercise of autonomy. Even very old hospitalized patients are able to express their health values, underscoring the need to elicit such choices directly from the patient, unless that patient lacks decision-making capacity.[16]

### Beneficence

The principle of beneficence refers to the clinician's responsibility to provide benefit or help the patient (i.e., "to do good"). Beneficence is the essence of the patient–doctor relationship. Promotion of good health, curing disease, and relieving pain and suffering are all key elements in the principle of beneficence. Conversely, medical interventions that provide no benefit should be avoided.

## Nonmaleficence

The principle of nonmaleficence states that throughout the physician–patient relationship, the physician shall "at the least, do no harm." It is incumbent upon all clinicians to determine the goals of the intervention and to weigh these goals against the potential risk of an adverse outcome. Factors, such as advanced age, concurrent disease states, comorbidities, and expected prognosis must be considered in the equation. When available, the clinician may use formal algorithms to assess risk. For instance, preoperative cardiac risk stratification can help the clinician determine the risk of an adverse cardiac event from surgery. A short life expectancy may suggest that a particular screening test or procedure is not likely to have its expected benefit. In essence, the duty of nonmaleficence is balanced against the duty of beneficence when weighing risks and benefits.

## Justice

Justice refers to the duty to treat patients fairly. Justice can be viewed along two dimensions: access and allocation.[17] Access refers to whether those who are entitled to healthcare resources can obtain them. Allocation refers to the determination of how resources are distributed. The distribution of rights and responsibilities among the members of a society in a manner governed by consistent moral norms is often referred to as distributive justice.

In a microenvironment, such as a hospital or nursing home, conflicts involving the principle of justice may revolve around the use of scarce, expensive, or labor-intensive medical interventions in frail, elderly patients with limited life expectancies. On a macroenvironmental, national scale, justice may be the central principle in determining whether Medicare should cover a particular procedure or in determining who should have control over allocation decisions in managed care organizations.[18]

## Other Principles

In addition to the principles outlined in the previous sections, there are other ethical principles that are common in geriatrics, particularly in communal settings, such as assisted-living facilities or nursing homes, in which elderly residents not only obtain medical care but consider the facility their home. The principle of community, which refers to the duty to balance individual need with communal need, takes on great importance in such settings. Not only is personal autonomy important, but also individual dignity, a closely related but distinct value, is greatly valued. Also closely related to autonomy, the principle of authenticity refers to the ability to choose a lifestyle consistent with one's own values, beliefs, and habits.[19]

◆◆ **In Western society, the principle of autonomy has come to dominate other ethical principles, but this may not be true of all cultures.**

---

### CASE 1

#### Alice Oliver (Part 2)

The case of Mrs. Oliver represents a classic conflict between the duty to respect the patient's autonomy and the duty to do good (beneficence) and avoid harm (nonmaleficence). Mrs. Oliver is unable to exercise her autonomy without the cooperation of the care team in providing her food, but the team feels that supplying her choice of diet would violate the duty to avoid harm. Having identified the ethical principles that are at odds with each other, you must now systematically evaluate alternatives for resolution.

1. How would you go about devising a methodology for examining the ethical dilemma(s) in this case?
2. Is there a morally right and a morally wrong decision?

---

## Structure for Deliberating Ethical Dilemmas

There are several models for systematically evaluating and analyzing dilemmas in medical ethics. One of the most commonly used models is the "four topics" model devised by Jonsen et al.[20] This is a case-based approach that allows an organized review of the facts and issues in a given case, according to four topics: medical indications, patient preferences, quality of life, and contextual features (Fig. 8.1).

Each topic represents a systematic means of organizing the questions related to the corresponding ethical principles. Under the topic "medical indications" are questions that determine how the facts of the case determine what constitutes beneficence and nonmaleficence. The topic "patient preferences" contains questions that establish the patient's autonomy and how that autonomy fits into the ethical problem at hand. "Quality of life" contains questions that further elucidate what is considered beneficence and what is considered nonmaleficence, according to the patient's own values. "Contextual features" contains grouped questions that tease out other influences on the case and incorporate principles, such as loyalty and fairness.

Once the facts of the case are organized, it is important to identify the ethical dilemma(s), if any. Only when the ethical questions are framed is it possible to formulate potential solutions. Frequently, ethical dilemmas have more than one morally permissible alternative. If the ethics consultant or ethics committee has been asked to participate, it may be their role to outline these alternatives. Nonetheless, it generally falls to the healthcare team and patient to determine which alternative will be followed.

An additional step in the deliberation of an ethics case is to learn how to avoid the same situation in the future. By performing a root cause analysis, the healthcare team might modify communication, protocols, procedures, the organizational structure and other contributing factors, thereby reducing the probability of a similar crisis arising in the future.[21]

◆◆ **An ethical conflict may have more than one morally acceptable solution.**

What appears at first to be an ethical dilemma may ultimately emerge as an interpersonal dispute among family members or between staff and family members.[22] Patients may have several family members, often their children, who may disagree with each other, their parents, or with the healthcare team over decisions, large and small, sometimes making medical management time consuming and difficult. In these cases, typical ethical deliberation may not always be enough. Mediation,[23] negotiation,[24] or other alternative methods of conflict resolution may be more useful and appropriate.

◆◆ **It is sometimes difficult to differentiate an ethical dilemma from an interpersonal conflict, and they may occur together.**

| MEDICAL INDICATIONS | PATIENT PREFERENCES |
|---|---|
| **The Principles of Beneficence and Nonmaleficence** | **The Principle of Respect for Autonomy** |
| 1. What is the patient's medical problem? History? Diagnosis? Prognosis?<br>2. Is the problem acute? Chronic? Critical? Emergent? Reversible?<br>3. What are the goals of treatment?<br>4. What are the probabilities of success?<br>5. What are the plans in case of therapeutic failure?<br>6. In sum, how can this patient be benefited by medical and nursing care, and how can harm be avoided? | 1. Is the patient mentally capable and legally competent? Is there evidence of incapacity?<br>2. If competent, what is the patient stating about preferences for treatment?<br>3. Has the patient been informed of benefits and risks, understood this information, and given consent?<br>4. If incapacitated, who is the appropriate surrogate? Is the surrogate using appropriate standards for decision making?<br>5. Has the patient expressed prior preferences, e.g., Advance Directives?<br>6. Is the patient unwilling or unable to cooperate with medical treatment? If so why?<br>In sum, is the patient's right to choose being respected to the extent possible in ethics and law? |
| **QUALITY OF LIFE** | **CONTEXTUAL FEATURES** |
| **The Principles of Beneficence and Nonmaleficence and Respect for Autonomy** | **The Principles of Loyalty and Fairness** |
| 1. What are the prospects, with or without treatment, for a return to normal life?<br>2. What physical, mental and social deficits is the patient likely to experience if treatment succeeds?<br>3. Are there biases that might prejudice the provider's evaluation of the patient's quality of life?<br>4. Is the patient's present or future condition such that his or her continued life might be judged undesirable?<br>5. Is there any plan and rationale to forgo treatment?<br>6. Are there plans for comfort and palliative care? | 1. Are there family issues that might influence treatment decisions?<br>2. Are there provider (physicians and nurses) issues that might influence treatment decisions?<br>3. Are there financial and economic factors?<br>4. Are there religious or cultural factors?<br>5. Are there limits on confidentiality?<br>6. Are there problems of allocation of resources?<br>7. How does the law affect treatment decisions?<br>8. Is clinical research or teaching involved?<br>9. Is there any conflict of interest on the part of the providers or the institution? |

• **Figure 8.1** Four topics for ethical analysis. (From Jonsen AR, Siegler M, Winslade WJ. *Clinical Ethics: A Practical Approach to Ethical Decisions in Clinical Medicine.* 5th ed. New York: McGraw-Hill; 2002.)

---

**CASE 1**

**Alice Oliver (Part 3)**

Mrs. Oliver's nutrition may be viewed in a dual manner. Because nutrition is considered basic to life and comfort, the team has an obligation defined by the principle of beneficence to provide it. There is, however, a therapeutic component as well, because the food must be provided in a form and texture suitable to Mrs. Oliver's swallowing disorder. You tell the team that although Mrs. Oliver is refusing the recommended therapeutic form of the nutrition, they are still fulfilling the duty of beneficence and respecting her autonomy by providing her thin liquids, although the risk may be greater. In other words, the duties of autonomy and beneficence outweigh the duty of nonmaleficence. As long as Mrs. Oliver understands the increased risk she is assuming, it is ethically permissible to provide her with thin liquids. It is your responsibility, in conjunction with the care team, to establish that Mrs. Oliver has adequate information and decisional capacity to make this decision.
1. Is there another morally acceptable alternative to this case?

## Informed Consent

Informed consent is the foundation for the exercise of autonomy. It has become increasingly central to both the ethical and legal regulation of American medicine and the clinician–patient relationship since the concept was first used in 1957.[25] In representing the means by which the principles of autonomy, beneficence, and nonmaleficence are balanced and incorporated into medical decision making,[26] informed consent requires disclosure and comprehension of information, as well as voluntary and competent decision making[27] (Box 8.1).

## Disclosure

Patients require enough information to make clinical decisions. Some states measure the adequacy of disclosure according to the standard determined by what a reasonable clinician would disclose, whereas others measure adequacy by what information a reasonable patient would need to make the decision.[28]

Disclosure should allow the patient to weigh not only the risks and benefits of the proposed intervention but also the comparative risks and benefits of alternatives, including the status quo or doing nothing. The information should be provided in a language and educational level the patient can understand.

## Voluntariness

When patients are sick, they are often vulnerable as well. There may be conflicting values, not only among the patient's own values but also among the patient's, family's, and other caregivers' values. It is important therefore that the clinician ascertain that the decision is not coerced, that it truly represents the free will of the patient.

## • BOX 8.1   The Elements of Informed Consent

### Disclosing Information

Steps for disclosure: Before launching into a long narrative about the decision at hand, find out what the patient knows: "Can you tell me what you know about Alzheimer disease?" The answer will reveal the extent of the patient's understanding and appreciation. This information is a useful guide for further discussion and disclosure. After disclosing information ask, "what else?" and then wait at least 10 seconds before speaking again.

**Doctor means teacher, and consent means to feel together. A good physician is an empathetic teacher**.

### Assuring Voluntariness

Steps to ensure voluntariness: An environment, such as a nursing home or assisted-living facility, can affect a person's sense of freedom and choice. Most people do not recognize the subtle effect their day-to-day environment has on their voluntariness. Open-ended questions can elicit whether this is a problem: "Do you feel like you have a choice?" Give the person time to make a decision (unless it is an emergency).

**Remind a person that he or she is free to choose and give time to choose**.

### Assessing Competency

Steps to assess competency: In situations in which a patient is refusing what a physician considers "standard of care," a competency assessment is essential, but it can be the source of discord. Reassure the patient that the final choice is his or hers: "I am not here to argue. My duty as a doctor is to be a good teacher for you about your health and the options you have. I just want to make sure I've done an adequate job teaching you." Then assess the patient's understanding, appreciation, and reasoning by using the format of the open-ended questions described in Box 8.2.

**Competency derives from the ability to make a decision. Evidence of impaired decision-making capacity may be the first sign of clinically significant cognitive impairment**.

(From Karlawish JHT. *Getting Competent at Assessing Competency*. Presented at the 2003 Annual Meeting of the American Geriatrics Society.)

---

Simply asking patients whether they feel they have a choice or asking how much time they will need to make a choice may ensure voluntariness. Sometimes family members and friends may need to be excluded from the discussion to allow patients to freely express themselves. Overt threats from family are an obvious impediment to the free expression of choice, but subtle coercion or abuse may also occur.

The clinician may also exert undue pressure on the patient, interfering with the patient's perceived ability to express his or her free will. A patient may be afraid of disappointing the clinician or, worse, of being abandoned by the clinician if he or she does not consent. The patient's fear of abandonment may not mean the complete departure of the clinician from the clinician–patient relationship but the fear that the clinician may not be fully committed to all the patient's needs should the patient choose to pursue a course contrary to the clinician's recommendation.[29] Therefore the disclosure process should include information regarding the management of the patient and an assurance of support should he reject the proposed intervention.

### Decisional Capacity

Although disclosure of information and voluntariness are necessary for informed consent, the patient must also be able to use the information meaningfully to render an informed decision. The cognitive ability to process information and render a reasoned decision is referred to as decisional or decision-making capacity.

Most authors tend to use the term *competence* as a legal term, referring to the individual's soundness of mind to make most routine decisions. When a court rules that an individual is incompetent, that individual is determined to lack sufficient cognitive function to make most routine decisions. This is often accompanied by the appointment of a guardian and results in limitations in the individual's exercise of basic rights. The term *capacity* is used clinically on a case-by-case basis to denote the capability to render a specific decision. A patient may have the capacity to make some decisions but not others. In everyday practice and even among state laws, the distinctions of these terms often break down, leading to the use of the terms *capacity* and *competence* interchangeably.

The prevalence of cognitive impairment because of dementia or delirium raises difficult questions about the patient's capacity to participate in the process of informed consent. Cognitive impairment does not necessarily preclude the ability to render all medical decisions, nor is an abnormal cognitive screen score, by itself, an indication of incapacity.[30]

The clinician should determine decisional capacity on a case-by-case basis as part of the process of obtaining informed consent. A patient, who, because of dementia, is incapable of participating in decision making about a lower extremity vascular procedure, may nevertheless be able to clearly express a decision about resuscitation. Thus the inability to provide informed consent for one intervention does not indicate incapacity for other decisions. Likewise, the presence of mental illness, such as depression, should not, by itself, suggest that the patient cannot participate in decision making,[31] although there is evidence that the judgment of acutely ill adults may be sufficiently impaired in many cases to interfere with decision making,[32] but this simply underscores the importance of using a systematic assessment of decisional capacity specific to the decision at hand. Although not strictly necessary, there are a number of available tools for this purpose.[33]

**⇒⇒ The presence of dementia does not, by itself, indicate that the patient lacks decision-making capacity.**

The set of standards that has evolved for assessing decision-making capacity includes the following components: (1) understanding of information that is disclosed in the informed consent process, (2) appreciation of the information for one's own circumstances, (3) reasoning with the information, and (4) expressing a choice[34,35] (Box 8.2).

Understanding represents the ability to comprehend the information provided and to restate it in terms that make this evident. To demonstrate understanding, it is helpful to ask the patient to repeat, in his or her own words, the information the clinician has provided, so it is clear that the patient fully comprehends the information.

Appreciation represents the ability to recognize that the information applies to oneself. A patient may clearly articulate information about a proposed procedure, but assert the procedure is not needed because of an erroneous belief that he does not have the condition for which the procedure is indicated. This would suggest that the patient's appreciation is impaired.

Reasoning involves the ability to use and apply logic to information. This refers to the patient's ability to infer the consequences of a choice and to weigh the respective merits of various choices. The ability to consider the risks and benefits of a procedure or to weight the risks between two or more procedures is an example of reasoning.

---

**• BOX 8.2** Model Questions for Assessing Capacity

**Ability to Choose**

1. Have you made a decision about the treatment options we discussed?

**Ability to Understand Relevant Information**

2. Please tell me in your own words what I have told you about
   - The nature of your condition
   - The treatment or diagnostic test recommended
   - The possible benefits from the treatment/diagnostic test
   - The possible risks (or discomforts) of the treatment/diagnostic test
   - Any other possible treatments that could be used, as well as their benefits and risks
   - The possible benefits and risks of no treatment at all
3. We have talked about the chance that [X] might happen with this treatment? In your own words, can you tell me how likely do you think it is that [X] will happen?
4. What do you think will happen if you decide not to have treatment?

**Ability to Appreciate the Situation and its Consequences**

5. What do you believe is wrong with your health now?
6. Do you believe it is possible that this treatment/diagnostic test could benefit you?
7. Do you believe it is possible that this treatment/diagnostic test could harm you?
8. We talked about other possible treatments for you—can you tell me, in your own words, what they are?
9. What do you believe would happen to you if you decided you did not want to have this treatment/diagnostic test?

**Ability to Reason**

10. Tell me how you reached the decision to have [not have] the treatment/diagnostic test?
11. What things were important to you in making the decision you did?
12. How would you balance those things?

(Modified from Ganzini L, Volicer L, Nelson WA, et al. Ten myths about decision-making capacity. *J Am Med Dir Assoc*. 2004;5:263-67. Also from Grisso T, Appelbaum PS. *Assessing Competence to Consent to Treatment: A Guide for Physicians and Other Health Professionals*. New York, NY: Oxford University Press; 1998.)

---

Expressing a choice refers to the ability of the patient to make and state a decision. The inability to express a choice renders assessment of the other criteria for competency unnecessary, but the ability to express a choice is, by itself, inadequate to judge competency. The inability to express a choice should not be confused with the refusal to make a choice when understanding, appreciation, and reasoning have been demonstrated to be intact. The latter essentially represents an endorsement of the status quo. For example, a patient who has carefully considered a discussion about do-not-resuscitate (DNR) orders but asks that the clinician return for further discussion in a week has implicitly consented to resuscitative efforts and declined to authorize a DNR order.

How rigorously one applies these criteria to the decision-making process depends on the characteristics of the proposed intervention and the concordance between the patient's decision and the clinician's advice. For instance, few would argue that these criteria should be extensively applied to the question of drawing blood to determine basic electrolytes. In contrast, high-risk procedures or interventions with complex benefit/risk equations might require a stricter application of these criteria. Moreover, when a patient disagrees with the clinician's advice, particularly when the risk/benefit ratio of treatment is clearly favorable, a higher standard may be applied.[36]

❖ The process of obtaining informed consent for a given procedure is the appropriate means of determining decision-making capacity.

---

**CASE 1**

**Alice Oliver (Part 4)**

To respect Mrs. Oliver's autonomy, it is the responsibility of you and the care team to establish that she has adequate information to make this decision, that she is making the decision of her own free will, and that she has capacity to make the decision. Once the criteria for informed consent are met, it is ethically permissible to provide thin liquids despite her increased risk of aspiration.

Although it is not necessary, some institutions may require the patient to sign a written "refusal to consent" form, indicating in writing that the patient is adequately informed about the risks of deviating from the team's recommendations.

1. Is it ever morally acceptable to override a patient's wishes?
2. What can be done if a healthcare provider continues to have personal moral objections to a patient's autonomously derived decision?

---

## Disclosure of Medical Error

A medical error may be defined as a commission or omission of an action with potentially negative consequences for the patient that would have been judged wrong by skilled and knowledgeable peers at the time it occurred, independent of whether there were any negative consequences.[37] Preventable adverse errors may be more common in elderly patients owing to the clinical complexity of their care, the number of medications prescribed, and their increased use of healthcare.[38] This may be particularly true in nursing homes.[39] The release of the Institute of Medicine's report on medical error, *To Err Is Human*, focused attention on the problem of medical error and resulted in calls for increased transparency in healthcare.[40] A national survey of risk managers conducted in 2002 revealed that more than half of respondents would disclose a death or serious injury, but respondents were less likely to disclose preventable harms than nonpreventable harms.[41]

Whether medical error should be disclosed was first introduced as a moral dilemma by Hilfiker in 1984.[42] Since then, disclosure of unanticipated outcomes of care, including medical error, has grown to be recognized as an ethical obligation of both physicians and nurses.[43-45] The ethical basis for disclosure involves not only respect for the patient but also support for patient autonomy and maintenance of the confidence and trust in the relationship with the clinician. According to the American Medical Association's Code of Medical Ethics, clinicians involved in a medical error should (1) disclose the occurrence of the error, explain the nature of the (potential) harm, and provide the information needed to enable the patient to make informed decisions about future medical care; (2) acknowledge the error and express professional and compassionate concern toward patients who have been harmed in the context of health care; (3) explain efforts that are being taken to prevent similar occurrences in the future; and (4) provide for continuity of care of patients who have been harmed during the course of care, including facilitating transfer of care when a patient has lost trust in the physician.[46] Although counterintuitive, there is some evidence that a policy of open communication and disclosure of medical error may reduce liability payments.[47]

## Extraordinary Versus Ordinary Care

When working with a patient to make medical decisions, clinicians should be cautious about the use of terms such as *extraordinary* or *heroic*. The term *extraordinary care* often appears in the writings of Roman Catholic theologians and refers to treatments that are very expensive, are possibly painful or uncomfortable, may provide an equivocal chance of success, and are not routinely used.[48,49] There is no consensus on this definition and it is inadequately informative to allow for moral decision making. Treatments, such as dialysis, that were once considered extraordinary are now routine. Treatments that may be considered routine under usual circumstances, such as antibiotics for pneumonia, may be considered extraordinary in some terminally ill patients. Because the distinction between extraordinary or heroic care versus ordinary care is not well demarcated, it is best to avoid the terms altogether. It is better to discuss the benefits, risks, and burdens of the specific treatments in question and to thereby assist the patient in making rational and informed medical decisions. If the patient's religious or theological beliefs will influence decision making, it may be helpful to suggest the participation of appropriate clergy with expertise in such matters.

◆◆ **When discussing advance directives with patients, it is better to discuss specific life-sustaining treatments rather than globally referring to "heroic" or "extraordinary" measures.**

---

### CASE 1

#### Alice Oliver (Part 5)

Several days later, Mrs. Oliver suffers a second stroke. This time, the hemiparesis appears to be denser. She is now confused. The dysphagia worsens, and she is unable to take food by mouth without coughing. As you try to explain possible therapeutic options to her, you realize that she may not be able to understand what you are saying. The social worker tells you that she has three children outside in the waiting room. You wonder who will now make decisions.

1. How do you determine who is the decision maker when a patient loses decision-making capacity?
2. How do you weigh competing wishes among multiple family members?

---

## Advance Directives

Advance directives are verbal or written directions provided by an individual outlining what medical decisions are to be made on that individual's behalf when that person no longer possesses decisional capacity. When it has been determined that a patient lacks the capacity to make decisions about medical interventions, healthcare providers, family, and caregivers often struggle to determine who should make the decision and what is the right decision. The process of making medical decisions on behalf of an incapacitated patient is known as substituted judgment. Many states have laws governing who is entitled to exercise substituted judgment when the patient no longer possesses decision-making capacity. For instance, the laws of the State of New York includes the Family Health Care Decisions Act, which allows designated family members or a close friend to render substituted judgment on behalf of a

patient who has lost decisional capacity, in the absence of a healthcare proxy or formally appointed healthcare agent.[50]

The US Supreme Court decision *Cruzan vs. Director, Missouri Department of Health*[51] established a federal right to withdraw or withhold life-sustaining treatment and established that a state can set a standard of evidence for the previously expressed wishes of patients who lack decision-making capacity that is "clear and convincing," a standard between preponderance of the evidence and beyond a shadow of a doubt.[52] This does not have to be written, but it is far more prudent to create a written record of such wishes than to rely on the memory of family members or caregivers during a time of crisis. These advance directives ensure that the voice of the patient will be heard when the patient is no longer able to participate in making critical medical decisions.

Because it is left to the states to set the standards for advance directives, it is important to understand the laws governing such documents and how they are used. In some states, an individual without decision-making capacity retains the right to have life-sustaining treatment withheld or withdrawn, but the evidence of such intent must be clear and convincing. Other states may have legislation allowing family members to withhold or withdraw life-sustaining treatment for incapacitated patients under lesser standards.

There are two common categories of written advance directives. One document appoints a surrogate or agent to make medical decisions should the individual lose decision-making capacity. This is known as a healthcare proxy, a durable power of attorney for healthcare, a designation of healthcare surrogate, or an appointment of a healthcare representative. The second, the living will, is a written statement of preferences for care when decision-making capacity is lost. Some advance directives may combine features of both types of documents.

The living will limits the patient's actionable preferences to the conditions delineated in the document, often to coma, persistent vegetative state, and irreversible terminal illness. It is difficult, if not impossible, to anticipate the variety of other medical conditions, such as severe dementia, that might affect the incapacitated patient in the future. The risk exists that the stipulations in the living will might not apply to the circumstances at hand. Some have even suggested that the concept of the living will should be abandoned in favor of the durable power of attorney for healthcare.[53] Such documents may also include language indicating future preferences, but by appointing an agent who is familiar with the patient's values, the document allows greater flexibility for the surrogate to make medical decisions when unanticipated circumstances arise.

Although different state legislatures have adopted different variations of these forms, a statutory form or other statement of preferences completed in one state will generally be recognized in another. The Federal Patient Self-Determination Act[54] requires healthcare organizations to ask patients whether they possess advance directives, to provide written information regarding the individual's rights under state law, and to educate the staff and community about advance directives.

Although hospital admission may be used as an opportunity to elicit healthcare preferences and complete advance directives, the stressful period at the onset of an acute illness is not the optimal time to discuss potentially difficult choices. It is more advisable to complete advance directives in a period of good or stable health. Questions about advance directives and an offer to help the patient complete them should be incorporated into a comprehensive geriatric assessment or the periodic examination. Medicare now reimburses clinicians for advance care planning, including completion of advance directives.[55]

A recently developed healthcare directive is the physician order for life-sustaining treatment (POLST), devised to address the preferences of patients with serious illnesses.[56] Technically, not an advance directive, POLST is a set of orders, based on the patient's current condition and anticipated trajectory, stipulating which interventions, when the need arises, should be provided or withheld. Typically, POLST contains orders related to attempting resuscitation and provision of antibiotics, fluids, and nutrition. It is specifically designed to be transferred from one setting to another, a transitional period when patients are often vulnerable to errors resulting from inaccurate transmittal of information about medications, therapies, and advance directives[57] (Fig. 8.2). The name and content of the POLST paradigm may vary from state to state. For instance, New York has adopted Medical Orders for Life-Sustaining Treatment (MOLST), North Carolina has adopted Medical Orders for Scope of Treatment (MOST), and Montana has adopted Provider Orders for Life-Sustaining Treatment (POLST).

It is customary in many hospitals and nursing homes for a social worker or other nonclinician to complete the POLST and present the completed form to the clinician for signature. It is preferable that a clinician, with knowledge of the patient's condition, values, and preferences, complete the form, because it is, after all, a set of medical orders. Furthermore, because patients' preferences and conditions may evolve, clinicians must review the POLST with the patient or surrogate periodically and when the patient's condition changes.

◆◆ **Because patients' experiences and values may change, it is advisable to periodically review advance directives to ascertain concordance with patients' current wishes, thus allowing for revision when necessary**.

## Futility

Futility is often invoked when a proposed treatment is highly unlikely to provide benefit. Others have proposed that the uses of the term *futility* in clinical medicine are too varied and diverse to allow for a precise definition.[59,60]

The principle of beneficence, the obligation to do good, infers that actions that have no reasonable likelihood of providing benefit should not be initiated or offered. Alternately expressed, an intervention that is unlikely to achieve its intended outcome should not be undertaken.

The meaning of the term *futile* depends on the intended outcome of a given intervention. For instance, the literature of comprehensive geriatric assessment (CGA) includes studies that demonstrate improved diagnostic accuracy, improved functional status, improved affect or cognition, reduced prescribed medications, decreased nursing home use, increased use of home health services, reduced hospital admission, reduced medical care costs, prolonged survival, or improved comfort.[61,62] One cannot say that CGA is futile for a given patient without explicitly indicating which are the outcomes in question.

Despite the availability of clinical practice guidelines and other tools of evidence-based medicine, clinicians may have difficulty assigning a statistical probability that denotes futility. One suggestion is that futility can be presumed if a treatment has not worked in the past 100 cases and will "almost certainly" not work if it is tried again.[63] There is no consensus about this definition, and there is evidence that as an expression of probability, *futility* means different things to different clinicians.[64] Other studies have shown that clinicians assign a wide variety of probabilities to define *futile*.[65]

Because futility may refer to a multitude of goals, sometimes perceived differently by patient, provider, and family, there is the risk that wielding the term inevitably results in the introduction of subjective and biased value judgments. Jecker and Schneiderman[66]

NEW YORK STATE DEPARTMENT OF HEALTH

# Medical Orders for Life-Sustaining Treatment (MOLST)

**THE PATIENT KEEPS THE ORIGINAL MOLST FORM DURING TRAVEL TO DIFFERENT CARE SETTINGS. THE PHYSICIAN OR NURSE PRACTITIONER KEEPS A COPY.**

LAST NAME/FIRST NAME/MIDDLE INITIAL OF PATIENT

ADDRESS

CITY/STATE/ZIP

☐ Male ☐ Female

DATE OF BIRTH (MM/DD/YYYY)          eMOLST NUMBER (THIS IS NOT AN eMOLST FORM)

## Do-Not-Resuscitate (DNR) and Other Life-Sustaining Treatment (LST)

This is a medical order form that tells others the patient's wishes for life-sustaining treatment. A health care professional must complete or change the MOLST form based on the patient's current medical condition, values, wishes, and MOLST Instructions. If the patient is unable to make medical decisions, the orders should reflect patient wishes, as best understood by the health care agent or surrogate. A physician or nurse practitioner must sign the MOLST form. All health care professionals must follow these medical orders as the patient moves from one location to another, unless a physician or nurse practitioner examines the patient, reviews the orders, and changes them.

**MOLST is generally for patients with serious health conditions. The patient or other decision-maker should work with the physician or nurse practitioner and consider asking the physician or nurse practitioner to fill out a MOLST form if the patient:**

- Wants to avoid or receive any or all life-sustaining treatment.
- Resides in a long-term care facility or requires long-term care services.
- Might die within the next year.

**If the patient has an intellectual or developmental disability (I/DD) and lacks the capacity to decide, the doctor (not a nurse practitioner) must follow special procedures and attach the completed Office for People with Developmental Disabilities (OPWDD) legal requirements checklist before signing the MOLST. See page 4.**

### SECTION A  Resuscitation Instructions When the Patient Has No Pulse and/or Is Not Breathing

Check **one:**

☐ **CPR Order: Attempt Cardio-Pulmonary Resuscitation**
CPR involves artificial breathing and forceful pressure on the chest to try to restart the heart. It usually involves electric shock (defibrillation) and a plastic tube down the throat into the windpipe to assist breathing (intubation). It means that all medical treatments will be done to prolong life when the heart stops or breathing stops, including being placed on a breathing machine and being transferred to the hospital.

☐ **DNR Order: Do Not Attempt Resuscitation (Allow Natural Death)**
This means do not begin CPR, as defined above, to make the heart or breathing start again if either stops.

### SECTION B  Consent for Resuscitation Instructions (Section A)

The patient can make a decision about resuscitation if he or she has the ability to decide about resuscitation. If the patient does NOT have the ability to decide about resuscitation and has a health care proxy, the health care agent makes this decision. If there is no health care proxy, another person will decide, chosen from a list based on NYS law. Individuals with I/DD who do not have capacity and do not have a health care proxy must follow SCPA 1750-b.

☐ Check if verbal consent (Leave signature line blank)

SIGNATURE          DATE/TIME

PRINT NAME OF DECISION-MAKER

PRINT FIRST WITNESS NAME          PRINT SECOND WITNESS NAME

**Who made the decisions?** ☐ Patient ☐ Health Care Agent ☐ Public Health Law Surrogate ☐ Minor's Parent/Guardian ☐ §1750-b Surrogate*

### SECTION C  Physician or Nurse Practitioner Signature for Sections A and B

PHYSICIAN OR NURSE PRACTITIONER SIGNATURE*          PRINT PHYSICIAN OR NURSE PRACTITIONER NAME          DATE/TIME

PHYSICIAN OR NURSE PRACTITIONER LICENSE NUMBER          PHYSICIAN OR NURSE PRACTITIONER PHONE/PAGER NUMBER

### SECTION D  Advance Directives

*Check all advance directives known to have been completed:*

☐ Health Care Proxy ☐ Living Will ☐ Organ Donation ☐ Documentation of Oral Advance Directive

**\*If this decision is being made by a 1750-b surrogate, a physician must sign the MOLST.**

DOH-5003 (12/18) p 1 of 4

• **Figure 8.2** Medical orders for life-sustaining treatment (MOLST). (© New York State Department of Health.)

**THE PATIENT KEEPS THE ORIGINAL MOLST FORM DURING TRAVEL TO DIFFERENT CARE SETTINGS. THE PHYSICIAN OR NURSE PRACTITIONER KEEPS A COPY.**

LAST NAME/FIRST NAME/MIDDLE INITIAL OF PATIENT                                    DATE OF BIRTH (MM/DD/YYYY)

| SECTION E | Orders For Other Life-Sustaining Treatment and Future Hospitalization When the Patient has a Pulse and the Patient is Breathing |
|---|---|

Life-sustaining treatment may be ordered for a trial period to determine if there is benefit to the patient. **If a life-sustaining treatment is started, but turns out not to be helpful, the treatment can be stopped. Before stopping treatment, additional procedures may be needed as indicated on page 4.**

**Treatment Guidelines** No matter what else is chosen, the patient will be treated with dignity and respect, and health care providers will offer comfort measures. *Check one:*

☐ **Comfort measures only** Comfort measures are medical care and treatment provided with the primary goal of relieving pain and other symptoms and reducing suffering. Reasonable measures will be made to offer food and fluids by mouth. Medication, turning in bed, wound care and other measures will be used to relieve pain and suffering. Oxygen, suctioning and manual treatment of airway obstruction will be used as needed for comfort.

☐ **Limited medical interventions** The patient will receive medication by mouth or through a vein, heart monitoring and all other necessary treatment, based on MOLST orders.

☐ **No limitations on medical interventions** The patient will receive all needed treatments.

**Instructions for Intubation and Mechanical Ventilation** *Check one:*

☐ **Do not intubate (DNI)** Do not place a tube down the patient's throat or connect to a breathing machine that pumps air into and out of lungs. Treatments are available for symptoms of shortness of breath, such as oxygen and morphine. (This box should not be checked if full CPR is checked in Section A.)

☐ **A trial period** *Check one or both:*
    ☐ **Intubation and mechanical ventilation**
    ☐ **Noninvasive ventilation (e.g. BIPAP), if the health care professional agrees that it is appropriate**

☐ **Intubation and long-term mechanical ventilation, if needed** Place a tube down the patient's throat and connect to a breathing machine as long as it is medically needed.

**Future Hospitalization/Transfer** *Check one:*

☐ **Do not send to the hospital unless pain or severe symptoms cannot be otherwise controlled.**

☐ **Send to the hospital, if necessary, based on MOLST orders.**

**Artificially Administered Fluids and Nutrition** When a patient can no longer eat or drink, liquid food or fluids can be given by a tube inserted in the stomach or fluids can be given by a small plastic tube (catheter) inserted directly into the vein. If a patient chooses not to have either a feeding tube or IV fluids, food and fluids are offered as tolerated using careful hand feeding. **Additional procedures may be needed as indicated on page 4.** *Check one each for feeding tube and IV fluids:*

☐ **No feeding tube**    ☐ **No IV fluids**
☐ **A trial period of feeding tube**    ☐ **A trial period of IV fluids**
☐ **Long-term feeding tube, if needed**

**Antibiotics** *Check one:*

☐ **Do not use antibiotics.** Use other comfort measures to relieve symptoms.

☐ **Determine use or limitation of antibiotics when infection occurs.**

☐ **Use antibiotics** to treat infections, if medically indicated.

**Other Instructions** about starting or stopping treatments discussed with the doctor or nurse practitioner or about other treatments not listed above (dialysis, transfusions, etc.).

**Consent for Life-Sustaining Treatment Orders (Section E)** (Same as Section B, which is the consent for Section A)

_____ ☐ Check if verbal consent (Leave signature line blank) _____
SIGNATURE                                                                                                            DATE/TIME

_____
PRINT NAME OF DECISION-MAKER

_____      _____
PRINT FIRST WITNESS NAME      PRINT SECOND WITNESS NAME

**Who made the decisions?** ☐ Patient ☐ Health Care Agent ☐ Based on clear and convincing evidence of patient's wishes
☐ Public Health Law Surrogate ☐ Minor's Parent/Guardian ☐ §1750-b Surrogate*

**Physician or Nurse Practitioner Signature for Section E**

_____    _____    _____
PHYSICIAN OR NURSE PRACTITIONER SIGNATURE*    PRINT PHYSICIAN OR NURSE PRACTITIONER NAME    DATE/TIME

**\*If this decision is being made by a 1750-b surrogate, a physician must sign the MOLST.**

DOH-5003 (12/18) p 2 of 4        **This MOLST form has been approved by the NYSDOH for use in all settings.**

• **Figure 8.2, cont'd**

**THE PATIENT KEEPS THE ORIGINAL MOLST FORM DURING TRAVEL TO DIFFERENT CARE SETTINGS. THE PHYSICIAN OR NURSE PRACTITIONER KEEPS A COPY.**

LAST NAME/FIRST NAME/MIDDLE INITIAL OF PATIENT                                                                    DATE OF BIRTH (MM/DD/YYYY)

## SECTION F    Review and Renewal of MOLST Orders on this MOLST Form

The physician or nurse practitioner must review the form from time to time as the law requires, and also:

- If the patient moves from one location to another to receive care; or
- If the patient has a major change in health status (for better or worse); or
- If the patient or other decision-maker changes his or her mind about treatment.

| Date/Time | Reviewer's Name and Signature | Location of Review (e.g., Hospital, NH, Physician's or Nurse Practitioner's Office) | Outcome of Review |
|---|---|---|---|
| | | | ☐ No change<br>☐ Form voided, new form completed<br>☐ Form voided, **no** new form |
| | | | ☐ No change<br>☐ Form voided, new form completed<br>☐ Form voided, **no** new form |
| | | | ☐ No change<br>☐ Form voided, new form completed<br>☐ Form voided, **no** new form |
| | | | ☐ No change<br>☐ Form voided, new form completed<br>☐ Form voided, **no** new form |
| | | | ☐ No change<br>☐ Form voided, new form completed<br>☐ Form voided, **no** new form |
| | | | ☐ No change<br>☐ Form voided, new form completed<br>☐ Form voided, **no** new form |
| | | | ☐ No change<br>☐ Form voided, new form completed<br>☐ Form voided, **no** new form |
| | | | ☐ No change<br>☐ Form voided, new form completed<br>☐ Form voided, **no** new form |
| | | | ☐ No change<br>☐ Form voided, new form completed<br>☐ Form voided, **no** new form |
| | | | ☐ No change<br>☐ Form voided, new form completed<br>☐ Form voided, **no** new form |
| | | | ☐ No change<br>☐ Form voided, new form completed<br>☐ Form voided, **no** new form |

DOH-5003 (12/18) p 3 of 4

• **Figure 8.2, cont'd**

**THE PATIENT KEEPS THE ORIGINAL MOLST FORM DURING TRAVEL TO DIFFERENT CARE SETTINGS. THE PHYSICIAN OR NURSE PRACTITIONER KEEPS A COPY.**

LAST NAME/FIRST NAME/MIDDLE INITIAL OF PATIENT
DATE OF BIRTH (MM/DD/YYYY)

## Requirements for Completing the MOLST for Individuals with Intellectual or Developmental Disabilities

Completing the MOLST for individuals with I/DD who lack capacity to make their own health care decisions and do not have a health care proxy:

- The law governing the decision-making process differs for individuals with I/DD. Surrogate's Court Procedure Act (SCPA) Section 1750-b must be followed when making a decision for an individual with I/DD who lacks capacity and does not have a health care proxy.

- MOLST may only be signed by a **physician**, not a nurse practitioner.

- Completion of the **MOLST legal requirements checklist for individuals with I/DD**, including notification of certain parties and resolution of any objections, is **mandatory prior to completion of MOLST**. The checklist is available on the NYS OPWDD website.

- The checklist should be completed when an authorized surrogate makes a decision to **withhold or withdraw life sustaining treatment (LST)** from an individual with I/DD. There are specific medical criteria, included in Step 4 of the checklist. The individual's medical condition must meet the specified medical criteria **at the time the request to withhold or withdraw treatment is made**.

- **Trials** – whether or not a new checklist is required following an unsuccessful trial of LST depends on the parameters of the trial, as specified in Step 2 of the checklist. If Step 2 of the checklist has provided that a trial for LST is to end after a specific period of time or the occurrence of a specific event, it may not be necessary to complete a new checklist following the trial. However, if a trial period is open ended, and the authorized surrogate subsequently decides to request withdrawal of the LST, a new checklist would be required.

- The checklist and 1750-b process apply to individuals with I/DD, regardless of their age or residential setting.

DOH-5003 (12/18) p 4 of 4

• **Figure 8.2, cont'd**

suggest that even quantitative expressions of probability cannot escape value judgments, such as the worth of taking particular chances or the quality of a patient's life.

There are certainly situations in which futility is obvious. Initiating resuscitative efforts on a nursing home resident found in bed in the morning, pulseless and cold, with the beginnings of rigor mortis is clearly futile if restoring cardiac function is the goal. Repairing a fractured hip in a bed-ridden, severely demented elderly woman may also be viewed as futile if the proposed goal is ambulation. Other situations are not so clear. For instance, the literature on the efficacy of acetylcholinesterase inhibitors for treating dementia is mixed and controversial, with clinicians staking out both sides of the treat/do not treat divide.[67,68] A clinician, who is unconvinced of the efficacy of these drugs, may indeed consider treatment with them to be futile, whereas others may consider these drugs to be the current standard of care.

Using futility as the basis for withholding treatments or the discussion of treatments must be done with great caution. Age alone rarely, if ever, provides a rationale for determining that an intervention is futile, although it may be factored into calculations of risk and longevity at times. Until potential goals of treatment are articulated and understood, preferably early in the course of illness, introducing futility into the conversation is unlikely to be productive.[69]

## Attempted Resuscitation and Do-Not-Resuscitate Orders

The use of closed chest cardiac massage to resuscitate an individual experiencing cardiac arrest was originally described in 1960.[70] Originally restricted to acute care facilities under specific circumstances, it is now widely accepted as a method for preventing death from cardiac arrest.

In 1974 the National Conference on CPR and Emergency Cardiac Care wrote, "The purpose of CPR is the prevention of sudden, unexpected death. CPR is not indicated in certain situations, such as in cases of terminal, irreversible illness." Discussion with the patient or family was not mentioned in the document. In 1980 the conference reiterated the purpose of CPR but noted, "The patient's family should understand and agree with the decision, although the family's opinion should not be controlling." This time, despite the comments about the family, there were no comments about the patient's wishes.[71]

Much has evolved since the original description of CPR in 1960. Because of the success of the procedure in treating sudden cardiac arrest, many cities have promoted training the general population in techniques of basic CPR. Many office buildings and airports now maintain automatic external defibrillators. Far from being reserved for only "sudden, expected death," the initiation of CPR is almost inevitable in healthcare institutions if specific orders to withhold CPR have not been entered. Most states have passed legislation specifying how orders to withhold CPR can be authorized. In the absence of a DNR order, it is presumed that the individual consents to CPR.

Studies examining the efficacy of CPR are often flawed, resulting from insufficient elderly subjects, differing endpoints, and differing reports on postresuscitation neurological status. Nonetheless, age alone has been shown to be a poor predictor of response to attempted CPR and should not be used as the lone determinant.[72]

In one study of out-of-hospital arrests, CPR in the elderly was found to be effective only in witnessed arrests that were not associated with asystole or electromechanical dissociation (now known as pulseless electrical activity).[73] Another study confirmed this, demonstrating that despite a reduction in success with increasing age, survival was greater for both octogenarians and nonagenarians whose presenting systems were pulseless ventricular tachycardia or ventricular fibrillation rather than asystole.[74]

In in-hospital cardiac arrests, age alone has also not been shown to be a determining factor of success. One study conducted in an intensive care unit (ICU) demonstrated survival to discharge in 7% of those suffering arrests, but only 5% survived more than 6 months. No patient who had asystole survived, but of those surviving 6 months, mental status remained unchanged. Interestingly, of the survivors, most stated they would decline future CPR.[75] Another study demonstrated that only 9 of 52 elderly patients who survived a cardiac arrest by 1 week went on to survive a full month, and only 5 of 37 previously independent patients remained independent after surviving cardiac arrest. Success was correlated with proper selection, presenting rhythm, and shorter response time, rather than age alone.[76] A subsequent study revealed poor outcomes in elderly patients with hypotension, pneumonia, renal failure, cancer, coma, intubation, pressors, and previous homebound status. All survivors experienced a decrease in functional status.[77]

Survival after cardiac arrest in the nursing home has been found to be rare,[78,79] leading one study to conclude, "We favor a more radical proposal: that CPR not be offered to NH [nursing home] residents."[80] Another study, although conceding that survival after cardiac arrest in nursing homes was unlikely, found that with appropriate selection and effective response, the survival of certain groups was comparable with that of elderly persons suffering out-of-hospital cardiac arrest. The study recommended that resuscitative efforts be withheld for unwitnessed arrests or arrests in which the presenting rhythm is asystole or electromechanical dissociation.[81]

Because most attempts at CPR in frail, elderly patients are unsuccessful, it may be misleading to discuss "resuscitation," which implies that the effort will be successful. Using the term *resuscitative effort* or *attempted resuscitation* may be more accurate. It is also important to differentiate the DNR order from the remainder of the care plan. A DNR order applies only to a cardiac arrest and is not equivalent to "do not treat."

Although consent to resuscitation is generally presumed in the absence of a DNR order, does this mean that it is also presumed that CPR will always be initiated in the absence of a DNR order? Does offering a DNR order equate to offering resuscitation under all other circumstances? Opinions vary on this point, but it is our opinion that the decision to initiate a resuscitative effort remains a medical decision that should be undertaken only if clinically indicated. It would make little sense to attempt resuscitation on a nursing home resident with end-stage dementia who experiences an unwitnessed cardiac arrest and presents with asystole. Likewise, it would not seem logical to initiate CPR on a ventilator-dependent ICU patient whose cardiac arrest was preceded by a gradual drop in blood pressure and vital signs, despite maximum doses of pressor agents and other supportive measures. Such actions must be consistent with state law and institutional policies and procedures. Furthermore, clinicians in training and nurses may feel uncomfortable making such decisions and opt instead for attempting resuscitation, despite its expected futility.

When a patient with a DNR order undergoes surgery, additional issues must be considered. In the controlled environment of an operating room, cardiac arrest, should it occur, is more likely to be reversible, because it would be witnessed in a controlled environment and managed quickly by a team experienced with such events. Because the likelihood of a successful resuscitation may be higher, it may be reasonable to offer a temporary suspension of a DNR order during the period in the operating room.[82] Some surgeons and anesthesiologists may even refuse to proceed without such contingencies.

---

**CASE 2**

**Discussion**

After Mr. Peterson's death, the nurses express their discomfort to you for withholding CPR in the absence of a DNR order. They ask whether they have breached hospital policy or state law in doing so.

From a purely pragmatic standpoint, it might be difficult for a nurse at the bedside or a first-year intern to make the decision to withhold CPR in the absence of a DNR order. Furthermore, state law or hospital policy might mandate the initiation of CPR in the absence of a valid DNR order, despite its apparent futility. Consequently, although it may be ethically permissible to withhold CPR when clearly futile, the legal obligation may be otherwise.

---

## Assisted Suicide and the Double Effect

Social attitudes toward the morality of assisted suicide have been evolving. In January 2006 the US Supreme Court blocked federal efforts to reverse Oregon's legalization of physician-assisted suicide. The 1997 Oregon Death with Dignity Act provides legal guidelines allowing physicians to provide lethal doses of medications to terminally ill patients who request them.[83] Since then, several states and a number of countries have legalized guidelines for providing physician-assisted suicide.[84] Nonetheless, assisted suicide remains controversial and has not achieved universal acceptance. Among the arguments against it is that the availability of good palliative and end-of-life care remains elusive, thus leaving for some patients assisted suicide as the only apparent avenue for relief from pain and suffering.[85] Regardless of one's position on assisted suicide, it is widely agreed that clinicians must do a better job in providing palliative care to patients experiencing physical or psychological suffering to reduce the possibility that a patient might have to consider such a difficult question.

In providing pain and symptom management to the dying patient, clinicians may worry that dosages of narcotics that will successfully relieve pain and discomfort might also hasten death, the so-called "double effect." In fact, there is little in the medical literature to support the notion that narcotics, when properly used at end of life, will hasten death.[86] In a small subset of patients who experience accelerating pain just before death despite conventional dosing of narcotics, it is possible that doses of narcotics adequate to relieve pain may also hasten death, even if by only a small time interval. Under these theoretical and probably unusual circumstances, the double effect must be approached like other circumstances requiring informed consent.[87] The following questions should be considered: (1) Is the patient's suffering proportionately severe to warrant the risks of intervention? (2) Has the patient or legal surrogate been fully informed of all likely outcomes of the intervention, both intended and expected, and is he or she aware of all the alternatives? (3) Is the intervention the least harmful one available given the patient's clinical circumstances and personal values?[88]

## Nutrition and Hydration

Whether nutrition and hydration are the obligatory fulfillment of basic human needs or purely medical interventions at the end of life has been debated vigorously in the ethics literature.[89,90] The matter is not settled, and the clinician must take care to understand state laws and explore the patient's values regarding these issues. When discussing the possibility of withdrawal or withholding of food and fluids with patients, the clinician should have some knowledge of the medical consequences of the decision. For instance, there is little evidence that tube feeding in advanced dementia improves outcomes, such as aspiration pneumonia, survival, pressure sores, infections, or comfort.[91,92] Both the American Geriatrics Society and AMDA—The Society for Post-Acute and Long-Term Care Medicine—have recommended that feeding tubes not be offered to patients with advanced dementia.[93,94] There is also evidence that food and fluid beyond that requested by terminally ill cancer patients may provide only a minimal role in providing comfort.[95] Nonetheless, the quality of informed consent for placement of gastrostomy tubes has been shown to be inadequate,[95] and using terminology such as *starvation* is unjustified and unnecessarily provocative.[96] Whether interventions such as a feeding tube or intravenous fluids should be offered when the clinician believes they will provide little benefit remains a thorny issue. It may be more appropriate to focus on those palliative interventions that will provide comfort to the patient and prepare the patient and family for the end of life rather than offer ineffective interventions.

On the flip side of the ethical quandaries involved in nutrition is the matter of voluntary cessation of nutrition, known as voluntary stopping eating and drinking (VSED). At end of life, patients may voluntarily choose to stop eating and drinking as a means of hastening death.[97] For a capacitated patient, this may be a rational choice. In institutional settings, it may be distressing to staff to observe a patient willingly being deprived of food and water. A difficult ethical dilemma may arise should a patient, who has written VSED into an advance directive and subsequently loses decisional capacity because of progressive cognitive impairment, asks for food or water. Should this void the advance directive regarding VSED? Should the patient, despite having advanced dementia, be considered to have sufficient decisional capacity to change the directive? It could be argued that there is a difference between the "then-self" and the "now-self."[98] To whom shall caregivers be obligated? Alternately, it could be argued that the threshold for establishing decisional capacity in this case requires only that the patient demonstrate willingness to eat and drink again, an admittedly low threshold. In either case, methodic ethical deliberation, which includes the voice of the patient, is necessary to determine what is ethically permissible.

## CASE 3

### Edward Gilliam (Part 1)

Mr. Gilliam is an 86-year-old widower who visits your office for a routine checkup. He apologizes for his lateness, explaining that he got lost driving to the office, a route he has driven for many years. His past medical history is significant for hypertension, diabetes, and osteoarthritis. You have received a consultation report from his ophthalmologist indicating a diagnosis of age-related macular degeneration. On Mini-Mental State Examination, he scores 25/30, a decline of 3 points since the previous year's examination. A report from a neuropsychological examination is equivocal, indicating the presence of significant but mild deficits in memory and executive function. You recommend to Mr. Gilliam that he cease driving. He responds that he has been driving for almost 70 years and insists he drives safely. He mentions that driving affords the freedom to "come and go as I please."

#### Case Analysis

When assessing a patient's ability to drive when possibly suffering from dementia, the ethical principle of autonomy conflicts with a potentially broader obligation to ensure reasonable safety, not only of the patient but of the public. There is evidence that self-report is an unreliable indicator of driver safety, a result of both denial and limited insight,[99] thus throwing into question the patient's capacity to exercise his autonomy. Although the clinician may not have a direct duty of nonmaleficence to the community, it has become increasingly evident that visits such as this may provide an opportunity for the clinician to prevent injuries or fatalities to the public. There is also evidence that although clinicians may be able to identify potentially hazardous drivers, the clinical assessment may be inadequate to accurately identify such drivers.[100] Although laws may vary from state to state, it is ethically permissible and, arguably, obligatory for the clinician to take the necessary steps to establish driver safety or, by appropriate reporting, allow relevant state agencies to make such determination.

## Cultural and Religious Considerations

Western medical ethical principles are based largely on the perceived rights of individuals, such as privacy, liberty, and self-determination. These underlie the principle of autonomy and, implicitly, its primacy among medical ethical principles. Some religious and cultural traditions may, however, present alternate social norms. Either patient or clinician may come from a non-Western cultural tradition, possibly leading to ethical conflicts stemming from different ethical principles. This may make resolution particularly challenging, given that the usual methodology for analyzing, deliberating, and resolving ethical conflicts assumes agreement on underlying principles. It must be remembered that the extent to which a patient chooses to exercise or cede autonomy is, itself, an autonomous decision. It is important that the clinician keep an open mind to alternative values stemming from unfamiliar cultural and religious traditions and incorporate these into the process of ethical deliberation.[101]

**♦♦ Do not make assumptions about the patient's moral preferences based only on the religion stamped on the chart.**

## Emerging Ethical Challenges

### Genetics and Precision Medicine

The rapid advancement of genetic analysis technology now allows genetic testing at the metaphoric push of a button. Genetic testing has at least three utilities: to establish a diagnosis in symptomatic individuals, to assess risk of a disease in asymptomatic individuals, and to guide pharmacologic therapy, when pharmacologically impacted by specific gene groups.[102] This new frontier in medicine promises to introduce new and novel ethical concerns regarding disclosure, privacy, and other related issues. There is already debate about the merits of disclosing genetic predisposition to Alzheimer disease, for instance.[103] What if that information is an incidental finding from the genetic testing for another purpose? Should the patient be told? Does that patient want to know? What kinds of consent and safeguards are necessary? These and other ethical considerations will undoubtedly emerge as this diagnostic tool becomes more widespread.

### Telehealth and Other Technological Innovations

Technological innovations, such as telehealth, wearable devices, and various internet applications are introducing new ethical challenges. Wearable devices, although while potentially improving the ability of clinicians to collect valuable physiologic information on patients over time, store large amounts of personal information that may be accessible by third parties. How to balance the benefits of this technology against privacy concerns remains to be resolved.[104]

Assuring privacy and confidentiality are also significant issues in the provision of telehealth services. Whereas telehealth may increase access for vulnerable, functionally and cognitively impaired older adults, that the clinician is remote and often unseen may potentially introduce ethical questions about the definition of the clinician-patient relationship, consent, and fidelity. As telehealth service gain more commercial appeal, conflicts of interest need to be resolved as well.[105]

## Summary

Medical ethics provides a structure for assessing the moral propriety of clinical decisions, particularly when patients' and clinicians' values conflict and collide. Most healthcare institutions now have ethics consultants or ethics committees to assist patients and clinicians in resolving difficult ethical dilemmas. By understanding principles of medical ethics and the structure for methodical analysis of ethical dilemmas, the clinician can resolve most common dilemmas that often arise in the care of the older patient and will inevitably arise as advances in medical care and technology present new challenges.

### Web Resources

*AMA Journal of Ethics*—an electronically published journal exploring ethical issue in medical care for clinicians and students alike: https://journalofethics.ama-assn.org/home.

*Journal of Medical Ethics*—An international journal reflecting the entire field of medical ethics, both practice and research: https://jme.bmj.com/.

Physician Orders for Life-Sustaining Treatment Program: www.polst.org.

Caring Connections, a national hospice and palliative care organization. Provides resources for end-of-life planning, including advance directives from each state: www.caringinfo.org.

## Key References

7. Beauchamp TL, Childress JF. *Principles of Biomedical Ethics*. 7th ed. New York, NY: Oxford University Press; 2012.

20. Jonsen AR, Siegler M, Winslade WJ. *Clinical Ethics: A Practical Approach to Ethical Decisions in Clinical Medicine*. 8th ed. New York, NY: McGraw-Hill; 2015.

34. Grisso T, Appelbaum PS. *Assessing Competence to Consent to Treatment: A Guide for Physicians and Other Health Professionals*. New York, NY: Oxford University Press; 1998.

35. Sessums LL, Zumbrzuska H, Jackson JL. Does this patient have medical decision-making capacity? *JAMA*. 2011;306(4):420–427.

**References available online at expertconsult.com.**

# 9

# Financing and Organization of Healthcare

JULIE P.W. BYNUM AND GEOFFREY J. HOFFMAN

## OUTLINE

## OBJECTIVES

*Upon completion of this chapter, the reader will be able to:*

- Understand the nature and spectrum of publicly funded social services available to older adults in the community.
- Describe the major public sources of funding for health services for older adults: Medicare, Medicaid, Older Americans Act, Title XX of the Social Security Act, and the Department of Veterans Affairs.
- Describe the out-of-pocket expenses older adults can expect to pay for both acute and long-term care.

- Understand the transitions in payer as a person moves from independent to assisted living and nursing home care.
- Describe the basic coverage provided by Medicare's Parts A, B, C, and D and by secondary insurance.
- Describe the range, limitations, and proportions of long-term care costs paid by four sources: patient and family personal funds, Medicare, Medicaid, and private insurance.
- Understand changes that are occurring in the healthcare market that affect older adults.

## Overview of System of Care for Older Adults

The American healthcare system is complex and expensive; older adults and the clinicians serving them may struggle to understand the available services and how they are paid. One important role for primary care providers is to help older adults access the resources they need at a cost they can afford. The goal of this chapter is to provide the basic knowledge of the organization and funding of healthcare that will enable primary care providers to play this critical role for patients.

### CASE 1

#### Jacob Miller (Part 1)

Jacob Miller is an 82-year-old man who lives by himself in a two-story home and has high blood pressure and gout. He does not drive so he gets out only a limited amount but can manage public transport. His daughter lives out of town and wonders what they can do to make him safer in his home.

Would Mr. Miller be eligible for any home-based services and what would you suggest?

## Unique Financial Challenges of Older Adults

Although not true of all older patients, one characteristic typically associated with older age is that the person has left the workforce and is therefore relying on savings, pensions, or other fixed sources of income. The 1965 introduction of the Medicare entitlement program, under Title XVIII of the Social Security Act, led to an enormous drop in the percentage of elderly people living in poverty. However, this population still faces financial challenges; the median annual income for older persons in 2017 was $32,654 for males and $19,180 for females.[1] In 2010, 13.4% of older adults' total expenditures went to purchase medical care, nearly two-thirds more than the proportion (8.2%) spent by all consumers, according to the Administration on Aging.[1]

In addition to living on a fixed income, over time older adults may accumulate chronic medical conditions and functional impairments that are leading drivers of healthcare costs. Some 75 cents out of every dollar spent on healthcare goes toward treating chronic conditions. The costs are even greater when a person has more than one chronic condition. In the United States, per capita spending for people with five or more chronic conditions is nearly 14 times greater than for those with no conditions, and 71% of healthcare spending is for patients with two or more chronic conditions. Individuals with chronic conditions also have limitations in activities of daily living (ADLs) related to health and independence. These functional impairments lead to older adults requiring not only medical care but also other types of long-term services and supports. The healthcare system on which older populations rely therefore includes not only medical services, but also social services that address long-term functional needs.

## Fundamentals of Public Funding of Healthcare for Older Adults

Beginning in the 1930s and through the 1960s, the financial challenges facing older adults and their access to medical care were important policy issues. After several prior efforts and lengthy national debate, the Social Security Act with Titles XVIII and XIX were passed in 1965, which established the Medicare and Medicaid programs. Another less well known 1965 legislation established the Older Americans Act (OAA), the objective of which is to be the vehicle for organizing, coordinating, and providing community-based services for older adults. The OAA led to the creation of the Administration on Aging (AoA). Then in 1975, Title XX of the Social Security Act was enacted as a mechanism for providing block grants to states to support social services, including social justice programs for children and elders. Subsequently, several laws have made revisions to the components of the healthcare and social service systems affecting older adults. Most recently, the Patient Protection and Affordable Care Act (ACA) signed into law in 2010 aimed to improve coverage of the uninsured through the expansion of Medicaid and the value of care by introducing new payment models with incentives for better coordination and quality of care. The ACA did not make changes to the underlying structures of Medicare and Medicaid.

These funding streams as set by law define how we typically categorize services for older adults. Federal, state, and local governments provide the funding and infrastructure for community resources that make housing, food, and transportation accessible and affordable. Acute medical services are primarily covered by Medicare, with some older adults also having private insurance,

Medicaid, or Veterans Health Administration benefits. Long-term care, often referenced as long-term services and supports, includes a broad array of services that are not covered by Medicare. Long-term care is funded through various sources, although mostly out-of-pocket payment unless the individual has purchased private long-term care insurance or is Medicaid-eligible, because Medicaid covers both acute and long-term care.

◆◆ **The Older Americans Act and the Social Services Block Grant program are the two leading federal sources of funding for social or community-based programs that facilitate older adults' ability to remain in the community and in their homes for as long as possible.**

## Financing the Healthcare System

### Community-Based Services

In addition to medical care, many other services are available to support the health and wellbeing of older adults. First among these are the services to make housing, food, and transportation accessible and affordable and to protect vulnerable populations from exploitation or abuse. The OAA and the Social Services Block Grant program are the two leading federal sources of funding for these programs. In the Social Services Block Grant program (Title XX), states are given discretion for using the funds for social programs that prevent, reduce, or eliminate dependency, neglect, or abuse and assure appropriate referral to institutional or home-based services. The OAA has a number of different provisions that are implemented mostly through the AoA.

The AoA funding spans four areas—health and independence, caregiving services, protection of vulnerable older adults, and consumer information access and outreach. In 2019 the AoA budget was $2.1 billion, 44% of which went to nutrition programs, 19% to community-based supportive services, and 9% to family caregiver services.[2]

Operationally, AoA has created a network of Area Agencies on Aging (AAA), and state or tribal agencies that organize and deliver the services locally. These agency programs include Meals on Wheels, congregate meals, adult day service, and adult protective services, as well as legal and elder abuse services. The common denominator among the programs is that they facilitate older adults' ability to remain in the community and in their homes for as long as possible by providing social supports, while avoiding exploitation. Locating these services can be daunting but online resources, such as the Eldercare Locator, maintained by the Department of Health and Human Services (www.eldercare.acl.gov) are helpful (Fig. 9.1).

### CASE 1

#### Jacob Miller (Part 2)

Unfortunately, Mr. Miller falls in the bathroom in spite of the current efforts to keep him safe at home. You learn that he has been evaluated in the emergency room and sent home with narcotics for back pain. Now that he is home, he is afraid of falling again and because of pain is not able to get out of the house on his own. His daughter brings him to your office for follow-up. Investigating the cause of the fall, you find out that Mr. Miller has been feeling dizzy lately and his blood pressure while sitting is 120/80 mmHg but drops to 110/65 mmHg with symptoms of dizziness when he

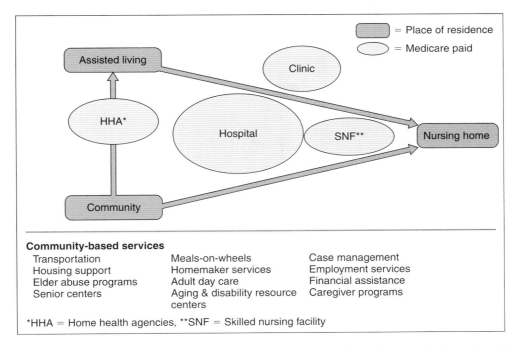

• **Figure 9.1** Overview of acute care, residential, and community-based services that make up the healthcare system for older adults.

stands. After a complete medical evaluation, you decide that he needs to have his blood pressure medications changed and the narcotics will have to be reduced as his pain improves.

What additional services can Mr. Miller receive in this new situation?

## Federal Insurance Coverage for Older Americans

Federal spending on healthcare for older adults includes funding from Medicare, Medicaid, the Administration on Aging, the Social Services Block Grant program, and the Veterans Health Administration (Table 9.1). Since enactment in 1965, Medicare and Medicaid have undergone continual changes in the details of the programs but their fundamental structures have remained the same. Medicare is an entitlement program established to cover the acute care needs of people who have reached the age of 65 years (or younger people who have end-stage renal disease or amyotrophic lateral sclerosis or receive Social Security Disability Insurance [SSDI] payments). As an entitlement, Medicare is available to everyone age ≥ 65 years who has paid Medicare payroll taxes for at least 10 years in his or her lifetime (or whose spouse has) regardless of income or ability to pay. Medicaid, in contrast, was established to provide coverage for people who have insufficient income to pay for services whether because of poverty or a disabling condition that limits ability to work.

The funding sources of Medicare and Medicaid are quite different. Medicare is paid for through two trust funds: The Hospital Insurance Trust (HI) fund, which pays for the majority of Part A spending, is financed primarily through a dedicated payroll tax paid by employers and their employees and collected by the federal government. Part A services include inpatient hospital care, skilled

nursing facility care, home healthcare, and hospice. The Supplemental Medical Insurance (SMI) Trust Fund pays for Medicare Part B and Part D services; this fund is supported through general federal tax revenues and by beneficiaries who pay a monthly premium. Part B covers physician services, outpatient hospital care, some home healthcare, preventive services and lab tests, and durable medical equipment; Part D is the prescription drug benefit. There is also Medicare Part C, called Medicare Advantage, a managed care option offered through private insurance companies that provide all Parts A and B and typically Part D coverage. Part C is not separately financed; its financing is obtained from the two trust funds and from the monthly standard Part B premium (and, for some beneficiaries, an additional premium required by their Part C plan). In summary, Medicare is paid by federal payroll taxes, general federal revenues, and premiums, deductibles, and copayments from patients.

◆◆ **Medicare is an entitlement program that is available to everyone age > 65 years who has paid payroll tax in his or her lifetime (or whose spouse has).**

Medicaid is jointly funded by the federal and state governments to provide acute and long-term care to low-income Americans. Because Medicaid was created to cover low-income individuals, the contributions made by patients are much lower, although there are some copayments. Federal law stipulates program eligibility for some populations (elderly or disabled beneficiaries, children, pregnant women, some parents, and working disabled) with incomes and assets below specified cutoffs. Historically, the federal government has reimbursed states a specified percentage of Medicaid program expenditures for these designated beneficiaries under a matching formula. States may opt to cover additional populations and to increase the income cutoffs for Medicaid eligibility. Many of the policy debates that arise with Medicaid revolve around state

| TABLE 9.1 | Summary of Federal Spending and Eligibility on Healthcare for Older Adults | |
|---|---|---|
| **Program** | **2019 Budget (Dollars) (Percent of HHS Total)** | **Eligible Elderly Population (Percent of Total Users Elderly)** |
| Dept. of Health and Human Services (HHS) | 1,216.0 billion (100%) | |
| Medicare | 629.8 billion (52%) | Age 65 years and paid payroll tax 10 years or disabled receiving Social Security Disability support (85%) |
| Medicaid | 412.0 billion (34%) | Low-income and certain populations (children, pregnant women, disabled, aged) (10%) |
| Administration on Aging | 2.1 billion (0.2%) | Age >65 years (100%) |
| Social Services Block Grants | 307 million (0.2%) | Determined by state |
| Veterans Health Administration | 80 billion (36% of Dept. of Veterans Affairs budget) | Veterans |

budgetary constraints and efforts to control costs through changes in coverage rules. Medicaid is particularly important for primary care geriatrics because so many elderly nursing home residents ultimately spend down their assets to qualify for Medicaid and transition to dependence on Medicaid for payment of their long-term care services. In fact, 30% of Medicaid's spending is directed toward long-term care and although older adults and disabled make up only 23% of beneficiaries, they account for 64% of total Medicaid spending.[3]

❖ **Medicaid was established to provide health insurance coverage for people who have insufficient income to pay for services, whether because of poverty or a disabling condition that limits ability to work.**

## Veterans Health Administration

The Veterans Health Administration (VHA) is a large integrated health system that provides acute care, social services, and long-term care to 6 million veterans a year (with 9 million eligible) with a budget of nearly $80 billion per year funded by the Department of Veterans Affairs. In 2017 the average age of VHA beneficiaries was 61 years. The VHA has been a leader in developing the geriatrics workforce and conducting aging-related clinical research. Their medical centers and outpatient clinics offer acute care, geriatric assessment, home-based primary care, caregiver support, and nursing and community-based care options. Eligibility for VHA care is determined by whether the individual has service-connected disabilities.

❖ **The Veterans Health Administration offers elderly veterans geriatric assessment, home-based primary care, caregiver support, and nursing and community-based care options in addition to acute care.**

## Patient's Perspective on Payment for Healthcare

From the perspective of the patients, the array of coverage and funding streams does not necessarily align with their experience of healthcare, which may lead to confusion. For example, a single home care agency may provide a physical therapist in the home after a hip fracture but also provide a long-term homemaker. The therapy is paid by Medicare as an acute service but a long-term homemaker would be an out-of-pocket expense or covered by Medicaid (if the patient is eligible). Similarly, a nursing home may provide on the same hallway both postacute rehabilitation services (skilled nursing facility level of care) paid by Medicare and long-term residence for those with chronic, severe impairment, which may be paid by Medicaid, private insurance, or out of pocket. Understanding the scope of services within and across care settings paid for by each funder is important for advance care and financial planning (Fig. 9.2).

Older adults who are still working at age 65 years need to clarify how their employer's insurance works with Medicare. Most older adults, even those that are employed, are enrolled in Medicare Part A when they turn age 65 years because it is usually premium free. However, if the employer's coverage meets Medicare standards, delaying Part B and Part D enrollment may be possible, saving the costs of these premiums. Although there are financial penalties for delaying enrollment in Part B and Part D for individuals turning 65 years of age, these are waived if the employer's coverage meets Medicare standards.

## Acute Care

### Medicare Part A

**Hospitalization.** Medicare covers any medically necessary hospitalizations, with the hospital receiving a prospective payment based on a determination of the average expected cost of the stay for a specific diagnosis (called a Diagnosis-Related Group [DRG]—adjusted reimbursement), and a $1364 deductible (as of 2019) that the patient pays. Note that any physician visit made to a patient during a hospitalization is billed under Part B, so the patient pays 20% of each physician visit as a coinsurance payment. Tests, laboratories, and medications are included in the DRG-adjusted reimbursement. Some hospitals use "observation" status to keep a patient in the hospital as an outpatient, while determining if full hospitalization is needed. These stays are billed under Part B and the patient pays

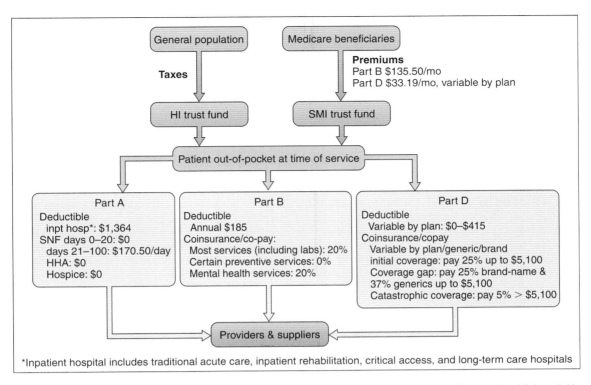

• **Figure 9.2** Medicare beneficiary out-of-pocket expenditures for Medicare services in 2019. *HHA*, Home health agencies; *HI*, hospital insurance; *SMI*, supplemental medical insurance; *SNF*, skilled nursing facility.

20% of the stay and will not be eligible for a posthospitalization skilled nursing facility stay.

**Postacute rehabilitation.** After hospitalization, many patients benefit from a period of rehabilitation before going home. Inpatient rehabilitation hospitals accept patients with certain diagnoses who are able to participate in 3 hours of rehabilitation per day. These stays are paid similarly to acute hospital stays. Skilled nursing facilities (SNFs) also deliver postacute rehabilitation as a separate service line in a facility that also delivers long-term care. SNFs are also paid under a prospective payment system similar to the hospitals. After a qualifying 3-day hospital stay, the patient incurs no cost for the first 20 days, but patients pay a daily rate ($170.50, as of 2019) for days 21 to 100, after which the Medicare benefit expires and patients pay for all costs. The covered length of stay in a SNF is dependent on the patient's medical stability and progress in rehabilitation therapies. A stable patient whose therapy progress has reached a plateau will no longer receive Medicare coverage for care in a SNF, even if he or she has not reached the 100-day limit.

**Home healthcare.** For patients who are certified as being homebound by a doctor, Medicare-reimbursed home healthcare agencies provide nursing visits; physical, occupational, or speech therapy; social work; and intermittent home health aide services for up to 60 days without any out-of-pocket charge to patients. These services must be ordered by a clinician to serve a medically necessary need, such as rehabilitation after a hospitalization, monitoring blood pressure, or pain response with new medications, or to provide home safety evaluation or therapy after a fall. Home healthcare does not cover homemaker services, such as shopping, cleaning, or laundry.

**Hospice.** The hospice benefit is also provided at no cost to the patient except for a small copayment for prescriptions and a 5% coinsurance for inpatient respite stays. When enrolling in hospice, two clinicians certify that life expectancy is less than 6 months and the patient agrees to forego curative treatment for his or her terminal illness but retains coverage for nonterminal conditions. Effective January 2016, Centers for Medicare and Medicaid Services (CMS) began reimbursing physicians for advance care planning discussions with patients.

**Durable medical equipment (DME).** Many health conditions or impaired-function states require supplies, devices, or equipment for management. Medicare covers these DME products with a 20% coinsurance requirement. Diabetic supplies are obtained through this benefit, as well as wheelchairs and mobility devices, but they require certification by a clinician that they are medically necessary.

### Medicare Part B

Medicare Part B covers professional fees (visits to clinicians), as well as services that occur on an outpatient basis. Physician services are billed using Common Procedural Terminology codes familiar to all practicing clinicians and paid according to the Resource-Based Relative Value Scale (RBRVS), which attaches a dollar amount to each service delivered. This system applies for both inpatient and outpatient visits and the patient is responsible for 20% of the bill. Outpatient hospital services, such as ambulatory surgery, same-day procedures, laboratory tests, and diagnostic tests, are also subject to the 20% coinsurance. Changes introduced under ACA have reduced patient payment responsibility: certain preventive services (such as the welcome to Medicare visit, Annual Wellness Visit, and screenings) are now free to patients.

Outpatient mental health services that previously had a 40% coinsurance have now been reduced to 20%, similar to other physician services. In 2019 the annual premium for Part B is set at $135.50 per month or around $1600 annually for most beneficiaries.

◆ **Medicare Part B provides coverage of professional fees (such as visits to physicians), as well as services that occur on an outpatient basis and requires older adults to pay a monthly premium plus a 20% copayment.**

### Medicare Part D

Beginning in 2006 under the Medicare Modernization Act, a prescription benefit was added to Medicare. Individuals have the option of enrolling with independent prescription drug plans (PDPs) to which they pay premiums, coinsurance, and copayments. Although the federal government pays for Part D, the administration of each PDP is separate, leading to many plan options and choices for patients; this complexity has led to a great deal of confusion. Part D was designed to limit out-of-pocket expenditures by providing coverage up to a limit of drug spending but then started covering again once the drug cost reached what is called a catastrophic level. This gap in coverage, which was experienced by nearly one-third of all Part D enrollees in the first year of the drug benefit, became known as the donut hole. Provisions in the ACA aimed to phase out the donut hole coverage gap over time. The coverage gap begins after the beneficiary and the drug plan have spent a certain amount for covered drugs. In 2019 the beneficiaries entered the coverage gap when they spent $3820 on covered drugs ($4020 in 2020). Starting in 2019, once Part D plan beneficiaries reached the coverage gap, they paid no more than 25% of the plan's cost for covered brand-name prescription drugs. Some plans may offer higher savings in the coverage gap. In 2019 Medicare paid 63% of the price for generic drugs during the coverage gap, and for 2020 and beyond, Medicare will pay 75% of the price. In 2019 Part D catastrophic coverage began when the beneficiary spent $5100 out of pocket ($6350 in 2020). Once beneficiaries leave the coverage gap, they automatically have "catastrophic coverage." Individuals only pay a small coinsurance amount or copayment for covered drugs for the rest of the year.

### Medicare Advantage (Part C)

In 1981 Medicare created an alternative to the traditional fee-for-service Parts A and B plans to allow beneficiaries to participate voluntarily in managed care, under a program later renamed Medicare Advantage (MA). In these plans Medicare pays an organization (e.g., a health maintenance organization, a preferred provider organization), usually organized by a private insurance company, a risk-adjusted sum per member per month to cover all of the Medicare-reimbursed services for enrolled beneficiaries. The federal government current per-member per-month payments to insurance companies are generous, resulting in good benefits (often including preventive dental care, vision, and hearing assistance coverage), making MA popular with many older adults. These plans usually integrate Part D prescription benefit coverage into their benefits. By 2018 about 34% of Medicare beneficiaries were in MA plans. MA plans are organized in specific geographic areas by county. More than one MA plan may be offered in a single area, resulting in competition among plans. Plans may not be available in all areas, especially in rural counties. Evaluation of the MA payment mechanisms demonstrated that plans were being paid disproportionately higher than the cost of providing similar services

under traditional Medicare. Reducing this differential was one of the cost-saving mechanisms in the ACA.

### Secondary Payers

Even after paying for Medicare premiums, patient cost-sharing (deductibles, coinsurance, and copayments) can impose significant financial burdens for older adults. In 2016 more than one-quarter of Medicare beneficiaries spent at least 20% of their incomes on premiums plus cost-sharing, with total out-of-pocket costs averaging over $3000; these costs are particularly burdensome for low-income older adults.[4] About one-quarter of beneficiaries enrolled in traditional Medicare choose to buy additional coverage through private insurance called Medigap plans that pay this additional cost-sharing and may offer additional coverage. Although annual premiums for Medigap plans are costly (averaging $2000 in 2016), patients may feel they are worth the cost if they expect to have extensive use of medical services (for instance, a hospital stay with a deductible of $1300). There are 10 standardized plan options and a multitude of vendors from which to choose, and plans vary in terms of their "wraparound" coverage of cost sharing. Also, some large employers provide Medigap coverage to their retirees. For low-income older adults, Medicaid serves a similar purpose as Medigap, covering what Medicare does not. Those individuals, labeled "dual eligible beneficiaries," can get help with out-of-pocket costs (premiums and cost-sharing) with the amount of coverage depending on individuals' incomes, state-specific resources criteria, and whether individuals are enrolled in Part A and B.

---

**CASE 1**

**Jacob Miller (Part 3)**

Mr. Miller, like many people older than 80 years, lives alone and likely could benefit from socialization and the intermittent monitoring that attending a senior center can bring. You can advise that the daughter contact the local Area Agency on Aging to find out what local senior centers and transportation are available. In addition, you can order a home safety evaluation under the Medicare home health benefit at no cost to him. A one-time home safety evaluation is available to all Medicare beneficiaries whether they are homebound or not.

After the fall, however, he would meet the criteria of being homebound and can receive nursing (for medication management) and physical therapy (for gait management) in the home. At this point, it would be advisable also to have a social work evaluation to determine if other types of supportive services, such as Meals-on-Wheels, are now indicated to keep him in his home.

---

## Long-Term Services and Supports

Unfortunately, some individuals require supports, such as daily supervision or assistance with their ADLs, that cannot be provided solely by family and friends. Today, these people have more options about how to receive their care, whether in a facility or while remaining in their home. Families and clinicians, however, are sometimes caught unaware that older patients will be responsible for these costs. Long-term services and supports are not covered by Medicare or traditional insurance plans, and the costs are high. Some people believe that in-home caregiving would be a less expensive alternative, but when 24-hour care or nursing care is needed the costs are equivalent (Table 9.2 compares the cost of various long-term care services). Medicaid, unlike Medicare, covers

| TABLE 9.2 | Median Cost for Long-Term Care Services in the United States in 2018 | |
| --- | --- | --- |
| Service | Description | Estimated Annual Expense |
| **Home** | | |
| Homemaker Services (licensed)—provides "hands-off" care, such as helping with cooking and errands. Also called personal care or companions | National median hourly rate: $21 | 15 hours/week × 52 weeks per year = $16,380 |
| Home Health Aide Services (licensed)—provides "hands-on" personal care but not medical care in home, such as help with bathing, dressing, and transferring | National median hourly rate: $22 | 15 hours/week × 52 weeks per year = $17,160 |
| **Community** | | |
| Adult Day Healthcare—provides social and other support services in a community-based protective setting during part of the day | National median daily rate: $72 | 250 business days per year = $18,000 |
| **Facility** | | |
| Assisted Living (one-bedroom, single occupancy)— provides "hands-on" personal care and some medical care for people who cannot live alone but do not need a nursing home | National median monthly rate: $4000 | 12 months per year = $48,000 |
| Nursing Home (semiprivate room)—provides 24-hour skilled nursing support | National median daily rate: $245 | 365 days per year = $89,425 |
| Nursing Home (private room)—provides 24-hour skilled nursing support | National median daily rate: $275 | 365 days per year = $100,375 |

(Modified from Genworth Companies. Genworth 2018 cost of care survey. Available at https://www.genworth.com/aging-and-you/finances/cost-of-care.html)

long-term services and supports; however, this coverage is restricted to low-income older adults with extremely limited resources (<$2000 in assets). Even although eligibility is limited, states have been creating new approaches for providing community-based, in-home services in an effort to offer an alternative to costly long-term nursing home placement.

---

### CASE 1

**Jacob Miller (Part 4)**

You meet with Mr. Miller 4 years later. He did quite well with in-home services for several years. Lately, however, he has been declining, with continued falls, weight loss, and seeming to make multiple medication errors. Your thorough evaluation reveals that he has developed dementia. He was planning to move in with his daughter, but unfortunately he had a stroke before the move could occur. He is now in the hospital with significant functional impairments, including an inability to swallow and cognition difficulties. His caring daughter asks for your advice about the options for rehabilitation and long-term care. She is particularly concerned because she works full time and cannot provide the ADLs needed, and after several years of in-home care the finances are very tight.
1. What type of postacute rehabilitation (home-based, inpatient rehabilitation, or skilled nursing facility) would Mr. Miller be eligible for and what would the cost implications be of each of these?
2. How many days of coverage would he receive under his Medicare benefit for rehabilitation?
3. At the end of the Medicare coverage, what is the likely course for Mr. Miller's long-term care?

## Residential Services

### Nursing Home

Residence in a nursing home is an experience faced nearly entirely by older adults. Some 84% of nursing home residents are older than 65 years. Yet only approximately 4% of the elderly population resides in nursing homes and a smaller percentage in assisted living. Nursing homes provide 24-hour supervision and nursing care for people who have ADL impairments, such as difficulties with bathing, dressing, feeding, and toileting, or who have behavioral or cognitive issues that preclude safe community residence. Traditional nursing homes are organized like hospitals but innovative efforts, such as those implementing the Greenhouse Model, which uses small, residential-style homes in community neighborhoods, attempt to bring in homelike features.

Many people enter nursing homes after a 3-day hospital stay so that Medicare will pay up to the first 100 days for postacute rehabilitation. If the person stays beyond eligibility for Medicare postacute services, however, payment becomes the individual's responsibility. When an older adult stays long enough to use nearly all of his or her own assets (a home can be protected if a spouse is still living in it), then the person can apply for Medicaid; however, each state has different criteria for Medicaid spend-down eligibility, so rules will vary considerably by state.

### Assisted Living

For people who are less impaired and can still live in their own space given adequate supervision, assisted living is an option. Assisted living facilities are highly variable in the services provided (and variable in state-level regulation) but typically have at least one nurse on duty for 24 hours a day and provide housekeeping, meals, medication dispensing, and (for extra fees) assistance with ADLs. Many state Medicaid programs provide some coverage for assisted living, but it can be challenging to obtain information about or coverage for these types of assistance.

### Continuing Care Retirement Community

Continuing care retirement communities (CCRCs) are a newer option that offers older adults residential care over their remaining life span as they move from independent living to assisted living and to nursing home care within a single community. Typically, members pay large entrance fees followed by monthly fees, although financing models vary widely. Entrance fees can range from $100,000 to $1,000,000, with monthly fees ranging from $3000 to $5000.[5]

### Other Types of Residential Care

There are residential care alternatives, such as board and care homes, and some states have adult foster care programs. These types of residential care programs should not be confused with senior housing, which is subsidized but does not necessarily include any additional medical or social service support.

## Home-Based Services

### Privately Hired Services

Many people who stay in their homes privately hire homemakers, nursing assistants, and even nurses in the home. These services are typically charged on an hourly basis so the cost depends on the needs of the individual. Companies have emerged that manage a staff of caregivers so that individuals can access trained and vetted caregivers by the hour. These companies are separate from the home health agencies that provide Medicare and Medicaid home care services. As previously noted, for short periods Medicare does pay for these home healthcare services for patients who are considered homebound but not as a long-term care management strategy.

### Medicaid Waiver Programs

States are increasingly investing their Medicaid dollars into home- and community-based care programs that allow Medicaid recipients to receive long-term care services outside of institutional settings. Being in the community is usually preferred by patients and is typically less expensive for the states. Many examples and innovative programs are developing in the United States. The Program for All Inclusive Care (PACE) began as a waiver program and is now available across the country. In PACE, people who are eligible for nursing home level of care can opt to enter a PACE program that combines their Medicare and Medicaid benefits to provide care that is centered on a day-hospital model with robust community support and care coordination. The PACE provider takes on the financial risk for both the acute and long-term care of the participant. To "rebalance" spending to direct a greater proportion of Medicaid dollars toward home and community-based services as opposed to costly institutionalization, many states have applied for Medicaid waivers to broaden the long-term services and supports that are available; these services can include homemaker, home health aide, adult day healthcare, and respite care services that can support older adults and their family caregivers and are not typically available under Medicare and traditional Medicaid.

## Changing Landscape of Organization and Finance of Healthcare

Among the most sweeping changes in the ACA were those that served to broaden coverage of the uninsured through an expansion of Medicaid and those that precluded use of preexisting condition clauses for insurance policies. These efforts to cover the uninsured had little direct impact on Medicare beneficiaries. However, there were several key elements of the law that affected older adults.

There are two main themes that cut across most of the new payment models rolled out after the ACA: a focus on reimbursing providers for quality not just quantity of services and developing reimbursement strategies that encourage care coordination. In traditional fee-for-service (FFS), healthcare providers are paid for a service whether performed well or not. A common example is the high number of hospital readmissions within 30 days of a hospital discharge under the Medicare program. Under FFS, the hospital would simply be paid for both hospitalizations, limiting the financial incentive to prevent readmission. One innovation to address this issue is to pay with a "bundle" that includes the entire episode (the hospitalization and a period after). Hospitals will have higher margins if the readmission rate is low, and there are several initiatives to improve providers' ability to manage care transitions clinically.

Better care coordination is seen as an opportunity to improve management of the complex, chronically ill patients who account for a large portion of spending. The primary care initiatives are finding new ways to pay primary care providers for the out-of-visit work that care coordination requires. The accountable care organization (ACO) combines both themes by rewarding providers who hit thresholds of quality while reducing their costs, but the ACO can do so only if the clinicians work together across all settings because the ACOs are accountable for the total costs of care, not only those in one setting.

Further, the changing landscape of healthcare includes a focus on vulnerable populations who might most benefit from improvements in coordinated care. These include the approximately 11 million older adults who are dually eligible for Medicare and Medicaid, or dual eligibles. Although they represent just 20% of the Medicare and 15% of the Medicaid populations, they account for 30% and 40% of those respective programs' spending. Coordinating care and reducing costs for this population is complicated by the complexity of aligning differing benefit, payment, and administrative designs in Medicare and Medicaid. The ACA created the Medicare-Medicaid Coordination Office and tasked it with improving access to high-quality and cost-effective care. More recently, CMS introduced a large-scale financial alignment demonstration project using an ACO model to target quality of care and spending for the dual eligible population.

## Summary

The United States has a complex array of federal, state, and local programs to support the medical care and social needs of older adults. Navigating these programs is challenging and costly for patients, their families, and providers, imposing financial and other resource burdens. There are significant and concerning gaps in coverage for long-term services and supports under Medicare, and restrictive eligibility criteria for coverage of these services available under Medicaid. As the population ages, requiring better approaches to providing high-value care, new legislation to address the long-term costs of Medicare and Medicaid is expected in the coming years.

### Web Resources

Administration on Aging, Eldercare Locator: www.eldercare.acl. gov.

Kaiser Family Foundation: www.kff.org.

Medicare & You 2019: https://www.medicare.gov/sites/default/ files/2018-09/10050-medicare-and-you.pdf.

MedPAC: Medicare and Payment Basics: www.medpac.gov/ payment_basics.cfm.

## Key References

1. Administration on Aging. *2018 Profile of Older Americans.* Available at: https://acl.gov/sites/default/files/Aging%20and% 20Disability%20in%20America/2018OlderAmericansProfile. pdf. Accessed July 22, 2019.
2. Congressional Research Service. *Older Americans Act: Overview and Funding.* November 14, 2018. Available at: https://www.everycrsreport.com/files/20181114_R43414_ a56f21f163603a64b9976dda14e0adef4a8027ef.pdf. Accessed August 19, 2019.

**References available online at expertconsult.com.**

# 10

# Billing and Coding

PETER A. HOLLMANN

## OUTLINE

*Additional online-only material indicated by icon.*

## OBJECTIVES

*Upon completion of this chapter, the reader will be able to:*

- Understand the relevant coding systems for billing: ICD, CPT, HCPCS Level II.
- Understand that coding and billing rules may vary based on benefits and payer.

- Understand the structure of evaluation and management codes in CPT and the Centers for Medicare and Medicaid Services (CMS) documentation guidelines.

Whether you are in solo practice, pay all your own practice expenses, and earn only what you bill, or whether you are an employee of a large group or institution, you are generating income based on billing. Although there are some payment methods that are not fee-for-service systems, most medical care provided by professionals in the United States is paid for using a fee-for-service payment methodology. This means you, or someone on your behalf, is submitting a bill to the patient or insurance company (including Medicare) for the services you perform. Because it is a fee-for-service system, you will need to state the name of the service you performed and your charge for that service. An orderly payment system requires a set of rules so that you are aware of your required behavior and the payers are aware of their requirements. The first rule of order is that there is a nomenclature system for every service. Use of this system is referred to as coding.

The rules of coverage, payment, coding, and billing can seem daunting. Further stress is added by the knowledge that your livelihood may be on the line or that billing performed incorrectly can have adverse legal and financial repercussions. If you do not bill personally, you are still responsible for the work of your agents. Try to remember that if you are able to care effectively for the complex geriatric patient, you have more than adequate brain power to handle billing and coding processes. As with patient care, a team approach is useful. When available, seek out the expertise of people who regularly perform billing functions.

This chapter is not intended to be a treatise on all important aspects of practice management and does not include topics such as when to refer patients to a collections agent for unpaid bills, accounting methods for tracking accounts receivables, or claims appeals. Nor will the chapter explain details of payment systems and delivery systems, such as capitation and accountable care organizations, even though the type of system may affect coding and billing practices. However, the chapter is intended to provide a solid foundation and educational resources for issues related to billing and coding.

## Coding Systems

There are three key coding systems. The first is the diagnostic classification system known as International Classification of Diseases, Clinical Modification (commonly called ICD-10). The World Health Organization creates ICD versions, but the clinical modifications are from the US National Center for Health Statistics; thus ICD-CM versions do vary by country. ICD also includes ICD-PCS, a procedural code set. Hospitals use ICD-PCS for inpatient procedure coding, but professionals use the American Medical Association's Current Procedural Terminology (CPT) and the Centers for Medicare and Medicaid's Healthcare Common Procedure Coding System, Level II (known as HCPCS). Hospitals also use CPT and HCPCS for outpatient procedure reporting.

CPT is the backbone of professional procedure reporting, but HCPCS is used to supplement CPT because CPT does not maintain codes for all items, such as a drug or device (e.g., durable medical equipment) classification system; also, Medicare may need codes that are very specific to its benefits as defined in law. Unfortunately, none of the systems use the terminology that clinicians use when communicating with each other in conversation. With the advent of electronic records, problem lists are now in "ICD speak" and finding the official term for a condition can be frustrating at times. Fortunately, few medical professionals will need to memorize the entire coding lexicon; the key is to understand and be familiar with high-volume codes.

ICD is organized by types of diseases (e.g., infection, cancer, cardiovascular) and has codes for symptoms or reasons for an encounter that are not diagnoses (e.g., Z00.00 is the diagnosis code for a routine general medical examination, and R06.00 is the code for dyspnea, unspecified). CPT is arranged by major categories and then subdivided by body system and anatomically. Major sections are evaluation and management (the office and facility visits often called cognitive services), anesthesia, surgery, radiology, pathology and laboratory, and medicine. The last category is a broad mix of services and includes diagnostic tests, such as electrocardiograms and codes for immunization administration and the vaccine itself. Evaluation and management services, commonly referred to as E and M (or E/M), are usually the bulk of services performed by geriatric providers who may report them. Physicians, nurse practitioners, clinical nurse specialists, and physician assistants may use E/M, but physical therapists and nutritionists have their own evaluation, assessment, and treatment codes in the medicine section. The medicine section also includes the procedures used by mental health professionals, whether physician or nonphysician, and includes psychological testing codes.

All sections are relevant to professionals and it is important to gain familiarity with the range of codes. For example, although a bladder volume scan is not technically imaging and is certainly not surgery, it is in the urodynamics subsection of CPT, which is within the surgery/urinary system section. If a code for a common service cannot be located, one should not conclude that a code does not exist; it is more likely that one needs to look harder to locate it. However, there are some important exceptions. For example, removing sutures that were placed by a clinician from another practice would be considered E/M; there is no suture removal code (unless performed under anesthesia). A mental status examination is part of the physical examination of E/M, and not in the neuropsychological testing sections. HCPCS codes are used for drugs administered, such as for a steroid injection into a joint. Medicare also uses HCPCS codes for specific benefits. For example, an influenza shot administration has CPT codes, but Medicare requires that HCPCS G code G0008 is reported. This is because the CPT administration code is agnostic to the vaccine given and not all vaccines are covered by Medicare (outside of the Medicare Part D drug benefit). It is strongly advised that all medical professionals maintain access to current editions of these coding resources. CPT changes annually and HCPCS changes quarterly.

◈ **Keep up to date with annual changes to procedure coding and Medicare benefits.**

## Knowing Payer, Benefits, Medicare Contractor, Specialty/Licensure, and Group Rules

Geriatrics professionals tend to think traditional Medicare. However, there are Medicare Advantage plans (Medicare Part C) and many retirees have "commercial" insurance. Others age > 65 years are eligible for Medicare but are still working and maintain coverage from their employer. Commercial insurance is employer-based insurance. These payers may cover more than Medicare or require participating providers to report services differently. This is usually because of benefits differences (i.e., what is covered by the plan). Generally speaking, all payers follow the same basic coding rules. The most common example of variation can be seen with the annual physical. Even with the Medicare Wellness Visit benefit, there is no annual physical per se and for years, a major point of differentiation for Part C plans was coverage of preventive services that Medicare did not cover. A commercial plan and some Medicare Advantage will typically require use of the CPT Comprehensive Preventive Medicine services codes such as 99397 to report the comprehensive preventative service, commonly referred to as the annual physical. This code will be denied when submitted to traditional Medicare. However, so much of this service is covered as part of the Annual Wellness Visit that, practically speaking, it is not truly a noncovered service where one may charge the beneficiary directly.

Medicare Part B, the part that covers professional services, is administered by multiple contractors (companies Medicare pays to process claims and enforce rules). The rules of different contractors tend to be consistent, but in some cases where national rules have not been promulgated or there is potential for variable interpretation, there can be differences. Even if the policies are the same, enforcement may be divergent. These disparities can occur in some high-volume services. A contractor may define E/M medical decision-making level of complexity as requiring a change in the medication regimen, whereas another may not have such a requirement. The contractor's website is a good source of information concerning these issues.

A healthcare professional's specialty or license type will dictate both coding and coverage rules. For example, physical therapists and physicians in most cases will not be using the same codes. Physicians may specify E/M whereas the physical therapists uses 97161–97164 for their assessments. However, a physician who performs a timed "get up and go" test may meet criteria to report it as a physical performance test 97750 if it takes at least 8 minutes and a separate report is created; otherwise the test is considered to be part of a physical examination. In mental health coding, there is a great deal of overlap between the various professions. At times very similar services are reported differently by different professions. Physicians do not report the CPT medical nutrition therapy services when counseling a patient on obesity; they report E/M as specified in CPT guidelines, and for certain patients in Medicare, physicians may use G codes for intensive behavioral therapy for obesity. Specialty type as well as license type is relevant. In E/M, a new patient is one who has not received a reported face-to-face service from a professional in the exact same specialty and subspecialty within the same group. Therefore if an internist refers a patient to a geriatrician within his or her group for an opinion or assistance in management and a joint medical record is used, the patient is nonetheless a new patient to that geriatrician; this means that a new patient E/M code is used as compared with the established patient code. However, if the geriatrician sees the internist's patient in the role as covering physician in the office, the geriatrician is acting on behalf of his or her colleague and the patient is therefore considered an established patient. It is important to be aware of the different specialty classification listings by payer and to be aware of Taxpayer Identification numbers and National Provider Identification (NPI) numbers that define groups, if you are in a group and billing. Some professionals may be in multiple groups and must pay special attention to this. Be aware of all the details in how you are registered with any payer, which is usually addressed when originally signing a participation agreement (or in Medicare registering in PECOS, the Medicare provider enrollment, chain, and ownership system). Keep your information up to date.

## Claims, Claims Edits, and Modifiers

Billing usually means submitting a claim to a payer. The claims-processing systems use edits, although not all payers use the same edits. Edits are processing rules used by the claims system (i.e., a computer). Some edits are in place to prevent coding errors. For example, if two skin lesions are removed and the same procedure code is reported twice, it will be assumed this was an erroneous duplicate entry unless a modifier code is appended to the second procedure code to designate that two separate services were performed (i.e., that two skin lesions were removed). The most common modifier relevant to geriatrics professionals is modifier 25, which indicates that the E/M was distinct and not part of a simultaneously performed surgical service. For example, if a patient with osteoarthritis is seen for an intraarticular steroid injection and no significant separate assessment was performed, no E/M should be reported. However, if another condition was treated, or the patient required a distinct history and examination to determine that osteoarthritis was present and to determine if the injection was warranted, modifier 25 is appended to the E/M code.

Edits also exist for a medical necessity match for services, such as laboratory tests. A claim for a thyroid-stimulating hormone test may be paid if the diagnosis is hypothyroidism but denied for a diagnosis of migraine. The edit may determine the insurance coverage or patient cost sharing. A diagnosis code that designates a service as preventive may result in no patient cost sharing, whereas the same service with a different diagnosis may have cost sharing. Such is the case with lipid testing in Medicare. A unique example, but commonly performed scenario, is when Advance Care Planning is done with an annual wellness visit. Advance Care Planning usually has standard Part B cost sharing, but when provided at an annual wellness visit and submitted with modifier -33, there is no cost sharing. These claims-processing rules/edits have greater variability between different payers and are often the source of a bill not being paid as expected.

## Evaluation and Management Services

These are the most commonly performed services by geriatric physicians, advanced practice nurses (registered nurse practitioners [RNPs] and clinical nurse specialists [CNSs]) and physician assistants (PAs). The codes are divided by place of service with separate categories for office/clinic, hospital inpatient, hospital observation, nursing facility, emergency department, home, and domiciliary care facility. The last category is potentially a point of confusion because the designation of being a type of a facility or being home varies by state regulation. In some places an assisted living facility is a facility; in other places an assisted living facility is classified as a person's home by regulation. It is important to note that the place of service is where the patient was seen, so if a patient was brought from a nursing facility to the physician's office, the office visit codes are used. Some services are further divided by new or established patients. A new patient is one who has not had a face-to-face service with the provider, or with a member of the provider's group in the same subspecialty, within the past 3 years, even if the provider has a record on the patient and saw him or her 4 years earlier. This concept does not apply to certain types of E/M, such as inpatient and nursing facility services. In these locations, the applicable concepts are admission and follow-up. In 2018 a code specific to cognitive assessment and care planning services (CPT 99483) was created. It does not have the standard E/M structure. In 2013 Transitional Care Management codes were introduced and these are a visit plus care management for 30 days when a patient leaves the hospital or nursing home. These, too, are structured differently.

E/M codes have levels. Some types of services have five levels (e.g., established patient office visits), whereas other sites of care (e.g., hospital inpatient) may have only three levels. The level of E/M service is tied to how much one gets paid for the service. For example, a level-3 established patient office visit in Medicare in 2092 paid just over $75, and a level-4 visit paid just over $110. If a physician saw 15 level-4 patients a day but billed 15 level-3 visits and did that every day for a year of practice, the physician would have underbilled by more than $100,000. The physician's overhead would not have changed; therefore his or her take-home pay is reduced by the underbilled amount.

Getting the level correct presents the largest source of coding consternation. The rules have been viewed as unduly complex and with the advent of checklists in electronic records, the rules can be applied in a manner that is clinically irrelevant. For many years the levels of E/M in CPT have been determined by three key components: history, examination, and medical decision making. For reporting in 2021, CPT has simplified Office and Other Outpatient Visits to be based upon medical decision making or total time on the date of the encounter. Some services, such as a hospital inpatient admission, require that all three components be at a minimum level, whereas others, such as an established patient visit, require that two of three components be at a minimum level. CMS created documentation guidelines (DGs) to clarify its interpretation of CPT's key components. The DGs are structured in a manner to make an audit tool possible. Electronic record systems designers have picked up on this and have embedded these rules into some templates, so that the record system will suggest the code to report. Letting the record system do the E/M coding should be avoided. Even a coding professional can only go by your documentation and does not necessarily fully understand the medical decision making applied. However, having professionals who manage a compliance program review your coding is helpful.

◆◆ **The clinician that treats the patient best understands decision making and the code level to report.**

Only the treating clinician knows what history and examination elements were required (medically necessary) for the patient's problem, and only the clinician understands the true level of medical decision making. An absurd example of coding by DGs or by using a literal interpretation of CPT related to the two of three (history, examination, or medical decision making) requirement for an established patient. For example, if a physician did a careful and complete history and examination and documented it like a medical student would, then the 2/3 requirement is met. Why even consider the differential diagnoses, treatment options, and patient/caregiver counseling? The coding requirement has been met. Of course, it has not really been met because without medical decision making there is no context for what an appropriate history or examination is.

However, the DGs do offer some guidance and education on correct coding. CPT also has clinical examples in an appendix and notes typical times of E/M services. This can be very helpful. To some degree, E/M services are all relative (i.e., a physician can have his or her median visit in mind as a standard, code it carefully using DGs, and then code up or down from there depending on how the other visits measure against the standard). This works with one major caveat—what is a median service for a geriatrician may be a rare high level of complexity service for another practice type. Compare a day in a walk-in treatment center of evaluating minor complaints that really do not even require a physician's care with the typical patient schedule in a frail elderly practice. The "set point" for the walk-in clinic may be a level-2 office and for the geriatrician, a level-4 visit. Physicians also need to remember to code based on the service performed. Even complicated patients can have simple visits. There are three major problems for geriatrics with E/M: a ceiling effect, all services are face to face with the patient, and the code structure reflects the single problem acute care orientation that plagues too much of medical training and care delivery. The 2021 changes will improve this situation for a subset of E/M services.

## Documentation Guidelines and Current Procedural Terminology Definitions

CPT defines history and examinations with levels labeled "problem focused," "expanded problem focused," "detailed," and "comprehensive." Medical decision making is "straightforward," "low-complexity," "medium-complexity," or "high complexity." Medical decision making is composed of three components: (1) number of diagnoses or treatment options, (2) amount and/or complexity of data to be reviewed, and (3) risk of complications and/or morbidity or mortality. (Medical decision making is slightly modified for office visits in 2021.) There is additional detail in the E/M guidelines section of CPT. The history and examination descriptions do lend themselves to quantification based on the traditional parts of the history and examination; medical decision making does not lend itself to such simplistic quantification. However, clinicians can understand it. Straightforward decision making is the type of decision making that is largely irrelevant; the problem required reassurance at most as it is self-limited. High complexity decision making will typically be about high-risk decisions to treat or not to treat and involve consideration of lots of data or many diagnoses and treatment options. The CMS DGs were written in 1995 and modified in 1997 to allow for single system (specialty oriented)

examinations. CMS provides educational resources on DGs at www.cms.gov/Outreach-and-Education/Medicare-Learning-Network-MLN/MLNEdWebGuide/EMDOC.html. Medicare contractors created counting systems for medical decision making, but there is no national system as each contractor used slightly different criteria. A common service in geriatrics is 99214, an office visit for moderately complicated care of an established patient. Table 10.1 gives a summary of the 1997 rules for two levels of a history ("detailed" applies to 99214). Table 10.2 gives CMS examples of quantifying risk. Table 10.3 puts together the DGs into a cheat sheet to help one remember the components in a 99214. Because the CPT changes for 2021 only apply to office visits, these tables are still correct for home services or assisted living facility services at a level-4 established patient. An example of the type of patient that would warrant a 99214 is an 82-year-old female brought to the office by a family member. The patient has hypertension, is on an angiotensin-converting enzyme inhibitor, has

**TABLE 10.1  CMS 1997 Documentation Guidelines for History**

| History Extent | HPI | PFSH | ROS |
|---|---|---|---|
| Expanded Problem Focused | Brief | n/a | Problem Pertinent |
| Detailed | Extended | Pertinent | Extended |

- ROS and PFSH may be noted in HPI
- ROS and PFSH can be noted as "no changes"
- ROS and PFSH can be obtained on patient form if confirmed

| | |
|---|---|
| Brief HPI: | 1–3 elements[a] |
| Extended HPI: | 4 or more elements |
| Pertinent ROS: | the system directly related to the HPI |
| Extended ROS: | direct and limited number of additional systems (2–9) |

[a]Elements: location, quality, severity, duration, timing, context, modifying factors, associated signs/symptoms.
*HPI*, History of present illness; *PFSH*, past, family, and social history; *ROS*, review of systems.
(From Centers for Medicare and Medicaid Services. 1997 Documentation Guidelines for Evaluation and Management Services. Available at www.cms.gov/Outreach-and-Education/Medicare-Learning-Network-MLN/MLNEdWebGuide/Downloads/97Docguidelines.pdf.)

**TABLE 10.2  CMS Documentation Guidelines for Risk**

| Risk Level | Examples |
|---|---|
| Low | 2 or more self-limited |
| | 1 stable (e.g., HTN) |
| | minor acute (e.g., UTI) |
| Moderate | 1 illness w/exacerbation |
| | 2 chronic stable |
| | 1 acute with systemic risk (e.g., pyelonephritis) |

*HTN*, Hypertension; *UTI*, urinary tract infection.
(Modified from Centers for Medicare and Medicaid Services. 1997 Documentation Guidelines for Evaluation and Management Services. Available at www.cms.gov/Outreach-and-Education/Medicare-Learning-Network-MLN/MLNEdWebGuide/Downloads/97Docguidelines.pdf.)

**TABLE 10.3** Summary of Elements for 99214 (Until 2021), 99336, and 99349

| History | Detailed: | 4 HPI | | 2−9 ROS | 2/3 PFSH | |
|---|---|---|---|---|---|---|
| Examination | Detailed: | 5 systems with 2 elements each to 2 systems with 6 elements each (12 total) | | | | |
| MDM | Moderate: | Multiple diagnoses | Mod data | | Mod risk | |
| Time | | | | | | 99214 (until 2021): 25 minutes face to face. 99336, 99349: 40 minutes face to face |
| Key components | | | | | | 2/3 required (until 2021 for 99214, but ongoing for 99336, 99349) |

*HPI,* History of present illness; *KEY Components:* history, exam, medical decision making; *MDM,* medical decision making; *PFSH,* past, family, and social history; *ROS,* review of systems.
(From Centers for Medicare and Medicaid Services. 1997 Documentation Guidelines for Evaluation and Management Services. Available at www.cms.gov/Outreach-and-Education/Medicare-Learning-Network-MLN/MLNEdWebGuide/Downloads/97Docguidelines.pdf.)

**TABLE 10.4** Changes in E/M CPT Guidelines for 99214 Effective 2021

| | Through CPT 2020 | Effective CPT 2021 |
|---|---|---|
| History | Detailed | As appropriate |
| Examination | Detailed | As appropriate |
| Medical decision making | Moderate | Moderate (elements revised) |
| Number of key components | 2/3 | Not applicable: use medical decision making or time |
| Time | 25 minutes face-to-face IF counseling and coordination of care were more than half the time | 30−39 minutes, if using time as the basis of code selection |

*CPT,* Current Procedural Terminology; *E/M,* evaluation and management services.

chronic pain from osteoarthritis as well as mild dementia, and was recently prescribed a nonsteroidal antiinflammatory drug by another physician. She now is experiencing confusion. (Note: The actual findings or treatment decision process may require a higher level of service.) These guidelines can create a ceiling effect given that some patients are at the next to highest level based on complexity, but coding at the highest level, unless time based with counseling and coordination of care being the main service, may require a fundamentally irrelevant review of systems or a physical examination that is not required to be comprehensive by patient care needs. There can be inadequate differentiation within the levels in which geriatricians normally operate. The office visit revisions of 2021 are specifically designed to address this. In 2021, coding based upon medical decision making may be level 4 for this patient but could be level 5 if the mental status changes are substantial, related to acute changes in renal function or congestive heart failure or may warrant consideration of hospitalization. In addition, total time on the date of the encounter could be the basis of code selection, even if counseling and coordination of care did not take up more than 50% of the face-to-face time of the visit. So, if visit preparation that day, plus time in the office, plus a follow-up call to the family/caregiver that day after diagnostic studies were resulted came to a total of 60 minutes, it could be a level-5 visit. Table 10.4 shows the change in rules for 99214.

❖❖ **When addressing multiple conditions, the number of conditions creates additive and interactive complexity to decision making.**

## Medical Necessity

The array of scoring points and rules in the DGs can easily obscure the fact that all services reported must be necessary. CPT introduces the level of the key components with an important phrase: "which requires." Copied and pasted notes, excessive history or examination findings, or other verbiage not relevant to the problem(s) treated at that encounter do not fulfill any documentation requirement.

❖❖ **All services must first be medically necessary.**

## Time and Face-to-Face Services

Time is money and although some codes are based on time, most are not. E/M gives typical times for each code, but time is used as the basis of E/M code selection only when counseling and care coordination dominate the service, meaning it takes up >50% of the time spent face to face with the patient. A lot of time is not face to face. Each E/M service accounts for some time doing things, such as reviewing a laboratory test, but a lengthy phone call with a family member caregiver is not accounted for and may not be charged to the family member except in limited cases. In the hospital and nursing facility, time does include unit time, not just time in the patient's room. Even though CPT discusses time with respect to the "patient and/or family," payers require that the patient be present for the service. Therefore a family conference in the physician's office about care planning for a nursing facility patient is reported neither as an E/M office visit nor as a nursing facility visit. However, if the same conference occurs on the patient's unit, the patient was seen for a portion of the service, and the parties are the surrogate decision makers, the visit does count as a covered visit. If a patient with dementia is seen and then sits quietly in the examination area while the discussion with the family takes place, that time also counts; however, if the patient stays home, that time does not count.

**◆◆ Consider using time to determine E/M level when counseling and coordination dominate.**

In 2021 for office and other outpatient visits, many of the shortcomings in the rules related to time are addressed. Time may be used as the basis of code selection, whether or not counseling and/or coordination of care dominated the service. Face-to-face and non—-face-to-face time is counted. It is based only on the time of the date of the encounter, even though the valuation (payment level) of the service assumes some time and work will take place before and after the date of the visit. Time is listed as a range and there is a prolonged service code when the maximum time range of the highest-level code (99205, 99215) is exceeded by 15 minutes or more. The ranges are not minimum requirements to report the code unless time is being used as the basis of code selection. For example, although the time for 99214 is 30 to 39 minutes, if medical decision making is the basis for code selection, 99214 may be reported when total time is less than 30 minutes, but medical decision making was moderate. Because total time is used, the total time may not be known when the patient leaves the office. There could be calls back to the patient that day or calls to other clinicians, the hospital, or the emergency department that are part of the encounter.

**◆◆ Effective 2021, keep track of total time on the date of the encounter, if using time as a basis of selecting the office visit code for a specific visit.**

There are some services that completely lack any face-to-face contact with the patient; these include care plan oversight (e.g., CPT 99375 or G code G0181), certifying a home care plan (G0180), and family therapy without the patient present (90846), although the last example does require face-to-face time with the family members. The most relevant of these services is the care management family, which reflect total time over a calendar month for patients who have a care plan. These are Care Management (99490, 99491) and Complex Care Management (99487, 99489), and Behavioral Health Integration Care Management (99484). There are codes for management of patients with physiologic monitoring in the home, team-based psychiatric collaborative care, and interprofessional consultation. There is a lot more to E/M than there was before 2013 when the importance of non—face-to-face care management and collaborative care gained greater recognition. Prolonged service codes 99354-99359 (and a new code in CPT 2021) are reportable when the time of the E/M service greatly exceeds the typical time. These are important services to understand given the high amount of extra time related to care coordination and counseling inherent in geriatric care.

## Medicare Coding Rules Compared with CPT Codes and Guidelines

### Report All Services

There are some key areas where CMS/Medicare does not align with CPT. The issue of annual physicals is described in a previous section. There are many preventive services that are commonly performed that have HCPCS codes and when added up are very significant to the economic health of a practice. They include the annual wellness visits, alcohol misuse screening and counseling, depression screening, tobacco cessation services, obesity services, and cardiovascular risk reduction counseling. These all are G code services and the CMS website has descriptions of each service and rules related to them. The other most significant difference between CMS/Medicare and CPT is the recognition of CPT consultation codes. These codes are invalid for Medicare, which instead requires use of the codes that would be reported per CPT if the service was not by referral. A particularly odd result of this policy is that a hospital inpatient consult of a high level (e.g., 99254) is to be reported with a code that CPT intends for use only for the admitting physician or professional (e.g., 99222). Also odd is the required use by consultants of an office code (99201—99215) for patients in a hospital on observation status.

## Charges and Charging for All Services Performed

As mentioned, it is important to know more than a few E/M codes. A nurse visit to check blood pressure is a 99211. There is a warfarin anticoagulation management code outside of the E/M section. Prolonged services may occur with regularity. Critical care is not restricted to any specialty and can occur even in the office or nursing facility. If a discharge takes more than 30 minutes, the lower-paying, less intensive service should not be reported. There are laboratory test, surgical procedure, machine test, and drug codes. It pays to learn about the Medicare and other payer rules. Pay attention to charges. The physician is usually paid the lesser of the charge or the allowance, so if the physician charges $50 for a service for which Medicare or another payer will pay the physician $75, the physician will get $50. The Medicare fee schedule is updated annually, and many payers will pay a percentage (higher or lower) than Medicare; therefore the Medicare fee schedule is a useful reference point. The physician's charges are what he or she actually charges, so when there is patient cost-sharing the physician is expected, generally, to attempt collection up to the allowed amount. This does not preclude writing off charges selectively, when the patient truly cannot pay. It does mean billing Medicaid as a secondary payer, even if no additional payment is expected.

**◆◆ Not all payers follow Medicare and may pay for more than CMS does.**

## Working as a Team — "Incident to," Shared Visits, and Teaching

A nurse visit (99211) can be billed by a physician because it is incident to that physician's care. There was a time when RNP, CNS, and PA services had to be reported by the physician, but now these professionals are given provider status of their own, depending on state scope-of-practice laws. However, when these professionals are providing care for an established patient under an established treatment plan and are employed by the physician or by the party that employs the physician and the physician is in the office suite, the physician may report the service in Medicare, even if the physician had no face-to-face time with the patient for that encounter. Because the other professionals are paid 85% of the physician fee schedule, correct use of this mechanism is like a 18% raise for these professionals. Not all services can be reported this way; for example, nursing facility visits cannot be "incident to." There is also "shared visit" reporting. This is when a physician and the other professional both see the patient and the physician reports a single service for the combined services of the two (e.g., in a hospitalized patient cared for by a hospitalist team of physicians and RNPs). It does require physician involvement, not just a countersignature. A similar concept is applied for teaching physicians who may use portions of the work of the trainee or student, so long as the physician independently verifies or is present for the key portions of the service.

◆ **"Incident to" reporting, when allowed, is equivalent to a nearly 20% raise.**

## Charging the Patient or Family

Not everything is covered by insurance, including Medicare. Special caution is required if billing a Medicaid beneficiary. Patient-responsibility balances for copayments or deductibles should be collected, but what about noncovered services? It was common practice until Medicare's inclusion of annual wellness visits to charge Medicare beneficiaries for noncovered annual physicals. Now there is not much left in such a visit that is not covered, even if the physician does not bill the annual wellness visit because a required element was not performed. However, if a family requests a conference in the physician's office to discuss whether mother needs a nursing home and mother is not present, that is not covered, is not part of the usual follow-up of a past visit and can be charged to the family. It is important to inform the family of this fact, why it is the case, and what you will charge. It is always advisable to use a CMS approved Advance Beneficiary Notice (ABN) form (available on the CMS website), even though it is really intended for services that are covered or not based on specific circumstance, such as removing a benign skin lesion for cosmetic reasons as compared with removal because the lesion was getting traumatized. It is advisable for recurrent issues that are atypical or uncertain to be reviewed with the local payer, Medicare contractor, or billing experts because the billing process is not always as straightforward as it may seem. Completing certain forms, copying charges, and consultations with an attorney related to guardianship are all issues sometimes faced by practices that are not covered by insurance. However, if the form is a certification for durable medical equipment, the patient cannot be charged for its completion.

## Global Periods and Per-Day Services

Geriatricians may perform some services with a global period longer than the date of service. For example, a lesion excision has a 10-day global period and payment includes any related E/M over those days and suture removal. If a rural geriatrician or hospitalist provides all the postoperative care for a patient, the correct code to report is the surgical procedure code. The surgeon uses a modifier

designating that the care did not include postoperative care and the geriatrician uses a modifier indicating only postoperative care was provided. Some codes are per visit and some are per day. Two visits to a hospitalized patient in one day are reported with a single hospital inpatient code. The work of both visits is added up, and the single best hospital visit code and possibly a prolonged service code is used. Be sure to record unit time for all visits if using prolonged services codes. All services related to an admission are reported by the admission code. If a physician sends a patient to the hospital from the office and admits the patient that day, reporting the initial hospital care service, then the office visit is not reported. An exception is transfers from the hospital to a nursing facility. A hospital discharge service and an initial nursing facility service may both be reported on the same day if two separate visits occur. As noted earlier, many care management services are for a calendar month or a 30-day period.

## Value-Based Programs and Migration Away from Fee for Service

Medicare has the Merit-based Incentive Payment (MIP) program. This program requires reporting on quality measures and there are percentage deductions or increases paid based upon performance. There are advanced alternative payment mechanisms such as Accountable Care Organizations (ACO) where there is a bonus or payback for related to total cost of care and quality targets. These programs include risk adjustment, and accurate ICD 10 coding is essential to determine the condition in the Hierarchical Condition Category (HCC) classification system, which in turn determines the Risk Adjustment Factor (RAF). Medicare Advantage programs depend upon this for their payment from Medicare and are very concerned with accurate condition coding. Medicare Advantage plans, hospitals, and others have quality payment programs that affect anyone who interacts with this organizations. These payments or penalties can be very meaningful. The Center for Medicare and Medicaid Innovation also has programs related to building advanced primary care in some regions. The impact of these programs is growing steadily. Newer programs will shift payment away from volume-based fee for service to value-based payments and mechanisms that will recognize systems of care. It is difficult to anticipate what coding and billing issues will arise. It is advisable to be aware of these trends and stay informed.

## Participation Status

Upon getting a provider number, and annually, Medicare allows physicians and other professionals to address their participation status. Being nonparticipating is not as simple as billing and collecting charges from the patient. If a professional paid on the physician fee schedule elects to not participate but accepts assignments (i.e., lets Medicare pay them directly on a claim in return for the professional not billing the beneficiary a balance), the professional receives 95% of the allowance. If the professional does not accept assignment he or she may not attempt to collect more than 109.25% of Medicare's maximal allowed charge for the service. If the professional opts out of Medicare, the contract is between the professional and the patient, but if the professional has opted out for all Medicare patients and the patient cannot get reimbursed by Medicare for the professional's services, the patient may receive Medicare-covered services from others.

## Resources

This chapter gives an overview of important aspects of coding and billing. Each year, or more often, new codes, rules, and programs are created. It is important to keep up to date. For Medicare, the CMS website has a great deal of information. One can even subscribe to update notices from MedLearn Matters. The Medicare Part B contractor website will have important information. Having a current CPT code set publication is advised and CPT has other useful educational publications. Specialty societies and professional organizations will often educate members on new issues and have basic coding courses at annual meetings. Billing companies and other practice management professionals are potential sources of information.

## Summary

Coding and billing require knowledge of terms and rules. There is some variation by payer or program, but there are many basic principles, such as correct use of CPT, that are general. These rules can be sufficiently understood by clinicians but do warrant some educational efforts to allow professionals to be properly paid for their services.

### Web Resources

Physician Center—starting point for many links, including MedLearn Matters educational products: www.cms.gov/Center/Provider-Type/Physician-Center.html.

Medicare Learning Network Preventive Services: www.cms.gov/Outreach-and-Education/Medicare-Learning-Network-MLN/MLNProducts/PreventiveServices.html.

Medicare guides related to Care Management services: https://www.cms.gov/Medicare/Medicare-Fee-for-Service-Payment/PhysicianFeeSched/Care-Management.html.

Centers for Medicare and Medicaid Services' Quality Payment Program: https://www.cms.gov/Medicare/Quality-Payment-Program/Quality-Payment-Program.html.

Centers for Medicare and Medicaid Services Advance Beneficiary Notices: www.cms.gov/Medicare/Medicare-General-Information/BNI/ABN.html.

Centers for Medicare and Medicaid Services' Guidelines for Teaching Physicians, Interns, and Residents: https://www.cms.gov/Outreach-and-Education/Medicare-Learning-Network-MLN/MLNProducts/MLN-Publications-Items/CMS1243499.html.

American Medical Association—CPT Medical Billing, Coding and Insurance: https://www.ama-assn.org/amaone/cpt-current-procedural-terminology.

# 11

# Hospital Care

JEFFREY D. SCHLAUDECKER, CHRISTOPHER R. BERNHEISEL, AND HILLARY R. MOUNT

## OUTLINE

*Additional online-only material indicated by icon.*

## OBJECTIVES

*Upon completion of this chapter, the reader will be able to:*

- Leverage the admission process to the hospital as an opportunity for a review of health status for older adults.
- Describe ways that perioperative care of older adults in the hospital is different from the care of younger patients.
- Apply preventative measures in the hospital to reduce risks to hospitalized older patients.

- Apply selective interventions to improve hospital outcomes and decrease unplanned readmissions and adverse patient outcomes.

Nosocomial infections, loss of independence, functional status decline, medication interactions, polypharmacy, overtreatment, falls, cognitive loss, delirium, misinformed handoffs, and poor care transitions are just some of the complications that can occur during the hospitalization of an older adult. Although advances in medical and surgical care have decreased morbidity and mortality related to many diseases, the hospital remains a place of potential peril for older patients. Care provided to older adults in the hospital should strive to limit exposure to iatrogenic complications, maintain functional status, and provide patient- and family-centered care that is evidence based and disease focused.

The risk of an older adult developing a new activity of daily living (ADL) disability during a hospitalization is estimated to be at least 30%, and about half of new disabilities occurring in older adults develop during a hospitalization.[1] Frail elders with limited functional reserves at baseline fare even worse. Unfortunately, 1 year after hospital discharge, less than half of older adults have returned to their prehospitalization level of functioning.[2] Certainly, hospitalization may be necessary to provide treatment for acute illness in older adults. It has been estimated that 7% to 15% of the 1 million older adults with Medicare who are hospitalized each year experience a preventable adverse event. Knowledge of the many causes of functional decline in the hospital and actions aimed at functional status preservation are paramount for any practitioner caring for hospitalized older patients.

◆◆ **Because of severe physiologic stressors and nosocomial exposures, hospitalization is best thought of as an intervention to use carefully in the care of older adults.**

---

**CASE 1**

**Robert Johnson (Part 1)**

You are called by a local emergency department about your 81-year-old patient, Mr. Johnson, who has suffered a mild stroke and fractured his hip during a related fall. Mr. Johnson has been your patient for about 7 years when he relocated to be near his adult children. Since losing his wife 3 years ago, Mr. Johnson's visits to your office have been sporadic, and he is under the care of several subspecialists for his macular degeneration, presbycusis, hypertension, and mild diastolic congestive heart failure. Cognitive testing was borderline during a visit 1 year ago, and a geriatric depression screen was positive, but he declined pharmacologic interventions and counseling at that time. The decision is made to admit Mr. Johnson to the hospitalist service and obtain a consultation from the orthopedic service.

What factors in his history need to be relayed to the team that will be caring for him in the hospital?

---

## Communication Is Essential in the Hospital

Caring for older adults in the hospital should involve an interprofessional group of care providers. Optimal geriatric hospital care is provided by case managers and geriatric social workers to assist in coordinating discharge needs, dieticians working to find food that is the correct caloric density and texture, nurses and nursing assistants providing direct patient care who are often the first to notice a patient change, consulting physicians, hospitalists, advance practice providers, pharmacists, physical therapists, occupational therapists, and speech and language pathologists all working together to bring optimal care to older adults and their families. These team members all must communicate with each other and with the patient and family during the hospitalization. The gathered information must additionally be communicated in an efficient and accurate way to the receiving facility that will take over care once the patient has left the hospital. This can include a rehabilitation facility, a skilled nursing facility, a long-term acute care hospital, a family member's home, or the patient's own residence.

Since the term *hospitalist* was first used in 1996 to describe the growing number of physicians whose primary site of practice was within the hospital, the field has expanded rapidly.[3] In urban areas today, hospitalists provide the majority of nonsurgical care to hospitalized adults in the United States.[3] The hospitalist is often the primary care coordinator and communicator among the many team members involved in the care of an older adult in the hospital.

Hospitalists are generally at least as efficient and effective as nonhospitalist providers, but the field has highlighted the critical need for excellent communication within all members of the healthcare team, including the family. In addition, it is critically important for the hospitalist to communicate across locations of care at the time of admission and discharge, including with both primary care providers and accepting physicians at skilled nursing facilities or rehabilitation units.

◆◆ **Primary care physicians, hospitalists, caregivers, and all members of the healthcare team caring for a hospitalized geriatric patient need to ensure maximal communication.**

## Hospital Design and Systems Change to Benefit Older Adults

Much as pediatric hospitals underwent changes in design to better reflect the unique needs of their young patients, specific areas in many hospitals today are designed to optimally meet the needs of older adults.

In 1992 with funds from the John A. Hartford Foundation, New York University began broadly field-testing nursing care models, including the geriatric resource nurse (GRN) program. This project became known as Nurses Improving Care for Health System Elders (NICHE) and aimed to create a better care environment for the hospitalized elderly patient by improving nursing practice.[4] Nursing leadership is integral to good care of older adults, and the NICHE program provides resources, project management support/mentoring for NICHE-based hospital initiatives, evidence-based clinical protocols that address "never events," and shared information, knowledge, and expertise to more than 300 participating hospitals.[5]

Acute care for the elderly (ACE) units have demonstrated improved functional outcomes without increased costs or length of stay.[4] This model of comprehensive inpatient geriatric care incorporates (1) hospital environment modifications, (2) minimization of adverse effects of hospitalization, (3) early discharge planning, and (4) patient-centered care protocols.[5]

The benefit of ACE units is also being expanded hospital wide. The concept of a mobile acute care for the elderly (MACE) unit has also been described. The main goals of the MACE unit are to bring the interdisciplinary, patient-centered team approach to hospitalized older adult patients throughout a hospital, rather than having the team located solely on one geographically based unit. A 2010 study found that among more than 8000 older adults, those being treated via MACE service (compared with those admitted to an ACE or a traditional unit) had lower length of stay and lower costs but no change in in-hospital mortality or 7- or 30-day readmission rates.[4]

◆◆ **The use of specialized acute care for the elderly units can improve outcomes by modifying the hospital environment to be less disruptive to older adults.**

## Hospital Physical Design

In addition to a redesign of care processes and procedures for caring for older hospitalized adults, the physical environments of hospitals are additionally being designed to allow for improved care.[6] Hospital design that focuses on the needs of older adults and their families has improved the hospital campus, the unit, the room, and the amenities available. Design features can include reserved or valet parking and benches along walkways, handrails, matte floor finishing or low-pile carpeting, low-color-contrast floors with clear contrast with walls, sound-absorbing materials in rooms with available assistive listening devices, choice of chairs with armrests, automatic faucets and doors, and easy-to-see and easy-to-activate call systems.[6]

### Patient- and Family-Centered Geriatric Hospital Care

Because many older adults rely on additional support for successful aging, geriatric hospital care must embrace the principles of patient- and family-centered care. As defined by the Institute for Patient- and Family-Centered Care, the core principles include respect and dignity, collaboration, participation, and meaningful information sharing.[7] Family is defined as broadly as possible to include any person that an older adult may rely on for support, whether emotional, physical, or financial.[7] Partnership with family during the hospitalization of older adults is paramount to a successful admission, and every attempt to involve family at the highest level desired by the patient should be sought. Minimizing barriers to family participation in healthcare should always be a paramount goal of excellent care.

## The Admission Process: Opportunities for Health Status Updates

When an older adult requires admission to the hospital, communication among providers inside and outside the hospital is critically important. The primary care physician and/or the nursing home physician and the family must all be involved to ensure a meaningful admission. For patients living in long-term care settings, often the nurses and/or patient care attendants/nursing assistants have valuable information about symptom development, and attempts to contact these care providers should be undertaken. Because older adults vary widely in their functional and health status, critical decisions about treatment should never be based solely on the patient's age. The in-hospital medical team will need guidance from community-based providers to accurately assess the older patient's baseline functional status.

At the time of admission, the hospital provider should perform a review of systems that focuses on geriatric syndromes and other issues common to older adults, including cognition and functional independence in ADLs and instrumental activities of daily living (IADLs). Vaccine status, especially about pneumococcal, seasonal influenza, and herpes zoster should also be ascertained. The time of admission to the hospital is also an excellent time for a medication review for both accuracy and necessity of all medications, both prescribed and over the counter. The presence of advance directives and documentation of a surrogate decision maker is also among information that should be incorporated into the admission record. Advance directives should also be discussed, updated, and documented.

❖ **The admission process provides an opportunity to review medications and ensure appropriate indications for all prescriptions, as well as ascertain vaccine status, code status, alcohol use, and elder abuse risk factors.**

## Elder Abuse

Screening for elder mistreatment among asymptomatic populations has not been evaluated, but the presence of elder abuse has been estimated to be nearly 10% with higher rates in those with dementia.[8] Elder abuse can broadly be defined as physical, psychological, or sexual abuse; material exploitation of money or property; or neglect and failure to meet a dependent older person's needs. The possibility of nonaccidental trauma or neglect of an older adult admitted to the hospital should be entertained by the clinician based on a high index of suspicion.[8] Identification of social support and appropriate referral to area Adult Protective Services agencies should be made whenever elder abuse is suspected (see Ch. 33).

## Alcohol Abuse

During the admission to the hospital, a discussion on alcohol use should be completed. The prevalence of older adults with alcohol-related problems has been reported to be between 2% and 22%, depending on the definition used.[9] Screening tools for younger adults usually focus on work or legal difficulties that arise from drinking, and these consequences are rarer in older adults with harmful drinking patterns.[9] The Alcohol Use Disorders Identification Test (AUDIT) or the three question AUDIT-C were both accurate for screening older adults for alcohol misuse (see Ch. 34).

## Frailty as a Risk for Poor Hospital Outcomes

Frailty is a geriatric syndrome defined as a state of increased vulnerability to both acute and chronic stressors as a consequence of reduced physiologic reserve.[10] Frailty is associated with functional decline, loss of independence, and mortality. The identification of this syndrome should be readily considered for any older adult being admitted to the hospital (see Ch. 29). The concept of frailty is relevant for providers of geriatric hospital care because it provides a ready explanation for the different stress tolerances of older adults. Stressors in the hospital are summative and can include not only the inciting medical or surgical event, but also sleep deprivation, medication side effects, sensory deprivation, and caloric deficiencies resulting from restrictive diets, nothing-by-mouth status, or general illness.[10–12] For men and women older than age 60 years, 10 days of bed rest results in a similar loss of muscle mass as a decade of normal aging.[13] To help lessen the impact of hospitalization on older adults, physical activity (especially resistance training), nutritional consultations and supplementation, and vitamin D supplementation when appropriate should be strongly considered.[11]

❖ **Stressors in the hospital are summative and include the inciting medical or surgical event, and also sleep deprivation, medication side effects, sensory deprivation, limited mobility, and caloric deficiencies resulting from restrictive diets, nothing-by-mouth status, or general illness.**

## Perioperative Care of the Elderly Patient in the Hospital

Nearly one-third of all patients undergoing a surgical procedure are now older than age 65 years, with the percentage expected to increase further over the next 15 years as the population continues to age.[13] Studies have shown 21% of elderly patients will suffer from at least one perioperative complication following a nonthoracic surgery, potentially leading to prolonged hospitalization, increased mortality, and long-term morbidity.[14,15] Because of the heterogeneity of elderly patients, a patient-centered approach in close conjunction with the surgical team is required to reduce the risk of complications and adverse outcomes. Comprehensive guidelines exist for the perioperative care of older adults, including those collaboratively created by the American College of Surgeons and the American Geriatrics Society (AGS).[16] These guidelines include a risk calculator that uses patient and procedure information to estimate a multitude of risks such as sepsis, discharge to a nursing facility, renal failure, and hospital length of stay (https://riskcalculator.facs.org/RiskCalculator/).[17]

Collaborative management with surgeons is essential to optimize outcomes for older adults. Comanagement between surgeons and medical providers in the perioperative period is collaborative and a learnable skill. One program available to medical providers is the AGS CoCare: Ortho[TM]. This modular educational program provides a foundation for geriatric comanagement of common conditions, as well as topic-specific content on discharge planning and other key topics.[18]

---

### CASE 1

#### Robert Johnson (Part 2)

Mr. Johnson was admitted to the hospital yesterday for his focal weakness and hip fracture. He was seen by a neurologist, who expects continued recovery of left leg weakness that is the result of a small ischemic stroke. He was put on nothing-by-mouth status at the time of admission and the orthopedic surgeon is planning on taking him for operative repair later this afternoon. In what ways can his care be optimized at this point in the hospitalization?

---

## Establishing Goals of Care

The preoperative evaluation of elderly patients begins with a frank discussion on goals of care (Fig. 11.1). Survival and longevity may be the most important outcomes for a younger population, but it may not be the primary goals for every elderly patient. A more important outcome may be related to the patient's functional status following the surgery. A full discussion of all the potential outcomes is necessary, with an honest discussion of prognosis of recovery related to functional status and the potential loss of independence. Older adults may elect to forgo emergent interventions if the outcome would likely lead to loss of

independence and functional status, and instead may elect for more conservative measures. The role of the medical clinician in the preoperative evaluation is to help review all of the options for the patient, including for palliative care. The preoperative evaluation provides an excellent opportunity to better define end-of-life decision making for the patient, especially for those surgical interventions that carry significant risks for the elderly patient. Patients should be encouraged to discuss their decisions with family members and their healthcare power of attorney to prevent undesired interventions in the future. Evidence-based tools exist to help guide providers, patients, and families through these discussions (https://www.hipxchange.org/SurgicalQPL).[19]

## Emergent Surgery

In general, patients who have acute surgical emergencies may proceed to the operating room (OR) with the assumption that any potential risk would be less than the potential benefit of the surgery. This may not be as true for elderly patients, and goals of care still must be addressed even in the emergent situation. A lifesaving surgical intervention that leads to loss of independence may not match the goals of care for an elderly patient, and palliative care is an important option to provide the patient. The emergent evaluation includes a brief discussion on preoperative functional status to help assess functional reserve along with the goals of care for the individual patient. Older adults who undergo emergent surgeries have a higher risk of adverse outcomes and long-term morbidity that may lead to loss of independence especially in those with low preoperative functional status.

❖❖ **Perioperative care in the hospital must be based on goals of care and should strive to ensure evidence-based use of risk stratification, medications, and early mobilization to prevent prolonged hospitalizations and nosocomial infections.**

## Cardiac Evaluation

### Active Cardiac Conditions

For elective surgeries, the clinician must inquire about any active cardiac conditions. Active cardiac conditions include all of those conditions that would warrant urgent treatment whether the patient was planning a surgical intervention or not: acute coronary syndrome, myocardial infarction within 30 days, significant arrhythmias, and severe valvular disease.[20] The time frame for delaying the surgical intervention depends on the cardiac event and the intervention. There is a paucity of evidence for the correct timing of surgery

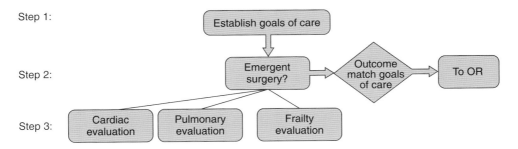

- **Figure 11.1** Preoperative evaluation. (Modified from Fleisher LA, Beckman JA, Brown KA, et al. 2009 ACCF/AHA focused update on perioperative beta blockade incorporated into the ACC/AHA 2007 guidelines on perioperative cardiovascular evaluation and care for noncardiac surgery: a report of the American College of Cardiology Foundation/American Heart Association Task Force on Practice Guidelines. *Circulation* 2009;120(21):e169–e276.)

following medical intervention. Decisions are based on best available evidence and consensus statements (Fig. 11.2).

A vital component of the perioperative care of patients with a history of a recent cardiac event is the management of antiplatelet therapy. Dual antiplatelet therapy should be continued for at least 12 months following acute myocardial infarction. Elective noncardiac surgeries should be delayed at least 30 days following a bare metal stent and 6 months following placement of a drug-

eluting stent. If risks of withholding the surgery exceed potential in-stent stenosis, surgery can be considered 3 months after drug-eluting stent placement.[21] In each of these situations, the patient should be continued on aspirin and the P2Y12 inhibitor held perioperatively.

Primary care doctors must work closely with their surgical colleagues to weigh the risk of bleeding against the risk of coronary artery disease, with strong consideration to continue aspirin for

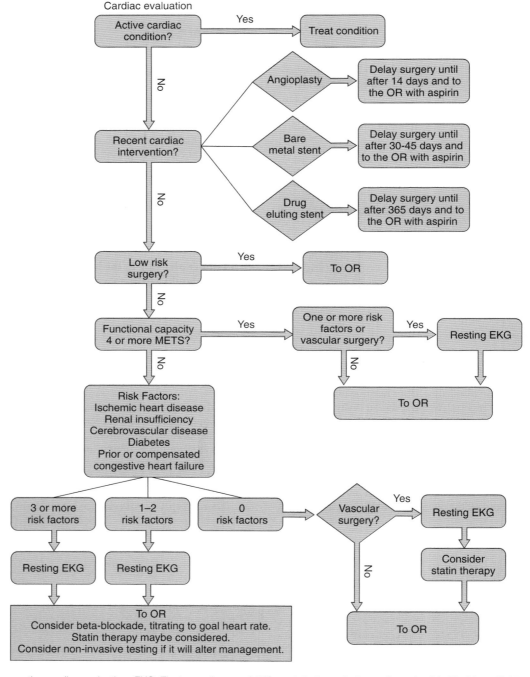

• **Figure 11.2** Preoperative cardiac evaluation. *EKG*, Electrocardiogram; *METs*, metabolic equivalents of a task. (Modified from Fleisher LA, Beckman JA, Brown KA, et al. 2009 ACCF/AHA focused update on perioperative beta blockade incorporated into the ACC/AHA 2007 guidelines on perioperative cardiovascular evaluation and care for noncardiac surgery: a report of the American College of Cardiology Foundation/American Heart Association Task Force on Practice Guidelines. *Circulation* 2009;120(21):e169–e276.)

secondary prevention of coronary heart disease in the perioperative period. The procoagulant, proinflammatory state, following surgery, places patients at a significantly higher risk for cardiac in-stent stenosis with potential catastrophic results, with an odds ratio of 3.1 peaking 10 days after surgery.[22] Restenosis has been reported with withdrawal of aspirin even after 2 years from stent placement.[23,24] The Perioperative Ischemic Evaluation 2 study (POISE-2) was a large trial comparing the perioperative continuation of aspirin versus stopping of aspirin 3 days prior and restarting 7 days after noncardiac noncarotid surgery.[20] Perioperatively stopping aspirin did not show any benefit in reduction of mortality, myocardial infarction, or venous thrombosis. For those patients who were started on aspirin perioperatively, there was a statistically significant incidence of major bleeding events with a hazard ratio of 1.34. Based on this available data, patients with known coronary artery disease, with or without stents, should be continued on aspirin perioperatively. Patients already on aspirin who are felt to be at higher risk for ischemic events should be continued on aspirin, but patients who are not previously on aspirin should not be started on aspirin preoperatively because of the associated increase of major bleeding without any identified benefit.

## Low-Risk Surgery

Patients undergoing low-risk ambulatory surgical procedures (e.g., endoscopic procedures or cataract, simple breast, or ambulatory surgeries) do not have a higher 30-day risk of cardiac events compared with peers.[25] With the lack of apparent increased cardiac risk, patients may proceed to the OR without any additional evaluation for low-risk surgeries.

## Risk of Major Adverse Cardiac Event

For patients who are undergoing intermediate or high-risk surgery, an evaluation for the risk of major adverse cardiac event should be performed using a validated risk assessment tool.[21] Three tools are recommended by the 2014 American College of Cardiology (ACC)/American Heart Association (AHA) perioperative guidelines: Revised Cardiac Risk Index (RCRI), the National Surgical Quality Improvement Program (NSQIP) surgical risk calculator (http://www.riskcalculator.facs.org/RiskCalculator/), and American College of Surgeons NSQIP Myocardial Infarction and Cardiac Arrest calculator (https://qxmd.com/calculate/calculator_245/gupta-perioperative-cardiac-risk). Patients with a risk of < 1% (0−1 risk factors by RCRI) may proceed to the OR without any additional evaluation. Patients with a calculated risk of ≥ 1% may require assessment for coronary ischemia to further risk stratify.

## Cardiac Functional Assessment

Cardiac functional assessment is of vital importance, especially in the older adult population who can have a broad range of activity and functional levels. Functional capacity can be estimated by history, using published scales, such as the Duke Activity Status Index, or simple history of activity tolerance according to metabolic equivalents (METS).[26] Patients who are able to perform physical activities at or higher than 4 METS (metabolic equivalents of a task) may proceed to the planned procedure without additional evaluation.[21] Those patients who are unable to achieve 4 METS are at higher risk for perioperative cardiac event and require additional discussion concerning the potential surgical risks. Additional testing to further risk stratify may be necessary, along with consideration for consultation by cardiology.

## Cardiac Risk Reduction Through Medical Interventions

### Beta-Blockade

There have been multiple studies looking at beta-blockade in the perioperative period, with conflicting results.[27−30] Early studies showed significant promise for the prevention of acute myocardial infarction; unfortunately, follow-up studies have not consistently demonstrated this benefit.

More recent studies confirmed the cardioprotective benefit of perioperative beta-blockade but demonstrated the increased risk of stroke and death. The differences between the studies provide insight into the mechanism of risk for perioperative beta-blockade and provide guidance for initiating beta-blockade. The avoidance of hypotension and bradycardia appears vital to reduce the risk of ischemic stroke. Patients on beta-blockade chronically should be continued perioperatively. For those patients with RCRI of ≥ 3 or who are found to be at intermediate or high risk for perioperative cardiac ischemia by an alternative scoring system, it would be reasonable to start beta-blockade before proceeding to the OR if it can be initiated at a low dose and titrated slowly up to goal before surgery. The exact timing for initiating beta-blockade has not been established, but based on the results of available data, same-day initiation with rapid titration should be avoided.[29]

### HMG-CoA Reductase Inhibitors (Statin Therapy)

The only prospective randomized trial on perioperative statin use was a small study of 100 patients investigating the perioperative use of atorvastatin for vascular surgery.[31] Patients were placed on 20 mg atorvastatin for a total of 45 days and a minimum of 2 weeks before the surgery with a composite outcome of death from stroke and acute coronary syndrome. A statistically significant difference in composite outcome was reached in the atorvastatin arm versus placebo at 6 months (8% vs. 26%). Multiple retrospective studies have also shown reduced perioperative cardiac events with the use of statins in both vascular and nonvascular studies. Based on the limited evidence available, the 2014 American College of Cardiology Foundation/AHA Guidelines find the use of statins "reasonable" for patients undergoing vascular surgery and "may be considered" for patients undergoing "elevated risk procedures."[21]

## Perioperative Pulmonary Complications

Perioperative pulmonary complications (PPCs) are encountered frequently following noncardiothoracic surgeries and contribute significantly to perioperative and long-term morbidity and mortality. The American College of Chest Physicians includes atelectasis, pneumonia, respiratory failure, and exacerbation of underlying chronic lung disease as PPCs. An incidence of 5.5% to 6.8% is found when using rigorous methods to define PPC.[15,32] PPCs are an even stronger predictor than perioperative cardiac complications for longer term perioperative mortality in the elderly, with a hazard ratio of 2.41.[33] Despite being a stronger predictor for adverse outcomes and having a similar frequency as perioperative cardiac events, perioperative pulmonary evaluation and PPCs prevention are often placed at a lower priority by clinicians and patients. Because advanced age is a risk factor for PPCs, clinicians who care for the elderly need to have increased awareness and diligence in evaluating and preventing PPCs.

## Preoperative Pulmonary Evaluation

The preoperative pulmonary evaluation starts with identification of risk factors for developing PPCs (Box 11.1). Of the risk factors

• **BOX 11.1** **Pulmonary Risk Factors**

Age >60 years
Chronic lung disease
   COPD
   Restrictive lung disease
   Pulmonary arterial hypertension
Smoking
Congestive heart failure
Poor functional status
ASA classification ≥2
Perioperative delirium
Surgery >3 hours
Abdominal surgery, thoracic surgery, neurosurgery, head and neck surgery, vascular surgery, aortic aneurysm repair, emergency surgery
General anesthesia
Albumin <3.5 g/dL

*ASA*, American Society of Anesthesiologists; *COPD*, chronic obstructive pulmonary disease.(From Owens WD, Felts JA, Spitznagel EL Jr. ASA physical status classifications: a study of consistency of ratings. *Anesthesiology* 1978;49:239–243.)

listed, a history of chronic obstructive pulmonary disease (COPD) and age >60 years are the two highest predictors of the development of PPCs. The risk for PPCs increases with each decade, with odds ratios of 2.09 for patients age 60 to 69 years and 3.04 for patients age 70 to 79 years.[33] Another important risk factor is functional status, which predicts both overall mortality and risk for PPCs with an odds ratio of 2.51 for developing PPCs if patients are unable to perform any ADLs and 1.65 if they require assistance for some of their ADLs. Those patients who are identified as having any risk factors for PPCs should proceed to additional evaluation and undergo preoperative and postoperative interventions to reduce risk.

Pulmonary function tests (PFTs) have an important role in the evaluation and risk analysis for patients undergoing cardiothoracic surgery, but evidence has not demonstrated benefit for noncardiothoracic surgeries, even in the setting of stable COPD, because the test results do not add any additional value beyond what is obtained in the history and examination.[33] Based on available evidence, the American College of Physicians (ACP) does not recommend the routine use of chest x-ray studies for a preoperative pulmonary evaluation.[33]

Low albumin is a very powerful predictor of perioperative mortality and long-term morbidity in addition to a predictor of PPCs. Patients with an albumin lower than 3.5 g/dL had an incidence of 27.6% of PPCs compared with an incidence of 7.0% in patients with normal albumin.[30] Unfortunately, nutritional support strategies, such as total parenteral nutrition (TPN), in the perioperative period have not demonstrated any benefit over regular diet.[34]

## Interventions to Reduce Pulmonary Complications

Evidence-based interventions to reduce PPCs are limited, with studies either not rigorously designed or not demonstrating significant benefit. PPCs are cut in half with either deep breathing exercises or incentive spirometry (IS) in the perioperative period.[35] The results seem to be superior if the patient receives education before the surgery.[36] For patients who are unable to participate in breathing exercises, continuous positive airway pressure (CPAP) has been demonstrated to reduce PPCs.[37]

Time-to-surgery is another potential risk factor for both pulmonary complications, as well as increased mortality, bed sores, length

of stay, and other complications. In appropriate patients, advocating for earlier surgery can potentially limit complications and lower mortality by up to 20% in hip fracture patients.[38,39] Smoking cessation has also been investigated as a method to reduce PPCs, with some evidence showing benefit.

## Postoperative Considerations

### Venous Thromboembolism Prevention

Venous thromboembolism (VTE) is considered the top preventable etiology for hospital death, with the postoperative state placing patients at even higher risk than hospitalized general medical patients. Table 11.1 summarizes the most recent guidelines from the American College of Chest Physicians.[40] Frequent and clear dialogue with surgical colleagues to balance postoperative bleeding risk with thromboembolism risk is essential (see further discussion in the section Preventative Measures in the Hospital).

### Postoperative Anemia

There are very few studies that evaluate transfusions for patients in the postoperative period. A study in 2011 compared a liberal transfusion cutoff of a hemoglobin of 10 g/dL to a restrictive transfusion cutoff hemoglobin of 8 g/dL performed on patients following hip replacement surgery.[41] In this trial, patients were transfused at the randomized predefined transfusion cutoffs or if they demonstrated symptomatic anemia (such as orthostatic hypotension, chest pain believed to be cardiac in origin, tachycardia that did not respond to fluids, or signs of congestive heart failure). At 30 days, the groups did not differ in mortality, functional status, cardiac events, infectious events, VTE, stroke, or congestive heart failure. Based on this trial, the American Association of Blood Banks (AABB) recommends a transfusion cutoff of 8 g/dL hemoglobin unless signs and symptoms of anemia are present.[42]

## Preventative Measures in the Hospital

Assuring patient safety in the hospital setting is a nationwide challenge. The geriatric population is at a higher risk of complications in the hospital for multiple reasons, including longer length of stays, more frequent hospitalizations, higher numbers of medical problems, and more severe illness at presentation.[43–45] More than 50% of elderly patients will experience at least one complication related to their hospitalization. These complications lead to longer length of stay per hospitalization, higher costs, and higher rates of institutionalization at discharge.[43,46] Nearly 17% of Americans age ≥65 years spent at least one night in the hospital in 2018. In 2014 Medicare spending on inpatient hospital stays was $147 billion.[46] A proactive approach should include preventative measures targeted at common complications.[46]

### CASE 1

#### Robert Johnson (Part 3)

Mr. Johnson underwent successful hip replacement 9 days ago. His neurologic deficits from the acute stroke have almost totally resolved, but his son calls your office to report that Mr. Johnson is extremely confused and has been very agitated in the evenings, requiring restraints to keep him from removing his own Foley catheter and intravenous lines. He has not been eating well at all, and the son also reports that his father is being treated for a deep venous thrombosis in his leg, a urinary tract infection, and pneumonia.

What things might have been done to prevent Mr. Johnson's postoperative delirium and other illnesses?

## TABLE 11.1 Venous Thromboembolism Prophylaxis

| Patient Category | Method of VTE Prophylaxis | Duration |
|---|---|---|
| Hospitalized patients | High risk for VTE (Padua Prediction Score ≥4): LMWH or UFH or fondaparinux<br>High risk for VTE and bleeding or high risk for major bleed: mechanical thromboprophylaxis with GCS<br>Low risk (Padua Prediction Score <4): No pharmacological or mechanical prophylaxis | Duration of hospitalization |
| Critically ill hospitalized patients | Routine use of LMWH or UFH<br>If bleeding or high risk for major bleed: mechanical thromboprophylaxis with GCS | Duration of hospitalization |
| Major orthopedic surgery (elective hip replacement, hip fracture repair, elective knee replacement) | LMWH is first line, with UFH, fondaparinux, rivaroxaban, apixaban, adjusted dose vitamin K antagonist, and aspirin as alternatives<br>Administer with IPC | 10–35 days (aim for 35 days when possible) |
| Knee arthroscopy | No risk factors: early and frequent ambulation<br>Additional risk factors: LMWH | Until ambulatory |
| Elective spine surgery | No risk factors: IPC and early and frequent ambulation<br>Risk factors (high-risk VTE, cancer): UFH, LMWH once hemostasis established or IPC with GCS | Until ambulatory |
| Major GYN surgery (any nonlaparoscopic) | If for *benign* disease:<br>Very low risk (<0.5%; Rogers score <7; Caprini score 0): Ambulation<br>Low risk (1.5%; Rogers score 7–10; Caprini score 1–2): IPC<br>Moderate risk (3.0%; Rogers score >10; Caprini score 2–4) and not at high risk for bleed: LMWH, UFH, or IPC<br>High risk (6.0%; Caprini score 5 or higher): LMWH or UHF with IPC<br>Malignancy: LMWH or UFH TID and IPC | Until hospital discharge<br>For *high-risk* patients (major cancer surgery or prior VTE)—Continue prophylaxis for 28 days posthospital discharge |
| Minor or entirely laparoscopic GYN surgery | Low-risk patient: Early ambulation<br>High-risk patient: LMWH, UFH or IPCs w/ GCS | Until hospital discharge |
| General abdominal-pelvic surgery | Very low risk for VTE (Rogers score <7; Caprini score 0): No intervention other than ambulation<br>Low risk (Rogers score 7–10; Caprini score 1–2) recommend mechanical prophylaxis by IPC<br>Moderate risk for VTE (Rogers score >10; Caprini score 3–4) not at high risk for bleeding complications: LMWH or UFH or mechanical prophylaxis by IPC. If LMWH or UFH are contraindicated, can consider low-dose aspirin, fondaparinux, or mechanical prophylaxis<br>Moderate risk for VTE (Rogers score >10; Caprini score 3–4) at high risk for bleeding complications: Mechanical prophylaxis by IPC<br>High risk for VTE (Caprini score ≥5) not at high risk for major bleeding complication: LMWH or UFH with mechanical prophylaxis by IPC<br>High risk for VTE (Caprini score ≥5) at high risk for major bleeding complication: Mechanical prophylaxis by IPC | General: Hospitalization<br>High VTE-risk undergoing surgery for cancer: 4-week duration with LMWH |

*GCS,* Graduated compression stockings; *IPC,* intermittent pneumatic compression; *LMWH,* low-molecular-weight heparin; *UFH,* unfractionated heparin; *VTE,* venous thromboembolism.
(From Gutterman D, Akl E, Guyatt G, Schuünemann HJ, Crowther M, and the American College of Chest Physicians Antithrombotic Therapy and Prevention of Thrombosis Panel. Executive summary: Antithrombotic therapy and prevention of thrombosis (9th ed). American College of Chest Physicians evidence-based clinical practice guidelines. *Chest* 2012;141;7S-47S.)

## Delirium Prevention

Delirium affects 8% to 30% of hospitalized patients aged >65 years, leading to longer hospital stays and almost $4 billion in Medicare expenditures (2004 data).[47] Patients with delirium have a higher mortality rate, higher rate of institutionalization, and a higher incidence of dementia.[48] Prevention begins with a thorough history and physical examination to identify risk factors for delirium. Once the at-risk patient is identified, all available preventative measures should be implemented (see Ch. 17).

Studies evaluating actionable steps to prevent delirium are few, but a 2006 Cochrane review identified the need for further studies because of the large scope of the problem.[49–52] It is clear that a multidisciplinary approach is effective[50] and that education of all patient-care team members is key to implementing preventative measures.[49,51] When available, specialized ACE units should be used because they have been shown to decrease hospital stays, reduce costs, and maintain functional status with no change in overall outcomes or readmission rates.[53] Despite studies showing that ACE units may decrease length of stay and improve outcomes in patients with delirium, small studies are inconclusive on the ability of ACE units to prevent delirium in high-risk patients.[54,55]

The Hospital Elder Life Program (HELP) is an innovative program improving hospital care for older adults through comprehensive interdisciplinary geriatric assessment.[56] The HELP program includes maintaining cognitive and physical functioning, assisting with hospital transitions to maximize independence at discharge, and strategies to prevent unplanned hospital readmissions. With robust evidence supporting decreased length of stay, prevention of functional decline, reduced nursing home placement, decreased hospital falls, and delirium prevention, the HELP program saves about $10,000 per patient per year in healthcare costs.

Preventative measures in the hospital must address a range of risk factors. Interventions include addressing and minimizing environmental risk factors, avoiding medicines that may predispose to delirium, screening high-risk patients, and ensuring optimal pain control (see Ch. 17). A useful patient-centered tool is recruiting family members or other visitors to aid in cognitive stimulation (reorienting, reminiscence, etc.). Family members may also be able to help in bringing any of the patient's sensory aids (glasses, hearing aids, dentures, etc.) to the hospital.

## Fall Prevention

Patient falls in the hospital are a serious concern, leading to injuries, longer hospital stays, decreased functional status, higher rates of institutionalization, more malpractice claims, and increased medical costs.[57,58] On average, patients who fell stayed 12 days longer and had charges $4233 higher than controls, after adjustment for potential clinical and nonclinical confounders.[58] Efforts to prevent falls intensified in most hospitals after a change in Medicare reimbursement policy in 2008. At that time, the Centers for Medicare and Medicaid Services included hospital falls in a group of eight hospital-acquired diagnoses that were deemed preventable. Now hospitals are not reimbursed for a higher-paying diagnosis-related group (DRG) after a fall in the hospital.[57]

Fall prevention begins with a thorough assessment of the patient on admission. Risk factors for falls can be divided into four main categories: mechanical, physical, cognitive, and environmental (see Ch. 20). An action plan for fall prevention may benefit all patients, but the cost effectiveness of this in hospitalized patients is unknown.[59] Ideally, prevention should target the patient's specific risk factors (see Ch. 20).[60–62] Vitamin D supplementation may decrease the risk of falls by as much as 20%,[63,64] and the AGS's guidelines for fall prevention give a strong recommendation for at least 800 IU of vitamin D per day in deficient or high-risk patients. A more recent (2010) randomized controlled trial evaluating a preventative health information technology tool (fall prevention tool kit [FPTK]) developed by a Massachusetts group showed a significant decrease in falls in the intervention group.[65]

It is important to balance the desire to decrease fall rates with the need for continued mobility.[57,66,67] Provider and patient fears of falling have the potential to cause more harm if preventative measures are too restrictive and safe mobility is not encouraged.

❖ **Delirium, falls, venous thromboembolism, skin breakdown, respiratory illnesses, and many other infectious diseases have modifiable risk factors that should be targeted in the hospital**.

## Sensory Deprivation

The hospitalized elderly patient is particularly vulnerable to complications related to sensory deficits. At baseline, the elderly are more likely to have auditory, visual, taste, or balance problems. Without the necessary sensory aids these patients are at a higher risk of delirium, falls, medication administration errors, hospital-acquired disability, institutionalization, and readmission. Visual deficits in particular have a greater effect on balance in the elderly than in younger patients.[68] It is important to assess the elderly patient on admission for these deficits and request that family or friends bring any necessary aids to the hospital. Glasses, hearing aids, and ambulatory aids help the patient stay mobile and cognitively engaged in his or her care.

## Venous Thromboembolism Prophylaxis

VTE prophylaxis should be a priority in all hospitalized patients because VTE is responsible for 10% of US hospital deaths each year.[69] The risk of VTE is increased in the hospitalized patient as a result of infections, immobility, and procedures. The Institute of Medicine (IOM) defines failure to provide adequate VTE prophylaxis to hospitalized patients when indicated as a medical error.[70]

All patients should be assessed for risk of VTE on admission.[71] No single risk assessment tool has been prospectively validated for use in deciding on appropriate prophylaxis. Hospitalization for acute medical illness is a risk factor for VTE and in the presence of other risk factors (Table 11.2) should prompt initiation of appropriate prophylaxis (see Table 11.1).[71,72] Pharmacologic prophylaxis should not be used if the risk of bleeding outweighs the risk of thrombosis.[71] Mechanical prophylaxis is a reasonable alternative or adjunct but may limit activity and increase risk for falls and skin breakdown.

## Skin Care

Appropriate skin care in the hospital is an important part of caring for the elderly because they are more susceptible to skin injury. Proactive care includes providing adequate skin moisturization with avoidance of maceration, shearing, tearing, or pressure damage. It is important to identify skin lesions or breakdown on admission and to include appropriate skin care in the treatment plan (see Ch. 30).

Activity should be encouraged with the appropriate level of supervision or aid as needed. Bed-bound or immobile patients should have pressure-reducing support products applied to cushion bony prominences (sacrum, heels, etc.). These patients should be repositioned at least every 2 hours to decrease risk of pressure ulcers. Staff education on skin care and appropriate repositioning techniques is important to minimize damage. Use of proper protective dressings to prevent infection, pressure-reducing mattresses to minimize pressure damage, and wound care specialist consultation may all be appropriate to tailor treatment.

Optimal nutrition and hydration are key to skin health and healing. Avoiding overly restrictive diet orders when possible, encouraging between-meal supplements, and avoiding medicines that impair taste or smell can help maximize nutrition.

❖ **Maintaining optimal nutrition and mobility in the hospital are hallmarks of excellent geriatric hospital care.**

| TABLE 11.2 | Risk Factors for Venous Thromboembolism | |
|---|---|---|
| Stasis | Age Over 40 Years | |
| | Immobility >3 days | |
| | Congestive heart failure | |
| | Stroke | |
| | Paralysis | |
| | Spinal cord injury | |
| | Hyperviscosity | |
| | Polycythemia | |
| | Severe chronic obstructive pulmonary disease | |
| | Anesthesia | |
| | Obesity | |
| | Varicose veins | |
| Hypercoagulable state | Cancer and cancer therapy | |
| | High estrogen states (including HRT) | |
| | Inflammatory bowel | |
| | Nephrotic syndrome | |
| | Sepsis | |
| | Smoking | |
| | Pregnancy and postpartum period | |
| | Inherited or acquired thrombophilia | |
| Endothelial damage | Surgery | |
| | Prior VTE | |
| | Central venous catheterization | |
| | Trauma | |
| Venous compression | Tumor | |
| | Hematoma | |
| | Arterial abnormalities | |

*HRT*, Hormone replacement therapy; *VTE*, venous thromboembolism.
(Modified from Anderson FA Jr, Wheeler HB. Venous thromboembolism: risk factors and prophylaxis. *Clin Chest Med.* 1995;16:235; and Bergqvist D, Pineo GF, Geerts WH, et al., and the American College of Chest Physicians Prevention of Venous Thromboembolism Panel. American College of Chest Physicians evidence-based clinical practice guidelines (8th ed). *Chest* 2008;133(6 Suppl):381–S.)

## Respiratory Illness Prevention

Hospitalized patients are susceptible to respiratory problems because of decreased mobility, exposure to other infected patients, prolonged supine positioning, pain, and other factors. Preventative measures include use of lung expansion maneuvers (incentive spirometry and deep breathing exercises) and encouraging appropriate mobility.[73] Continue home inhalers when possible to maintain baseline control of preexisting pulmonary disease. It is important to achieve adequate pain control to facilitate good lung expansion and mobility.

Older adults are particularly prone to aspiration events that can lead to pulmonary complications, such as pneumonitis or pneumonia.[74] To minimize risk for aspiration, encourage the patient to get up to a chair for meals, monitor for signs of oral motor dysfunction (cough, excessive throat-clearing, etc.), encourage mobility, and avoid psychoactive medications. Providing good oral care, avoiding unnecessary acid-blocking medications, and removing nasogastric tubes as soon as possible leads to decreased pulmonary complications.[74,75]

## Preventing Infections in the Hospital

Infections are a major source of hospital complications in the elderly. Two of three infected hospital patients in 2005 were elderly.[76] Patients >70 years were 10 times more likely to get a hospital-acquired infection than those <50 years.[77] Possible contributing factors to this susceptibility include poor functional status, malnutrition, greater severity of illness, and decreased reserve.

Decreasing hospital-acquired infections starts with strict adherence to standard precautions and hand washing.[78] When additional isolation protocols (contact, droplet, etc.) are needed these should always be followed. Judicious use of intravenous catheters, urinary catheters, and other invasive monitoring devices decreases risk of infection. It is also critical to follow guidelines based on likely pathogens and hospital-specific sensitivities to avoid excess dosing, which increases the risk for resistant organism isolation and *Clostridium difficile* infection.[79] Probiotics have been used to prevent antibiotic-associated diarrhea and *C. difficile* colitis.[80,81] A 2017 Cochrane review concluded that moderate certainty evidence suggests that probiotics are effective for preventing *C. difficile* infection[82] (see Ch. 49). It is important to remember that alcohol-based hand hygiene products are not as effective against the spores of *C. difficile;* therefore the Centers for Disease Control and Prevention recommends use of soap and water with this patient population.[78,83,84]

Recognizing infection in the elderly can also be challenging. Infection may be present without fever or leukocytosis. Subtle changes in behavior, alertness, or mood may be the only warning that an infection has set in, requiring a higher level of awareness when working with the hospitalized elder.

## Preventing Alcohol Withdrawal

Alcohol withdrawal in the hospital is a potentially life-threatening problem. At least one-third of elderly patients exhibit high-risk drinking habits.[85] It is important to ask about alcohol use on admission and anticipate the effects of withdrawal to prevent serious complications.[86] The revised Clinical Institute Withdrawal Assessment Scale (CIWAS-Ar) should be used to monitor these patients. Orders for oral chlordiazepoxide or lorazepam should be scheduled for the high-risk patient (Box 11.2) or as needed for low-risk individuals. A score of ≥8 is used as a cutoff for

---

**• BOX 11.2  Risk Factors for Moderate-Severe Alcohol Withdrawal**

- History of delirium tremens or severe alcohol withdrawal
- Age >30 years
- Concurrent illness
- History of heavy, sustained drinking (>60 g, >1 pint liquor, >96 oz beer/day)
- Presentation with withdrawal symptoms >2 days since last drink
- History of seizures

administering more medication.[87] Because multiple problems may mimic withdrawal symptoms, it is important to rule out other possible explanations such as infection, delirium, or withdrawal from other medications, including opioids and benzodiazepines.

## Selective Interventions to Improve Outcomes

### Maintaining Nutrition

Nutritional status affects healing time, immune system function, energy levels, and strength, all of which are vital to recovering from hospitalization. Baseline malnutrition leads to higher complication rates, increased mortality, longer hospital stays, and a greater than 300% increase in hospital costs.[88] It is important to identify poor nutritional status and actively manage nutrition in the hospitalized elderly patient.

Risk factors for malnutrition before becoming hospitalized include age > 60 years, poor access (if living alone and inadequate social or financial support), lower education level, fatigue, depression, pain, dysgeusia, dysphagia, lack of teeth or ill-fitting dentures, malignancy, polypharmacy, and medication side effects.[89–93]

Assessment of nutritional status involves a detailed physical examination and, in some situations, laboratory investigation. Multiple screening tools exist with variable utility.[94] Sarcopenia is defined as having a muscle mass > 2 standard deviations below the mean for a healthy young adult as assessed by imaging (dual-energy x-ray absorptiometry or bioelectrical impedance), but is often estimated by physical examination when data are not available.[95] Laboratory evaluation is not necessary in most settings because a thorough history and physical examination identify most malnourished patients. If indicated, laboratory evaluation can include serum albumin (half-life 20 days), prealbumin (half-life 2 days), transferrin (half-life 10 days), cholesterol panel, and electrolytes.[96,97] In certain settings, such as preoperative monitoring, the albumin level or prealbumin (also known as transthyretin) may be measured serially with physical examination and calorie counts to aid in identifying improved nutrition before scheduling surgery.[97,98]

All hospitalized patients benefit from maximizing nutrition, but this is particularly important for the malnourished elderly patient, and interventions to boost nutrition should be tailored to the needs of the patient. These include assistance with meals, getting up to a chair for meals, avoiding diet restrictions unless imperative to the patient's treatment, and offering nutritional supplements.[99–102] If the patient has any swallowing difficulties, a diet with the appropriate consistency of solids and liquids should be provided. If the patient has new oropharyngeal dysfunction, a speech therapy consultation may be beneficial. Offering supplements between meals is superior to merely adding cans to meal trays. Nutrition consultation may be of benefit in malnourished patients requiring restricted diets or requiring other routes of feeding (nasogastric tube, J-tube, TPN, etc.). Eliminating restrictive diets (low salt, low fat, etc.) except for when use is clearly clinically necessary is also important. For example, despite a past history of coronary artery disease, a 90-year-old woman hospitalized for pneumonia and eating only 50% of meals should be on a regular diet to maximize food choice and caloric density.

Pharmacologic interventions to improve nutrition status include avoiding medicines that alter taste or smell (Box 11.3).[103,104]

Appetite-stimulating medicines may be tried, but strong evidence supporting their efficacy is lacking. Mirtazapine has been used for dual-indications in depression and poor appetite.[105] Megestrol acetate shows benefit in cachectic or cancer patients, but side effects include increased edema, congestive heart failure, deep vein thrombosis, and adrenal insufficiency.[106,107] There was no demonstrated increase in muscle mass with megestrol acetate in a small study of veterans aged > 65 years, and its use should be avoided in hospitalized elders.[108] Dronabinol and medical marijuana are used primarily in patients with acquired immunodeficiency syndrome or cancer to boost appetite, and the older patient may be more susceptible to side effects, including altered mental status; thus the use of dronabinol and medical marijuana should be avoided.[109]

### Mobility and Functional Decline

Hospital-associated disability refers to multiple deficits induced or accelerated by hospitalization. This disability leads to greater institutionalization, increased mortality, and greater overall healthcare costs.[110,111] More than 30% of hospitalized elderly aged > 70 years leave the hospital with the loss of at least one ADL.[112] Using aggressive preventative measures can avoid or slow decline related to hospitalization. It is important to assess and document the patient's ability to perform ADLs, as well as IADLs, on admission. Those with dependence in any of these are at marked increased risk for hospital-associated disability.[113–115]

Preventative measures include encouragement of early mobilization, providing ambulation-assist devices as needed, staff education, and environmental modifications. Barriers to mobility, such as restricted activity orders and hospital equipment (intravenous lines, urinary catheters, etc.), should be removed if not absolutely necessary. Family members should be included in the care plan to help encourage ambulation and assist the patient throughout the day. Early referral to physical therapy and occupational therapy helps ensure structured daily activity. Staff and families in all locations should be educated on the importance of encouraging

---

**• BOX 11.3** Medicines Impairing Taste and Smell

Allopurinol
Alcohol
Angiotensin-converting enzyme inhibitors
β-Lactam antibiotics
β-Adrenergic blocking agents
Calcium channel blockers (except diltiazem)
Chemotherapeutic drugs
Hydrochlorothiazide
Levodopa
Losartan
Lovastatin
Metronidazole
Nicotine skin patches
Nifedipine
Nitroglycerin
Nonsteroidal antiinflammatory drugs (NSAIDs)
Opiates
Spironolactone
Terbinafine
Tetracycline

(Modified from Ackerman BH, Kasbekar N. Disturbances of taste and smell induced by drugs. *Pharmacotherapy* 1997;17(3):482–496; and Ciancio SG. Medications' impact on oral health. *J Am Dent Assoc.* 2004;135(10):1440–1448.)

ambulation, identification of functional decline, and ways to avoid hospital-associated disability.

## Glycemic Control in the Hospital

Hospitalized diabetic patients are frequently switched from oral agents to insulin therapy on admission to the hospital. Multiple hospital system policies endorse tight glycemic control using a basal-bolus insulin regimen, a recommendation that followed studies showing improved infection rates in hospitalized patients with strict glucose management, but no change in mortality.[116] A subsequent metaanalysis of these trials showed a decreased risk of infection with tight glycemic control mainly in surgical or intensive care unit patients, but a higher risk of hypoglycemia.[116] Target glucose levels recommended by the American Diabetes Association, American Association of Clinical Endocrinologists, and other prominent US guidelines are < 140 to 180 mg/dL (7.8–10.0 mmol/L) for fasting levels in general noncritically ill hospitalized patients, with all random glucoses under 180 mg/dL (10.0 mmol/L).[117,118] The ACP recommends avoiding strict control in noncritically ill patients (diabetic or not) with a target range of 140 to 200 mg/dL.[119]

The elderly patient is more vulnerable to complications with tight glycemic control (see Ch. 41).[120–122] Nutritionists recommend a diet that is nutrient dense, with a low glycemic index and high fiber, to optimize care in elderly diabetic patients. Hypoglycemia puts the patient at risk of falls, delirium, cognitive decline, and fatigue leading to decreased mobility and thus should be avoided.

❖ **Tight glucose control in the hospital offers few, if any, benefits for older hospitalized adults, is based on limited evidence, and is fraught with potential devastating side effects**.

## Care Transition Initiatives and Unplanned Hospital Readmissions

Care transitions refer to the movement of patients between healthcare providers or settings. Transitions including outpatient visits, office visits between medical subspecialists, and the movement into and out of the hospital during the admission and discharge processes are particularly fraught with potential errors and dangers. Confusing medication lists, discharge instructions unclearly written or written at inappropriately high health literacy levels, and a lack of connection to receiving providers in the primary care office or skilled nursing facility all have potential to adversely affect the patient's health and trigger an unplanned readmission. One study noted that up to 40% of patients aged > 85 years are admitted to a skilled nursing facility before returning home, which further increases the risk for errors with these additional transitions. Increasing pressure to decrease length of stay threatens to further increase errors.

Almost one in five Medicare beneficiaries is readmitted to the hospital within 30 days, and almost one-third are readmitted within 90 days. Following the 2010 Patient Protection and Affordable Care Act (ACA)—which introduced the prospect of financially penalizing hospitals based on readmission rates within 30 days after hospitalizations for acute myocardial infarction, congestive heart failure, and pneumonia—readmission rates have modestly been reduced.[123] These associated costs to the healthcare system are immense, and many readmissions are potentially avoidable.[124,125] Readmitted individuals are likely to have multiple medical comorbidities and a longer initial length of stay. Among older adults readmitted within 30 days, age > 80 years, depression, and poor patient education on discharge are all linked to higher rates of unplanned readmission.[126] Community-dwelling elderly Medicare beneficiaries readmitted within 30 days also had significantly increased 1-year mortality rates (39% vs. 12%).[126] Decreasing unplanned readmissions is crucial for both improving patient care and reducing unnecessary cost expenditures, and several care transition initiatives are currently active and building evidence of effectiveness.

## Project BOOST

The Society of Hospital Medicine (SHM) created Project BOOST (Better Outcomes by Optimizing Safe Transitions) as a year-long mentorship program that aims to improve hospital discharges and reduce unplanned readmissions. Created with input from national leaders on care transitions, hospitalist leaders, payers, and regulatory agencies, Project BOOST also targets improved patient satisfaction and improved information flow between outpatient and hospitalist providers to identify particularly high-risk patients and to improve the preparation of patients and families for discharge.[127] A 2013 analysis of 11 participating Project Boost hospitals revealed a reduction in 30-day rehospitalizations from 14.7% to 12.7%.[128]

Project BOOST has five main elements:
1. Comprehensive evidence-based intervention
2. Implementation guide to help interdisciplinary teams redesign workflow
3. Longitudinal technical assistance for 1 year, including train-the-trainer materials for nurses, case managers, physicians, and social workers
4. BOOST collaboration of site webinars and teleconferences
5. An online resource center with benchmark data

## The Naylor Transitional Care Model

Whereas SHM's Project BOOST aims to alter the healthcare system at large and primarily targets physicians and providers, the Naylor Transitional Care Model and the Coleman Care Transitions Intervention (see following section) both focus more on the patient's role in enhanced self-management. The Naylor model involves interdisciplinary care coordination of master's degree–equipped advanced practice nurses (APNs) working with discharging physicians to provide up to 8 weeks of discharge support to medically complex and high-cost patients.[129] Following in-hospital visits by the APN, the program includes comprehensive discharge planning, as well as weekly home-visit follow-up and frequent phone support. The Naylor model has been shown to significantly improve physical function, enhance patient quality of life, and reduce rehospitalizations.[129]

## The Coleman Care Transitions Intervention

Similar to the Naylor model, the Coleman Care Transitions Intervention seeks to empower patients through one hospital visit and one home visit by a "transition coach." An empowered patient is encouraged to have increased knowledge of medication management, follow-up plans, knowledge of disease-specific "red flags" that suggest worsening conditions, and enhanced personal record keeping. The designated Coleman transition coach, who is usually a nurse, social worker, or community health worker with added training, works with patients to prevent unplanned readmissions of medically complex older adults and improve care transitions.[130] The following components make up the Coleman Care Transitions Intervention:

1. A patient-centered personal health record that facilitates interdisciplinary communication during care transitions
2. A discharge preparation checklist of activities designed to empower patients and caregivers before hospital discharge
3. In-hospital transition coach meeting to assist patients and caregivers in asserting their role in managing care transitions
4. Transition coach follow-up at skilled nursing facility or home and phone calls to enhance continuity

A study of 158 community-dwelling older adults found that the Coleman model of a transitions coach to empower patients and caregivers to make their preferences known significantly reduced readmission at 30, 60, and 90 days, and also increased patient understanding of health condition and medication regimen.[130]

◆◆ **Optimal care transitions and safe discharges to prevent unplanned readmission and adverse patient outcomes are critical for good geriatric hospital care.**

## The Ideal Discharge for the Elderly Patient

One critical element of a successful hospitalization for an older adult is a safe care transition and an accurate discharge summary. SHM has identified several key elements of an ideal discharge that must be included (Table 11.3). The ideal hospital discharge for the elderly patient focuses on patient education about follow-up, medication changes, patient instructions on activity, advance directives, code status, and an accurate discharge summary for providers.

---

**CASE 1**

**Discussion**

Mr. Johnson's postoperative delirium and nosocomial complications are unfortunately a common occurrence during hospitalization of older adults. At the time of admission, there were a multitude of risk factors for a prolonged and complicated hospitalization, including potential cognitive impairment, vision and hearing impairment, medical comorbidities, and

---

**TABLE 11.3  Ideal Discharge for the Elderly Patient**

| Element | Particulars | Required | Optional |
|---|---|---|---|
| Patient-centered medication education | • Written schedule (new, modified, unchanged, and discontinued medications) | X | |
| | • Purpose and cautions for all medications | – | X |
| | • Clinical pharmacist consultation (if cognitive impairment or > 3 medication changes) | X | |
| | • Close follow-up plan for hazardous medications (warfarin, diuretics, corticosteroids, hypoglycemic medications, narcotics, cardiovascular medications) | – | |
| | | – | |
| | | – | |
| | | X | |
| Cognition | • Description of mentation (lucid, forgetful, significant dementia) | X | |
| Patient instructions | • Written at sixth-grade level | X | X |
| | • 24/7 call-back number | X | |
| | • Teach-back to confirm patient understanding | – | |
| Provider identification | • Identify referring and receiving provider | X | |
| | • Communicate immediate follow-up issues | X | |
| Follow-up plan | • 2 weeks or sooner for hazardous medications or fragile clinical condition | X | |
| | • Testing or provider appointments | X | |
| Code status | • Code status and other pertinent end-of-life issue stipulations | X | |
| Discharge summary | • Presenting problem | X | |
| | • Primary/secondary diagnosis | X | |
| | • Key findings/test results | X | |
| | • Brief hospital course | X | |
| | • Discharge medicine reconciliation | X | |
| | • Condition at discharge, including functional and cognitive status | X | |
| | • Discharge destination and rationale | X | |
| | • Anticipated problems and suggested interventions | X | |
| | • Follow-up appointments | X | |
| | • Pending lab testing | X | |
| | • Recommendations of any subspecialty consultants | X | |
| | • Documentation of patient education and confirmation of patient/caregiver understanding | X | |

(Developed by the Society of Hospital Medicine HQPS Committee, 2005. Available at www.hospitalmedicine.org/AM/Template.cfm?Section = QI_Clinical_Tools&Template = /CM/ContentDisplay.cfm&ContentID = 10303.)

social isolation. Limited primary care supervision with multiple subspecialist physicians raises the likelihood of polypharmacy. Certainly operative intervention was warranted on Mr. Johnson's fracture, but his prolonged time not eating before surgery certainly could have increased his already frail health status. These limitations in physiologic reserves, combined with delirium, restraints, decreased mobility from a stroke, and poor nutritional intake all set the stage for nosocomial infections and a prolonged hospital stay. Mr. Johnson would benefit from a seamless transition to his next location of care, likely a skilled nursing facility, through the assistance of an evidence-based care transition program that can ensure a smooth handoff between providers and an accurate and timely discharge summary.

## Summary

Providing safe and effective care of older adults in the hospital is a challenging proposition. The need for disease-specific interventions and procedures targeting the incident illness must be balanced with the potential hazards lurking in hospitals. Potentially preventable unplanned readmissions are related to increased mortality and loss of functional independence. An interdisciplinary approach to geriatric hospital care that involves social workers, nurses, case managers, collaborating physicians, patients, and families/caregivers is essential. Safer care transitions through evidence-based interventions and accurate medical records should be the goal of all involved in the care of elderly patients in the hospital.

### Web Resources

www.hospitalmedicine.org/BOOST. Society of Hospital Medicine Project BOOST (Better Outcomes by Optimizing Safe Transitions)

https://nicheprogram.org/about/mission Nurses Improving Care for Healthsystem Elders

https://www.hospitalelderlifeprogram.org Hospital Elder Life Program (HELP): A comprehensive patient-care program that ensures optimal care for older adults in the hospital

## Key References

5. Landefeld CS, Palmer RM, Kresevic DM, et al. A randomized trial of care in a hospital medical unit especially designed to improve the functional outcomes of acutely ill older patients. *N Engl J Med*. 1995;332:1338–1344.

47. Inouye SK. Delirium in older persons. *N Engl J Med*. 2006;354:1157–1165.

112. Covinsky KE, Pierluissi E, Johnston CB. Hospitalization-associated disability: "She was probably able to ambulate, but I'm not sure." *JAMA*. 2011;306(16):1782–1793.

124. Jencks SF, Williams MV, Coleman EA. Rehospitalizations among patients in the Medicare fee-for-service program. *N Engl J Med*. 2009;360:1418–1428.

***References available online at expertconsult.com.***

# 12

# Long-Term Care

GWENDOLEN T. BUHR AND HEIDI K. WHITE

## OUTLINE

*Additional online-only material indicated by icon.*

## OBJECTIVES

*Upon completion of this chapter, the reader will be able to:*

- Identify the most common postacute care and long-term care (LTC) options and list the services provided by each.
- Accurately assess and recommend level of care needs, incorporating information from family, caregivers, therapists, and other members of the interprofessional team.
- Describe the various LTC medical practice models and the role of physicians, nurse practitioners, and physician assistants in each.
- Summarize the role of the medical director in the nursing home.

- Identify and explain five common clinical challenges in LTC medicine.
- Describe the process of evaluating decision-making capacity in older adults and apply shared decision making to clinical situations in LTC.
- Describe how principles of quality improvement and individualized care can be applied in LTC.

## CASE 1

**Mary Lewis (Part 1)**

Mary Lewis is a 91-year-old female with hypertension, osteoarthritis of her back causing chronic low back pain, depression, and anxiety. Recently her son died so she is lonelier because they spent a lot of time together. She lives in her own home, but her back pain no longer allows her to tend her garden, which she previously enjoyed. Recently she gave up driving because her depression and anxiety made this more difficult. Her daughter thinks it may be time for her to move out of the house but is not sure what alternative setting would be best.

- What suggestions for alternative living arrangements do you have for the daughter?
- What questions should you ask to assess Mrs. Lewis's needs?

## The Growing Need for Long-Term Care

The United States is an aging society. The population older than age 85 years, which is the group that most frequently uses long-term care (LTC), is projected to grow by 208% between 2015 and 2050, much faster than the population as a whole.[1] By 2050 the number of people aged 45 to 64 years available to act as caregivers will drop from seven people to every person over 80 years to three people.[1]

Older persons face a number of challenges that place them at risk for needing LTC:

- Functional disability increases exponentially as people age, and the presence of functional limitations is a major reason for needing LTC services. Some 46% of persons older than age 75 years have difficulty in physical functioning.[2] The number of older adults needing help with personal care increases as people age from 4% of those between 65 and 74 years, to 9% between 75 and 84 years, and 20%, 85 years and over.[2]
- Dementia is another major risk factor for needing LTC, and its prevalence rises steeply with age. The number of Americans living with Alzheimer dementia (AD) is projected to increase from 5.8 million people in 2019 to 13.8 million in 2050.[3] The prevalence of AD and other dementias is 3% among Americans aged 65 to 74 years, 17% for those aged 75 to 84 years, and 32% among those aged 85 years and older.[3] In fact, 75% of people with AD will be living in a nursing home (NH) by age 80 years compared with only 4% for the general population.[3] Furthermore, two thirds of older adults dying of dementia do so in a NH, a much higher figure than for other chronic diseases.[3] Behavioral symptoms are a major reason caregivers of older adults with dementia choose to place them in a NH.[4]
- Older persons are more likely to live alone than younger persons and therefore lack a potential live-in caregiver. Currently, 32% of people older than age 75 years live alone,[1] and 55% of women older than age 85 years live alone.[5] Furthermore, more older Americans are divorced than earlier generations, often resulting in poorer quality relationships with adult children who are then less likely to act as caregivers.[6] In 2018, 14% of women and 11% of men 65 years and older were divorced compared with 3% and 4% in 1980.[5] Finally, a greater number of older adults are childless and overall have fewer children than in prior generations.[6]
- Adult children often do not live near enough to their parents to enable them to provide the daily or weekly hands-on care needed. Many potential family caregivers are also caring for their young children as a result of delayed childbearing and longer life expectancies. Therefore older adults will increasingly rely on paid caregivers.
- Poor caregiver health is another reason for entry into LTC.[4] Some 74% of caregivers of people with AD reported being concerned about their own health because of caregiving. Some 59% of family caregivers of people with AD report high to very high levels of emotional and physical stress, 30% to 40% report symptoms of depression, and 44% have anxiety.[3] The prevalence of caregiver burden, depression, and anxiety is greater among caregivers of people with AD than caregivers of older adults without dementia.[3]

## Types of Long-Term Care

LTC offers a critically important care option for many of the frailest and most vulnerable older adults. LTC can be defined broadly as medical or nonmedical care that is provided in the community, congregate housing, residential care facilities (e.g., assisted living), and NHs to meet health or personal care needs during a short or long period of time.

Table 12.1 summarizes the most common types of LTC. The breadth of LTC is apparent from the table, but what the table does not highlight is that most LTC is provided in the home by unpaid family members and friends. An estimated 40 million family caregivers were providing care in 2013.[1]

◆◆ **Long-term care can be defined broadly to include medical or nonmedical care that is provided in the community, congregate housing, residential care facilities (e.g., assisted living), and nursing homes to meet health or personal care needs during a short or long period of time.**

### Nursing Homes

NHs house two types of residents: (1) short-stay postacute care residents, who were admitted for rehabilitation usually after a hospitalization, and (2) long-stay residents who are receiving chronic disease care or palliative care. The percent of older adults living in NHs increases with age—1% for persons age 65 to 74 years to 3% for persons age 75 to 84 years to 9% for persons age 85 years and over.[2] NH residents are mostly White (75%), female (68%), and elderly (85%, ≥65 years).[11] The racial makeup of the NH population should become more diverse in the future as the population of older adults changes in the United States.[1] NH residents often have multiple chronic illnesses: Hypertension (76%), dementia (49%), depression (53%), and heart disease (39%) are the most common.[7] Most NH residents have functional limitations. For example, in 2016, 87% to 97% needed assistance with bathing, dressing, walking, toileting, or transferring in and out of bed.[7] Most NHs (69%) are for profit and chain affiliated (58%). Almost all NHs are Medicare and Medicaid certified and most NH residents have Medicaid as the primary payor source.[7]

### Residential Care/Assisted Living Communities

RC/AL communities go by a variety of names depending on state regulations, including assisted living residences, board and care homes, congregate care, enriched housing, homes for older adults, personal care homes, and shared housing. In 2016 most RC/AL communities were for profit (81%) and chain affiliated (57%).[7]

**TABLE 12.1** Types of Long-Term Care in the United States[1,7-10]

| Type | Definition and Description | Approximate Number of Providers and Patients Served | Average Cost/Predominant Source of Payment |
|---|---|---|---|
| Nursing homes (NH) | • Federally regulated<br>• Provide room, meals, personal care, 24-hour nursing care, medication management, social and recreational activities, and medical care to residents with chronic conditions<br>• Physician involvement: moderate (required visit every 60 days and as medically necessary) | 1,340,485 residents; 1,656,232 beds | $245 per day (semiprivate) $275 per day (private)/ Medicaid (62%), private pay or LTC insurance (25%), Medicare short-stay postacute care (14%) |
| Residential care/ assisted living (RC/AL) communities | • Regulated by the states under a variety of names (including personal care homes, group homes, board and care homes, and others)<br>• Provide room, meals, supervision, assistance with medications, some personal care, and may include some nursing oversight<br>• Many charge a base rate with added fees for additional services<br>• Physician involvement: low (required yearly and as medically necessary) | 996,100 units; 28,900 facilities | $132 per day/primarily private pay, Medicaid (17%) |
| Adult daycare or adult day service centers | • Provide meals, recreation, health-related services (e.g., medication management; weight, blood pressure, and diabetes monitoring), transportation, assistance with ADLs, and exercise in a group environment for individuals with cognitive and/or functional impairments<br>• Physician involvement: minimal (often initial medical summary required) | Generally licensed or certified by states; 286,300 recipients; 4600 centers | $72 per day/Medicaid (66%) |
| Program of All-Inclusive Care for the Elderly (PACE) | • Provides comprehensive long-term services and supports to individuals age ≥55 years who live in a PACE service area, are eligible for NH care, and are able to live safely in the community<br>• Care coordinated by an interprofessional team composed of a primary care physician, RN, MSW, PT, OT, RT, dietician, PACE center manager, home care coordinator, personal care attendants, and a driver at a day health center<br>• Physician involvement: variable according to the needs of the participant but a physician is often on site and may visit people in their homes | 50,000 participants in 263 centers in 31 states | Average monthly payment for dual-eligible $3620; Medicare and Medicaid risk adjusted capitation payments; 90% are dually eligible for Medicaid and Medicare, 9% are Medicaid only, 1% are Medicare only |
| Specialized dementia units | • Either RC/AL or NH that provides specialized care for people with dementia—often a separate secured unit, trained staffing, special programming, a modified physical environment, and family involvement<br>• Physician involvement: variable depending on whether it is RC/AL or NH | 14% of RC/AL communities and 15% of NHs have specialized dementia units within a larger facility; 9% of RC/AL only serve dementia residents | See NH and RC/AL costs |
| Home care/personal care | • Home health aide or homemaker/companion that provides nonmedical care (help with ADLs, cooking, shopping, laundry) to enable older adults with chronic illnesses to remain at home<br>• Physician involvement: minimal | 12,200 home health agencies served 4,455,700 patients; 778,457 home health aides in the United States | $22 (home health aide) $21 (homemaker) per hour/private pay, Medicaid (10%) |

*ADLs,* Activities of daily living; *MSW,* master's level social worker; *NH,* nursing home; *OT,* occupational therapist; *PT,* physical therapist; *RN,* registered nurse; *RT,* recreational therapist.

Some 46% were small (4–10 beds), but these facilities served only 8% of the overall RC/AL population. The majority of residents (52%) lived in large (26–100 beds) or (32%) in extralarge (>100 beds) facilities.[7] Some 48% of RC/AL communities were Medicaid certified. Nearly all RC/AL communities provide basic health monitoring, personal care, social and recreational activities, dietary and nutritional services (83%), and personal laundry and housekeeping services. RC/AL facilities must offer assistance with medications, but this may include assistance with self-administration or staff administering medications. Most also offer transportation to medical appointments and case management, and physical, occupational, or speech therapy (71%), whereas fewer offer social services (10%), or mental health or counseling services (54%).[7] Many of the services require additional fees. RC/AL communities employ mostly aides (83%) and fewer registered nurses (RNs) (39%) or licensed practical or vocational nurses (LPNs or LVNs) (36%).[7] More RC/AL communities than NHs offer dementia care in a distinct unit or wing or in a facility specializing in dementia care (23%).[7] Residents are typically White (81%), female (71%), and age ≥75 years (82%).[7] The majority of RC/AL residents need assistance with bathing (64%) and walking (57%), and almost half need assistance with dressing (48%) and toileting (40%).[7] RC/AL residents often have multiple chronic illnesses: Hypertension (51%), dementia (42%), arthritis (42%), depression (31%), and heart disease (34%) are the most common.[7] These demographic descriptors indicate that considerable overlap exists between the population of RC/AL communities and NHs.

## Continuing Care Retirement Communities/Life Plan Communities

An attractive option for LTC available to middle- and upper-income Americans is the continuing care retirement community (CCRC), also known as Life Plan Communities. The Life Plan Community contains independent living units, assisted living, and NH care on the same campus; it guarantees access to LTC services in exchange for substantial admission and monthly fees.[13] The Life Plan Community provides 24-hour security, social and recreational activities, a common dining room with some meals provided, housekeeping, transportation, and fitness programs. The reasons for joining include access to and a guarantee for medical care, maintaining independence, and not being a burden on family. A recent survey of 80 Life Plan Communities and more than 5000 residents across the United States found that Life Plan Community residents have greater life satisfaction, a more positive outlook about the future, more social contacts and less loneliness, more physical and intellectual activity, and a higher sense of purpose compared with older adults in general.[12] In addition, most residents reported that their social, intellectual, and physical wellness had improved since moving to the Life Plan Community.[12] Disadvantages of Life Plan Communities include the high cost, concentrating the experience of disability and death into a small age-segregated community, and loss of autonomy in decisions to move to higher levels of care if necessary.[11]

## Program for All-Inclusive Care for the Elderly

PACE is a community-based model that aims to keep persons who are age 55 years or older and are certified by their state to need NH care living in the community. Enrollees must have the desire to remain at home and be able to do so safely.[14] An interprofessional team provides individualized, coordinated care, primarily carried out in a medical daycare setting. For most PACE participants (95%), a comprehensive service package enables them to receive care at home rather than in a NH.[14] The average PACE participant is 76 years old, and 70% are women.[14] The majority need assistance with their activities of daily living (ADLs): 26% with one to two ADLs, 25% with three to four ADLs, and 35% with five to six ADLs. PACE participants have multiple chronic illnesses; vascular disease, heart failure, diabetes, depression, polyneuropathy, and dementia are the most common.[14] Financing is through capitated monthly payments from Medicare and Medicaid, Medicaid only, or for persons who do not qualify for Medicaid, from private sources.[14] PACE operates as both a provider and an insurer, and is obligated to pay for whatever healthcare services its participants need—including hospitalization, NH care, and other costs by non-PACE providers. Thus the program has a strong incentive to prevent hospitalizations and maintain participant health. In fact, research shows that PACE participants have reduced hospital admissions, rehospitalizations, and emergency department (ED) visits compared with other dually-eligible beneficiaries aged >65 years.[14] The PACE program has also been shown to reduce caregiver burden and have high caregiver and participant satisfaction.[14]

## Adult Daycare or Adult Day Service Centers

Adult daycare or adult day service centers provide care for adults in a community-based group setting. Services offered by most centers are social activities, transportation, meals and snacks, personal care, and therapeutic services.[8] The centers most commonly operate during normal business hours, affording caregivers respite 5 days per week. Adult day centers generally can be categorized into one of three types: (1) social, (2) medical/health, and (3) specialized (such as for participants with dementia or developmental disabilities).[8] In 2016 a minority of adult daycare centers were for profit (45%) or chain affiliated (43%) in contrast with NH and RC/AL communities.[7] Adult daycare centers have more social workers and activities staff hours per participant than NHs or RC/AL.[7] Adult day participants are younger (37% age <65 years, and only 16% age >85 years) and more racially diverse (23% Hispanic, 15% Black, and 20% other) than those in other LTC settings; fewer had ADL dependencies; and they were more balanced with respect to gender (58% women).[7] Most adult day centers are Medicaid certified (77%).[7]

## Community Services and Supports/Aging in Place

Most people prefer to live in their own homes as long as possible. There are many support services that can aid this effort. When available, family caregivers provide much of the care at home. Food can be supplemented by organizations such as Meals on Wheels, a publicly funded program by the Older Americans Act that provides nutritious home-delivered meals to older adults living in poverty. The program not only combats hunger, but also eases social isolation and addresses safety concerns such as falls. For older adults who are able to get out of their home, many senior centers provide congregate meals through similar funding, while also allowing older adults to socialize with friends and neighbors.

In addition to single-family houses, older adults can find independent living senior apartments, some of which the Department of Housing and Urban Development subsidize. Some of these apartments may provide meals, housekeeping, personal care assistance, transportation, social activities, and laundry. They can also facilitate access to other services and programs available from other community-based agencies. Many of these services may have an extra cost.

Another way that older adults can age in their own homes is to join or create a Village (vtvnetwork.org), which are nonprofit organizations within communities designed to help with transportation, shopping, home repairs, and social and educational activities, as well as coordinated access to affordable services or discounted service providers. There is an annual cost to membership. Also for a fee, older adults or their families can hire a geriatric care manager to help with coordination of care and identification of needs and community resources.

Although there can be challenges concerning the funds necessary to maintain life at home, the Affordable Care Act strengthened and expanded the Money Follows the Person Medicaid program. The goals of the program are to increase the use of home and community—based services (HCBS) and reduce the use of institution-based services. The program has successfully transitioned over 63,337 Medicaid beneficiaries through 2015 to the community from institutions and shown sustained improvement in quality of life.[15] In 2016, 45% of Medicaid spending went to HCBS, a percentage that is increasing over time.[1]

---

### CASE 2

#### Albert Thompson (Part 1)

Albert Thompson is an 89-year-old nursing home resident with advanced Parkinson disease and mild dementia. A nurse calls you because she noticed that he hardly ate or drank anything for dinner. She reports that a certified nursing assistant (CNA) obtained Mr. Thompson's vital signs; his temperature was 100.4° F, blood pressure 110/60 mmHg, pulse 80 beats/min, and respirations 18 breaths/min. When you try to ask further questions, the nurse is unprepared. She has not assessed the patient herself. She does not have his current medication or problem list. She seems to be frazzled and mentions she has only been working in the building for 3 weeks. She suggests strongly that you send the patient to the ED.

1. What additional information would you most like to have? What steps can be taken short of sending this patient to the ED for evaluation?
2. Because you are also the medical director of this facility, what steps can you suggest to better prepare nurses to assess and manage patients with providers over the telephone?

---

## Medical Care Provider Practice Patterns in Long-Term Care

Because exposure to LTC remains limited in medical school and residency programs, expertise in LTC medical practice is typically obtained through experience, a geriatric fellowship program, or through curriculum offered by the AMDA—The Society for Post-Acute and Long-Term Care Medicine. AMDA offers an online educational program to support the society's competencies for attending physicians practicing in LTC settings.

NHs are required by law to have a medical director; RC/AL communities are not, but a few do have them. The medical director is a physician who oversees and guides care in a LTC facility.[16] The primary functions are summarized in Table 12.2. AMDA has a certification program that uses an experiential

model in which practicing physicians who are providing LTC and medical director duties can be certified by completing educational requirements through participation in a geriatric fellowship program, continuing medical education, AMDA-sponsored courses in medical direction, and/or other continuing education programs.

> ◆◆ **AMDA has a certification program that uses an experiential model in which practicing physicians who are providing LTC and medical director duties can be certified.**

Physicians who practice in NHs do so within a variety of practice models. The traditional model has been as an adjunct to an office-based practice. In the last decade new practice models have arisen: the LTC-only practice and the house-call practice. With these, there has been a call to recognize that NH medicine is emerging as a specialty in its own right, similar to the hospitalist.[17] Physicians working in this specialty have been referred to as skilled nursing facility specialists (or SNF-ists), NH physician specialists, or LTC specialists. The NH physician specialist spends a substantial portion of time in the delivery of NH care and is proficient in NH regulations and the medical management of common syndromes faced by NH residents.

> ◆◆ **The nursing home physician specialist spends a substantial portion of time in the delivery of nursing home care and is proficient in nursing home regulations and the medical management of common syndromes faced by nursing home residents.**

Nurse practitioners (NPs) provide primary care to NH residents as NH employees, as members of primary care practices, or as employees of health maintenance organizations. NPs are advanced practice registered nurses (APRNs) who obtain graduate education, post-master's certificates or doctoral degrees, and then obtain certification through a national certifying examination or through state certification mechanisms. The NP scope of practice varies by state. In many states NPs diagnose, order, and interpret diagnostic tests, as well as initiate and manage treatments, including prescribing medications and controlled substances, under the exclusive licensure authority of the state board of nursing.[18] However, federal NH regulations require each patient to have a physician and only allow certain tasks to be delegated to advance practice providers.

Physician assistants (PAs) must follow these same federal regulations in NHs. They are nonnurse providers whose training typically consists of 1 year of basic science classes and 1 year of clinical rotations. PA educational programs prepare them to take medical histories, perform physical examinations, order and interpret laboratory tests, diagnose illness, develop and manage treatment plans for their patients, prescribe medications, and assist in surgery. They must pass a national certification examination. The PA scope of practice varies by state, but is generally governed by medical boards and largely determined at the physician or practice level; most commonly, a physician can delegate to PAs anything that is within the physician's scope of practice and the PA's training and experience.[19]

Optum CarePlus (formerly Evercare) is a Medicare Advantage program specifically for long-stay NH residents that extensively uses NPs or PAs. The NPs or PAs work as employees of the managed care company and provide more intensive primary care than is typical. They are assigned to work in specific NHs, usually one or two, carrying a caseload of approximately 100 residents.[20] The NH residents continue to have their primary care physician, who Evercare pays on a fee-for-service basis, including

| TABLE 12.2 | Functions and Duties of a Nursing Home Medical Director |
|---|---|

| Function | Duties |
|---|---|
| Administrative | • Communicate regularly with the administrator and DON<br>• Participate in administrative decision making<br>• Recommend, approve, and inform medical staff about relevant policies and procedures<br>• Participate in licensure and compliance surveys |
| Professional service | • Organize and coordinate physician services and the services provided by other professionals as they relate to patient care to ensure the quality and appropriateness of services |
| Quality assurance and performance improvement | • Participate in monitoring and improving the quality of medical care in the facility, so as to ensure that it is effective, efficient, safe, timely, patient centered, and equitable<br>• Participate in the QAPI program, ensuring that it encourages self-evaluation, anticipates and plans for change, and meets regulatory requirements<br>• Help the facility use QAPI results, as appropriate, to update and improve policies, procedures, and practices |
| Staff and personal education | • Participate in education of facility staff<br>• Sustain own professional development through continuing education |
| Employee health | • Participate in the surveillance and promotion of employee health, safety, and welfare, specifically regarding infectious disease issues |
| Community relations | • Help articulate the facility's mission to the community |
| Resident rights | • Participate in establishing policies and procedures to ensure that resident rights are respected. This includes their right to request practitioners to limit, withhold, or withdraw treatment(s) |
| Contextual factors | • Acquire and apply knowledge of social, regulatory, political, and economic factors that relate to patient care and related services |
| Person-directed care | • Support and promote person-directed care |

*DON,* Director of nursing; *QAPI,* quality assessment and performance improvement.
(Modified from AMDA. The nursing home medical director: Leader and manager (White Paper A11). Columbia, MD: AMDA; 2011. Available at https://paltc.org/amda-white-papers-and-resolution-position-statements/nursing-home-medical-director-leader-manager.)

payment for time spent in family or care-planning conferences (which is not ordinarily reimbursed under Medicare). The NP also educates the NH staff through formal and informal in-service training. Because the NP or PA is present in the NH frequently under this model, this person monitors residents closely and develops relationships with the staff, which facilitates early identification of acute illnesses. They are salaried employees of the managed care company; therefore NPs and PAs can spend more time in preventive and early intervention direct care that might not otherwise be reimbursed by Medicare. In addition, the managed care program can pay the NH for "intensive service days," when an ill resident might otherwise need to be hospitalized. As a result, sites have fewer hospitalizations and ED visits than traditional care models and higher patient/family satisfaction with the care.[20] More recently, Medicare selected Enhanced Care and Coordination Providers in seven states to implement clinical and education evidence-based models to reduce avoidable hospitalizations in an effort to improve care and quality of life. Again, increasing the presence of APRNs in nursing facilities to provide consistent medical care and staff engagement had a positive effect on reducing hospitalizations among facility residents.[21] The shortage of primary care physicians and the flexibility of practice in LTC setting—unlike the 10- or 15-minute appointment in traditional ambulatory care—has led to more LTC-focused practices relying on advance practice providers to provide a substantial portion of the care in concert with physicians.

Federal regulations require that NH residents be seen by the physician for the initial comprehensive visit and then every 30 days for the first 90 days. Thereafter patients must be seen every 60 days and when medically necessary. Other than the initial comprehensive visit, the routine (regulatory) visits can be alternated between the medical doctor (MD) and NP or PA. Patients in the NH are generally seen by their primary care providers in their residence. This is in contrast to the RC/AL communities, in which the practice norm is for the resident to be transported to his or her provider's office, although models of care where providers come to the RC/AL are growing.[22] Because RC/AL communities are regulated by the states, regulations differ depending on the state of residence, but most commonly only a yearly physician visit is required.

Providing quality individualized care is heavily dependent on communication with both the patient and the family. NH admission is the best time to make initial contact with the responsible family member, including those of patients who are cognitively intact and in full capacity to make decisions. Clear communication is also crucial when a patient's condition changes—ideally before the situation becomes urgent. Patients are generally appreciative when asked if the physician can speak with a family member regarding their care. Hearing the patient and family concerns, their understanding of diagnoses and prognosis, and expectations for personal involvement in care can help to direct the care plan.

**❖ Hearing the patient and family concerns, their understanding of diagnoses and prognosis, and expectations for personal involvement in care can help to direct the care plan.**

Goals of care and advanced directives should be established or reviewed as soon as possible after admission to a LTC setting. It is important to address advance directives at the time of admission and when the resident's condition deteriorates. Tools have been developed to assist clinicians in identifying residents appropriate for palliative and hospice care (www.eprognosis.org). Enhancing the role of palliative care in NHs will also help align decisions about hospitalization with the individual's overall goals of care.

Much of the care delivery in LTC occurs via telephone—more so than in other clinical settings. Many of the telephone calls occur after hours and on weekends to on-call providers who may not be familiar with the patient or the facility. Most telephone calls report a clinical problem. For example, in one study of a typical NH, the problems that were most frequently reported by phone were falls, pain, agitation, abnormal blood glucose, and fever, with the calls typically prompting a clinical action, such as ordering a medication or treatment, clinical observation by the nursing staff, or diagnostic studies.[23] A consistent communication structure, like SBAR (situation, background, assessment, recommendation), can ensure effective and efficient communication.

## Nursing Homes

Nurses are the foundation of care in the NH. Most nurses employed in NHs are LPNs or LVNs. Their work largely consists of administering medications, collecting data on patients, determining the need for interventions, implementing care plans, supervising nursing assistants, and communicating with medical care providers. The LPNs/LVNs work under the direction and supervision of RNs and physicians in a limited and focused scope of practice. RNs commonly fill administrative or supervisory roles in the NH, such as charge nurse or director of nursing.

The interprofessional team is the cornerstone of care in the NH. The interprofessional team is made up of nurses, medical providers (physicians, NPs, and PAs), social workers, the NH administrator, dietician, activities coordinator, consultant pharmacist, CNAs, environmental service workers, and therapists (occupational, speech, and physical). These individuals pool their expertise and collaborate so that patients receive better care. Every NH resident is required to have an assessment that identifies his or her abilities and needs and a comprehensive, individualized care plan developed by the interdisciplinary team (IDT) that maximizes the patient's abilities and meets the patient's needs. Care planning conferences are held with the patient and/or family and the IDT soon after admission and at least every 90 days to design and update the care plan.

❖ **The interprofessional team is the cornerstone of care in the nursing home**.

CNAs fill a critical role in the NH, providing most of the basic patient care. They assist residents with ADLs, provide skin care, take vital signs, answer calls for help, and are expected to monitor the residents' wellbeing and report significant changes to nurses. Of the 1.2 million CNAs in the United States, the vast majority are female with a high school or less education (74.4%), middle-aged with a family income of less than $30,000.[24] There is considerable racial diversity, with 53% of CNAs being White, 38.7% Black, and 9.3% Hispanic or Latino in origin.[24] According to the US Bureau of Labor Statistics, as of 2018 the median hourly pay rate was $13.72; strong growth in the available positions is expected over the next 10 years. Most became CNAs because they like helping people, but when surveyed 65.8% revealed that they might leave the facility in the next year because of poor pay or because they found a better job.[24] Being a CNA is hard work; 56.2% report being injured at work in the previous year.[24]

Staff turnover is a major challenge facing NHs in the United States; it is costly and a major factor contributing to quality problems. Turnover rates for licensed nurses tend to hover around 30% and can be much higher for nursing assistants. Recommendations for increasing staff recruitment and retention include increased training, increased pay, the provision of health insurance benefits, improving the work environment by nurturing positive relationships between CNAs and their supervisors, fostering respect among the workforce, and providing opportunities for advancement.[25]

## Residential Care/Assisted Living Communities

The RC/AL communities care model grew out of the hospitality industry rather than the health industry. Consequently, the goals of RC/AL communities are to provide a homelike environment emphasizing privacy and freedom and to foster independence and autonomy. RC/AL requirements differ depending on the state, but in general they are considered nonmedical facilities and are not required to have nurses, CNAs, or medical directors. RC/AL practice offers a wider variation of services than NHs with respect to staffing available, range of patients served, and cost of care. Small RC/ALs (≤10 beds) tend to have a licensed nurse who does assessments and provides care oversight but may be on site as little as 8 hours a week; larger RC/ALs often have at least one full-time nurse. In most states, certified medication aides rather than nurses pass medications, with regulations varying as to whether they "administer" the medications or "assist residents with self-administration." When RC/AL residents need skilled nursing or rehabilitative services, these typically are provided either by home health agencies or by temporary transfer to a SNF, although some larger facilities have begun offering some rehabilitative services in-house.

---

**CASE 2**

### Albert Thompson (Part 2)

Later that week you are again called about Mr. Thompson by a different nurse. This nurse indicates that Mr. Thompson rolled out of bed and hit his head on a side table. He has a bruise on his forehead. An ice pack has been applied. His vital signs are normal. They heard the fall and went immediately to the room. There was no loss of consciousness. He is moving all extremities. With help he was able to get up, walk to the bathroom with his walker, and then return to bed. He is complaining of a mild headache. Because he is on warfarin you suggest that he be sent to the ED for evaluation and a computed tomography scan of his head. However, the nurse says that the patient has discussed with his doctor his desire not to return to the hospital and this is documented.

- Describe an appropriate course of management.
- What should be done to assess and manage this patient's future risk for falling?

---

## Common Clinical Challenges

The main focus in LTC settings is on maintaining function and quality of life rather than on the diagnosis and treatment of individual medical conditions. What follows are a few medical conditions unique to the LTC environment, especially prevalent in LTC residents, or more challenging because of the congregate living situation.

❖❖ **LTC is a unique environment and patient population where the main focus is on maintaining function and quality of life rather than on the diagnosis and treatment of individual medical conditions.**

## Distinguishing Between Dementia, Delirium, and Depression

Residents in LTC facilities are especially at risk for delirium. The essential features of delirium are inattention, acute onset and fluctuating course, and a change in cognition with associated features of disturbances in the sleep-wake cycle, mood swings, and disturbed psychomotor behavior (e.g., hyperactive, hypoactive, mixed, or unclassifiable). In contrast, dementia is a chronic slowly progressive disorder of cognitive decline in one or more cognitive domains that interferes with functional performance. Depression is characterized by gradual onset of depressed mood or loss of interest or pleasure. Delirium with psychomotor agitation or retardation can appear very much like depression, emphasizing the importance of conducting a structured bedside evaluation. Notably, attention is generally intact with depression.

Delirium that began during a hospitalization can persist for weeks or months and predispose to geriatric syndromes such as dehydration, pressure ulcers, urinary retention, malnutrition, aspiration, and falls.[26] Often it is unrecognized—one study of long-stay LTC residents found that 21.3% developed delirium over a 6-month period, but nursing staff identified only half of cases.[27] Antipsychotics are commonly prescribed for delirium; however, a systematic review of hospitalized patients found that there was no difference in length of stay, delirium duration, or mortality between patients treated with placebo and those given antipsychotics, including haloperidol or second-generation antipsychotics.[28] Therefore antipsychotics should be reserved for treatment of severe agitation that poses a risk to safety. Instead nonpharmacologic programs consisting of orientation activities, hydration and snacks, and evening relaxation strategies (including hand or foot massage, quiet music, and a warm drink to aid in sleep) are feasible in the NH[29] and have been shown to be effective at reducing delirium incidence, falls, and costs.[30] It is imperative to prevent delirium because it can lead to higher risk of dying, long-term functional decline, hospital readmission, and permanent NH placement.[31]

The Minimum Data Set (MDS) version 3.0, a federally mandated assessment of all residents in Medicare- and Medicaid-certified NHs, uses the following three validated, objective instruments to assess LTC residents for depression, dementia, and delirium:
- The Patient-Health Questionnaire (PHQ)−9, a valid, simple tool for identifying and following patients with depression
- The Brief Interview for Mental Status (BIMS), a valid screen for cognitive impairment
- The Confusion Assessment Method (CAM), a widely used and validated screening instrument for delirium

## Neuropsychiatric (Behavioral and Psychological) Symptoms of Dementia

Neuropsychiatric symptoms can include apathy, depression, agitation, aggression, anxiety, confusion, psychotic symptoms (hallucinations and/or delusions), resistance to care, disinhibition, and changes in sleep pattern. Virtually everyone with dementia, and even those with mild cognitive impairment, will develop neuropsychiatric symptoms at some point during their disease. Although it is true that antipsychotic drugs are an important treatment for patients with certain mental health conditions, the US Food and Drug Administration has warned that antipsychotic medications are associated with an increased risk of death when used in elderly residents with dementia. Therefore these medications must be used judiciously and only if the resident's behavioral symptoms constitute a danger to the resident or others. The Centers for Medicare and Medicaid Services (CMS) created the National Partnership to Improve Dementia Care in Nursing Homes, which is focused on reducing the number of long-stay NH residents who are receiving antipsychotic medications. Since its inception, the prevalence of antipsychotic use has decreased from 23.9% in 2012 to 14.6% in 2018, a 39% decrease.[32]

To treat challenging behaviors, interventions that do not involve medications are key. A systematic review of interventions for aggressive and agitated behaviors found that nonpharmacologic interventions are more efficacious than pharmacologic interventions.[33] Multidisciplinary assessments and care addressing unmet needs, massage and touch therapy, and music combined with massage and touch therapy were clinically effective treatments. Nonpharmacologic strategies to treat neuropsychiatric symptoms should be individualized and based on the resident's level of cognition and physical function and long-standing personality and interests. Individualized music through headphones allows a heterogeneous group of residents to listen to music that connects to their long-term memories and resonates with positive emotions without adding to background noise that may agitate others. Resources are available to help with implementation of these types of programs (https://musicandmemory.org/). Other nonpharmacologic strategies that have shown benefit include aromatherapy with lavender or lemon balm, pet therapy, physical exercise, light therapy, Snoezelen multisensory therapy, recordings of family members (stimulated presence therapy), and person-centered bathing solutions (www.bathingwithoutabattle.unc.edu).

A multidisciplinary national dementia care expert panel devised the DICE approach to neuropsychiatric symptoms. DICE stands for describe, investigate, create, and evaluate.[34] With this approach, when a behavior occurs, it is described in detail, including the physical and social context. Next, the behavior should be investigated and a broad differential should be considered—for example, physical pain, hunger, constipation, urinary retention, fatigue, poor sleep, anxiety, fear, depression, the caregiver approach, institutional routines, medication side effects, over-/understimulation, functional limitations, or infection are some. The interprofessional team should create a plan to prevent and respond to the behaviors with nonpharmacologic interventions and monitor for effectiveness. If psychotropic medications are employed, they must be carefully monitored, the target behavior should be carefully documented and tracked, and the psychotropic medication must undergo gradual dosage reductions according to CMS guidelines.

## Infections and Antibiotic Stewardship

The hallmarks of infection in younger people may not be apparent in older LTC residents. For example, fever as typically defined is absent in more than half of LTC residents with a serious infection, prompting the Infectious Diseases Society of America to define fever in LTC as a single oral temperature >100° F (37.8° C); or repeated oral temperatures >99° F (37.2° C) or rectal temperatures >99.5° F (>37.5° C); or an increase in temperature of

>2° F (>1.1° C) over the resident's baseline temperature.[35] Infection should be suspected in residents with a decline in functional status, new or increasing confusion, new incontinence, falling or deteriorating mobility, reduced food intake, or failure to cooperate with staff. However, restraint should be used with respect to antibiotic prescribing because inappropriate antibiotic use in the NH contributes to high rates of antibiotic-resistant pathogens, such as methicillin-resistant *Staphylococcus aureus* and vancomycin-resistant *Enterococcus*, and to antibiotic-induced *Clostridium difficile* colitis. CMS recently called attention to this with new requirements for NHs to have an infection prevention and control program that includes a system for preventing, identifying, reporting, investigating, and controlling infections. In addition, the NH must have an antibiotic stewardship program and employ someone with specialized training in infection prevention and control.

LTC facility residents with infections may become dehydrated. Hypodermoclysis is the infusion of fluid into the subcutaneous tissue of the leg, abdomen, or chest. It should be considered as an alternative to intravenous (IV) hydration for treating mild/moderate dehydration because it causes no more complications than IV fluid administration and is cheaper, more comfortable, can be easily done in people with poor veins, and requires less nursing time.[36]

Before treating a suspected infection, the resident's advance directives should be reviewed because some LTC residents elect not to treat infections near the end of their life. Some of the most common infections in LTC include the following.

### Urinary Tract Infection

The urinary tract is one of the most common sites of infection in LTC residents. However, urinary tract infection (UTI) is often overdiagnosed because asymptomatic bacteriuria is also common. Asymptomatic UTI should not be treated because treatment results in antibiotic resistance, drug side effects, increased cost, and no improvement in morbidity or mortality.[37] It is often difficult, however, to differentiate between symptomatic and asymptomatic UTI because of the high prevalence of communication barriers, chronic genitourinary symptoms, and behavioral symptoms in these settings. Pyuria does not distinguish between symptomatic and asymptomatic UTI either, because it is present in 90% of cases of asymptomatic bacteriuria and 34% of persons without bacteriuria. Thus the absence of pyuria can rule out a UTI but the presence of pyuria lacks specificity. The Centers for Disease Control and Prevention (CDC) has created criteria for defining symptomatic UTI,[38] and the surveyor guidance is in line with these recommendations. For residents who do not have an indwelling catheter, minimum criteria for initiating antibiotics include $> 10^5$ CFU/mL (positive) or pending urine culture and dysuria alone or two or more of the following: fever as defined earlier, new or worsening urgency, frequency, suprapubic pain, gross hematuria, costovertebral angle tenderness, urinary incontinence, or shaking chills. For residents with an indwelling catheter or a suprapubic catheter, minimum criteria for initiating antibiotics include the presence of $> 10^5$ CFU/mL (positive) or pending urine culture and one or more of the following: fever as defined earlier, new costovertebral tenderness, rigors, or new onset of delirium.[39]

### Norovirus

Noroviruses are the most common cause of outbreaks of acute gastroenteritis in LTC. Norovirus infection typically presents with watery diarrhea and vomiting; although it is generally self-limited, it can cause significant morbidity and mortality in the LTC population. Norovirus occurs year round, but most outbreaks occur between December and February. Noroviruses are highly contagious, and transmission occurs with person-to-person contact, contact with contaminated food or water, or contact with contaminated objects. The incubation period is 24 to 48 hours, and symptoms often last for 24 to 72 hours, but in frail older adults symptoms can be prolonged, often leading to dehydration. It is imperative that measures be employed to prevent and control norovirus outbreaks, including isolation of infected people; using gowns, masks, gloves, and hand hygiene with soap and water when caring for affected people; minimizing staff working at multiple facilities; requiring affected staff to stay out of work for at least 48 hours after symptoms resolve; and disinfection and sterilization of fomites.[40]

### Clostridium Difficile Colitis

Another common and more serious cause of diarrhea in LTC is *C. difficile* infection. Risk for *C. difficile* colitis increases with antibiotic exposure, proton pump inhibitors, staying in healthcare settings (hospitals and NHs), and advanced age. A large prevalence of LTC residents have asymptomatic colonization with *C. difficile* (up to 51%), and the incidence of *C. difficile* infection unrelated to recent hospitalization has been reported as high as 50%.[41] To prevent and control *C. difficile*, the CDC recommends that clinicians prescribe antibiotics judiciously, test for *C. difficile* when LTC residents have diarrhea (defined as three or more unformed stools in <24 hours) without an obvious alternative explanation (laxative use or a norovirus outbreak), isolate residents with *C. difficile* immediately, wear gloves and gowns when caring for residents with *C. difficile*, and clean room surfaces with bleach or another Environmental Protection Agency–approved, spore-killing disinfectant after a resident with *C. difficile* has been treated. It is important not to test people who do not meet the criteria for diarrhea because this can lead to false-positive diagnoses in the setting of high prevalence of asymptomatic carriage. Recurrence of *C. difficile* infection after treatment is at least 25%.[41]

### Influenza

Outbreaks of influenza in LTC occur sporadically, even when high levels of resident immunization have been achieved. LTC residents are at high risk for serious influenza complications, such as myocardial infarction, heart failure, and pneumonia. Influenza vaccination is recommended annually for all residents and staff. Vaccination of LTC staff has been effective at preventing resident influenza-like illness and mortality.[42]

When there is influenza activity in the local community, surveillance for influenza should be performed among all residents, staff, and visitors. A high index of suspicion is often required because frail older adults may have atypical signs and symptoms and may not have fever. A nasopharyngeal swab should be obtained at the onset of a suspected respiratory viral infection outbreak (defined as two or more ill residents), from which identification of influenza virus or other common viruses will confirm an outbreak. Infection prevention and control measures, antiviral treatment, and antiviral chemoprophylaxis should be instituted at the first sign of an outbreak. Infection prevention and control measures include standard and droplet precautions.

### Pneumonia

Pneumonia is the most common infection leading to hospitalization and mortality among LTC residents. The American Thoracic Society and Infectious Diseases Society of America guidelines on the diagnosis and treatment of community-acquired pneumonia have recommendations pertinent to LTC.[43] These include use of the Pneumonia Severity Index, a validated clinical prediction rule for prognosis that indicates which residents should be transferred to the hospital for management if this is aligned with the resident's goals. In addition, during influenza season, if there have been cases of influenza in the community, a rapid influenza molecular assay is advised. Poor mouth care causes up to half of the cases of pneumonia in LTC, and control of gingivitis and dental plaques will reduce incidence rates. Mouth Care Without a Battle (mouthcarewithoutabattle.org) is an evidence-based approach to person-centered mouth care for residents with dementia.

## Pressure Ulcers/Injury

Pressure injuries are caused by unrelieved pressure on the skin, usually over bony prominences, such as the ischium, sacrum, trochanter, and heel. Pressure injuries are associated with increased pain, disfigurement, and increased infection risk. CMS has NH quality measures for pressure ulcers. In 2018 the prevalence of pressure ulcers was 7.3% in US NH residents at high risk for pressure ulcers because of malnutrition or mobility limitations prohibiting them from changing position on their own.

## Pain Management

Pain is common in residents in LTC and is often unrecognized and untreated or undertreated, especially in racial and ethnic minorities and cognitively impaired residents.[44,45] Dementia can be a significant barrier to recognizing and appropriately treating pain. There is no evidence that persons with dementia have less pain, although they are less likely to report it. However, with careful observation, pain can be detected by listening to the resident's verbal expression and/or watching for evidence of inflammation or nonverbal signs, such as facial grimacing. Empirically treating pain in residents with moderate to severe dementia has been shown to reduce neuropsychiatric symptoms.[46]

## Falls and Fall Risk

Falls are a common cause of loss of independence, injury (e.g., hip fracture and head injury), and death among older adults residing in LTC. Conditions contributing to increased risk include impairment of gait, balance, or vision; medications such as benzodiazepines, selective serotonin reuptake inhibitors, and antipsychotics; orthostatic hypotension; arthritis; Parkinson disease; and cognitive impairment. A history of falls is a strong predictor of future falls. The most common types of interventions include environmental adaptations and assistive technology (e.g., lighting, handrails, raised toilet seats, assistive devices), medication review and targeted modification, increasing the number of staff, providing staff training, and exercise. Most studies are of low quality; therefore it is unclear if fall-prevention interventions are effective.[47] For residents with low vitamin D, the prescription of vitamin D can reduce the rate of falls.[47]

After a resident has fallen, the resident should be evaluated with vital signs (including orthostatic blood pressure) and examined for possible musculoskeletal or neurologic injury, and the resident's medical provider should be notified. The resident should be observed for at least 72 hours for delayed signs or symptoms of injury and for complications such as a subdural hematoma. The provider should assess the resident to (1) identify and address risk factors and treat the underlying medical conditions contributing to

falls, (2) determine if the resident sustained an injury, and (3) determine if medications that may increase fall risk can be decreased or eliminated. Although all falls and injuries resulting from falls cannot be prevented, an interprofessional effort and multifactorial approach toward managing falls and fall risk may reduce incidence rates.

---

### CASE 1

#### Mary Lewis (Part 2)

Before Mrs. Lewis's daughter could make any alternative care arrangements, Mrs. Lewis became ill and required hospitalization. After her hospital stay, she went to a local nursing facility for rehabilitation. During this stay, the daughter was able to consult with the facility social worker and arrange transfer to a senior apartment complex that provides two meals a day in a dining room, transportation services, and housekeeping.

Mrs. Lewis has now been living in that setting for 3 years. During that time, she has developed vascular dementia and her mobility has declined. With the help of a case manager, the daughter has secured care through a home care agency for 10 hours each day, but her mother is alone at night.

The daughter called you a few days ago because her mother fell and spent 6 hours on the floor because she was not wearing her alert button around her neck. Thankfully she was not injured but the daughter is concerned that it is time again for more care. Her mother keeps "firing" the home care workers, and the agency is running out of people to send. The daughter is concerned that her mother will not understand or accept her need for more care and another move.

1. How might you determine whether Mrs. Lewis has capacity to decide about whether she should move to higher level of care?
2. If she is not capable of making this decision herself, how should you talk to her and her daughter about the need for a change?

---

## Common Challenges

The variable capacities of the residents to make decisions, as well as the congregate living situation, create distinctive considerations. Providers are constantly balancing the principles of autonomy and beneficence for their LTC residents and the desire to strive for the greater good.

### Determining Capacity

When residents are unable to function safely where they live but are reluctant to move, the physician may be called upon to determine their capacity to make a decision, especially when a resident's preferred decision does not appear to be in his or her best interest. Capacity includes the ability to (1) express a choice, (2) understand and make a decision, (3) appreciate one's own situation and the consequences of the decision, and (4) rationally manipulate information to make comparisons and weigh options. Capacity is decision specific and exists on a continuum such that it depends on the complexity and degree of risk involved in the particular decision at hand. Individuals may be perfectly able to make simple decisions but lack capacity to make more complicated decisions.

◆◆ **Capacity is decision specific and includes the ability to express a choice, understand and make a decision, appreciate one's own situation and the consequences of the decision, and rationally manipulate information to make comparisons and weigh options.**

Allowing as much decision-making capacity as possible is important in the LTC setting. For residents to make informed decisions, they must have capacity to make the decision in question, be provided with adequate information and alternatives, and be free from coercion. Shared decision making values mutual participation by the resident, family members, and providers and takes into account the resident's unique beliefs.

## Advance Care Planning

In the LTC setting, medical providers often interact with substitute decision makers chosen by the resident through advance directives (referred to as a healthcare proxy or power of attorney) or appointed by a court (referred to as a guardian). When a resident has not appointed a decision maker, family member(s) serve in this capacity, as determined by state law according to the proximity of relationships. Physicians should encourage families to designate one person as the primary spokesperson and decision maker. However, it is ideal for all family members to be in agreement when a key decision is made; thus family meetings are often helpful. Physicians should also help families understand substituted judgment, the process of making a decision according to what the resident would have decided if he or she were capable. However, when the decision makers do not know the wishes of the resident, they can be directed to make decisions in the resident's best interest.

## Abuse and Neglect

The World Health Organization defines elder abuse as "a single, or repeated act, or lack of appropriate action, occurring within any relationship where there is an expectation of trust which causes harm or distress to an older person." Elder abuse is common and often goes unreported. One in six Americans over the age of 60 years has experienced some form of abuse, and the prevalence is higher in institutional settings where residents are dependent on others for assistance and commonly have neuropsychiatric conditions. There are six types of elder abuse in long-term care in descending order of prevalence: psychological, resident-to-resident, physical, financial, neglect, and sexual abuse.[48,49] Resident-to-resident abuse most commonly occurs between two residents in a NH or assisted living facility and can be verbal or physical altercations. Clinicians should screen for elder abuse; in fact, they are mandated to report confirmed cases of elder abuse, and in most states must also report cases of suspected elder abuse. Signs of elder abuse include bruises on the extremities or back; changes in personality, anxiety, or depression; and fear or flinching that cannot be otherwise explained. A NH must report allegations of abuse or neglect to the State Survey Agency immediately in cases of serious bodily harm and within 24 hours if there was not serious bodily harm. Frontline staff play pivotable roles in recognizing and reporting cases, as well as prevention. Clearly interventions to decrease elder abuse are a key area for future research.

## Measuring and Promoting Quality of Care and Quality of Life

### Federal Structures That Promote Nursing Home Quality

NHs are required by federal law to collect clinical assessment data on each resident on admission, with any significant change in

---

**• BOX 12.1  Nursing Home Compare Quality Measures of the US Centers for Medicare and Medicaid Services**

**Measures Applied to Short-Stay (Postacute Care) Residents**

Percentage who were rehospitalized after a nursing home admission
Percentage who have had an outpatient emergency department visit
Percentage who got antipsychotic medication for the first time
Rate of successful return to home and community from a skilled nursing facility (SNF)
Rate of potentially preventable hospital readmissions 30 days after discharge from a SNF
Medicare spending per beneficiary (MSPB) for residents in SNFs
Percentage who self-report moderate to severe pain
Percentage who improved in their ability to move around on their own
Percentage whose functional abilities were assessed and functional goals were included in their treatment plan
Percentage who experience one or more falls with major injury during their SNF stay
Percentage with new or worsened stage II–IV pressure ulcers
Percentage assessed and given, appropriately, the influenza vaccination during the current or most recent influenza season
Percentage assessed and given, appropriately, the pneumococcal vaccine
Percentage who newly received an antipsychotic medication, but do not have evidence of a psychotic or related condition, such as schizophrenia, bipolar disorder, Tourette syndrome, Huntington disease, hallucinations, or delusions

**Measures Applied to Long-Stay Residents**

Percentage experiencing one or more falls with major injury
Percentage with a urinary tract infection
Percentage who self-report moderate to severe pain
Percentage of high-risk residents with stage II–IV pressure ulcers
Percentage of low-risk residents who are regularly incontinent of bowel or bladder
Percentage who have had a catheter inserted and left in their bladder
Percentage who are physically restrained on a daily basis
Percentage whose need for help with daily activities has increased
Percentage whose ability to move independently worsened
Percentage who had a weight loss of ≥5% in the last month or ≥10% in the last two quarters
Percentage who have depressive symptoms
Percentage assessed and given, appropriately, the influenza vaccination during the current or most recent influenza season
Percentage assessed and given, appropriately, the pneumococcal vaccine
Percent who newly received an antipsychotic medication, but do not have evidence of a psychotic or related condition, such as schizophrenia, bipolar disorder, Tourette syndrome, Huntington disease, hallucinations, or delusions
Percentage who got an antianxiety or hypnotic medication
Number of hospitalizations per 1000 long-stay resident days
Number of outpatient emergency department visits per 1000 long-stay resident days

(From Centers for Medicare & Medicaid Services. MDS 3.0 quality measures user's manual. Available at www.cms.gov/Medicare/Quality-Initiatives-Patient-Assessment-Instruments/NursingHomeQualityInits/Downloads/MDS-30-QM-Users-Manual-V60.pdf.)

---

status, and at quarterly intervals. These assessments are gathered and reported using the MDS, now in version 3.0, from which quality indicators are derived that measure and monitor the care. The data are transmitted to state and federal regulators in a national database called Online Survey, Certification, and Reporting (OSCAR), which has made it possible to compare NH performance across the country.

Selected quality indicators for every Medicare- and Medicaid-certified NH in the country are available to consumers through the Nursing Home Compare section of the CMS website (www.medicare.gov/NursingHomeCompare). Box 12.1 provides a list of currently published quality indicators. The assumption is that the availability of this public data will foster consumer-driven pressure to improve and maintain quality within NHs.

The CMS contracts with a Quality Improvement Organization (QIO) in each state to provide NHs, as well as hospitals and other healthcare providers, with expertise and tools to enact quality improvement initiatives that use quality indicators derived from MDS data. For example, QIOs have worked with NHs to reduce pressure ulcer occurrence, reduce the use of physical restraints, and improve transitions between hospitals and NHs. The QIO website contains a wealth of information and resources to support quality improvement processes in NHs (https://qioprogram.org/nursing-home-resources/). Effective quality improvement hinges on using a structured process that emphasizes small cycles of change and subsequent evaluation, education, and involvement of key front-line staff, agreement on what needs to improve, and expert coaching through the process of change, including dissemination of impactful interventions.

State government entities are responsible for surveying NHs annually to ensure compliance with state and federal regulations. They use these data to determine how to apply their efforts during the survey process within a given facility. The review process relies heavily on the interpretation and enforcement of federal regulations often referred to as F-tags. For example, F-tag 841 is the federal regulation that codifies the functions of a medical director. CMS provides guidelines to help surveyors interpret the code and apply it in meaningful ways to individual NHs. Survey results, which are available publicly through Nursing Home Compare, provide another means of measuring quality.

Currently federal Quality Assessment and Assurance requirements (483.75[o]) mandate that facilities maintain a Quality Assessment and Assurance committee that meets at least quarterly to address quality-related concerns and deficiencies. In addition, Section 6102(c) of the Affordable Care Act requires CMS to establish Quality Assessment and Performance Improvement (QAPI) standards and provide technical assistance to NHs on best practices to meet these standards. This marks an additional step moving NHs toward using process improvement procedures as an ongoing methodology to assess needs, implement change, and measure outcomes.

CMS recently updated the federal regulations that allow SNFs to receive Medicare and Medicaid reimbursement for services. These new regulatory requirements have incorporated antibiotic stewardship and greater emphasis on assessment and planning for psychiatric conditions. These initiatives lend themselves to quality improvement through process improvement methodology and highlight the need for physicians and medical directors to be engaged with other professionals in the NH to enhance care. In addition, CMS initiated a new Medicare payment system for skilled nursing facilities in October 2019 in an effort to better account for the complexity of clinical care needed to effectively provide rehabilitative services.

## Quality of Life

Promoting quality of care is an important aspect of what needs to be accomplished in NHs, but enhancing quality of life is an equally important goal, especially for the substantial proportion of individuals who spend months and years of their lives in NHs. Quality of life encompasses both staff and residents. Measuring quality of life can be a challenge, but the measurement should incorporate issues such as choice and control over ADLs, access to outdoor environments, the quality of interpersonal interactions, privacy, the promotion of function/physical activity, and participation in care planning. The application of available research has served to promote quality of life in NHs; for example, the use of physical restraints has declined and is no longer accepted as an effective means of preventing injury.[50] Similarly, restrictive diets (to control diabetes, cholesterol levels, and salt intake) are being abandoned because they have been associated with poor nutritional intake.[51] Not surprisingly, many residents and their families will choose quality of life over length of life by refusing treatments that are restrictive, unpleasant, or of dubious benefit, such as dialysis for declining renal function or statins for hypercholesterolemia.

## Approaches to Quality Enhancement

Early recognition of changes in condition can improve care outcomes. INTERACT (Interventions to Reduce Acute Care Transfers; https://pathway-interact.com/) is a quality improvement program to reduce hospital transfers from the NH. The interventions are designed to improve the identification, evaluation, and communication about changes in resident status early so that the condition can be stabilized and treated in the NH rather than the hospital. The program consists of the SBAR form and progress note that aid communication with providers, decision support tools that guide notification of the clinician, and the stop and watch early illness identification tool that directs direct care providers to notice any change when caring for a resident and to notify the nurse promptly. Also included in the program are advance care planning tools and quality improvement tools. This program has been found to be effective in reducing hospitalizations from the NH.[52]

Improving transitions between the hospital, NH, and community settings for both short-term and long-term residents is essential to quality across the continuum of care. Unplanned hospital admission rates are being closely scrutinized by hospitals and NHs, which means NHs and LTC physician providers have a growing opportunity to work in collaboration across these settings to identify and solve transition problems and implement best practices. Patients transitioning in or out of the NH should include the following: (1) appropriate information on the problem that prompted the transfer or a discharge summary; (2) contact information for the NH, primary care physician, the resident's legal healthcare representative, and other service providers, such as home health and durable medical equipment; (3) updated medication and allergy lists; (4) physical and cognitive functional status; (5) advance directives; and (6) the goals/expectations of patient, family, and provider.[53] In addition, personal contact between nurses and physicians or advance practice providers in each setting is advisable.

## Innovative Models

A substantial number of stakeholders are advocating for wholesale change within NHs and the broader arena of LTC services. As a result of this groundswell of interest in change, a variety of new models have evolved. Many of these models involve creating homelike environments and using technology.

## The Green House Model

The Green House model is based on three core values—real home, meaningful life, and empowered staff. Small residential-style houses are created in community neighborhoods, often alongside the founding traditional NH. Core elements include private rooms for

10 to 12 residents (called elders) with private full baths, a personal (locked) medicine cabinet, a communal hearth area (with open living room, dining room, and kitchen), a dining table that seats all elders and caregivers, fenced outdoor space, and lots of windows. There is 24-hour access to food. Pets are encouraged and accommodated. The care is provided by self-managed universal workers called Shahbazim that are consistently assigned rather than by CNAs and LPNs. The Shahbazim do all of the caregiving tasks, including the cooking in the open kitchen, cleaning, laundry, ordering, and scheduling. A nurse is available 24 hours a day. There is relatively little research on the outcomes of the Green House model, but existing evidence has shown positive results related to privacy, dignity, autonomy, food enjoyment, and improved resident and family satisfaction.[54] Although hugely popular, the movement is growing slowly because of the need for new construction rather than remodeling of existing institutions, and concerns about cost.

## Eden Alternative

Originating in the early 1990s, the Eden Alternative (www.edenalt.org) is an international not-for-profit organization dedicated to transforming care environments into habitats for human beings that promote quality of life for all involved. This program is known for bringing plants and animals into the NH environment, along with an appreciation for a homelike community that takes into account both residents and caregivers.

## GRACE Team Care Model

Geriatrics Resources for Assessment and Care of Elders (GRACE) Team Care was initially developed and implemented more than a decade ago by the Indiana University School of Medicine's Center for Aging Research, but has since been adapted across the United States. This interprofessional model involves a NP and social worker completing an in-home assessment that is then reviewed by a larger team, including a geriatrician, pharmacist, and mental health liaison. The team then develops a personalized care plan that includes evidence-based protocols for 12 common geriatric syndromes, such as falls, sensory impairments, and cognitive impairment. The plan is implemented by the NP and social worker in consultation with the primary care provider. A particular emphasis is support for care transitions between emergency facilities, hospitals, skilled nursing, and home settings. A randomized controlled trial of this model indicated improved quality and outcomes for the low-income older population.[55] For high-risk older adults, cost of chronic and preventative care was offset by reductions in acute care costs.[56] Such models are necessary to meet the complex care needs of older adults who remain in community settings.

## Technological Innovation

Technology is providing new ways to address old problems in LTC. Global positioning systems (GPS) allow caregivers to track the location and movements of people in their care. GPS allows the individual freedom to move about a facility, home, or neighborhood with the capability of alerting the caregiver if the client moves outside a particular geographic area. Personal emergency response systems allow individuals with chronic conditions or physical frailty to summon help in urgent situations, such as a fall. Devices often come with a wearable button to press that calls a caregiver or health professional. Many devices will sense a change in plane such that pushing a button is not necessary when a fall occurs. Medication

reminders come in a variety of forms providing alerts and opening specific pill containers minimizing the possibility of medication errors. Many telephone adaptions are available to help older adults with a variety of limitations, such as hearing and memory, to be able to successfully use phone communication. Wireless home monitoring can help caregivers monitor the use of appliances, especially whether appliances have been appropriately turned off. Telehealth monitoring and video visits allow older adults to transmit personal health data, such as blood pressure, pulse, pulse oximetry, weight, and many other parameters, easily and quickly to healthcare providers to better manage chronic and acute conditions and to receive instructions that can help avoid difficult trips out of the home to clinics or emergency facilities. Technology will help to address the growing workforce gap while allowing greater independence, more convenience, and ease of access to healthcare services.

### CASE 1

#### Discussion

It is common for primary care providers to be asked for recommendations on level of care needs.

Part 1. As Mrs. Lewis's provider, you can help her daughter determine an appropriate level of care by asking questions regarding instrumental ADLs and ADL performance, financial resources, and personal preferences. The local Area Agency on Aging will have resources that would help the daughter to identify appropriate care. Alternatively, a geriatric care manager available through private practice, health insurance benefits, or health system resources may be available to help the daughter in assessing the needs of her mother and determining what settings may be accessible given the available financial resources.

Part 2. Mrs. Lewis is capable of expressing an opinion about where she wants to live. However, your interview reveals that she does not appreciate the potentially dangerous outcomes she narrowly avoided during her recent falls or the extent of her cognitive and physical limitations. She remains resistant even to the help she now has in her home and does not want anyone "watching" her at night. You explain that it is your opinion that she needs to be in an environment with around-the-clock supervision, that you recommend assisted living, and that you are instructing her daughter to begin searching for appropriate options. You would like for Mrs. Lewis to visit the facilities with her daughter to participate in the decision-making process.

Even though Mrs. Lewis is not able to make this decision on her own, it is important to gain her assent to this transition and offer as much autonomy as is reasonable after the daughter has identified financially feasible options that are close to the daughter's residence. It is also very helpful for you as the primary provider to take responsibility for this decision so that Mrs. Lewis does not blame the daughter for making the decision against her wishes.

### CASE 2

#### Discussion

Part 1. Patience and kindness are always the best professional approach, whether face to face or on the telephone. Calmly and with appropriate explanation ask Mr. Thompson's nurse to call you back with the following information: Has the patient been coughing? Does the patient have any dysuria, or changes in urinary frequency, urgency, or new incontinence? What allergies does he have? What medications is he taking currently? What do the recent provider notes indicate about this patient? What are his care directives?

When she calls you back, she tells you that he has been having dysuria, and a urine sample was sent to the lab earlier that day. The urinalysis is positive for nitrites, leukocyte esterase, with many white blood cells and bacteria.

He was successfully treated with ciprofloxacin 3 months ago and has no allergies. You decide to start ciprofloxacin while waiting for culture results.

The next morning you meet with the director of nursing to discuss implementing a program to better prepare new nurses to assess and communicate about problems and concerns. You mention that AMDA has Know-It-All-Before-You-Call cards that can be purchased and made available on each nursing unit. The training will include key physical examination data and medical history to gather on common problems before calling the provider.

Part 2. Falls require both an immediate assessment and management plan and a subsequent evaluation process aimed at minimizing risk and preventing future falls. Over the phone, you decide to ask the nurse to perform neurologic checks every 15 minutes for the first hour, then hourly for 3 hours, then every 4 hours for 48 hours. The nurse should call you if there is any change in alertness, worsening confusion, worsening headache, or asymmetry to Mr. Thompson's strength or coordination. Given his wishes to not go to the hospital, the nurse will give him acetaminophen 650 mg now for the headache and obtain an international normalized ratio in the morning.

Each nursing home has a formal process for reviewing falls, assessing patients, and implementing interventions to prevent falls. It is important that the provider also participate in the evaluation and intervention plan. The nurse tells you the patient is afraid he will no longer be allowed to enjoy a beer as he usually does each night. In fact, the next day the care team would like your colleague, his usual physician, to discontinue the order that allows him to have alcohol. The physician objects because this will adversely affect his quality of life. You encourage the nurses to check positional blood pressures, and he is documented to be orthostatic. The nurse encourages fluids, and on recheck the following week he is no longer orthostatic. In response to this information, as medical director you suggest that the care team discuss with Mr. Thompson the possibility of abstaining from alcohol when he is ill, in an attempt to limit his risk for falls. Mr. Thompson agrees and so does his primary physician.

## Summary

LTC is a rewarding field of practice for a primary care provider that incorporates a complex skill set, including an understanding of the health system, care processes, and medical knowledge. Collaborative practice is a key professional quality for successful LTC practice—both within the LTC organization and with other professionals in hospital, hospice, home health, and ambulatory settings—so that care is optimal and transitions are not plagued by unintended consequences. In addition, LTC practitioners must partner with the residents for whom they care and their families, helping them to understand the complexities of the environment and to have the optimal experience possible given the challenges of their health problems and prognosis.

### Web Resources

https://paltc.org. AMDA The Society for Post-Acute and Long-Term Care Medicine is the professional association of medical directors, attending physicians, advance practice providers, and others practicing in the LTC continuum.

bathingwithoutabattle.unc.edu. A significant portion of LTC residents exhibit aggressive behaviors during bathing. This website contains information on a CD and video package that teaches individualized approaches for bathing.

mouthcarewithoutabattle.org. To address resistance to mouth care, this evidence-based program teaches person-centered daily mouth care for residents with cognitive and physical impairment.

https://qioprogram.org/nursing-home-resources/ Quality Improvement Organizations provide key resources for anyone interested in improving the quality of life and quality of care for those living in nursing homes.

https://pathway-interact.com/. INTERACT (Interventions to Reduce Acute Care Transfers) is a quality improvement program that focuses on the management of acute change in resident condition to reduce the frequency of transfers to the hospital.

www.medicare.gov/NursingHomeCompare. Nursing Home Compare contains quality of care information on every Medicare- and Medicaid-certified nursing home in the country.

www.pioneernetwork.net. The Pioneer Network is the leading advocacy organization of the culture change movement.

www.edenalt.org Eden Alternative is an organization dedicated to transforming care environments into habitats for human beings that promote quality of life for all involved.

https://musicandmemory.org/ Music and memory is an organization that brings personalized music into the lives of the older population or infirm through digital music technology.

## Key References

1. Houser A, Fox-Grage W, Ujvari K. *Across the States: Profiles of Long-Term Services and Supports*. Washington, DC: AARP Public Policy Institute; 2018. Available at: https://www.aarp.org/content/dam/aarp/ppi/2018/08/across-the-states-profiles-of-long-term-services-and-supports-full-report.pdf. Accessed August 23, 2019.
16. AMDA. *The Nursing Home Medical Director: Leader and Manager*. Columbia, MD: AMDA; 2011. Available at: https://paltc.org/amda-white-papers-and-resolution-position-statements/nursing-home-medical-director-leader-manager. Accessed November 01, 2019.
31. Kosar CM, Thomas KS, Inouye SK, Mor V. Delirium during postacute nursing home admission and risk for adverse outcomes. *J Am Geriatr Soc*. 2017;65:1470−1475.

35. High KP, Bradley SF, Gravenstein S, et al. Clinical practice guideline for the evaluation of fever and infection in older adult residents of long-term care facilities: 2008 update by the Infectious Diseases Society of America. *Clin Infect Dis*. 2009;48(2):149−171.
37. Genao L, Buhr G. T. Urinary tract infections in older adults residing in long-term care facilities. *Ann Longterm Care*. 2012;20:33−38.
52. Ouslander JG, Bonner A, Herndon L, Shutes J. The interventions to reduce acute care transfers (INTERACT) Quality improvement program: an overview for medical directors and primary care clinicians in long term care. *J Am Med Dir Assoc*. 2014;15:162−170.

**References available online at expertconsult.com.**

# 13

# Home Care

JOHANNA L. BELIVEAU AND MICHAELA PREISS

## OUTLINE

## OBJECTIVES

*Upon completion of this chapter, the reader will be able to:*

- Describe the types of healthcare services available to older adults at home.
- Understand the basic payment mechanisms for these services.
- List evidence-based outcomes of home care for older adults.
- Recognize the limitations of the existing evidence base on home care.

- Identify key elements of recent legislation affecting medical home care.

## CASE

### Mrs. K (Part 1)

Mrs. K is an 83-year-old woman with hypertension, type 2 diabetes mellitus, congestive heart failure, and osteoarthritis who lives alone and has missed two clinic appointments with you in the last 6 months. She comes to your office today with her daughter Linda, who is visiting from California. Linda is concerned because Mrs. K seems to be "letting things go" around the house lately and has not filled her medication prescriptions for the last few months. Mrs. K denies any recent acute illness or injury, but says she has been afraid to leave the house "for a while now" since she tripped on a garden hose and almost fell 8 months ago. Medications include aspirin, metformin, lisinopril, furosemide, and acetaminophen. Physical examination is remarkable for a blood pressure of 156/87 mm Hg without postural change and symmetric 2 + pitting edema of both legs to mid-shin, which is new since her last visit with you. Lungs are clear to auscultation. Her gait is slow with a wide base and unsteady turning radius. She is unable to rise from the chair without using her arms to push herself up. Cognitive testing reveals mild short-term memory impairment but preserved judgment and executive function. Laboratory studies show a serum creatinine of 1.3 mg/dL, potassium 4.2 mg/dL, and hemoglobin (Hb)A$_{1C}$ of 10.2%. Thyroid function tests are normal. You are concerned about

her poorly controlled hypertension and diabetes, as well as her gait and memory impairment, so you decide to refer her to a Medicare-certified skilled home care agency for services.

1. What home care services do you request for Mrs. K?

## What Is Home Care?

Home care in its most general sense refers to any diagnostic, therapeutic, or social support service provided to patients in their homes.[1] These services may range from a visiting nurse assessment of cardiovascular status and medication teaching and management, to a physician or nurse practitioner evaluating and treating pulmonary edema, to a speech therapist providing language rehabilitation, to an aide assisting with mobility and activities of daily living, to a medical social worker helping caregivers identify and coordinate community services to help keep patients in their home instead of moving into institutional long-term care. Table 13.1 shows the array of home care services available.

| TABLE 13.1 | What Is Home Care? | | |
| --- | --- | --- | --- |
| **Skilled Home Care** | **Medical/Other House Calls** | **Personal Care** | |
| Nursing | Primary care home visits | Bathing | |
| Therapy | Podiatry | Dressing | |
| Physical | Dentistry | Feeding | |
| Occupational | Optometry | Toileting | |
| Speech | Hospital at Home | | |
| Medical social work | Home hospice | | |

Medicare is the major insurer for older adults in the United States and covers "part-time or intermittent" skilled care as outlined in Table 13.1. Furthermore, Medicare pays for skilled home care only if a patient is homebound (i.e., leaving the home requires considerable and taxing effort, and absences from home are infrequent or of brief duration).[2] Note that a home healthcare service will not qualify as "skilled care" if it could safely be done by patients themselves or a nonmedical person without supervision from a nurse or therapist listed earlier.[2] Therefore Medicare does not cover personal care unless it is in the context of skilled care. A patient who requires assistance only for activities of daily living, and does not have a need for skilled care, must find some other way to obtain and/or pay for these services. Medicaid covers personal care at home, usually for a few hours per day, several days per week. This allows patients with mental illness and/or physical, developmental, or intellectual disabilities to receive their healthcare in a community setting or at home, as opposed to a traditional medical institution.[1] However, strict financial eligibility criteria may exclude many older adults who are not impoverished. In addition to these formal services that are directly funded by various insurance payors, informal unreimbursed care provided by family and friends is crucial to keeping patients at home, and represents a silent but enormous economic force in the US healthcare system.[3] In this chapter, we describe the two most common types of formal home care: Medicare skilled home care and medical house calls. We also briefly describe Hospital at Home, an emerging model of acute care in which intensive home-based medical management substitutes for a hospital inpatient admission, and the Independence at Home demonstration project included in the Patient Protection and Affordable Care Act of 2010.

Fig. 13.1 depicts the continuum and overlap of the various major types of home care. The light gray circle on the left represents the population of older adults who receive primary care services from physicians and other medical providers. Most of these patients are seen in the office, but some of them receive primary care visits at home (dark gray circle), and are sometimes referred for skilled home care (gold bar) for additional home-based rehabilitation or medical management and monitoring. Some patients experience acute illness (gold circle), which is managed at home through medical house calls or Hospital at Home, often in conjunction with skilled care (intersection of gold bar with light gray, dark gray, and gold circles).

❖❖ **Medicare does not cover personal care (bathing, toileting, dressing) at home unless it is in the context of skilled care; informal care to meet these needs is crucial to keeping patients at home, and has tremendous economic implications for caregivers and society in general.**

## CASE

### Mrs. K (Part 2)

Mrs. K is referred to skilled home care and is visited by a nurse and a physical therapist at home. The nurse monitors her blood pressure and reports it back to you weekly so that you can adjust her medications. She helps Mrs. K and her daughter organize a pillbox that Mrs. K can fill weekly with telephone prompting as needed from her daughter. She also provides written materials and "refresher" teaching on diabetes self-management and monitoring. Meanwhile, the therapist evaluates Mrs. K's home and suggests several practical options for minimizing safety risks, such as installing grab bars in the bathroom (not paid for by Medicare) and securing some loose carpeting at the base of the stairs. The therapist also works with Mrs. K twice a week to increase her lower extremity strength, balance, and steadiness, and teaches her a home exercise program with written materials that she can use to continue exercises on her own. After about 5 weeks of this level of home care, Mrs. K is ambulating more safely and confidently, and her $A_{1C}$ (drawn by the nurse during a visit for blood pressure monitoring) returns at 9.2%. She is discharged from skilled care, but misses another office appointment with you because she remains fearful of walking outside her home and forgets that she has a medical appointment.
1. What options are available for ongoing medical primary care for Mrs. K?

## Who Needs Home Care?

Homebound patients who have a skilled need may receive home care from a Medicare-certified home health agency. These patients generally have medical or functional conditions that are likely to

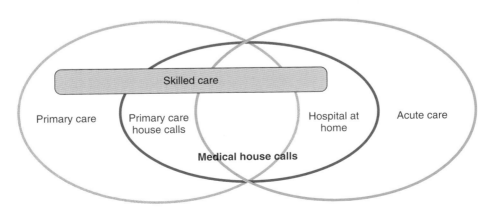

• **Figure 13.1** Types of medical home care.

improve with treatment over a short period (1–2 months), and have difficulty leaving their homes to access office-based treatment for these conditions. Examples of such skilled needs include nursing care of wounds (surgical, venous stasis, or pressure), physical and occupational therapy after hip fracture, speech therapy after a stroke, or monitoring of blood pressure and renal function during adjustment of medications for uncontrolled medical conditions (diabetes, hypertension, heart failure). Importantly, nursing visits solely for the purpose of drawing blood are not considered a skilled need. While a patient is receiving skilled care, Medicare also covers personal care services, including assistance with bathing and dressing.

Another important group of patients who can benefit from home care may not be homebound by Medicare's skilled home care definition, but are medically complex or have medical conditions refractory to the usual office-based management. Although these patients may not be eligible for skilled home care, a targeted medical house call by a physician or nurse practitioner to assess adherence, functional conditions, caregiver/patient dynamics, and other barriers to effective care can provide invaluable context for the medical provider, and open up new opportunities to work with the patient to optimize care. In fact, one study comparing office-based medical and psychiatric evaluations with in-home assessments showed that a substantial minority of patients had important problems that were discovered only on the home visit, and almost all patients had problems identified at home that increased the risk of morbidity or significant functional decline.[4]

Finally, a subset of older adults are frail, medically complex patients who do not have a need that qualifies for skilled home care, but are unable to access office-based primary care because of functional impairment. This population is particularly appropriate for medical house calls provided by physicians, nurse practitioners, or physician assistants for ongoing management of their chronic diseases.

◆◆ **Medical house calls by physicians, physician assistants, or nurse practitioners can be useful as an adjunct to office-based care or as primary care for appropriate patients.**

## How Is Home Care Delivered?

A physician must certify that a patient is homebound and has a skilled need for a Medicare-certified agency to receive reimbursement for skilled services. Since 2011, Medicare has required a face-to-face medical visit at the time of initial certification to confirm the necessity of skilled home care. The face-to-face visit may occur in any setting, and must occur in the 90 days before or 30 days after the initiation of skilled home care services. A nurse practitioner, physician assistant, or trainee physician may perform the visit on behalf of the certifying physician, but the certifying physician must personally sign a document confirming the face-to-face visit. Nurse practitioners and physician assistants may not sign home care certification orders, although they can sign orders for durable medical equipment, such as canes, walkers, and bedside commodes.

The typical certification period for Medicare skilled home care is 60 days. If a patient receiving speech, physical, or occupational therapy is making progress at the end of this time and still has significant potential for rehabilitation, the physician can recertify that the patient is still homebound and still has a skilled need requiring home care. Similarly, if a skilled nursing need remains active, nursing services can also be reordered. There is no requirement for a

face-to-face visit for recertification, and there is no limit on the number of times that a patient may be recertified, as long as these two fundamental conditions (skilled need and homebound) are met. In fact, there are two notable exceptions to the usual expectation that skilled services will be short term: chronic urinary catheters and pernicious anemia requiring vitamin $B_{12}$ injections. For these two conditions, Medicare will cover ongoing skilled care, including monthly nursing visits for injections or catheter changes, as well as personal care and "as-needed" nursing visits.

A related but distinct form of home care is medical home visits, or house calls. Medical house calls comprise a small but growing proportion of provider visits. A 2016 study estimated that between 2006 and 2011, the total number of home visits conducted by physicians increased slightly from 917,202 to 980,703, a 6.9% increase, whereas the visits themselves were performed by a smaller percentage of total physicians (5.1% vs. 4.5%). In 2011 family physicians made more home and domiciliary care visits than any other specialty.[5] These medical house calls occur in a variety of practice structures. Some office-based medical providers make occasional routine or urgent home visits to selected patients, whereas other providers have dedicated house call sessions integrated into their regular office schedule. Still others have mobile practices that exclusively make house calls, either as private practice models or as part of larger academic or institutional practices.[6]

Finally, Hospital at Home is an intensive form of home care in which physicians, nurses, other providers, and home caregivers collaborate to provide hospital-level care in a patient's home for common, uncomplicated acute illnesses that can be diagnosed and treated safely, efficiently, and effectively in the home. Conditions that have been demonstrated to be appropriate for Hospital at Home treatment include community-acquired pneumonia, exacerbations of chronic obstructive pulmonary disease or congestive heart failure, cellulitis, deep venous thrombosis, pulmonary embolism, volume depletion, dehydration, urinary tract infection, and urosepsis.[7] A 2009 metaanalysis showed that patients receiving Hospital at Home care were more satisfied with care than those receiving inpatient care, and that Hospital at Home care was less expensive than usual acute inpatient care. In addition, there was a remarkable 38% reduction in the risk of death at 6 months for Hospital at Home patients compared with controls at 6 months.[8] Although much of the literature on Hospital at Home was originally generated in nations with robust single-payer healthcare systems, a successful Hospital at Home program has been developed over the past 2 decades in the United States, and several related dissemination projects are underway in Veterans Affairs (VA) hospitals and Medicare managed care settings.[9]

◆◆ **Although not yet widely available outside of select VA and managed care systems, Hospital at Home improves health outcomes at lower costs than usual inpatient care for appropriate patients with targeted conditions.**

---

**CASE**

**Mrs. K (Part 3)**

You decide to start making primary care medical house calls to Mrs. K as a result of her difficulty getting to her appointments with you because of her gait and memory impairment.
1. How are home care providers reimbursed?

## Who Pays for Home Care?

In 2018 home health care accounted for 3% of total national healthcare expenditure, or $102.2 billion. Medicare and Medicaid paid for 75% of this total and the remaining amount was covered by a combination of commercial insurers, social services block grants, V A programs, and out-of-pocket payments by patients.[10] Again, the economic contribution of the informal caregiver cannot be overstated. A 2014 RAND Corporation study found that the estimated cost of informal caregiving for older adults is $522 billion annually, with informal caregivers spending approximately 30 billion hours per year caring for their older adult family members and friends. Replacing this unpaid informal caregiving with paid skilled caregiving would cost $642 billion each year.[3]

As a provider ordering home care services, clinicians should know that Medicare reimburses home health agencies for skilled care based on the clinical characteristics of the patient, with an emphasis on the specificity of the primary diagnosis. Skilled services are provided in accordance with a plan of care developed and certified by a physician who is overseeing the patient's medical care. In addition, the physician who signs the skilled care certification can be reimbursed specifically for these activities (certification, code G0180, or recertification, code G0179), as long as the patient has seen that physician at least once in the 6 months before the episode of home care. Physicians and other medical providers may also bill for care plan oversight (CPO; code G0181) if the time spent communicating with other healthcare professionals (nurses, therapists, consultants, etc.) in a calendar month during an episode of skilled home care adds up to at least 30 minutes. CPO does not include time spent in the presence of the patient communicating with other professionals, but does include the time it takes to document data collection and medical decision making.

Medical house calls are reimbursed by Medicare and most commercial insurers based on the medical necessity of the home visit. Providers must document a medical reason for seeing the patient in a house call instead of an office visit. Inconvenience or lack of transportation is not a medical justification for a home visit. Furthermore, Medicare does not reimburse provider expenses incidental to the provision of house calls, such as mileage or public transportation fares. Although reimbursement rates vary with geographic region, they are generally slightly higher for home visits than for office visits of comparable evaluation and management complexity. Table 13.2 lists the codes and typical visit duration expected for various levels of home visits.

❖❖ **Certification or recertification of home care orders and CPO are reimbursable activities.**

## Does Home Care Work?

Because the term *home care* is used to describe a broad range of services, it is challenging to synthesize the evidence that peppers the medical literature. However, several relevant studies of home-based preventive care and medical home visits in the United States and Europe throughout the 1990s and early 2000s demonstrated improvements in healthcare use (particularly nursing home placement[11,12]; satisfaction of patients, caregivers, and physicians[13–17]; quality of life[13,14]; and end-of-life care[18]) and particularly when the interventions were longitudinal, multidimensional, and/or targeted to an appropriate population. Notably, the funding mechanisms for most of these interventions did not rely primarily on traditional fee-for-service reimbursement, because such reimbursement is typically insufficient to establish or maintain the home-based primary care services.

## Healthcare Reform and Home Care

### Medicare Certified Home Health

On January 1, 2020, the Centers for Medicare and Medicaid Services (CMS) implemented a new payment structure for Medicare-certified home care agencies. This is the first major reform since the home health prospective payment system (PPS) went into effect in 2000. Consistent with national trends, the new patient-driven groupings model (PDGM) is designed with value over volume in mind.[19] This is a major shift for home care agencies who were highly incentivized under PPS for the volume of therapy services provided and significant changes will be required for agencies to be successful under the PDGM model. A much greater emphasis is placed on patient characteristics, such as primary diagnosis, to determine the level of resources (revenue) required to adequately provide care.

As the certifying physician, it is important to provide complete, accurate, and specific diagnosis information and supporting documentation to fully capture patient complexity under PDGM. If a primary diagnosis is vague or unspecified, it will be rejected for payment and returned to the home health agency for more definitive coding. Table 13.3 lists the top five diagnoses considered vague or unspecified. Frequent collaboration and communication between

| TABLE 13.2 | Healthcare Common Procedure Coding System Codes for Home Visits | | | | | |
|---|---|---|---|---|---|
| Home Visit, New Patient | Domiciliary Care, New Patient | Typical Time for Code (min) | Home Visit, Established Patient | Domiciliary Care, Established Patient | Typical Time for Code (min) |
| 99341 | 99324 | 20 | — | — | — |
| 99342 | 99325 | 30 | 99347 | 99334 | 15 |
| 99343 | 99326 | 45 | 99348 | 99335 | 25 |
| 99344 | 99327 | 60 | 99349 | 99336 | 40 |
| 99345 | 99328 | 75 | 99350 | 99337 | 60 |

| TABLE 13.3 | Patient-Driven Groupings Model Unspecified Diagnoses for Home Care |
|---|---|
| Code | Description |
| M62.81 | Muscle weakness, generalized |
| R26.89 | Other abnormalities of gait and mobility |
| M54.5 | Low back pain |
| R26.81 | Unsteadiness on feet |
| R53.1 | Weakness |

the physician and home care agency is critical to ensuring timely completion of all Medicare requirements to render appropriate services to beneficiaries.

## Medical House Calls

In March 2012 the Independence at Home (IAH) Act, section 3024 of the Patient Protection and Affordable Care Act of 2010, became law. The IAH Act mandated a demonstration study of an innovative payment methodology for medical house calls that marked a major change in Medicare reimbursement of care for the frail, medically complex older adults that spend the greatest amount of the Medicare budget. Mobile multidisciplinary teams of primary care providers must demonstrate improved outcomes for these patients by providing or coordinating care across different settings, including hospitals and nursing homes. Each team will work with existing community networks of pharmacies, medical supply companies, home care agencies, and hospices to provide patient-centered care to people at home. Healthcare technology that supports effective and secure communication about patients among providers and facilities is a fundamental part of the IAH infrastructure, as is around-the-clock access to skilled telephone triage and urgent visits as needed to prevent unnecessary hospital use. The following characteristics define IAH teams selected for the demonstration project:

1. They will provide home-based comprehensive care to functionally disabled Medicare beneficiaries with multiple chronic illnesses and prior high healthcare costs.
2. They must show a 5% minimum annual savings for Medicare, compared with predicted costs based on the target population's historical use.
3. They will share in any savings to Medicare above this first 5%, to use for program development including technology or other clinical services.
4. They must meet three minimum performance standards (patient and family satisfaction, patient care quality measures to be established by the Centers for Medicare and Medicaid Services, and the 5% savings noted earlier).
5. They will retain all current traditional Medicare coverage and will be completely voluntary on the part of the patient.

Subsequent legislation has extended the IAH demonstration past its original 3-year scope and, as of 2017, 14 home-based primary care sites were participating in the project. The first 5 years of the demonstration did not show significant reductions in total Medicare expenditures relative to similar beneficiaries. However, IAH practices made several organizational changes to care delivery. This may have contributed to fewer total emergency department visits and potentially avoidable hospital admissions. More information is available at https://innovation.cms.gov/innovation-models/independence-at-home.

❖❖ **Interdisciplinary teams providing coordinated, around-the-clock patient-centered care have the opportunity to change the face of Medicare for the type of community-dwelling, frail, medically complex older adults who expend the majority of the Medicare budget.**

## Summary

For the aging population of the United States, home care remains an important form of healthcare that can complement or replace office or hospital-based care. The current reimbursement system allows many older adults to benefit from both medical home visits and skilled home care services provided by allied health professionals, but economic and demographic projections suggest that continued innovations in home healthcare delivery and reimbursement are sorely needed. Careful evaluation of patient care and economic outcomes over time should lead to the patient-centered, safe, efficacious, timely, equitable, and cost-effective care that all patients want and deserve.

### Web Resources

*Health Care Spending and the Medicare Program*—Medicare Payment Advisory Commission Data Book, June 2019: http://www.medpac.gov/docs/default-source/data-book/jun19_databook_entirereport_sec.pdf?sfvrsn = 0.

National Health Expenditures 2018 High lights Fact Sheet: https://www.cms.gov/files/document/highlights.pdf.

National Association of Home Care and Hospice: www.nahc.org.

## Key References

3. Chari AV, Engberg J, Ray KN, and Mehrotra A. The opportunity costs of informal elder-care in the United States: new estimates from the American time use survey. *Health Serv Res.* 2015;50:871–882.
5. Sairenji T, Jetty A, & Peterson LE. Shifting patterns of physician home visits. *J Prim Care Commun Health.* 2016;7(2),71–75.
7. Leff B, Burton L, Mader SL, et al. Hospital at home: feasibility and outcomes of a program to provide hospital-level care at home for acutely ill older patients. *Ann Int Med.* 2005;143:798–808.
12. Stuck AE, Egger M, Hammer A, et al. Home visits to prevent nursing home admission and functional decline in elderly people: systematic review and meta-regression analysis. *JAMA* 2002;287(8):1022–1028.
14. Hughes SL, Weaver FM, Giobbie-Hurder A, et al. Effectiveness of team-managed home-based primary care: a randomized multicenter trial. *JAMA* 2000;284(22):2877–2885.

*References available online at expertconsult.com.*

# 14

# Rehabilitation

J. MARVIN MCBRIDE, PAUL THANANOPAVARN, AND VICTORIA S.T. TILLEY

## OUTLINE

*Additional online-only material indicated by icon.*

## OBJECTIVES

*Upon completion of this chapter, the reader will be able to:*

- Assess a patient's rehabilitation needs using a standardized approach.
- Appreciate the roles and skill sets of different members of the rehabilitation team.
- Understand the different environments in which rehabilitation can be accomplished.

- Recognize the various assistive devices available to meet a patient's needs.
- Appreciate the implications of Medicare, Medicaid, and insurance coverage for rehabilitation services and the impact on patient access to those services.

## Introduction

In the medical context, rehabilitation (literally "make fit again" from the Latin) is traditionally defined as activity intended to improve a person's function when that function has been impaired by illness or injury. In the older adult, this definition is often expanded to address functional impairment from age-related debility, as well as efforts at preventing functional decline, sometimes referred to as prehabilitation. With increasing age, the incidence of many of the illnesses and injuries that may result in an indication for rehabilitation also increases, and many of these older patients will have multiple medical comorbidities complicating their care. The common theme in geriatric medicine of decreasing

physiologic reserves with age certainly applies in the context of rehabilitation, effecting all organ systems. Cognitive impairment is a common medical comorbidity that can result in a need for rehabilitation and also complicate the ability to rehabilitate. Older patients may also have financial limitations, difficulty accessing transportation, may be isolated from social support systems, and live in a variety of settings from their homes to assisted living facilities to nursing homes, all of which can influence access to care and the treatment plan. Frailty and sarcopenia are frequent comorbidities in the oldest-old and can significantly impair a patient's ability to rehabilitate. A person's expected longevity, goals of care, and motivation must also be considered in developing a plan of care.

❖ **Clinicians with a strong understanding of the basic precepts of geriatric medicine who partner with a multidisciplinary rehabilitation team are well positioned to provide optimal rehabilitative care to the older patient.**

In the context of increasing demand for clinicians with interest and experience in the field, primary care providers (PCPs) have opportunities to serve as attending clinicians for comprehensive outpatient rehabilitation facilities, skilled nursing facilities, long-term acute care hospitals, and (as of 2020) inpatient rehabilitation facilities, in addition to their usual practice of ordering and monitoring rehabilitation for their patients in the outpatient setting (Table 14.1). In an inpatient rehabilitation setting a physiatrist, a physician specialist in physical medicine and rehabilitation, will serve as the attending physician and in other settings may be available as a consultant. Many other skilled healthcare disciplines are commonly part of the rehabilitation interdisciplinary team (see Ch. 2, Table 2.1).

## World Health Organization Disability Assessment Framework[1]

It can be helpful to have a standard intellectual framework to guide assessment of a patient and to develop an appropriate rehabilitation treatment plan. The World Health Organization (WHO) provides such a framework for understanding disability through the terms *impairment, activity limitation,* and *participation restriction.* Impairment is the loss of function of a body part. Activity limitations are the functional activities that are lost because of an impairment. Participant restriction results from this loss of basic functional activity that restricts the person's ability to fully participate in life's situations, such as living independently, fulfilling societal obligations, and enjoying recreational activity.

❖ **Rehabilitation is most comprehensive and successful when all levels of impairment, activity, and participation are addressed.**

**TABLE 14.1** **Rehabilitation Environments**

| Environment | | Rehabilitation Services | Medicare Coverage |
|---|---|---|---|
| **Hospital** | | | |
| | General medical-surgical hospital | Evaluation, may provide minimal therapy | Part A |
| | Inpatient rehabilitation facility | 3 hours per day of multidisciplinary therapy | Part A |
| | Long-term acute care hospital | Up to 1 hour per day | Part A |
| **Nursing home** | | | |
| | Skilled nursing facility | Up to 1 hour per day, 5 days/week | Part A |
| | Long-term care nursing home | Up to 1 hour per day, less than daily | None for room, board, nursing care Part B for provider services, labs, etc. |
| **Domiciliary** | | | |
| | Assisted living facility (including Memory Care) | Up to 1 hour per day, less than daily | Part A if homebound and services rendered by home health agency<br>Part B if not homebound and services rendered by outpatient rehab provider |
| **Home (including congregate independent living settings)** | | | |
| | | Up to 1 hour per day, less than daily | Part A if homebound and services rendered by home health agency<br>Part B if not homebound and services rendered by outpatient rehab provider at home |
| **Outpatient** | | | |
| | Outpatient rehabilitation clinic | Up to 1 hour per day, less than daily | Part B |
| | Comprehensive outpatient rehabilitation facility | Varies | Part B |
| | Program for all-inclusive care for the elderly (PACE) programs | Varies | Part B |
| **Community-based programs** | | | |
| | | Group exercise, stretching, balance classes | Not covered |
| | Evidence-based programs offered in community settings<br>Senior centers<br>Adult daycare | Otago, A Matter of Balance, STEADI, etc. | |

## The Comprehensive Functional Assessment

When beginning rehabilitation, a patient receives a comprehensive functional assessment, including evaluation of ongoing medical comorbidities, premorbid functional status, current function, living situation and equipment, caregiver support, and patient functional goals.

## Ongoing Medical Comorbidities

Attention to delirium prevention, reasonable glycemic and blood pressure control, avoidance of orthostatic hypotension, constipation and urinary retention, control of pain and nausea, and management of cardiopulmonary disease are critical to successful rehabilitation.

## Premorbid Functional Status

A patient with a high baseline level of function with few medical problems before injury or illness has potential to recover a high level of independence with proper rehabilitation. In other cases, older patients with multiple ongoing medical, neurologic, or musculoskeletal impairments will have a more difficult course of rehabilitation and different goals. For example, a frail older adult who is bedbound with severe dementia and multiarticular arthritis at baseline would have little potential for significant functional gains with rehabilitation.

## Current Functional Status

After an injury or illness, the person's current functional status will determine the type and intensity of rehabilitation necessary to improve quality of life and independence. The assessment begins with a comprehensive physical examination that focuses on the cardiopulmonary system to assess ability to tolerate exercise; the neurologic examination with assessment of cognitive function, strength, and coordination; and the musculoskeletal examination focusing on the condition of the joints and spine, including the presence of pain. In the older population, the function of the bowel and bladder also need close assessment because dysfunction in these areas may interfere with therapy and may lead to more dependence. Functional status is typically described in a fairly standard way across disciplines and environments; the Functional Assessment Standardized Items (FASI)[2] is an example of one formal assessment tool. It includes seven self-care and six mobility items, each scored for the patient's level of need for assistance from 1 (dependent) to 6 (independent)—the total score thus ranges from 13 (dependent in all items) to 78 (independent in all items) (Table 14.2).

❖❖ **A person's functional status before injury or illness is one of the most important factors in determining rehabilitation potential and goals.**

## Living Environment and Equipment

Establishing the specifics of a patient's home environment early in the rehabilitation process is necessary to help determine the therapeutic goals that will need to be achieved for a patient to return home safely. For example, how many stairs are there to get in the house and are there handrails? Are all bedrooms and full baths upstairs or can the person live on the ground level? For patients who are expected to require mobility in a wheelchair, consideration for a ramp to enter the house and measurements of doorways and bathrooms must be made to ensure wheelchair accessibility. Older patients may have equipment and assistive devices, such as walkers, wheelchairs, commodes, and orthotic braces that will need evaluation by a therapist to ensure they are in proper working condition and appropriate for use.

## Social and Caregiver Support

Depending on the severity of a patient's functional impairments, a caregiver or support system may be needed to assist the patient in the home setting. For example, a patient who is just a few weeks after the repair of a hip fracture may only need some help with instrumental activities of daily living (IADLs), such as driving and shopping, whereas a patient with a major stroke or spinal cord injury may require caregivers who are able to provide physical assistance for all activities of daily living (ADLs). Older patients who are dependent for all of their care require an extensive and dedicated family support system or paid caregivers to remain in the home. If this support system is not available, placement in an assisted living facility or long-term care nursing home may be necessary.

## Perception of Impairment

Often the primary reason for a physical impairment may appear obvious. However, there may be cases where the underlying cause for an activity limitation may not be readily apparent. One may assume, for example, that an older person hospitalized for sepsis may have trouble getting out of bed because of deconditioning from hospitalization; however, asking the patient the reason why he or she is not able to get up and walk may reveal a new impairment, such as acute knee pain from gout, which will need to be treated to allow progress with therapy.

## Rehabilitation Goals and Plan of Care

To develop a patient-centered rehabilitation plan, the provider must ask the older person about short- and long-term functional goals because this will affect the focus of therapy and prescription of equipment. For example, for an older man with bilateral below-the-knee amputations, the clinician may ask if his goal is to walk again with prosthetic legs or to use a wheelchair for future mobility. The patient's answer will determine if the therapy team should work on gait training with prosthetics or if the focus should be on transfers and mobility in a wheelchair. The patient's motivation and functional goals may also influence the site of postacute rehabilitation. A motivated patient with high-level functional goals may be accepted into an intensive inpatient rehabilitation program, whereas a patient with limited goals and tolerance to therapy may be more suited for subacute rehabilitation in a skilled nursing facility. At the end of the assessment, the provider should review the findings of the assessment with the patient and caregivers and ensure they understand the plan of care and potential outcomes of rehabilitation. Patients with complex impairments such as a spinal cord injury, limb amputation, or brain injury may benefit from a consultation with a rehabilitation medicine physician or physiatrist to help coordinate multiple therapies, counselors, and equipment needs in addition to providing education on treatment goals and prognosis for functional recovery.

TABLE
14.2 **Functional Assessment Standardized Items**

**Self-care Items:**

| | |
|---|---|
| Eating | The ability to use utensils to bring food and/or liquid to the mouth and swallow food and/or liquid once meal is placed before patient |
| Oral hygiene | The ability to use suitable items to clean teeth or use dentures |
| Toileting hygiene | The ability to maintain perineal hygiene, adjust clothes before and after voiding or having a bowel movement |
| Shower/bath self | The ability to bathe self, including washing, rinsing, and drying self; does not include transferring in/out of tube/shower |
| Upper body dressing | The ability to dress and undress above the waist, including fasteners |
| Lower body dressing | The ability to dress and undress below the waist, including fasteners; does not include footwear |
| Putting on/taking off footwear | The ability to put on and take off socks and shoes or other footwear that is appropriate for safe mobility |

**Mobility items:**

| | |
|---|---|
| Sit to lying | The ability to move from sitting on side of bed to lying flat on the bed |
| Lying to sitting on side of bed | The ability to move from lying on the back to sitting on the side of the bed with feet flat on the floor, and with no back support |
| Sit to stand | The ability to come to a standing position from sitting in a chair, wheelchair, or on the side of the bed |
| Chair/bed-to-chair transfer | The ability to safely transfer to and from a bed to a chair (or wheelchair) |
| Toilet transfer | The ability to get on and off a toilet or commode |
| Walking | Once standing, the ability to walk at least 10 feet. Additional measures for walking 50 feet with two turns and walking 150 feet |

**Score**

| | |
|---|---|
| 6. Independent | Patient completes the activity by him/herself with no assistance from a helper |
| 5. Setup or clean-up assistance | Helper sets up or cleans up; patient completes activity. Helper assists only before or following the activity |
| 4. Supervision or touching assistance | Helper provides verbal cues and/or touching, steadying or contact guard assistance as patient completes activity |
| 3. Partial/moderate assistance | Helper does less than half of the effort. Helper lifts, holds, or supports trunk or limbs, but provides less than half of the effort |
| 2. Substantial/maximal assistance | Helper does more than half of the effort |
| 1. Dependent | Helper does ALL of the effort. Patient does none of the effort to complete the activity. Or the assistance of two or more helpers is required for the patient to complete the activity |

The total score ranges from 13 to 78. A lower score indicates increased dependency; a higher score indicates greater independence.

## CASE 1

### Ms. Walker (Part 1)

Ms. Walker is a 70-year-old, functionally independent woman with a medical history significant only for osteopenia, who slipped on a throw rug in her bathroom and fell on her right side. She sustained a right femoral neck fracture requiring a right hemiarthroplasty for surgical fixation and now has posterior hip precautions. Postoperatively, she is having significant right hip pain and requires physical assistance to stand and take a few steps with a rolling walker. She lives alone in a two-story house and is concerned about her ability to return home and being a burden on her family who live out of state. She has been transferred to a skilled nursing facility for subacute rehabilitation, where you are seeing her for her admission assessment.

How can a fall and hip fracture affect a patient's function and independence?

How does the type of hip fracture and operative approach to fixation affect hip precautions and rehabilitation course?

What are some of the potential medical complications after hip surgery?

What are important considerations for discharge to a home environment?

# Hip Fracture Rehabilitation

Falls and hip fractures are a significant cause of functional impairment in the older adult population and cause significant morbidity and mortality. More than 300,000 hip fractures occur annually in the United States[3] and the yearly incidence is expected to increase as the population ages. The rehabilitation of a patient with a hip fracture can be understood using the WHO disability framework and a comprehensive functional assessment (Tables 14.3 and 14.4).

## Rehabilitation of Persons After Hip Fracture

Hip fractures in the older adult most commonly occur at the femoral neck or intertrochanteric regions on the femur. The anatomy and vascular supply of the proximal femur influence the surgical approach and therefore the rehabilitation of a hip fracture. The primary blood supply for the head of the femur is through the femoral neck and can be compromised with a fracture through the neck region. Often these patients will need replacement of the femoral head and neck with a hemiarthroplasty, and if the acetabulum is degenerated, a total joint arthroplasty. Hemiarthroplasty or total joint arthroplasty require opening the joint capsule, which can lead to hip dislocations. In contrast, a patient with an intertrochanteric femur fracture usually has the vascular supply of the femoral head and neck intact, therefore an intramedullary femoral nail and screw is usually sufficient. The hip joint capsule is not compromised so hip dislocation precautions are not required.

## CASE 1

### Ms. Walker (Part 2)

Ms. Walker required a hip hemiarthroplasty and has posterior hip precautions orders for her rehabilitation. For the next 4 to 6 weeks, she has restrictions on her movements that could lead to a posterior hip dislocation.

Hip fracture patients with hemiarthroplasty or total joint arthroplasty postrepair instructions include no flexion of the hip past 90 degrees, crossing of legs, and no leg internal rotation. Functionally, the patient will be unable to bend down to put on socks and shoes or stand up from a low bed or toilet seat because these actions will cause the hip flexion past 90 degrees. When in bed, she may need a triangular abduction pillow to prevent leg adduction. She will need occupational therapy to teach her to perform lower body ADLs with a sock-aid, reacher, or dressing hook and physical therapy to stand up without bending forward (Fig. 14.1). She may need an elevated toilet seat and handlebars to assist in maintaining precautions. For gait training, she may be using a rolling walker or standard walker because this device provides a wide base of stable support and may be able to progress to less restrictive devices as her balance and strength improve (Fig. 14.2). Adequate pain control is important to allow progress with therapy avoiding oversedation and delirium. Scheduling an analgesic approximately 30 minutes before therapy is frequently helpful. Nursing care will include inspection of the surgical incision, monitoring for bleeding and infection, frequent repositioning, and elevation of heels to prevent skin pressure injury. Venous thromboembolism (VTE) precautions can be tailored to the patient's risk factors. Anticoagulation using low-molecular-weight heparin, warfarin, or oral anticoagulant such as apixaban or rivaroxaban can be used. For some low-risk patients, aspirin may be an acceptable option with ongoing close monitoring for signs or symptoms of VTE.[4]

**TABLE 14.3   Case 1, Hip Fracture: World Health Organization Disability Framework**

| Term | Definition | Case Example | Intervention |
|---|---|---|---|
| Impairment | Loss of body part or function | Femoral neck fracture | Surgical fixation |
| Activity limitation | Loss of ability to perform an activity | Inability to walk and perform lower body ADLs | Physical therapy, occupational therapy, assistive devices |
| Participation restriction | Loss of ability to participate in a life situation | Inability to care for self at home | Short-term rehab in a skilled nursing facility |

*ADLs,* Activities of daily living.

**TABLE 14.4   Case 1, Hip Fracture: Comprehensive Functional Assessment**

| | |
|---|---|
| Medical comorbidities | To progress with rehabilitation, active medical issues must be identified and managed. In the postoperative setting after a hip fracture, this may include addressing pain, delirium, cardiac or pulmonary decompensation, constipation, urinary retention, venous thromboembolism risk, and pressure ulcers |
| Premorbid functional status | Independent in activities of daily living (ADLs) |
| Current functional status | Requires assistance to take a few steps with a rolling walker |
| Living environment and equipment | Two-story house—will need to clarify if she could live there safely if she is not able to climb stairs. Equipment—rolling walker for now—to be determined closer to discharge |
| Social and caregiver support | Lives alone, family out of state—will need to clarify the degree to which they can help and patient's ability to pay for home health aides if needed |
| Perception of impairment | Consistent with osteoporotic fracture of femoral neck |
| Rehabilitation goals | Return to living independently, with modifications to home or relocation if necessary |

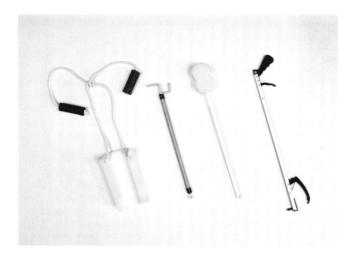

• **Figure 14.1** "Hip kit": sock aid, dressing hook, sponge, and reacher.

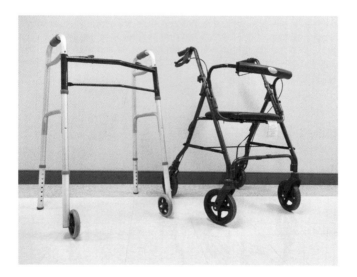

• **Figure 14.2** Rolling walkers.

---

**CASE 1**

**Ms. Walker (Part 3)**

Ms. Walker is walking well enough after 2 weeks in the postacute setting to return home. Because she lives independently, planning with her family began early during her admission. An assessment of her home determined she can be independent downstairs until she is able to climb her stairs independently. Assistive devices, such as an elevated toilet seat, hospital bed, and appropriate gait device, are ordered. Initially, she will continue her rehabilitation through a home health agency, which can provide physical therapy, occupational therapy, nursing follow-up, and (very limited) personal care assistance. Once she has progressed with her independence and endurance, evidence strongly supports that she should transition to outpatient therapy to ensure her return to her previous activities.[5]

---

**CASE 2**

**Mrs. Kane (Part 1)**

Mrs. Kane is a 70-year-old woman, independent at baseline with mobility and self-care, wakes up in the morning with new-onset right-sided weakness and the inability to speak. Her husband calls 911 and she is hospitalized but is unable to receive thrombolytic or intravascular therapy. Magnetic resonance imaging reveals an acute infarct in the distribution of the left middle cerebral artery and no extracranial vascular stenosis. Electrocardiographic monitoring reveals normal sinus rhythm; echocardiogram reveals no structural abnormalities. Laboratory studies are only significant for a low-density lipoprotein cholesterol of 180 mg/dL. The primary medical team allows for permissive hypertension and begins aspirin and a high-potency statin. Speech therapy assesses moderately severe expressive aphasia, cognitive deficits, and dysphagia and recommends a pureed diet with thickened liquids after video swallow study. Physical and occupational therapy assess that because of her right-sided flaccid hemiplegia and right foot drop, she is requiring moderate assistance to stand and is unable to use her right arm for basic ADLs. Nursing documents urinary incontinence, but low postvoid residual volumes. Her husband is willing to care for the patient in their handicapped-accessible home, but first would like her to receive the most intensive therapy available to improve her function.

How would you organize the rehabilitation of this patient to address her impairments, loss of functional activities, and loss of societal participation?

What are the rehabilitation interventions that can improve her function?

In what type of setting can her rehabilitation care be delivered in an interdisciplinary manner?

## Stroke Rehabilitation

A patient with a severe stroke will require intensive therapy to regain or compensate for loss of function in multiple aspects of human activity. She will need a coordinated approach from multiple rehabilitation professionals to provide proper medical, psychological, therapeutic, equipment, and social supportive services for her to be able to return home safely with her husband (Tables 14.5 and 14.6).

Medically, ischemic stroke patients are managed comprehensively to enhance stroke recovery and prevent recurrent stroke, and monitored closely for complications such as hemorrhagic conversion, seizures, and aspiration pneumonia. Blood pressure goals during acute hospitalization for ischemic stroke remain controversial[6]; however, systolic blood pressures > 200 mmHg may prevent the patient from participating in therapy, and cautious reduction is reasonable to facilitate rehabilitation. The Fluoxetine for Motor Recovery After Acute Ischaemic Stroke (FLAME)[7] trial demonstrated that the selective serotonin reuptake inhibitor (SSRI) fluoxetine may be of benefit in enhancing motor recovery; however, other SSRIs may be indicated and better tolerated in the older adult population. Poststroke depression is also common, affecting up to one third of stroke patients who may benefit from antidepressant and psychological counseling.[8]

Motor recovery often progresses in stages, starting with flaccid hemiparesis, followed by increased reflexes, tone, and spasticity either in flexion or extension patterns across a limb. In some cases, spasticity may decrease as muscle strength and control return. Key aspects of improving motor recovery are the need for the therapy to be individually tailored, progressive, activity specific, and of sufficient intensity and repetition to demonstrate functional gains.[9]

**TABLE 14.5** Case 2, Stroke: World Health Organization Disability Framework

| Term | Case Example | Intervention |
|---|---|---|
| Impairment | Left MCA stroke with right hemiplegia, expressive aphasia, dysphagia | Primary stroke treatments and secondary stroke prevention |
| Activity limitation | Unable to transfer and walk, perform ADLs using right arm and legs, communicate needs, swallow normal foods and liquids, functional incontinence | Physical, occupational, and speech therapy. Assistive devices, timed-toileting program. SSRI treatment |
| Participation restriction | Unable to mobilize, help with self-care and communicate needs to husband to safely return home | Inpatient rehab for intensive interdisciplinary therapy and family training |

*ADLs,* Activities of daily living; *MCA,* middle cerebral artery; *SSRI,* selective serotonin reuptake inhibitor.

**TABLE 14.6** Case 2, Stroke: Comprehensive Functional Assessment

| | |
|---|---|
| Medical Comorbidities | Hyperlipidemia |
| Premorbid functional status | Independent in activities of daily living (ADLs) |
| Current functional status | Hemiplegic requiring assistance for bed mobility, transfers, and self-care. She has aphasia and dysphagia |
| Living environment and equipment | Handicapped-accessible home. Equipment to be determined closer to discharge |
| Social and caregiver support | Lives with supportive husband |
| Perception of impairment | Consistent with major stroke |
| Rehabilitation goals | Return to living with husband in their own home |

One example of a type of occupational therapy approach that may benefit Mrs. Kane in Case 2 is constraint-induced movement therapy, which forces her to use the hemiparetic arm by constraining the unaffected arm.[10] She may require hand splints to prevent finger flexion contractures and special orthotics to help grip utensils. Gait training with physical therapy may require the use of assistive devices and orthotics along with individualized intensive training. Because Mrs. Kane is unable to use her right side, she will require her left arm to provide support and balance. This often begins by using a fixed handrail, then progressing to a hemiwalker, which has a large base of support but is difficult to advance forward because of size (Fig. 14.3). With training she may be able to walk with a more maneuverable four-point or single-point cane (Fig. 14.4).

⚫⚫ **Poststroke depression is also common, affecting up to one third of stroke patients who may benefit from antidepressant and psychological counseling.**

Patients with stroke with lower extremity involvement may experience either hypotonicity or hypertonicity in the affected side. Hypotonicity presents as lower extremity weakness with instability at the knee and foot drop because of difficulty initiating ankle dorsiflexion. They will also have difficulty with initiating a step because of weakness in the hip flexors. Hypertonicity may appear in a flexion or extension pattern. The extension pattern presents as overexcitation of the extensor muscles, so the patient may have difficulty with bending the knee when taking a step and foot drop because of strong plantar flexors. A flexion pattern presents in the opposite way, so the patient will have difficulty extending the knee to put weight on it and will

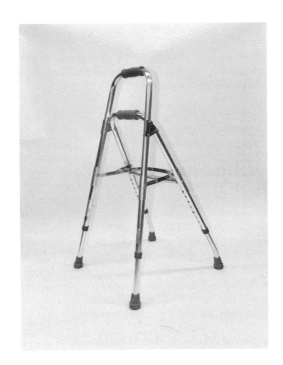

• **Figure 14.3** Hemiwalker.

have anterior hip tightness. Individuals are unique in their recovery and how they may present.

Shoe orthotics, ankle-foot orthoses (AFOs), and knee-ankle-foot orthoses (KAFOs) can be helpful and necessary to assist

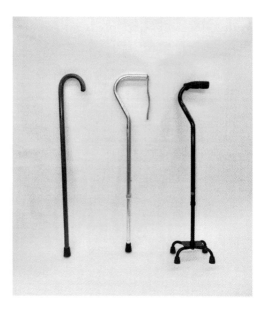

• **Figure 14.4** Canes.

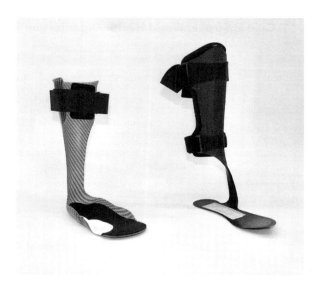

• **Figure 14.5** Ankle-foot orthoses.

someone in ambulation and recovery. An AFO can help Mrs. Kane's gait in two ways—it can assist in dorsiflexion of the foot to prevent the toe from contacting the ground during swing phase and provide plantar flexion assistance during stance phase, which provides a force that pushes the knee posteriorly to help prevent the knee from buckling. A KAFO can provide additional support around the knee to increase stability (Fig. 14.5).

❖ **The decision as to the exact type of orthotic to prescribe is best done in a team approach with the rehabilitation physician, physical therapist, and orthotist.**

Evaluation of dysphagia should occur early in the poststroke period as aspiration. Symptoms of oral dysphagia include pocketing of foot or liquid, reduced mastication, and difficulty with oral secretion management. Symptoms of pharyngeal dysphagia include coughing or clearing of the throat with swallowing, a change in respiration with swallow, and a wet vocal quality. A speech-language pathologist will use varying consistencies of food and liquid to evaluate for dysphagia and aspiration. For high-risk patients, visual examination of swallowing mechanics using a modified barium swallow with fluoroscopy or fiberoptic endoscopic visualization of the swallowing structures in the throat can be sensitive tests to rule out aspiration and help guide safe food and liquid consistencies. Patients who are unable to swallow any food or liquid without aspiration may need to consider alternative means of nutrition, such as a gastrostomy tube.

❖ **Evaluation of dysphagia should occur early in the poststroke period because aspiration pneumonia can cause significant morbidity and mortality in neurologically impaired patients.**

Aphasia is a common symptom of stroke and can present with impaired ability to produce and/or understand written and spoken language. Many aphasias are associated with strokes affecting the left brain. Lesions to the Broca area in the left frontal lobe present with nonfluent aphasia with relatively spared comprehension, and

damage to the Wernike area in the posterior superior temporal gyrus presents with fluent aphasia with impaired comprehension, paraphasic errors, and neologisms. A speech language pathologist can use various techniques, including melodic intonation therapy (which can use melody and rhythm to improve spoken language) and vision action therapy (which teaches the use of hand gestures for communication). Severe cases may need assistive devices such as picture and symbol communication boards and specialized electronic devices.[11]

Stroke patients benefit most from close medical care and multiple therapy specialists coordinated in an interdisciplinary manner. Interdisciplinary care is closely coordinated between rehabilitation specialists resulting in synergistic outcomes that otherwise could not have been accomplished by multiple disciplines working in their separate domains. An example would be the coordinated interventions needed to address the patient's urinary incontinence. The rehabilitation physician would evaluate the patient to rule out urinary tract infection, detrusor instability, and urinary retention. Physical therapy would work on transfers out of bed and gait training to the bathroom. Occupational therapy would focus on toilet transfers and toileting skills, whereas speech therapy may work on enhanced communication skills for the aphasic patient to indicate toileting needs. The rehabilitation nurses will help the patient practice those skills with a timed toileting program. The social worker may order special equipment and services for the home and set up family training. This type of interdisciplinary therapy is a core feature of inpatient rehabilitation, which requires frequent team meetings with all disciplines to coordinate the patient's intensive therapy and family training. Other rehabilitation settings, such as skilled nursing facilities and home health therapy, provide multidisciplinary therapy but may be less coordinated than inpatient rehabilitation.

## CASE 2

### Mrs. Kane (Part 2)

Mrs. Kane's rehabilitation progress results in sufficient functional recovery so that she can return home for the next phase of her rehabilitation. Intense interdisciplinary rehabilitation in an inpatient rehabilitation facility (IRF) maximized her neurologic gains that mostly occur in the first 2 months after a stroke.[12] In addition, her successful return to home is the result of her relatively young age, high baseline functional status, and supportive caregiving from her husband. It will be important to continue with therapy intervention as Mrs. Kane transitions home. Although gains may slow in pace, they can still occur with continued intervention and participation in home and community-based exercise programs. Her need and modifications for assistive devices may also change as she progresses, so this should be monitored to assist with safe transitions.

With advanced age, the prognosis for good functional recovery after stroke declines. Patients older than 85 years are more likely to become dependent for ADLs if they have premorbid dependence, hemiplegia, and cognitive impairments.[13] Older patients with these less favorable prognostic factors may often be more appropriate for subacute rehabilitation in a skilled nursing facility for prolonged but less intense therapy with the potential that many will transition to long-term care.

| Grade | Definition |
|---|---|
| 0 | No increase in tone |
| 1 | Slight increase in muscle tone, manifested by a catch and release at the end of range of motion (ROM) |
| 1+ | Slight increase in muscle tone, manifested by a catch, followed by minimal resistance throughout the remainder of the ROM |
| 2 | More marked increase in tone, but affected limb is easily flexed |
| 3 | Considerable increase in tone, passive movement is difficulty |
| 4 | Affected part rigid |

**TABLE 14.7 Modified Ashworth Scale (Spasticity Grading)**

## CASE 2

### Mrs. Kane (Part 3)

Mrs. Kane returns home with her husband. She received continued therapy through home health and has now transitioned to outpatient physical and occupational therapy. One month later she presents to your office with increased right-sided tone, spasticity, and shoulder pain that is interfering with her functional mobility, self-care, therapy, and care of her hand. On examination, the right shoulder demonstrates restricted and painful range of motion (ROM) in all planes. Her elbow is flexed, and her hand is clenched tight in a fist. Spasticity is graded 3 on the modified Ashworth scale.

What is the approach to addressing poststroke spasticity?

What is the differential diagnosis and management options for poststroke shoulder pain?

## Spasticity

Spasticity is an upper motor neuron syndrome defined as a velocity-dependent increase in stretch reflexes that may lead to overactivity of a muscle. Consequences of untreated spasticity include pain, diminished function because of difficulties in positioning and movement, and the development of contractures and pressure ulcers. Spasticity is commonly graded using the modified Ashworth scale (Table 14.7).

Hemiplegia and spasticity can lead to a painful shoulder with restricted movement along with arm and hand tightness. The differential diagnostic possibilities for poststroke shoulder pain include shoulder subluxation, bursitis/tendonitis, adhesive capsulitis, and neurogenic pain or reflex sympathetic dystrophy. Therapeutic interventions may include ROM exercises, gentle mobilization, facilitation of agonist motions, massage, shoulder taping, and arm supports to prevent subluxation, such as a hemilap tray on the wheelchair and a GivMohr or similar supportive sling that supports the hemiplegic arm while avoiding shoulder internal rotation contractures (Fig. 14.6). Additional interventions may include topical and oral pain medications or corticosteroid injections. Spasticity may be helped by oral medications, such as baclofen, tizanidine, or diazepam; however, all of these medications can have central nervous system effects that can lead to sedation and falls. As an alternative, targeted neuromuscular blockade of selected spastic muscles using botulinum toxin injections has been shown to improve tone and upper extremity activity capacity after

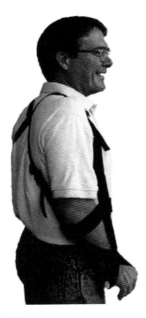

• **Figure 14.6** GivMohr sling.

stroke; however, the effects only last a few months and the treatment is expensive.[14]

## CASE 3

### Mr. Pace (Part 1)

Mr. Pace is a 69-year-old man with hypertension, type 2 diabetes, and chronic obstructive pulmonary disease (COPD) with a 50 pack-year history of cigarette smoking who presents to the hospital with chest pain and shortness of breath. Evaluation reveals an anterior ST-elevation myocardial infarction (MI) for which he undergoes left anterior descending coronary angioplasty and placement of a drug-eluting stent. Ventriculogram demonstrates a left ventricular ejection fraction of 25%. After medical optimization, Mr. Pace is now medically ready for discharge but continues to have fatigue and shortness of breath with exertion.

How can comprehensive cardiac and pulmonary rehabilitation programs improve Mr. Pace's morbidity, mortality, and function?

## Cardiac and Pulmonary Rehabilitation

The incidence of cardiovascular disease increases with age and can lead to significant morbidity, mortality, and disability.[15] After a cardiac event such as an MI, a patient may develop shortness of breath, exertional angina, and deconditioning. Fearful of another cardiac event, the patient may become more sedentary, which exacerbates muscle weakness and cardiopulmonary decline. Cardiac rehabilitation decreases cardiovascular mortality and hospital admissions and improves health-related quality of life.[16] Medicare benefits include comprehensive cardiac rehabilitation programs for beneficiaries who have experienced an MI in the preceding 12 months; have undergone coronary artery bypass grafting (CABG), heart valve repair or replacement, coronary angioplasty, or heart or heart-lung transplant; or who have stable angina or chronic heart failure. Cardiac rehabilitation usually involves three phases: Phase 1 includes graded exercises to improve basic mobility and self-care skills in the hospital to ensure the patient is stable and that it is appropriate to return home; phase 2 consists of outpatient monitored exercise and risk factor reduction in a multidisciplinary structured program; and phase 3 is the maintenance program.

Phase 2 of cardiac rehabilitation programs includes medical evaluation and treatment of heart disease, lifestyle education, psychosocial management, and physical exercise training. Lifestyle education includes a review of a patient's dietary and physical activity habits along with psychosocial counseling that evaluates issues such as depression, anxiety, social/family, and sexual function that may affect rehabilitation and wellbeing.

The physical exercise training component of cardiac rehabilitation typically starts with a treadmill stress test to rule out ongoing ischemia and malignant dysrhythmias and to establish a baseline level of cardiopulmonary fitness and maximum heart rate. The training program is progressive with target heart rate and exercise duration increasing as the patient becomes more fit. With exercise, the heart becomes a stronger pump while skeletal muscle is able to use circulating oxygen more efficiently. There is development of more coronary collaterals and a decrease in atherosclerotic plaque formation and platelet aggregation, which help contribute to a decrease in mortality.[17]

Patients with cardiac and pulmonary disease may also benefit from a pulmonary rehabilitation program. Medicare benefits include pulmonary rehabilitation for beneficiaries with moderate to very severe COPD. Patients with COPD often develop a downward spiral of shortness of breath that leads to inactivity and deconditioning that further exacerbates dyspnea and dysfunction. Progressive cardiopulmonary exercise is central to pulmonary rehabilitation—although intrinsic lung function may not improve, pulmonary rehabilitation improves symptoms, exercise performance, and quality of life in persons with COPD.[18] For older patients with limited cardiopulmonary reserve that need help with energy conservation, a four-wheeled rollator walker may provide a platform to carry items, such as portable oxygen, and provide a seat to take rest breaks. Rollators have hand brakes to prevent them rolling away but are still less stable than two-wheeled walkers and must be used with caution with patients with gait instability or significant cognitive impairment.

◆◆ **Cardiac rehabilitation decreases cardiovascular mortality and hospital admissions, and improves health-related quality of life.**

**CASE 3**

**Mr. Pace (Part 2)**

Mr. Pace unfortunately is readmitted to the hospital with a painful, purple, and pulseless right foot with signs of gangrene. He undergoes right below-the-knee amputation and is motivated to walk again.

What are the rehabilitation interventions necessary for a patient to regain mobility and potentially walk again after an amputation?

## Lower Extremity Amputation Rehabilitation

Complications of diabetes and peripheral vascular disease account for the majority of lower limb amputations in older adults. Compared with younger patients, older vascular amputees have less functional reserve, strength, and balance to quickly regain mobility to use a prosthesis. Vascular supply is often compromised in the entire leg or in both legs, which can result in below-the-knee amputations (BKAs) being converted into above-the-knee amputations (AKAs) and bilateral lower extremity amputations.

In the immediate period after a lower limb amputation, the focus is on healing and protecting the incisional wound, treating postsurgical and phantom pain, and controlling limb edema. A limb protector should be prescribed to protect the healing incision from inadvertent trauma in the event of a fall. Limb protectors can also be used in bed to promote knee extension as knee flexion contractures can make fitting and walking with a prosthesis difficult.

For incisional pain, caution should be used with narcotics that can lead to delirium. Phantom sensation and pain can often be tempered by massaging or tapping the residual limb, compression, or using neuropathic pain medications such as gabapentin or nortriptyline.[19] Use of mirror therapy where the patient sees the intact limb in the place of the missing limb can also help with phantom pain.[20]

Edema in the residual limb can be controlled with elastic wraps or shrinker socks because excess edema can impair wound healing and exacerbate pain. Proper teaching about the use of elastic wraps is important because these bandages can inadvertently "choke" the limb if applied inappropriately. Shrinker socks can be worn continuously to help control edema and shape the residual limb to receive a prosthesis.

Early rehabilitation will emphasize upper extremity strengthening and mobility using an appropriate assistive device and the intact leg to perform basic mobility and ADLs. The patient's ability to stand on one leg, cardiopulmonary fitness to walk with assistive device, and intact cognition are predictors of potential walking ability with a prosthesis.[21] Lower extremity amputees require a high level of balance and coordination to walk with a prosthesis, and energy costs are high. Compared with a nonamputee patient, a person with a BKA requires 40% more energy to walk, whereas a person with an AKA requires up to 100% more energy.[22] Because of these energy costs, it is rare to see a very old or debilitated person walk with an AKA or bilateral lower limb amputation. The physical therapist (PT) and prosthetist can help determine the type of prosthetic component needed based on the patient's expected functional level (Fig. 14.7).

Patients who are unable to use a prosthetic may require a wheelchair. Manual wheelchairs can be set up to be partially propelled using the intact leg and both arms. Other options to consider in a wheelchair are elevating leg rests for knee contraction prevention and edema control, detachable arm rests to facilitate slide board transfers, proper seat cushion to prevent pressure ulcers, customizable seat back to compensate for postural deformities, and lightweight frame and components to allow easier propulsion for the patient and caregivers. Patients who do not have the strength or endurance to propel a manual wheelchair may benefit from a power wheelchair, provided they have sufficient cognitive abilities and arm dexterity to use a joystick. Power wheelchairs have many customizable options but are heavy, difficult to transport, expensive, and require extensive documentation for insurance reimbursement. Power scooters are a less expensive option that may be lighter and easier to transport and disassemble, but scooters have a larger turning radius making them difficult to operate in tight spaces. Seating is usually less customizable, and transfers in and out of scooters are more difficult than wheelchairs (Fig. 14.8).

## Durable Medical Equipment

Medically necessary durable medical equipment (DME) such as prosthetics and orthotics, walkers, manual and power-based wheelchairs, bedside commodes or elevated toilet seats, hospital beds, patient lifts, and oxygen equipment may be partially covered by Medicare Part B. Use of such equipment while a patient is in a hospital, IRF, or skilled nursing facility (SNF) is covered under Medicare Part A payments to the facility. In other settings, DME can be ordered by a physician or nonphysician provider (NPP—the Medicare term for a nurse practitioner or physician assistant) and obtained from a Center for Medicare and Medical Services (CMS)—approved DME provider. The medical necessity criteria for Medicare are strict and the application process can be exacting, so a good working relationship between the clinician and the DME provider can be very helpful to the process. Medical necessity criteria for DME under Medicaid are much less stringent. The specific requirements vary depending on the item, but Medicare requires a prescription, may require a certificate of medical necessity (CMN) and/or a "7 element order," and may require a face-to-face visit with the provider within the 6 months before delivery of the DME. Other payors have similar but distinct requirements. DME that

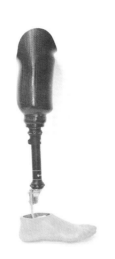

• **Figure 14.7** Below-the-knee prosthesis.

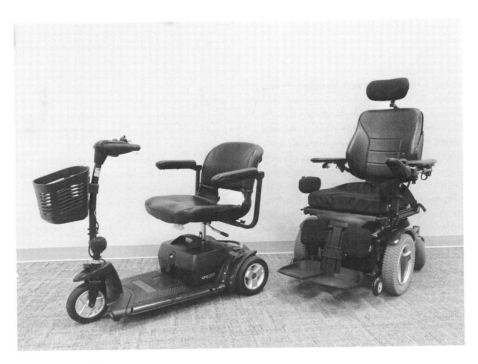

• **Figure 14.8** Scooter and Power wheelchair.

requires customization, for example, power wheelchairs with modifications owing to limited patient function, or wheelchairs with narrower or lower bases for smaller patients, will require more extensive justification. Medicare has established national coverage determinations (NCDs) that specify the medical necessity criteria for many DME items; those not listed in a NCD may be subject to local coverage determinations established by the Medicare DME regional contractor for your region of the country. These are accessible online in the Medicare Coverage Database.[23] DME suppliers will typically have a good understanding of what documentation is required. It will often be helpful to have PT and occupational therapist (OT) evaluations to document the medical necessity of an item, although ultimately it is the clinician who is responsible for certifying the medical necessity of an item.

## Prevention and Prehabilitation

Prevention is an important element in managing the health and outcomes of older adults. According to the WHO: "Physical inactivity is one of the leading risk factors for noncommunicable diseases and death worldwide" and "physical inactivity burdens society through the hidden and growing cost of medical care."[24] Prevention of falls has been an area of particular focus in the United States as one in four adults over the age of 65 years falls each year, and the estimated healthcare cost of treating falls-related injuries is estimated at $50 billion annually.[25] There is strong evidence that fall risk can be determined and falls can be prevented with appropriate screening and intervention.[26] The Centers for Disease Control and Prevention has developed the Stopping Elderly Accidents, Deaths, and Injuries Initiative (STEADI) for use in primary care practices to help screen for falls and determine an appropriate course of care (see Web Resources). Physical inactivity and home environment are two determinants of fall risk. Referrals to a PT and an OT may be needed to intervene in assessing and developing exercise programs, helping to prescribe and fit appropriate DME, and assessing home safety. Otago is an evidence-based home exercise program provided by PTs for frail adults that has proven to significantly decrease fall risk.[27] Community-based organizations, such as senior centers, YMCAs, and Park and Recreation programs, also offer evidence-based fall prevention programs such as A Matter of Balance, Stepping On, Tai Ji Quan: Moving for Better Balance, YMCA Moving for Better Balance, and others (see Web Resources for the National Council on Aging National Falls Prevention Resource Center website) (also see Ch. 20).

Patients planning elective hip or knee replacements can also benefit from rehabilitation therapy before the surgical procedure.[28,29] ROM and strength are important predictors of postoperative outcomes for total hip and knee replacements. PTs can assess functional ROM and strength of the muscles supporting the joint and help maximize function before surgery. PTs can also help educate the patient on what to expect postoperatively with exercises, possible DME needs, and therapy postdischarge. A home assessment by the therapist can help the patient plan for what he or she will need to be able to do postoperatively, so the patient can return home safely. Providing information and education before surgery can help the patient and caregivers plan for a smoother transition postoperatively.

## Rehabilitation for Persons With Vestibular Disorders

Dysfunction of the vestibular system often presents as vertigo, the inaccurate sensation of (often whirling) motion. Because of

distinctions in etiology and therapy, vestibular disorders are typically divided into those with a peripheral etiology—arising from the labyrinth or vestibular nerve—and those with a central etiology—arising from the brainstem or cerebellum. Vestibular rehabilitation is most likely to be beneficial in the case of unilateral peripheral vestibular disorders,[30] but at least anecdotally it may have some benefit in bilateral peripheral disorders and central vestibular disorders as well. These programs use a variety of techniques but typically promote activities that trigger vertigo in a safe environment to encourage central adaptation, train the person to use alternative visual-spatial clues, and encourage activity to combat the "fear of falling" (see Ch. 21).

## Rehabilitation for Persons With Parkinson Disease

Because of hypokinesia and rigidity, patients with Parkinson disease often have difficulty with posture, balance, gait, and speech, and can benefit from physical, occupational, and speech therapy to address these multiple functional deficits. Given the progressive and often prolonged nature of this illness (often several decades), the specific deficits addressed in therapy will change as disease moves from early/mild stages to end-stage disease. It is therefore appropriate for rehabilitation therapy to be engaged with a patient with Parkinson disease multiple times over the course of the illness. Moderate to vigorous intensity activity, including cardiovascular, progressive resistance, balance, and stretching exercises early in diagnosis and continued as the disease progresses is beneficial.[31,32] Dual task activities, facilitation techniques, and rhythmic activities such as Tai Chi and dance slow progression of symptoms.[33] The Lee Silverman Voice Treatment (LSVT) LOUD and BIG programs were developed specifically for the voice and motor deficits in Parkinson disease, and named in honor of Lee Silverman, a woman with Parkinson disease who was the inspiration for the program's development. Therapists who wish to offer these copyrighted programs must be trained and certified by LSVT Global. LSVT LOUD focuses on improving speech volume, whereas LSVT BIG focuses on improving fine and large muscle movement. There is a significant evidence base supporting the effectiveness of these programs,[34,35] and they are frequently prescribed by neurologists specializing in movement disorders. The LSVT programs may also be effective in some other disorders, including stroke and atypical parkinsonian syndromes (see Ch. 52).

**It is beneficial for rehabilitation therapy to be offered to patients with Parkinson disease multiple times over the course of their illness.**

## Impact of Healthcare Policy and Reimbursement

Rehabilitation treatment exists within the context of specific models of care, and the development of current systems of care, the distribution of resources, and an individual patient's access to care are clearly driven by both historical and current health policy and reimbursement schemes. In the United States, reimbursement models in geriatric rehabilitation have been primarily influenced by CMS policy and Medicare reimbursement, with less influence by the Veterans Administration and even less influence by commercial payors. Historically, rehabilitation services were reimbursed by Medicare primarily on a fee-for-service basis, but the perfect storm of increasing numbers of Medicare beneficiaries, increasing longevity, increasing utilization of services per beneficiary, and inexorable upward pressure on unit prices has resulted in unsustainable upward expenditure trends. Attempting to mitigate those trends, Medicare and other payors have instituted multiple broad changes in reimbursement models, as well as engaging in multiple experimental initiatives that have changed the environment in which geriatric rehabilitation occurs. The details are complex and changing rapidly but can be broadly understood as attempting to optimize value—achieving maximal benefit at the minimal cost in the context of what the system and nation consider affordable. In the general medical-surgical hospital setting, facility reimbursement (which includes therapy services) per the diagnosis-related group (DRG) prospective payment system or on a per-diem basis has resulted in a shift in the work of therapy professionals from actual rehabilitation to patient evaluation with some attention to minimizing functional decline during hospitalization, with rehabilitation therapy typically deferred to other settings. The high cost of IRFs (despite their superior clinical outcomes for stroke and other diagnoses) has resulted in significant restrictions as to which patients and conditions are considered best served by IRFs compared with other levels of care.

SNF care has most recently been reimbursed by Medicare on a prospective payment basis using five "resource utilization groups," which were driven primarily by the number of minutes of rehabilitation therapy provided. That model changed October 1, 2019, to a patient-driven payment model, which will be based primarily on the patient's diagnoses and characteristics (similar to the hospital DRG model) rather than by therapy minutes. This may cause a significant disruption to the system—the impact is unpredictable, but may result in a decrease in SNF utilization, with a corresponding increase in home health and/or outpatient therapy service utilization.

Outpatient therapy services were placed under a total reimbursement cap in fiscal year (FY) 2017. This was removed in FY 2018 but signals a concern regarding total expenditures in this area that will likely result in further reimbursement changes in the near future. Overall, the trend is clear: Medicare and other payors can be expected to incentivize patients and providers to use the least expensive level of care possible, while expecting no worse patient outcomes.

The tools currently used to assess patient functional status in IRF, SNF, and home health agencies and reported to CMS are different in each setting, which makes it challenging to compare patient characteristics and outcomes. IRFs currently use the functional independence measure (FIM), SNFs use the Minimum Data Set version 3.0 (MDS 3.0), and home health agencies use the home health outcome and assessment information set (OASIS). The FASI tool mentioned earlier in the chapter has been tested by CMS for Medicaid beneficiaries receiving home and community-based services, and CMS is considering requiring this (or a similar tool) across the continuum of care in the future instead of the current FIM, MDS, and OASIS.

The Medicare "bundled payments for care improvement" is a voluntary initiative that bundles payments for episodes of care for certain DRGs for facilities and providers across some or all of the continuum of care. There are four models that vary in detail, but the intent is to incentivize providers and health systems to increase value by optimizing the mix of inpatient hospital, IRF, SNF, home health agency, and outpatient rehabilitation services care to result in the best clinical outcome at the lowest cost. Lower extremity total joint replacements were the episodes most commonly selected. Recently published analysis of the first 5 years of this program showed decreased total Medicare expenditures, primarily because of decreased postacute care expenditures, with equivalent quality outcomes, but decreased patient satisfaction.[36]

Population management models of care in which health systems (physician group practices, physician-hospital organizations, accountable care organizations [ACO], etc.) assume management and financial responsibility for specific patients are growing in size because Medicare Advantage plans encourage risk assumption by providers and CMS encourages providers to enter into alternative payment models, such as ACOs to avoid the bureaucratic complexity and threatened Medicare fee schedule cuts of the Merit-Based Incentive Payment System. These models have the potential to dramatically change the healthcare environment by integrating the currently separate entities responsible for parts of the continuum of care, or at least aligning their incentives more closely. In these models, instead of the hospital, IRF, SNF, home health aide, or outpatient rehabilitation department each attempting to maximize revenue and minimize costs within their respective silo, they become simply costs to the larger system, whose revenue is determined by the number and complexity of patients for which it assumes care (see Ch. 9).

## Summary

Rehabilitation medicine is an essential aspect of quality care for older adults that can help clinicians improve function and quality of life for older individuals who have lost function because of illness, injury, or age-related debility. Accurate assessment of an older person with impaired function, access to a multidisciplinary team that optimizes that person's function and quality of life, while managing the complex medical problems and overcoming other barriers to care, provides a powerful example of the best that medicine can offer.

### Web Resources

1. American Academy of Physical Medicine and Rehabilitation: https://www.aapmr.org

2. American Geriatric Society: https://www.americangeriatrics.org

3. American Occupational Therapy Association: https://www.aota.org

4. American Physical Therapy Association: https://www.apta.org

5. American Speech-Language-Hearing Association: https://www.asha.org

6. Medicare Coverage Database: https://www.cms.gov/medicare-coverage-database/

7. National Council on Aging National Falls Prevention Resource Center: https://www.ncoa.org/center-for-healthy-aging/falls-resource-center/

8. STEADI: https://www.cdc.gov/steadi/index.html

## Key References

5. Davis AM, Perruccio AV, Ibrahim S, et al. The trajectory of recovery and inter-relationships of symptoms, activity, and participation in the first year following total hip and knee replacement. *Osteoarthr Cartilage*. 2011;19(12):1413—1421.

9. Winstein CJ, Stein J, Arena R, et al. Guidelines for adult stroke rehabilitation and recovery: a guideline for healthcare professionals from the AHA/ASA. *Stroke*. 2016;47(6): e98—e169.

16. Anderson L, Thompson DR, Oldridge N, et al. Exercise-based cardiac rehabilitation for coronary heart disease. *Cochrane Database of Syst Rev*. 2016;(1):CD001800.

18. Spruit MA, Singh SJ, Garvey C, et al. An official American Thoracic Society/European Respiratory Society statement: key concepts and advances in pulmonary rehabilitation. *Am J Respir Crit Care Med*. 2013;188(8):e13—e64.

26. US Preventive Services Task Force. Interventions to prevent falls in community-dwelling older adults: US Preventive Services Task Force recommendation statement. JAMA. 2018;319(16):1696—1704.

*References available online at expertconsult.com*.

# 15

# Palliative Care

DANIEL STADLER AND AMELIA CULLINAN

## OBJECTIVES

*Upon completion of this chapter, the reader will be able to:*

- Understand the difference between palliative care and hospice.
- Be familiar with the basics of pain management, including pain assessment and treatment.
- Be familiar with the most common nonpain symptoms encountered in palliative care.

- Create a basic framework for structuring conversations with patients and families that includes breaking bad news and negotiating the goals of palliative care.
- Respond to and manage requests for hastened death.
- Assist patients with their transition to hospice care.

## What Is Palliative Care?

Advances in medicine and public health have led to increased life expectancy and fewer instances of sudden or unexpected death at younger ages. Death today occurs much more frequently in old age following a lengthy period of chronic illness, functional dependency, and (all too often) physical and psychosocial suffering. Palliative care offers patients and families relief from some or all of these stressors.

The Center to Advance Palliative Care (CAPC) defines palliative care as healthcare for people with serious illness, which is focused on providing relief from symptoms and stress—and improving quality of life and comfort—for both the patient and the patient's loved ones. Palliative care provides support for patients, families, and healthcare providers through:
- symptom assessment and treatment;
- assistance with decision making regarding the benefits and burdens of various therapies;

- help in establishing goals of care; and
- collaborative and seamless transitions between models of care (such as hospital, home, nursing homes, and hospice).

For the geriatric patient, palliative care is most appropriately centered on limiting functional and cognitive impairment, minimizing caregiver burnout, and relieving the burden of physical and psychological symptoms.

In contrast with hospice, which is generally offered once life-prolonging treatments are no longer appropriate, palliative care can be offered simultaneously with disease-modifying, life-prolonging, or even potentially curative treatments for patients with serious illness.

A central tenet of palliative care is the concept that no one individual or discipline can provide all the care needed by a patient facing serious, life-limiting disease. Specialty palliative care is typically provided by an interdisciplinary team of physicians, nurse practitioners, physician assistants, nurses, social workers, chaplains, and other healthcare professionals—all of whom have a specific role and skill set. Palliative care can be delivered in any setting where a patient receives care, ranging from longitudinal outpatient clinics, hospitals, in-patient hospice, and home consultations (Fig. 15.1).

## When to Refer to Specialty Palliative Care

A referral by a primary clinician to palliative care should be considered when it is felt that the needs of a patient and family facing serious illness cannot be entirely met by the existing resources. Palliative care teams have the training, expertise, and time necessary to engage with patients and families around the complex issues that arise when facing a life-limiting disease.

◆◆ **Reasons to refer to specialty palliative care**

- **Refractory symptoms**
- **Difficulty with medical decision making**
- **Healthcare team moral distress or burnout**
- **Patient and/or family distress**
  - **Maladaptive coping styles: pessimism, high regret, passivity, tendency to blame others**
  - **Marital or familial conflict**
  - **History of severe psychiatric illness or suicidal ideation/attempts in patient or family**
  - **Limited/absent familial or community supports**

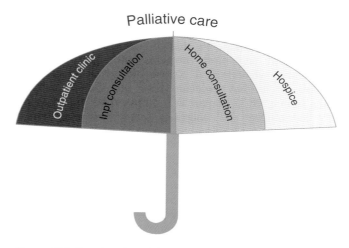

• **Figure 15.1** Domains of specialty palliative care.

- **Death anxiety**
- **Spiritual distress (i.e., "God is punishing me")**
- **History of ineffective coping in response to past stressors**
- **Lack of trust in healthcare providers**

## How to Refer to Palliative Care

Patients and their loved ones are often resistant to the idea of palliative care because it brings up the uncomfortable, and often taboo, subject of death and dying. Frequently, people associate a palliative care referral with "giving up."

Rather than waiting until late in the disease course to refer, consideration should be given to early referrals. This allows the palliative care team to be seen as an addition to the existing care team and not just associated with the last days of life. We recommend couching the referral in the context of the patient's expressed needs. For example:

- Identify and name the patient and family's specific challenges: "So, we've talked about how stressful things have been for you lately.... " Then align the referral to those needs: "... and there's a team who have been really helpful to me when patients and families need extra support."
- Anticipate resistance and offer a different perspective to patients and families: "Some people worry that palliative care is just for people who are at the end of life, or that it's the same as hospice. The truth is that palliative care teams help people at many different stages of illness."
- Explain the purpose of palliative care: "Palliative care focuses on providing comfort, reducing stress, and improving quality of life for patients and loved ones...."
- Highlight the services provided: "Palliative care can assist with managing symptoms, spiritual and psychological care, decision-making, coordination of care, and so on."

## Core Principles of Communication in Serious Illness

Before the onset of serious illness, the "right" medical thing to do is often obvious to both patients and their clinicians. In-depth discussion about goals are generally not necessary. When patients are facing serious illness, however, decisions are increasingly preference sensitive; an intervention that one individual would find intolerably burdensome regardless of the benefit might be an acceptable risk for another.

This is especially true among older patients—some request a "do whatever is necessary" approach, others seek to avoid risk of further debility, others express a readiness to die after a long life well lived. The key to a successful palliative care plan is having the skills and knowledge to meaningfully engage in conversations with patients and their families to determine which of these approaches is most appropriate for them.

In this chapter, we highlight several types of conversations a clinician may engage in with a patient about their serious illness. In one, the conversation is hypothetical, and the clinician is trying to ascertain what goals and values would drive the patient's decisions if serious illness develops. In another, the clinician is breaking bad news to a patient, while still presenting the information in a way that is helpful and useful to that particular individual. In another, the clinician discusses the impending approach of end of life, with the goal of determining the best next steps to support the patient through this final stage. Although the content of these discussions is different, the same key principles should be emphasized.

**Core principles of communication about serious illness:**

- **Invite key family and friends to participate**
- **Allow adequate time and do not appear rushed—sit down**
- **Listen more and talk less**
- **Explore understanding of illness and correct misperceptions**
- **Deliver clear prognostic information tailored to patients' preferences, medical literacy, hearing impairment, etc**.
- **Expect and respond to emotion**
- **Elicit values and goals before discussing possible next steps**
- **Confirm understanding—ask "Have I got this right?"**
- **Make recommendations that align treatment plans with patient's values**

The Serious Illness Conversation Guide (Fig. 15.2) provides a framework and suggested patient-tested language to incorporate these principles into discussions with patients. It can be used routinely in advance of diagnosis, early in the course of a serious illness, or later when serious end-of-life decision needs to be made.[1]

**Recommended points in disease trajectory to explore seriously ill patients' values and goals:**

- **At diagnosis**
- **After major hospitalizations or onset of significant complications**
- **Institutionalization**
- **Every 5 years**

These conversations can be directed by different members of an interprofessional team. For example, a nurse or social worker can elicit a patient's understanding of illness and information preferences, and then team up with a physician or an advance practice registered nurse for delivery of desired prognostic information.

After eliciting the patient's values and goals, the clinician should then frame a recommendation for the patient's care going forward. It is important not to skip this step because it affirms to the patient that the clinician is both there to help and is listening. Clinicians should begin their recommendation by summarizing what they understand to be important to the patient, and explicitly aligning those goals with the recommended plan.

---

**CASE**

**Roberta Smith (Part 1)**

Roberta Smith is a 68-year-old woman with hypertension and hyperlipidemia. She is scheduled to establish care with Dr. Martinez today as her new primary care provider. Roberta is a retired teacher who lives alone. Widowed for 5 years, she has 4 children, several of whom live close by. She does not have an advance directive.

1. What are the primary palliative care tasks Roberta's new primary care provider should consider doing during the initial visit with Roberta?

---

## Advance Care Planning

Serious illness typically affects more than the body; some combination of fatigue, confusion, medication side effects, and delirium can render a person unable to make the complex decisions needed at this challenging time. Advance care planning is the process through which individuals identify the goals, values, and priorities that should guide those decisions if a time comes when they are unable to fully participate in the process. Those priorities are then typically formalized or documented through the generation of advance directives. Primary care providers are strongly encouraged to routinely engage in these discussions with all their complex or geriatric patients early on in the provider-patient relationship.

There are several components to standard advance directives:

Durable power of attorney for healthcare (DPOA-HC). The DPOA-HC (also known as the healthcare agent or proxy) is a person legally designated by the patient to make healthcare decisions in the event that the patient is unable to do so. In general, this is a person who knows the patient well and has a deep understanding of the patient's values and goals. All individuals should be encouraged to name a DPOA-HC, but particular emphasis should be given to older patients or patients with serious illness. A patient who has no legal spouse or children—or a patient who would not want a spouse or child acting on his or her behalf—should be counseled to name a DPOA-HC as quickly as possible. Patients should be encouraged to discuss their thoughts, priorities, and values about health and debility with all their loved ones, but particularly and in some detail with their designated healthcare agent (Box 15.1).

**Choosing a DPOA-HC**

**A good healthcare agent is someone who:**
- **has an intimate day-to-day awareness of the patient's circumstances;**
- **knows what provides meaning and purpose to the patient's life;**
- **knows what quality of life the patient would consider to be worse than death;**
- **can distinguish one's own preferences from those of the patient; and**
- **can easily be contacted in the event of a healthcare decline and is able to (on occasion) attend healthcare visits, via telephone if needed.**

Statements of values/wishes/priorities. These are recorded statements that articulate the key values, priorities, and specific actions an individual wants to have guide any decision making in the face of serious illness. These can take many forms; some are standardized and others are very informal.

Examples include:
- The serious illness conversation (see earlier)
- A living will
- "Five wishes" documents
- Personally written essays
- Transcriptions or summaries of conversations
- Audiotaped or videotaped statements or conversations

Sometimes these statements are very specific, articulating particular actions to be taken or avoided, such as, "I want a brief trial on a ventilator," or "I never want to live permanently in a nursing home." Others are simply a description of values and priorities, such as "Being able to care for myself independently is the thing that gives my life meaning. If it is unlikely that I will be able to do this, I do not want steps taken to prolong my life." It is well demonstrated that an individual's perspective on what makes life worth living can change over time. Individuals in their 60s who state that life without the ability to drive or live alone is intolerable may feel differently about this in their 80s, when this loss of independence seems less problematic. For this reason, it is suggested that these conversations or written statements be revisited

# Serious illness Conversation Guide

## PATIENT-TESTED LANGUAGE

**SET UP**

"I'd like to talk about what is ahead with your illness and do some thinking in advance about what is important to you so that I can make sure we provide you with the care you want – **is this okay?**"

**ASSESS**

"What is **your understanding** now of where you are your illness?"

"How much **information** about what is likely to be ahead with your illness would you like from me?"

**SHARE**

"I want to share with you **my understanding** of where things are with your illness..."

*Uncertain:* "It can be difficult to predict what will happen with your illness. **I hope** you will continue to live well for a long time but I'm **worried** that you could get sick quickly, and I think it is important to prepare for that possibility."
OR
*Time:* "**I wish** we were not in this situation, but I am **worried** that time may be as short as __ (*express as a range, e.g. days to weeks, weeks to months, months to a year*)."
OR
Function: "**I hope** that this is not the case, but I'm **worried** that this may be as strong as you will feel, and things are likely to get more difficult."

**EXPLORE**

"What are your most important **goals** if your health situation worsens?"

"What are your biggest **fear and worries** about the future with your health?"

"What gives you **strength** as you think about the future with your illness?"

"What **abilities** are so critical to your life that you can't imagine living without them?"

"If you become sicker, **how much are you willing to go through** for the possibillity of gaining more time?"

"How much does your **family** know about your priorities and wishes?"

**CLOSE**

"I've heard you say that __ is really important to you. Keeping that in mind, and what we know abot your illness, **I recommend** that we __ . This will help us make sure that your treatment plans reflect what's important to you."

"How does this plan seem to you?"

"I will do everything I can to help you through this."

SI-CG 2017-04-18 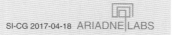 ARIADNE LABS

• **Figure 15.2** The Serious Illness Conversation Guide (2015–2017 Ariadne Labs: A Joint Center for Health Systems Innovation (www.ariadnelabs.org) between Brigham and Women's Hospital and the Harvard T.H. Chan School of Public Health, in collaboration with Dana-Farber Cancer Institute. Licensed under the Creative Commons Attribution-NonCommercial-ShareAlike 4.0 International License. http://creativecommons.org/licenses/by-nc-sa/4.0/)

## • BOX 15.1  Establishing a Durable Power of Attorney for Healthcare

- Most states have forms by which an individual can legally designate a durable power of attorney for healthcare (DPOA-HC) through a simple process. An attorney can also assist but this is generally not necessary.
- As long as the patient has capacity to make complex healthcare decisions, the DPOA-HC has no more access to information or authority over healthcare decisions than any other individual.
- Typically, a patient will designate one individual as primary DPOA-HC and an alternate individual who will step in if the primary agent is unable or unwilling to fulfill the role. Sometimes two or more individuals will be named. In that case, unless specified differently, both must agree on a decision before it can be implemented.
- If at some point a patient becomes unable to make complex medical decisions, a healthcare provider formally "activates" the DPOA-HC. From this point the DPOA-HC becomes the person healthcare personnel communicate with regarding which interventions to pursue and signs consent forms as needed. Sometimes the activation is temporary because of transient impairment and the DPOA-HC is "deactivated" at some later point. At other times the DPOA-HC functions as the decision maker until the death of the patient
- The designation of a DPOA-HC does not preclude other friends and family members from participating in decision making. Just as a patient might ask certain individuals to sit in on a meeting or attend an appointment to offer counsel, so too the DPOA-HC can invite others to participate. But if there is disagreement and/or inadequate time to pursue consensus, the DPOA-HC has the final say.

intermittently throughout a person's life, generally every 4 to 5 years, or at times of a major change in condition or function.

Provider orders for life-sustaining treatment. Despite many efforts to ensure that patients' values and wishes drive decision making, all too often these conversations and documents go unheeded and patients receive aggressive, life-prolonging interventions regardless of the expected outcome. To counter this, a national initiative has developed whereby clinicians formally sign a series of orders directing how care should be provided in the setting of acute injury or illness. There are several order forms available throughout the United States. Examples include the POLST (provider orders for life sustaining treatment) and the MOLST (medical orders for life sustaining treatment).

In general, these forms identify the patient's overall goals of treatment as either aggressive, limited, or comfort-focused. They further identify specific actions to be taken regarding the use of cardiopulmonary resuscitation (CPR), hospitalization, antibiotics, hydration, and nutrition. A provider can complete one of these order forms for any patient, but particular attention is generally given to the most vulnerable. An affirmative answer to the "surprise" question, "Would the provider be surprised if the patient died within 2 years?" is often used to identify patients who would most benefit from a document of this kind.

### CASE

#### Roberta Smith (Part 2)

After discussion with Dr. Martinez and then with her family, Roberta completes her advance directives. She names her daughter Sarah as her DPOA-HC and her son Anthony as the alternate. She writes in her advance directive that she finds meaning and purpose in her relations with her family and her ability to be useful to others; she does not ever want to be a

burden to her family. She asks that actions be taken to prolong her life, as long as there is a reasonable chance that she will be able to live independently and care for herself without significant help.

Two years later, Roberta, who is now age 70 years, is admitted to the hospital after falling at home. She was found on her kitchen floor by a neighbor—confused, in pain, and unable to stand. In the emergency department, she provided a rambling history, and x-rays revealed a nondisplaced femoral neck fracture. When asked to consent to an open reduction with internal fixation, she simply repeats "When it's my time, it's my time."

## Capacity, Competency, and Surrogacy

Competency or incompetency is a determination adjudicated by the legal system when an individual's ability, capacity, and/or authority to make decisions is in question. This is most typically addressed when a petition for a legal guardian has been placed. A legal guardian is a surrogate assigned by the state through the justice system. It requires a formal petition and hearing before a judge to be established or revoked and can provide the surrogate with authority over finances, residency, property, and so on, as well as healthcare decisions. Guardianship is generally pursued whenever the overall care needs of an individual are particularly complex or when there is dissension among family members about how to proceed.

Capacity refers to a patient's ability to make a specific decision or type of decision at a specific time. A patient with early dementia may have the capacity to agree to a simple intervention, such as an x-ray but may not have the capacity to make complex decisions such as consenting to a major surgery or CPR. A patient with delirium may not have the capacity to make healthcare decisions for a period but can regain that capacity at a later point. The task of establishing capacity falls to healthcare providers. If the determination is controversial, complex, or unclear, a referral to psychiatry can aid in this process.[2]

⚹⚹ **Elements of a capacity assessment**

**An individual is determined to have capacity to make a specific decision if all of the following factors are present:**
- **The individual can accurately explain the nature of his or her condition and the risks associated with it.**
- **The individual can explain the potential risks and benefits associated with electing or declining the intervention in question.**
- **The individual can explain the alternatives to the intervention in question and the risks and benefits associated with them.**
- **The individual makes the same decision consistently over time.**

If an individual is deemed by a healthcare provider to lack the capacity to make a specific health-related decisions (see Pearl: Elements of a capacity assessment), that authority passes to the DPOA-HC if one has been formally designated. In the absence of a formally designated DPOA-HC, states have different laws guiding whom to consult. Most laws designate close family members as the default decision maker. Often, these surrogate decision makers' right to make decisions for the patient is limited to a set period of time while guardianship is pursued.

## Symptom Management

Palliative care clinicians are frequently called upon to assist with symptom management for patients facing serious illness. Some of the most common symptoms that may accompany serious illness are pain, nausea, dyspnea, anxiety, delirium, anorexia, and fatigue. A detailed discussion on the management of all these is beyond the scope of this chapter and some of this material is addressed elsewhere in the text. Table 15.1 can be used as a simple reference for first- and second-line pharmacologic agents in the treatment of difficult symptoms. Note that apart from these agents, attention should always be given to nonpharmacologic interventions and treatment of the underlying cause of the symptom in question.

## Assessing and Treating Pain in Older Adults

Pain is an unpleasant sensory and emotional experience associated with actual or potential tissue damage.[3] Nearly 50% of severely ill hospitalized patients report that they have pain.[4,5] Pain in older patients may be poorly controlled because they may underreport pain or may have difficulty communicating, and physicians may undertreat pain because of concerns about side effects in older patients.[6]

## Pain Assessment

The treatment of pain begins with a thorough and complete assessment. Assessment of pain involves multiple components, and practitioners must consider each to best understand the nature and character of a patient's symptoms.

The first step of assessment is to inquire about the location of the pain, as well as whether it radiates to any other part of the patient's body. A description of the pain to determine if its origin is nociceptive, neuropathic, or some combination of both should be obtained, as well as questions as to when the patient's pain began; this information is required because chronic pain is often treated differently than acute pain. For a useful mnemonic device for assessing pain, see Box 15.1.

A crucial component of pain in older adults relates to its impact on function and independence. Symptoms that limit patients' activities of daily living (ADLs)[7] should trigger clinicians to engage community-based services. In cases where the patient cannot provide a thorough history because of conditions, such as dementia or aphasia, this information can be obtained from nursing staff and the patient's family. The clinician's physical examination should

**TABLE 15.1 Pharmacologic Management of Common Symptoms in Serious Illness**

| Symptom | First-Line Agent | Second-Line Agent |
|---|---|---|
| Mild pain | Acetaminophen | Low-potency opioids<br>Adjuvants |
| Moderate pain | Low-potency opioids | Higher doses of low-potency opioids<br>High-potency opioids<br>Adjuvants |
| Severe pain | High-potency opioids | Higher doses of high-potency opioids<br>Adjuvants |
| Dyspnea | Moderate-potency opioids | High-potency opioids |
| Cough | Moderate-potency opioids | High-potency opioids |
| Nausea/vomiting | Promethazine<br>Prochlorperazine<br>Ondansetron | Benzodiazepines<br>Typical antipsychotics |
| Delirium | Trazodone | Typical and atypical antipsychotics |
| Fear/anxiety | Lorazepam<br>SSRIs | Atypical antipsychotics |
| Itching | Antihistamines | Steroids |
| Anorexia | Mirtazapine | Steroids |
| Fatigue | Methylphenidate | Steroids |
| Hiccups | Chlorpromazine<br>Metoclopramide | Typical antipsychotics |

*SSRIs*, Selective serotonin reuptake inhibitors.

be used to confirm any suspicion generated during the history taking. Conditions to note include groaning, grimacing, protecting a body part, muscle spasm, gait impairment, agitation, abnormal joint alignments—to name just a few.[8]

## Treatment of Pain

The basic and most widely used approach to management of pain is illustrated by the World Health Organization's "pain ladder."[3] The first step, for patients with mild pain, encourages the use of nonopioid medications, such as acetaminophen or nonsteroidal antiinflammatory drugs (see following section).[9] If a patient's pain increases to a moderate level or remains poorly controlled with milder medication, the next step involves adding or substituting a weak opioid medication, such as hydrocodone. The third step, for patients with severe pain, or pain as yet uncontrolled with milder agents, advises the use of a strong opioid (e.g., morphine, hydromorphone).

Adjuvants are medications that can be combined synergistically with typical analgesic agents to improve symptoms, reduce the analgesic dose needed, and minimize side effects. The term *adjuvant* refers to the fact that these medications are drugs with a primary indication other than pain, but they have analgesic properties in some painful conditions.[10] Adjuvant analgesics include antidepressants, corticosteroids, local anesthetics, anticonvulsants, muscle relaxants, osteoclast inhibitors, N-methyl-D-aspartate (NMDA) receptor blockers, alpha-2 adrenergic agents, and radiopharmaceuticals, to name only a few.[11]

When prescribing medications for older patients, the issue of cost and accessibility must be taken into account. Analgesic medications can be expensive, particularly for patients on fixed incomes. Clinicians should inquire how patients pay for their prescriptions to ensure that they have the means to obtain the necessary medications. Although opioid abuse and diversion is less common among older patients, care should always be taken to ensure that patients use these medications appropriately and to minimize the risk to the patient and the community at large.

## Management of Nonpain Symptoms

Patients with chronic illness may have multiple nonpain symptoms during the course of their illness; some of the more common nonpain symptoms that may accompany chronic illness are nausea, dyspnea, depression, anxiety, agitation, anorexia/cachexia, fatigue, and pruritis. Discussion of all of these topics is beyond the scope of this chapter, but we will briefly focus on the first three.

### Nausea

Multiple physiologic processes underlie the sensation of nausea, so therapy is best directed at the mechanism behind the symptom. The three main areas related to the sensation of nausea are the brain's chemoreceptor trigger zone, the vomiting center, and the gastrointestinal (GI) tract.[12,13] The main classes of medications used for nausea and vomiting are the dopaminergic antagonists, anticholinergics, antihistamines, and serotonin antagonists. Anticholinergic agents, such as scopolamine, work in the vestibular system and in the vomiting center, but these agents should be used with caution in older patients because of their numerous side effects. Serotonin agents, such as ondansetron and granisetron, are particularly good for patients with chemotherapy-induced nausea and unlike many antinausea medications are not typically sedating. Other agents used in the treatment of nausea are steroids (which act by reducing edema in the bowel wall and brain), octreotide (which reduces GI secretions by reducing blood flow), and benzodiazepines and antipsychotics (which reduce stimulation of the vomiting center).

### Depression

Depression in patients facing serious illness is extremely common but often difficult to diagnose. Characteristics of depression, such as insomnia, weight loss, anorexia, and fatigue may not be reliable because they may be symptoms of the underlying disease. A question such as "How are your spirits?" is often the best way to determine if there is cause for concern.

The treatment of depression should always be multifocal. Counseling, spiritual support, exercise, and meaningful work are all associated with relief of symptoms and should be considered. With regard to medications, serotonin reuptake inhibitors (SSRIs) can be very effective but may generally take 4 to 6 weeks before an effect is seen. If a patient has a shorter life expectancy, a stimulant, such as methylphenidate, can demonstrate improvement within days, although the risk of adverse effects with these agents is greater than with SSRIs.

### Dyspnea

One of the most distressing symptoms for patients and their families is that of dyspnea or shortness of breath. The sensation of dyspnea is subjective and does not necessarily correlate with oxygen or carbon dioxide levels. The most effective way to improve dyspnea is to determine its underlying cause and then treat it. The differential diagnosis for breathlessness is broad, and includes pulmonary edema, anemia, bronchospasm, bronchial obstruction, anxiety, pulmonary embolism, pneumonia, and inability to clear airway secretions. Each of these has its own particular treatments, which should be provided as appropriate.

Regardless of the cause of dyspnea, several interventions can be helpful in providing relief to patients. Nonpharmacologic therapies, such as reducing room temperature, repositioning the patient, introducing humidity, a bedside fan, and supplemental oxygen are low risk and often helpful. Small doses of morphine (2—4 mg by mouth in an opioid-naïve patient) can be very effective in relieving dyspnea. Benzodiazepines can relieve the anxiety associated that frequently accompanies a sense of breathlessness. Opioids and benzodiazepines should be used with caution to avoid oversedation and apnea.

---

**CASE**

**Roberta Smith (Part 4)**

Roberta is started on scheduled tramadol for several days and then the dose is gradually reduced. Her physical and mental condition stabilize, and she is discharged to a rehabilitation facility where she makes marked improvement and returns home after a few weeks.

During the next several years, Roberta has increasing difficulty ambulating and has several falls although none with serious injury. Five years after her hospitalization, Dr. Martinez observes worsening rigidity, a shuffling gait, and a new resting tremor; he schedules an appointment to inform Roberta that she has Parkinson disease.
1. How would you tell Roberta about her diagnosis?

---

## Breaking Bad News and Discussing Prognosis

One of the most important components of palliative care is breaking bad news. The core principles for conversations about serious illness and the Serious Illness Conversation Guide, as referenced earlier in this chapter, can help guide a clinician through this difficult conversation. Later in this chapter we present a specific format, based on the work of Robert Buckman MD, which describes the process in more detail.

### Plan the Meeting

Decide who should attend the meeting. Will the patient respond better with a large supportive group, or is it best to keep it small? Should specific family members or friends attend? Should other specialists be present to provide input? Will the presence of other members of the team, such as a chaplain or social worker, help? Arrange for an appropriate time and place that ensures privacy, is free from interruptions, has boxes of tissues available, and the capacity for all attendees to sit down.

### Explore What the Patient Already Knows

Although the news may have been presented previously, it may not have been absorbed or well understood. Questions, such as, "What have you been told about your condition?" or "What have you heard about what the future holds?" can be extremely helpful in determining the patient's and family's degree of understanding, receptivity to the information, and medical literacy.

## Establish What the Patient Wants to Know

Some patients do not want to know much about their illness and prognosis; they find it so profoundly disturbing that they become incapable of taking action. Many geriatric patients will request that a close family member or loved one function as the repository of information and decision maker, preferring to take a more passive role. Individuals with cognitive impairment may not have the capacity to process serious information—offering bad news may only serve to upset them. Questions such as, "How much do you want to know about your illness?" or "Who should I talk to about what is going on with your health?" are open-ended questions that can help the team determine how much detail to provide and to whom.

## Give the News

Sentences such as, "I'm afraid I have some bad news," or "The results are not what we hoped," are helpful in warning patients and families that difficult information is forthcoming. The medical information and prognosis should then be given using simple language free of medical jargon; consider leading with a succinct summary, such as "Your cancer is no longer curable" before delivering additional detail as desired by the patient. Often, clinicians seek to soften the impact of the information, which can lead to confusion and false hope: stating that "the biopsy shows cancer" is preferable to "the biopsy suggests cancer" or "the biopsy might be cancer." It is also important to avoid phrases, such as "there is nothing else we can do," which can suggest that the provider in uninterested, unwilling, or unable to treat the patient's symptoms if the underlying disease is incurable.

## Pause and Respond to Emotions

After providing bad news, clinicians are frequently and understandably tempted to immediately move the discussion toward developing an action plan. This is strongly discouraged. After hearing bad news, people are often in shock and are unable to process the information—let alone make a plan. The patient and loved ones may demonstrate a wide variety of reactions (anger, denial, sorrow, blame, resignation, and calm acceptance are all common), which need to be explored before moving forward. Anticipating these responses, and calmly showing empathy and understanding, is critical to maintaining the healthy therapeutic relationship that will be needed in the days ahead. After presenting the bad news, it is generally best to pause and see how the patient and family respond. After they have responded, phrases, such as "It makes so much sense that you would feel this way," or "I deeply wish this was not the case," can go a long way in helping patients feel understood, less alone, and able to move forward. The NURSE mnemonic (Table 15.2) offers discrete skills for use in responding to and modulating patients' or families' emotions.[14] Often, more than one statement or skill will be needed to help a patient or family member feel ready to move on with the conversation.

## Making a Plan

Hearing that there are practical steps to take can help make the situation less distressing. Clinicians should avoid being too vague

| TABLE 15.2 | Skills for Responding to Emotion |
|---|---|
| **N**aming | "I can see how sad this makes you." |
| **U**nderstanding | "Of course, this is devastating news." |
| **R**especting | "I can see how much you love your family." |
| **S**upporting | "I'm going to be with you through all of this." |
| **E**xploring | "Can you give me a sense of what you're thinking?" |

### • BOX 15.2  Tips for Determining Prognosis

- The speed of functional decline to date often indicates the speed of decline in the future
- Formal prognostic tools can be helpful. Consider consulting:
  - Palliative Performance Index
  - Karnofsky Performance Scale
  - Palliative Prognostic Index
  - ePrognosis
  - GO-FAR (Good Outcome Following Attempted Resuscitation)

### • BOX 15.3  Tips for Discussing Prognosis

- Rather than avoiding giving a prognosis, choose prognostic information appropriate to the patient's diagnosis
  - Time-based: Use ranges such as "months to a few years," "weeks to months," "days to weeks," or "hours to days."
  - Uncertainty: "Best case/worst case/most likely" is useful in acute illness, such as CVA; "you could get very sick, very quickly" is useful in diseases prone to exacerbations, such as COPD or CHF.
  - Functional: "This is as strong as you will feel" is useful in slowly progressive disease, such as frailty or dementia.
- Use "I hope" and "I worry" to frame different possible outcomes, or "I wish" to soften difficult news.
- Acknowledge the imprecision and that you may be wrong; the purpose of prognostic information is to help patients and families prepare, not to be spot-on accurate.

*CHF*, Congestive heart failure; *COPD*, chronic obstructive pulmonary disease; *CVA*, cerebrovascular accident.

("Let's watch to see what develops") or overwhelming patients with a complex multistage plan. Recommending one or two key next steps (e.g., a referral to a specialist, a follow-up test, or a new medication) is generally the best course. Most important is to establish a follow-up visit in the not-too-distant future. By this time, patients and families may have had time to absorb the information and generate specific questions. Begin that session by briefly repeating the news, asking how the patient and family are adjusting, and inviting questions and the need for any clarifying information (Boxes 15.2 and 15.3).

## CASE

### Roberta Smith (Part 5)

Dr. Martinez arranges to meet with Roberta and her family to inform them of the diagnosis of Parkinson disease and the expected time and course of progression. Roberta and her family are understandably distressed but find comfort in a named diagnosis. Dr. Martinez refers Roberta to a neurologist and together they develop a treatment plan that includes medication and other forms of disease management support for Roberta and her family.

Seven years later, as expected, Roberta has declined further. She has been hospitalized several times for falls and infections. She is still living at home but depends on her daughter for most household tasks. She has recently started having difficulty bathing herself or getting to the toilet, and her daughter has suggested that she should no longer live alone. Particularly upsetting to Roberta is the fact that she can no longer babysit her young grandson. At the end of a routine visit with you, Roberta says, "I am becoming such a burden to my family and I am basically worthless to everyone. There's no point in going on—don't you have some pill I can take to get this over with?"

1. How would you respond to Roberta's question?

## Requests for Hastened Death

At times, the suffering and burdens of a condition will appear so great that a patient will begin to consider whether death would be preferable and approach a healthcare provider about taking some action to hasten death. These conversations call upon a clinician's highest levels of discernment and compassion. Sometimes, these thoughts are a manifestation of psychiatric illness and suicidality; other times, they are a rational and thoughtful response to serious debility and illness.

## Responding to a Request

In general, three principles should guide the initial response whenever a patient raises the subject of foreshortening life:

1. Empathize—Regardless of the affect or word choice, when a patient approaches a healthcare provider with thoughts about hastening death, it is certain that the patient is experiencing a deep sense of loss and suffering. Statements, such as, "I am so sorry you are feeling this way" or "It makes so much sense that you would feel this way," can be immeasurably helpful.
2. Explore—Nothing conveys compassion more than curiosity and good listening. Further, it is through this exploration that the provider can begin to determine the best next steps. Questions such as, "What makes you feel this way?", "How long have you been thinking about this?", "Have you spoken with other people about it?", "Do you have a specific plan?", and "How can I be most helpful to you?" should guide the early response.
3. Align—Many patients feel that these concerns are beyond the scope of the typical provider/patient relationship. It is important for the provider to assure support of the patient through this process, regardless of the outcome. A statement, such as the following can be immensely comforting: "I am not sure where this will lead, but I want to assure you that I am committed to working with you, supporting you through this, and doing whatever I can to relieve your suffering."

Many times, this simple empathic response is all the patient is really seeking. After a few questions, it becomes clear that the patient is not seriously considering a specific action, but rather was feeling understandably frightened and only in need of reassurance. At other times, the patient is seriously and rationally thinking about taking action and is looking to better understand what options if any are available.

## Physician-Assisted Death

Some states have "physician-assisted death" laws that permit physicians to prescribe medications to aid in hastening a patient's death without the threat of prosecution. In most states, patients must have a terminal illness and a prognosis of less than 6 months to live, as well as meeting other specific qualifications, such as making written or verbal requests for medication. Some state laws require a court decision before such medication can be prescribed by a physician.

However, because laws, patient qualifications, and reporting requirements vary from state to state, it is especially important for clinicians caring for older patients or patients with life-limiting illnesses to be informed about physician-assisted death regulations in the state where they practice. Although it is recommended that clinicians consult a legal professional in individual cases to ensure that they are protected from liability and all state reporting requirements are met, knowledge of state law regarding physician-assisted death will help clinicians to provide patients and their loved ones with appropriate information and options (Box 15.4).

A detailed description and implementation strategy for different approaches to hasten death is beyond the scope of this text. However, several principles should guide providers as they engage with the patient about these concerns, regardless of the path taken.[15]

1. Be alert for suicidality borne out of mental illness. Indications that this may be the case include:
   - Marked and active psychiatric illness
   - Inconsistency with the patient's previously known values
   - An impulsive and/or violent plan
   - Lack of consideration for the impact on family and loved ones
   - Lack of support from family and loved ones
   - Cognitive impairment
   - A reasonable chance of clinical improvement

   If the provider feels that the patient's statements are rooted in significant psychopathology, a more definitive and immediate response is generally required. This typically involves engaging the psychiatric community and may also include psychiatric hospitalization, active counseling, engagement with loved ones to assure a safety plan, and/or medication adjustment.

---

**• BOX 15.4  Hastened Death—Definitions and Terminology**

- **Euthanasia:** The intentional killing of a person, at that person's voluntary and competent request, typically by the administration of drugs and for reasons of mercy. (Illegal in the United States, legal in other selected countries)
- **Physician-assisted suicide or physician-assisted death:** The provision of medication by a physician to a terminally ill patient in response to the patient's voluntary and competent request to assist the patient to commit suicide by self-administration of the medication. (Legal in selected US states)
- **Withdrawal of life prolonging treatment:** The discontinuation of life-prolonging interventions in response to a patient or surrogate's voluntary and competent request. (Legal throughout the United States)
- **Voluntary stopping of eating and drinking (VSED):** The voluntary and deliberate refusal to eat and drink by a competent and capacitated person with the primary intention of hastening death. (Legal throughout the United States)
- **Palliative sedation:** The lowering of a terminally ill patient's consciousness using sedating medications, if necessary to the point of death, with the intent not to hasten death, but to limit patient awareness and suffering when suffering is otherwise intractable and intolerable. (Legal throughout the United States)

2. Explore and address reversible causes wherever possible.

Sometimes, a physical symptom is at the heart of the patient's request and treating that symptom can provide both physical and existential relief. At other times, patients need clarification about a misconception. Often patients perceive themselves as a burden to family, when in fact the family feels privileged to be providing care. Sometimes patients have a confused understanding of their illness or prognosis and simply need clarification about what to expect. Misunderstandings about financial concerns and the cost of care can also inform these beliefs and may simply need further explanation.

3. Slow it down.

After the provider has determined that no immediate steps are required to ensure the patient's safety and actions have been taken to reverse symptoms and misconceptions, the next step is to ensure that the patient's desire for hastened death persists over time. In general, this is done by setting up a time to discuss this further, often with other friends or family members present. A provider might say something such as, "I would like you to take some time to think about this further and discuss it with your family before we make any concrete plans. Would it be OK to set up a time for you to come back with your family when we can all meet and talk some more?" The amount of time between these visits will vary depending on a range of factors, but it is important to allow enough time for patients to seriously reconsider their concerns—but not so long that the provider appears insensitive to the underlying suffering.

4. Support family and friends.

A central tenet of palliative care directs us to provide support toward both the patient facing serious illness and the people who care for that individual. It is not infrequent, particularly in geriatric cases, that family members seem to suffer more than an individual who may be facing the long-anticipated end of a long and fruitful life. This is particularly true in cases involving requests for hastened death. The patient may in fact be feeling some gratification at the prospect of the end to pain and debility; some people even experience a sense of empowerment in finally being able to take control of their life after a long period of dependency. Friends and family members on the other hand may struggle with a sense of giving up too early or loss of identity as caregiver—or simply grieving the anticipated loss of their loved one. The legacy of suicide that can pass through families is of particular concern here and attention should be taken toward clearly distinguishing these situations from one borne out of psychiatric illness and despair. It is strongly encouraged to include friends and family members early in the decision-making process to ensure their support of the process and to investigate their coping strategies. The inclusion of social work or chaplaincy here can be invaluable. Asking the patient (if they are able and willing) to record some statement explaining the decision is often useful in helping others to understand and support the process and to distinguish it from suicide borne out of depression and disordered thinking.

5. Refer to hospice and/or palliative medicine.

The needs of a patient and family during the dying process requires many people with varying skill sets and ample time.

Perhaps no situation illustrates this more than requests for hastened death. Engaging palliative care specialists to assist in the discernment process and overseeing the process going forward can be invaluable. Engaging hospice as soon as a decision is made to proceed ensures that adequate expertise and access to symptom management, caregiver support, crisis prevention, and bereavement can be provided.

6. Reiterate the ability to change plans at any time.

The process of deciding to proceed with hastening death can at times be complex and lengthy and involve multiple people. Patients may feel obliged to proceed despite second thoughts or misgivings because they do not feel able to call off what has been a lengthy process. The care team should reiterate frequently than many people do change their mind and offer frequent opportunities for the patient to express concerns.

---

**CASE**

**Roberta Smith (Part 6)**

After several discussions with her daughter, Roberta comes to accept that she is not perceived as a burden and in fact her family feels a deep sense of gratitude in being able to support and care for her. She accepts Sarah's offer to move into Sarah's home. A POLST document is completed specifying that CPR should not be performed in the event of cardiac arrest, but short and limited hospitalizations should be arranged in the event of an acute decline.

Over the next 2 years, Roberta's condition continues to decline steadily. She is unable to perform any of her ADLs and has trouble swallowing. She has been admitted to the hospital repeatedly, with increasingly brief periods between acute events. At a discharge follow-up appointment, Dr. Martinez meets with Roberta and Sarah together to consider a referral to hospice.

1. How should you frame your recommendation about a transition to hospice?
2. What things should be done to prepare Roberta and her daughter for a smooth transition to hospice?

---

## Transitioning to Hospice

### The Hospice Benefit

Hospice is an insurance benefit provided to patients who are believed to have a prognosis of 6 months or less. The goal of hospice is to optimize symptom management and psychosocial support while not prolonging life. It is usually provided by an interdisciplinary team, which typically includes physicians, nurses, social workers, home health aides, and chaplains. The team has a holistic approach to supporting not just the patient, but also the family and/or caregivers. Hospice can be delivered wherever a patient resides—in a nursing home, assisted living facility, dedicated inpatient hospice facility, or in a patient's home. The hospice agency is responsible for providing any needed interventions to optimize patients' comfort, including nursing care, medications, oxygen, and durable medical equipment, such as hospital beds and commodes. In the event that the hospice team is unable to assure the patient's comfort where they reside, the hospice benefit provides for transitioning a patient to a higher level of care, called general inpatient (GIP), which is typically delivered in either hospitals, nursing facilities, or inpatient hospice facilities, and which provides intravenous medications and continuous nursing care.

## Making a Recommendation for Hospice

Hospice recommendations are often the most challenging to make because patients and families are resistant to the word "hospice" and often have significant misconceptions about what it offers. It may be helpful to start the conversation by summarizing the needs and values identified by the patient, which align with a hospice plan of care, then explaining that "There's a service that can help with what you have said is important to you—it's called hospice." This can be followed up by exploring if they have heard of hospice before and even explicitly naming the resistance that some patients have about it: "Some people worry that hospice is just for patients who are imminently dying." The clinician can then correct misconceptions, elicit questions, and teach about what hospice has to offer (see other section in this chapter on the differences between palliative care and hospice) (Box 15.5).

### • BOX 15.5    Hospice Referral Checklist

- Consider stopping routine labs, vitals, weights, and so on
- Simplify the medical regimen
  - Consider discontinuation of life-prolonging medications
  - Consider discontinuation of preventative medications
- Discontinue unnecessary follow-up appointments and limit the number of providers involved in care
- Discontinue procedures or testing that will not increase the patient's comfort
- Start prn (as needed) crisis medications (remember to anticipate the potential loss of an oral route of administration)
- Order a foley catheter and hospital bed prn
- Consider spiritual care and/or social work referral
- Anticipate bereavement challenges

## Summary

Palliative care for older adults differs from the traditional hospice model in that it is offered simultaneously with life-sustaining treatments. It consists of managing pain and other symptoms, clarifying goals of care, and ensuring continuity across systems of care. Pain management in palliative care involves clear assessment and then establishing a regimen that meets the patient's overall pain needs. Treating nonpain symptoms, such as nausea, dyspnea, and depression, is a cornerstone of palliative care, and this treatment is best served by having a clear understanding of the underlying pathology. When communicating bad news or having conversations to negotiate goals of care, it is important to have a method of approach for these often-difficult conversations.

### Web Resources

CAPC: https://www.capc.org/

National Hospice & Palliative Care Organization: https://www.nhpco.org/

Fast Facts: https://www.mypcnow.org/fast-facts/

ePrognosis: https://eprognosis.ucsf.edu

GO-FAR (Good Outcome Following Attempted Resuscitation) Score: https://www.mdcalc.com/go-far-good-outcome-following-attempted-resuscitation-score

## Key References

1. Bernacki RE, Block SD. Communication about serious illness care goals: a review and synthesis of best practices. *JAMA Int Med.* 2014;174(12):1994–2003.
2. Sessums LL, Zembruska H, Jackson JL. Does this patient have decision-making capacity? *JAMA.* 2011;306(4) 420–427.
14. Campbell TC, Carey EC, Jackson VA et al. Discussing prognosis: balancing hope and realism. *Cancer.* 2010;16: 461–466.
15. Block SD, Billings JA. Patient requests to hasten death: evaluation and management in terminal care. *Arch Intern Med.* 1994;154:2039–2047.

**References available online at expertconsult.com.**

# Geriatric Syndromes and Common Special Problems

*What does it matter if he can't remember them, as long as they remember him?*

**Wife of 94-year-old patient (of RH), about their great grandchildren's visits**

*Body and mind, like man and wife, do not always agree to die together.*

**CHARLES C COLTON, c 1780-1832, churchman and writer, in Lacon 1, 324**

*Perhaps being old is having lighted rooms inside your head, and people in them, acting.*

*People you know, yet can't quite name.*

**PHILIP LARKIN, 1922-1985, English author, in The Old Fools**

*Better by far you should forget and smile*

*Than that you should remember and be sad.*

**CHRISTINA ROSSETTI, 1830-1874, in Remember**

*Memory is history recorded in our brain; memory is a painter, it paints picture of the past and of the day.*

**GRANDMA MOSES, 1860-1961, Painter, in My Life's History, ed. Aotto Kallir**

*The humor of the dementia clinic:*

*(RH to a patient) "...and what State are we in?"*

*(Patient) "Confusion!?"*

*...AND...*

*Wife of patient with dementia to RH, who has started to discuss medication to calm her husband:*

*She: "Are you going to zap him? Make a zombie of him?"*

*RH: "No, no—of course not."*

*She (interrupting): "Well you need to zap him—he's awful, blows his nose on the table cloth, drinks out of the saucer, and the language—no, doc, you need to zap him!!!"*

*When I meet a man whose name I can't remember, I give myself two minutes; then, if it is a hopeless case, I always say, "And how is the old complaint?"*

**BENJAMIN DISRAELI, 1804-1881, Queen Victoria's favorite prime minister**

*I am a very foolish, fond old man,*

*Fourscore and upward, not an hour more of less;*

*And, to deal plainly,*

*I fear I am not in my perfect mind*

**WILLIAM SHAKESPEARE, 1564-1616, in King Lear, IV, 7**

*He that conceals his grief finds no remedy for it.*

**TURKISH PROVERB**

*Wine is only sweet to happy men.*

**JOHN KEATS, 1795-1821, in To. . . (Fanny Brawne)**

*It provokes desire, but it takes away the performance. Therefore much drink may be said to be an equivocator with lechery.*

**WILLIAM SHAKESPEARE, 1564-1616, in Macbeth, II:3**

*I smoke 10 to 15 cigars a day; at my age you have to hold on to something.*

**GEORGE BURNS, 1896-1996, US comedian**

*As men draw near the common goal*

*Can anything be sadder*

*Than he who, master of his soul,*

*Is servant to his bladder*

**ANON, in The Speculum, Melbourne, 1938**

*The ultimate indignity is to be given a bedpan by a stranger who calls you by your first name.*

**MAGGIE KUHN, 1905-1995, activist and founder of the Grey Panthers**

*Old people, on the whole, have fewer complaints than the young, but those chronic diseases which do befall them never leave them.*

**HIPPOCRATES, c 460- c 357 BC, in Aphorisms**

*So we'll go no more a-roving*

*So late into the night,*

*Though the heart be still as loving,*

*And the moon be still as bright.*

*For the sword outwears its sheath,*

*And the soul wears out the breast,*

*And the heart must pause to breathe,*

*And Love itself have rest.*

*Though the night was made for loving,*

*And the day returns too soon,*

*Yet we'll go no more a-roving*

*By the light of the moon.*

**GEORGE GORDON, LORD BYRON 1788-1824, "So We'll Go No More A-Roving"**

# 16

# Emergency Care

PHILLIP D. MAGIDSON AND ROBERT S. ANDERSON JR.

## OBJECTIVES

*Upon completion of this chapter, the reader will be able to:*

1. Identify key differences between the practice of emergency medicine and geriatric primary care.
2. Appreciate inherent challenges and risks faced by older adults cared for in the emergency department setting.
3. Recognize the capabilities and practice patterns of emergency departments and emergency medicine providers in addressing nonurgent needs of older adults.

4. Understand key considerations in caring for older adults in the primary care setting with chest pain, shortness of breath, abdominal pain, or traumatic injury and when to refer these patients to the emergency department.

◆◆ **The number of older adults presenting to emergency departments continues to increase despite a decrease in inpatient capacity**.

## The Role of Emergency Medicine

Emergency medicine (EM) was not officially recognized as a medical subspecialty by the American Board of Medical Subspecialties until 1979—just over 10 years after the first geriatric fellowship was established.[2,3] The evolution of this specialty and the services, providers, and patients of the emergency department (ED) has been significant over the past 50 years. Before the 1970s, EDs were often poorly equipped, single rooms in the hospital basement, with poorly trained or supervised clinicians providing a majority of the care. As this subspecialty has developed with highly trained providers and an increase in the availability of diagnostic and therapeutic

resources, there has been a concomitant growth of utilization of the ED by patients, as well as decrease in inpatient services. Since the early 1990s, ED visits have increased at rates significantly greater than population growth with nearly 146 million visits in 2016.[4,5] This growth represents a 62% increase since the early 1990s. The reason for this growth is likely multifactorial with the aging population, increase of availability of technology in the ED, and difficulty in obtaining timely or urgent primary care all contributing.[6,7] Over that same time period, however, the number of inpatient hospital beds has decreased by nearly 18%.[8] Despite the ED serving as a safety net for many without access to routine care for chronic conditions, the actual expertise of EDs and emergency medicine providers (EMP) is caring for acute disease processes. In fact, the American College of Emergency Physician's (ACEP) *Definition of Emergency Medicine* defines EM as "the medical specialty dedicated to the diagnosis and treatment of unforeseen illness or injury."[9] Given the focus of this subspecialty and considerable volume of patients, frequency of interruptions in the ED setting compared with the primary care setting, older adults with more subacute or chronic complaints who can be managed in the outpatient setting by those more skilled in chronic, outpatient management, ought to be—specifically by primary care providers (PCPs). The challenge can be knowing when and how to engage EM and ED resources. This chapter's goal is to help further prepare the PCP to address this challenge.

◆◆ **Given the focus of EM and the practice environment of the ED, older adults with subacute or chronic disease processes are better cared for in the outpatient setting.**

## Goals of Care Are Best Considered Before Emergency Care

Among older adults, 75% visit an ED in the last 6 months of life with more than 50% visiting in the last month of life.[10] By the nature of EM, there is an overarching focus on providing aggressive resuscitative interventions for those acutely ill even if those interventions may not be consistent with a patient or family goals of care. Even though over 90% of EM physicians believe goals of care discussions are within the scope of their practice, 66% of providers report difficulty initiating these discussions with insufficient time, lack of patient relationship, and patient expectations as commonly cited barriers.[11] This further emphasizes the importance of these discussions in the primary care setting, especially in older adults with advanced disease nearing the end of life. Of course, it is most critical that there be communication of these preferences to the EMP either verbally, with a call to the EMP or in writing with a medical orders for life-sustaining treatment (MOLST) or provider orders for life-sustaining treatment (POLST) form.

## Training Differences Between Primary Care Providers and Emergency Medicine Providers

To most in the healthcare field, it is no secret that certain medical subspecialties attract different personalities. However, even beyond this self-selective process, other factors such as unique problem-solving strategies that developed in residency training, further differentiate providers in different fields and their approach to patient care. Perhaps more unique to EM is the ability to evaluate an undifferentiated patient while synthesizing limited data points and doing so quickly with significant distractions. One method of doing this is through heuristic decision making. Heuristic decision making is a decision-making strategy that focuses on few, yet relevant predictors. In fact, many clinical decision rules routinely used in EM, such as the pulmonary embolism rule-out criteria (PERC), the HEART Score, or the quick sequential organ failure assessment (qSOFA) look at very specific decision points while ignoring some other available information. This heuristic decision-making model tends to lead to high sensitivity with lower specificity.[12,13] Providers in primary care tend to have more familiarity with patients, access to more longitudinal information, and more time to make clinical decisions and hence use a more deductive approach. There is also an expectation within primary care to make a definitive diagnosis, even if not immediately, that is frequently shared by the provider and patient. This is in contrast with EM where the EMP may be working to simply rule out life-threatening pathology whereas the patient, like in the primary care setting, is hopeful for a definitive diagnosis.

◆◆ **The practice of primary care and EM differ in training, approach to risk tolerance, available information, and interruptions during the patient evaluation.**

## Risk Intolerance in Emergency Medicine

EMPs tend to practice more defensive medicine with one study examining defensive medicine practices showing EM physicians, compared with other high-risk subspecialties, order more tests than indicated, by their own self-reports.[14] Despite this practice, EM physicians are just slightly more likely to have an annual malpractice claim compared with all physicians. Nevertheless, malpractice claim rates among EM physicians are still about 50% higher than those in adult primary care subspecialties.[15] The cause of this is likely multifactorial. Contributory reasons likely include longer and more established relationships between PCPs and their patients, higher risk diagnoses considered in the ED, ED crowding, and less complete and thorough documentation in EM.[16] Given these considerations and the complexity of older adults, this patient population receives considerably more diagnostic testing and medical consultation in the ED setting compared with younger adults.[17-19]

## Reasons for Referral to the Emergency Department

Common reasons that older adults visit the ED for nonemergent conditions, both self-referred and at the encouragement of their PCP, as well as associated challenges are displayed Table 16.1. It is important for the PCP to understand how many of these conditions are addressed in the ED as this may help to prevent unnecessary referrals and help to modulate patient and family expectations.

One of the first steps in identifying a true medical emergency and need for urgent referral to the ED is determining if there is an active or impending insult to the patient's airway, breathing, or circulatory status. This first step, known as evaluating the airway, breathing, circulation (ABCs), is important for all PCPs and EMPs alike when faced with a potential medical emergency. Evaluation for acute neurologic disease (as evidenced by new "disability") has led to the modification of ABCs to ABCDs. Table 16.2 reviews specific abnormalities to the ABCDs that should prompt referral to the ED.

## The Emergency Department

◆◆ **In the ED, older adults stay longer, require more diagnostic tests/social services, and are more likely to be admitted than younger patients.**

### Epidemiology

In 2016 patients age $\geq 65$ years accounted for $> 23$ million ED visits or nearly 16% of all ED visits in the United States, and the likelihood of coming to the ED via ambulance and emergency medical services (EMS) increases with age. In fact, $> 40\%$ of patients age $\geq 75$ years arrive via ambulance. Furthermore, older

| TABLE 16.1 | Common Avoidable Emergency Department Referrals | |
|---|---|---|
| **Reason for Visit** | **Associated Problems** | **Alternative Approaches** |
| Asymptomatic anemic patient presenting for transfusion | Routine blood transfusions in the ED can be challenging as EMPs, who are not familiar with the patient, may pursue a workup that is not necessary (if the cause is known). In addition, many EDs have policies mandating hospitalization for patients who are transfused. | Outpatient infusion center appointments or routine visits with hematology who develop familiarity with a patient and have the capacity to transfuse in the outpatient setting. |
| Refills for controlled substances | Almost no PCP would refer their patient to the ED for a refill; however, challenges arise when a patient's PCP may be unavailable. Covering providers or office staff may refer patients to the ED who are requesting refills on controlled substances. With a heightened awareness of high-risk prescribing and some laws governing said prescribing from the ED, EMPs are less willing to provide said prescriptions.[20] | Have a plan in place with covering providers on how to handle these requests. Consider prewriting prescriptions for when patients are scheduled to need a refill and leave these with office staff so they may be available to patients even if the PCP is not. |
| Nonemergent, advanced imaging | Although the ED may be operating 24/7, not all services are available. Advanced imaging studies, such as CT scans, MRIs, and ultrasounds may not be available at all times. Patients who arrive with requests for such imaging may find themselves discharged without the test or hospitalized for an outpatient imaging study. | Encourage nonemergent outpatient imaging studies whenever possible; if the ability to make such arrangements is not possible, confirm with the EMP the availability of the imaging modality before sending the patient to the ED. |
| Asymptomatic hypertension | Acutely aggressive management of a hypertensive patient should generally only occur in the setting of end-organ dysfunction. Patients sent to the ED for asymptomatic hypertension are unlikely to receive any acute interventions. In fact, ACEP has a clinical policy statement on said condition that most EMPs follow, which discourages aggressive treatment or intervention.[21] | Titration of home blood pressure medications in the office, over the phone, or via a home visit is just as, if not more productive than, an ED visit. Educate patients about best practices for isolated, elevated blood pressure reading. |
| Dental complaints without systemic infection | Unfortunately, EMPs are generally no better positioned to care for routine dental concerns than a PCP's office. In a patient protecting his/her airway without signs of systemic infection, most EDs simply provide analgesia and referral to dental services. | In a well-appearing older adults without systemic infectious complaints, direct referral to dental services is likely more appropriate than referral to the ED. |

*ACEP*, American College of Emergency Physicians; *CT*, computed tomography; *ED*, emergency department; *EMPs*, emergency medicine providers; *MRI*, magnetic resonance imaging; *PCP*, primary care provider.

| TABLE 16.2 | Warning Signs for Emergent Decompensation |
|---|---|
| | **Emergent Abnormalities** |
| Airway | Airway edema, stridor, semi- or complete unconsciousness |
| Breathing | Bradypnea (<10 breaths per minute) or extreme tachypnea (>32 breaths per minute), new hypoxia with oxygen saturation <93% in patients without lung disease or oxygen saturation <88% in patients with lung disease. |
| Circulation | Signs of end-organ hypoperfusion, such as cyanosis, change in mental status, cool extremities with decreased pulses, or a heart rate <50 beats per minute or >120 beats per minute or systolic blood pressure <100 mmHg. |
| Disability | New or decreased mental status, pupil abnormality or new, focal neurologic deficit. Frequently measured via the 15-point Glasgow coma scale. |

adults are more likely to be classified as having a higher acuity when they do present to the ED with the initial acuity classification increasing by age.[5] Older adults have 20% longer length of stays in the ED, up to 50% more diagnostic studies, and are 400% more likely to require social services than younger patients.[22–24] These patients are also significantly more likely to be admitted both to the general inpatient wards and to intensive care units (ICUs). Of older adults discharged from the ED, there is considerable functional decline, as well as significant ED recidivism.[19,25] Moreover, older adults who are seen in the ED have high rates of adverse outcomes after an initial visit with one study suggesting a 34% 1-year mortality.[26]

Despite the challenges associated with caring for older adults in the ED and increased morbidity and mortality linked with such visits, most older adults have PCPs and many have consulted them before presentation to the ED. One study reported that 32% of patients with a PCP and a nonurgent medical issues were unable to access PCP resources and therefore presented to the ED.[6] In some instances, the PCP has referred the patient to the ED for evaluation, which provides an opportunity for the development of cross-discipline collaborative efforts to identify both appropriate and inappropriate ED referrals and ways to improve communication between the EMP and the PCP.[25,27–29]

## The Physical Environment of the Emergency Department

Very few EDs are designed with older adults in mind. EM, like the space in which it is practiced, focuses on identifying time-sensitive disease and injury within the confines of a fairly rapid triage, diagnosis, and treatment process. In addition, there is a continual effort to see more patients quickly as data show a positive correlation between ED crowding and ED mortality.[30] In this environment, patients who are more medically complex and have complicated medical histories, as well as extensive medication lists and sensory or communication impairments, are at a disadvantage.[27,31]

The risk of delirium is significant for older adults in EDs. With limited natural light, continuous flow of patients and ongoing activity, and inconsistent access to nutrition, the ED may not only be deliriogenic but many older adults with delirium are not identified as such while they are being cared for in the ED.[32,33] This unrecognized delirium has significant morbidity and mortality implications in the older adult population. In addition, the boarding of patients in the ED after the decision to admit to hospital (a matter of routine in many EDs) can further complicate the care of more complex, older adults.[34] For these reasons, avoidance of the ED by older adults should be considered preferable when alternatives are possible.

## The Geriatric Emergency Department

A collaborative effort between professional societies in EM, geriatrics, and nursing led to the publication of *Geriatric Emergency Department Guidelines* in 2014.[24] The purpose of these guidelines was to help identify best practices in the care of older adults and has paved the wave for the ACEP to begin to offer formal accreditation for meeting and exceeding these standards.[35] These geriatric emergency departments (GEDs) generally offer older adults enhanced services within four domains[31]:

1. Staffing patterns: specifically, GEDs are more likely to have nursing with additional training in the care of older adults, as well as improved social work support and geriatric case management. With an increase in the need for social services in these patients, strong interdisciplinary teams are crucial and frequently found in GEDs. Some work has shown availability of increased social support for older adults in the ED can decrease readmission rates.[36]
2. Environmental enhancements: the physical space in many GEDs can offer patients and families more comfortable patient care areas during the ED visit. Availability of adaptive equipment, including audio amplification systems, magnification for reading, nonslip flooring, handrails, comfortable seating for family, and greater access to mobility aids both during the ED visit and at discharge are some examples.[37]
3. Geriatric-specific policies/procedures: as a component of achieving ACEP GED accreditation, there is a requirement to have established, geriatric-specific policies or interventions in place. To that end, many GEDs have a wide range of older adult–specific interventions, such as a formal medication reconciliation process, cognitive screening, frailty evaluation, and functional and fall assessments.[38,39]
4. Staff education and training: most GEDs report a specific mission of formally preparing their workforce to care for older adults. In general, nurses and physicians working within or holding a leadership role within GEDs have undergone and participate in continual education on best practices in caring for older adults.[31]

◆◆ **GEDs provide staffing, environmental enhancements, procedures, and training specific to older adults and their needs.**

When referring an older adult to the ED, it is important to understand that all EDs, whether a specific GED or not, can provide excellent care to all patients, including older adults. However, GEDs do offer older patients and their families a unique focus on specialized care that may enhance the patient experience and provide the highest-value, evidenced-based geriatric emergency care.

## Transitions in Care

Older adults are more likely than any other group of patients to be transferred between facilities.[40,41] Up to one-quarter of nursing home (NH) residents are transferred to the ED annually.[42] Despite this high frequency of transfers of care, numerous studies have shown vital information, including patient symptomatology, medication lists, baseline cognitive status, code statuses, and goals of care, are missing in up to 90% of patients transferred between the ED and NHs.[43–46]

This lack of information transfer is not without consequence, both for the patient and the health system. One study examining changes in medication regimens between acute and long-term care (LTC) facilities identified adverse drug events resulting 20% of the time.[47] In addition, studies suggest poor communication between LTC facilities and the ED results in the increase of unnecessary ED utilization, as well as inpatient and postacute care services.[40,48]

In considering best practices for improving transitions of care between the community and the ED, a number of different strategies have been used, including use of the electronic medical record to send messages between ED and outpatient providers, standardized handoff tools, clear communication of advanced directives and use of the POLST or MOLST, and use of a geriatric nurse coordinator or discharge planner.[40,49,50] Other methods aimed at reducing transitions of care and the many associated challenges include alternative models of care, such as the programs of all-inclusive care for the elderly (PACE), as well as the implementation of hospital at home (HaH) programs. Good evidence suggests programs such as HaH can reduce costs, improve patient satisfaction, and reduce adverse events and functional decline when applied to appropriate patient populations.[51–53]

## Common Emergency Department Conditions

### Chest Pain

**CASE 1**

**Mr. Allen (Part 1)**

You see Mr. Allen, a 72-year-old male, in your clinic for chest pain. The patient's wife had called the clinic earlier, reporting her husband woke up with new chest pain. The patient says he had been feeling more tired than usual the day before. However, he woke up this morning with chest pain that seemed to be worse when he was getting ready for the day. He describes it as a pressure with radiation to his right arm. He has never had this pain before. The patient has a history of hypertension and well-controlled diabetes. His vital signs are normal. He appears somewhat uncomfortable as you observe him walking to the examination room, at which time he endorses recurrence of the chest pain. The pain resolves when he sits down on the examination table. His physical examination is otherwise unremarkable.

ST-segment elevations and the patient is taken emergently to the cardiac catheterization lab where a right main coronary artery occlusion is found. The patient was admitted, had a successful drug-eluding stent placed, and was discharged home in good condition after a brief inpatient stay.

Chest pain accounts for over 7 million ED visits annually, a complaint more common in older adults.[5] The differential diagnosis for chest pain is broad and the decision for the PCP to refer to the ED can be challenging. However, it is likely most PCPs (and ED providers alike) will consider acute coronary syndrome (ACS) early in older patients with chest pain as over half of all myocardial infarctions occur in adults age > 65 years.[54] Although atypical signs and symptoms of ACS in older adults, such as weakness, general malaise, and back pain, are more common than in younger adults, chest pain with radiation to both arms, pain similar to previous ischemic episodes, and changing patterns of chest pain over 24 hours are very suggestive of an ischemic process.[55,56] A patient with these complaints reported to the PCP in the office should have an urgent electrocardiogram (ECG) with comparison to prior ECGs if possible, and urgent referral to the ED, if consistent with previously established goals of care. Initiation of goals of care discussion in this situation may not be practical. Acute treatment by the PCP can include full dose aspirin between 160 mg and 325 mg, which has demonstrated consistent mortality benefits.[57]

Acute aortic dissection, although a rare entity, can be devastating with mortality rates reaching nearly 60% for some specific subtypes.[58] Even in older adults, chest pain is by far the most common presenting complaint. A sudden onset of chest pain should raise the clinical suspicion for acute dissection.[58] Although conventional teaching of obtaining a chest radiograph may be tempting, especially in the outpatient setting, nearly 40% of patients with acute aortic dissections do not have classic "widened mediastinum" and over 12% have a completely normal film.[58] Therefore a high clinical suspicion for this disease should warrant referral to the ED for prompt evaluation. Again, laying the groundwork for goals of care before the ED visit is important.

Pulmonary embolism (PE) is a particular consideration in patients with a prior history of PE or deep venous thrombosis who present with chest pain. In older adults, with an eventual diagnosis of PE, syncope and hypoxic are more common than in younger adults.[59]

Another cause of chest pain in older adults includes herpes zoster, a condition that can be readily be identified in the office when considered. With an increase in reliance on laboratory values and diagnostic imaging a good skin examination should not be neglected by the PCP or EMP alike. Gastroesophageal reflux disease (GERD) is also common among older adults, but should be a diagnosis of exclusion with an initial presentation of chest pain in a patient without a history of GERD.

## CASE 1

### Mr. Allen (Part 2)

You are most concerned about ACS given the patient's presentation and history. The ECG you obtain shows new T-wave inversions. The patient's baseline functional status is good. As your staff calls an ambulance, you administer 324 mg of aspirin by mouth. In the ED, repeat ECG shows inferior

## Shortness of Breath

Similar to patients presenting with chest pain, the causes of acute shortness of breath are vast. In patients in the outpatient setting with this complaint, it is important to consider the aforementioned ABCDs in helping to triage the patient to outpatient or acute ED treatment. Significant irregularities to the ABCDs should lead to prompt ED referral.

Decompensated heart failure (HF) is the most common reason for older adults to be admitted to the hospital.[60] The decision to refer older adults to the ED for HF should be based on the ability of the PCP to identify the causative reason, the degree of decompensation, and anticipated interventions. For example, patients who report running out of their medications with minimal symptoms should not be referred to the ED without at least an attempt to resume an outpatient regimen. Studies have shown in older adults hospitalized, there can be significant and sometimes dangerous or unnecessary medication changes. Attempts to restart outpatient regimens without a visit to the ED may help mitigate this risk.[61]

For PCPs with access to an outpatient diuresis infusion center, there is evidence to suggest referral to treatment in these centers can reduce congestive heart failure (CHF) hospitalizations.[62] For patients where outpatient management may not be possible or decompensation is greatly impacting the ABCDs, referral to the acute hospital may be warranted. As previously discussed in this chapter, older adults tend to have extensive workups in the ED. Given this, if a known or highly suspected cause of a CHF exacerbation is suspected, communication with the EMP may help reduce unnecessary ED diagnostic testing and length of stay for these patients.

◆◆ **Consider the use of clinical decisions tools, such as the CURB-65 score, to determine the need for referral to the ED for older adults with pneumonia** (Table 16.3).

Pneumonia is a common cause of shortness of breath in older adults, occurring at a rate four times that of the general population.[63] The diagnosis of pneumonia can frequently be made in the outpatient setting by reviewing vital signs, examination, and basic laboratory findings, as well as imaging studies. The decision to refer a patient for further evaluation and treatment for pneumonia can be guided by well-established clinical decision tools, including the PORT score and CURB-65 score for pneumonia severity.[64,65] These tools can help predict lower risk patients who can be managed in the outpatient setting; however, they do require obtaining laboratory values.

The natural history of chronic obstructive pulmonary disease (COPD) is such that frequent exacerbations are not uncommon. Many of these are triggered by viral or bacterial infections but other factors (including HF, weather changes, tobacco use, or other systemic illness) can cause decompensation in stable COPD patients.[66] Mild exacerbations can generally be safely managed in

## TABLE 16.3    CURB-65 Score and Interpretation

| CURB-65 PARAMETERS | |
|---|---|
| Confusion | 1 point for yes |
| BUN >19 mg/dL | 1 point for yes |
| Respiratory rate ≥ 30 breaths/min | 1 point for yes |
| Systolic BP <90 mmHg or diastolic BP ≤ 60 mmHg | 1 point for yes |
| Age ≥ 65 years | 1 point for yes |

| CURB-65 Score | 30-day Mortality |
|---|---|
| 0-low risk, consider home treatment | 0.60% |
| 1-low risk, consider home treatment | 2.7% |
| 2-short inpatient hospitalization or closely supervised outpatient treatment | 6.8% |
| 3-Severe pneumonia; hospitalization recommended | 14.00% |
| 4 or 5-Severe pneumonia; hospitalize and consider ICU level care | 27.80% |

*BP*, Blood pressure; *BUN*, blood urea nitrogen; *ICU*, intensive care unit.

the outpatient setting with an increase in home medications or short course of systemic steroids or antibiotics. Patients with more serious exacerbations may require referral to the ED and subsequent hospitalizations.[67] The challenge is identifying which patients may require such a referral.

During the initial examination, tachypnea, pursed lip breathing, or accessory muscle use suggests advancing respiratory disease. Altered mental status or a change in mental status is strongly suggestive of hypoxia or hypercarbia and is a true medical emergency.[68] Further evaluation in the outpatient setting of patients where referral to the ED is less clear can include pulse oximetry, chest x-ray to evaluate for concurrent pneumonia, and blood gas sampling. Although obtaining an arterial blood gas in the clinic can be challenging, venous blood gas pH and carbon dioxide ($CO_2$) measurements may be easier to acquire and have shown excellent correlation with arterial values in patients with COPD exacerbations.[69] Significant $CO_2$ and findings of acidosis should prompt referral to the ED.

If the patient's initial presentation of shortness of breath is coupled with either a normal pulmonary examination or normal oxygenation, ACS (discussed earlier), PE, or metabolic derangement should be considered.

A PE will frequently present with a normal lung examination although a thorough physical examination, including evaluating for asymmetric lower extremity swelling or pain, should increase suspicion for this diagnosis. Hypoxia and cyanosis are more commonly seen in older adults than in younger patients and, coupled with a nonfocal pulmonary examination, should prompt referral to the ED for evaluation for PE.

Diagnostic studies that can be considered in the outpatient clinic include a chest x-ray and d-dimer. The classically taught Westermark's sign and Hampton's hump are fairly specific for the diagnosis of a PE but both have low sensitivity.[70] In lower risk patients where PE is being considered, a D-dimer may be ordered. It is important for the PCP to recognize an age adjusted D-dimer should be used when interpreting these test results in older adults because falsely elevated D-dimers are more common in older adults. In general, age times 10 mcg/L with a lower limit of 500 mcg/L is what is reported in the literature.[71] This age-adjusted approach increases the specificity in older adults. In patients with a higher pretest probability of PE, computed tomography (CT) angiography or ventilation/perfusion (V/Q) scans should be undertaken. Although these can be arranged on an outpatient basis, timely completion of these tests in an acutely dyspneic older adult generally warrants ED referral.

In stable patients diagnosed with an acute PE, some literature in younger adults suggests that initiation of anticoagulation in the outpatient setting can be accomplished safely.[72] In select patients, initiation of outpatient anticoagulation and avoidance of an ED referral or the acute hospital setting may be appropriate.[73]

## Abdominal Pain

Behind chest pain and shortness of breath, acute abdominal pain is the third most common reason older adults visit the ED.[5] The potential for a broad differential coupled with physiologic changes of aging make identification of life-threatening abdominal disease processes challenging, especially in a timely manner.[74]

The PCP should have a fairly low threshold to refer older adults with undifferentiated abdominal pain to the ED for evaluation or to obtain advanced imaging. Many of the classic signs or symptoms of systemic disease, such as a fever response (blunted in 20%–30% of older adults) or an elevated white blood cell count, may not be seen.[75,76] The triad of anorexia, fever, and right lower quadrant pain seen in appendicitis is present in just 20% of older adults.[77] Abdominal pain with associated back pain, hypotension, and a pulsatile mass is generally seen in less than 50% of older adults with an abdominal aortic aneurysm.[78,79] Similarly, Charcot triad of cholangitis, including fevers, right upper quadrant pain, and jaundice, is present in as few as 30% of older adults with the disease.[80,81]

◆◆ **Classic signs or symptoms of systemic disease, such as fever, leukocytosis, and localized pain, are less commonly seen in older adults with significant intraabdominal pathology.**

As a component of the workup of many of these patients, imaging, including x-ray, ultrasound, and CT, will be obtained. The use of intravenous (IV) contrast is preferred in patients with undifferentiated abdominal pain, although the prevalence of impaired renal function has limited its use in older adults. There is, however, considerable new data and work that suggest the risk of contrast induced nephropathy (CIN) has been overestimated.[82–84] Given the diagnostic utility of IV contrast in the older adults with abdominal pain and new data suggesting contemporary contrast medium may pose less of a risk of CIN, it is important for all providers, including those in the outpatient setting, to consider its use.

Although both benign and serious intraabdominal pathology should be considered in older adults with acute abdominal pain, providers should consider extraabdominal causes of abdominal pain in these patients. Table 16.4 outlines the differential diagnosis for extraabdominal causes of abdominal pain in older adults.

## TABLE 16.4 Abdominal Pain Mimics

| Organ System | Nonabdominal Cause of Pain |
|---|---|
| Cardiac | Angina or myocardial ischemia, pericarditis or myocarditis, HF |
| Pulmonary | Lower lobe pneumonia, pneumothorax, PE |
| Neurologic | Peripheral nerve tumor |
| Metabolic | Diabetic or alcoholic ketoacidosis, adrenal insufficiency, hypercalcemia, uremia |
| Hematologic | Acute leukemia, rectus sheath hematoma |
| Infectious | Herpes zoster, cellulitis, uterine or bladder prolapse, urinary retention |
| Toxicologic | Iron or heavy metal overdose, opioid withdrawal, antibiotic side effects |

*HF*, Heart failure; *PE*, pulmonary embolism.

## Trauma

### CASE 2

#### Mrs. Guiterrez (Part 1)

A 65-year-old female calls your office, concerned about a headache she continues to have after a fall yesterday. The patient, whose only history is osteoarthritis and atrial fibrillation for which she takes a beta blocker and oral anticoagulant, says she tripped over her cat yesterday in the kitchen. She reports falling and striking her head on a cabinet. She remembers the entire incident and is confident she did not lose consciousness. She was able to get herself up and continued through her day, albeit a little shaken. That evening she developed a left-sided headache that has persisted until this morning.

Trauma care in older adults presents unique challenges to the PCP and EMP alike. Many older adults can sustain serious injury with seemingly minor traumas, and medical providers frequently fail to recognize such injuries in a timely fashion.[85–88] This coupled with numerous biologic and physiologic changes of aging accounts for why the risk of mortality from trauma in older adults is twice that of younger patients.[89]

Falls are the leading cause of death from trauma in older adults and the rate of death from falls has increased over 30% since 2007, with traumatic brain injury being the most common direct cause.[90,91] In evaluating older adults in the primary care office or over the phone who have reported a fall, it is important for the PCP to consider the following when determining if urgent/emergent evaluation is warranted:

1. Vital signs may be falsely reassuring in older adults after a traumatic injury. Even small abnormalities in heart rate, blood pressure, or subtle changes in mental status are associated with poorer outcomes and increased mortality.[92,93] Patients with such abnormalities should be referred to the ED, ideally a regional trauma center, for complete evaluation.

2. The seriousness of rib fractures in older adults is greatly underappreciated, even by EMPs. With each additional rib fracture in older adults, mortality increases by 19% and the risk of pneumonia by 27%.[94] For this reason, chest wall trauma (even if minor) with suspected or confirmed rib fractures warrants referral to the ED and full trauma evaluation. Aggressive multimodal pain management, including acetaminophen, nonsteroidal antiinflammatory drugs such as ibuprofen, topical analgesics such as lidocaine patches, adjunctive opioid therapy, and, in some cases, catheter-based analgesia such as paravertebral nerve catheters, may be used.[95]

3. Patients with new difficulty bearing weight after a fall, even with negative x-rays, should undergo more advanced imaging and likely ED referral. Although plain radiographs are good at identifying most hip injuries, occult fractures may be missed. CT or magnetic resonance imaging may be required in such patients, and therefore referral to the ED or trauma center is likely indicated.[96]

◆◆ **Older adults are frequently undertriaged with respect to traumatic injuries. Referral to the ED or local trauma centers for even seemingly minor trauma in this patient population should be strongly considered.**

An additional challenge in caring for older adults with trauma surrounds the evaluation of those patients on anticoagulation (AC). Although the decision to prescribe ACs to older adults is beyond the scope of this chapter, suffice it say their use within this population, both traditional vitamin K antagonists such as warfarin and direct oral anticoagulants, is prevalent. The decision to obtain radiographic imaging, particularly head CTs, is an important choice that may be required of PCPs when evaluating patients in the clinic or fielding phone calls from patients or family members.

There is considerable evidence that even minor head trauma in older adults on AC increases the risk of immediate and delayed intracranial hemorrhage (ICH).[97–99] Such ICH is not without significant consequence. By some estimates, the mortality rate of older adults with a fall-related ICH approaches 15%.[100] For this reason, referral to the ED and trauma centers for older adults on AC with head injuries, even minor, should be liberal.

Even in the absence of fracture or other serious injury, older adults who are victims of trauma should receive very careful evaluation, including for changes in gait, ability to perform activities of daily living, availability of home resources, and the potential need for physical therapy and occupational therapy. This multidisciplinary approach is another reason referral to the ED or local trauma centers should be strongly considered in these patients.

### CASE 2

#### Mrs. Guiterrez (Part 2)

Although the patient denies any focal neurologic complaints, you remain concerned about her persistent headache in the setting of anticoagulation. You encourage the patient to go to the ED and she reluctantly agrees. You speak with the ED physician and express you concerns about an acute ICH. Shortly after the patient arrives in the ED, she is quickly taken for a head CT that shows subarachnoid hemorrhage. Her anticoagulation is reversed and she is admitted to the neurosurgery service for continued care.

## Summary

Geriatric patients may present to the PCP for the evaluation of urgent or emergent complaints. Challenges associated with the identification of time-sensitive illness or injury in this patient population includes atypical presentations, subtle vital sign abnormalities, and resource availability. Communication between EMPs and PCPs is an essential component in improving the transitions of care between the outpatient and acute setting and perhaps the surest way to align patient and provider expectations when caring for the acutely ill geriatric patient.

## Key References

4. Institute of Medicine. *Hospital-Based Emergency Care: At the Breaking Point*. Washington, DC: National Academies Press; 2007.
6. Afilalo J, Marinovich A, Afilalo M, et al. Nonurgent emergency department patient characteristics and barriers to primary care. *Acad Emerg Med*. 2004;11(12):1302−1310.
16. Ferguson B, Geralds J, Petrey J, Huecker M. Malpractice in emergency medicine—A review of risk and mitigation practices for the emergency medicine provider. *J Emerg Med*. 2018;55(5):659−665.
32. Han JH, Wilber ST. Altered mental status in older patients in the emergency department. *Clin Geriatr Med*. 2013;29(1): 101−136.
91. Allen CJ, Hannay WM, Murray CR, et al. Causes of death differ between elderly and adult falls. *J Trauma Acute Care Surg*. 2015;79(4):617−621.

**References available online at expertconsult.com.**

# 17

# Delirium

**BENJAMIN S. COOLEY, SOPHIA WANG, AND BABAR A. KHAN**

## OUTLINE

*Additional online-only material indicated by icon.*

## OBJECTIVES

*Upon completion of this chapter, the reader will be able to:*

- Discuss the definition, burden, neuropsychiatric sequalae, and pathophysiology of delirium among hospitalized older adults.
- Understand the delirium vulnerability-trigger interaction model, use this model to characterize the vulnerability of hospitalized older adults for developing delirium, and identify the precipitating factors that trigger delirium among these vulnerable individuals.
- Recognize the importance of using primary prevention to decrease the burden of delirium in hospitalized older adults

and the value of proactively screening to identify at-risk persons at the time of hospital admission.
- Discuss the evidence for nonpharmacologic and pharmacologic prevention and management of both hypoactive and hyperactive delirium.
- Describe a multicomponent hospital system to decrease the burden of delirium and to discuss implementation strategies and future directions in the prevention, assessment, and management of delirium.

---

### CASE 1

#### Joyce Smith (Part 1)

Joyce Smith is an 81-year-old woman with mild cognitive impairment thought to be secondary to Alzheimer disease. She lives at home with her daughter. She is independent in all of her basic activities of daily living (ADLs), but dependent on her daughter for shopping, finance management, and transportation. Ms. Smith comes to your office with her daughter and says everything is fine. Her daughter tells you she is having delusions that her neighbors are stealing her mail and poisoning her food. She has been losing weight and can no longer stand up from her chair on her own. She also complains of dyspnea on exertion. The remainder of her physical examination is normal.

What is the differential diagnosis for Ms. Smith's paranoid symptoms?

## Definition Prevalence of Delirium

The terms *delirium* (from *de* — "away from" and *līra* — "tracks or furrow"), *acute confusional state, acute brain failure,* and *encephalopathy* have all been used to describe the neuropsychiatric syndrome characterized by an acute onset disturbance in attention and cognition.[1] The syndrome is defined by a change in consciousness, with a reduced ability to focus, sustain, or shift attention that occurs over a short period of time and tends to fluctuate over the course of the day.[2,3] In the right patient and circumstances, delirium can be caused by a wide variety of medical illnesses, medication side effects, and intoxications or withdrawal from substances.[4]

The collection of these core and associated symptoms can be used to divide delirium into hypoactive, hyperactive, or mixed types.[5–7] Historically, hypoactive delirium was thought to have the worst prognosis. However, a recent prospective study in

• BOX 17.1    Delirium Symptoms

- Acute change in mental status
- Fluctuating course
- Attention disturbance
- Memory disturbance
- Orientation disturbance
- Perceptual disturbance
- Thought disturbance
- Sleep disturbance
- Consciousness disturbance
- Speech disturbance
- Psychomotor activity disturbance

---

**CASE 2**

**Judith Murray (Part 1)**

Judith Murray, an 84-year-old woman with a history of hypertension, is in the emergency department (ED) after having fallen and broken her hip. She is a widow who has been living in her house in a rural area. She has children who live elsewhere and see her only once or twice per year, and they report she has no problems with her ADLs, but they cannot assess her instrumental ADLs. She is taking no routine medications. Her labs on hospital admission show evidence of dehydration with sodium of 152 mmol/L and a blood urea nitrogen (BUN)/creatinine ratio of more than 20:1. The nurse has administered the Mini-Mental State Examination (MMSE) and the Geriatric Depression Scale (GDS). The patient scored 21/30 on the MMSE and 7/15 on the GDS. She had no evidence of attention deficit or fluctuating mental status.

What is Ms. Murray's probability of developing postoperative delirium?

---

geriatric patients with delirium showed no difference in outcomes between the different subtypes.[8] The neuropsychiatric symptoms of delirium can range from apathy and withdrawal, to paranoia, hallucinations, and combativeness. One study suggested that these psychotic features present in nearly 50% of cases of delirium, with a greater prevalence associated with hyperactive delirium and in younger patients.[9] Many of the neuropsychiatric symptoms seen in delirium are shared across various brain disorders, such as dementia, depression, mania, and psychosis. The core features that differentiate delirium from these other brain-based disorders are inattentiveness, altered level of arousal, and an acute and fluctuating nature of symptoms. Box 17.1 summarizes the various categories of delirium neuropsychiatric symptomatology.

## Pathogenesis

The pathophysiology of delirium can be viewed via a complex systems approach, as a disruption at multiple levels. Seven core non-mutually exclusive areas have been hypothesized in the development of delirium: neuroinflammation, neuronal aging, oxidative stress, neurotransmitters, neuroendocrinology, diurnal dysregulation, and network dysconnectivity.[4,10,11] Understanding these core areas and their implication for the etiology and management of the delirium is critical.[12]

Neuroimaging studies of patients with delirium suggest that the prefrontal cortex, basal forebrain, anterior thalamus, and nondominant parietal and fusiform cortex are involved in inducing delirium symptoms.[13–15] Neural network studies using electroencephalography (EEG) and functional magnetic resonance imaging (fMRI) suggest that delirium is a result of inefficiency and disintegration in the connections between various remote brain regions, including the dorsolateral prefrontal cortex and posterior cingulate cortex, as well as changes in functional connectivity with subcortical regions.[16,17] Neurophysiologic and metabolic changes that modify cerebral neurotransmission are also considered to be a cornerstone of delirium pathogenesis.[18–22]

Common stressors include medications, alcohol and medication withdrawal, infection, hypoxia, hypoperfusion, trauma, and surgery.[15,20,23] Circadian rhythm disruption with associated alterations in melatonin secretion is implicated in, and may even precede, symptoms of delirium.[24] The neurotransmitter dysfunction centers around cholinergic deficiency and dopaminergic excess,[20,23,25] although multiple other neurotransmitter disruptions play a role in various types of delirium.[4] Thus delirium should be viewed as a complex system failure, with a "final common pathway" leading to disrupted neural networks and neurotransmitter dysfunction.[23,26]

## Prevalence

Delirium is common in older adults in the outpatient setting, in long-term care facilities, upon presentation to the ED, during hospitalization stays (most notably in the intensive care unit [ICU] and perioperative settings), upon discharge from the hospital, and at the end of life.[1,11] Overall, patients age $\geq 65$ years accounted for 37% of all hospital discharges and 43% of hospital days.[27] The prevalence of delirium among the hospitalized older adults varied from 10% to 52%,[28–53] depending on the reason for hospitalization (Table 17.1), and this increases to 32% to 86% in those with dementia.[54] Of patients with delirium, 65% have the hypoactive type, 25% the hyperactive type, and 10% a mixed type.[55]

With the aging of the US population, the incidence and prevalence of age-related diseases, including delirium, is projected to increase.[56,57] According to the US Centers for Medicare and Medicaid Services, hospital spending costs are expected to grow by an average of 5.7% per year between 2020 and 2027.[58] The healthcare system is currently spending between $38 and $152 billion annually in delirium-related costs,[59] and with the rise in aging-related diseases this expenditure is likely to significantly increase.[57]

| TABLE 17.1 | Prevalence of Delirium Among Hospitalized Older Adults | |
| --- | --- | --- |
| **Setting and Population** | | **Delirium Prevalence Range** |
| Older adults hospitalized for medical illness[28–35] | | 11%–41% |
| Postoperative: older adults undergoing surgical repair of hip fracture[36–39] | | 40%–52% |
| Postoperative: older adults undergoing elective major noncardiac surgery[40–45] | | 10%–39% |
| Postoperative: older adults undergoing cardiac surgery[46–53] | | 13%–44% |

# Short- and Long-Term Impact of Delirium

Delirium in the older adult population increases the risk of death.[20,60,61] According to one study, the presence of delirium in hospitalized patients increases the risk of death 2-fold and the risk of institutionalization 2.5-fold.[60] These increases in risk are independent of age, gender, comorbidity, severity of illness, and preexisting dementia. Those with hypoactive delirium are thought to have a worse prognosis than the other subtypes.[62] Coexistence of delirium with dementia increases the risk of rehospitalization and long-term care admission compared with patients with dementia or delirium alone.[25,54]

There are also increased economic costs associated with delirium in older adults. After adjusting for severity of illness and length of stay, one study found that delirium itself predicted an increased cost of $18,000 over a 30-day ICU stay.[63] Without the increased mortality associated with delirium, the cost would rise by 20%.[63] Significant economic impact is also found hospital-wide, with costs up to 51% higher for older hospitalized patients with cognitive impairment (dementia and delirium) compared to older adults without cognitive impairment.[64,65]

Delirium has traditionally been thought of as an abrupt change from baseline that typically is short term, which resolves with resolution of the underlying causes. However, recent literature suggests that delirium may have devastating long-term cognitive, psychiatric, and functional sequelae in certain vulnerable populations, such as ICU survivors. Postintensive care syndrome (PICS) is defined as long-term cognitive, psychiatric, and functional deficits after ICU hospitalization.[66,67] Delirium is a major risk factor for PICS, which can affect both younger and older adults. Long-term cognitive deficits are also being studied in the postoperative population.[66] For elective operations, preoperative cognitive impairment coupled with postoperative delirium appears to predict poor postoperative cognitive functioning.[68] Studies of noncardiac surgery have shown that postoperative delirium predicts short-term postoperative cognitive decline.[68–70] There is ongoing discussion about the definition of postsurgical cognitive dysfunction and how this fits into conceptualizations of neurocognitive decline and delirium among the older adult population.[69,71,72]

## Risk Factors and Precipitating Factors

Delirium among hospitalized older adults is the result of a complex interaction between various degrees of insult severity and different levels of patient vulnerability.[73] This vulnerability-trigger interaction, or two-hit hypothesis, is responsible for the wide range (10%–86%) of delirium prevalence rates reported among hospitalized older adults. Finding a single factor responsible for the onset of delirium is rare.[1,11] Using the vulnerability-trigger interaction model, clinicians can categorize the contributing factors of delirium into two groups: first, the cluster of predisposing or vulnerability factors (Table 17.2), and second, the cluster of precipitating or trigger factors (Table 17.3).

Potent anticholinergic medications, such as oxybutynin for urinary incontinence or diphenhydramine for sleep, can be critical precipitating and predisposing factors in the development of delirium. The most common anticholinergic medications that are used in older adults are summarized in Table 17.4. The concept of total anticholinergic burden has been used to reflect the cumulative anticholinergic activities of all medications taken by an individual patient.[78,79] Thus both a single drug with strong anticholinergic properties and a combination of multiple drugs with a relatively small anticholinergic effect might contribute to the development of delirium in older adults.[74,76,80,81]

Various methods are used to determine the anticholinergic activity of a given drug and thus the anticholinergic burden faced by a particular patient. These include the use of a drug's in vitro affinity to the muscarinic receptor,[56] clinical expert opinion regarding a drug's clinical anticholinergic adverse effects,[75,76] and serum anticholinergic activity (SAA) measurement secondary to the intake of a single or multiple drugs.[74,77] Table 17.4 integrates the results of different studies to categorize the anticholinergic activities of medications into drugs with definite central anticholinergic activity, assigned a score of 2 or 3, and those with possible central anticholinergic property with a score of 1. Based on recent evidence, each definite anticholinergic drug increases the risk of cognitive impairment by 46% over 6 years.[82] In addition, with each 1-point increase in the anticholinergic burden score, there is a decline in MMSE of 0.33 point over 2 years and a 26% increase in the risk of death.[83]

---

**CASE 1**

### Joyce Smith (Part 2)

In your office, you obtain laboratory results for a urinalysis, metabolic profile, and chest x-ray study; they are normal. You prescribe risperidone 0.5 mg at night and send Ms. Smith home with her daughter after providing reassurance and family education. However, Ms. Smith continues to complain of shortness of breath, and the delusions about her neighbors persist. The next day she "runs away" from home, and the police find her wandering in the neighborhood. She is brought to the ED for assessment, and a computed tomography (CT) scan of her head and a chest radiograph are negative. Pulse oximetry shows mild hypoxia, which is corrected by oxygen. Her risperidone dose is increased to 0.5 mg twice a day. She is also started on trazodone 50 mg daily by the ED physician, and she is given codeine for off-and-on cough complaints. She is sent home with her daughter for follow-up in your office.

If Ms. Smith does not currently have delirium, what is her current risk for developing delirium in association with hospitalization for an acute illness?

---

**CASE 1**

### Joyce Smith (Part 3)

A week later you receive a call from Ms. Smith's daughter who reports that her mother is now very lethargic and is difficult to keep awake. You instruct the daughter to take her mother back to the ED to be evaluated. She again is hypoxic but also tachycardic and tachypneic and is found to be somnolent and obtunded. In consultation with the ED physician you obtain a CT pulmonary angiogram, which shows a large right-sided pulmonary embolism with several small chronic emboli in the left lung.

What is the most urgent next therapeutic intervention?

---

## Diagnosis and Assessment of Delirium

It is challenging to effectively create care systems and train clinicians on where delirium is recognized and diagnosed. This is evident from the fact that between one-third and two-thirds of delirium cases remain undiagnosed.[61] To differentiate between

**TABLE 17.2    Predisposing Factors for Delirium Among Older Adults Hospitalized for a Medical or a Surgical Illness**

| Risk Factor | Odds Ratio (OR) Range[a] | The Delirium Vulnerability Scale |
|---|---|---|
| Cognitive Impairment:<br>• Chart diagnosis of dementia<br>• MMSE <24<br>• Prior history of delirium | <br>3.5—5<br>2—4<br>4 | Choose one score only<br>3 points<br>2 points<br>1 point |
| Current history of depression | 2—4 | 1 point |
| Current history of alcohol abuse | 3—6.5 | 2 points |
| Current and untreated hearing loss | 2 | 1 point |
| Current and untreated vision loss | 2—3.5 | 1 point |
| Need assistance in two basic activities of daily living | 2.5 | 1 point |
| Current use of anticholinergic | 1.5—2.7 | 2 points |
| Dehydration defined by BUN/creatinine >21:1 | 1.8—2 | 1 point |
| Sodium abnormality (Na <130 or Na >150) | 2—4 | 1 point |
| Vascular risk factors: history of:<br>• Hypertension<br>• Congestive heart failure<br>• Diabetes mellitus<br>• Cerebrovascular accident<br>• Atrial fibrillation | <br>2.3<br>1.3—2.9<br>1.3<br>2.2<br>1.4 | Choose a score of 1 point if at least one risk factor was present<br>(maximum score is also 1 point) |
| Admitted for | | |
| • Urgent surgical repair of hip fracture<br>• Elective aortic aneurysm repair | 3<br>6 | 2 points<br>3 points |
| Total Points | | _____ [range 0—17] |
| Interpretation:<br>• 0—1 point<br>• 2—3 points<br>• 4—7 points<br>• >7 points | Risk category<br>Low<br>Mild<br>Moderate<br>Severe | Probability of developing delirium[b]<br><5%<br>5% to 20%<br>21% to 40%<br>>40% |

*BUN,* Blood urea nitrogen; *MMSE,* Mini-Mental State Examination.

[a]OR estimates were based on review of the literature.

[b]Delirium probability estimates for each risk category were based on a literature review[31,34,35,38,40,43,45,50–54,76,78,90] and the authors' clinical and research experiences. The delirium vulnerability scale has not been validated in a prospective cohort study.

**TABLE 17.3    Precipitating Factors for the Development of Delirium During Hospitalization for Medical or Surgical Illness[50,51,73,74]**

| Precipitating Factor | Odds Ratio (OR) |
|---|---|
| Use of physical restraints | 4.4 |
| Malnutrition | 4 |
| Using more than three new medications during hospitalization | 2.9 |
| Use of bladder catheterization | 2.4 |
| Exposed to any iatrogenic event | 1.9 |
| Intraoperative hypotension (at least 31% drop in mean perioperative BP or a SBP ≤80 mmHg | 1.4 |
| Postoperative Hct <30% | 1.7 |
| Untreated postoperative pain | 5.4—9 |
| Use of anticholinergic drug | 1.5—2.7 |

*BP,* Blood pressure; *Hct,* hematocrit; *SBP,* systolic blood pressure.

**TABLE 17.4 Medications With Central Anticholinergic Activity**

| Score = 3<br>High Anticholinergic Activity | Score = 2<br>Moderate Anticholinergic Activity | Score = 1<br>Mild Anticholinergic Activity |
|---|---|---|
| Amitriptyline | Amantadine | Alverine |
| Amoxapine | Belladonna | Alprazolam |
| Atropine | Carbamazepine | Atenolol |
| Benztropine | Cyclobenzaprine | Bupropion |
| Brompheniramine | Cyproheptadine | Captopril |
| Carbinoxamine | Loxapine | Chlorthalidone |
| Chlorpheniramine | Meperidine | Cimetidine |
| Chlorpromazine | Methotrimeprazine | Clorazepate |
| Clemastine | Molindone | Codeine |
| Clomipramine | Oxcarbazepine | Colchicine |
| Clozapine | Pimozide | Diazepam |
| Darifenacin | | Digoxin |
| Desipramine | | Dipyridamole |
| Dicyclomine | | Disopyramide |
| Dimenhydrinate | | Fentanyl |
| Diphenhydramine | | Furosemide |
| Doxepin | | Fluvoxamine |
| Flavoxate | | Haloperidol |
| Hydroxyzine | | Hydralazine |
| Hyoscyamine | | Hydrocortisone |
| Imipramine | | Isosorbide |
| Meclizine | | Loperamide |
| Methocarbamol | | Metoprolol |
| Nortriptyline | | Morphine |
| Olanzapine | | Nifedipine |
| Orphenadrine | | Prednisone |
| Oxybutynin | | Quinidine |
| Paroxetine | | Ranitidine |
| Perphenazine | | Risperidone |
| Promethazine | | Theophylline |
| Propantheline | | Trazodone |
| Quetiapine | | Triamterene |
| Scopolamine | | |
| Thioridazine | | |
| Tolterodine | | |
| Trifluoperazine | | |
| Trihexyphenidyl | | |
| Trimipramine | | |

Based on the following methods: (1) the drug's in vitro affinity to the muscarinic receptor,[75] (2) the opinion of clinical experts regarding the drug's clinical anticholinergic adverse effects,[75,76] and (3) the patient's serum anticholinergic activity (SAA) secondary to the intake of a single or multiple drugs.[74,77]

| TABLE 17.5 | The Confusion Assessment Method Diagnostic Instrument* |
|---|---|

| Diagnostic Features | Definitions and Characteristics |
|---|---|
| 1. Acute onset and fluctuating course | Presence is indicated by a positive response to one or more of the following questions:<br>• Is there evidence of an acute change in mental status from the patient's baseline?<br>• Did the (abnormal) behavior fluctuate during the day, that is, tend to come and go, or increase and decrease in severity? |
| 2. Inattention | Presence is indicated by a positive response to the following question:<br>• Did the patient have difficulty focusing attention (e.g., being easily distractible) or have difficulty keeping track of what was being said? |
| 3. Disorganized thinking | Presence is indicated by a positive response to the following question:<br>• Was the patient's thinking disorganized or incoherent, such as rambling or irrelevant conversation, unclear or illogical flow of ideas, or unpredictable switching from subject to subject? |
| 4. Altered level of consciousness | Presence is indicated by any answer other than "alert" to the following question:<br>• Overall, how would you rate this patient's level of consciousness? (alert [normal]), vigilant [hyperalert], lethargic [drowsy, easily aroused], stupor [difficult to arouse], or coma [unarousable]) |

*Delirium is defined as present if the patient has 1 + 2 + (either 3 or 4).
(Modified from Inouye SK, vanDyck CH, Alessi CA, et al. Clarifying confusion: The Confusion Assessment Method. A new method for detection of delirium. *Ann Intern Med* 1990;113:941−948. Confusion assessment method: Training manual and coding guide, Copyright 2003, Hospital Elder Life Program, LLC. With permission.)

dementia, delirium, and other psychiatric illnesses with similar neuropsychiatric symptom profiles, clinicians need to be familiar with the core diagnostic features of delirium and understand that having a diagnosis of dementia does not rule out delirium.

There are several bedside tools available for delirium assessment.[84,85] A recent review of delirium assessment tools looks at ability to both detect delirium and assess the severity.[86] Eleven tools underwent a methodologic quality review, and six of these tools were found to meet criteria as high-quality and valid methods of detecting and assessing the severity of delirium: The Confusion Assessment Method (CAM)-Severity, Confusion State Examination, Delirium-O-Meter, Delirium Observation Scale, Delirium Rating Scale, and Memorial Delirium Assessment Scale.[86]

CAM[3] is the most widely used tool and has the most evidence supporting its use as a bedside assessment. Table 17.5 provides the CAM diagnostic algorithm for identifying delirium. The CAM has a sensitivity of 94% to 100%, a specificity of 90% to 95%, a positive likelihood ratio of 9.6 (95% confidence interval [CI], 5.8−16.0), and a negative likelihood ratio of 0.16 (95% CI, 0.09−0.29).[3,87] The CAM-Severity (CAM-S), the CAM ICU-7,[88] and the S-PTD[89] have also been validated in specific populations.[86]

◆◆ Delirium is associated with increased mortality, poorer functional status, limited rehabilitation, increased hospital-acquired complications, prolonged length of hospital stay, increased risk of institutionalization, and higher healthcare expenditures.

After diagnosing delirium, a clinician can use the vulnerability-trigger interaction model to identify the underlying modifiable and nonmodifiable triggers. In one study of delirium among hospitalized older adults with a medical illness, fluid and electrolyte abnormalities were the possible trigger in 40% of the cases, infection in 40%, drug toxicity in 30%, metabolic disorders in 26%, sensory and environmental problems in 24%, and low perfusion in 14%.[31] Among hospitalized older adults undergoing surgical repair of a hip fracture, 62% of the delirium cases had several triggers, with the most common ones being environmental, infection, medications, and fluid-electrolyte disturbances.[90]

◆◆ Delirium is diagnosed if a patient has an acute change in mental status with inattention accompanied by disorganized thinking or a change in alertness.

Table 17.6 provides a simple approach for delirium assessment. This approach is based on both the authors' clinical experiences and review of the literature.[84,91] The suggested assessment for delirium requires an in-person interview with the patient to identify the presence of emergent risk factors, such as hypoxia, hypotension, or sepsis. This is followed by a comprehensive history and chart review to identify potential contributions to the development of delirium, including dehydration, electrolyte abnormalities, organ failure, infectious processes, or new sedative or anticholinergic drugs. Currently, there is no routine recommendation for brain imaging or more invasive diagnostic tests unless one suspects a new focal central nervous system process based on physical examination or chart review.

◆◆ A thorough history, physical examination, chart review, and laboratory testing should be completed to identify reversible causes of delirium. In general, brain imaging, lumbar puncture, and electroencephalograms are not part of the routine workup for delirium unless there are focal neurologic signs or concerns of subclinical seizure activity.

## CASE 2

### Judith Murray (Part 2)

Ms. Murray undergoes hip replacement surgery. On postoperative day 2, her thought process is illogical and incoherent, but she is able to recognize her family members. She repeatedly attempts to remove her oxygen mask and Foley catheter, and to get out of bed. Overnight, the on-call physician orders lorazepam 1 mg IV to control her symptoms of agitation, which paradoxically seems to worsen her symptoms.

Could this syndrome have been prevented? Once it develops, what are the safest and most effective strategies to manage the patient's delirium-induced agitation?

| TABLE 17.6 | Identifying and Managing the Causes and Contributing Factors of Delirium in a Hospitalized Patient | |
|---|---|
| **Assessment** | **Treatment** |
| Vital signs (pulse, BP, T, RR, and pulse oximetry)<br>Physical examination to diagnose and treat<br>   infectious process or other acute medical conditions<br>   (pneumonia, pressure ulcers, MI, CVA, etc.)<br>Urinalysis<br>Cr, Na, K, Ca, glucose<br>CBC with differential<br>Review old and new anticholinergic medications<br>Review old and new sedating medications<br>Review the need for Foley catheter, IV lines, and other<br>   tethers | General measures:<br>• Encourage sleep, orientation, and activity<br>• Personalize the environment<br>• Treat medical conditions, such as dehydration, electrolyte disturbances, and infection<br>• Discontinue catheters, IV lines, and other tethers if benefit does not outweigh harm<br>• Discontinue sedating and anticholinergic medications when possible and appropriate<br>• Identify and treat acute pain<br>• Prevent and/or treat constipation<br><br>Interventions for agitation:<br>• Consider professional sitter<br>• Assess the impact of agitation on patient safety and disconnect Foley and other tethers if<br>  possible<br>• If history of alcohol use, consider lorazepam 0.25–0.5 mg PO/IM/IV q 4–6 hours PRN<br>• If safety an issue, and sitter ineffective, and being treated for a reversible medical condition,<br>  consider haloperidol 0.25 mg PO/IM/IV q 4 hours PRN (maximum dose <3 mg/day,<br>  reevaluating every 24 hours and discontinuing haloperidol before discharge<br><br>Interventions for lethargy:<br>• Protect skin; check regularly for skin breakdown<br>• Decrease dose of hypnotics and of other sedative medications |

(From Khan BA, Zawahiri M, Campbell NL, et al. Delirium in hospitalized patients: implications of current evidence on clinical practice and future avenues for research—a systematic evidence review. J Hosp Med. 2012;7(7):580-589; Bush SH, Lawlor PG, Ryan K, et al. Delirium in adult cancer patients: ESMO clinical practice guidelines. *Ann Oncol.* 2018;29:iv143-iv165.)

*BP,* Blood pressure; *CBC,* complete blood count; *CVA,* cerebrovascular accident; *IV,* intravenous; *MI,* myocardial infarction; *RR,* respiratory rate; *T,* temperature.

## Prevention and Management of Delirium

A number of reviews and guidelines have been published regarding the prevention and management of delirium in specialty populations[92] and hospitalized older adults.[93–98] These reviews indicate that prevention and interdisciplinary system-based interventions constitute an effective and promising program to reduce the burden of delirium.[93] A recent metaanalysis of delirium prevention programs showed that implementation of well-designed programs could reduce the incidence of delirium by 11.5%.[93] Important interventions to prevent delirium include orientation activities for the cognitively impaired, early mobilization, prevention of sleep deprivation, minimizing the use of psychoactive drugs, ensuring use of prescribed eyeglasses and hearing aids, and treating volume depletion.[99]

Preventive interventions can be categorized into nursing policy interventions and physician-ordered interventions (Table 17.7). These interventions concentrate on modifying specific vulnerability or trigger factors, such as the management of cognitive impairment, sleep deprivation, anticholinergic burden, pain, constipation, and restraints. Using such a preventive interdisciplinary program reduces absolute risk by 5% to 31%, with the number needed to treat to prevent one case of delirium ranging from 3 to 20.[100] A cost-effectiveness analysis of the multicomponent interdisciplinary interventions to prevent delirium, evaluated in the National Institute for Health and Care Excellence guidelines,[97] showed that such interventions are cost effective when applied to older medical patients at intermediate or high risk of developing delirium.

Other preventative system-based approaches have been studied and implemented widely. Most notably, the ABCDE bundle,[101] a set of evidence-based strategies for minimizing delirium in mechanically ventilated patients, resulted in a 50% decreased odds of delirium in the intervention group. Similarly, the pain, agitation, delirium (PAD) guidelines also provide useful information on prevention and management of delirium in critical care settings.[102] The Hospital Elder Life Program, a well-examined hospital-wide program for reducing the incidence of delirium in older adult patients, integrates these threads of prevention evidence.[103] A recent metaanalysis of studies that implemented this program showed that its implementation can decrease the incidence of delirium in half, reduce the rate of falls by 42%, save money in hospital and long-term care costs, reduce lengths of stay, and prevent institutionalization.[103]

There is limited evidence for the use of antipsychotics for the prevention of delirium in hospitalized older adults.[104] A recent multicenter randomized clinical trial of prophylactic haloperidol versus placebo showed no change in the incidence of delirium in older adults.[105] In a study of critically ill patients, prophylactic haloperidol did not improve survival at 28 days,[106] nor did it appear to prevent the conversion of subsyndromal delirium to delirium.[107] Furthermore, the majority of patients undergoing major surgery do not benefit from pretreatment with haloperidol to reduce postoperative delirium.[108] There has also been interest in the use of alpha-2 agonists, particularly dexmedetomidine in the ICU, for the prevention and management of delirium.[109–111] Interest in these agents has focused on alternative methods of sedation, which may spare patients exposure to more well-known deliriogenic agents, such as opioids and benzodiazepines, as well as using lower doses to reduce delirium incidence.[112–114] Other studies have not found a significant benefit with dexmedetomidine, and in fact raise concern that it may conversely increase risk of adverse events, including hypotension and bradycardia.[115]

**TABLE 17.7    Interventions to Prevent Delirium**

| Factor | Nursing Policy Interventions |
| --- | --- |
| Sleep | Maintain 4 to 6 hours of uninterrupted sleep each night<br>If the patient complains of insomnia consider the following:<br>• Decrease the environmental noise at night<br>• Provide a drink of hot milk<br>• Provide a back rubbing for 15 minutes<br>If these fail then consider using a hypnotic drug |
| Orientation | Orient patient about the date, place, and reason for hospitalization<br>Keep a clock and calendar inside the patient's room<br>Keep light on from 7 AM (sunrise) to 7 PM (sundown) |
| Environment | Encourage patient's family to bring personal items<br>Encourage patient's family to bring hearing aid and glasses<br>Encourage low-stimulating family visits |
| Activity | Evaluate the appropriateness of restrictive activity order |
| Tethers | Evaluate the necessity of using Foley catheter, restraint, IV line, and monitors |
| Pain | Identify and manage adequately |
| Constipation | Identify and manage adequately |
| | **Physician-Ordered Interventions** |
| Cognitive impairment | Continue or start cholinesterase inhibitors and/or memantine if patient has possible or probable Alzheimer disease<br>Avoid, discontinue, or substitute all anticholinergic medications |
| Anticholinergics | Avoid, discontinue, or substitute all anticholinergic medications |
| Benzodiazepines | Avoid or assess the need for these drugs then taper off, except in alcohol/sedative-hypnotic withdrawal |
| Pain | Maintain pain level of ≤3/10<br>Scheduled acetaminophen then scheduled narcotic if necessary<br>Avoid meperidine, tramadol, codeine |
| Constipation | Scheduled sorbitol or stimulant (if narcotics are used for pain control) |
| Insomnia | Melatonin 3 mg 2 hours before bed. Trazodone 12.5–25 mg QHS PRN insomnia |
| Mobility | Eliminate Foley catheter and physical restraints and order early mobilization if appropriate |
| High risk for alcohol withdrawal | Consider scheduled short-acting benzodiazepine |
| Dehydration | Maintain BUN/creatinine <20/1<br>Maintain normal level Na. |

(From Khan BA, Zawahiri M, Campbell NL, et al. Delirium in hospitalized patients: implications of current evidence on clinical practice and future avenues for research—a systematic evidence review. J Hosp Med. 2012;7(7):580-589; Bush SH, Lawlor PG, Ryan K, et al. Delirium in adult cancer patients: ESMO clinical practice guidelines. *Ann Oncol.* 2018;29:iv143-iv165.)
*BUN,* Blood urea nitrogen; *IV,* intravenous.

❖❖ **The clinician's primary objective should be the prevention of delirium because once delirium symptoms have developed, the older patient is at risk for poor clinical outcomes.**

Once delirium develops, managing it effectively can be challenging. Given the heterogeneity of delirium etiologies, it is critical to thoroughly investigate and take the underlying etiologies into consideration when developing a robust treatment plan.[12] Successful management of delirium (see Table 17.7) depends on the accurate delivery of two types of interactive therapies:

• Treatment of the underlying causes, such as dehydration, infection, and/or the exposure to one or more of the anticholinergic medications and providing safe and appropriate pharmacologic and nonpharmacologic care[97,116]
• Supportive care targets the two types of delirium: hyperactive (agitation) and hypoactive (lethargy). For agitated delirium, the cornerstone of treatment is to provide safe and supportive

care that allows the management of the underlying causes of delirium. Such supportive care includes access to a trained professional sitter, involvement of family and caregivers[96]

Although controversial, there may be a role of antipsychotics in the management of delirium symptoms,[117] given largely mixed results regarding the role of antipsychotics in delirium management.[118–123] Only in settings where the risks and benefits have been fully analyzed, and the safety of staff and patient is in jeopardy, might administration of low-dose haloperidol (less than the total of 3 mg/day) be helpful. Although generally safe for older adults at low doses,[124] antipsychotic use raises both short- and long-term concerns. Immediate effects that require monitoring include excessive sedation, extrapyramidal symptoms, and QTc prolongation, whereas long-term effects may encompass metabolic syndrome, tardive dyskinesia, and increased risk of all-cause mortality.[123,125] If antipsychotics are used judiciously for management of hyperactive delirium in the hospital setting, all efforts should be made to remove these medications as quickly as possible to reduce long-term side effects.[126,127] In contrast, hypoactive delirium treatment focuses on frequent reorientation, correction of sensory impairments, skin protection, mobilization, and minimization of sedative medication.[128]

### CASE 1
#### Discussion

Ms. Smith's presentation is a typical example of delirium as the only manifestation of a life-threatening emergency. She is eventually found to have a pulmonary embolism, and with treatment of this underlying cause, her delusions, inattention, and lethargy disappear, and her risperidone can be reduced and eventually stopped.

### CASE 2
#### Discussion

Ms. Murray appears to have preexisting, undetected, mild dementia, which places her at increased risk for a postoperative delirium. A thorough workup for the cause of her delirium reveals she has a urinary tract infection. After starting an antibiotic, as well as discontinuing benzodiazepines and anticholinergic medications, you arrange for a one-to-one sitter to stay with Ms. Murray in her hospital room and prescribe haloperidol 0.25 mg IV q 6 hours as needed to manage her agitation.

## Summary and Future Directions

Major areas of current delirium research include the identification of new processes to target those at risk for developing delirium, prevention of delirium, novel approaches to the assessment of delirium, and more effective approaches for the management of delirium. Other important areas of study include the characterization of biomarkers and the implementation of more robust systems-based delirium prevention protocols. Biomarkers, imaging, and EEG readings[129,130] may be leveraged to identify those at risk and diagnose delirium more reliably. Studies focused on neurotransmitters and biomarkers of delirium suggest that melatonin and other markers may be early predictors.[20,24] Additional studies are examining the role of biomarkers associated with neurocognitive disorder diagnoses, such as amyloid beta-42, total and phosphorylated tau, *APOE4*, brain-derived neurotrophic factor, and ubiquitin. Disease markers for postoperative delirium have also been analyzed for use in detection of older adults at risk for delirium.[131–133]

Decreasing the burden of delirium in older adults requires the implementation of a specialized delirium program that includes three crucial components: (1) instituting a standardized screening to identify patients with a high vulnerability for the development of delirium (using the delirium vulnerability scale); (2) educating nurses, physicians, and other healthcare personnel to recognize and diagnose delirium and identify its triggers; and (3) structuring a consultation service that provides in-depth recommendations to prevent and manage delirium. Members of the consultation service should include at least a physician (geriatrician, geriatric psychiatrist, or a specialized hospitalist), nurse, and an administrator.

### Web Resources

American Delirium Society. www.americandeliriumsociety.org.
ICU Delirium and Cognitive Impairment Group at Vanderbilt University Medical Center. www.icudelirium.org.
European Delirium Association. www.europeandelirium association.com/
Hospital Elder Life Program www.hospitalelderlifeprogram.org.

## Key References

1. Maldonado JR. Acute brain failure. *Crit Care Clin*. 2017;33:461-519.
4. Maldonado JR. Delirium pathophysiology: an updated hypothesis of the etiology of acute brain failure. *Int J Geriatr Psychiatry*. 2017;33:1428-1457.
86. Jones RN, Cizginer S, Pavlech L, et al. Assessment of instruments for measurement of delirium severity. *JAMA Intern Med*. 2019;179:231.
93. Khan A, Boukrina O, Oh-Park M, Flanagan NA, Singh M, Oldham M. Preventing delirium takes a village: systematic review and meta-analysis of delirium preventive models of care. *J Hosp Med*. 2019;14:E1-E7.
96. Marcantonio ER. Delirium in hospitalized older adults. *N Engl J Med*. 2017;377:1456-1466.
103. Hshieh TT, Yang T, Gartaganis SL, Yue J, Inouye SK. Hospital elder life program: systematic review and meta-analysis of effectiveness. *Am J Geriatr Psychiatry*. 2018; 26:1015-1033.

*References available online at expertconsult.com.*

# 18

# Alzheimer Disease and Other Dementias

KAHLI ZIETLOW AND ELEANOR MCCONNELL

## OUTLINE

*Additional online-only material indicated by icon.*

## OBJECTIVES

*Upon completion of this chapter, the reader will be able to:*

- Recognize the medical, financial, and social impacts of Alzheimer disease and other dementias on patients and caregivers.
- Describe the signs, symptoms, and diagnostic approach to the following common cognitive disorders of older persons: Alzheimer disease, vascular dementia, frontotemporal dementia, Lewy body dementia, Parkinson dementia, and mild cognitive impairment.
- List both modifiable and nonmodifiable risk factors for development of cognitive impairment and dementia and strategies for prevention.

- Conduct and interpret a diagnostic evaluation of a patient with cognitive complaints using history taking, cognitive testing, laboratory studies, and brain imaging.
- Implement a person-centered care approach to dementia care, including shared decision making, medication use, nonpharmacologic management of behavioral symptoms, and working with community resources to enhance wellbeing.

### Mr. Frank (Part 1)

Mr. Frank is a 78-year-old retired mechanic with a past medical history notable for hypertension and atrial fibrillation. He presents to your clinic for a new patient evaluation, but he arrives almost 90 minutes late without an explanation for his tardiness. He drove himself to the appointment. He recently relocated to the area to be closer to his family, a brother and niece. He lives alone in an apartment. He has a high school level of education and retired 6 years ago. He is unable to name any of his medications, but brings a printed list from his prior doctor's appointment 11 months ago, including warfarin. From limited records available in the electronic medical record, it seems he had a labile international normalized ratio (INR). He is uncertain of the last time he had bloodwork done. On examination, his oral hygiene is poor, but he is otherwise well nourished and appropriately groomed. He is oriented to self, location, and year, but names the month incorrectly. His examination is otherwise unremarkable.

What signs is Mr. Frank displaying that are concerning for a possible cognitive disorder? What would be your next steps in management of Mr. Frank?

## Spectrum of Cognitive Aging

Normal cognitive aging is characterized by both improvements in some intellectual abilities, such as vocabulary and general knowledge, and declines in other abilities, such as neural processing speed, mental flexibility, and memory. These normal aging changes can result in occasional forgetfulness, mild word-finding difficulties, and awareness of a decline in mental acuity that may cause older adults to seek medical evaluation.[1] Patients may report increased reliance on appointment books or calendars, lists, and phone reminders, but suffer no functional deficits. On objective cognitive tests they will generally score in the "normal" range. Such patients should be provided education and reassurance.

Pathologic cognitive changes exist on a spectrum (Fig. 18.1). Preclinical disease is defined as biochemical or structural neurologic changes that may be detectable through advanced imaging and/or biomarker tests, but do not manifest as clinical symptoms. Preclinical Alzheimer disease (AD) likely occurs decades before the onset of symptoms. Mild cognitive impairment (MCI) refers to a disorder in which patients or family members report cognitive symptoms, and where decline in memory or other cognitive function is observed, but where functional ability is preserved.[2] Patients may score just below the cutoff of "normal" ranges on brief cognitive measures. MCI occurs because of a variety of etiologies, and may or may not be a precursor of eventual dementia. Some patients with MCI will improve in response to approaches, such as altering pharmacotherapy or improved management of chronic diseases.[3] MCI is categorized according to the type of cognitive impairment present, and can include amnestic, dysexecutive, or mixed types.[4] Amnestic MCI is much more likely to progress to AD, with conversion rates of 10% annually.[5] Dementia is characterized by progressive deterioration in multiple domains of cognitive function, including memory, judgment, problem solving, and/or use of language, that interferes with a persons' day-to-day function. Estimates of how long older adults live with dementia after being diagnosed vary from an average of 3 to 9 years, with more recent estimates pointing out important differences by ethnic group and presence of comorbid illness.[6]

The most recent edition of the *American Psychiatric Association's Diagnostic and Statistical Manual* (DSM-5) has updated terminology, and now refers to dementias as major neurocognitive disorders, and encourages specification of the underlying etiology. MCI is now referred to as mild neurocognitive disorder.[7] In this chapter, we will continue to use the terms *dementia* and *MCI*.

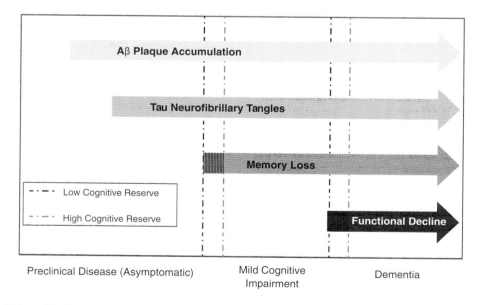

• **Figure 18.1** Hypothetical model of the pathogenesis of Alzheimer disease. Amyloid β plaque and tau neurofibrillary tangles begin forming and accumulating many years before onset of symptoms. Patients with higher cognitive reserve (e.g., through higher educational attainment) can tolerate higher plaque and tangle burden before demonstrating symptoms.

❖ Pathologic cognitive dysfunction exists on a spectrum of preclinical changes, mild cognitive impairment (MCI), and dementia. MCI is classified by primary cognitive domain affected (e.g., amnestic, dysexecutive). Amnestic MCI is much more likely to progress to Alzheimer disease.

## Prevalence

Dementia is underrecognized and underdiagnosed in primary care, and therefore exact prevalence rates are difficult to obtain.[8] The Centers for Disease Control and Prevention estimates that over 5 million people age ≥65 years (approximately 10.3%) in the United States have dementia, and this number is expected to grow to over 13 million by 2060.[9] The prevalence of dementia increases with age, and there are significant variations in prevalence across age and ethnicity, with Asian and Pacific Islanders having the lowest prevalence, followed by non-Hispanic White persons, Native Americans, Hispanic persons, and Black persons (Table 18.1).

## Impact of Dementia

The progressive decline in multiple cognitive domains has profound effects on the patient's overall function and wellbeing, as well as the health and wellbeing of family members and caregivers.[10,11] Patients experience frustrations because of memory loss, difficulty managing challenges that arise in their day-to-day lives, and impaired ability to communicate with others. As the persons' ability to manage basic activities of daily living (ADLs) wanes, threats to safety and independent living arise, and patients may become socially isolated. Deficits in communication or unmet needs may manifest as behavioral symptoms. Dementia also impacts primary care providers and their approach to chronic disease management, as the patient's ability to self-manage illness is impaired. In addition to patient-level and provider-level impact, there is a growing societal impact of dementia. The economic burden of dementia care is growing rapidly worldwide, with an estimated $268 billion annual cost in the United States and Canada alone in 2015, up 26% since 2010. Approximately 20% of that cost is for medical care, and the remaining cost is evenly distributed among social and community care agencies and family caregivers.[12]

Progression of dementia and symptom experience is variable according to disease type and environmental factors, and this uncertainty creates challenges for patients, their families, and caregivers,[13] underscoring the importance of taking a comprehensive and person-centered approach to the care of those living with dementia. Staging systems have been developed using functional criteria, such as the Clinical Dementia Rating (CDR) scale,[14] and by specifying cut-points on brief cognitive assessments, such as the Folstein Mini-Mental State Exam (MMSE) or the Montreal Cognitive Assessment Instrument (MoCA).[15] Although no universally accepted staging system exists, monitoring progression of dementia can help clinicians, patients, and families anticipate stage-specific symptoms that differ over the course of the illness, and recognize both preserved and lost abilities that form the foundation for effective caregiving strategies. In some cases, dementia stage also helps predict response to pharmacotherapy. Table 18.2 summarizes the most common symptoms according to domain of cognitive function and stage of illness.

## Mild Dementia

In the early stage of illness, also described as "mild" dementia, which is associated with a CDR score of 1 or an MMSE of 20 to 26, patients typically experience symptoms associated with poor memory, such as forgetting key events, repetitive questioning, and misplacing familiar objects. Impaired judgment may lead to safety risks or vulnerability to scams or financial exploitation. Impairments in executive function may lead to difficulty following directions, managing complex tasks such as paying bills, and may also result in a loss of spontaneity or sense of initiative. One of the hallmarks of AD is a lack of insight into loss of abilities (anosognosia), which can result in the person seeming defensive or indifferent to his or her level of impairment and its consequences.[16] However, during this stage of dementia, individuals are generally still able to maintain their basic ADLs and some instrumental ADLs (IADLs). Many people with mild dementia continue to live independently or with minimal support. Individuals may retain capacity to provide consent for simple medical procedures, assign a healthcare power of attorney, participate in advanced care planning, and work with their family or lawyers to address their financial and legal affairs.

## Moderate Dementia

During the intermediate stage of illness, which corresponds to a CDR score of 2 or an MMSE of 12 to 19, patients will typically experience worsening memory loss and executive function. Difficulty with use of language will emerge, including problems

**TABLE 18.1  Dementia Prevalence Estimates by Racial and Ethnic Group in United States, 2014**

| Racial Ethnic Group | PERCENTAGE OF POPULATION ESTIMATED TO HAVE DEMENTIA BY AGE GROUP | | |
| --- | --- | --- | --- |
| | Age 65–74 y | Age 75–84 y | Age 85 + y |
| Asian-Pacific Islander | 2.8% | 11.7% | 32.2% |
| Black | 6.0% | 19.2% | 43.1% |
| American Indian and Alaska Native | 3.8% | 13.8% | 34.6% |
| Hispanic | 4.7% | 17.1% | 40.2% |
| Non-Hispanic White | 3.7% | 12.6% | 33.6% |

(From Matthews KA, Xu W, Gaglioti AH, et al. Racial and ethnic estimates of Alzheimer's disease and related dementias in the United States (2015-2060) in adults aged ≥65 years. *Alzheimers Dement.* 2019;15(1):17-24, see Fig. 3.)

**TABLE 18.2  Symptoms and Preserved Abilities of Alzheimer Dementia by Disease Stage**

| | Mild | Moderate | Severe |
|---|---|---|---|
| **Memory** | | | |
| Symptoms | • Loss of short-term memory; may recall some aspects of important events<br>• May lose enjoyment in reading because of difficulty following a story line | • Forgets entire events have occurred, some long-term memories remain<br>• Repetitive questioning may become troublesome for caregivers | • Complete loss of short-term memory<br>• May not recognize familiar individuals<br>• Long-term memories fade |
| Preserved abilities | • May benefit from simple reminders, routines, and habits<br>• May still derive enjoyment from reminiscing | • May still enjoy reminiscing with the assistance of visual or verbal stimulation | • Implicit memory may still be preserved<br>• Familiar environments and persons may be comforting |
| **Executive Function** | | | |
| Symptoms | • Difficulty acting on desired goals, resulting in irritation<br>• Judgment may be poor<br>• Social graces may suffer<br>• May demonstrate anhedonia or apathy | • Problem-solving ability very limited<br>• Angry outbursts<br>• Impulsive<br>• Difficulty in new situations<br>• Requires reminders or physical support to complete ADLs | • Requires assistance with all ADLs<br>• Cannot independently set goals or act upon them<br>• Gradual loss of motor abilities, including dysphagia |
| Preserved abilities | • Decision-making capacity is likely to be intact<br>• Comprehension may increase if information presentation is adapted | • Capacity for simple, every-day decision making may be preserved, even if capacity for complex decision making is lost | |
| **Language and Communication** | | | |
| Symptoms | • Some word-finding difficulties | • More pronounced difficulty understanding written or spoken language<br>• Difficulty making needs known | • Gradual loss of speech |
| Preserved abilities | • Can engage in conversations, but may require environmental supports, such as those recommended by speech and language pathologists | | • Ability to communicate needs nonverbally through emotional expression or other cues (e.g., grimacing to indicate pain) |
| **Sensory/Perceptual** | | | |
| Symptoms | • Difficulty with interpreting complex visual figures or displays | • May develop hallucinations or delusions | • May react poorly to noxious stimulation from the environment |
| Preserved abilities | • Ability to follow and enjoy simplified visual displays | | • May enjoy individually enhanced sensory environments<br>• Tactile stimulation may be preferable to auditory or visual |
| | • May respond positively to interventions, such as personalized music | | |

Symptoms and preserved abilities by cognitive domain across various stages of Alzheimer dementia. *ADLs*, Activities of daily living.

with reading and writing, as well as communicating needs effectively. People at this stage of illness will have difficulty learning new things or coping with new situations, and may lack the ability to think logically, leading to irritation or angry outbursts. They may display impulsive behaviors, leading to safety challenges, such as wandering, risky driving, or unsafe gun handling. Difficulties in carrying out multistep tasks, such as dressing or bathing, will occur, even though the physical ability to complete each task component is preserved, and this will result in gradual dependence on others for performance of ADLs and IADLs. Symptoms such as hallucinations, delusions, or paranoia may emerge.[16] The middle stage is a time when caregiver burden may be particularly problematic;

however, with appropriate support, caregivers and people living with dementia may be supported in the home, without the need to transition to residential long-term care.[17] Patients with moderate dementia will generally remain verbal, recognize close family members, and may still be able to reminisce about distant memories and enjoy pleasant events.

## Severe Dementia

Late-stage dementia, CDR of 3 or MMSE less than 12, may last 1 year or longer. During the late stage of dementia, individuals lose the ability to communicate verbally, may develop sleep dysregulation, and will lose other motor functions that can result in mealtime difficulties, dysphagia, and weight loss. In addition, patients will gradually lose their desire to eat or drink, which is often distressing for family members. Dysmobility, affecting balance, walking, and ability to transfer, will occur, and many people eventually become bedridden. Dysmobility can also result in functional incontinence.[16] The combination of incontinence and dysmobility greatly increases risk for development of pressure ulcers and the need for an increased level of care. Patients will gradually experience a complete loss of language, and may only be able to communicate with facial expressions, such as grimacing or smiling. Death from severe dementia typically results from malnutrition or infections because of aspiration pneumonia or pressure ulcers.[18]

## Pathophysiology of Alzheimer Disease

AD accounts for over two-thirds of all cases of dementia. The pathophysiology of AD is complex. The hallmark pathologic characteristics of AD are amyloid beta (A$\beta$) plaques and tau fibrillary tangles. A$\beta$ peptides are a natural by-product of cerebral metabolism and are of variable lengths. Certain peptide lengths (i.e., A$\beta_{42}$) are more prone to aggregation. An imbalance between production and clearance of A$\beta$ peptides, as well as tendency for aggregation, leads to the formation of harmful plaques. A number of genetic factors affect the length, production, and clearance of A$\beta$ and thus can affect propensity for developing the disease. Tau, a naturally occurring protein that stabilizes axonal microtubules, also becomes hyperphosphorylated and pathologically aggregates, producing neurofibrillary tangles.[19] Plaques and tangles cause a number of downstream effects, including synaptic dysfunction, mitochondrial damage, vascular damage, and inflammation. Drugs targeted at removal of plaques and tangles have not been effective in reversing clinical dementia.[20] This suggests that, although plaques and tangles are necessary for the development of AD, removal of these structures is insufficient for treatment. Because the neuropathology of AD develops over multiple decades, it may be that clinical trials have failed because they occurred too late in the disease course.

## Risk Factors for Alzheimer Disease and Other Dementias

### Nonmodifiable Risk Factors

After age, genetics and family history are the strongest risk factors for the development of AD. Patients have a 10% to 30% increased risk of developing AD if they have a first-degree relative with AD. However, this risk is attenuated if the relative developed AD after the age of 85 years.[21] Large-scale studies have not demonstrated convincing differences in the rates of AD or all-cause dementia by gender; however, men are at higher risk of developing vascular dementia.[22]

Early-onset AD accounts for < 1% of all cases of Alzheimer and is linked to autosomal dominant mutations in one of three genes: amyloid precursor protein *(APP)*, presenilin 1 *(PSEN1)*, and presenilin 2 *(PSEN2)* (Table 18.3). The *APP* gene produces the amyloid precursor protein, which is implicated in the development of A$\beta$ plaques. *APP* is carried on chromosome 21, hence those born with trisomy 21 (Down syndrome) have a significantly elevated risk of AD; approximately half of all adults with trisomy 21 who live to age 60 years will develop AD.[23]

*APOE* is the gene most highly associated with development of late-onset AD (LOAD), that is, AD occurring after the age of 65 years. *APOE* encodes apolipoprotein E, a protein that mediates cholesterol transportation and metabolism. The *APOE* gene has three alleles: $\epsilon$2, $\epsilon$3, and $\epsilon$4. $\epsilon$2 is relatively rare in the general population (<2% $\epsilon$2 homozygotes) and is protective against the development of AD.[24] $\epsilon$3 is neutral with regard to risk of AD, whereas $\epsilon$4 increases the risk of AD significantly. Approximately 15% to 25% of the population carries at least one $\epsilon$4 allele. Data from the large-scale Rotterdam study in the Netherlands found $\epsilon$4 homozygotes had an almost 10-fold increase in risk of developing AD.[25] However, it is important to note that *APOE* is not a causative gene for development of AD. Even $\epsilon$4 homozygotes will not absolutely develop dementia, and at least one-third of patients develop AD without an $\epsilon$4 allele. Because the relationship between *APOE* and development of AD remains unclear, and because there are limited interventions for patients at high risk for LOAD, routine genetic testing for *APOE* subtype is not recommended for clinical use at this time. As in-home genetic testing becomes more widely available to the lay-public, providers should be aware that tests for "dementia risk" are being commercially offered. Providers should be prepared to address concerns about tests that report positivity for genes implicated in the pathogenesis of dementia.

Low level of educational attainment is another risk factor for dementia; likely patients with lower levels of educational attainment have poorer cognitive reserve and thus a lower threshold to tolerate amyloid plaque burden or other degenerative changes. Finally, a number of comorbid illnesses are associated with increased risk of dementia, including chronic kidney disease, atrial fibrillation, and depression. Dementia and depression have a bidirectional relationship. An occurrence of depression in one's lifetime is associated with a doubling in risk for development of dementia. Depression occurring in later life (e.g., after the age of 60 years) is commonly associated with development of dementia, and may be a prodromal symptom of AD. Patients with dementia also have high rates of depressive symptoms, particularly during mild-moderate stages of disease. There is no high-quality evidence to show treatment of depression ameliorates risk of developing dementia.

## Potentially Modifiable Risk Factors

A variety of risk factors contribute to the development of AD and other dementias. These are summarized in Fig. 18.2. Many of

| TABLE 18.3 | Genes Implicated in the Development of Alzheimer Disease |
|---|---|
| **Gene** | **Comment** |
| *APP* | >30 known mutations associated with EOAD; located on chromosome 21; associated with elevated risk of AD in Down syndrome |
| *PSEN1* | >150 known mutations associated with EOAD |
| *PSEN2* | <20 known mutations associated with EOAD |
| *APOE* | Three known alleles:<br>$\epsilon$2 — protective of LOAD<br>$\epsilon$3 — Neutral risk of LOAD<br>$\epsilon$4 — Increased risk of LOAD |

*AD,* Alzheimer disease; *EOAD,* early-onset Alzheimer disease; *LOAD,* late-onset Alzheimer disease.

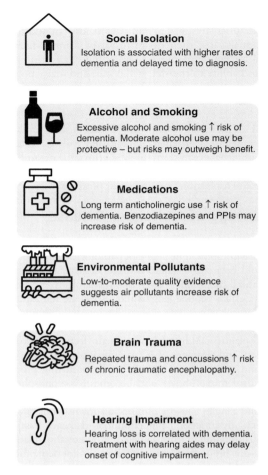

**Hypertension**
High quality evidence demonstrates correlation between mid-life hypertension and dementia.

**Cardiovascular Disease**
High cholesterol, atherosclerosis, and cerebrovascular disease are all associated with ↑ risk of dementia.

**Obesity**
Mid-life obesity increases risk of dementia. Conversely, late-life weight loss may precede onset of dementia.

**Diabets**
Diabetes is associated with ↑ risk of dementia. Poor glucose control is associated with worse cognitive decline.

**Sedentary Lifestyle**
Patients who engage in at least a low to moderate level of physical activity have ↓ risk of cognitive decline.

**Sleep Disorders**
OSA is associated with ↑ risk of dementia. Sleep disturbance is associated with dementia but causal relationship is unknown.

**Social Isolation**
Isolation is associated with higher rates of dementia and delayed time to diagnosis.

**Alcohol and Smoking**
Excessive alcohol and smoking ↑ risk of dementia. Moderate alcohol use may be protective – but risks may outweigh benefit.

**Medications**
Long term anticholinergic use ↑ risk of dementia. Benzodiazepines and PPIs may increase risk of dementia.

**Environmental Pollutants**
Low-to-moderate quality evidence suggests air pollutants increase risk of dementia.

**Brain Trauma**
Repeated trauma and concussions ↑ risk of chronic traumatic encephalopathy.

**Hearing Impairment**
Hearing loss is correlated with dementia. Treatment with hearing aides may delay onset of cognitive impairment.

• **Figure 18.2** Potentially modifiable risk factors for development of dementia. *OSA*, Obstructive sleep apnea. Icons available from The Noun Project (http://thenounproject.com). From left to right: "Sphygmometer" by Vectors Point, PK; "Single House" by Seona Kim, KR; "Heartbeat" by Clockwise, IN; "Alcohol" by Adrien Coquet, FR, "Weight Scale" by Semmel Zenko; "Medication" by Chameleon Design, IN; "Glucose Meter" by LAFS, RU; "Pollution" by Chattapat, TH; "Chair" by Hermine Blanquart, FR; "Brain" by Matthew S Hall, US; "Sleep" by H Alerto Gongora, CO; and "Hearing" by Ben Davis, RO.

these risk factors are based on observational studies and thus based on only moderate quality evidence. It is important to note that, in addressing risk factors of dementia, risks and benefits of interventions must be carefully balanced. For instance, although there is strong evidence to suggest treatment of mid-to-late life hypertension is associated with decreased risk of cognitive impairment,[26] older adults are also at significant risk of orthostatic hypotension and falls because of arterial stiffening and comorbid conditions that can cause autonomic neuropathy. Similarly, although avoiding hyperglycemia is important, decreased renal clearance of insulin and other pharmacologic agents may increase risk of life-threatening hypoglycemia. Addressing risk factors for dementia should be done in a patient-centered manner that accounts for comorbid conditions and does not compromise patient safety.

Hearing loss is correlated with risk of dementia, but the causal relationship is not clear.[27] One large observational study suggested that treatment of hearing loss may delay diagnosis of dementia, but the study had numerous limitations as it was based on insurance claims data.[28] Regardless, treating hearing loss has been shown to improve quality of life, prevent social isolation, and improve

functional status, and thus addressing hearing loss should remain a priority in patients with cognitive impairment.

## Diagnostic Approach

### Screening for Cognitive Impairment

The US Preventative Services Task Force (USPSTF) guidelines state that there is insufficient evidence to recommend for or against screening for cognitive impairment in asymptomatic older adults.[29] Because there are limited options for treatment of dementia, the benefits of screening the general population are unclear. However, given the high prevalence of MCI and dementia, providers should maintain a high index of suspicion. Although there are no targeted treatments for dementia, accurate, early diagnosis allows patients and their caregivers to address symptom management, identify resources to preserve functioning, and engage in appropriate preparations, including financial and legal, advanced care planning, and obtaining caregiver support. Providers should understand the warning signs that may indicate a patient is experiencing cognitive dysfunction and have a low threshold to perform additional evaluation.

## Initial Assessment: History and Physical Examination

Primary care providers are often the first point of contact for patients with cognitive dysfunction.[30] Concerns may be raised by patients; alternatively, a friend or family member may raise concerns or the provider may note aberrant behavior that arouses suspicion for a cognitive disorder. Box 18.1 summarizes warning signs providers or family members may notice that should trigger a workup for cognitive problems.

When patients complain of cognitive symptoms or exhibit warning signs of dementia, providers should perform a thorough history, including duration of cognitive complaints. Because cognitive impairment and dementia often have insidious onset, family members may have difficulty recognizing early clinical signs. Providers can ask about specific tasks or points in time to help establish a more definitive time course, for example, "When did you give up paying the household bills?" Or, "Did you notice any memory changes in your grandmother last summer?" Providers should also perform a thorough neuropsychiatric review of systems, medication reconciliation, and a social history, including level of education, literacy evaluation, substance use, and living situation. Patients' past medical history should be carefully reviewed, with attention to cardiovascular disease and neurologic disorders, including prior traumatic brain injury. Family history may be helpful in identifying specific etiologies, particularly in younger patients. Finally, providers should inquire about the patient's functional status. Understanding baseline functional status and tracking changes over time can help to track disease progression, and also helps primary care providers to identify appropriate resources and supports as patients accumulate deficits. Whenever possible, collateral history should be obtained from a family member or friend, as patients with cognitive impairment often lack insight into their deficits and may be unreliable historians. A multidisciplinary team, including nurses, social workers, and physical, occupational, and speech therapists, can enhance both assessment and management.

Providers should also perform a thorough physical examination. Certain findings, such as parkinsonism, frontal release signs, or focal neurologic deficits, may point to specific etiologies (see Differential Diagnosis, later). Evidence of cardiovascular disease, such as carotid bruits or skin changes consistent with peripheral arterial disease, may suggest concurrent vascular dementia. In patients with dementia, providers should perform a thorough skin examination, note hygiene and grooming, and look for evidence of neglect or injury. Patients with dementia are among the highest risk for elder abuse, with some studies estimating half of all dementia patients will encounter some form of elder abuse in their lifetime.[31]

## Cognitive Testing and Specialty Referrals

Patients with cognitive concerns or warning signs for cognitive impairment/dementia should have a brief cognitive test administered. There are a wide variety available, and providers should use a tool based on their own preference and patient-specific factors. Some of the most common brief cognitive assessment tools are summarized in Table 18.4.

Neuropsychological testing (NPT) can provide additional diagnostic information to aid in diagnosis if the clinical picture is unclear.[32] Referral to neuropsychologists may be appropriate if there is a large discrepancy between clinical presentation and performance on a brief cognitive screen (for instance, a patient with significant functional deficits or memory concerns but a high score on a brief cognitive screen, or vice versa). NPT is also appropriate if there is concern that an affective disorder is confounding performance on cognitive testing, to evaluate potentially rare etiologies of dementia, or in patients with very high or very low levels of education. Patients who are highly educated may experience a ceiling effect on brief cognitive tests and perform well even if they have experienced significant cognitive decline. Conversely, patients with low educational attainment and/or low health literacy may perform poorly on such tests without experiencing changes in baseline cognition. Patients with rapidly progressive disease should be referred to a neurologist for urgent evaluation.

**◆◆ Neuropsychological testing can be useful in patients with discrepancies between clinical presentation and performance on cognitive testing or in patients with very high or low educational attainment. Neurology referral is indicated for dementia present in young patients (i.e., age <60 years) and/or for rapidly progressive dementia.**

## Diagnostic Evaluation of the Person With a Suspected Cognitive Impairment

In patients with a history consistent with cognitive impairment and abnormal cognitive testing, a limited laboratory and imaging workup should be performed to exclude reversible causes of cognitive impairment or confounding conditions that may worsen cognition.

The American Academy of Neurology recommends testing vitamin $B_{12}$ levels and thyroid functioning in all adults with cognitive impairment.[33] Addressing vitamin $B_{12}$ deficiency and/or thyroid dysfunction is unlikely to completely reverse cognitive impairment, but may lead to improvements. Human immunodeficiency virus (HIV) and *Syphilis* serologies are recommended if the patient has risk factors for contracting sexually transmitted infections. Routine bloodwork, including a basic metabolic panel, liver function tests, and a complete blood count, are appropriate if a patient has not undergone this testing recently. Although

---

### • BOX 18.1   Potential Warning Signs for Cognitive Disorders

Inappropriate with clinical staff
Unable to maintain simple conversation
Frequently repeating oneself
Getting lost in familiar locations
Clothing is soiled, in poor condition, or inappropriate to season
Compromised personal hygiene
Unexplained changes in weight
Frequently missed appointments
Impairments in memory
Changes in functional status
Difficulty maintaining daily routine
Increasing reliance on others
Allowing family members to speak for them during appointments
Not properly filling or taking medications

(Modified from Volkmer A, Spector A, Warren JD, Beeke S. Speech and language therapy for primary progressive aphasia across the UK: A survey of current practice. *Int J Lang Commun Disord.* 2019;54:914–926.)

| TABLE 18.4 | Brief Objective Measures of Cognitive Impairment | | | |
|---|---|---|---|---|
| Tool | Available in Public Domain? | Administration Time | Comments | Sensitivity and Specificity[c] |
| MMSE | No | 10–15 minutes | Suffers from ceiling effect in highly educated individuals | Sensitivity: 81%<br>Specificity: 89% |
| MoCA | Yes[a] | 10–20 minutes | Available in >50 languages, including version for visually impaired. Most sensitive tool for detecting mild cognitive impairment | Sensitivity: 91%<br>Specificity: 81% |
| SLUMS | Yes | 10–15 minutes | Primarily validated in male veterans | Sensitivity: 84%–100%<br>Specificity: 87%–100% |
| AD8 | No[b] | <5 minutes | Administered by informant or patient. Highly variable specificity across a number of studies | Sensitivity: 73%–97%<br>Specificity: 17%–90% |
| **Mini-Cog** | No[b] | <5 minutes | Clock draw + 3-item recall creates a dichotomous result (impaired/nonimpaired) and does not generate a score that can be tracked over time | Sensitivity: 76%–100%<br>Specificity: 54%–85% |

A summary of brief cognitive screening tools that can be used in primary care clinic.

[a]MOCA is copyrighted and now requires most administrators to complete paid training before use. Exceptions include students, trainees, and neuropsychologists.

[b]AD8, Mini-Cog may be used for clinical purposes free of charge.

[c]Sensitivity and specificity based on distinguishing dementia from cognitively intact. (From Wilterdink JL. *Mental Status Scales to Evaluate Cognition.* 2019 [cited October 15, 2019]. Available at: https://www.uptodate.com/contents/mental-status-scales-to-evaluate-cognition.)

*AD8,* Ascertain Dementia 8; *MMSE,* Folstein minimental status exam; *MoCA,* Montreal Cognitive Assessment; *SLUMS,* St. Louis University Mental Status Exam.

electrolyte abnormalities such as hyponatremia and hypocalcemia can adversely affect cognition,[34] these metabolic derangements usually present acutely. Other bloodwork should only be ordered on a case-by-case basis if a patient exhibits specific risks or exposures (e.g., heavy metal screening).

Neuroimaging is indicated in many, but not all, patients presenting with cognitive impairment. Patients with neurologic abnormalities on examination, a history of falls or trauma (even minor trauma), patients on anticoagulants, and patients with atypical features (such as age <65 years and/or rapidly progressive disease) should undergo imaging with either a brain computed tomography (CT) or magnetic resonance imaging (MRI). MRI has higher resolution to detect subtle pathologies but may be difficult for some patients to tolerate. In contrast, patients without neurologic deficits who present with insidious and slowly progressive memory loss, without risk factors for intracranial hemorrhage, do not necessarily require brain imaging.

Recently, a variety of advanced imaging techniques have become available. Advanced structural MRI techniques allow for volumetric assessment of specific brain structures, such as the hippocampus, to assess for location-specific atrophy. Positron emission tomography (PET) and single-photon emission computerized tomography scans may demonstrate localized hypometabolism in affected areas of the brain. Specialized PET tracers targeting amyloid and tau are an area of evolving research that may allow for more accurate diagnoses of dementia subtypes.[35] However, in the United States, such imaging techniques are not typically covered by patient insurance, and outside of research purposes the clinical utility of these advanced imaging techniques is unclear.

❖❖ **Evaluation of cognitive dysfunction includes a thorough history, including medication review, functional status, and collateral history from a trusted family member or friend, a complete physical examination, and an objective measure of cognitive function. Laboratory workup includes thyroid-stimulating hormone (TSH), vitamin B₁₂, HIV, and *Syphilis* serologies if risk factors are present. Neuroimaging is indicated in most but not all cases.**

## Early Detection

Because pathologic changes of AD are hypothesized to develop decades before the onset of clinical symptoms, there is enormous interest in detecting preclinical disease in asymptomatic individuals.[36] It may be that these patients would benefit the most from targeted treatments to prevent the neurodegenerative changes that ultimately lead to clinical manifestations. In addition to the advanced imaging techniques described earlier, there is interest in identifying biomarkers that can predict eventual onset of AD. Low levels of cerebrospinal fluid (CSF) Aβ peptide and elevated levels of CSF tau and phosphorylated tau are promising targets. However, the role of biomarkers in the prediction of AD is an area of evolving research, and no blood or CSF test is currently recommended for clinical use.

## Differential Diagnosis

There are a number of disorders that may cause cognitive complaints. Common etiologies are summarized in Table 18.5. In addition to normal aging, MCI, and dementia, a number of other factors can cause cognitive dysfunction. Providers should be aware of the broad differential for cognitive complaints, and perform appropriate testing and evaluation based on individuals' unique history and risk factors.

TABLE 18.5

# Cognitive Disorders in Older Adults

| Diagnosis (% of Dementias Attributable) | History | Physical Examination Findings | Imaging Findings | Comment |
|---|---|---|---|---|
| Normal aging changes (n/a) | Delayed retrieval (forgetting names, dates), slower processing (takes longer to learn new things). No functional limitations | None | Mild generalized cortical atrophy, mild ventricular enlargement No focal findings | Patients may have white matter disease and/or prior lacunar infarcts related to HTN, DM, and cardiovascular disease, etc., but unrelated to memory complaints |
| Mild cognitive impairment (n/a) | Cognitive deficits beyond what is expected for age across one or more domains | None | Variable depending on etiology Atrophy of medial temporal lobe and/or hippocampus (pre-Alzheimer disease) | Clinical course highly dependent on etiology. Amnestic MCI most likely to progress to dementia (50%) Neuropsychologic testing may help to clarify diagnosis |
| Alzheimer disease (67%) | Progressive memory loss and other cognitive deficits | Essentially normal in early stages Moderate: Patients may develop apraxia, aphasia | Medial temporal, parietal lobe, and/or hippocampal atrophy on MRI Positivity on amyloid PET scan | Patients will occasionally present with unusual variants based on atypical neuroanatomic pathology; for example, fixed delusions or behavioral manifestations (dysexecutive variant) or prominent visual symptoms (posterior cortical atrophy) |
| Vascular dementia (20%, includes mixed dementia) | Prominent vascular risk factors, possible history of stroke/TIA, possible stepwise disease progression. Executive dysfunction may be prominent early symptom | Variable depending on distribution of disease | Cortical and subcortical infarcts and white matter disease | Commonly present in conjunction with Alzheimer disease —known as mixed dementia |
| Lewy Body dementia and Parkinson dementia (15%) | Fluctuating cognition, well-formed visual hallucinations, REM sleep disorder, falls, sensitivity to neuroleptics | Orthostatic hypotension, postural instability, hyposmia, bradykinesia, resting tremor, rigidity | No specific findings on MRI Positivity on dopamine transporter PET scan | Parkinson dementia occurs in patients with preexisting Parkinson disease of at least 1-year duration, followed by onset of cognitive deficits |
| Frontotemporal dementia (<5%) | Two variants: Behavioral variant (50%) presents with progressive personality and behavioral changes Primary progressive aphasia presents with progressive language impairment | Frontal release signs | Frontal and temporal lobe atrophy | Executive function and episodic memory generally preserved in early stages of disease |
| Chronic traumatic encephalopathy (CTE, unknown) | History of multiple concussions and/or traumatic brain injury, most commonly in former athletes or military personnel. Concurrent behavioral changes and psychiatric disease common | None | Nonspecific white matter changes | Tauopathy in cortical and perivascular regions of the brain. CTE can only definitely be diagnosed by autopsy; there is currently no definitive clinical criteria for diagnosis |
| Rapidly progressive dementia (<1%) | Memory symptoms progressive over weeks to months | Variable depending on etiology: Myoclonus/startle reflex suggestive of prion disease | Variable depending on etiology | Rapidly progressive dementias are rare and merit urgent referral to a neurologist Specialized testing should be based on patient-specific risk factors |
| Delirium (n/a) | Identifiable toxic, metabolic, or infectious etiology and/or precipitants (e.g., acute hospital admission). Rapid onset | Inattention, disorganized thinking, and/or altered level of consciousness. Fluctuating course | No specific findings | EEG will demonstrate acute slowing Generally reversible with correction of precipitant(s) |

*DM,* Diabetes mellitus; *EEG,* electroencephalogram; *HTN,* hypertension; *MCI,* mild cognitive impairment; *MRI,* magnetic resonance imaging; *PET,* positron emission tomography; *REM,* rapid eye movement; *TIA,* transient ischemic attack.

Depression may cause attentional deficits and apathy that mimic dementia. Patients undergoing cognitive evaluation should be concurrently screened for mood disorders. Obstructive sleep apnea may similarly cause daytime somnolence and deficits in short-term memory. Normal pressure hydrocephalus, subclinical seizures, and subdural hematomas (SDH) may also lead to cognitive impairment. It is important to note that SDH may occur in patients with minimal trauma and without a history of head injury. Untreated hearing and vision impairment may also mimic cognitive impairment and confound cognitive evaluations.

Finally, because of age-related changes in physiology and metabolism, older adults are vulnerable to medication side effects that can cause a number of cognitive complaints. In particular, anticholinergic medications block acetylcholine receptors, mimicking the synaptic dysfunction that occurs in a number of dementia disorders. Anticholinergic agents are found in a number of prescription and over-the-counter (OTCs) medications, including cold medications and OTC sleep agents. Providers should perform a thorough medication reconciliation, including OTCs, and patients should be counseled to avoid potentially inappropriate medications. Other medications implicated in short-term cognitive dysfunction include benzodiazepines, psychotropic medications, and opioids. The American Geriatrics Society (AGS) maintains the "Beers List" of potentially inappropriate medications in older adults, which is updated annually and can help providers critically evaluate their patient's medication list and reduce unnecessary polypharmacy.[37]

## Disclosing the Diagnosis

Data show that, on average, patients with dementia often do not receive a diagnosis until 2 years after initial presentation, and up to half of clinicians purposely withhold a diagnosis of dementia.[38] Clinicians may delay revealing the diagnosis for a number of reasons, including uncertainty about diagnosis, concerns about lack of available treatment options, and concern about psychological distress related to the diagnosis. However, a multinational survey of adults across the United States and Europe demonstrated that the overwhelming majority (nearly 90%) would want to know if they or a loved one was suffering from dementia. After cancer, AD was the second biggest health fear identified, so it is important that providers demonstrate compassion and empathy while disclosing the diagnosis.[39]

When disclosing the diagnosis, a trusted family member or friend should be present, both to provide emotional support to the patient and because the patient's limitations may impair his or her ability to retain information. It may be helpful to give the diagnosis within a framework of stages of cognitive impairment, explaining to the patient where he or she lies in the spectrum.[40] Ask the patient and family member what they know about dementia, and be prepared to address misconceptions. Assure the patient that, although there is no cure, there are a variety of treatment options available, but refrain from providing minutiae of specific treatments at this early stage. Instead, focus on goals that enhance wellbeing, such as preserving independence and preventing rapid cognitive decline. Emphasize the longitudinal nature of the disease, and provide reassurance that you will continue to be a partner in his or her care. It is likely that the patient will require multiple close follow-up visits to process the new diagnosis and develop a comprehensive treatment and safety plan. Consider early referral to local patient and caregiver support groups, if available. For technologically savvy patients and caregivers, online resources, including the Alzheimer's Disease Education and Referral Center (ADEAR) or Alzheimer's Association, can provide additional education and support.

## Preventing Dementia

The pathophysiology and development of cognitive impairment and dementia is complex. Dementia is thought to arise from a number of both modifiable and nonmodifiable risk factors and includes complex interplay between genetic and environmental factors that remains an area of ongoing research. Because the neurodegenerative changes that lead to dementia arise over decades, it is challenging to perform high-quality research isolating single causative factors. Given the natural course of neurodegenerative changes leading to dementia, it is likely that interventions beginning in middle age or earlier, and sustained throughout adulthood, would be most effective in reducing risk of dementia.

Table 18.6 summarizes strategies for prevention of dementia and the strength of supporting evidence, as outlined from updated World Health Organization 2019 guidelines.[41] There is currently insufficient evidence to demonstrate that treatment of depression or hearing loss improves cognitive outcomes, although it is important to address these conditions for other reasons, including improvement in quality of life.

In patients with MCI, cholinesterase inhibitors are not effective at either treating symptoms or preventing progression to dementia. Emerging evidence shows that engaging in computer-assisted cognitive training has benefits on global cognitive functioning, as well as attention, memory, and learning.[42] Speech language pathologists also offer cognitive training that may be beneficial for patients with insights into their deficits.

Providers should be aware of a number of pseudoscientific products and services that may be offered to patients in the hopes of

| TABLE 18.6 | Strategies for Prevention of Dementia | |
|---|---|
| **Recommendation** | **Quality of Evidence** |
| Engage in physical activity | Moderate |
| In adults with **mild cognitive impairment**, engage in physical activity to slow cognitive decline | Low |
| Tobacco cessation | Low |
| Do not exceed maximum daily recommended amount of alcohol intake | Moderate[a] |
| Follow a healthy diet based on WHO recommendations[b] | Moderate[c] |
| Follow a Mediterranean diet | Moderate |
| Maintain a healthy weight | Low |
| Participate in cognitively stimulating activities or cognitive training | Low |
| Treatment of hypertension | High |
| Treatment of *diabetes mellitus* | Moderate |
| Treatment of dyslipidemia | Low |

Strategies for Prevention of Dementia, as based on World Health Organization (WHO) 2019 Guidelines for Risk Reduction of Cognitive Impairment and Dementia.
[a]14 units of alcohol per week for men, 7 units of alcohol per week for women.
[b]Components include: 5 daily servings of nonstarchy vegetables, <10% dietary intake of free sugars, <30% dietary intake of fats (preferentially unsaturated fats), <5 g daily intake of salt.
[c]Strength of evidence is variable based on individual dietary components.

preventing dementia. For instance, a number of commercially available supplements claim to prevent dementia. There is currently no evidence to support the use of any supplements or herbal products for improving cognitive performance or preventing dementia. Fish oil, omega-3 fatty acids, vitamin B complexes, and vitamin E specifically lack evidence to support their use in preventing dementia. There is currently no evidence to support cannabis in the prevention or treatment of dementia[43]; the role of cannabis in the treatment of behavioral and psychosocial symptoms of dementia (BPSD) is an area of ongoing research. Although cognitively-stimulating activities may improve cognitive functioning, patients and providers should be wary of commercial products specifically advertised to prevent dementia.

---

**CASE**

**Mr. Frank (Part 2)**

Mr. Frank has been in your care for several years now. He has moved to an assisted living residence, where the staff helps him with bathing and dressing. His brother and niece visit him weekly. You receive a phone message from his niece saying that she is concerned that her uncle is going downhill rapidly, following a fall he had last week. After the fall, he was taken to the emergency room where they determined Mr. Frank had no fractures or intracranial hemorrhage. However, since returning back to the facility, he is no longer eating as usual, seems very agitated during mealtimes, and the administrative staff have indicated that he may be required to leave the facility because his behavior is disruptive for other residents in the dining room.

What could be causing Mr. Frank's new agitation? How would you evaluate and manage Mr. Frank?

---

## Treatment Overview

No disease-modifying or curative drug therapies exist for MCI, AD, or other dementias; treatment is therefore symptomatic. A growing evidence base confirms the potential to improve quality of life through a person-centered approach that focuses on maximizing wellbeing, managing comorbid illness,[44] and capitalizing on preserved abilities,[45] including the ability to form and preserve meaningful relationships. Although medications are available, they are primarily symptomatic and do not alter disease course. Furthermore, their effects are modest and must be balanced with the risk of adverse effects. Adopting a person-centered approach to care[46] and attending to the wellbeing of people living with dementia and their caregivers through the use of nonpharmacologic interventions are the foundations of dementia care.

## Person-Centered Care Framework

The AGS position statement on person-centered care provides a framework for managing primary care of people living with dementia. Table 18.7 displays how these components of person-centered care can be operationalized across the course of illness. Additional processes that support person-centeredness include active information exchange among all parties involved in care, ongoing education and training for patients and caregivers (both formal and informal) to support the person's autonomy, informed decision making and self-determination, and ongoing evaluation to ensure that the person's goals are being addressed.[46] Decision-

making capacity is task specific, and mastering techniques to communicate key information to people with cognitive dysfunction is key to supporting and preserving autonomy whenever possible. Providers can support a person's decision-making capacity by being aware of and adapting to the person's literacy level, adjusting for sensory deficits, addressing anxiety, and providing time to process information critical to making an informed decision.[47]

## Pharmacotherapy

Currently, only two classes of medications are approved by the US Food and Drug Administration for treatment of AD: cholinesterase inhibitors (including donepezil, galantamine, and rivastigmine) and the N-methyl-D-aspartate (NMDA) receptor inhibitor, memantine. The benefits from these medicines are typically small, and vary according to the cause of dementia and illness stage. All of these agents carry the risk of clinically significant adverse effects. Cholinesterase inhibitors may cause gastrointestinal distress and weight loss, urinary urgency, bradycardia, syncope, and sleep disturbances (including vivid, troublesome dreams). Memantine has fewer side effects but is associated with dizziness and possibly hallucinations and increased agitation. Thus clinicians, patients, and family caregivers need to carefully weigh the benefits and risks of pharmacotherapy and monitor carefully for adverse effects.

According to a metaanalysis, comparing donepezil to placebo over 12 to 26 weeks of therapy, patients at all stages of illness showed small improvements in cognition, function, and global clinician rating scores, with no effect on behavioral symptoms, quality of life, or healthcare utilization. There was a small advantage of titrating therapy from 5 mg to 10 mg daily. Patients experienced higher rates of side effects but no additional clinical benefit at 23 mg per day.[48] Similarly, a metaanalysis of memantine demonstrated small benefits in global clinical impression ratings, cognition, and function, and behavioral symptoms for those with moderate to severe illness. These effects are observed regardless of whether the patient received concomitant cholinesterase inhibitor therapy.[49] Trials of pharmacotherapy are appropriate for patients with AD, vascular dementia, Lewy Body dementia, and Parkinson dementia. However, these medicines should not be used for those with frontotemporal dementia because they may worsen symptoms.[50] Dosing and titration guidelines for acetylcholinesterase inhibitors are shown in Table 18.8. Cholinesterase inhibitors are contraindicated in patients with baseline bradycardia or cardiac conduction disease, and should be used with caution in patients taking medications that alter atrioventricular node function. Galantamine is contraindicated in patients with severe hepatic impairment (Child-Pugh score >10), with dose reduction recommended for mild-moderate hepatic impairment (Child-Pugh score 5–9). These medicines frequently cause genitourinary and gastrointestinal side effects. They should be avoided in patients with urge type incontinence, chronic diarrhea, or when risk of side effects outweighs benefits.

## Family Caregiver Education and Support

Unpaid family caregivers provide the majority of care for people living with dementia. Without adequate preparation and support, the stresses of the caregiving role can threaten the health and wellbeing of both caregivers and patients. Caregivers from Black and Latino backgrounds are particularly vulnerable to caregiving stress, and are more likely to have unsatisfying relationships with

**TABLE 18.7   Person-Centered Care Approach Applied to Care of People Living With Dementia**

| Key Component | Early Stage | Middle Stage | Late Stage |
|---|---|---|---|
| Develop a personalized, goal-oriented care plan, based on a thorough medical, functional, and social assessment | • Conduct a functional assessment, including sensory status, language abilities<br>• Establish stage-appropriate, personally meaningful goals<br>• Encourage advance care planning, including naming a surrogate decision maker | | • Engage with family members and surrogate decision makers to interpret patient's nonverbal communication |
| | • Discuss advantages and disadvantages of pharmacotherapy to help with cognitive or behavioral symptoms and monitor regularly for side effects | | • If on ChE-I, consider discontinuation |
| Periodically review the person's goals and care plan to assess ongoing effectiveness and to address evolving goals | • Refer to community resources to promote the person's ongoing connection with and engagement in personally meaningful activities<br>• Assess and address caregiver stress<br>• Consider referral to senior centers or adult day programs to promote social engagement<br>• In-home care services may be helpful | | • Personalized music programs may be helpful<br>• Hospice consultation may be indicated |
| Engage an interprofessional team that adapts its composition in response to the needs of the person living with dementia | • Care managers to refer to resources in community<br><br>• SLP referral to teach caregivers supported communication approaches | • Care managers: assist with symptom management, respite services<br>• SLP consultation for assistance with supported communication approaches and feeding techniques | • Care managers: assistance managing symptoms, referral for respite services<br>• Palliative care or hospice consultation for symptom management and end-of-life care |
| | • PT/OT: in-home safety evaluation and customization of activities | • OT consultation to maximize functional independence | • OT sensory stimulation approaches to promote wellbeing |
| | • Pharmacy to assist with deprescribing and simplification of medication regimen<br>• Specialty referrals (psychiatry, dementia care clinics) for management of BPSD | | |
| A specified team leader to facilitate information transfer, care coordination, and continuity | • Primary care provider or specialty-trained care manager, such as nurse specialist or social worker | • Primary care provider or specialty-trained care manager | • Primary care provider or hospice team |

*BPSD*, Behavioral and psychological symptoms of dementia; *CHe-I*, acetylcholinesterase inhibitors; *OT*, occupational therapy; *PT*, physical therapy; *SLP*, speech language pathology.

**TABLE 18.8   Acetylcholinesterase Inhibitor Dosing**

| Drug | Initial Dose | Recommended Dose | Minimum Therapeutic Dose | Formulations |
|---|---|---|---|---|
| Donepezil | 5 mg daily | 10 mg daily | 5 mg daily | 5, 10, 23 mg |
| Galantamine IR | 4 mg BID | 12 mg BID | 8 mg BID | 4, 8, 12 mg |
| Galantamine ER | 8 mg daily | 24 mg daily | 16 mg daily | 8, 12, 24 mg |
| Rivastigmine | 1.5 mg BID | 6 mg BID | 3 mg BID | 1.5, 3, 4.5, 6 mg |
| Rivastigmine patch | 4.6 mg daily | 9.5 mg daily | 9.5 mg daily | 4.6, 9.5, 13.3 mg |

*BID*, Twice daily.

Acetylcholinesterase inhibitor dosing and suggested titration intervals. (From US Department of Veterans Affairs. *Pharmacy Benefits Management Services.* 2018 [cited October 15, 2019]. Available at: https://www.pbm.va.gov/.) Note that medications doses can be increased every 4 weeks as patient tolerates.

healthcare professionals, underscoring the importance of appreciating cultural perspectives on caregiving.[51] Caregivers benefit from systematic preparation for their role.[52] The following interventions are supported by evidence: (1) education on the disease itself, and how to manage symptoms,[53] (2) support groups that can be delivered in-person or virtually through teleconference,[54] (3) training on problem solving around behavioral symptoms and consultation for particular challenges in care,[55,56] and (4) respite care services.[57] Caregiver support programs can be located through the Alzheimer's Association or through local Area Agency on Aging networks (see Web Resources).

Primary care teams should systematically assess for caregiver stress or burden using tools, such as the Zarit Burden Inventory[58] or more recently developed short forms of this instrument.[59] Providers should additionally assess caregivers for unmet needs and be prepared to offer referrals to supportive services or educational resources in response. Patients and caregivers should be encouraged to prepare for office visits ahead of time by writing down concerns, and telephone consultations or separate visits with caregivers may be helpful. When available, social workers may also be able to help patients and caregivers address transportation, financial, and/or legal needs that arise over the course of illness. In-home primary care services for dementia patients have been shown to reduce caregiver burden and improve both patient and caregiver quality of life, although such services are only available sporadically and often have long wait lists.[17] Importantly, caregiver burden is related to use of residential long-term care services, so focusing on caregiver wellbeing may support aging in place.

## Promoting Safety

### High-Risk Medications

Adverse medication effects are common among older adults with dementia.[60] Providers should work collaboratively with patients and families to promote drug safety. Early after the diagnosis, providers should clarify whether patients are managing medications alone. If so, patients and families can use a number of strategies to aid the patient in properly taking medications. Families may periodically check pillboxes to ensure medications are being filled and administered properly. Simplified regimens (e.g., only once-a-day medications), smartphone reminders, or pharmacy-delivered prepackaged pill boxes may aid with compliance. The standardized assessment instrument "Medicog"[61] can help providers assess whether patients have capacity to self-manage a pillbox. As dementia progresses, patients will eventually require additional oversight of medication administration. Importantly, avoiding adverse drug events can help patients preserve cognition. Consider working with a clinical pharmacist to deprescribe medications,[62] particularly those of questionable benefit or with a narrow therapeutic index. Providers should carefully weigh the risks and benefits of particularly high-risk medications, such as anticoagulants, opioids, insulins, and sulfonylureas.

### Driving

Driving safety and cessation are among the most contentious topics in dementia care because driving has both practical and symbolic meaning for older adults. Data demonstrate that the discussion of driving cessation is best received if cast in the context of disease-specific recommendations, conducted within a trusting relationship, and if patients themselves remain involved in the decision making.[63] AGS and the National Highway and Traffic Safety Administration have prepared a guide for clinicians to assess driving fitness and information regarding state-by-state reporting requirements for clinicians.[64] Deficits in executive function, working memory, attention, and visuospatial awareness may all be indicators that a patient is no longer safe to drive. Formal driving assessments by occupational therapy and/or local departments of motor vehicles may help make a determination

that patients can no longer safely drive. Providers should be familiar with their state-specific reporting laws for suspected impaired driving.

### Gun Safety

An estimated 42% of older adults either own firearms or live in households where firearms are present.[65] The primary safety risk for people living with dementia from firearms is suicide because both dementia and depression are risk factors. Presence of guns also carries a risk of harm to family or intruders. Primary care clinicians should inquire about access to firearms and counsel patients and family members about options for enhancing safety through relocation, secure storage, and devices that disable the firearm.[65]

### In-Home Safety

Family and caregivers benefit from coaching to address common home safety hazards, particularly coaching that aligns to the caregivers' health literacy level and uses principles of self-efficacy.[66] Specific areas requiring attention include removing unused medications, prevention of injuries in the bathroom, protecting against injuries in the kitchen, and injuries associated with leaving the home unattended.[67] Physical and occupational therapists can perform in-home assessments to address specific safety and falls risks, and recommend appropriate adaptive equipment. In addition, patients and caregivers should have a plan for natural disasters such as fire or severe weather. Patients should have a disaster care plan in place that addresses possibilities such as power outages or need for evacuation. The Federal Emergency Management Agency provides guidance on developing a disaster plan.

### Nutrition

Adequate nutrition can be threatened by a number of dementia-related impairments across the stages of illness, and therefore routine screening for malnutrition is recommended.[68] During early stages, patients may forget to throw out spoiled food or miss mealtimes without adequate social cueing. Executive dysfunction may impair grocery shopping or meal preparation. Fire hazards, such as leaving the stove on, should be addressed proactively as part of an in-home safety evaluation.

In moderate stages of dementia, patients will likely need their meals prepared by others, and patients may require prompting to remember to eat. Meal delivery services, including Meals on Wheels, may be an option for patients with limited social support. Oral nutritional supplements can promote weight gain, but do not improve functional status or survival.[69] Maintaining good oral health may improve intake and helps prevent aspiration. In more advanced stages of disease, swallowing dysfunction may occur, and careful positioning and handfeeding may be required. Use of enteral feeding is not supported by evidence.[70] Instead, hand-feeding by a caregiver provides socialization and pleasure in the late stages of AD. Patients will eventually lose their thirst and hunger drives and refuse even hand-feeding. This is part of the natural progression of the disease course, and families should be reassured that patients are not "starving" or uncomfortable as a result.

### Finances and Scams

Older adults with cognitive impairment are at risk of a number of adverse financial outcomes. They may miss bill payments and accrue late fees, overpay bills or services, misplace cash, or inadvertently give away personal information, such as account numbers or social security numbers. In addition, older adults with cognitive impairment are often maliciously targeted by scam artists in person, on the telephone, or online. In the United States, adults with dementia should consider freezing their credit to protect themselves from identity theft. A trusted family member or attorney should be provided access to bank accounts to monitor for suspicious activity. If patients have problematic behaviors, such as giving money away or misplacing cash, consider removing debit cards, credit cards, and checkbooks from the home and only allowing the patient to carry a small amount of cash at a time. Payment information that is stored in online browsers or websites should be deleted. Family members may eventually need to seek a financial power of attorney to manage finances in the best interest of the patient. If there is no family member willing or able to take on this role, a financial surrogate may need to be appointed by the court system. However, the patient should continue to participate in financial discussions and decision making as their cognition allows.

## Management of Comorbid Conditions

### Depression in Dementia

Prevalence studies estimate that > 10% of patients with AD and as many as half of patients with vascular dementia meet criteria for major depression.[71] Screening for depression in patients with dementia may be challenging. In early stages of dementia, providers can continue to use validated tools for screening for depression in older adults, such as the personal health questionnaire (PHQ-9), geriatric depression scale, or the Koenig depression scale.[72–74] However, as the disease progresses, patients may not be able to provide reliable answers to screening questions. Instead, caregivers or providers may note depressive symptoms, such as anhedonia, crying spells, apathy, and changes in sleep or appetite.

There is limited evidence for nonpharmacologic treatment of depression in dementia. Cognitive behavioral therapy and counseling may be effective for patients with mild dementia who can still meaningfully participate. Exercise has been shown to be effective for treating depressive symptoms.[75] Pharmacologic treatment should be pursued in patients with moderate-to-severe symptoms that are causing distress; selective serotonin reuptake inhibitors are considered first-line therapy.

### Delirium

Delirium is defined as an abrupt change in mental status, resulting in confusion and alterations in awareness. DSM-5 criteria include the presence of acute onset of mental status changes and/or fluctuating course, inattention, and the presence of either disorganized thinking or alterations in consciousness.[7] Delirium is often precipitated by acute illness, a change in environment, a metabolic disturbance, a medication effect, or other contributing factors. A preexisting history of cognitive impairment is a major risk factor for developing delirium. In older adults with dementia at baseline, it may be challenging to detect sudden changes in mental status, underscoring the importance of documenting patients' baseline functional and cognitive status.

If a patient with dementia is admitted to the hospital, a primary care provider or caregiver can provide valuable information about the patient's baseline cognition, so changes can be rapidly detected and addressed.[76] Delirium is distressing for patients and family members, increases hospital length of stay, risk of nosocomial infections and falls, risk of institutionalization, and is associated with increased mortality.[77] Providers of patients with dementia should be vigilant in screening for and treating delirium as it occurs. Importantly, incident delirium is often associated an irreversible decline in cognition in patients with dementia. No pharmacologic treatment for delirium exists, and treatment consists of managing precipitating factors.

## Preventive Care in Dementia

Particularly in the mild dementia, patients should continue to receive standard-of-care treatment for their medical illnesses. There is some evidence to suggest that excellent control of blood sugar, hypertension, and other comorbidities may slow cognitive decline. Patients should also receive all recommended vaccinations. Cancer screenings can be considered in patients with mild dementia if aligned with their goals of care. As dementia progresses to moderate-severe stages of illness, the benefit of aggressive management of cardiovascular risk factors is unclear. Emphasis should shift to keeping patients safe—for example, administration of insulin may be deemed too high risk. Providers should check in with patients and caregivers early and often to clarify goals of care, with a gradual shift toward keeping patients comfortable and in a safe environment.

❖❖ **Office visits can be traumatic for patients living with dementia. Work with the patients and caregivers to plan for visits in advance by writing down questions and concerns, and encourage a care partner to accompany the patient at each visit, to promote understanding of recommendations and follow-through.**

## Dementia Care Management Issues

### Advanced Care Planning

Discussions around advance directives and designation of a healthcare agent and a financial decision-making surrogate are best undertaken in the early stages of illness when the patient can most clearly articulate preferences and goals and when decision-making capacity remains intact. In addition, providers, patients, and caregivers should partner to develop plans for transportation, medication administration, housing, and other anticipated needs that will arise as the disease progresses.

### Behavioral and Psychological Symptoms of Dementia

BPSD, also known as neuropsychological symptoms of dementia, are common. There are a variety of manifestations, from crying spells and agitation to hallucinations or apathy. BPSD leads to increased caregiver burden and institutionalization.

Behavioral symptoms are best understood as an attempt to express an unmet physical or psychosocial need, and treatment centers on identifying and addressing these needs, or preferably, anticipating the unmet need before it arises. A general approach to behavioral symptom management has been described using the acronym DICE: describe, investigate, create, and evaluate, to guide both family and paid caregivers to develop problem-solving skills that underpin all symptom management interventions.[78] Other nonpharmacologic techniques for addressing BPSD include distraction, redirection, and managing behavioral triggers.[79] Patients should also be evaluated for superimposed delirium, which should be treated if present.

Family or staff caregivers may require assistance from behavioral health experts or psychiatrists to fully understand and manage symptoms. As noted previously, memantine has been shown to have some effect on behavioral symptoms, generally in moderate stage disease, but has not been shown to reduce agitation. Cholinesterase inhibitors have not been shown to improve BPSD. Pharmacotherapy for behavioral symptoms generally has more risks than benefits, but has a limited role in patients with troublesome symptoms that do not respond to nonpharmacologic interventions. Pharmacologic therapy for BPSD is beyond the scope of this chapter; it should be provided under the care of a specialist with experience in the management of BPSD.

❖ **Behavioral and psychological symptoms of dementia (BPSD) are distressing for patients and families, and require an individualized approach to assessment and management. These symptoms often communicate unmet physical or psychosocial needs. Connecting caregivers with experts in behavioral analysis, such as psychiatrists or specialized dementia care clinics, may be necessary to adequately address BPSD.[80]**

## End-of-Life Care

As function and ability to communicate decline, patients will require progressively more care from family or paid caregivers. Quality of life and avoiding unnecessary or futile medical interventions are key foci of care. When quality of life was studied by interviewing proxy respondents among nursing home residents, awareness of self and enjoyment of activities declined as illness progressed.[81] These proxy respondents identified a variety of approaches that they believed enhanced quality of life for their loved ones, including being able to engage socially at mealtime or outside the facility, engaging in activities that are consistent with the patient's life history, use of personalized music, maintaining relationships with staff, having preferences for medical care respected, attending to physical care to promote hygiene, and environmental features that promote comfort and respect. Use of tools, such as those provided through the physicians' orders for life-sustaining treatment (POLST) paradigm, can facilitate avoiding unnecessary care.

Hospice care, although associated with better pain control and greater family satisfaction with end-of-life care, is underused in dementia, in part because of the difficulty of predicting whether someone with dementia has a life expectancy of ≤ 6 months. Indications for hospice care in severe dementia include severe dysmobility, loss of communication abilities, and development of malnutrition or dysphagia. Patients with a score of ≥ 7

on the functional assessment staging scale are also generally eligible for hospice care.[82] Regardless of whether hospice care is sought, clinicians should pay particular attention to pain assessment and management and should consider deprescribing medications that do not have a clear indication. Even dementia-specific treatments, including cholinesterase inhibitors and memantine, are likely of little to no benefit in latest stages of dementia, and providers should explore discontinuation with family members.

## CASE

### Discussion

During Mr. Frank's initial presentation, a number of warning signs for possible cognitive impairment are present, including his late arrival, poor oral hygiene, and inability to articulate his medications. However, without understanding the patient's baseline cognition, biopsychosocial situation, and functional status, it is impossible to say whether Mr. Frank is experiencing a pathologic change in his cognition consistent with mild cognitive impairment or dementia. Immediate next steps would be obtaining collateral history from a trusted friend or family member. Administering a brief objective cognitive test would be helpful, but it cannot be interpreted without appropriate clinical context, including a complete history and physical examination. If Mr. Frank has evidence of a cognitive disorder, important next steps would be addressing immediate safety concerns. You should assess the risk and benefits of continuing anticoagulation and, if appropriate, consider a pill box, frequent monitoring of INR, and other measures such as enlisting family assistance to ensure proper medication administration. Other safety issues, including ensuring adequate access to nutrition, financial security, and a driving evaluation, would all be important early steps in Mr. Frank's care. In addition, Mr. Frank will require ongoing management of his chronic medical conditions and age-appropriate preventative care. Frequent follow-up appointments in short intervals will help to accomplish these care goals, ensure patient safety, and develop a rapport with the patient and his family.

The call from Mr. Frank's niece raises a variety of important questions for his management, including distinguishing whether his new symptoms are caused by progression of dementia versus whether his symptoms can be explained by unrecognized pain, delirium, or a combination of the two. Because Mr. Frank is living in an assisted living facility, you will need to arrange for an in-person assessment of Mr. Frank to evaluate his current health status and to develop a plan for addressing his new symptoms. Ideally, the assessment is conducted at the assisted living residence to observe his behavior and interactions with staff. Furthermore, Mr. Frank may become more agitated during transportation to a clinic visit. Options to obtain the in-residence assessment include performing a house-call, or involving a home health agency to obtain a registered nurse assessment and to obtain necessary laboratory studies.

In addition to evaluating the patient for delirium and potential precipitating causes such as pain or dehydration, consider using the DICE model to guide your assessment of his symptoms, and ongoing communication with additional team members, including Mr. Frank's family, the assisted living staff, and the home health agency staff if they are involved. Keep in mind that Mr. Frank may not be able to respond to conventional pain assessment tools, but observational instruments, such as the pain assessment in advance dementia (PAIN-AD), have demonstrated reliability for patients with moderate to severe dementia.[83] Table 18.9 summarizes the results of Mr. Frank's assessment and indicates that he has pain upon sitting that is likely caused by a postfall coccygeal bruise. Managing his pain effectively should relieve the behavioral symptoms and result in a return to baseline.

| TABLE 18.9 | Case Study—Using DICE to Assess Mr. Frank |
|---|---|

| DICE Component | Findings |
|---|---|
| Describe | Looks relaxed while lying in the bed and walking, but when sitting, immediately becomes restless and grimaces frequently<br>No inattention nor fluctuation in cognitive status |
| Investigate | Physical examination reveals bruising around coccyx, pain on palpation, but no deformity. He is able to drink and eat independently, but seems more willing to eat or drink while standing |
| Create | Initiate scheduled acetaminophen to control pain and physical therapist referral for special cushioning. Pursue other nonpharmacologic approaches to pain management (ice, heat)<br>Offer finger foods and drinks while standing up in dining room |
| Evaluate | Monitor behavioral response to acetaminophen, including reduction in grimacing, agitation, and food intake<br>If agitation does not improve, consider evaluation by psychologist or other behavioral specialist |

## Summary

Cognition changes as we age, such that older adults experience delays in processing and recall. These changes may be distressing to patients, but are not indicative of pathologic cognitive dysfunction. Rather, they represent the normal aging process. Cognitive disorders exist on a spectrum. Preclinical changes manifest as subtle neurostructural changes or changes in biomarker levels without clinical signs or symptoms; this stage of disease is a focus of ongoing research. Mild cognitive impairment is defined as cognitive changes beyond what is expected from normal aging but with preserved function, and may or may not be a precursor of eventual dementia. Dementia is defined as cognitive dysfunction across multiple domains with impaired functioning. AD is the most common cause of dementia. Early detection of dementia can help patients and caregivers make appropriate long-term arrangements and allow for interventions that may slow cognitive decline, although there are no disease-modifying treatments available. Treatment should be person centered, encompass the patient's psychosocial context, and focus on enhancing wellbeing. Attention should be particularly paid to addressing safety issues, assessing and addressing caregiver support needs, and focusing early on advanced care planning.

### Web Resources

Administration on Community Living Eldercare Locator: www.eldercare.gov/

Alzheimer's Association: https://www.alz.org/

Department of Veterans Affairs resources for Alzheimer's and Dementia Care: https://www.va.gov/GERIATRICS/pages/Alzheimers_And_Dementia_Care.asp

Department of Veterans Affairs Shared Decision-Making Resources: https://www.va.gov/GERIATRICS/Guide/LongTermCare/Making_Decisions.asp

National Institute on Aging Alzheimer's Disease Education and Referral (ADEAR) Center: https://www.nia.nih.gov/health/about-adear-center

Physician's Orders for Life Sustaining Treatment (POLST) form and website: https://polst.org/faq/

Veterans Affairs videos for caregiver: https://www.ruralhealth.va.gov/vets/resources.asp

University of California Los Angeles caregiver education videos: https://www.uclahealth.org/dementia/caregiver-education

US Department of Veterans Affairs. *Pharmacy Benefits Management Services*. 2018 [cited October 15, 2019]. Available at: https://www.pbm.va.gov/.

## Key References

19. Querfurth HW, LaFerla FM. Mechanisms of disease. *N Engl J Med*. 2010;362(4):329−344.
30. Robinson L, Tang E, Taylor JP. Dementia: timely diagnosis and early intervention. *BMJ*. 2015;350:h3029.
42. Lee L, Weston WW. Disclosing a diagnosis of dementia: helping learners to break bad news. *Can Fam Physician*. 2011;57(7):851−852.
48. American Geriatrics Society Expert Panel on Person-Centered Care. Person-centered care: a definition and essential elements. *J Am Geriatr Soc*. 2016;64(1):15−18.

**References available online at expertconsult.com.**

# 19

# Depression

DANIELLE GOLDFARB, OMAIR H. ABBASI, AND WILLIAM J. BURKE

## OUTLINE

## OBJECTIVES

*Upon completion of this chapter, the reader will be able to:*

- Understand the impact of depression on a patient's general medical condition and quality of life.
- Identify risk factors for depression and suicide, and interventions for each.
- Describe the differences in presentation between late-life depression and early-onset depression.
- Assess for various types of depression, including major depression, subsyndromal or minor depression, persistent depressive disorder, and depression secondary to substance use or a general medical condition.

- List common screening tools and lab tests to be performed when considering a diagnosis of depression.
- Discuss treatment options for depression, including medications, psychotherapy, electroconvulsive therapy (ECT), and rapid transcranial magnetic stimulation (rTMS).
- Identify cases that need referral to a psychiatrist or emergent psychiatric intervention.

## Prevalence and Impact

People age $\geq 65$ years make up 16% of the total US population.[1] In 2035 the United States will reach a new milestone when, for the first time in history, adults age $> 65$ years will outnumber children age $< 18$ years (78 million vs. 76.7 million, respectively).[2] Depression is common in older adults with estimated prevalence rates of 1% to 3% in the community and up to 10% to 15% in primary care settings.[3–5] Depression comprises the largest category of psychiatric disorder in older adults and is currently the fifth leading cause of disability as estimated by disability-adjusted life years.[6] Meanwhile, depression in older adults, or late-life depression (LLD), is underdiagnosed and undertreated, and there is limited availability of geriatric psychiatrists. By the year 2030, it is estimated that there will be approximately 2640 geriatric psychiatrists in the United States, or 1 per 5682 older adults with a psychiatric disorder.[7] It is therefore imperative that primary care providers (PCPs) are able to detect and treat depression in older adults.

There is a common misconception that depression occurring in late life is a normal part of aging, or a normal reaction to stressors, such as retirement, the loss of loved ones, medical ailments, and loss of independence. In fact, an enduring finding in epidemiologic studies is that only a small number of older adults living in the community admit being depressed.[8] Rates of depression are higher in older adults who require more care or are in institutional settings. Some 14% of patients receiving in-home care[9,10] and between 14% and 20% of nursing home residents[11,12] meet criteria for depression. However, only a small percentage of older patients with depression receive proper treatment for their symptoms; those most likely to receive inadequate or no treatment for their depression are male, Black, Latino, and those with a preference for counseling over antidepressant treatment.[13,14]

Depression in older adults is often associated with significant morbidity and mortality. Schulz et al. followed a group of > 5000 individuals age > 65 years and found that those with higher baseline depressive symptoms were 1.5 times more likely to die.[15] The mortality rate coincided with the level of depression even when controlling for other factors. Another study following > 7000 community-dwelling older adults over 9 years found that depressive symptoms at baseline were associated with increased mortality independent of cardiovascular events.[16] LLD is related not only to increased mortality but also increased morbidity. Older patients who were depressed at baseline and underwent certain cardiac procedures were found to have increased postoperative mortality compared with nondepressed counterparts.[17] Older patients who report depressive symptoms are also more likely to report a lower quality of life, higher level of chronic pain, and increased disability.[18] LLD is also associated with significant economic burden, including direct and indirect costs. Medically ill patients with depression have increased total healthcare costs, including greater healthcare utilization, medications, and nonmedical resources, such as social services. One study found that depressed patients with heart failure and diabetes had almost double the healthcare costs of nondepressed patients ($20,046 vs. $11,956).[19] Snow and Abrams[20] provide a comprehensive review of the indirect costs of LLD, which include productivity losses incurred by the patient, family, employer, and society. The greatest driver of indirect costs is unpaid, informal caregivers, typically family and friends, who are serving as primary caregivers of older adults with depression, estimated at $9.1 billion,[21] which is $16.1 billion in year 2019, using the US government consumer price index data.[22]

◆◆ **Depression is a significant illness that affects level of functioning, quality of life, cost of care, and mortality. It is not a normal part of aging and is the fifth leading cause of disability among older adults in the United States.**

## Risk Factors and Pathophysiology

LLD shares much in common with depression occurring earlier in life but has unique, distinguishing characteristics in presentation, etiology, and risk factors. Biologic, psychological, and social influences together are implicated in LLD. In younger adults, the stress-diathesis model is one of the more popular explanations for why people develop depression. This theory suggests that both genetic vulnerability and psychosocial factors play important roles. In contrast, there is less consistent evidence for genetic predisposition as a major contributor to LLD, with studies showing little correlation between family history and late-onset depression.[23] However, other neurobiologic factors are important. For example, compromises in brain neurocircuitry, particularly in frontolimbic pathways, have a strong association with many depressive disorders in late life. This may explain the high incidence of depression in patients with neurologic conditions affecting these pathways, such as stroke, cerebrovascular disease, Parkinson disease (PD), and Alzheimer disease (AD).[24]

Although the biologic processes of LLD may separate it from early-onset depression, the stress diathesis model is still useful in emphasizing the importance of psychosocial risk factors[23] (Box 19.1). These risk factors in turn can be modified by other factors, including a patient's coping skills and the presence of ongoing stress outside of the context of the psychosocial risk factor. As well, the concept of resilience has gained increasing research attention with respect to its role in LLD development and outcomes.[25] It should also be recognized that most individuals with a given risk factor will not meet depressive diagnostic criteria. Rather, the risk factors should be considered when suspecting depression and in the formulation of treatment.

**CASE**

### Ms. Smith (Part 1)

Ms. Smith is a 68-year-old White female who lost her husband to cancer 15 months ago. Ms. Smith's daughter accompanies her to the office and states that since the loss of her husband, Ms. Smith has become short-tempered with her family. She skips family dinners and when she does attend, she tearfully discusses the loss of her husband. The daughter also mentions that Ms. Smith has refused to pack her husband's personal belongings and that they remain in the closet. Ms. Smith admits that she has feelings of bitterness about losing her husband and cannot seem to stop thinking about him. She often feels that if she had done something differently, her husband may have lived. Ms. Smith's daughter feels that her mother has refused to heal and is concerned about depression.

What is your current differential diagnosis for Ms. Smith?
What additional questions would you want to ask?

## Diagnosis of Late-Life Depression

Diagnosing depression in older adults can be a challenge. Although the *Diagnostic and Statistical Manual of Mental Disorders, Fifth Edition* (DSM-V) diagnostic criteria for major depressive disorder (MDD) are the basic construct for depression in the older population, there are distinctions in how depression may present. Older depressed individuals have a higher tendency to have somatic complaints (primarily gastrointestinal), illness anxiety, and irritability but are less likely to have low self-esteem or guilt compared with younger persons.[26] In addition, older depressed patients tend to have a higher rate of psychotic and severe (melancholic) depression with more weight loss and decreased appetite.[27] It is not uncommon in the clinical setting that an older depressed adult denies depressive or mood symptoms during history-taking and on questionnaires, but older adults instead report a multitude of physical symptoms. When, upon further investigation, the somatic complaints are out of proportion to medical illness, the clinician should suspect depression may be present. Querying family members or friends of the patient is important to clarify whether depression may be playing a role, and those individuals may report that the patient has lost interest in activities or has had a change in affect. There may also be a chronologic correlation between new or worsening physical complaints and the onset of an identifiable stressor that alerts the provider to consider depression as a diagnosis.

Two other subtypes of depression of importance are persistent depressive disorder (formerly dysthymic disorder) and minor or subsyndromal depression. Persistent depressive disorder was characterized initially in the DSM-V and considered a consolidation of dysthymic disorder and chronic depressive disorder. Persistent depressive disorder is a more chronic, less severe form of MDD. Diagnostic criteria for persistent depressive disorder are characterized by duration longer than 2 years with two or more of the following symptoms: poor appetite or overeating, sleep disturbance, low energy or fatigue, difficulty with concentration, indecisiveness, feelings of hopelessness, and low self-esteem (DSM-V). Unlike MDD, persistent depressive disorder is associated with a younger age of onset,[28] and presenting symptoms are similar to younger cohorts. Although persistent depressive disorder is unlikely to begin in late life, it may persist from midlife into late life.[29]

Subsyndromal depression was previously known as minor depression in the DSM-IV-TR and revised to "Other specified depressive disorder, depressive episode with insufficient symptoms" in the DSM-V. Subsyndromal depression is diagnosed when the number of depressive symptoms is between two and four symptoms, which is below the number needed to establish a diagnosis of MDD. Several epidemiologic studies have shown subsyndromal depression to have a two to three times higher prevalence than MDD in older adults, with a point prevalence of approximately 9.8% in community-dwelling older adults and as high as 35% of primary care geriatric patients.[30] Furthermore, this form of depression becomes more prevalent with advancing age[31] and therefore often cooccurs with medical comorbidities; when additional external factors exist, such as loneliness, decreased mobility, spousal death, and financial stressors, the constellation often leads to increasing functional disability, similar to that of MDD, and increased mortality.[32] One study identified vision loss as the medical illness most readily associated with this form of depression.[33] Given the potential increased morbidity and mortality associated with undetected, untreated subsyndromal depression, primary care physicians and specialists alike should consider the use of validated, age-specific depression screening tools (to be discussed later) to support diagnosis and treatment.

⏺⏺ **Depressed patients who are age 65 years and older are more likely to present with somatic complaints or illness anxiety rather than guilt or low self-esteem.**

**Older people may develop masked depression in which there is a lack of reported depressed mood. Assessing for anhedonia and corroborating history with family members is vital.**

**There is a higher incidence of subsyndromal depression than major depressive disorder in older adults.**

## Differential Diagnosis

### Normal Grief and Bereavement

Diagnosing depression can be particularly difficult in the setting of bereavement where the overlap of symptoms typical of normal grieving and major depression can be extensive. However, multiple studies have shown that the two can be differentiated and that persons who develop LLD after loss of a loved one have distinctive outcomes. What differentiates any normative process from psychopathology is its effect on functioning. Typically, the bereaved individual does not become functionally impaired or is minimally impaired. Grief and bereavement also do not typically involve active suicidal thinking; rather, the bereaved may have passive thoughts about "joining" their loved one. Although it is not uncommon for grieving individuals to feel that they have seen their loved one in a crowd or hear the deceased calling their name, florid psychosis in the form of prolonged auditory or visual hallucinations and delusions should raise suspicion of another underlying psychiatric disorder. Cultural background plays a major role in the length of time an individual will grieve, but it is generally expected that a person will begin recovery within 1 year after his or her loss.

### Complicated Grief

An evolving concept in the study of grief is complicated grief, a protracted, severe form of grieving in which a person experiences strong feelings of anger or bitterness about the loved one's death, feelings of emptiness, a persistent longing to be with the loved one, recurring intrusive thoughts about the loss, and reclusiveness from family and friends.[34] Complicated grief occurs in 7% to 20% of bereaved individuals in the general population,[35,36] with higher estimates of 25% in older adults.[37] Criteria and terminology for complicated bereavement were revised in the DSM-V, which provided provisional criteria for persistent complex bereavement disorder (PCBD), listed in Section III, Conditions For Further Study (DSM-V). A diagnosis of PCBD requires that symptoms must persist for at least 12 months. A working group for the International Classification of Disease-11 proposed the inclusion of a diagnosis of prolonged grief disorder,[38] which requires symptoms to be present for at least 6 months.

Complicated grief differs from clinical depression in that the former's presenting symptoms are more focused on the loss. Although both diagnoses carry some level of dysfunction, the distinction is important because persons experiencing complicated grief have inconsistent responses to antidepressants and psychotherapeutic treatments useful for MDD.[39] Shear and colleagues developed complicated grief therapy (CGT), as specific therapy in this condition.[40] CGT combines features of cognitive behavioral and interpersonal therapy in which patients revisit the loss of their loved one under guidance of a therapist to bring resolution. The therapist also aids the individual to engage in situations and activities that were once avoided because of the loss. Preliminary studies show that CGT has better results than standard interpersonal therapy for treatment of complicated grief[40] and specifically in an older adult population.[41]

### Depression and Cognitive Impairment

A particular challenge occurs when depression overlaps with cognitive impairment. In one scenario, depression may arise simultaneously with cooccurring cognitive dysfunction. This presentation has a variety of names, including depressive pseudodementia and dementia syndrome of depression. The initial view was that patients developed cognitive deficits as one element of a severe neurovegetative state related to a depressive disorder and that, as the depression resolved, so did cognitive impairments. What is apparent now is that this clinical presentation includes a number of conditions that can be distinguished largely by their outcomes. Astute history taking is crucial to delineate the timeline of symptom onset because the classic presentation described earlier is one of the truly reversible causes of dementia. It is now known that even those who have an excellent response to depression treatment and initial resolution of cognitive symptoms have an increased risk of developing dementia in ensuing years.[42] In recent decades, more attention has been paid to depression as a risk factor or prodromal feature of neurodegenerative dementing diseases. For example, some patients develop a late-life depressive disorder without cognitive decline and, over time, gradually become cognitively impaired and eventually progressing to dementia.

An interesting study further explored the relationship between depression and dementia by examining if depression that first occurred in midlife carried a different prognosis than that developed for the first time in the senium. The risk of developing dementia was increased by 20% when midlife depressive symptoms were present, by 70% when only late-life symptoms were present, and by 80% when depressive symptoms were present at both times.[43] When these risks were evaluated by type of dementia, subjects with LLD had only a twofold increase in risk of AD. However, patients with depressive symptoms in both midlife and late life had a more than threefold increase in vascular dementia risk. The authors concluded that depression occurring either in midlife or in late life is associated with a higher risk of developing dementia and that the pattern is important. New depression in late life is more likely to be part of an AD prodrome, and recurrent depression is more strongly associated with vascular dementia.[43] One longitudinal study found somewhat contrasting results. Following more than 10,000 individuals over a 28-year period, the authors found that those reporting depression in late life had a higher risk of developing dementia; whereas midlife depression was not associated with risk of later dementia.[44]

Besides major depression in older adults, more subtle depressive symptoms and other mild psychiatric symptoms in late life have been found to be associated with later development of mild cognitive impairment (MCI) and dementia. The term *mild behavioral impairment* has been proposed as a diagnostic construct describing this transitional syndrome of mild psychiatric symptoms and persistent behavioral changes with minimal to no cognitive or functional impairment.[45] Data analyzed from the National Alzheimer's coordinating centers volunteers, which maintain longitudinal clinical and neuropathologic data from Alzheimer disease centers across the country, found that depression was present in 24% of individuals before onset of MCI. In a prospective cohort study of cognitively healthy older adults, the presence of various neuropsychiatric symptoms (NPS), including depression, agitation, apathy, anxiety, and/or irritability, significantly predicted incident MCI risk compared with older adults without such NPS.[46] Another common pattern is the subset of patients with minimal to MCI or mild dementia who develop depressive symptoms after the onset of cognitive symptoms. At times this reflects the overlap in symptoms that dementia and depression share: decreased energy, problems with concentration, sleep disruption, psychomotor changes, and loss of interest.[47] Families often ascribe these changes to depression; however, apathy is frequently one of the most common behavioral and psychological syndromes that affects those with early AD.

Technological advances have helped to begin to elucidate the neurobiologic changes potentially linking AD and depression. Although it is well established that cerebral amyloid deposition begins decades before the clinical symptoms of AD, the presence of AD neuroimaging and fluid biomarkers in LLD is garnering more recent interest. A cross-sectional neuroimaging study exploring the deposition of amyloid and tau protein using positron emission tomography scans found a higher binding rate in patients with a diagnosis of MDD. Moreover, these protein depositions were found in the posterior cingulate and lateral temporal areas of the brain known to be involved in AD.[48] In addition, a study by Gerritsen et al. exploring depression and its correlation with changes in hippocampal and entorhinal volumes noted that patients experiencing a first episode of depression in late life exhibited volume loss in entorhinal rather than hippocampal structures, the latter being seen in early-onset depression.[49] Elevated levels of cerebrospinal fluid and neuroimaging AD biomarkers have been found in individuals with LLD and other mood symptoms in various prospective cohort studies of cognitively normal older adults.[50–52] Although this preliminary evidence for an underlying biologic correlation between AD and depression is intriguing, further studies are needed before a definite connection can be established.

❖❖ **Depression and dementia are frequently intertwined in older people, with high rates of depression in patients with dementia, and depression itself being a risk factor for dementia.**

## Depression Secondary to a General Medical Condition

A common caveat in the DSM-V regarding a psychiatric diagnosis is that "the symptoms are not caused by the direct physiological effects of a substance or a general medical condition." Given that comorbid illness itself is a risk factor for depression, it is difficult to differentiate whether a physical illness is causing depression or indirectly adding to it as a risk factor.

This relationship has been extensively explored in the setting of stroke with depression being both a risk factor[53] and result of stroke. Approximately 20% of stroke survivors develop MDD and another 20% develop subsyndromal depression.[54] Numerous potential pathophysiologic factors have been implicated, including inflammatory processes, genetic and epigenetic variations, white matter disease, cerebrovascular deregulation, altered neuroplasticity, and changes in glutamate neurotransmission.[55] Those that develop poststroke depression tend to have a greater functional decline in activities of daily living (ADLs),[56] less recovery of function,[57] greater impairment of cognition,[58] and increased mortality[59] compared with nondepressed stroke patients. Adequate treatment of poststroke depression improves outcomes in both ADLs and cognitive impairment.[60,61] In addition, preventative treatment after stroke with antidepressants may reduce incidence of significant morbidity and mortality. A multicenter randomized controlled trial (RCT) compared escitalopram to placebo or problem-solving therapy (PST) for prevention of depression 1 year after acute stroke. Patients receiving placebo were five times more likely to develop poststroke depression compared with escitalopram, and those receiving PST were two times more likely.[62] A follow-up study showed patients given escitalopram were more likely to develop depression 6 months after discontinuation of treatment whereas patients receiving PST or placebo were not.[63]

Even in the absence of clinical stroke, cerebrovascular mechanisms are associated with depression and have been proposed as a distinct subtype of depression, characterized clinically by symptoms, including prominent psychomotor retardation, apathy, and disability; vascular lesions on neuroimaging; a poor response to treatment; unstable remissions; and a higher risk of developing dementia.[64] Alexopoulos[65] first described the vascular hypothesis for LLD, postulating that cerebrovascular disease plays a critical role in provoking and perpetuating depressive symptoms as a result of structural damage to frontal–subcortical circuits. The diagnosis of vascular depression remains controversial because of a lack of definitive biologic or neuroanatomic substrates and is invoked primarily by neuroimaging findings of white matter hyperintensities on T2 weighted or fluid attenuated inversion recovery magnetic resonance imaging (MRI), subcortical lacunes, microinfarcts, microhemorrhages, along with frontal and hippocampal gray atrophy.[66] White matter hyperintensities on MRI are correlated with a decreased response to antidepressants.[67,68] Meanwhile, increased cerebral blood flow in the middle and posterior cingulate following antidepressant treatment is associated with decreases in depressive symptoms in older adults.[69] Likewise, preexisting vascular burden may be a determining factor in whether executive dysfunction improves in older depressives in response to treatment.[70,71] In addition, inflammatory markers (C-reactive protein), fasting glucose, diabetes mellitus,[72] and the metabolic syndrome, which all have effects on vascular functioning, have been independently associated with the onset of depressive symptoms in older adults.[73]

Other chronic medical illnesses with high rates of depression are arthritis, heart disease, and cancer; in these, the level of functional disability is strongly associated with depression.[74] The most robust data available are in patients with heart disease. Cardiac conditions, such as heart failure and acute myocardial infarction (MI), are strongly correlated with depression; approximately 20% to 40% of individuals with these conditions have MDD.[75] Patients who develop depression shortly after an MI have increased mortality.[76] In fact, patients with ischemic heart disease taking selective serotonin reuptake inhibitors (SSRIs) have a reduced rate of MI.[77] One metaanalysis found that markers of cerebral and peripheral microvascular dysfunction were associated with incident late-life depression.[78] Although heart disease and the other aforementioned conditions correlate with depression, further studies are needed to elucidate the pathophysiologic mechanisms.

◆◆ **Both stroke and heart disease have a strong correlation with depression.**
**Treatment of comorbid depression with antidepressants can significantly improve morbidity and mortality.**

Delirium is a condition that is misdiagnosed as depression up to 40% of the time.[79] Although hyperactive delirium may present with agitation and bizarre behavior, hypoactive delirium displays symptoms similar to depression, including apathy, indecisiveness, and psychomotor retardation, accompanied by memory and functional impairment. The clinical setting for these misdiagnoses is most often the inpatient setting where a patient suddenly begins to refuse interventions or participation in care, and the assumption is that the patient has "given up." Delirium should be suspected if both mood and cognitive symptoms occur with rapid onset (hours to days) and have a fluctuating course. Cognitive screening tests can be serially administered to document changes in cognition. The primary treatment for delirium is to find the underlying cause. Antidepressants have no role in this setting.

## Substance-Induced Depression

According to a 2012 report from the Institute of Medicine approximately 5.6 to 8 million older adults had one or more mental health or substance use conditions. This number is expected to increase 80% by the year 2030.[80] Substance abuse, although not as common among older adults, is an important problem in late life that can lead to significant morbidity and mortality. As a result, mood disorders related to substance use should always be included in the differential diagnosis. Alcohol is overwhelmingly the most common misused substance in late life, although with baby boomers aging, marijuana use may become common. Patterns of substance-related inpatient hospitalizations for older adults are changing as well. Though alcohol remains the primary substance triggering inpatient admission, other substances (including cocaine/crack, marijuana/hashish, heroin, nonprescription methadone, and other opiates and synthetics) have increased over time as the primary substance for older adults.

According to the DSM-V criteria, when considering substance-induced depression secondary to drug abuse or dependence, it is important to have chronologic evidence of mood symptoms "developing during, or within a month of, substance intoxication or withdrawal." In some cases, a patient may be using a substance to "self-medicate" the underlying mood disorder. It is important to elicit a history to establish if the mood symptoms were present during extended periods of sobriety.

In addition to substance abuse, iatrogenic depression may also occur from commonly prescribed medications, such as benzodiazepines, opiates, and steroids. Although beta-blockers have received much attention for possibly inducing depression, this association is inconsistent.[81] Regardless of type of medication, if depression begins within 1 month of starting a medication, especially if a patient has no history of prior depression, it can be presumed that it may be medication induced. If depression is possibly secondary to a newly prescribed drug, the medication should be discontinued or substituted, and the patient monitored for mood improvement.

## Assessment

As with diagnosing any illness, thorough history taking is crucial to a correct depression diagnosis. In evaluating an older patient, collateral sources, such as the patient's spouse, family members, and/or professional caregivers, can provide key information, especially in the context of cognitive impairment. This should not, however, be performed in lieu of speaking to the patient but rather to correlate the patient's concerns with others' observations. When taking a history, the clinician should pay close attention to the chronology of the patient's symptoms, especially regarding changes in level of functioning associated with said symptoms. Although older depressed patients may be preoccupied with physical ailments, a connection may be found between symptoms and an acute or chronic stressful event. Significant areas of questioning should include the patient's socialization pattern, ADLs, and level of physical activity. Appetite and weight loss are of high importance because these can be severe in geriatric depression and may even cause failure to thrive. In addition, asking about psychotic symptoms (e.g., delusions and hallucinations) is also important because psychotic depression typically requires intensive pharmacotherapy with an antidepressant and antipsychotic or electroconvulsive therapy.

It is important to screen for bipolar disorders by asking about a history of mania (Box 19.2). Presentation of bipolar depression is virtually identical to unipolar depression, and only properly inquiring about a previous manic episode will differentiate the two. It is also important to avoid antidepressant treatment in bipolar patients, where mood stabilizers, such as lithium and lamotrigine, would be first-line treatment.

• BOX 19.2 **Abbreviated Criteria for Identifying a Manic Episode**

- A distinct period of time (at least 7 days) where a person's mood becomes persistently elevated, expansive, and/or irritable. During this time the patient also displays at least three of the following symptoms:
  a. Inflated self-esteem and grandiosity—Patient may start challenging authority at the workplace. May become suspicious that others are talking about or plotting against him or her.
  b. Decrease in need for sleep—Patient may sleep for only 3 hours per night without experiencing any tiredness during the day. Make sure to ask about daytime naps to rule out underlying sleep disorder.
  c. Increase in distractibility—Patient may have difficulty focusing on one task at a time.
  d. Increase in goal-directed activity—Patient may take on multiple projects at once.
  e. Impulsivity—Patient may partake in risky behaviors without considering the consequences.
  f. Rapid thinking or racing thoughts—Patient may have multiple unrelated thoughts at the same time and find it difficult to express these thoughts to others.
  g. Talkativity—Patient finds oneself speaking rapidly, often forcing others to interrupt.

**Considerations**

- Emphasize to the patient that these symptoms have to be both persistent and present together as an episode. Many depressed patients experience some of these symptoms between episodes of depression or from a comorbid anxiety disorder.
- Verify that the patient was not using illicit substances during these episodes.
- In questionable cases, a collateral source can help in establishing a diagnosis.

## CASE

### Ms. Smith (Part 2)

You ask about Ms. Smith's medical history. Ms. Smith states that she feels she may have some form of cancer but is unsure. She reports that she "feels tired and sore all the time" and that "there must be something wrong with me." Her daughter reports that Ms. Smith has worried about having cancer since the loss of her husband. Ms. Smith has had a thorough medical workup regarding the possibility of cancer and was provided with the report; however, she continues to worry. Ms. Smith does take ibuprofen occasionally for muscle aches but otherwise is not taking any medications on a regular basis and has no other past medical history. She admits to being treated for depression in the past with nortriptyline after divorcing her first husband 35 years ago. She denies other past psychiatric history. Ms. Smith also drinks about 4 oz of wine with dinner twice a week. She denies any other substance use. When asked about suicidal thinking, Ms. Smith admits she occasionally longs to join her husband, but denies any thoughts about ending her life.

What screening tests may you want to administer?
What lab tests would you want to order?

Outside of the presenting complaint, additional inquiries regarding the patient's substance use—past and present—are essential because substances play a role in mood regulation, have long-term effects on the brain, and can negate the effects of psychotropic treatment. Medications should also be reviewed, including correlation between onset of symptoms and the start or change in a medication.

Depression rating scales can be useful in identifying depression in an older patient. A commonly used scale is the 15-item version of the Geriatric Depression Scale (GDS).[82] The GDS is unique in that it does not emphasize physical symptoms of depression (e.g., sleep and appetite changes) but focuses on psychological factors to suggest the presence of depression. A score of ≥ 5 suggests a need for further evaluation. The GDS can be administered in 5 to 10 minutes or can be given to the patient to fill out. Other commonly used depression scales include the 9-item Patient Health Questionnaire (PHQ-9)[83] and the Beck Depression Inventory (BDI). Both the PHQ-9 and the BDI have the option of being completed by the patient. The PHQ-9 more closely follows DSM-V diagnostic criteria for MDD. A score of ≥ 10 on the PHQ-9 indicates the possibility of MDD. An even more rapid, simplified screening test is the 2-item PHQ-2 questionnaire, which asks simply about lack of interest and depressed mood yet has a sensitivity of 83% and specificity of 92% for detecting depressive disorders.[84]

It is very important to test cognitive functioning during any assessment for depression using standard rating scales. As mentioned earlier, the relationship between mood and cognition is complex. Although more commonly tested scales, such as the Montreal Cognitive Assessment[85] and the Mini-Mental State Exam (MMSE) require some time to execute, a more rapid test, such as the Mini-Cog screening test, can be useful.[86] In this test, the patient is provided three words that he or she is asked to remember. The patient is then instructed to draw a clock depicting a given time. The administrator of the test monitors the patient's accuracy in drawing the numbers on the face of the clock, the structure of the clock itself, and the appropriate lengths of the minute and hour hands. After completing this task, the patient is asked to repeat the three words provided previously. This abbreviated form of cognitive testing has screening utility similar to the MMSE.[87]

In addition to the score a patient receives, the patient's behavior during testing can provide some clues as to whether depression may be present. Depressed patients often show little effort during examination, readily answer, "I don't know," and have inconsistent memory loss and performance within the examination. In addition, they may respond well to semantic prompts during recall, and their recognition memory may be relatively intact.[88]

❖❖ **It is essential to screen for cognitive dysfunction during evaluation of a patient for depression. The Mini-Cog (described in text) is an efficient screening tool with screening utility similar to the MMSE.**

## Suicide

Suicide can be a difficult topic to broach with patients; however, it is an important aspect of any psychiatric evaluation (Boxes 19.3 and 19.4). If asked, a majority of older adult patients will reveal suicidal thinking if it is present, yet physicians do not address this topic with their most ill and most disabled patients.[89] Although the number of suicide attempts is highest in middle-aged adults and suicide rates in older adults have been trending down over the last several years,[90] suicide nonetheless has special significance in older adults. The most vulnerable population segment is White males; in this group, US suicide rates peak at 49 of 100,000 in the oldest age segment.[91] The rate of suicide among the oldest White males is four times the national age-adjusted rate.[90]

In comparison with younger age groups, in which 1 in 200 suicide attempters die by their own hand, the ratio for completed suicides in older adults is 1 in 4. This could be because younger adults are more likely to attempt suicide impulsively or as a communicative act, whereas older patients make more lethal attempts that

## • BOX 19.3  Suicide Prevention

The following strategies are recommended:
1. Screening for depression
2. Limiting access to means for suicide (e.g., asking about and removing firearms from the home)
3. Addressing issues concerning aging, psychosocial losses, and increasing dependence on others
4. Inquiring about community and family support
5. Close follow-up after initiating mental health treatment

(From Erlangsen A, Nordentoft M, Conwell Y, et al. Key considerations for preventing suicide in older adults: consensus opinions of an expert panel. *Crisis* 2011;32(2):106-109.)

## • BOX 19.4  Approaching a Patient About Suicide— Mastering the Dialogue

1. Break the ice: "When someone is feeling low or depressed, it is not uncommon to have thoughts that life is not worth living or of no longer wanting to be around. Do you ever experience this type of thinking?"
2. Identify the presence or absence of a plan: "Occasionally, when people have this type of thinking, they might also have thoughts about wanting to end their life. Have you ever found yourself thinking this way?"
3. Have the patient expand in detail: "Have you ever thought of a way that you might take your life?" (Providing examples, such as overdosing, etc., is not shown to be harmful and may actually help the patient in providing details.)
4. Establish intent: "Have you ever tried to harm yourself in the past?" "Do you have any thoughts about doing so now?"

they have planned over time.[90] Older patients are also often frail, isolated, and live alone, allowing for little chance of rescue or survival after a suicide attempt. An analysis of Medicare claims of emergency department (ED) visits for deliberate self-harm identified a low percentage of mental health diagnoses coded during emergency treatment and lack of timely follow-up mental health treatment.[92] Less than half (47.2%) of individuals aged 65 to 69 years received a mental health diagnosis in the ED, whereas only 12.2% aged 75 to 79 years did. Furthermore, major risk factors for geriatric suicide (e.g., male gender and high lethality method) did not increase the likelihood of being given a mental disorder diagnosis coded during the ED visit for self-harm. About one-quarter of the Medicare beneficiaries presenting to the ED with self-harm were not hospitalized but rather discharged to the community, and, of those discharged, only 39% received outpatient mental health-care within 30 days. These facts may seem rather daunting, but awareness of this issue allows for interventions, including preventative strategies. Although it is not possible to accurately predict who will attempt suicide, retrospective studies of suicide attempts in persons age 65 years and older have identified several potential risk factors. Psychiatric illness is present in most suicides of older adults (71%–97%) with depression being the most common diagnosis.[90] Importantly, whereas 94% of suicide attempters who are 65 years or older have been seen by a health professional in the past 12 months, only 4% are diagnosed with a mood disorder before the attempt; 51% were diagnosed after the attempt.[93] Older patients are more likely to turn to their PCP than to seek treatment from a mental health specialist, emphasizing the importance of screening for both mood disorders and suicidal ideation by these services. It has been shown that although antidepressants have been associated with increased suicidal ideation or gestures in young adults, they actually significantly decrease its likelihood in older depressed patients,[94] making early identification and treatment imperative.

◆◆ **Older patients with depression and suicidal ideation are more likely to turn to their PCP than to seek treatment from a mental health specialist. Antidepressants significantly decrease suicidal ideation or gestures in older depressed patients.**

In addition to depression, other identifiable factors may alert the PCP to carefully screen for suicide. Important is the patient's current physical health, with studies showing a three- to ninefold increase in risk for suicide depending on the number of cooccurring ailments. Chronic severe pain is particularly important in older men, showing a strong correlation with suicidal thinking. Social factors also play a role, particularly those that may be more common in late life, such as increasing dependence, financial stress, grieving the loss of loved ones, and disruption of social support from family members.[91] An identified protective factor in older adults is "social connectedness." Maintaining social relationships has been shown to decrease mortality by half in older patients[95] and is on par with other healthy habits, such as quitting smoking or losing weight in its health-protective effects.[96] When involvement and collaboration with the patient's family, friends, and professional caregivers (i.e., nursing home staff) is encouraged, this process may also be able to provide additional information regarding the patient's potential suicide risk.[96]

With the time constraints faced by many PCPs, collaborative care models for mental health suggest that treatment management, including measures for suicide prevention, can be facilitated by use of designated care managers or other forms of mental health support workers collaborating closely with PCPs and psychiatric consultants. Studies also show that telephone encounters may substitute for face-to-face interventions for mental health follow-up.[97] In addition to these preventative measures, it is recommended that patients with a history of chronic suicidal ideation or previous suicide attempts be referred to a psychiatric provider. In cases where there is significant concern about a patient's safety, prompt referral to the ED for further mental health evaluation and possible psychiatric hospitalization is necessary.

## Laboratory Testing and Neuroimaging

Laboratory testing is an integral part of assessment for depression. It is not used to arrive at a primary psychiatric diagnosis, but rather to rule out other causes for a patient's mood symptoms. There are many medical conditions that affect mood and may mimic depression. These should be ruled out before initiating antidepressant treatment. Common ailments presenting as depression and their respective lab tests are listed in Table 19.1.

The American Psychiatric Association (APA) does not recommend neuroimaging in the routine clinical diagnostic evaluation of psychiatric disorders except in an exclusionary capacity to rule out neoplasm, hematoma, hydrocephalus, or other treatable neurologic causes or to detect the presence of cerebrovascular disease or atrophy.[98] With regard to depression, neuroimaging is recommended for preelectroconvulsive therapy (pre-ECT) clearance to rule out contraindicated brain pathologies. Given the APA guidelines, neuroimaging, with computed tomography or MRI, may be considered in older patients with late onset first episode depression without obvious psychosocial stressor precipitant, with associated neurologic signs, or with treatment-resistant depression.

| TABLE 19.1 | Medical Conditions and Corresponding Lab Tests | |
|---|---|
| **Medical Condition** | **Lab Test** |
| Hypo-/Hyperthyroidism | TSH/Free T4 |
| Vitamin deficiency | Serum B₁₂, MMA, 25-OH vitamin D, folate |
| Anemia, infection | Complete blood count with differential |
| Urinary tract infection | Urinalysis |

*MMA*, Methylmalonic acid; *T4*, thyroxine; *TSH*, thyroid-stimulating hormone.

## CASE

### Ms. Smith (Part 3)

Ms. Smith scores a 12 on the 15-item GDS. You also administer a MMSE, and Ms. Smith scores 27/30, losing points only for serial 7s. Ms. Smith's electrolytes and liver function tests are within normal limits. You note, however, that Ms. Smith has an elevated thyroid-stimulating hormone (TSH) of 24.4 and a low free thyroxine (T4) of 0.4. Other lab tests, including vitamin B₁₂, folate, and complete blood count, are within normal limits.

What are Ms. Smith's treatment options?
What are some good and bad prognostic factors for Ms. Smith?

## Treatment

There is limited high-quality evidence to inform our understanding of the specific efficacy of pharmacologic treatment of depression in older adults. Depression trials, including patients of any age, depend on careful subject selection to ensure comparability of treatment groups. This is much more challenging in older patients where heterogeneity is inherent, not only psychiatrically but also in terms of medical and psychosocial comorbidities. Another characteristic of placebo-controlled trials of antidepressants in older adults has been high placebo response rates.[99] As in other antidepressant studies, drug–placebo differences are greatest in patients with more severe illness.[100] Trial design also plays an important role in contributing to variable outcomes. Moderators that could affect LLD outcomes, such as psychosocial interventions incorporated into trials, are not consistently measured.[99] Furthermore, antidepressant studies have frequently been criticized for their lack of real-world applicability in terms of the types of patients treated and the clinical setting used in the research study.[101]

Metaanalyses of available studies show mixed evidence of antidepressant efficacy. A metaanalysis by Nelson et al.[102] showed overall improved outcome with antidepressant treatment over placebo; however, the level of improvement varied and was modest. A crucial step in initial LLD monotherapy treatment is ensuring that adequate dose and duration is attempted before switching or augmenting, yet this approach has not been routinely carried out in the primary care setting.[103] The National Institute of Mental Health–sponsored Sequenced Treatment Alternatives to Relieve Depression (STAR*D) study,[104] a clinically based, nonplacebo-controlled study, analyzed remission rates with a stepwise algorithm for depression treatment in psychiatric and primary care settings. This large-scale study found that approximately 30% of depressed adults of all ages treated in medical and mental health settings developed a complete remission of all depressive symptoms

when initially treated with the antidepressant citalopram. In addition, 45% to 50% of patients showed response (i.e., had a 50% improvement in symptoms) to that first treatment. In those that did not remit, switching to another antidepressant or augmenting citalopram with buspirone or bupropion increased the remission rate to more than 50%. A post hoc analysis of STAR*D showed no significant difference in remission rates between older participants (those >55 years of age) and their younger counterparts[105] and no differences in depression outcomes by treatment setting (mental health vs. primary care clinic). This reinforces the effectiveness of detecting and treating geriatric depression in all settings.

In about one-third of depressed older patients, depression persists despite treatment, which is called treatment-resistant late-life depression and defined as depression that has not responded to two therapeutically dosed antidepressant medications or has relapsed during treatment.[106] When sustained remission is not achieved with antidepressant monotherapy in LLD, there is limited empirical data to guide next steps.

Efforts have been made to explore factors that may influence treatment outcome. Some suggest that the age of onset of LLD (>55 vs. >65 years of age) plays an important role in outcome, with later onset of depression leading to a decreased likelihood of improvement.[107] Poor outcomes with pharmacotherapy have also been associated with high anxiety at the time of depression onset and age of first episode.[108] Certain executive function deficits in depressed older adults are associated with decreased antidepressant treatment response and greater risk of relapse.[109]

There has been greater interest since 2010 of studying potential moderators in LLD treatment outcomes. A patient-level metaanalysis by Nelson et al.[110] of 10 placebo-controlled trials of second-generation antidepressants (including citalopram, escitalopram, paroxetine, fluoxetine, venlafaxine) in LLD found that patients with a longer illness duration (>10 years) and moderate to severe depression had greater treatment benefit compared with placebo. Antidepressants were not effective for patients with shorter duration of illness. More research on the interplay between moderators, neuroanatomic models, neuroimaging findings, and antidepressant outcomes is crucial to guide treatment in LLD.

Keeping these issues in mind, when antidepressants are used judiciously and with realistic expectations, they can be effective, with numbers needed to treat of 13 for response and 20 for remission.[102]

## What Agent to Choose?

Overall, there are no significant differences in treatment efficacy between available antidepressants. A recent review of available evidence demonstrates that SSRIs and serotonin norepinephrine reuptake inhibitors (SNRIs) remain first-line treatment for LLD.[111] Drug selection in LLD is largely based on other factors, such as those noted in Box 19.5.

### SSRIs

SSRIs are among the most commonly prescribed drugs in medicine. SSRIs are generally well tolerated although they have both common and less well-known side effects that are important to consider when prescribing for older adults (Box 19.6). With a majority of serotonin receptors being located in the gut, the most common initial side effects of SSRIs tend to be gastrointestinal (GI) and transient. A temporary decrease in initial dosing minimizes GI side effects for most patients while serotonin receptors in the gut are downregulated. Later emerging GI side effects include

Choice of antidepressant should be made based on the following factors:
- Safety
- Side-effect profile
- Ease of discontinuing treatment
- Ease of administration (once-daily vs. twice-a-day dosing)
- Safety in frail patients
- Few dosage adjustment steps
- Minimal drug interaction potential

- Gastrointestinal upset
- Jitteriness
- Hyponatremia
- Drug–drug interactions (because of effects on CYP450 liver enzymes)
- Gastrointestinal bleeding
- Extrapyramidal side effects (tremors, parkinsonism, bruxism)

constipation with paroxetine and diarrhea with sertraline. The latter can be quite persistent with an onset that is delayed enough that it is often poorly recognized as a cause. In addition, SSRIs can have an activating effect when initially prescribed, which may result in insomnia or jitteriness. Changes in dose and time of administration are usually sufficient to address these issues.

SSRIs have known effects on a number of hepatic CYP450 enzymes, importantly CYP2D6, which is involved in the metabolism of several commonly used medications. Paroxetine and fluoxetine have the highest inhibitory effects on CYP2D6, whereas escitalopram, citalopram, and sertraline have little practical impact on the P450 system. For this reason, one of the latter drugs is often chosen as initial therapy for older adults, who are often taking other medications.

A particularly important side effect of the SSRIs (and the SNRIs) in older patients is hyponatremia, caused by the syndrome of inappropriate secretion of antidiuretic hormone (SIADH). Case control and retrospective studies have suggested an incidence of between 10% and 40%.[112] Risk factors include old age, female sex, low weight, diuretic use, and lower baseline sodium levels.[113,114] In a majority of instances, onset of SIADH is within 2 weeks of starting treatment with an SSRI.[114,115] It is important to realize that most hyponatremic patients have very nonspecific symptoms, such as fatigue, anorexia, and confusion. Only a minority will have persistent, severe hyponatremia that can result in seizures, coma, and death. Checking serum sodium after 2 weeks can be considered in patients starting an SSRI who have additional risk factors or who are taking other medications associated with antidiuretic hormone secretion (e.g., thiazides, nonsteroidal antiinflammatory drugs [NSAIDs]).[114]

⏵⏵ **Checking serum sodium after 2 weeks in patients starting an SSRI who have additional risk factors or who take medications associated with antidiuretic hormone secretion is recommended.**

SSRIs are also associated with an increased risk of upper GI bleeding, particularly in patients taking concomitant NSAIDs, aspirin, or oral anticoagulants. Estimates of the risk of these events

have varied widely, but most recent estimates have suggested the risk is fairly low with a number needed to harm over a year of treatment being 411 for SSRIs alone and 106 for SSRIs used with NSAIDs.[116] Although the mechanism for this bleeding risk has focused on the known effect of SSRIs on serotonin depletion in platelets, with subsequent impairment of platelet aggregation, a more important effect may be the ability of NSAIDs or aspirin to directly increase gastric acidity.[117] This latter effect may explain why the risk of GI bleeds occurs in the upper GI tract, as well as the fact that proton-pump inhibitors can reduce the bleeding risks.[117] Bleeding events can occur within the first month of treatment[118] but may occur over a much greater time frame (e.g., median time to bleeding in 101 spontaneous reports was 25 weeks). In instances where SSRIs and SNRIs are given with an NSAID, the time to a potential bleeding episode may reflect the time necessary for the peptic ulceration to occur.[117] If a patient is on a blood thinner such as warfarin, it is recommended that the patient's international normalized ratio be checked more frequently during the start of treatment and at dose changes.

Use of SSRIs can occasionally result in the induction or exacerbation of neurologic symptoms, including parkinsonism, dyskinesias, akathisia, and bruxism.[119] Nevertheless, SSRIs and SNRIs can be useful to treat depression in PD and are well tolerated.[120] When SSRIs are used in patients with PD, studies show there is an approximately 3% chance of developing an exacerbation of extrapyramidal symptoms, primarily tremors.[121] Treatment options include dose reduction, discontinuation, or the addition of a benzodiazepine or beta-blocker.

SSRIs have generally been considered to have a safe cardiovascular profile. However, the US Food and Drug Administration (FDA) has released recommendations regarding the dosing of citalopram based on its potential for dose-dependent prolongation of the QT interval.[122] The new FDA dosing guidelines call for a maximum dose of 40 mg per day in individuals up to age 65 years and a per-day maximum of 20 mg in those age >65 years. The FDA also suggests more frequent electrocardiogram (ECG) monitoring in patients with heart failure or bradyarrhythmia, or who are on concomitant medications that prolong the QT interval. The latter recommendations may be relevant for patients taking acetylcholinesterase inhibitors for dementia, many of whom develop bradycardia with treatment. Note that as of this time, the FDA directives do not extend to the s-enantiomer of citalopram, escitalopram, although a conservative approach might.

### SNRIs

SNRIs (duloxetine, venlafaxine, desvenlafaxine) inhibit the synaptic reuptake of both norepinephrine and serotonin. Although there is no conclusive evidence that the SNRIs are any more efficacious than SSRIs in treating depression in older adults,[123,124] this class does offer distinct benefits for chronic pain conditions with or without comorbid depression.[125] Venlafaxine predominantly affects serotonin uptake at doses <150 mg daily, and accordingly at those doses its side effects are typical of SSRIs.[126] Duloxetine has a more balanced effect on both serotonin and norepinephrine at clinically relevant doses and is indicated for a number of pain indications, including fibromyalgia, neuropathic pain associated with diabetic peripheral neuropathy, and chronic musculoskeletal pain.

### Other Antidepressants

Other options for treatment of depression in older adults include bupropion, which is mechanistically unique among antidepressants and the only agent with an additional indication for smoking cessation.[127] Bupropion has the additional benefits of having no sexual side effects, minimal weight gain potential, and negligible GI bleeding risk. On the other hand, it can be too activating for some patients, does not appear to be as effective for anxiety disorders, and has a moderate inhibitory effect on CYP2D6. Mirtazapine, also devoid of sexual side effects, is an alpha-2 antagonist and indirectly increases serotonin and norepinephrine transmission. It is also a potent inhibitor of histamine (H1) receptors, with subsequent effects on sleep and appetite. Sedation is greatest at lower doses (<15 mg daily) and is offset at higher doses by increased noradrenergic activity. Unlike the antidepressant effect, the impact on sleep is immediate, and, if not excessive, can provide for improved patient adherence. In one RCT, mirtazapine showed more pronounced improvement in depression when compared with paroxetine in the first few weeks of treatment, likely because of its effects on sleep, which is a major component of depression rating scales.[128] With both mirtazapine and bupropion, there is little information on long-term use and further study is needed.

**Tricyclic antidepressants.** Tricyclic antidepressants (TCAs) have been extensively studied, and there are numerous trials showing efficacy. However, TCAs have many safety issues and have a higher incidence of side effects particularly in older patients, the most prominent of which are various anticholinergic effects and cardiac effects, including increased heart rate, slowing of cardiac conduction, and orthostatic hypotension. ECGs should be monitored before and during TCA use, and careful measurement of orthostatic blood pressure is mandatory. The two TCAs with the best safety profile for older patients are the secondary amines nortriptyline and desipramine. Both of these drugs can be measured in the blood stream, and nortriptyline has a therapeutic window that can guide dosing.

❖ **Although TCAs are safe to use in older adults, it is important to monitor pulse, orthostatic blood pressure, cardiac conduction, and anticholinergic side effects.**

**Psychostimulants.** When the aforementioned treatments fail, psychostimulants are sometimes considered for monotherapy or adjunctive therapy in depressed older adult patients. One benefit with psychostimulants is that response to treatment is seen relatively quickly (i.e., within days). This may be helpful in cases where time to response is critical, such as with patients in rehabilitation programs or in end-of-life care. Trials, however, have been relatively short in total treatment time and number of patients treated.[129] Subsequently, long-term efficacy with this class of medications is unknown. There are several studies showing psychostimulants improving particular symptoms that may be seen with older depressed patients, such as apathy, fatigue, impaired executive functioning, and even gait dysfunction with a decreased incidence of falls.[129] However, these improvements do not necessarily correlate with overall improvement in depression and trials primarily included patients with comorbid medical conditions and hypoactive delirium. A 16-week double-blind, placebo-controlled RCT of 143 depressed older patients comparing combined treatment with citalopram and methylphenidate with either drug alone found that combined treatment led to more improvement in mood, as well as a higher rate of remission compared with either drug alone.[130] Precautionary measures when using psychostimulants include taking a thorough cardiac history because there is limited data about safe use of stimulants in older adults; however, recent reports of use in younger adults have been largely reassuring. Blood pressure and heart rate should be monitored regularly because both can be increased by psychostimulant use.

## Augmentation Strategies

Although monotherapy is preferred in older adults, the addition of another medication, also known as augmentation, is a reasonable consideration in TRD. However, there are limited high-quality trials of antidepressant augmentation strategies specifically targeting an older population. For an overview of available evidence of treatments for treatment-resistant LDD, see Knochel et al.[131] There are several reasons for the lack of evidence in older adults as previously mentioned, including frequent medical comorbidities, polypharmacy, and age-related changes in pharmacokinetics and pharmacodynamics.

## Lithium

Several geriatric studies support lithium augmentation in TRD in older adults, finding a response rate between 28% and 71%.[132–134] Lithium is fairly well tolerated in this older population. Despite the evidence, lithium augmentation is not favored because of drug titration and the need for careful ongoing monitoring.

## Second-Generation Antipsychotics

There has been increasing use of second-generation antipsychotic (SGA) augmentation in depression of all age groups, although there are few high-quality studies of SGA augmentation in LLD, and most are limited by small sample size. High dropout rates have been identified because of adverse effects, including sedation, dizziness, constipation, and orthostatic hypotension.[135] In 2005 the FDA issued a black box warning advising that all SGAs were associated with excess mortality in older patients, including an increased risk for sudden cardiac death, as well as cerebrovascular adverse events in older patients with dementia.[136]

In terms of SGA selection, aripiprazole and quetiapine have the most supportive evidence currently. Studies of aripiprazole have shown decreased depressive symptoms and increased remission rates in older patients.[136–140] Quetiapine has been shown to be effective in achieving higher remission and response rates when used as monotherapy in LLD, suggesting promise as a safe augmenting agent. In these trials, aripiprazole and quetiapine were well tolerated. The most common adverse effects were akathisia with aripiprazole and somnolence with quetiapine. However, when SGAs are used, clinicians must continue to closely monitor for side effects, including extrapyramidal symptoms and drug-induced parkinsonism.[141]

### Novel Treatments

Intranasal (IN) esketamine was approved by the FDA in 2019 for TRD when used in conjunction with a traditional oral antidepressant.[142] Studies support IN esketamine as a potential fast-acting and effective treatment in depressed patients.[143] In the geriatric population, clinical trials show the use of IN esketamine is safe and effective. Studies in older adults with TRD revealed significant reduction of depressive symptoms with only mild to moderate side effects, similar to those found in the general adult population.[144–146]

## Pharmacologic Treatment Considerations

Box 19.7 suggests tips to educate patients and their families about the treatment of depression. Regardless of which medication is chosen, frequent monitoring and dose titration are vital.

**Clinical Tips for Educating Patient/Family About Depression and Its Treatment**

1. Explain that major depressive disorder is a medical illness (like diabetes or hypertension) and review specific signs and symptoms and treatment with patient and family. Reinforce that the patient is not simply being treated for "sadness."
2. When reviewing history with the patient, the clinician may want to use phrases, such as "How long have you been fighting/struggling with depression?" rather than "How long have you been depressed?" This should allow the patient to take a more proactive stance against the ailment.
3. Educate the patient that antidepressants should not be taken on an as-needed basis. They should not be doubled-up on "bad days" nor skipped on "good days."
4. Clarify to the patient that antidepressants do not solve problems. Review and prioritize acute and chronic psychosocial stressors with family and patient to create an appropriate treatment plan (e.g., social work referral, psychotherapy).
5. Preemptively educate the patient and family about common initial side effects, such as jitteriness and gastrointestinal upset, stressing the transient nature of these symptoms and dosing strategies to avoid them.

When initiating treatment, it is important to note that although older patients can tolerate standard dosing of many antidepressants, they are more susceptible to side effects. As mentioned previously, SSRIs have a number of side effects that are transient in nature, such as jitteriness and nausea. Although these are not life threatening, they can certainly be uncomfortable for the patient and may lead to poor adherence or premature discontinuation of the medication. The general rule is to begin treatment at a low dose (e.g., start with 50% of the target dose) and titrate after 4 to 7 days to minimize initial side effects. Although the target dose for many older patients is lower than for younger adults, it is crucial to monitor the patient for both medication intolerance and improvement of depressive symptoms. If the patient reports no side effects with the initial dose, yet does not show any improvement of depression, then it is prudent to continue increasing the antidepressant until a trial of the maximum tolerable dose of the medication is achieved. Although susceptibility to side effects is a concern on initiation of an antidepressant, once older adult patients have been established on a tolerable dose of the medication, they have a rate of discontinuation with continued treatment similar to that of the general adult population.[147]

A patient who has responded to antidepressant treatment should be continued on treatment for approximately 1 year for a first depressive episode. After a second or third episode, however, it has been recommended to extend treatment after reaching remission, with some patients requiring lifelong treatment.[148] For example, one study comparing treatment with paroxetine versus placebo in combination with psychotherapy 2 years after a depressive episode showed a relative risk of reoccurrence 2.4 times higher with placebo than with paroxetine.[149] It is therefore vital to continue antidepressants after remission of a depressive episode, especially for patients with a history of relapse.

For those patients who do not respond to an initial adequate trial of pharmacotherapy, choices include switching antidepressants or augmentation. For most patients who have taken an SSRI as a first agent, a simple choice is to switch to an alternative SSRI or different class of medication, such as an SNRI, or bupropion. These switching options had equivalent outcomes in the STAR*D

trial. Alternatively, for a patient who has had a partial but incomplete response, augmentation with either buspirone or bupropion can be considered or a trial of cognitive behavioral therapy (CBT; see following section). In STAR*D, augmentation with these strategies appeared to be slightly more effective than switching to a new drug.

## Psychosocial Interventions

Although antidepressants are a useful modality for treating LLD, they are not the sole option. Psychosocial interventions are often very effective and may be particularly useful in patients with less severe major depression, minor depression, or dysthymia, where the evidence for use of antidepressants is less robust. However, just as with pharmacotherapy, data on efficacy are limited using these interventions. Interventions that have been explored in an older adult population and have evidence of efficacy include problem-solving therapy (PST), which focuses on teaching patients strategies to solve everyday problems and deal with crises; CBT, which focuses on behavioral activation and identifying and correcting automatic negative thought processes; and treatment initiation and participation therapy, which focuses on education about health and medication.[150] Of these, PST has been shown to be useful in patients with cognitive impairment who would be less amenable to explorative types of therapy. CBT has also shown utility, with or without the concomitant use of desipramine, for even severe forms of depression.

Neuroplasticity-based computerized cognitive remediation (nCCR) is a novel intervention developed to target executive dysfunction in treatment-resistant LLD.[151] Executive dysfunction is a predictor of poor treatment response to conventional antidepressants.[109] nCCR improves various cognitive functions and induces structural and functional brain changes.[151] One study found that compared with escitalopram, CCR in geriatric depression (CCR-GD) was similarly effective at reducing depressive symptoms but with a quicker response in 4 weeks compared with 12 weeks in escitalopram use. As well, CCR-GD showed improved executive function measures over escitalopram.[152]

Because of the heterogeneity of the older population, many individuals may have particular needs or additional psychosocial factors contributing to their depression. Case management is a valuable tool to aid with these concerns. Over the last decade, an initiative known as the Improving Mood, Promoting Access to Collaborative Treatment care model[153] has proven quite beneficial and is being implemented in many settings. In this model, a care manager (most often a nurse) is present in the clinic and is assigned to patients diagnosed with depression. The care manager educates the patient about depression, monitors for improvement and adherence, and provides regular follow-up and counseling. The care manager typically consults with a psychiatrist on a regular basis. This model of care has been extensively studied, including in a public health setting,[154] and shown to decrease overall cost of care and significantly improve patient treatment response over what would be considered standard care.

## Other Somatic Treatments

ECT is often overlooked as a possible intervention in treatment of LLD (Box 19.8). ECT is highly effective and can be particularly beneficial for patients with active suicidal ideation and psychotic depression. It has the lowest incidence of mortality among all procedures performed under general anesthesia. There are no absolute contraindications to the use of ECT. It has been shown to be more efficacious in LLD than in the general adult population. It results in more immediate response in symptoms and may be effective for those patients experiencing significant disability from their

## • BOX 19.8   Electroconvulsive Therapy

1. Useful when more rapid antidepressant effect is desired (failure to thrive, severe/psychotic depression, active suicidal ideation)
2. No absolute contraindications
3. Useful for frail older adult patients who may not be able to tolerate medications

depressive symptoms. ECT is also a useful alternative for frail older patients who may have multiple comorbid conditions and who are unable to tolerate antidepressant treatment. However, it should be noted that even after acute treatment and symptom improvement, there is an 85% chance of relapse in the first 6 months if the patient is not provided adjunctive maintenance pharmacotherapy. Therefore ECT is best seen as an acute intervention to hasten response. Primary side effects experienced by the older population are short-term memory loss and a possible increase in incidence of falls, particularly in nursing home patients.[155] Recent evidence continues to demonstrate that ECT is an efficacious, safe, and tolerable treatment in LLD.[156]

Another form of somatic treatment, rapid transcranial magnetic stimulation (rTMS), was FDA-approved in 2008. This treatment does not require anesthesia and can be performed on an outpatient basis. The only absolute contraindication of rTMS is the presence of implants or ferromagnetic devices in or near the head, and the most serious, although rare, adverse event is seizure, occurring in < 1 in 10,000 patients.[157] For the rTMS procedure, the patient is seated while magnetic pulses are used to stimulate the brain to induce change in mood. The procedure is typically prescribed as a total course of pulses delivered in 30- to 40-minute sessions daily over a period of 4 to 6 weeks. The patient is not sedated and can converse during treatments. Of the dozens of randomized rTMS trials in major depression, few have included older adults. Of those studying older adults, findings were variable in terms of rTMS efficacy; however, safety and tolerability have been demonstrated, and more studies are needed.[158] Given that the strength of the magnetic field falls off rapidly with distance and that many older adults have significant brain atrophy and white matter burden, this treatment modality may require higher doses in older patients than those used in younger adults for efficacy.[159] Of note, a pooled analysis of seven randomized trials comparing ECT (bilateral or lateral) with repetitive TMS in 275 patients with major depression found that ECT was superior in terms of remission rates (53% vs. 32%).[160]

### Exercise

Although numerous studies have attempted to evaluate physical exercise in improving depressive symptoms in depressed older people, findings are inconsistent, and evidence is not high quality. For a systematic review of available evidence, see Mura and Carta[161] who conclude that there is some promising research showing that combined exercise and antidepressant treatment is helpful in treatment-resistant late-life depression.

### CASE

#### Ms. Smith (Part 4)

You begin Ms. Smith on thyroid replacement therapy while simultaneously starting her on nortriptyline, 25 mg by mouth at bedtime. You also perform a baseline ECG. You explain to Ms. Smith and her daughter about the signs and symptoms of major depression and the use of antidepressants, including possible side effects and length of treatment. You also refer Ms. Smith for psychotherapy and educate her about its potential benefits when combined with antidepressants.

Ms. Smith returns to the clinic in 2 weeks and states that she has noticed some improvement in sleep, but she has not had much improvement in her other symptoms. She denies any side effects from the nortriptyline. You increase the dose from 25 mg to 50 mg and have her return in 4 weeks. At her next visit, you obtain a TSH level, which has returned to normal. Ms. Smith reports that she has been attending therapy once a week and has felt some resolution regarding the loss of her husband. She has started attending more family dinners and has been babysitting her grandchildren, which she enjoys. Under the direction of her therapist, she has made a scrapbook of her travels with her husband and has started sorting through some of his belongings, gifting a portion of them to her children. Her energy level has improved, and she has been going on walks with her daughter as well. On repeat administration, Ms. Smith scores a 3 on her GDS and a 29/30 on her MMSE.

#### Discussion

Ms. Smith originally presented with what seemed to be complicated grief. However, when exploring Ms. Smith's symptoms further and using standardized scales, it was noted that Ms. Smith was suffering from depression. It was also discovered that the patient was hypothyroid; however, because Ms. Smith meets criteria for depression and has a history of depressive disorder, it would be optimal to treat both her hypothyroidism and depression simultaneously. Nortriptyline was selected as the treatment here given her prior good response and her willingness to accept treatment with that agent. Remember that use of TCAs necessitates baseline ECG and monitoring of orthostatic blood pressures.

## Summary

Depression continues to be recognized as a major contributing factor to both morbidity and mortality in older adults. Simultaneously, there is a shortage of psychiatrists, and even more so geriatric psychiatrists, nationwide. Thus it is crucial that primary care physicians acquire the capabilities to both detect and treat depression. This is especially pertinent to identification of depression in older adults, which has unique presentations, prognoses, and higher likelihood of multiple medical comorbidities requiring a heightened sense of awareness. Furthermore, treatment of depression in older adults requires a different approach than that of younger depressed patients. In sum, depression is a treatable condition; if medication and psychosocial interventions are optimized, it can be overcome. The patient's overall health, function, and quality of life depend on appropriate treatment.

### Web Resources

The Institute of Medicine report on mental health care for older adults: www.iom.edu/Reports/2012/The-Mental-Health-and-Substance-Use-Workforce-for-Older-Adults.aspx.

National Institute of Mental Health pamphlet on depression in older adults: www.nimh.nih.gov/health/publications/depression/complete-index.shtml.

Searchable database of evidence-based interventions for mental health: www.nrepp.samhsa.gov.

## Key References

**91.** Conejero I, Olié E, Courtet P, Calati R. Suicide in older adults: current perspectives. *Clin Interv Aging.* 2018;13:691–699.

**105.** Kozel FA, Trivedi MH, Wisniewski SR, et al. Treatment outcomes for older depressed patients with earlier versus late onset of first depressive episode: a Sequenced Treatment Alternatives to Relieve Depression (STAR*D) report. *Am J Geriatr Psychiatry.* 2008;16(1):58–64.

**108.** Andreescu C, Reynolds CF III. Late-life depression: evidence-based treatment and promising new directions for research and clinical practice. *Psychiatr Clin North Am.* 2011;34(2):335–355, vii-iii.

**111.** Beyer JL, Johnson KG. Advances in pharmacotherapy of late-life depression. *Curr Psychiatry Rep.* 2018;20:34.

**150.** Kiosses DN, Leon AC, Areán PA. Psychosocial interventions for late-life major depression: Evidence-based treatments, predictors of treatment outcomes, and moderators of treatment effects. *Psychiatr Clin North Am.* 2011;34(2):377–401, viii.

**References available online at expertconsult.com.**

# 20

# Gait, Balance, and Falls

JOSEPH HEJKAL AND ALFRED L. FISHER

## OUTLINE

*Additional online-only material indicated by icon.*

## OBJECTIVES

*At the completion of this chapter, the reader should be able to:*

- Describe the burden of impaired mobility and falls in older adult patients.
- List the most common causes of falls and understand that multiple causes are often present at once.
- Develop a structured history and physical examination in a patient at high risk of falling.
- Be able to treat or refer appropriately for common causes of mobility impairment and falls.

## CASE

### Mr. McDonald (Part 1)

Mr. McDonald is a 68-year-old man who presents to clinic for frequent falls associated with gait changes over the past 2 years. He feels unsteady but not lightheaded or dizzy, and he cannot associate his falls with his environment (i.e., he has fallen outside, inside, in the bathroom, in the hallway, etc., without distinction) or postural changes. His worst injury has been a fractured rib about a year ago, and he denies any head trauma associated with these. He often holds on to nearby surfaces, but he does not use an assistive device. When he falls he cannot get back up on his own. He especially has trouble with stairs.

His medical history includes type 2 diabetes, not currently on medications, polyneuropathy, stage III chronic kidney disease, hearing loss, heavy tobacco use, and previous alcohol use disorder in remission.

What are the most common causes of gait dysfunction and frequent falls in older adult patients?

What are initial probing questions that could help tease out why this patient is falling?

## Prevalence and Impact

Older adults frequently report falls and mobility difficulty, with about 25% reporting a fall in the past year and one-third admitting to mobility problems.[1] Although both falls and reduced mobility have morbidity and mortality implications, older adults report worse life experience with ambulatory limitations with an isolated fall history:[1] For example, those with low mobility engage less often socially,[2] and they are at higher risk for depression. In addition, because mobility encompasses the spectrum of functional bodily movement from walking and climbing stairs to the basic act of transferring, low mobility contributes to functional dependence and may drive institutionalization.

❖❖ **Although falls cause injury and pose more risk, an abnormal gait and fear of falling cause more distress to patients.**

In addition, falls are associated with increased mortality[1] and may lead to a disastrous injury, such as hip fracture or subdural hematoma, which are associated with significant morbidity and mortality and can often be life altering for the individual. One-year hip fracture mortality rates are about 20% to 25%,[3] and survivors can often experience significant functional decline.[4] Those with subdural hematoma (acute, subacute, and chronic) also experience potentially serious consequences, including high rates of mortality and severe disability.[5]

## Risk Factors and Pathophysiology

Many organ systems impact balance, and the neuromuscular system is primary among these. This can be divided into (1) sensory input and transmission, (2) central processes (adaptive processing, executive planning, motor programs), and (3) motor output and transmission. Other involved organ systems include the cardiovascular system through support especially for brain perfusion, the skeletal system through the actions of joints, and even the urogenital system. Impairments in these systems, such as orthostatic hypotension, joint pain from arthritis, or bladder urgency leading to a poorly planned rush to the toilet can cause falls. The neurologic components will be reviewed later in some detail.

Three main sensory inputs help maintain balance. Proprioception is the ability to sense the position (and change in position) of a joint especially via the muscle spindles and Golgi tendon organs, with afferent signals from these ascending via fast Ia and Ib fibers to the dorsal columns—medial lemniscus pathway to the thalamus and through the posterior spinocerebellar tract to the cerebellum. Not only can these be susceptible to a variety of diseases that lead to peripheral neuropathy, or lesions in the spinal cord or brain, but aging itself leads to decreased proprioception.[6] The vestibular system (utricle, saccule, semicircular canals) senses the position and acceleration of the head in space and sends its impulses via cranial nerve VIII to the vestibular nuclei. This system is susceptible to various disorders of the inner ear, and vestibular function also declines with age.[7] Vision is the third main sensory modality that contributes to balance, and age-related diseases frequently lead to visual impairments. These diseases commonly include cataracts, glaucoma, macular degeneration, and refractive error whereas less common causes include central brain lesions leading to cortical visual impairment or compression of the optic nerve, chiasm, and tract pathways.

Within the brain, the frontal cortex is important for the planning, initiation, and execution of movement. The basal ganglia promotes appropriate movement, through both the initiation and suppression of movement and by executing motor programs. The cerebellum is particularly important for processing and responding to proprioceptive and vestibular input and for error correction. The brainstem is involved in vestibular processing and responses and maintaining posture, and it plays some role in integrating the other pathways.

The final essential component of the neural pathways involved in balance are the motor pathways. Most important in balance are the corticospinal and vestibulospinal tracts, which lead from the motor cortex or vestibular nuclei through the spinal cord. Peripheral nerves then relay the motor signaling to the innervated muscles with the final link between the nervous system and muscles being the neuromuscular junctions. Diseases affecting the spinal cord, peripheral nerves, neuromuscular junction, or muscles can compromise the involved motor pathways leading to declines in strength or coordination, which can compromise motor compensation.

Beyond the neural pathways that directly affect balance, clinical studies have identified a range of patient factors that are associated with falls, including increasing age, female sex, the presence of vertigo, slow gait speed, cognitive impairment, parkinsonism, frailty, polypharmacy particularly involving medications with central nervous system effects, previous falls, vision impairment, and other factors.[8–10] In addition to the aforementioned, pain, especially arthritic pain, is the most common cause of reduced mobility and abnormal gait in older adults.[11]

## Differential Diagnosis and Assessment

Ambulation and balance are complex tasks, with a myriad of disorders that affect them, so a systematic approach to eliciting the history can help make assessment cognitively manageable. As with most problems in older adult patients, causes are typically multifactorial (e.g., orthostatic hypotension in conjunction with peripheral neuropathy or underlying parkinsonism), so the range of conditions considered must be wide. In addition, environmental factors can also play a key role and can be easy to overlook in the office environment.

▸▸ **Think about factors other than impaired balance when assessing the falling patient, such as rushing to use the restroom, poor judgment, vision impairment, environmental clutter or hazards, or the presence of small pets.**

### History

Patients do not always spontaneously bring up mobility concerns or falls, so it is important to ask at least yearly—in fact, falls screening is part of the annual Medicare wellness visit.[12]

▸▸ **Ask these three questions to screen for fall risk:[12]**
**Have you fallen in the last year?**
**Do you worry about falling?**
**Do you feel unsteady when standing or walking?**

Factors that may lead patients to not spontaneously discuss falls or mobility limitations could include embarrassment, fear of placement in a nursing home, or the mistaken belief that these are part of aging and cannot be helped by providers.

#### Precipitants and Location

The timing of falls can provide important clues related to the cause. For example, if falls typically occur shortly after standing up, then orthostatic blood pressure changes may be related. If falls occur most often at night, then urinary incontinence, low lighting, poor proprioception, or the use of pharmacologic sleep aids might be contributing factors.

It can be particularly helpful to learn if the patient falls in certain locations. Clutter in the home or uneven ground in the yard may contribute. If the patient is embarrassed about the condition of the home, a history of clutter may be hard to elicit, and collateral informants can sometimes provide helpful insight. The sites of falls may point to other hazards in the home, such as stairs, uneven floors, rugs, electrical cords, small pets, or bathrooms. Targeting these environmental factors is often a critical component in the prevention of subsequent falls.

### Symptoms Often Seen Along With Falls

Symptoms of syncope or presyncope should lead to workup of orthostatic, cardiac, or neurocardiogenic causes as appropriate. Regardless of symptoms, orthostatic blood pressures should be obtained on a patient with falls because this can contribute to falls even in the absence of clear patient-reported symptoms.

Some patients feel unsteady on their feet, and this is worth delving into, with similar, open-ended questions about timing, precipitants, and the like. Frequent falls without feeling unsteady may suggest that the patient lacks awareness of his or her risk of falling or is unable to recall the events associated with past falls, or may suggest that sudden cardiac or neurologic changes precipitate the falls. Such a history should raise suspicion for underlying cognitive deficits or, more rarely, acute, transient changes in postural function, such as drop attacks or seizures.

The provider should also ask about visual problems, and whether the patient has regular vision exams. Cataracts, macular degeneration, and glaucoma are all common in older adults, can significantly compromise vision, and increase fall risk.

Other geriatric syndromes are also associated with falls and should be asked about and evaluated if present. Notably, cognitive impairment is associated with falls[8] and is usually not identified by the patient. New-onset, subacute cognitive changes could also raise the possibility of a chronic subdural hematoma related to a fall. Separately, urinary urgency or incontinence can lead to falls as a patient rushes to the restroom to avoid accidents. A history of incontinence and cognitive impairment along with typical gait features can also raise concerns about normal-pressure hydrocephalus as an underlying unifying diagnosis.

### Changes in Gait

Patients who fall often experience significant changes in how they ambulate, but other than describing it as "slow" or "unsteady" it can be hard for most patients or family members to describe gait changes in detail. Assessing how gait changes are affecting function can be more revealing. For example, fear of falling may lead to the limiting of activities out of caution. In some patients, this fear can lead to more disability than the falls themselves. A patient may also adapt by holding on to furniture or an assistive device. Sometimes an assistive device can also lead to restricted activity, because of an associated slower gait and an increase in the time needed to reach locations or to accomplish instrumental activities of daily living. Also, some adaptive devices, like walkers, can be difficult to maneuver in a tight environment, and this can limit where a patient can travel.

### Medical History and Drugs

Falls can also be a result of comorbid medical conditions or the effects or side effects of medications. As a result, the review of a patient's medical history can be revealing for contributing factors. Parkinson disease directly affects mobility as a result of rigidity, difficulty initiating movement, impairments in error correction, and in some individuals the development of autonomic insufficiency. The cardiac history could reveal risk factors for cardiac or orthostatic syncope, or reasons for early fatigue or claudication. Other diagnoses, and medications associated with them, could lead to suspicion for peripheral neuropathy. For example, diabetes could cause neuropathy, either on its own or from vitamin B12 deficiency associated with metformin use.

In addition, medication review is essential, including over-the-counter drugs. Essentially all central-acting medications, such as selective serotonin reuptake inhibitors and other antidepressants, opioids, anticonvulsants, benzodiazepines, and medications with anticholinergic side effects, are associated with higher fall risk. Medications associated with orthostatic blood pressure changes, especially alpha-blockers, nitrates, and diuretics, may be implicated. Similarly, significant alcohol use and the use of illicit substances should be assessed.

---

### CASE

#### Mr. McDonald (Part 2)

On examination, Mr. McDonald often looks to his wife to answer questions. Blood pressure is 155/68 mmHg and does not change with position. Vital signs are otherwise normal. General physical examination is normal. Motor examination is pertinent for a lack of rigidity and a mild resting tremor of the right upper extremity (RUE). Finger-to-nose and heel-shin testing demonstrate normal coordination. Pain sensation is slightly diminished in both feet. He has decreased vibratory sense on the right leg to the shin. Strength is slightly decreased in the left upper extremity, and his hip flexors are also slightly weak bilaterally. Visual acuity is 20/40 bilaterally with correction. Reflexes are more brisk on the left side. Cognitive testing demonstrates a Montreal Cognitive Assessment score of 18/30.

Gait testing demonstrates a wide base with everted feet and shortened stride length. He takes three steps to turn around. He is stable during the Romberg test but stumbles on a pull test.

What are the common causes of peripheral neuropathy that should be evaluated in his case?

What gait features are associated with frontal disorders (especially vascular disease or normal pressure hydrocephalus), subcortical disorders (especially parkinsonism), spasticity, weakness, or pain?

---

## Physical Examination

The physical examination largely focuses on a thorough neurologic examination, gait assessment, and a few other key systems, including the cardiovascular and pulmonary systems, and the lower extremities. Table 20.1 summarizes physical examination techniques and their associated disease processes.

### General Physical

Orthostatic vital signs should be obtained and the patient's body mass index (BMI) should be measured. An underweight BMI or temporal wasting may reflect poor nutrition or frailty, which can lead to poor muscle mass and strength. Many systemic diseases can lead to poor activity tolerance and could be uncovered by the cardiopulmonary examination, assessment for lower extremity edema, and assessing for peripheral vascular disease.

### Neurologic Examination

The provider should assess cognitive function with a brief, standardized test, such as the Mini-Mental State Exam, Mini-Cog, or Montreal Cognitive Assessment, even in the absence of reported cognitive changes, because abnormalities are common and often not reported. Recognizing cognitive deficits allows for better assessment of fall risk and it alerts the provider to the need for involving the patient's support system for confirming the history and for follow-through on recommendations.

❖ **Assess patients with abnormal gait for cognitive changes.**

Strength (especially of the proximal hip flexor/extensor musculature) should be assessed by testing hip flexion strength while the

**TABLE 20.1   Systems to Look at When Assessing the Falling or Gait-Impaired Patient**

| System | Examination Maneuvers/Findings | Abnormal Findings May Suggest |
|---|---|---|
| Nervous | Coordination (finger-to-nose, rapid alternating movements with dysmetria or dysdiadochokinesia) | Cerebellar dysfunction/ataxia, medications, alcohol |
| | Rigidity, tremor | Parkinsonism (drug-induced, vascular, or primary) |
| | Spasticity, hyperreflexia, increased tone, weakness | Lesions in brain or spinal cord, especially strokes or spinal myelopathy |
| | Abnormal cognitive testing | Contributing cognitive impairment, normal-pressure hydrocephalus |
| | Sensory testing (pinprick, light touch, vibratory and/or position sense) | Peripheral polyneuropathy, nerve entrapment, radiculopathy, focal cord or brain lesions |
| | Focal weakness (e.g., foot drop, Trendelenburg gait), without spasticity | Radiculopathy, anterior horn disease, mononeuropathy, nerve entrapments, focal cord or brain lesions |
| | Heart examination: arrhythmias, loud murmurs | Structural heart disease, syncope |
| Cardiovascular | Orthostatic hypotension | Autonomic insufficiency (related to autonomic neuropathy, parkinsonism), dehydration, medications |
| | Crepitus, restricted range of motion in lower extremity joints, pain | Osteoarthritis, previous trauma |
| Musculoskeletal/orthopedic | Effusions, synovitis, pain | Inflammatory rheumatologic disease, osteoarthritis in some cases |
| | Abnormal visual acuity | Refractive error, glaucoma, macular degeneration |
| Eyes | Abnormal visual fields | Stroke, pituitary tumor, glaucoma, macular degeneration |
| | Shuffling, en bloc turn, festination, bradykinesia | Parkinsonism (vascular, Parkinson disease, drugs, or a "Parkinson plus" disorder) |
| Gait examination/balance testing | Wide-based, cautious, "magnetic" gait with everted feet | Frontal dysfunction (often looks similar to parkinsonian gait), normal pressure hydrocephalus, cerebrovascular disease, alcohol abuse |
| | Steppage gait | Foot drop caused by peripheral neuropathy, radiculopathy, stroke |
| | Trendelenburg gait | Contralateral hip abductor weakness caused by nerve entrapment, radiculopathy, or CNS lesion |
| | Circumduction | Stiff knee, spastic knee extensors caused by CNS lesion |
| | Antalgic gait | Painful lower extremity |
| | Unsteadiness on pull test | Postural instability in parkinsonism; may be affected by many other balance disorders |
| Balance tests | Unsteady tandem gait | Parkinsonism, vestibular disorders, and peripheral neuropathy |
| | Unstable Romberg | Vestibular disorders, proprioceptive disorders |
| Objective gait tests | Timed up and go >12 s | High-fall risk |
| | Gait speed <0.6 m/s | High-fall risk |

*CNS,* Central nervous system.

patient sits and by observing the patient attempt to stand without using his or her arms. Resting muscle tone, presence or absence of tremors, and the passive range of motion of limbs should also be assessed (looking for increased tone, rigidity, and spasticity). Lower extremity spasticity, especially if combined with bowel or bladder difficulties, sensory abnormalities, or motor or sensory problems in the upper extremities, may suggest cervical myelopathy.

Sensation, especially in the feet, should be evaluated with multiple modalities (e.g., pinprick, vibration, and position sense). Balance testing via Romberg test, tandem walking, and sternal nudge or pull test is helpful. The Romberg test involves having the patient stand with feet together and eyes closed. The practitioner then assesses for sway or instability, standing behind the patient to steady him or her if needed. Excessive sway or stumbling indicates a deficit in either the proprioceptive or vestibular mechanisms of postural/balance maintenance. Tandem gait (walking with one foot directly placed in front of the other) provides somewhat similar information. Although tandem gait is classically used as an assessment for cerebellar dysfunction, it is also often abnormal in parkinsonism, vestibular disorders, and peripheral neuropathy.[13]

The pull test is performed with the patient in a comfortable stance (feet not together). The provider then firmly pulls the patient's shoulders backwards. Significant unsteadiness (multiple steps backwards, falling) is a sign of postural instability seen in patients with parkinsonism. Note that it is important to have adequate support when performing this test (e.g., having a strong person behind the patient to catch him or her in case of a fall).

Vision testing should be performed, generally with correction if the patient usually wears glasses. It is worth examining the other ocular cranial nerves as well, to look for nystagmus or other signs of ocular or vestibular dysfunction. Visual field testing by confrontation may be helpful if defects are suspected, but it is not a sensitive examination technique.

### Gait Assessment

A key component of gait assessment is directly observing the patient stand and walk. Often, subtle changes in the musculoskeletal or neurologic examination that would not be obvious on a seating examination become much more visible and relevant when the patient is walking.

**Standing.** It can be helpful to have the patient stand up from a sitting position with the arms crossed. An inability to stand without using the arms of the chair for leverage is an effective indicator of proximal muscle weakness.

**Gait Speed.** Speed can be directly measured by timing the patient while walking at a comfortable pace between two lines of tape 4 m apart. Slow gait speeds, specifically 0.6 m/s or less, is often seen in those at risk for subsequent falls. Alternatively, speed may be excessively rapid in those with cognitive impairment or executive dysfunction. Slow gait speed is also part of some criteria for the frailty syndrome, and is also independently associated with higher risk of mortality[14]—which provides an additional utility to the measurement.

**Stance.** A widened stance, typically at shoulder width or wider and sometimes with everted feet, often reflects a cautious gait and may be seen in normal pressure hydrocephalus (NPH), frontal disorders, cerebrovascular disease, or as a sequela of prior alcohol abuse.

**Step Patterns.** Observing step clearance can distinguish a normal gait from a shuffling or steppage gait with high knee flexion because of foot drop. An asymmetric rhythm might especially suggest an antalgic gait, in which a rapid step is taken when the painful limb is supporting the patient's weight. Other abnormalities that could be observed include circumduction, which is seen when the patient cannot flex the knee well because of spasticity, knee stiffness, or other causes, or a Trendelenburg gait, which is the collapse of hip during the swing phase because of contralateral hip abductor weakness. Stride length decreases with age, but it may be particularly short in frontal gait disorders and parkinsonism.

**Parkinsonian Characteristics.** Classic parkinsonian gait characteristics include shuffling, slow movements/bradykinesia, reduced arm swing, en bloc turning, freezing, kyphotic posture, and festination, which is a gait characterized by the uncontrollable gathering of speed. Importantly, these characteristics also resemble frontal gait disorders, such as NPH.

Online videos are available to familiarize providers with gait examination and the characteristics of various abnormalities. In particular, Stanford University and University of Utah both have produced videos demonstrating abnormal gait patterns, which can enhance a provider's ability to recognize them during a clinical exam (see the web resources at the end of this chapter for the URLs).

### Fall Risk Screening Tools

Specific tests that can help predict falls include the timed up and go (TUG) test and simple measures of gait speed. The TUG involves having the patient stand up, walk 10 feet at a comfortable pace, turn around, and return to the chair. If this takes longer than 12 seconds, the person is considered at high fall risk. A gait speed of less than 0.6 m/s while walking at normal gait speed over 4 m is also considered at higher risk.[10]

◆◆ **Because of its relationship with clinical frailty, slow gait speed predicts falls, functional decline, and death.**

---

**CASE**

### Mr. McDonald (Part 3)

The patient's physical examination shows a number of disparate neurologic findings and an abnormal gait with a wide base, everted feet, shortened stride length, and instability to sternal nudge. You consider both NPH and cerebrovascular disease as top possible diagnoses. You also look for diagnoses that might explain his neuropathy.

You order a computed tomography (CT) of the head, which demonstrates multifocal lacunar strokes in the basal ganglia, internal capsules, and thalamus bilaterally. A vitamin B12 level, folate level, serum protein electrophoresis, and free light chain assay are normal.

Name at least four pathologic factors that increase Mr. McDonald's fall risk.

What treatments would you suggest?

---

## Ancillary Tests

The use of any ancillary testing should always be guided by the results of the history and examination conducted as described earlier. For example, the evaluation of peripheral neuropathy should include vitamin B12 level testing, a diabetes screening test, such as the measurement of a fasting blood sugar or glycosylated hemoglobin, usually a serum protein electrophoresis with either serum free light chains or a urine protein electrophoresis, and in selected circumstances screening for other, more unusual causes such as thiamine deficiency.

Neuroimaging is often appropriate in the evaluation of gait and balance disorders and should be prompted by subacute or acute changes in gait, physical abnormalities that could be explained by cerebrovascular disease, including parkinsonism that could be related to basal ganglia infarcts, and in particular if there is concern for NPH. Of note, NPH often presents without the full classic triad of falls, urinary incontinence, and cognitive impairment, and an abnormal gait is the most common characteristic. If there is concern that a spinal cord lesion could be at play, such as cervical myelopathy, then imaging of the appropriate spinal levels is warranted.

Rarely, signs of peripheral neuropathy, especially with motor involvement, could prompt the use of subsequent testing, such as nerve conduction studies or an electromyogram (EMG). Vestibular testing should be pursued in a patient with persistent vertigo.

In the patient with a history of syncope, obtaining an electrocardiogram (ECG) is appropriate, and additional workup is guided by clinical suspicion based on history and examination findings. Ambulatory ECG monitoring and potentially echocardiography should be used if suspicion is high for cardiac etiology. If there is suspicion for seizures, then electroencephalogram (EEG) monitoring is indicated, and neuroimaging should be pursued for suspected seizures or observed focal neurologic deficits. Other diagnostic modalities include tilt table testing to confirm suspected vasovagal syncope when the diagnosis is not clear, or a monitored carotid sinus massage in a patient with suspected carotid sinus hypersensitivity.

## CASE

### Discussion (Mr. McDonald)

Your overall impression of Mr. McDonald's balance impairment is a multifactorial problem related to cerebrovascular disease, peripheral neuropathy because of diabetes and possibly to previous alcohol use, with additional risk because of his cognitive deficits, and mild visual impairment. You recommend a course of physical therapy for balance training and strengthening, evaluation by ophthalmology, and risk factor modification to prevent future strokes. On follow-up 3 months later, he has undergone physical therapy, and he feels steadier on his feet but still feels at risk. He has not continued to fall.

## Management

As with any disorder, treatment of an impaired gait is usually focused on the underlying pathophysiology. However, in geriatric patients, there are often two or three factors related to falls or mobility problems, and so there may be multiple targets for intervention.

### Exercise and Balance Training

Balance training, physical therapy, and exercise interventions have been shown to help prevent falls, and they are probably the best modalities for reducing the fall risks related to muscle weakness or neurologic injury. The use of Tai Chi is particularly well supported by clinical research. Structured exercise has also been shown to improve gait speed, which may improve overall mobility and independence above and beyond fall risk alone.

For the patient with osteoarthritis, a structured exercise program under the direction of a physical therapist, aquatic exercise (level of evidence [LOE] = A for both), and weight loss in overweight individuals improve pain and function (LOE = B).[15]

### Orthostatic Hypotension

If orthostatic hypotension is identified on examination, then a variety of techniques can help. Compression stockings can help improve venous return and may have a modest effect on symptoms (LOE = C).[16] Alternatively, multiple medications, including diuretics, antihypertensive medications, nitrates, and older antidepressants can lead to orthostatic hypotension, which is often improved with the discontinuation of unnecessary medications or switching to other medication classes. If episodes occur after meals, then adjusting to frequent, smaller meals can be helpful. Addition of blood pressure-supporting medications is also sometimes needed, and choice often depends on side effects. The most concerning, common side effects of fludrocortisone are hypokalemia, the potential to worsen heart failure in at-risk patients, and lower extremity edema. Midodrine is an $\alpha$-1 receptor agonist that acts to increase vascular tone, and has a distinct group of side effects, including the potential to cause urinary retention in men. Droxidopa is a norepinephrine prodrug that was US Food and Drug Administration–approved in 2014 for treatment of certain types of orthostatic hypotension. This medication appears to have few side effects other than increasing supine blood pressure, which is a side effect shared with midodrine and fludrocortisone.[17] Importantly, although compression stockings and medications may improve symptoms and quality of life, none of the earlier interventions has been shown to decrease falls, although midodrine has been shown to reduce episodes of vasovagal syncope (LOE = B).[18]

### Assistive Devices and Orthotics

A provider may recommend an appropriate assistive device and/or review the fit, condition, and use of a device already used. Physical therapists (PTs) and occupational therapists (OTs) also have particular expertise to recommend and fit devices. Patients often inherit or borrow devices from friends, neighbors, or family members. As a result, the height or other adjustable settings are often incorrect, or the device may be in poor condition because of age and prior use. The use of the device is also important to review, as patients may have never received or may have forgotten past training about device use. For example, the patient may place a cane in the wrong hand, which is an error in use that a provider can easily correct.

Many assistive devices can be useful in the setting of falls or mobility limitations. A cane provides another point of reference for feeling where a person is in relation to the ground, it provides another point of contact for stability, and it can offload a painful or weak limb. Walkers increase stability by adding a large area for additional support, and they can offload painful joints, too. They are often associated with poor posture, however. A front-wheeled walker is the most commonly used type in the geriatric population. Four-wheeled walkers are more helpful in those with generalized weakness or easy fatigability who may need a seat upon which to rest, or who need to carry an oxygen tank with them. However, because this type of four-wheeled walker easily rolls, and their brakes add complexity to use, they are less appropriate for those who are very unstable, and patients with dementia can have difficulty mastering the use of the brakes.[19]

❖❖ **PTs and OTs can help recommend an appropriate assistive device. The American Academy of Family Physicians has a nice overview at** https://www.aafp.org/afp/2011/0815/p405.html **(Accessed 8/20/19).**

Similarly, orthotics are helpful in selected cases. For example, an ankle-foot-orthosis maintains dorsiflexion in a patient with foot drop, thus reducing trip hazard and enabling a more natural gait. Shoe inserts or orthotic shoes may help in painful foot disorders, such as plantar fasciitis, or in the setting of abnormal foot anatomy.

Providers should observe the footwear typically worn by patient and advise changes when needed. For example, an at-risk patient may consistently wear high heels or shoes lacking support such as sandals.

### Medications

Deprescribing is a powerful tool for fall risk reduction. As mentioned earlier, many classes of medications are associated with increased fall risk, including antidepressants, anticonvulsants, benzodiazepines, sleep aids, and medications with high levels of anticholinergic effects. In particular, benzodiazepines have shown a strong link to falls in observational studies. As a result, the risks and benefits of continuing any of these medications should be assessed, and a plan to reduce, eliminate, or substitute higher risk medications can be put into place.

❖ **First, blame medications for falls. Review (or ask a pharmacist to review) the patient's medications, looking for those that increase fall risk and can be safely discontinued or substituted. Be sure to ask about over-the-counter medications too, because some medications, like older antihistamines, can contribute to fall risk.**

On the other hand, adding certain medications may be helpful, such as analgesics in those with osteoarthritic pain. Scheduled acetaminophen is commonly used, although recent studies have called into question its effectiveness with regard to pain relief for knee and hip arthritis.[20] Nonsteroidal anti-inflammatory drugs (NSAIDs) have an increased risk of side effects (hypertension, gastritis or ulcer, renal failure, vascular events) in older adults, so the risks and benefits should be weighed differently than in younger patients. In particular, topical NSAID treatments may offer benefit with fewer systemic side effects (LOE = A for benefit of both topical and oral NSAIDs). Corticosteroid or hyaluronic acid injections also may be helpful, especially over the short term. Interestingly, some of the benefit may be caused by the placebo effect of receiving an injection.[21] Opiates and tramadol appear to have little to no benefit in comparison to nonopiate therapy and placebo, respectively, in terms of pain or pain-related function.[22,23]

## Managing Environmental Factors

Environment often plays a strong role in falls, so interventions targeting these risks can often impact falls even in patients with medical factors that cannot be addressed (LOE = B).[24] For example, interventions can promote a safe home environment through steps, including removing throw rugs, installing grab bars, keeping hallways well-lit at night, reducing clutter, and targeting other trip hazards. OTs can be consulted through a home health referral to make a home visit and provide recommendations regarding home hazards and ways that they can be remedied through structural changes or addressing clutter. Patients who live alone may benefit from a wearable emergency response system, some of which can sense a fall with an accelerometer and automatically alert family or a service. Even more basic emergency response systems still provide patients the ability to summon help in the event of a fall with injuries or if they are unable to right themselves after a fall.

## Other Specific Findings

If a causal, underlying medical condition is found, of course, treatment should be directed there if possible. In particular, if NPH is suspected, a trial of gait observation before and after lumbar puncture is appropriate—a neurologist or neurosurgeon may help with this. Rarely, a vitamin deficiency, such as for vitamin B12, is responsible for peripheral neuropathy, and repletion can reverse the neuropathy.

Managing urinary symptoms, especially nocturnal frequency, can reduce fall risk, especially in cognitively impaired patients. This management could include the use of medications to reduce urge symptoms, or the enhanced management of lower urinary tract symptoms in men with an enlarged prostate. The use of incontinence products, such as briefs, can also reduce patient stress about potential accidents. For patients living in facilities, requesting staff to prompt the patient to toilet at 2- to 3-hour intervals during the day is recommended.

Osteoporosis screening should be performed in accordance with published guidelines, but finding an elevated fall risk can sometimes remind the practitioner that a hip fracture could be imminent without intervention and prompt screening and treatment.

## When to Refer to Specialists

Ear, nose, and throat referral may be appropriate in patients with persistent vertigo or nystagmus. Visual acuity worse than 20/40 with correction should prompt an ophthalmology consultation, to diagnose and treat the underlying condition. In particular, cataract surgery has been shown to decrease fall risk.[25] On the other hand, the use of bifocals for vision correction may increase fall risk because the patient's lower visual field, including peripheral vision, may be obscured because of the differing prescription. If visual field deficits are suspected but are not clear on confrontation exam, then an ophthalmology referral is also indicated for formal testing.

Specific gait abnormalities or examination findings will also warrant referral. If parkinsonism is evident on examination, as indicated by findings, such as rigidity, bradykinesia, and tremor, then referral to neurology or a movement disorder specialist (if available) can be beneficial. This is particularly true when the examination suggests a "Parkinson plus" syndrome, which involves both parkinsonism on examination and other neurologic findings, suggesting the involvement of other regions. For example, severe postural instability, autonomic dysfunction, or ataxia early in the disease course could suggest the presence of multisystem atrophy whereas difficulty with vertical gaze initiation could suggest the diagnosis of progressive supranuclear palsy. Significant parkinsonism with coexisting cognitive impairment should generally prompt referral, except possibly in late-stage Alzheimer disease, where parkinsonism is common, or in a clear case of Lewy body disease if the practitioner is comfortable diagnosing and managing this condition. Findings of severe arthritis changes or joint deformity often warrant orthopedic evaluation, and foot deformities or footwear concerns would lead to a podiatry referral. If available, frequent fallers can also benefit from a falls clinic.

## Guidelines

The US Preventive Services Task Force currently recommends exercise interventions in community-dwelling adults at elevated fall risk (LOE = A)[26,27] and multifactorial interventions that seek to identify and address a number of patient-specific contributing factors to falls—essentially what is described earlier—in selected patients (LOE = B). Despite earlier observational data, vitamin D supplementation should not be given for fall prevention in community-dwelling older adults (LOE = X),[26] based on negative results in later randomized trials, although it seems to have a role in the long-term care population and, of course, in vitamin D–deficient patients.

The Centers for Disease Control and Prevention (CDC)'s Stopping Elderly Accidents, Deaths, and Injuries (STEADI) initiative contains a useful toolkit to help integrate falls screening, assessment, and intervention into a primary care clinic workflow. Based on the 2011 joint American Geriatrics Society/British Geriatrics Society fall prevention clinical practice guideline, it offers a set of simple clinical screening tools and algorithms, as well as patient and provider education and training materials. Although its main focus is on community-dwelling patients, there is some data that STEADI tools may prevent falls after discharge from the hospital, as well.[28] See Fig. 20.1 for our application of the CDC's recommended algorithm for falls screening, assessment, and management, to the content covered in this chapter.

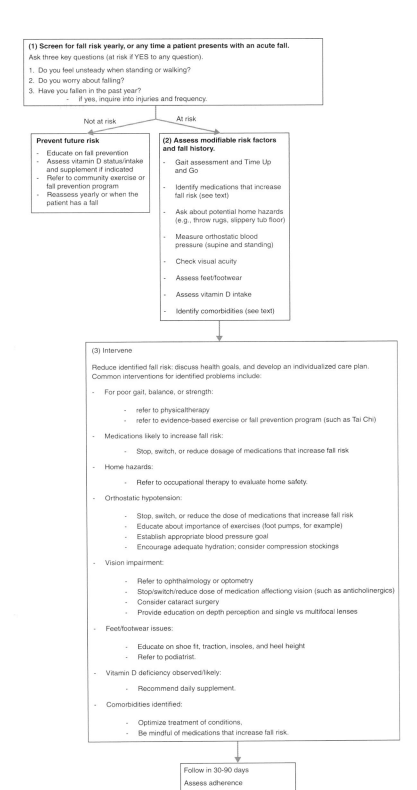

**(1) Screen for fall risk yearly, or any time a patient presents with an acute fall.**

Ask three key questions (at risk if YES to any question).

1. Do you feel unsteady when standing or walking?
2. Do you worry about falling?
3. Have you fallen in the past year?
   -    if yes, inquire into injuries and frequency.

Not at risk          At risk

**Prevent future risk**

-    Educate on fall prevention
-    Assess vitamin D status/intake and supplement if indicated
-    Refer to community exercise or fall prevention program
-    Reassess yearly or when the patient has a fall

**(2) Assess modifiable risk factors and fall history.**

-    Gait assessment and Time Up and Go

-    Identify medications that increase fall risk (see text)

-    Ask about potential home hazards (e.g., throw rugs, slippery tub floor)

-    Measure orthostatic blood pressure (supine and standing)

-    Check visual acuity

-    Assess feet/footwear

-    Assess vitamin D intake

-    Identify comorbidities (see text)

**(3) Intervene**

Reduce identified fall risk: discuss health goals, and develop an individualized care plan. Common interventions for identified problems include:

-    For poor gait, balance, or strength:

     -    refer to physicaltherapy
     -    refer to evidence-based exercise or fall prevention program (such as Tai Chi)

-    Medications likely to increase fall risk:

     -    Stop, switch, or reduce dosage of medications that increase fall risk

-    Home hazards:

     -    Refer to occupational therapy to evaluate home safety.

-    Orthostatic hypotension:

     -    Stop, switch, or reduce the dose of medications that increase fall risk
     -    Educate about importance of exercises (foot pumps, for example)
     -    Establish appropriate blood pressure goal
     -    Encourage adequate hydration; consider compression stockings

-    Vision impairment:

     -    Refer to ophthalmology or optometry
     -    Stop/switch/reduce dose of medication affecting vision (such as anticholinergics)
     -    Consider cataract surgery
     -    Provide education on depth perception and single vs multifocal lenses

-    Feet/footwear issues:

     -    Educate on shoe fit, traction, insoles, and heel height
     -    Refer to podiatrist.

-    Vitamin D deficiency observed/likely:

     -    Recommend daily supplement.

-    Comorbidities identified:

     -    Optimize treatment of conditions,
     -    Be mindful of medications that increase fall risk.

Follow in 30-90 days

Assess adherence

Address barriers to implementing care plan.

• **Figure 20.1** Algorithm for fall risk screening, assessment, and intervention in community-dwelling adults over the age of 65 years. This algorithm adapts the STEADI approach from the CDC (https://www.cdc.gov/steadi/pdf/STEADI-Algorithm-508.pdf) to the approach we outline in the chapter. We share the screen, assess, and multifactorial intervention process with the goal being to identify individuals either with falls or with a high risk of falls to then identify contributory factors that then become targets for intervention. See the relevant text sections for further discussion of individual steps or factors. *CDC*, Centers for Disease Control and Prevention; *STEADI*; Stopping Elderly Accidents, Deaths, and Injuries.

# Nursing Homes and Hospitals

## Long-Term Care

Patients are typically screened for fall risk on admission to nursing facilities, as the Minimum Data Set records both fall history and the amount of assistance needed for mobility. These encounters can be good opportunities for fall risk reduction strategies because residents of long-term care facilities have a higher rate of falls and injury. A variety of instruments may be used (e.g., the Berg Balance Scale), none of which have particularly strong predictive values in community dwellers, but some of these seem to have better predictive value in nursing home (NH) settings where fall rates are higher.[29,30]

Multifactorial, individualized interventions may be effective in preventing falls in long-term care settings,[31] although a recent Cochrane review found that this may apply best in the subacute setting (LOE = C).[32] Vitamin D supplementation does appear to reduce fall rates in NH residents, who have high baseline rates of deficiency (LOE = B).[32] Other interventions, such as medication review and exercise, have less clear benefits in this population.

## Hospitals

In hospitalized patients, various interventions have been tried without conclusive results.[33] The Cochrane review did not find evidence of effects of almost all interventions in NH settings or hospitals, including bed alarms, medication review, and physiotherapy, mostly because the quality of the available evidence was low.[32] The most promising intervention was multifactorial, targeted interventions (LOE = C). Nursing tools used to predict fall risk appeared to have no effect on outcomes compared with nurses' clinical judgment without involving a screening tool, although it is possible that such tools help allocate fall-prevention resources better, make evaluations less taxing, or can help less experienced nurses with the evaluation process. Of note, a multifaceted, multidisciplinary program with the main goal of decreasing inpatient delirium may also significantly decrease fall rates,[34] as may specialized inpatient geriatric units,[35] which also have a strong emphasis on delirium prevention. Delirium is associated with a higher fall risk, so a reduction in the prevalence or severity of delirium could account for a decline in falls. Bedrest and other forms of mobility restriction, sometimes used to prevent in-hospital falls, also have serious side effects, such as muscle atrophy and other adverse physiologic changes. More importantly, limiting mobility in the hospital leads to serious longer-term consequences, including decreased mobility after discharge. As a result, the use of mobility restriction in the hospital needs to be well justified, and then monitored to determine when the restriction can be discontinued.

When a patient does fall, either in a NH or hospital setting, it is important to have a systematic method for assessing the patient and for follow-up. Most institutions have established their own protocols. Box 20.1 summarizes one such approach and is also offered as a reference/checklist when fielding phone calls related to a patient who has fallen in a NH.

---

**• BOX 20.1  Postfall Assessment**

**Immediate**
- Call for help
- Basic life support: danger, responsiveness, airway, breathing, CPR, defibrillate if indicated (DR ABCD)

**Rapid Assessment**
- Pain: grimacing, bracing, restlessness
- Bleeding: skin bruising, edema
- Injury: deformity of leg, inability to move
- Immobilize cervical spine if suspect any head injury before moving

**Secondary Assessment**
- Vital signs (VS): blood pressure (sitting and standing), pulse, respirations, pulse oximetry, temperature, pain scale
- Check blood glucose
- Neurologic checks (hourly × 4, then q4h × 24h)

**History**
- Can patient communicate effectively? Obtain patient's description of fall events
- Obtain witnesses' reports of events
- Description of area where patient was found after fall
- Was patient using/not using assistive device or help of another person on falling?
- Any medication or over-the-counter meds used in past 24 hours or recent illnesses?
- Is the patient on anticoagulant, NSAID, aspirin, antiplatelet therapy, or known coagulopathy?[a]
- Any acute change in behaviors, increasing confusion, lethargy, vomiting, or headache?[a]

**Notification/Verification**
- Notify healthcare proxy if patient desires or does not have decision-making capacity
- Does the patient have an advance directive?
  - Yes—Determine appropriate action consistent with expressed wishes
  - No—To emergency room, clinic, or observe per provider recommendation

**Documentation**
- Complete fall report
- Review incident with clinical leadership
- Implement changes as indicated for future prevention

*CPR*, Cardiopulmonary resuscitation; *NSAID*, nonsteroidal anti-inflammatory drug.
[a]Computed tomography scan recommended.
(Modified from Clinical Excellence Commission. http://www.cec.health.nsw.gov.au/__documents/programs/falls-prevention/draft_revised_post_fall_algorithm_21_oct_2011.pdf.)

---

## Summary

Limited mobility and falls are usually multifactorial in older individuals, with neurologic and musculoskeletal etiologies being commonly involved. However, medications taken by the patient, comorbid medical conditions, and patient environmental factors can often play a central role, and are typically overlooked via the standard medical diagnostic approach. As a result, a more systematic approach to the evaluation of falls involving a detailed history and focused physical examination is more likely to identify opportunities for intervention. As a result, providers will likely find that there are usually many ways to intervene. Among the possible interventions are those that use exercise or Tai Chi to promote strength and balance, or the targeting of multiple contributing factors, are the most likely to be successful in reducing or preventing falls.

## Web Resources

CDC's STEADI initiative: https://www.cdc.gov/steadi
Stanford gait assessment: http://stanfordmedicine25.stanford.edu/the25/gait.html. Accessed 8.12.19.

University of Utah gait examination: https://neurologicexam.med.utah.edu/adult/html/gait_abnormal.html. Accessed 8.12.19.

## Key References

2. Rosso AL, Taylor JA, Tabb LP, Michael YL. Mobility, disability, and social engagement in older adults. *J Aging Health.* 2013;25(4):617−637.

4. Ehlers MM, Nielsen CV, Bjerrum MB. Experiences of older adults after hip fracture: an integrative review. *Rehabil Nurs.* 2018;43(5):255−266.

26. Force USPST, Grossman DC, Curry SJ, Owens DK, et al. Interventions to prevent falls in community-dwelling older adults: US Preventive Services Task Force Recommendation Statement. *JAMA.* 2018;319(16):1696−1704.

33. Hempel S, Newberry S, Wang Z, et al. Hospital fall prevention: a systematic review of implementation, components, adherence, and effectiveness. *J Am Geriatr Soc.* 2013;61(4):483−494.

**References available online at expertconsult.com.**

# 21

# Dizziness

MALLORY MCCLESTER BROWN AND PHILIP D. SLOANE

## OUTLINE

*Additional online-only material indicated by icon.*

## OBJECTIVES

*Upon completion of this chapter, the reader will be able to:*

- Describe the physiologic mechanisms that give rise to a complaint of dizziness, and discuss how these mechanisms relate to specific dizziness symptoms.
- Explain how dizziness in the older adult population may differ in comparison to younger adults, particularly with regard to clinical presentation.

- Use key data from the history and physical examination to create a differential diagnosis in a patient with a dizziness complaint.
- Identify and describe the presentation, prognosis, and treatment of the common causes of dizziness in the older adult population.

### CASE 1

#### Paula Crohn (Part 1)

Paula Crohn is a 78-year-old woman who presents to your office with new onset dizziness. She was on a boat over the weekend for the first time in many years when she had the sudden onset of dizziness. She describes a sensation of "heaviness" in her head. During this episode, she sat quietly and did not speak. She states that it resolved after approximately 15 minutes. She thought she may have a cold coming on.

However, since then she has continued to feel "off" for the past 4 days. The patient describes a continued sensation of dizziness and loss of balance. She denies changes in her vision and her hearing. She can watch television, sew, and engage with friends just fine but as soon as she moves in space, she feels "funny." She has not had a fall but feels like she might.

Past history is significant for a recent diagnosis of hypertension, seasonal allergies, essential tremor, and shoulder pain. Ms. Crohn does not

usually use an assistive device; however, she has taken to using her late husband's walking stick to help with balance. Medications include a low dose of hydrochlorothiazide, propranolol, and occasional use of celebrex.
1. What additional history questions might you ask to help in determining the underlying diagnosis?
2. What physical examination components could be used?
3. What is the differential diagnosis (in order of likelihood) for her dizziness based on what you have learned about this patient thus far?

### CASE 2

#### Nancy Suma (Part 1)

Nancy Suma is an 87-year-old female with a history of urinary incontinence, coronary artery disease, gout, and osteoarthritis who presents for follow-up of a fall that occurred 2 weeks ago while she was visiting family.

She hit her head during the fall; so family took her to the emergency department (ED). In the ED, a head computed tomography (CT) scan was complete and showed no acute infarct or hemorrhage, no obvious fracture but bilateral scalp swelling and a hematoma. She was admitted for observation for 2 days during which cardiac monitoring did not reveal any arrhythmia. Laboratories and vitals were also unrevealing throughout her stay. She continues to describe a sensation in which she "sees spots" with sudden movements. It is worse in the morning when she gets up, but remains throughout the course of the day, especially with standing. She has not thrown up since the hospitalization and her husband notes she has not been confused or more groggy than usual.

1. What additional history would you like to know?
2. What additional portions of the physical examination are particularly useful for her?
3. What is on your differential diagnosis for her dizziness (in order of likelihood)?

## Prevalence and Significance

Dizziness is a common problem addressed in primary care geriatrics and encompasses a variety of symptoms.[1] Its prevalence increases with age, affecting 20% to 30% of adults over the age of 65 years at some time,[2,3] more commonly women.[3] The likelihood of reporting dizziness increases by 10% for every 5 years of increasing age.[4] It is associated with substantial healthcare costs.[5]

The term *dizziness* can be used by patients and doctors to mean many different sensations, including[2]:

- Movement (spinning) of the patient or the room, which we call vertigo
- Disequilibrium or unsteadiness, which is worse when on the feet
- A lightheaded feeling, as though one were about to faint, which is termed presyncope
- A combination of two or more of the earlier sensations, which in older persons almost always includes an element of disequilibrium
- Other, for example, malaise, general weakness, headache, vision changes

Nearly 50% of patients with dizziness report a fear of falling.[6] This fear of falling leads to increased anxiety and consequently to restricted activity, which in turn leads to deconditioning, weakness, worsened disequilibrium, and substantial indirect healthcare costs (such as additional need for help in the home). On the other hand, falling can be a legitimate worry and can lead to such consequences as fractures and head trauma, loss of independence, and even death.[7] Therefore a challenging aspect of dealing with acute and (especially) chronic dizziness is promoting activity while at the same time seeking to minimize risk.

⇢⇢ **Multisensory or multifactorial dizziness is the most common cause of chronic dizziness in older persons.**

In the United States, dizziness accounts for 2.6 million (or 3.3%) of ED visits per year.[8] Its prevalence as a presenting complaint in primary care increases with age and is reported to be the most common presenting symptom of patients aged ≥ 85 years in primary care settings.[9] Two separate population-based studies have found that between 50% and 60% of patients with dizziness reported moderate to severe limitations on everyday life,[10,11] including becoming homebound and isolated, as well as more sedentary.[12]

## Risk Factors and Pathophysiology

The increased prevalence of dizziness with advancing age is the result of specific disease processes superimposed on normal aging physiology.[13] Postural stability involves the complex integration of visual, proprioceptive, somatosensory, and vestibular signals; therefore pathology of any of these signals may lead to the sensation of altered orientation in space, typically perceived as dizziness.[3] A brain that has insufficient information to be confident of where it is in space generates a sensation of dizziness. This can be caused by reduced sensory inputs or impairment of their integration. Well-described anatomic and physiologic changes associated with aging that make older adults susceptible to dizziness include a reduction in sensory receptors located in the inner ear (semicircular canals, saccule, and utricle), proprioceptive end organs, and retina. Vision and visual-vestibular reflexes are known to decline with advancing age. Because adults rely heavily on vision to compensate for vestibular and postural control deficits, a decline in vision contributes significantly to dizziness and subsequent imbalance in older individuals (Fig. 21.1).[3]

Given its multitude of possible etiologies, as well as commonly vague description, dizziness often poses a diagnostic dilemma. It is a subjective complaint, which cannot be measured, and it can be produced by several mechanisms simultaneously occurring. Dizziness is now understood to be a geriatric syndrome, caused and defined by multiple underlying factors and is recognized for its complexity.[5] Most patients with dizziness have a benign condition; however, a small number (<5%) harbor a serious and potentially life-threatening cause.[14]

## Approach to the Patient

### Clarifying the Symptom (When Possible)

Dizziness is often separated into four broad categories: vertigo, disequilibrium, near-syncope, and nonspecific or other causes.[7] One

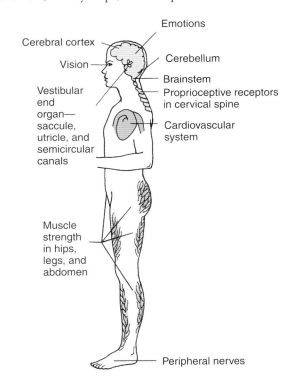

• **Figure 21.1** Components of the balance system.

challenge in diagnosis is that patients often have a hard time distinguishing among various symptoms, and the words they choose do not reliably indicate the underlying etiology.[1]

Distinguishing these is the first step in management, as it will indicate possible causal conditions. This relies largely on the history. Discriminatory questions include:

- "Please try to describe exactly what you feel when you are dizzy."
- "Does the room spin, as if you are on a roundabout?" (vertigo)
- "Do you feel light-headed, as if you are about to faint?" (presyncope)
- "Does it occur when you are lying down?" (if so, presyncope is unlikely)
- "Does it come on when you move your head?" (vertigo more likely)
- "Does it come and go?" (chronic, constant symptoms are more likely to be mixed or psychiatric in origin) (Bowker)

Vertigo is a sensation in which patients feel that their environment is moving. Although the sensation is often rotational, patients also may feel as though they are falling. It is usually episodic, begins abruptly, and is often associated with nausea or vomiting.

Disequilibrium is a feeling that a fall is imminent and is characterized by unsteadiness or imbalance that occurs only when erect and primarily involves the trunk and lower extremities rather than the head; the sensation disappears when sitting or lying.

Near syncope is a feeling that the person is about to pass out. This is distinguished from, but etiologically quite similar to, syncope, the medical term applied when the patient actually faints or blacks out (i.e., has a sudden and temporary loss of consciousness, with spontaneous recovery), because of insufficient oxygen delivery to the brain (via hypotension or other mechanisms). In contrast, patients with presyncope or near-syncope can remember manifestations (e.g., dizziness, blurred vision, weakness, the fall). When a patient complains of the feeling of being about to pass out, we typically think of something cardiovascular in nature. If it happens with standing, we think of postural hypotension, possibly from drugs, acute illness, or a vasovagal phenomena. If it happens while sitting or lying down, a cardiac arrhythmia may be involved.

❖ **Serious and potentially life-threatening causes of acute dizziness are usually cardiovascular (cardiac or cerebrovascular). Thus ruling out cardiovascular causes is critical, because they are the only things that affect prognosis.**

## The Clinical History

The first steps in obtaining a clinical history should involve identifying the dizziness subtype. Other key elements of the initial history include establishing the duration of the symptoms (acute or chronic), determining whether or not the dizziness occurs in episodes, and reviewing medications. These initial steps should markedly narrow the differential diagnosis and guide the remainder of the evaluation, in large measure because the different dizziness subtypes (vertigo, presyncope, and disequilibrium) are associated with different mechanisms and body system, therefore providing important clues to your differential diagnosis.[4] Table 21.1 describes how these initial questions can help identify likely diagnoses.

Symptoms can result from a disturbance in any number of balance control systems, including the visual pathways, vestibular apparatus, cardiovascular system, and central nervous system (CNS). The history can help identify the likely anatomic origin and should include character of the dizziness, timing, whether this is the first attack, the duration of this and any prior episodes, provoking factors, and accompanying symptoms (see Table 21.1). Hearing loss and tinnitus suggest a labyrinthine source, whereas cranial nerve deficits tend to localize pathology to the brainstem or peripheral nerves.[15] Unilateral hearing loss more likely indicates a peripheral cause whereas bilateral symptoms are more likely to be centrally caused. Symptoms, such as visual disturbance (accompanied by nystagmus) and limb ataxia suggest a brainstem or cerebellar lesion.

❖ **Classical hearing loss patterns in dizziness are as follows: low frequency, fluctuating is typical of Ménière disease; low frequency, unilateral, gradually decreasing suggests eighth nerve tumor.**

Timing of the symptoms is important. Common causes of brief dizziness (seconds) include benign paroxysmal positional vertigo (BPPV) and orthostatic hypotension, both of which typically are provoked by changes in head and body position. Attacks of vestibular migraine and Ménière disease often last hours. When episodes are of intermediate duration (minutes), transient ischemic attacks of the posterior circulation should be considered, as well as migraine.

Duration of symptoms can be divided into acute and chronic symptoms. Acute dizziness is defined by being present for 2 months or less whereas chronic dizziness is defined by a time course longer than 2 months. Acute dizziness is usually the result of an insult to one system and can often be treated in a similar way in both younger and older patients. Chronic dizziness is more commonly secondary to a multifactorial cause (often referred to as multisensory dizziness) and requires a treatment plan that addresses multiple systems.

❖ **The most common cause of acute dizziness in older persons is BPPV.**

The initial evaluation should create a differential diagnosis from which a plan for further evaluation, treatment, or observation can be developed.[16] Often, the goal of history-taking is to determine factors that may be modified to help in alleviating the symptom of dizziness. Physical deconditioning, visual problems, lack of use of proprioceptive aids (canes, handrails), medications, and psychological problems are among the most common treatable factors that can contribute to dizziness and its effective treatment.

Note that the most common cause of chronic dizziness in older adults is multisensory or multifactorial dizziness. This condition arises because maintenance of body equilibrium is the function of many different parts of the body, including the vestibular labyrinth, the cerebellum, the brainstem, the visual system, muscle strength, and proprioceptive fibers in the neck and lower extremities. Older persons often report chronic dizziness because of minor or old deficits in several of these systems. A typical case might be a patient who had labyrinthitis decades ago, with some residual impairment of vestibular function, but who only began to experience dizziness when cataracts developed, impairing visual compensation, and diabetes-related peripheral neuropathy impaired proprioceptive input. In such cases, the key role of the geriatrician is to help alleviate symptoms and to improve function. This involves looking for multiple factors and ways to address the symptoms at hand, not necessarily curing them. In the earlier case, for example, the treatment might include correcting cataracts,

## TABLE 21.1   Key Elements of the Initial Dizziness History

### Classify Dizziness Sensation

| Sensation | Description | Mechanism |
|---|---|---|
| Vertigo | Spinning, sense of rotation | Impairment of vestibular system |
| Presyncopal lightheadedness | Feeling one may pass out | Cerebral ischemia |
| Disequilibrium | Loss of balance | Multiple possible mechanisms: abnormal proprioception, cerebellar, motor, or vestibulospinal function |

Approximately half of dizziness in older adults cannot be clearly assigned to one type

### Determine Episodic Versus Chronic/Continuous Nature

| Temporal Nature | Common Causes |
|---|---|
| Episodic | If episodes last for minutes, think benign paroxysmal positional vertigo (BPPV), transient ischemic attack (TIA), cardiac arrhythmia, or orthostatic hypotension<br>If episodes last hours, think Ménière, vestibular migraine, panic disorder, TIA, or transient hypoperfusion<br>If episodes last $\geq$ 24 hours, think recurrent vestibulopathy, Ménière disease, or medication adverse effects |
| Continuous | Medications, psychological, labyrinthitis, vestibular neuronitis, or stroke (especially cerebellar) or multisensory dizziness |

### Identify Accompanying Symptoms

| Symptom | Possible Diagnosis |
|---|---|
| Ear fullness | Ménière disease, otitis media |
| Unilateral hearing loss | Labyrinthitis, Ménière disease, acoustic neuroma (rare) |
| Weakness or diplopia, dysarthria | Vertebrobasilar insufficiency, TIA, migraine |
| Stiff, sore neck | Cervical osteoarthritis with irritation of proprioceptive nerve fibers in facet joints |
| Tinnitus | Ménière disease, acoustic neuroma |

### Inquire About Factors that Worsen or Bring on the Dizziness

| Factor | Suggested Cause |
|---|---|
| Nervousness, worry, emotional stress | Psychological dizziness (e.g., anxiety, depression) |
| Looking upward | Cervical osteoarthritis |
| Rolling over in bed, bending over | BPPV, other vestibular pathology |
| After meals | Postprandial hypotension |
| Standing from Supine position | Postural hypotension |

providing a cane to aid proprioception, and strengthening lower extremity muscles through exercises (to help reduce both falls risk and fear of falling).

◆◆ **A key role of the geriatrician is to help alleviate symptoms and improve function. This involves testing all balance system elements, looking for multiple factors and ways to address (not cure) them.**

## Medication History

Many medications can induce dizziness as an adverse reaction, especially in geriatric patients (Table 21.2). These include anticonvulsants, aminoglycosides, anxiolytics, antidepressants, antihypertensives benzodiazepines, chemotherapeutics, neuroleptics, and nonsteroidal antiinflammatory drugs (NSAIDs). The mechanism varies. Medications that are used to treat cardiovascular disease, such as antiarrhythmics, diuretics, and antihypertensives, typically lead to orthostasis, which can increase fall risk. Antihistamines and some cold remedies also contribute to orthostatic hypotension. NSAIDs and aminoglycosides can be ototoxic, resulting in vestibular impairment and dizziness.[12,17] Polypharmacy increases the risk—one study suggested that patients taking more than five medications had at least a 25% increased risk of presenting with dizziness symptoms.[18]

## Differential Diagnosis

As described previously, the differential diagnosis for dizziness is broad and the underlying cause is often multifactorial. Common dizziness diagnoses and contributing factors in this age group include postural dizziness with or without postural hypotension, positional vertigo, cerebrovascular disease, a variety of acute and recurrent labyrinthine problems, neck problems, physical

| TABLE 21.2 | Common Medications That Cause Dizziness | |
|---|---|---|
| **Medication Class** | **Provocation Mechanism** | |
| Anticonvulsants | Ocular motility | |
| Anxiolytics | Orthostasis, CNS direct effect | |
| Antidepressants | Orthostasis, CNS direct effect | |
| NSAIDs | Ototoxicity | |
| Antiarryhtmics, diuretics, antihypertensives | Orthostasis | |
| Antihistamines and cold remedies | Orthostasis | |

*CNS,* Central nervous system; *NSAIDs,* nonsteroidal antiinflammatory drugs.

deconditioning, visual impairment, and medications. Often, multiple problems coexist, and secondary psychologic disability results.[13]

## Types of Dizziness Sensations

### Vertigo

Vertigo is a sensation in which patients feel that their environment is moving. Although the sensation is often rotational, patients also may feel as though they are falling. Vertigo is usually episodic, begins abruptly, and is often associated with nausea or vomiting when it is severe. It typically involves cranial nerves VII or VIII.

#### Benign Paroxysmal Positional Vertigo

BPPV is the most common vestibular disorder in older persons, occurring in up to 40% of patients experiencing dizziness. It is characterized by intense vertigo lasting a minute or so after movement. It often comes in bouts lasting for days to weeks, occurring several times in a several week period, and then not recurring for months to years. There is usually a latent period of 5 to 10 seconds between change in position and the onset of dizziness and nystagmus. The dizziness tends to subside once the position is resolved.[7] The patient may experience tinnitus but does not experience hearing loss.

It is a specific variety of vertigo characterized by fatigable nystagmus with a short latency period that can be best observed when the Dix-Hallpike maneuver is performed. Patients with BPPV typically present with brief episodes of vertigo associated with a change in head position, such as when turning over in bed or straightening up after bending over. Some 20 to 60 seconds of rotational dizziness after sitting the patient rapidly from a supine position with the head turned 30 degrees to one side or the other is the classic response. Rotational nystagmus is often seen at that time as well. Extending the neck to look and reach up may also produce symptoms in patients with BPPV.[15]

The precipitating factor may be a recent history of middle ear infection (bacterial or viral) or head trauma. More typically, however, BPPV is caused by small, dense calcific particles (otoliths) from the saccule or utricle of the inner ear breaking loose and migrating into the posterior semicircular canal where they amplify rotational movements in the plane of the canal.[4] Over time, particles are absorbed, scarred down, or otherwise dealt with so that symptoms abate.

Fortunately, BPPV usually resolves spontaneously. The Epley maneuver or canalith repositioning procedure can speed resolution.

The success rate for this treatment is about 90%.[15] If symptom control is required before the patient can obtain this treatment, a patient may trial meclizine, valium, or promethazine, but caution should be practiced in using these sedating drugs for older adults because they tend to cause dizziness between BPPV episodes and increase postural instability and falls risk.

#### Acute Labyrinthitis

Acute labyrinthitis is characterized by the sudden onset of severe vertigo often accompanied by visceral autonomic symptoms, including nausea, vomiting, and diaphoresis, and horizontal nystagmus. Hearing may be reduced or distorted in this clinical presentation. Some 50% of patients have a viral upper respiratory infection before onset. Vascular injury may also be a cause. The vertigo typically is severe for 1 to 5 days with several weeks of gradual improvement in older adults. Treatment is mostly supportive. Meclizine and promethazine may be helpful in the acute phase. In severe cases, 5 to 10 days of systemic steroids could be useful. Vestibular exercises have proven effective in reducing long-term disability.

#### Vestibular Neuritis

Vestibular neuritis is a similar clinical presentation, characterized by a sudden onset of vertigo that lasts several hours and that may be accompanied by severe nausea and vomiting. Tinnitus, without auditory impairment, may occur as a result of neuritis. It is thought to be caused by a viral infection of the vestibular nerve concomitant with or following a middle ear infection.[7]

#### Ménière Disease

Ménière disease is characterized by abrupt onset of severe paroxysmal vertigo lasting minutes to hours accompanied by fluctuating low-frequency hearing loss, roaring tinnitus, and aural fullness[15] along with nausea and emesis.[7] The hearing loss is unilateral and sensorineural. Before a vertiginous episode, the patient typically reports a feeling of ear stuffiness.

Ménière disease is caused by distension of the endolymphatic space within the cochlea of the inner part of the ear leading to displacement of inner ear structures. Fluid transport is thought to play an element in this etiology because the disease typically responds to salt restriction and diuretics, which are especially helpful in preventing recurrences. Ear, nose, and throat providers may be helpful in this management.

For acute symptoms, low-dose diazepam, 2 to 7.5 mg once, is generally more effective and less sedating than meclizine, 12.5 to 25 mg every 6 to 8 hours.[15] In severe recalcitrant cases, surgery for the treatment of endolymphatic hydrops may be helpful, but it then leaves the person without vestibular function on the treated side.

### Presyncope

The presyncope symptom complex denotes diffuse cerebral ischemia caused by hypoperfusion. It can be caused by cardiac causes (e.g., dysrhythmias or aortic stenosis), noncardiac causes (e.g., postprandial hypotension, vasovagal episodes, orthostatic hypotension, medications), or both.[3] The feeling arises because of a temporary decrease in blood supply to the brain, leading to cerebral hypoxia. Some medications and dehydration may aggravate symptoms. Beyond the common causes described later, anemia, viral infections, and cardiac arrhythmias may be other contributors to presyncope.

## Orthostatic Hypotension

Postural hypotension may be caused by pooling of blood in the lower extremities, medications, prolonged bed rest, dehydration, or autonomic dysfunction. Orthostatic hypotension is defined by the American Academy of Neurology as a systolic blood pressure decrease of at least 20 mmHg or a diastolic blood pressure decrease of at least 10 mmHg within 3 minutes of standing. Still, some older adults may experience dizziness because of diminished cerebral blood flow even without meeting the earlier criteria. In addition, there is a variant of orthostatic hypotension in which a dramatic blood pressure drop occurs between 10 and 30 minutes after assuming an upright posture (i.e., sitting upright or standing).

Treatment should be targeted at eliminating medications that impair venous tone and contribute to this presentation, and encouragement of physical activity and fitness training. Utilization of compression stockings may also be useful. Providing intravenous fluids to a patient who is dehydrated may be useful in reversing symptoms. In refractory cases, fludrocortisone 0.1 to 1.0 mg daily may help, beginning with 0.1 mg orally (PO) and increasing weekly until pedal edema or adverse effects develop.

## Vasovagal Episodes

Vasovagal attacks can produce lightheadedness, nausea, and pale, cold, and clammy skin without frank syncope. These "episodes" can be caused by emotional stress, such as fright, significant fatigue, gastrointestinal conditions, such as diarrhea and fecal impaction, micturition, and severe pain. They may also be induced when strong emotions initiated in the limbic system activate brainstem medullary vasodepressor centers. Parasympathetic hyperactivity causes a decrease in cardiac output, leading to a reduced cerebral blood flow, hypotension, and bradycardia.[15] Low-dose beta-blocker treatment can be effective, by lessening ventricular mechanoreceptor activation owing to their antisympathetic and negative inotropic effect.[4,19]

## Postprandial Hypotension

Postprandial hypotension, the decrease in systolic blood pressure of 20 mmHg or more within 1 to 2 hours of eating a meal may also cause dizziness.[20]

# Disequilibrium

Disequilibrium is described as a feeling that one is likely to fall and/or is unsteady or imbalanced when erect. The sensation primarily involves the trunk and lower extremities rather than the head. It disappears when sitting or lying.[15] Disequilibrium is generally a multisensory disorder. Its causes and contributing factors can include disorders of the musculoskeletal system, proprioceptive system, cerebellum, vision, vestibular system, peripheral neuropathy, or neurodegenerative disorders in combination or separately—indeed pretty much anything that can cause other dizziness symptoms that tend to be continuous rather than episodic.[4] Symptoms are often worse in the dark. Therapy typically involves use of a cane or walker to help in providing the patient with additional support. Physical therapy may also be useful.

# Other Causes of Dizziness

A number of other vague, difficult-to-categorize presentations exist. Patients may describe a sensation of floating, swimming, giddiness, or dissociation. In many instances (40%−60%), one of these "other" causes may accompany vertigo, presyncope, or disequilibrium in older patients.[12]

## Psychiatric Disorders

Mental health disorders, such as anxiety (including panic disorder), depression, somatization disorder, and substance abuse are among the most common causes of chronic dizziness in young adults. In older persons they are less common as primary causes, but anxiety and/or depression do often accompany dizziness as secondary or contributing factors. One study found that 37.5% of patients aged ≥ 60 years with chronic dizziness met the *Diagnostic and Statistical Manual-III* criteria for psychological disorders, with anxiety disorders, adjustment reactions, and depressive disorders being the most common diagnoses.[21] Typically a vague lightheadedness, continuous dizziness, or floating sensation is described. Treating the psychiatric condition may reduce the disability and provide some improvement in overall function.

## Acoustic Neuroma

Acoustic neuroma should be ruled out in any patient with a progressive unilateral sensorineural hearing loss. The hearing loss differs from that seen in Ménière disease in that it is high frequency and associated with extremely poor word recognition ability. It differs from the presentation of age-related hearing impairment in that it is unilateral and can progress rapidly. Balance is lost, but complaints are more of disequilibrium and do not seem to be related to position. Persons presenting with acoustic neuroma often complain of tinnitus in the affected ear and may have some neurologic symptoms if the tumor is compressing additional cranial nerves.[7]

## Cerebrovascular Disease

Disorders of circulation in the CNS often require neuroradiologic imaging with CT or magnetic resonance imaging (MRI) to confirm the diagnosis. Vertebrobasilar ischemia and cerebellar disorders are the most common CNS disorders associated with dizziness.[7]

Vertebrobasilar ischemia is a manifestation of cerebrovascular disease in which dizziness is accompanied by a sense of imbalance or disequilibrium. When dizziness is related to a transient ischemic attack or stroke, it is accompanied by the onset of neurologic symptoms such as diplopia, dysarthria, or weakness.

Ischemia of the labyrinth or the central vestibular nuclei within the brainstem may result in episodes of acute vertigo associated with focal neurologic deficits such as diplopia, hemiparesis, dysarthria, headache, and blurred vision.[15]

## Other Medical Diagnoses That Can Present as Dizziness

A number of other conditions may present with dizziness and should be considered when obtaining a history, especially if your initial evaluation does not identify a diagnosis or your initial treatment is not effective. These include anemia, metabolic disorders such as diabetes mellitus and thyroid disease, systemic infection, dehydration, trauma, cervical spine problems, neurovascular compression, and basilar insufficiency.

## CASE 1

### Paula Crohn (Part 2)

With pointed questioning about her symptoms, she reveals that the worst dizziness is with rolling over in bed. She also has symptoms when she looks up or moves her head quickly.

Physical examination reveals normal blood pressure values (125/70 mmHg), normal heart rate (80 beats per minute), and otherwise stable vital signs. Her general appearance is well, cardiovascular and respiratory exams are within normal limits. Neurologic examination reveals a positive Dix-Hallpike with notable nystagmus.

Ms. Crohn has experienced similar symptoms in the past.
1. What is your most likely diagnosis at this time?
2. What is the standard treatment that can be used for Ms. Crohn's condition?

## CASE 2

### Nancy Suma (Part 2)

Upon further review of her case, Ms. Suma has had notably difficult-to-control blood pressure with a number of incidents of hypotension followed by elevated blood pressure when medications were changed. She had a stent placed after an NSTEMI 5 years prior. She has not had an echocardiogram since that time, but had grade II diastolic dysfunction on that test.

Her husband reveals that Ms. Suma drinks only two glasses of water each day. She admits she tries to avoid fluids to avoid frequent trips to the bathroom and incontinent episodes. Your nurse repeats her blood pressure measurements in the sitting and standing positions and finds she is notably orthostatic with a change in pressure from 135/80 to 100/60 mmHg upon standing. Her examination reveals a grade III holosystolic murmur heard best at the left upper sternal border but a regular rhythm. She also has 1 to 2+ pitting edema bilaterally in her lower extremities.
1. At this point, what is the most likely diagnosis?
2. What tests or treatments may you consider next?

## Physical Examination

As the causes for dizziness can be so varied, an examination must be tailored to each patient.

This examination is likely to include review of vital signs, general characteristics of the patient, along with a thorough cardiopulmonary exam. Musculoskeletal examination may also be a useful component of the physical examination. Because dizziness can be secondary to a neurologic cause, a thorough neurologic examination is necessary and should include cranial nerve testing, cerebellar testing, and peripheral neuropathy screening. In addition, focus should be paid to hearing, vestibular function, and eye movements. Postural blood pressures, hearing screening, bilateral otoscopic examination, range of motion of the spine, examination of the heart and peripheral arteries, and a standardized depression screen should also be included as appropriate.

Eye movement and equality of this movement should be closely observed. Peripheral eye movement disorders (e.g., cranial neuropathies, eye muscle weakness) are usually disconjugate. Cerebellar, or central pathologies, may be indicated by difficulty in pursuit (ability to follow smoothly moving target) and saccades (ability to look back and forth between two targets). Spontaneous nystagmus, the involuntary back-and-forth movement of the eyes, should also be assessed. Nystagmus is most often of the jerky type, in which a slow drift (slow phase) in one direction alternates with a rapid saccadic movement (quick phase or fast phase) in the opposite direction that resets the position of the eyes. Except in the case of acute vestibulopathy (e.g., vestibular neuritis), if nystagmus is easily seen in the light (as opposed to darkness without ability to focus, as during an ophthalmologic examination), the cause is usually a central neurologic process. When a lesion effects the cerebellar pathway, two characteristic forms of nystagmus typically develop. One is downbeat

nystagmus, where nystagmus occurs vertically with a downward fast phase. The other is gaze-evoked nystagmus where there is horizontal nystagmus that changes direction with gaze. Peripheral lesions typically cause unidirectional horizontal or rotational nystagmus.[1]

The Dix-Hallpike maneuver should be attempted for all patients with brief episodes of dizziness and/or dizziness induced by changes in head position. The patient begins in a sitting position with the head turned to 30 degrees to the right or left. The examiner begins by holding the back of the head, then lowers the patient into a supine position with the head extended backward by about 20 degrees while watching the eyes. Posterior canal BPPV can be diagnosed confidently if transient upbeating-torsional nystagmus is seen. If no nystagmus is observed after 15 to 20 seconds, the patient is raised to a sitting position, and then the procedure is repeated with the head turned to the other side.[1]

## CASE 1

### Discussion

Ms. Crohn is likely experiencing an episode of BPPV, perhaps brought on by a viral middle ear infection in the context of a cold. However, in the setting of recently starting a new blood pressure medication, it is also important to rule out orthostatic hypotension and dehydration. The Epley maneuver can be used to help in treating her BPPV. Typically with time, symptoms will resolve. If symptom control is required, meclizine can be used but should be used with caution in older adults. Some patients may experience recurrences intermittently over several weeks that then resolve for a period of time.

❖❖ **Meclizine (antivert) often makes most dizziness symptoms worse in older persons.**

## Testing

No laboratory testing should be considered routine or mandatory in primary care patients with dizziness. Instead, test selection should be guided by the history and examination. Specific screening laboratory tests, which may be helpful in difficult cases of dizziness, include complete blood cell count, blood glucose, blood urea nitrogen, calcium, liver function, Venereal Disease Research Laboratory test, and thyroid function.

Hematologic studies and chemistry testing may be used to screen for systemic and metabolic causes such as anemia, hyperthyroidism, or syphilis.

Electrocardiography may identify cardiac rhythm abnormalities such as a complete heart block, atrial fibrillation or flutter, or a tachycardia. Prolonged ambulatory monitoring may also be necessary in looking for an intermittent rhythm abnormality especially in patients with presyncope.

Audiometry can be useful in investigating for hearing loss. This can help in identifying acoustic neuroma and/or Ménière disease.

Brain imaging can be used to evaluate for a mass lesion or identify a stroke. MRI is superior to CT imaging as small ischemic lesions that may not be seen on CT scan but can still be the clinical cause of the dizziness.

The Dizziness Handicap Inventory is a 25-item self-assessment instrument that measures the magnitude of functional, emotional, and physical problems associated with vestibular impairment. It can also be helpful in determining where the patient is with regard to quality of life and function. Note that this is only used for following chronic dizziness, but it serves as a good tool for monitoring progress (Table 21.3).

## CASE 2

### Discussion

Ms. Suma has a complicated past medical history but her cardiac history is most concerning. She is taking in little fluid, has notable edema in her bilateral lower extremities, and has known cardiac damage. She is most likely experiencing orthostatic hypotension, which probably led to the initial fall. However, with her seemingly new murmur on examination, you could consider repeating her echocardiogram to guide best management of her coronary artery disease and blood pressure.

## Management

Treatment of dizziness relies on the correct diagnosis and contributing factors. A number of causes of dizziness are reversible or treatable (adverse medication reactions, anemia, depression, cerumen impaction). Other causes, such as BPPV and vasovagal phenomena, are self-limited and benign. In other cases, and particularly in chronic dizziness or in persons with multiple chronic conditions and/or advanced age, dizziness results from multiple factors, and the key to therapy is identifying factors that can be treated. In all cases, the goal of treatment is to identify and effectively treat the underlying cause or, if the underlying cause cannot be reversed or cured, to improve function and minimize symptoms.

**TABLE 21.3   Dizziness Handicap Index**

| | | | Yes | Sometimes | No |
|---|---|---|---|---|---|
| 1. | P | Does looking up increase your problem? | | | |
| 2. | E | Because of your problem, do you feel frustrated? | | | |
| 3. | F | Because of your problem, do you restrict your travel for business or recreation? | | | |
| 4. | P | Does walking down the aisle of a supermarket increase your problems? | | | |
| 5. | F | Because of your problem, do you have difficulty getting into or out of bed? | | | |
| 6. | F | Does your problem significantly restrict your participation in social activities, such as going out to dinner, going to the movies, dancing, or going to parties? | | | |
| 7. | F | Because of your problem, do you have difficulty reading? | | | |
| 8. | P | Does performing more ambitious activities, such as sports, dancing, household chores (sweeping or putting dishes away) increase your problems? | | | |
| 9. | E | Because of your problem, are you afraid to leave your home without having without having someone accompany you? | | | |
| 10. | E | Because of your problem have you been embarrassed in front of others? | | | |
| 11. | P | Do quick movements of your head increase your problem? | | | |
| 12. | F | Because of your problem, do you avoid heights? | | | |
| 13. | P | Does turning over in bed increase your problem? | | | |
| 14. | F | Because of your problem, is it difficult for you to do strenuous homework or yard work? | | | |
| 15. | E | Because of your problem, are you afraid people may think you are intoxicated? | | | |
| 16. | F | Because of your problem, is it difficult for you to go for a walk by yourself? | | | |
| 17. | P | Does walking down a sidewalk increase your problem? | | | |
| 18. | E | Because of your problem, is it difficult for you to concentrate | | | |
| 19. | F | Because of your problem, is it difficult for you to walk around your house in the dark? | | | |
| 20. | E | Because of your problem, are you afraid to stay home alone? | | | |
| 21. | E | Because of your problem, do you feel handicapped? | | | |
| 22. | E | Has the problem placed stress on your relationships with members of your family or friends? | | | |
| 23. | E | Because of your problem, are you depressed? | | | |
| 24. | F | Does your problem interfere with your job or household responsibilities? | | | |
| 25. | P | Does bending over increase your problem? | | | |

Patients are asked to complete the previous survey as it pertains to their dizziness or unsteadiness in the setting of chronic dizziness. Scoring is 0 for an answer of no, 2 for sometimes, 4 for yes. Scores above 10 should be referred for further evaluation of balance and gait.
16—34 points (mild handicap) 36—52 points (moderate handicap) 54+ points (severe handicap).

## Pharmacologic Approaches

Medications are often overused in the treatment of dizziness. Indeed, symptom relief is often provided by withdrawal of medication rather than prescription of a new one. However, there is sometimes a benefit from the use of small doses of medication. Meclizine and other antihistamines may provide relief for acute peripheral vestibular issues, such as Ménière disease or acute labyrinthitis, but caution must be exercised. Symptomatic treatment of nausea with antiemetics may be useful in some cases. Particularly in older adults, all medications should be used with caution to avoid sedation, imbalance, hypotension, and other possible side effects.

## Vestibular Rehabilitation

Vestibular rehabilitation (VR) is a specialized form of physical therapy intended to alleviate both the primary and secondary symptoms of vestibular disorders. It is an exercise-based program designed to reduce vertigo and dizziness through habituation exercises, reduction of gaze instability, and/or reduction of imbalance and fall risk. It also addresses secondary impairments, such as fear of falling, that are a consequence of the dizziness.

The goal of VR is to use a problem-oriented approach to help the patient develop compensatory mechanisms to manage dizziness. Depending on the vestibular-related problem(s) identified, three principal methods of exercise can be prescribed: (1) habituation, (2) gaze stabilization, and/or (3) balance training.[22,23]

Habituation exercise is indicated for patients who report increased dizziness when they move around, especially when they make quick head movements, or when they change positions like bending over or looking up to reach above their head. The goal of habituation exercise is to reduce the dizziness through repeated exposure to specific movements or visual stimuli that provokes patients' dizziness. These exercises are designed to mildly, or at the most, moderately provoke the patients' symptoms of dizziness. Over time, the dizziness intensity can be lowered because of the brain learning to ignore the abnormal signal. Instructing a patient to move multiple times each day from sitting to lying on the back or from flat on the back to the left side are examples of a habituation exercise.

Gaze stabilization exercises are used to improve control of the eye movements so that vision is clear during head movement. These exercises are appropriate for patients who report problems seeing clearly because their visual world appears to bounce or jump around, such as when reading or when trying to identify objects in the environment, especially when moving about. Gaze stabilization exercises are a reasonable procedure for persons with unilateral vestibular disturbances, such as vestibular neuritis, or persons who have had tumors of the eighth nerve removed.

Such exercises may follow a protocol, such as that described here:
1. Hold the target "X" card in your hand about arm's length away and at eye level.
2. Keep your eyes focused on the target and turn your head slowly from side to side. Always keep the target steady and in clear focus. Move your head side to side as fast as you can without the target getting blurry or moving. Do this for 1 to 2 minutes without stopping.
3. Repeat the exercise, but instead of turning your head from side to side, move your head slowly up and down. Always

keep the target steady and in clear focus. Do this for 1 to 2 minutes without stopping.
4. Repeat this exercise with the large "M" target taped to the wall about 5 feet away. The M should be at eye level. First do the exercise with side-to-side head movements, and then do up-and-down head movements.[24]

Balance training exercises are used to improve steadiness so that daily activities for self-care, work, and leisure can be performed successfully. Exercises used to improve balance should be designed to address each patient's specific underlying balance problem(s), to strengthen balance-related muscles (such as the gluteals) and to reduce environmental barriers and fall risk. For example, the exercises should help improve patients' ability to walk outside on uneven ground or walk in the dark.

The purpose of these exercises is to improve an individual's compensatory mechanisms to overcome their dizziness to prevent injury. The brain interprets information gained from the vestibular or balance system. When there is an injury or abnormality in any portion of this system, the brain must be retrained or taught to interpret correctly the information it receives. The goal in repeating these exercises is for the brain to learn to tolerate and accurately interpret this type of stimulation. One must seek out and overcome those positions or situations that cause dizziness. Avoiding uncomfortable activities will only prolong or prevent convalescence.

One example of balance training exercises may be to practice walking.

An individual may work toward walking in a straight line. In a hallway or next to a wall, the patient would be instructed to practice walking in a straight line for 5 minutes with one foot in front of the other or "heel to toe" (with the heel of one foot touching the toe of the other foot). If this is too hard at first for the individual, then encourage practice walking "almost heel to toe" and gradually work to heel-to-toe touching.

## Surgical Therapy

Surgery is very rarely indicated for the treatment of dizziness. With the exception of the surgical removal of a tumor causing dizziness, few indications exist. In severe Ménière disease or refractory BPPV, ablative (intratympanic gentamicin ablation) or nonablative (endolymphatic sac decompression and posterior canal occlusion) may be considered.[4] Both procedures are thought to be very effective for the rare patient who requires this level of intervention for their Ménière disease. Hearing loss may occur in approximately 5% of patients who undergo these procedures.

## Patient Education

One of the consequences of having a disorder causing dizziness is that the symptoms frequently cause people to adopt a sedentary lifestyle to avoid bringing on or worsening dizziness and imbalance that occurs with movement. As a result, decreased muscle strength and flexibility, increased joint stiffness, and reduced stamina can occur, worsening disability and reducing quality of life. Patients should be educated on the pathophysiology and multifactorial nature of dizziness to help the patient understand the underlying diagnosis, treatment course, and general plan of care. Treatment strategies used in rehabilitation can be beneficial for the secondary problems.

Patients experiencing dizziness should be educated based on their specific condition. For example, postural dizziness can be managed by slowly rising from sitting to standing and allowing time to adjust to the positional change.

Geriatric patients should be advised to avoid over-the-counter medications without consultation of the doctor, as many of these agents can worsen or exacerbate dizziness.

## Summary

Dizziness is a common complaint in older adults. Many cases are chronic and multifactorial in nature. Chronic dizziness is different than acute forms as it often includes multiple systems, and treatment often aims to improve compensation and therefore function and quality of life.

## Key References

1. Walker MF, Daroff RB. Dizziness and Vertigo. In: Jameson J, Fauci AS, Kasper DL, Hauser SL, Longo DL, Loscalzo J. eds. *Harrison's Principles of Internal Medicine*. 20th ed. New York, NY: McGraw-Hill; 2018.
3. Eaton DA, Roland PS. Dizziness in the older adult, Part 1. Evaluation and general treatment strategies. *Geriatrics*. 2003;58:28−30, 33−36.
6. Lo AX, Harada CN. Geriatric dizziness: evolving diagnostic and therapeutic approaches for the emergency department. *Clin Geriatric Med*. 2013;29(1):181−204.

8. Weinstein BE, Devons CA. The dizzy patient: stepwise workup of a common complaint. *Geriatrics*. 1995;50(6): 42−46, 49.
15. Eaton DA, Roland PS. Dizziness in the older adult, Part 2. Treatment for the causes of the four most common symptoms. *Geriatrics*. 2003;58(4):46, 49−52.

**References available online at expertconsult.com.**

# 22
# Syncope

**LORRAINE S. SEASE**

## OUTLINE

*Additional online-only material indicated by icon.*

## OBJECTIVES

*Upon completion of this chapter, the reader will be able to:*

- Describe the physiologic mechanisms that give rise to a complaint of syncope.
- Use key history and physical examination data to create a differential diagnosis for the patient experiencing syncope.
- Identify and describe the presentation, prognosis, and treatment of the common causes of syncope in the older adult population.

## Prevalence and Impact

Syncope is an abrupt loss of consciousness with inability to maintain postural tone, followed by complete and spontaneous recovery.[1] The most immediate cause is cerebral hypoperfusion, but the etiologies are many. The prevalence rate, or cumulative incidence of syncope, varies widely between studied groups with the highest reported rates of >50% in women age >80 years. Recurrent syncope is also more common in older groups, especially those age >70 years. This group also experiences higher rates of hospitalization and death related to syncope.[2]

In the older adult, the search for a cause may be complicated by atypical presentation with falls and no clear memory of the event. Life-threatening cardiac etiologies and orthostatic hypotension are more common. The syncopal event itself is more likely to cause injury. Multiple etiologies or contributing factors may need to be addressed swiftly to prevent recurrence and further harm. A thorough history and physical followed by an algorithmic approach to evaluation should lead to an identified cause in almost 90% of cases (Fig. 22.2).

### CASE 1

#### Lucia (Part 1)

Lucia is a 67-year-old woman who visits your walk-in clinic after having passed out at her granddaughter's wedding reception. Upon questioning, she tells you that the reception was held outdoors, in 85° F heat. After standing for a long time in the sun, she felt flushed and a little nauseous. The next thing she knew she was lying on the ground.

Lucia's past medical history is significant for obesity and hypothyroidism. Her only medication is levothyroxine, at a stable dose for several years. Three months ago she was hospitalized overnight after an episode of chest pain. During that hospitalization she had a normal electrocardiogram (ECG) and a negative stress echocardiogram.

1. Based on this history alone, what are the most likely types of syncope and the possible causes or contributing factors?
2. Is Lucia at high risk for cardiac syncope?

## CASE 2

### George (Part 1)

George is a 70-year-old man who reports that he passed out while eating lunch with a friend. His friend is with him at the appointment. He was talking normally and feeling well when, according to his friend, George suddenly slumped over onto the table into his food. His friend called for help and estimates that within 10 seconds George had awakened and lifted his head, looking very pale. His speech and actions were sluggish for another minute or two, but soon he was feeling back to normal. George adamantly rejected calling an ambulance, so his friend agreed to bring him to your office for a same-day appointment.

You have been George's physician for the past 15 years and know that he is an active retiree with longstanding hypertension, hyperlipidemia, and well-controlled diabetes. His medications include lisinopril, hydrochlorothiazide, lovastatin, aspirin, metformin, and glipizide. His last ECG was 5 years ago and was normal. This is his first episode of syncope.

1. Which aspects of George's history put him at increased risk of syncope?
2. Based on the brief description of the syncopal event, what type of syncope do you suspect?
3. Which of George's medications could have contributed to the event?

## Risk Factors and Pathophysiology

The underlying pathophysiology leading to syncope is inadequate oxygenation of the cerebral cortex and reticular activating system, resulting in loss of consciousness. A variety of mechanisms lead to this outcome, but the final common pathway involves reduced blood flow or reduced oxygen-carrying capacity. Fig. 22.1 is a graphic identifying the main physiologic factors that can lead to inadequate brain oxygenation. The differential diagnosis is extensive; many diseases and conditions can lead to this outcome. They fall into these general categories: neurally mediated (reflex) causes, orthostatic hypotension, and cardiac causes.

There are changes in many older adults that make syncope more likely. Physiologic changes in blood pressure regulation increase risk. Changes in baroreflex sensitivity reduce ability to compensate with an increased heart rate or vasoconstriction when blood pressure drops.[3] Changes in the renin-aldosterone system can decrease the ability to retain salt and water, reducing intravascular volume and thus reducing cerebral blood flow. Atherosclerosis and increased endothelin production can impair dilation of cerebral blood vessels in the presence of reduced blood flow. Left ventricular dysfunction and cardiac valvular disease can both lead to reduced cardiac output and arrhythmias. Changes to the autonomic nervous system reduce the body's compensatory mechanism when blood pressure drops.

Other comorbidities and medications can increase risk of syncope. Any condition that decreases intravascular volume or cardiac output can contribute. This includes acute conditions, such as sepsis, hemorrhage, myocardial infarction, and dehydration, among others.[4] Chronic diseases that can contribute include coronary artery disease leading to carotid sinus hypersensitivity, autonomic insufficiency from Parkinsonism, and uncontrolled hypertension. Uncontrolled hypertension can actually increase risk of symptoms from orthostatic changes.[5]

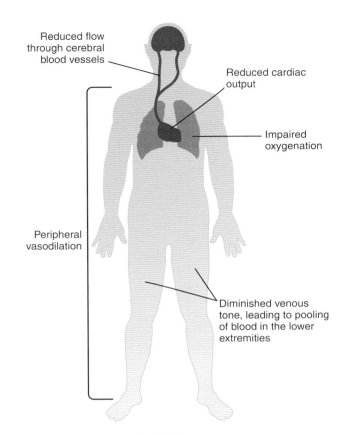

Reduced flow through cerebral blood vessels

Reduced cardiac output

Impaired oxygenation

Peripheral vasodilation

Diminished venous tone, leading to pooling of blood in the lower extremities

• **Figure 22.1** Mechanisms that lead to syncope.

## Differential Diagnosis and Assessment

The major causes of syncope are categorized as neurally mediated or reflex syncope, orthostatic, and cardiac (Table 22.1). There are numerous other conditions that may be diagnosed as syncope but do not meet the definition. Seizures, transient ischemic attack, cataplexy, psychogenic pseudosyncope, and intoxication all fit in the latter category.[1,6] Unexplained falls may actually be undiagnosed syncope and should be evaluated as such in the older patient.

❖❖ **Unexplained falls may actually be undiagnosed syncope and should be evaluated as such in the older patient.**

### Neurally Mediated Syncope

Neurally mediated syncope is considered the most common form in all ages, including the geriatric population.[7] This usually involves the initiation of reflexes that lower blood pressure through venous pooling in the legs, or slow the heart rate through stimulation of the vagus nerve. A variety of physiologic stimuli can trigger this reflex: urination, defecation, cough, gastrointestinal stimulation (especially pain), stimulation of the carotid sinus (e.g., by a tight collar), and intense emotions. Neurally mediated syncope is often considered a benign etiology, but given its high prevalence it can be responsible for a large burden of morbidity and mortality. Multiple contributing factors may lead to this form of syncope.

Vasovagal is the most common type of neurally mediated syncope. This typically involves prolonged standing, emotional

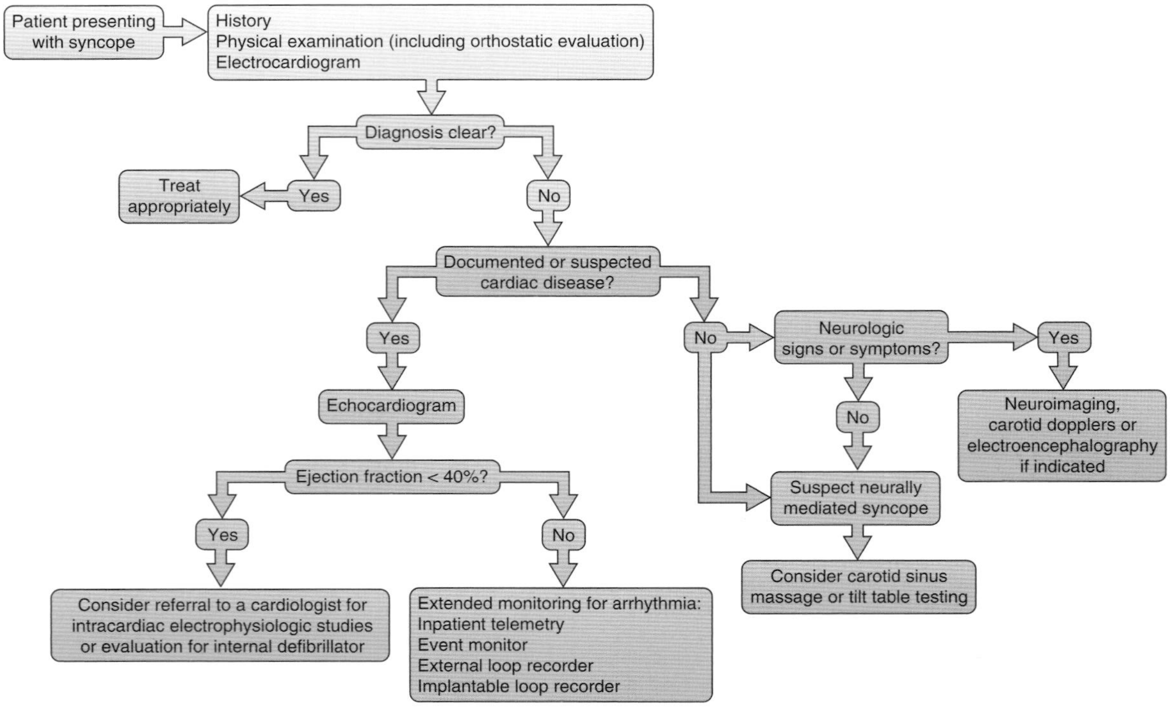

• **Figure 22.2** Syncope evaluation algorithm.

distress, or exertion in warm environments causing the peripheral venous pooling and a drop in blood return to the heart. As the heart recognizes a sudden decrease in preload, it tries to compensate by contracting harder. The quick increase in contraction activates mechanoreceptors in the ventricles that start a reflex mechanism causing the central nervous system to stimulate vasodilation and bradycardia. As the drop in cardiac output becomes more profound, syncope may occur. When suspecting a neurally mediated syncope, look for associated symptoms of nausea and/or vomiting, and a history that includes prolonged standing, hot environments, and/or unpleasant situations. You should be cautious to not assume this diagnosis in patients with known heart disease or repetitive episodes of syncope.

⬥⬥ **Neurally mediated syncope can usually be diagnosed by history and the initial evaluation alone.**

Carotid sinus hypersensitivity is common especially in older men. This is because manual stimulation of the carotid sinus can, in susceptible individuals, stimulate a drop in blood pressure or ventricular pause. A few individuals (e.g., those wearing tight collars) have true carotid sinus syncope, another form of neurally mediated syncope. Stimulation of the carotid sinus must actually reproduce the syncope and not just the fall in blood pressure or absent pulse. In most cases, the provocation of syncope with carotid sinus massage indicates a susceptibility to neurally mediated syncope rather than a diagnosis.

## Orthostatic Hypotension

Orthostatic hypotension is a drop in arterial pressure that occurs when an individual moves to an upright position. Typically, the autonomic nervous system rapidly compensates for this by increasing the

venous tone in the legs; when this system fails, syncope may occur. When the circulating blood volume is depleted, as in dehydration, orthostatic hypotension and syncope may occur even with appropriate autonomic compensation. This diagnosis should be considered in individuals who are on medications that can predispose to orthostasis, who are volume depleted because of illness or blood loss, or who have autonomic insufficiency from a neurologic disorder such as Parkinson disease. A typical case occurs soon after standing up or after prolonged standing in a hot, crowded environment.

The definition of orthostatic hypotension is a drop in systolic blood pressure of $\geq 20$ mmHg, or a drop in the diastolic pressure of $\geq 10$ mmHg, 3 minutes after assuming the upright position, or in head-up tilt table position of at least 60 degrees.[7] This is caused by reduced cardiac output when vasoconstriction upon standing is not adequate to maintain enough venous return to the heart. Neurodegenerative disorders can reduce the ability of sympathetic vasomotor neurons to release norepinephrine that is responsible for vasoconstriction. Some studies have demonstrated that syncope resulting from orthostatic cerebral hypoperfusion can occur even when the standard criteria for orthostasis are not met. Three general mechanisms can lead to this orthostatic syncope (or near-syncope) that does not meet the definition of orthostatic hypotension: early orthostasis, late orthostasis, and impaired cerebral perfusion with only mild decreases in systemic blood pressure. Atherosclerotic narrowing of the carotid and/or vertebral arteries may also increase the susceptibility to syncope from these mechanisms.

## Cardiac Syncope

Cardiac syncope occurs when cardiac output is reduced by arrhythmia, myocardial ischemia or infarction, or outflow obstruction, leading to decreased blood flow to the brain. Several studies have shown an increase in overall mortality and sudden death among patients with

TABLE 22.1

## Differential Diagnosis of Syncope

| Type of Syncope | Common Causes | Prevalence in Persons ≥ 65 Years | Additional Notes |
|---|---|---|---|
| Neurally mediated | • Vasovagal<br>• Situational—defecation, urination, coughing, eating<br>• Carotid sinus syncope | 44% | • Most common cause in older adults<br>• Precipitating factors and prodromal symptoms are clues |
| Orthostatic hypotension | • Autonomic failure from underlying disease—Parkinson, spinal cord injury<br>• Drug-induced—alcohol, vasodilators, diuretics, phenothiazines, antidepressants<br>• Volume depletion | 23% | • More likely to occur in the morning<br>• More common in older ages |
| Cardiac | • Arrhythmias—bradycardia, tachycardia<br>• Structural heart disease—valvular disease, acute infarction, hypertrophic cardiomyopathy, cardiac mass, tamponade | 15% | • Presence of chest pain or dyspnea is strong clue<br>• Less likely to describe nausea, sweating, blurred vision, awareness of impending syncope |
| Drug-induced | • Alcohol, vasodilators, diuretics, phenothiazines, antiarrhythmics, QT-prolonging drugs | 5% | • Drugs can affect susceptibility to all forms of syncope |
| Multifactorial | | 4% | • Generally thought to be more common, especially in older adults, but most studies attempt to identify one primary cause |
| Unexplained | | 10% | |
| Cerebral vascular disease | • Stroke<br>• TIA<br>• Seizure | None in this cohort | • Reported in 3%–32% of cases in other studies including all adults[26] |
| Psychogenic | • Pseudosyncope | None in this cohort | • Reported in 1%–7% of cases in other studies including all adults[26] |

(From Ungar A, Mussi C, Del Rosso A, et al. for the Italian Group for the Study of Syncope in the Elderly. Diagnosis and characteristics of syncope in older patients referred to geriatric departments. *J Am Geriatr Soc*. 2006;54(10):1531–1536.)

*TIA,* Transient ischemic attack.

cardiac syncope compared with patients with syncope from other causes.[1,6] A cardiac cause should be considered when syncope is preceded by palpitations or chest pain, or when it occurs during exertion. Patients with known severe structural heart disease should be considered to have cardiac syncope until proven otherwise.

## Drugs as a Cause of Syncope

Drugs should always be reviewed for contributing factors to syncope of all types. The use of three or more antihypertensives may increase risk of orthostatic hypotension.[8] The use of beta-blockers and thiazide diuretics may be more likely to contribute than angiotensin-converting enzyme inhibitors, angiotensin receptor blockers, or calcium-channel blockers.[9] Alcohol, vasodilators, diuretics, phenothiazines, and antidepressants can also lead to orthostasis. Antiarrhythmic drugs can lead to bradycardia, and QT-prolonging drugs may lead to torsades de pointes. Many drugs used in older adults can prolong the QT interval necessitating a thorough drug review on all patients with syncope.

## Conditions That Mimic Syncope

Other conditions may appear to be syncope but with thorough evaluation are categorized differently. Cataplexy, drop attacks, and some complicated migraines are examples. Seizures, transient ischemic attacks, and subclavian steal may cause neurologic changes leading to falls but do not meet the definition of syncope as transient loss of consciousness with rapid spontaneous recovery.

### CASE 1

#### Lucia (Part 2)

Lucia is lying on the examination table and appears comfortable, but tired. She is sipping water. She tells you that she "just got too emotional." Her initial vital signs were a pulse of 105 beats per minute and a blood pressure of 122/76 mmHg with no significant difference between the supine and upright positions. The other vital signs were normal. Your nurse has already placed an intravenous line and administered 1 L of normal saline at your request. You recheck Lucia's pulse and notice that it is down to the 80s and regular.

You find no abnormalities on Lucia's examination, including a comprehensive cardiac and neurologic examination. She is alert and well oriented. There are no signs of trauma from her fall. Her ECG shows normal sinus rhythm at 90 beats per minute, no conduction delays, and no signs of ischemia.

1. Based on the history, physical examination, and ECG, what other testing is warranted to diagnose her syncope?
2. What new findings, if any, make you think Lucia is at risk for cardiac syncope?
3. Will you hospitalize Lucia?

Upon entering the examination room, you find George sitting in his chair chatting with his friend and looking comfortable. He is fully alert and oriented. His vital signs are normal, including blood pressure in the supine and upright positions. There are no signs of trauma and his head, neck, and pulmonary examinations are normal. The cardiovascular examination is reassuring, with normal heart sounds, no murmur, and a regular rhythm. Carotid arteries are without bruits, and a comprehensive neurologic examination is negative.

The ECG reveals a heart rate of 72 beats per minute with a regular rhythm. Changes from his previous ECG include signs of left ventricular hypertrophy (LVH) and a new left bundle branch block.

1. What is the differential diagnosis for the etiology of George's syncope?
2. Based on the history and examination, what further testing is warranted to diagnose a cause of his syncope?
3. What findings indicate that George is at increased risk of syncope caused by cardiac arrhythmia?
4. Does George need any additional neurologic workup, such as computed tomography (CT) or magnetic resonance imaging (MRI) of the brain, or electroencephalography (EEG)?
5. Will you hospitalize George?

## Evaluation

The evaluation of the patient with syncope involves the parallel process of seeking a specific diagnosis and ruling out cardiac causes that are associated with a higher risk of sudden death. This can be done by taking a careful history, conducting a focused examination, and obtaining an ECG. However, patients without a diagnosis but who are at high risk of having cardiac disease should have additional studies (Table 22.2).

❖ **All syncope evaluations should begin with a detailed history, examination, and ECG.**

Historically, diagnostic testing for syncopal events has been applied inconsistently, and many evaluations did not result in an etiology. Syncope must first be accurately identified and differentiated from events, such as seizure, head injury, and coma. Once identified, the well-established guidelines for evaluation include specific algorithms that should lead to a diagnosis in close to 90% of cases.

## History and Physical Examination

A meticulous history and physical examination are inarguably the foundation of any syncope evaluation. Questions should help the clinician gain an understanding of the circumstances and symptoms that were present before, during, and after the attack, including association with position, particular situations, or activity. Witnesses of the syncopal event should also be questioned. The history alone can often diagnose syncope that is neurally mediated (vasovagal), caused by orthostasis, or drug-induced. Important aspects of the past medical history include a history of cardiac disease, neurologic disease, of metabolic disorder, a medication history, and an inquiry into recent ingestion of alcohol and

**TABLE 22.2**   **Diagnostic Evaluation of Syncope**

| Diagnostic | Level of Evidence[a] | Notes |
|---|---|---|
| History, physical examination, and electrocardiogram as initial evaluation on all patients | B | Electrocardiogram can be diagnostic; also used to risk-stratify for cardiac disease |
| Evaluation for orthostatic hypotension when suspected | B | Blood pressure measured supine and during active standing for 3 minutes |
| Tilt-table testing | B | To evaluate unexplained syncope in high-risk settings (occupational) or for recurrent syncope after cardiac causes ruled out |
| Electrocardiographic monitoring | B | When initial evaluation is suggestive but not diagnostic of arrhythmia as the etiology<br>Setting of monitoring chosen based on risk |
| Electrophysiologic study | B | For patients with known ischemic heart disease when arrhythmia is suspected<br>Not indicated if there is already an indication for a defibrillator |
| Echocardiography | B | To evaluate suspected structural heart disease or risk-stratify |
| Exercise testing | C | When syncope occurs during or soon after exercise |
| Psychiatric evaluation | C | When psychogenic cause is suspected |
| Neurologic evaluation | B | Not recommended for routine evaluation of true syncopal event<br>Use only if history and examination suggests neurologic cause, such as stroke or seizure |
| Routine comprehensive blood testing not recommended | B | Targeted blood tests reasonable based on clinical assessment |

(From Shen W-K, Sheldon RS, Benditt DG, et al. 2017 ACC/AHA/HRS Guideline for the evaluation and management of patients with syncope: a report of the American College of Cardiology/American Heart Association Task Force on Clinical Practice Guidelines and the Heart Rhythm Society. *J Am Coll Cardiol.* 2017;70(5):e39−e110.)
[a]Level of Evidence: A = high-quality evidence from at least one randomized controlled trial; B = moderate-quality evidence from randomized or nonrandomized controlled trials; C = limited data from studies with limitations of design/execution, or consensus of expert opinion.

nonprescription drugs. A comprehensive physical examination may provide clues to the presence of cardiac disease, underlying neurologic disorder, or vascular disease.

## Assessing for Orthostatic Hypotension

To test for orthostatic hypotension, have the patient lie supine for 3 minutes, after which the blood pressure and pulse are checked. Then have the patient stand for 3 minutes, during which the pulse and blood pressure are monitored. Orthostatic hypotension is said to be present if the patient experiences a drop of at least 20 mmHg in systolic blood pressure or at least 10 mmHg in diastolic blood pressure within 3 minutes after standing from the recumbent position. This can also be demonstrated using the tilt table in the head-up position at a minimum 60-degree angle.

Multiple variables can affect the blood pressure readings, including the time of day, ambient temperature, postural deconditioning, and medications. Some patients may not show the diagnostic drop in blood pressure until they have been standing for at least 10 minutes. For these reasons, it is important to repeatedly check for a significant orthostatic blood pressure reduction while keeping in mind when medications are taken, time of meals, and any other factors that may have contributed to the syncopal episode. Many patients who demonstrate a significant drop in blood pressure after standing will also have an increase in pulse rate, but it is not necessary for the diagnosis of orthostasis.

⁙ **Always consider medications as a possible contributing factor.**

## Ruling Out Cardiac Causes

Structural heart disease, defined as coronary heart disease, congestive heart failure, valvular disease, or congenital heart disease, is the only independent risk factor for a cardiac cause of syncope. ECGs and echocardiograms may not be diagnostic in many cases, but they can stratify patients' risk by identifying who has structural heart disease. The extent of the evaluation for a cardiac cause depends on the patient's risk status and the history of the event.

The ECG is an inexpensive and noninvasive test that can diagnose some cases of syncope and guide further testing in others. More important, the ECG is excellent at identifying who has structural heart disease. Abnormal findings include signs of previous myocardial infarction (i.e., Q waves or inverted T waves), bundle branch block, evidence of ventricular hypertrophy, atrioventricular blocks, bradycardias or tachycardias, premature ventricular contractions, pacemaker spikes, or significant ST abnormalities. Patients with syncope and any of these ECG abnormalities should receive cardiac testing, whereas there is poor diagnostic yield from further cardiac testing of patients with a normal ECG and no cardiac history.

Patients with a cardiac history or abnormal ECG should have an echocardiogram if the etiology of syncope is still unknown after the initial history and physical examination. Similar to the ECG, echocardiography will diagnose a few rare causes of syncope, such as critical aortic stenosis, hypertrophic cardiomyopathy, myxoma, or tamponade. In addition, the systolic function (i.e., ejection fraction) can be used as a marker of risk for arrhythmia. An ejection fraction of 40% or less places a patient at significantly higher risk of arrhythmia.

The continued search for arrhythmia in patients with undiagnosed syncope may include in-hospital telemetry monitoring, 24- or 48-hour Holter monitoring, external loop recorders, and implantable loop recorders. These should be reserved for the select group of patients with unexplained syncope who are at increased risk for arrhythmia based on history and initial workup. Syncope may have occurred during exertion, when supine, or preceded by palpitations. The generalized use of these studies is inefficient and expensive. The finding of arrhythmia correlating with syncope or syncopal events without arrhythmia is both prognostically important and should be considered a successful test. The implantable loop recorder deserves special mention because it can be used for up to 36 months after implantation, increasing the likelihood of identifying another syncopal event.[10] It can store data for 20 minutes before activation, allowing patients or their companions a longer time window to activate the device. Recent guidelines encourage early consideration of an implantable loop recorder in patients with recurrent unexplained syncope and without suspected structural heart disease.[6]

Cardiac stress testing is rarely diagnostic in the evaluation of syncope. It should be considered in patients who have syncope during or after exercise or who experience chest pain associated with syncope. These select patients may show cardiac ischemia or arrhythmias associated with exercise.

Intracardiac electrophysiologic studies are invasive and very expensive. They should be reserved for patients with known structural heart disease who have very high risk for arrhythmias because of depressed ventricular function.[1,6] This will most likely include patients with previous myocardial infarction. In this procedure, catheters are inserted from the femoral vein into the heart near the electrical conduction system. Atrial and ventricular pacing along with electrical stimulation are used to assess sinus node recovery time, sinoatrial conduction time, and atrioventricular node function. This allows detection of conduction abnormalities that can predispose to arrhythmia.

### CASE 2

#### George (Part 3)

Concerned that a cardiac arrhythmia may have caused George's syncope, you hospitalize him for cardiac monitoring and further risk stratification. The LVH and bundle branch block on the ECG, combined with his history of multiple cardiac risk factors, place him at high risk of having coronary heart disease and therefore of arrhythmia. His medication list is also worrisome because it contains drugs that could contribute to hypotension, electrolyte imbalances, and dizziness. A reflex-mediated situational syncope from swallowing is unlikely because George had no prodromal symptoms. The reassuring neurologic examination and lack of postictal symptoms eliminate the need for further neurologic testing at this time.

An echocardiogram shows an ejection fraction of approximately 40% with mild hypokinesis of the left ventricle and trace mitral valve regurgitation. You have George do a stress treadmill test along with the echocardiogram to make sure there is no reversible ischemia. George is able to exercise to about 80% of his maximum heart rate, but has to stop before goal because of fatigue. However, there are no signs of ischemia on the ECG or echocardiogram. George's serum sodium, potassium, chloride, blood urea nitrogen, creatinine, and magnesium are all within normal limits. His cardiac enzymes are also normal.

By this time George has been in the hospital for almost 24 hours on telemetry without event. You explain to George that you think he probably had a myocardial infarction at some point in the past couple years, and you are worried that he passed out from a cardiac arrhythmia. You decide to discharge him home with a 30-day event monitor and arrange for an appointment with a cardiologist. He is not to drive in the interim.

1. What evidence makes you more concerned about a cardiac arrhythmia?
2. What are your options to further investigate for a cardiac arrhythmia?
3. How do you defend your decision to hospitalize George? Could all of this have been done as an outpatient?

## Evaluation for Neurally Mediated Syncope

Many cases of neurally mediated syncope will be diagnosed by the initial evaluation alone, based on a classic history. When the etiology of syncope is unknown and the syncopal events have become repetitive or dangerous, tilt table testing and carotid massage can be useful as confirmatory tests. It is important that cardiac syncope be effectively ruled out by prolonged cardiac monitoring if there is known or suspected cardiac disease.

Tilt table testing evaluates whether a patient is susceptible to neurally mediated syncope. There are multiple protocols for tilt table testing, some including the use of drugs, such as isoproterenol or nitroglycerin, to increase susceptibility to syncope and improve the sensitivity of the test.[11] The procedure involves baseline measurement of blood pressure and heart rate while supine, then quickly bringing the patient to an upright position by tilting to approximately 60 degrees. A foot board is in place for support. The patient is then kept in the tilted position for 45 minutes to observe for syncope or presyncopal symptoms while continuing to monitor heart rate and blood pressure. Some protocols include giving isoproterenol or nitroglycerin after the patient has been asymptomatic in the tilted position for 10 to 15 minutes, followed by further monitoring. If syncope symptoms occur during testing and correlate with a quick drop in blood pressure or pulse rate, it is considered a positive test. Likewise, if syncope occurs without a change in vital signs, a neurally mediated syncope is less likely and other etiologies should be considered. Arguments against the use of tilt table testing include variable sensitivity of the procedure, questionable diagnostic yield, and reproducibility of the test.[12]

Standardized carotid sinus massage (CSM) in the supine and upright positions can help differentiate carotid sinus syndrome, or carotid sinus hypersensitivity, another risk factor for neurally mediated syncope. The carotid sinus is located in the common carotid artery at the branching point of the internal and external branches. Baroreceptors in the carotid sinuses respond to changes in pressure by stimulating the vagus nerve and causing inhibition of the sinus node of the heart or a reduction in blood pressure. A positive cardioinhibitory result is present if a cardiac pause (asystole) of 3 seconds or longer occurs during or immediately after CSM; a positive vasopressor result is present if the systolic blood pressure drops 50 mmHg or more and is accompanied by symptoms. To confidently diagnose carotid sinus syndrome as a cause of syncope, the syncopal event should be reproduced during the test. This procedure requires continuous heart rate monitoring, frequent blood pressure monitoring, intravenous access, and the availability of atropine and transcutaneous pacing. The presence of carotid bruits or known atherosclerotic disease of the carotids is a contraindication to the procedure because of the rare but real chance of harm from stroke.[13,14]

## Neurologic Evaluation

Neuroimaging and EEG have been used frequently in the routine workup of patients with unexplained syncope. Retrospective reviews have shown them to have a poor yield and high cost when used on unselected patients. In a review of 649 cases of syncope, 253 patients received EEG testing, and only 6 had abnormal results that explained the cause of syncope (i.e., a yield of 2%). All 6 of those patients had a history and physical examination that was consistent with seizure. In the same group, 283 patients had brain CT scanning, also with a yield of 2%; all had a history and examination consistent with acute stroke. Carotid Dopplers were done

in 185 patients, with a 0% yield.[15] As a result, published recommendations for syncope evaluation limit neurologic or cerebrovascular imaging and EEG testing to patients with symptoms or signs of acute stroke or seizure.[3]

## Psychiatric Evaluation

Some cases of recurrent syncope will not have a clear diagnosis after initial evaluation and should be considered for evaluation of pseudosyncope. Clues to a psychiatric origin include a history of anxiety or depression, repetitive syncope of unknown origin, a repeatedly negative cardiac workup, and multiple episodes of syncope without injury. In patients with suspected psychiatric disease, consulting with a psychiatrist is important both to identify or rule out a mental health diagnosis and to review the potential effects of psychotropic medications. Video recording and tilt table testing can also be helpful, because, if syncope is provoked, the physician can readily differentiate psychogenic (i.e., with no blood pressure or pulse changes) from neurally mediated syncope.[16]

---

### CASE 1

#### Lucia (Part 3)

The history of Lucia's syncopal event is confirmed by her husband and daughter. They explain that Lucia had been standing in the sun for over an hour even though they had encouraged her to take a rest in the shade. It had been a long day, full of excitement and emotion, in the hot sun, and possibly with a glass or two of champagne. The bride and groom were just getting ready to leave the reception when Lucia passed out. This confirms your theory that Lucia most likely experienced a situational neurally mediated syncope. You have her get up and walk around, making sure that she feels steady on her feet. Then you send her home with her family with instructions to drink plenty of fluids and follow up with her primary physician within a week.

---

### CASE 2

#### George (Part 4)

Two days later, George's wife calls you after he passed out again briefly while working in the yard. You are able to get the report from the event monitor and it shows that George had 30 seconds of ventricular tachycardia. You have George readmitted to the hospital immediately where an implantable cardiac defibrillator is inserted the following day.

---

## Management

Management of syncope involves first deciding on the appropriate setting for evaluation when it is not clear from your initial evaluation. The initial evaluation helps to estimate the patient's short-term risk of a severe event, including death. Patients without an established diagnosis of their syncopal event and with known or suspected cardiac disease are at high risk of death or a serious event and should be hospitalized for immediate evaluation. Others must be triaged based on risk factors. Numerous studies have looked at decision rules using age, history, symptoms, vital signs, laboratory results, and ECG results, among others, to help decide when patients should be hospitalized after presenting for evaluation of a syncopal event. The criteria most commonly cited are an abnormal ECG, shortness of breath, heart failure, abnormal vital signs, and

• BOX 22.1  Criteria That Suggest Cardiac Etiology of Syncope That Should Prompt Hospitalization

- Syncope while supine
- Syncope during exertion
- Palpitations before syncope
- Family history of sudden cardiac death at a young age
- History of previous myocardial infarction
- Signs of heart failure
- Abnormal electrocardiogram suggesting possible arrhythmic cause
- Persistent abnormal vital signs
- Known structural heart disease (e.g., severe aortic stenosis, hypertrophic cardiomyopathy)

(From Shen WK, Sheldon RS, Benditt DG, et al. 2017 ACC/AHA/HRS guideline for the evaluation and management of patients with syncope: a report of the American College of Cardiology/American Heart Association Task Force on Clinical Practice Guidelines and the Heart Rhythm Society. *J Am Coll Cardiol.* 2017;70(5):e39–e110; Brignole M, Moya A, de Lange FJ, et al. 2018 ESC Guidelines for the diagnosis and management of syncope. *Eur Heart J.* 2018;39(21):1883–1948.)

older age.[17–20] Box 22.1 lists the symptoms or signs of heart disease that should prompt hospitalization.

⧫⧫ **Consider hospitalization to evaluate patients with a high likelihood of cardiac syncope.**

First-time syncope in patients without known or suspected heart disease usually warrants the reduction of risk factors for further syncope. This includes reducing polypharmacy and medication misuse, treating underlying illness, and education regarding avoidance of triggers. Further treatment for patients with recurrent syncope or syncope in high-risk settings requires knowledge of the underlying mechanism of the syncopal event (i.e., type and cause of syncope).

## Treatment of Neurally Mediated Syncope

Lifestyle measures are the basis for treatment of reflex syncope. Awareness of the cause of the event and prodromal symptoms allow avoidance of triggers and possible prevention by abortive maneuvers. Education should also include information on drugs, including alcohol, that may increase susceptibility to syncope events. Physical counterpressure maneuvers can help increase blood pressure when prodromal symptoms occur; these include squatting, leg crossing, and hand gripping with arm tensing.[21] These isometric exercises can be taught easily to willing and functional patients to help them avoid or delay syncope. The exercises will be less useful in frail older adults.

## Treatment of Orthostatic Hypotension

Patients and their family members should be educated on how to treat symptoms of orthostasis to prevent recurrent syncope and falls. Fig. 22.3 outlines an approach. Acute water ingestion and use of physical counterpressure maneuvers can help. There are a variety of counterpressure maneuvers described, including crossing and squeezing the legs and buttocks, most likely the easiest and most doable for an older adult. Compression garments may be useful if accepted. An elastic abdominal compression wrap has shown some

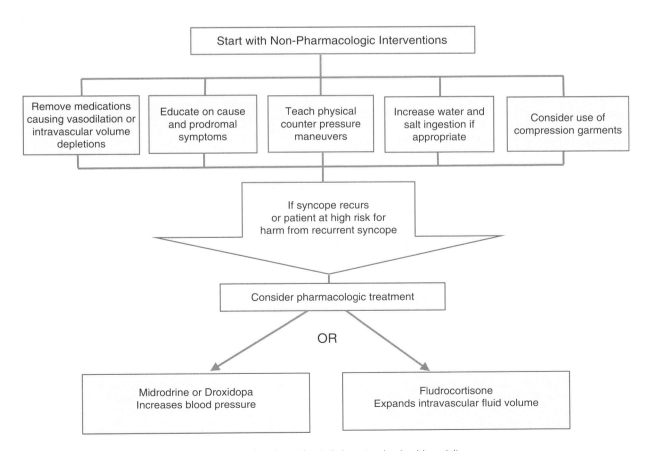

• **Figure 22.3** Management algorithm to prevent syncope related to orthostatic hypotension in older adults.

ability to help increase blood pressure whereas compression socks have shown little benefit.[22] These efforts aim to reduce venous pooling in the extremities to avoid a dangerous drop in blood pressure.

Education about lifestyle changes can make a significant difference in raising the standing blood pressure and preventing syncope. Increased intake of salt and fluids—including 2 to 3 L of fluid and 10 g of sodium per day—can help when cardiac disease or hypertension is not a contraindication. Sleeping with the head elevated > 10 degrees can help reduce nighttime polyuria, although effect on orthostasis is not consistent.[21]

There are now several pharmaceutic options to consider for management of orthostatic hypotension after education and lifestyle changes fail to prevent recurrence. They deserve consideration when risk of recurrent syncope and injury is high. Midodrine, an alpha-agonist, shows some benefit in reducing symptoms of orthostasis and increasing standing blood pressure. Fludrocortisone, a mineralocorticoid that expands fluid volume through its effect on the kidneys, is also used for these same effects although the evidence of its benefit is not as strong. More recently, droxidopa was approved for the treatment of orthostatic hypotension showing that it can reduce symptoms and increase standing blood pressure.[23] There are potential negative effects of all of these drugs, including supine hypertension and worsening of congestive heart failure. Patients or their caregivers must be educated on the need to take these at least 4 hours before lying down to avoid dangerous hypertension.

## Treatment of Cardiac Syncope

Patients with syncope related to structural cardiac disease should have disease-specific interventions. Underlying disease, such as acute myocardial infarction, pericardial tamponade, or aortic stenosis, should receive appropriate therapy. Treatment of arrhythmias should be targeted to the cause. As in all types of syncope, drugs that may contribute should be discontinued when possible. Cardiac defibrillators, catheter ablation, cardiac pacing, and antiarrhythmic drug therapy are additional treatment options.

Implantation of a cardiac defibrillator is indicated when syncope is caused by ventricular tachycardia or fibrillation and structural heart disease is present.[6] Severely depressed left ventricular ejection fraction alone, even without documented ventricular tachycardia, is also an indication for defibrillator placement. Unfortunately, patients are still at risk for recurrent syncope after defibrillator placement, but their risk of sudden cardiac death diminishes.

Catheter ablation should be considered in patients with syncope related to supraventricular tachycardia or ventricular tachycardia when there is no structural heart disease. Some cases of rapid atrial fibrillation may also be treated with catheter ablation. Antiarrhythmic drugs include rate-controlling and rhythm-controlling drugs; they are used as first-line treatment in many cases of atrial fibrillation or in conjunction with catheter ablation.

Cardiac pacemaker placement is indicated in the presence of syncope that has been correlated with bradycardia caused by sinus node disease. It should also be considered in patients with syncope who are found on monitoring to have asymptomatic pauses of $\geq$ 3 seconds, second-degree Mobitz II block, or complete atrioventricular block. Patients with bundle branch block who have abnormal electrophysiologic testing may also benefit from pacemaker placement.

## Treating Other Causes of Syncope

As noted previously, cerebrovascular disease is an uncommon cause of true syncope. When it does occur, treatment should be directed to the underlying disease, such as stroke. Psychogenic causes of syncope necessitate psychiatric evaluation and help with treatment. Explanation of the psychological cause and acknowledgment that the syncopal acts are involuntary can help the patient accept the possibility of the diagnosis. This is important to make referral for treatment successful.[16,24]

### CASE 1

#### Discussion

Lucia's case was fairly straightforward because of the circumstance of her event and her uncomplicated past medical history. After her initial medical history, examination, and ECG, you do not think the syncope is related to medications and you are fairly certain that she is at low risk for cardiac syncope. You believe that she was probably dehydrated from standing in the sun, and that a glass or two of champagne may have impaired her venous tone. As she became overheated and overcome by emotion, she was at risk for neurally mediated syncope. The nausea she experienced before passing out is consistent with this explanation.

The lack of cardiac or neurologic findings on examination was reassuring. She had no signs or symptoms of trauma that would necessitate radiographic evaluation. Her slower pulse rate after receiving some fluids again suggest she was dehydrated. The normal ECG along with no history of heart disease and a recently normal echocardiogram convince you that she does not have structural heart disease that would put her at increased risk for cardiac syncope. Therefore you feel confident diagnosing Lucia with situational syncope and sending her home with her family.

If similar syncopal events become a reoccurring problem for Lucia, you could consider tilt table testing to confirm your suspicion of her susceptibility to neurally mediated syncope. Educating her on prodromal symptoms and situations associated with neurally mediated syncope may help avoid injury.

### CASE 2

#### Discussion

George's case presents an example of syncope that cannot be diagnosed by history, examination, and ECG alone. You should be concerned about cardiac syncope from the beginning after hearing about the sudden nature of his syncope and the lack of prodromal symptoms. Other red flags from George's history include his medical history that puts him at high risk of cardiac disease, and his medications. The abnormal ECG provides additional evidence that cardiac causes should be considered. The echocardiogram helps to risk-stratify George because his low ejection fraction is an additional risk factor for arrhythmia.

In this case, cardiac stress testing is not done as part of the syncope workup but to further investigate the new diagnosis of cardiac disease. If you already knew about George's cardiac disease and abnormal ECG, then the echocardiogram and cardiac monitoring would have been sufficient.

Hospitalization was warranted for George because of the high suspicion of cardiac syncope and the need to further evaluate his cardiac disease. On discharge, George had a support system in place and would always have someone around who could call for help and activate the event monitor if he became symptomatic again. It would also be important to ensure that George's family is aware of steps they might take in the case of a cardiac event, including when to initiate cardiopulmonary resuscitation and use of an automated external defibrillator. Finally, do not forget to think of safety issues, such as driving, flying, operating heavy machinery, and risk of injury from falls.

## Summary

Healthcare professionals inconsistently use evidence-based guidelines in the evaluation and management of older adults with syncope regardless of setting. Syncope observation units for moderate-to high-risk patients have not been widely adopted and could improve care while also reducing cost.[25] More effective treatments to prevent recurrent syncope are needed. Future research needs include pharmacologic options and pacemaker placement for the treatment of some forms of neurally based syncope. Home blood pressure and heart rhythm monitoring are becoming more accessible and potentially useful to the clinician to help with diagnosis.

The multifactorial nature of syncope in older individuals makes it a challenging problem to diagnose and treat. Syncope may be misdiagnosed as falls, or neurologic events such as seizures may be miscategorized as syncope. There are excellent evaluation and management algorithms but they first require accurate identification of the event. This may require additional investigation and corroboration from family. For some patients, the etiology of syncope will never be clear. A comprehensive geriatric assessment using the interdisciplinary team will maximize chance of diagnosis and management to prevent recurrence.

## Key References

1. Shen WK, Sheldon RS, Benditt DG, et al. 2017 ACC/AHA/HRS guideline for the evaluation and management of patients with syncope: a report of the American College of Cardiology/American Heart Association Task Force on Clinical Practice Guidelines and the Heart Rhythm Society. *J Am Coll Cardiol.* 2017;70(5):e39−e110.
3. Lipsitz LA. Altered blood pressure homeostasis in advanced age: clinical and research implications. *J Gerontol.* 1989;44(6):M179−183.
6. Brignole M, Moya A, de Lange FJ, et al. 2018 ESC Guidelines for the diagnosis and management of syncope. *Eur Heart J.* 2018;39(21):1883−1948.
7. Freeman R, Wieling W, Axelrod FB, et al. Consensus statement on the definition of orthostatic hypotension, neurally mediated syncope and the postural tachycardia syndrome. *Clin Auton Res.* 2011;21(2):69−72.
21. Logan IC, Witham MD. Efficacy of treatments for orthostatic hypotension: a systematic review. *Age Ageing.* 2012;41(5):587−594.

**References available online at** expertconsult.com.

# 23

# Urinary Incontinence

CATHERINE E. DUBEAU

## OBJECTIVES

*Upon completion of this chapter, the reader will be able to:*

- Discuss the prevalence and impact of urinary incontinence (UI) in older persons.
- Describe how medical conditions and medications affect continence.
- Perform an initial evaluation of incontinence in an older person.

- Develop and implement an initial patient-centered treatment plan for incontinence incorporating multifactorial causes and tailored to the older person's goals of care.

---

Urinary incontinence (UI) is the symptom of involuntary leakage of urine, and is one of the major geriatric syndromes.[1] Other lower urinary tract symptoms commonly occur with incontinence (Table 23.1). The four main symptom types of UI in older persons are urge, stress, mixed urge and stress, and nonspecific.

## CASE

### Anna Roberts (Part 1)

You are seeing Mrs. Roberts for routine follow-up; her problem list includes hypertension, type 2 diabetes, chronic kidney disease stage 3, congestive heart failure, mild aortic stenosis, and knee osteoarthritis. She is 78 years old and ambulates with a cane. Her medications are lisinopril, amlodipine, furosemide, aspirin, atorvastatin, metformin, glipizide, and calcium with vitamin D. She complains of feeling more fatigued and is not sleeping well; her review of symptoms is otherwise negative. Her examination reveals a new 6-lb weight gain and 2+ peripheral edema. When asked about the weight gain, she admits to occasionally skipping doses of furosemide when she is going out for the day for fear of wetting herself. You are unsure if incontinence is new as she has never mentioned it before.

1. How will you assess Mrs. Roberts for the presence of incontinence, now and going forward? What factors are potentially contributing to her urine leakage?

## Prevalence and Impact

The prevalence of UI increases with age in both men and women, but it should never be accepted as a normal part of aging. Among women, the prevalence of UI is 15% to 30% in the community,[2] 50% among the homebound, and 70% in nursing home residents.[3] The prevalence in men is about one-third that

## TABLE 23.1  Lower Urinary Tract Symptoms

| Symptom | Description |
| --- | --- |
| Urgency | Compelling, often sudden need to void that is difficult to defer. |
| Urge incontinence | Leakage preceded by/associated with urgency. Common precipitants include running water, hand washing, going out in the cold, even the sight of the garage or trying to unlock the door when returning home. The need to "rush to the toilet" and length of time one can forestall an urgency episode are less useful symptoms because they reflect cognition, mobility, toilet availability, and sphincter control, as well as bladder function. |
| Stress incontinence | Leakage with effort, exertion, sneezing, or coughing. Leakage may be provoked by minimal or no activity when there is severe sphincter damage. Leakage coincident with cough, laugh, sneeze, or physical activity suggests failure of sphincter mechanisms. Leakage that occurs seconds after the activity, especially if difficult to stop, suggests a cough-induced uninhibited detrusor contraction. |
| Mixed incontinence | Presence of both urgency and stress UI symptoms. Patients vary in the predominance, severity, and/or bother of urge versus stress leakage. |
| Overactive bladder | Symptom syndrome (not a specific pathologic condition) consisting of urgency, frequency, and nocturia, with or without urge incontinence. |
| Frequency | Complaint of needing to void too often during the day, as defined by the patient. |
| Nocturia | Complaint of waking at night one or more times to void. If these voids are associated with UI, the term *nocturnal enuresis* may be used. |
| Slow (weak) stream | Perception of reduced urine flow, usually compared with previous performance. |
| Hesitancy | Difficulty in initiating voiding, resulting in a delay in the onset of voiding after the individual feels ready to pass urine. |
| Straining | Muscular effort either to initiate, maintain, or improve the urinary stream. |
| Intermittent stream | Sensation that the bladder is not empty after voiding. |
| Postvoid dribbling | Small amounts/drops of urine after voiding has stopped. More common in men. |

*UI*, Urinary incontinence.

of women until age 85 years, when the ratio becomes 1:1. The prevalence of moderate to severe UI (at least weekly or monthly leakage of more than just drops) is 23% among women aged 60 to 79 years and 32% in those 80 years and older.[2] Among nursing home residents, prevalence rates range from 43% to 77% (median 58%).[3] The severity of UI (i.e., greater frequency and/or volume of leakage) also increases with age.[4] UI severity often increases without treatment. One-third of middle-aged and younger-old women (aged 54–79 years) with baseline monthly UI progressed to leaking at least once a week over 2 years.[5] Little is known about the incidence and severity of UI over time in older men. The most common type of UI in older persons is urgency UI[2]; however, the prevalence of stress UI in men is rising with increased surgical treatment of prostate cancer. The evidence is inconsistent whether race and ethnicity are associated with UI prevalence in older women,[6,7] and there are no data on their impact in older men.

UI decreases health-related quality of life, and negatively impacts self-esteem, self-perception of aging, activities, and sexuality.[8] Although some older persons with UI curtail outside activities, many continue but are burdened by fear of embarrassment.[9] Among frail nursing home residents, UI adversely impacts social interactions, an important aspect of quality of life in this setting.[10]

Morbidity from UI includes urinary tract infections, skin breakdown, falls, and fractures. UI places significant burden on caregivers and can lead to depression and subsequent nursing home placement; indeed, approximately 6% to 10% of nursing

home admissions in the United States are attributable to UI.[11] UI results in significant economic costs for the affected individuals and the healthcare system. The estimated total national cost of overactive bladder (OAB) with urgency urinary incontinence (UUI) in 2007 was $65.9 billion, with projected costs of $76.2 billion in 2015 and $82.6 billion in 2020. This 2007 estimate was markedly higher than those reported in older studies and have nearly doubled for older persons in the last decade.[12] Over half of UI-related costs (56%) are consequence costs (e.g., from nursing home admissions and loss of productivity). Treatment and diagnosis account for approximately one-third of costs. Out-of-pocket expenses, predominantly for protective undergarments, are estimated to run from $750 to $900 yearly, or almost 1% of the median annual household income.[13]

Despite the significant personal burden of UI, at least half of older persons with UI never mention it to their care providers, and in turn physicians often do not ask patients about it or fail to offer specific treatment.

❖❖ **Screen all older persons for urinary incontinence.**

## Screening

Annual screening for UI is recommended for all older persons (Table 23.2). Although the link between screening and improved outcomes is weak, the rationale for screening is based on the high prevalence of UI, underreporting by patients, and known

## TABLE 23.2   Recommendations for Urinary Incontinence (UI) Screening

| Organization | Target Population | Recommendation | Level of Evidence/Grade of Recommendation/Rationale |
|---|---|---|---|
| USPSTF[57] | All older adults | Screen for UI as part of an overall prevention recommendations for older adults | Not provided |
| Women's Preventive Services Initiative[58] | All women | Screen annually for UI | Weak; detect UI before it significantly affects women's lives |
| World Health Organization[59] | All older persons | Routinely check for UI in older women and men | Rationale: at least half of women with UI do not report this issue to their general practitioner |
| ACOVE[60] | All persons age ≥ 75 years | 1. During an initial evaluation, all persons should have documentation of the presence or absence of UI  2. During annual evaluations, all persons should have documentation of the presence or absence of UI | N/A |

*ACOVE*, Assessing Care of Vulnerable Elderly; *USPSTF*, US Preventive Services Task Force.

quality gaps in treatment. Table 23.3 lists suggested screening questions.[14]

## CASE

### Anna Roberts (Part 2)

On further questioning, Ms. Roberts says that when she takes her "water pill" she "can't make it to the bathroom on time." She wears protective pull-ups instead of regular underwear, which she changes at least once during the day. She reports going to the bathroom at least three times during the night, which is affecting her sleep. She has no leakage when she coughs, denies dysuria, but reports more constipation lately. Her diabetic control has been good.

1. What type of incontinence does Mrs. Roberts have?
2. What additional evaluation and testing are needed before recommending therapy?

## Risk Factors

UI shares common risk factors with other geriatric syndromes, such as falls and functional dependence, suggesting common etiologic pathways.[15] These risk factors include lower and upper extremity weakness, sensory and affective impairment, and brain magnetic resonance imaging or computed tomography white matter signal abnormalities.[16] Along with age and functional impairment, the other main risk factors for UI are female gender, obesity, diabetes, stroke, depression, fecal incontinence, and hysterectomy.[2,17] Nursing home residents with UI are more likely than continent residents to have impaired mobility, dementia, delirium, and receive psychoactive medications.[18] Parity increases the risk of UI in younger women, but the impact attenuates with age.[2] Although there is some evidence for a genetic predisposition to UI,[19] this may not be a significant risk factor in older persons.

UI is common in persons with cognitive impairment, which is associated with a 1.5- to 3.5-fold increase in UI risk, especially for

## TABLE 23.3   Screening Questions for Incontinence

| Type of Incontinence | Question | Psychometrics |
|---|---|---|
| Any | "Have you had any problems with bladder or urine control?"  "Do you ever leak urine when you don't want to?" | Kappa 0.8 (95% CI, 0.3–0.9)  Percentage agreement 90% (95% CI, 84%–95%) |
| Stress incontinence | "Do you ever leak urine coughing, sneezing, lifting, walking, or running?" | Positive LR 2.2 (95% CI, 1.6–3.2)  Negative LR 0.39 (95% CI, 0.25–0.61)  Sensitivity 0.86 (95% CI, 0.79–0.90)  Specificity 0.60 (95% CI, 0.51–0.68)  Posttest probability decreases with age (from 87%–42%) |
| Urge incontinence | "Do you experience such a strong and sudden urge to void that you leak before reaching the toilet?" | Positive LR 4.2 (95% CI, 2.3–7.6)  Negative LR 0.48 (95% CI, 0.36–0.62)  Sensitivity 0.75 (95% CI, 0.68–0.81)  Specificity 0.77 (95% CI, 0.69–0.84)  Posttest probability increases with age (from 52%–91%) |

(From Holroyd-Leduc JM, Tannenbaum C, Thorpe KE, Straus SE. What type of urinary incontinence does this woman have? *JAMA*. 2008;299:1446–1456.)

*CI*, Confidence interval; *LR*, likelihood ratio (likelihood that a given test result would be expected in a patient with the target disorder compared with the likelihood that the same result would be expected in a patient without the target disorder).

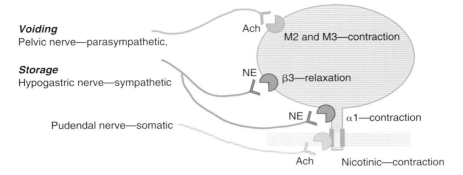

**Voiding**
Pelvic nerve—parasympathetic,

**Storage**
Hypogastric nerve—sympathetic

Pudendal nerve—somatic

Ach
M2 and M3—contraction

NE
β3—relaxation

NE
α1—contraction

Ach
Nicotinic—contraction

• **Figure 23.1** Physiology of micturition. *Ach*, Acetylcholine; *M*, muscarinic; *NE*, norepinephrine.

bothersome UI.[20] At the same time, UI is not inevitable even in frail cognitively impaired persons, because the association between cognitive impairment and UI is at least in part mediated by functional impairment and disability.[21]

## Pathophysiology

The lower urinary tract has two main functions, storage of urine and effective voiding. Key components of the bladder for continence are its detrusor smooth muscle and epithelial layer (the urothelium). Continence is mediated through the actions of the central and autonomic nervous systems (Fig. 23.1).[22] Storage occurs through sympathetic stimulation of alpha-adrenergic receptors in the smooth muscle sphincter causing contraction, and beta-adrenergic receptors in the detrusor causing relaxation. Voiding occurs with parasympathetic stimulation of muscarinic receptors in the detrusor. The urothelium contains rich and varied receptor signaling systems, which conduct information about bladder filling and sensation through the sacral spinal cord to pontine and subcortical areas.[23] The prefrontal cortex is an important center for suppressing urgency and forestalling voiding.[24] The micturition center in the pons coordinates the cortical inhibitory inputs with the afferent signaling from the detrusor to allow storage of a large volume of urine at a low pressure, and adequate bladder emptying through detrusor contraction and sphincter relaxation.[22] Maintenance of urethral closure during storage is augmented by support of the fascia and the levator ani.[25]

The main lower urinary tract pathophysiologic types of UI in older persons are:
- Urge, the inability to store urine because of uninhibited contractions of the bladder muscle (detrusor)
- Stress, the inability to store urine because of inadequate sphincter closure
- Mixed, a combination of urge and stress physiology
- Inability to void completely because of insufficient bladder contraction and/or bladder outlet obstruction

UI solely caused by impaired bladder emptying (sometimes called "overflow" incontinence) is uncommon even among frail older persons and older men with benign prostate disease.[26] OAB is a syndrome defined by the symptom of urgency, usually with frequency and nocturia, with or without urgency incontinence.[1] Frail older adults may have detrusor hyperactivity with impaired contractility (DHIC), in which urge UI coexists with impaired detrusor contractility (evidenced by an elevated postvoiding residual volume [PVR]), when no other cause of impaired emptying is identified).[27]

**◆◆ UI in older persons is multifactorial, resulting from interactions between lower urinary tract abnormalities, neurologic control of voiding, multimorbidity, medications, and functional impairment.**

A key difference between UI in younger and older persons is that in older persons, UI may be precipitated or worsened by factors outside of the lower urinary tract. These factors include mobility, environment (access to toilets), medical conditions (Table 23.4), medications (Table 23.5), mentation, manual dexterity, and motivation.

## Evaluation

Fig. 23.2 provides an outline of evaluation of UI in older persons. Once a patient acknowledges UI, the next step is to characterize and determine the type of UI symptoms (see Table 23.1), including the frequency and volume of leakage. A proxy for the latter can be the frequency of pad changes. Most UI is relatively slow in onset and should not be associated with pelvic pain. Acute onset of UI and/or the presence of suprapubic, lower abdominal, and/or pelvic pain are "red flags" for underlying neurologic or neoplastic disease, and should prompt quick referral to neurology and/or urology/gynecology specialists.

There should be an assessment of the bother and quality-of-life impact of UI for the patient and the caretaker. A recent consortium recommended the Urogenital Distress Index-6 because of its brevity, inclusion of a variety of UI symptoms and types of UI, as well as symptom bother, its well-established validity, sensitivity to change, and scholarly use.[28] It also can be used to assess the effect of treatment (minimum important difference in score = 11).[29] This can be done informally, or through specific questions and questionnaires. Some patients, especially women, may report little bother because they "manage fine with pads." It is important to ask such persons about their concerns about treatment, as they may be underestimating efficacy and overestimating invasiveness and adverse effects of treatments.

Other lower urinary tract symptoms, particularly slow stream, hesitancy, insufficient emptying, and postvoid dribbling, are less specific but may be bothersome to the patient and can be important to assess before treatment. Frequency may reflect high fluid intake overall and/or use of caffeinated drinks and alcohol.

The evaluation should include a review of past medical history and medications for factors that may contribute to UI and/or its severity. For some conditions (e.g., stroke), it is important to assess its relationship to the onset of UI, to determine whether the condition is related to UI. All patients with UI should be screened for

## TABLE 23.4 Medical Conditions Associated With Urinary Incontinence

| Condition | Effect on Continence |
|---|---|
| Cardiovascular disease | |
| • Arterial vascular disease | Detrusor underactivity or areflexia from ischemic myopathy or neuropathy |
| • Heart failure | Nocturnal polyuria |
| Gastrointestinal disease | Impaired emptying/urinary from constipation; fecal and urinary incontinence commonly coexist |
| Metabolic diseases | |
| • Diabetes mellitus | Uninhibited bladder contractions (DO) with UUI; detrusor underactivity caused by neuropathy; osmotic diuresis; altered mental status from hyper- or hypoglycemia; retention and overflow from constipation |
| • Hypercalcemia | Diuresis; altered mental status |
| • Vitamin B$_{12}$ deficiency | Impaired bladder sensation and detrusor underactivity from peripheral neuropathy |
| Musculoskeletal disease | Mobility impairment; DO with UUI from cervical myelopathy in rheumatoid arthritis and osteoarthritis |
| Neurologic conditions | |
| • Cerebrovascular disease, stroke | DO with UUI from damage to upper motor neurons; impaired sensation to void from interruption of subcortical pathways; impaired function and cognition |
| • Delirium | Impaired function and cognition |
| • Dementia | DO with UUI from damage to upper motor neurons; impaired function and cognition |
| • Multiple sclerosis | DO, UUI, areflexia, or sphincter dyssynergia (concomitant sphincter and detrusor contraction), depending on level of spinal cord/CNS involvement |
| • Normal-pressure hydrocephalus | DO with UUI from compression of frontal inhibitory centers; impaired function and cognition |
| • Parkinson disease | DO with UUI from loss of inhibitory inputs to pontine micturition center; impaired function and cognition; retention from constipation |
| • Spinal cord injury | DO with UUI, areflexia, or sphincter dyssynergia (depending on level of injury) |
| • Spinal stenosis | DO with UUI from damage to detrusor upper motor neurons (cervical stenosis); DO or areflexia (lumbar stenosis) |
| Obstructive sleep apnea | Nocturnal polyuria |
| Peripheral venous insufficiency | Nocturnal polyuria |
| Pulmonary disease | Conditions with chronic cough can worsen stress UI |
| Psychiatric disease | |
| • Affective and anxiety disorders | Decreased motivation |
| • Alcoholism | Functional and cognitive impairment; rapid diuresis and retention in acute intoxication |
| • Psychosis | Functional and cognitive impairment; decreased motivation |

(Modified from DuBeau CE. Urinary incontinence. In: Harper, GM, Lyons, WL, Potter JF eds. *Geriatrics Review Syllabus: A Core Curriculum in Geriatric Medicine*, 10th ed. New York, NY: American Geriatrics Society; 2019: p. 302.)

*CNS*, Central nervous system; *DO*, detrusor overactivity; *UI*, urinary incontinence; *UUI*, urgency urinary incontinence.

depression and functional status. If not previously done, patients should be assessed for functional impairment that can affect toileting (e.g., with chair rise or Timed Up and Go) and cognitive screening (e.g., MiniCog or Montreal Cognitive Assessment), which may be considered for the purpose of planning treatment.

All patients should have a physical examination assessing comorbid conditions that may be contributing to UI. An abdominal examination is neither sensitive nor specific for detecting bladder distension.

At the initial or subsequent primary care evaluation, all women should have a pelvic examination to check for vulvovaginal abnormalities. Signs of vaginal mucosal atrophy are thinning, pallor, loss of rugae, urethral caruncle, and inflammation (erythema,

petechiae, telangiectasia, and friability). A more detailed examination includes check for pelvic organ prolapse and a bimanual examination for masses or tenderness. To check for prolapse, use a split-speculum examination, removing the top blade of the speculum entirely. Insert and hold the bottom blade firmly against the posterior vaginal wall for support. Ask the woman to cough, looking for whether the urethra remains firmly fixed or swings quickly forward (urethral hypermobility) and for bulging of the anterior vaginal wall either to or through the level of the hymenal ring (anterior wall support defect, or cystocele). Check for a posterior wall support defect (rectocele) by turning the bottom blade of the speculum to support the anterior vaginal wall and having the patient

## TABLE 23.5  Medications Associated With Urinary Incontinence

| Medication | Effect on Continence |
| --- | --- |
| Alcohol | Frequency, urgency, sedation, delirium, immobility |
| $\alpha$-Adrenergic agonists | Outlet obstruction (men) |
| $\alpha$-Adrenergic blockers | Stress leakage (women) |
| ACE inhibitors | Associated cough worsens stress and possibly urgency leakage in older adults with impaired sphincter function |
| Anticholinergics | Impaired emptying, retention, delirium, sedation, constipation, fecal impaction |
| Antipsychotics | Anticholinergic effects plus rigidity and immobility |
| Calcium-channel blockers | Impaired detrusor contractility and retention; dihydropyridine agents can cause pedal edema, leading to nocturnal polyuria |
| Cholinesterase inhibitors | Urinary incontinence; potential interactions with antimuscarinics |
| Estrogen | Worsens stress and mixed leakage in women |
| Gabapentin, pregabalin | Pedal edema causing nocturia and nighttime incontinence |
| Loop diuretics | Polyuria, frequency, urgency |
| Narcotic analgesics | Urinary retention, fecal impaction, sedation, delirium |
| NSAIDs | Pedal edema causing nocturnal polyuria |
| Sedative hypnotics | Sedation, delirium, immobility |
| Thiazolidinediones | Pedal edema causing nocturnal polyuria |
| Tricyclic antidepressants | Anticholinergic effects, sedation |

(From DuBeau C. Urinary incontinence. In: Harper GM, Lyons WL, Potter JF eds. *Geriatrics Review Syllabus: A Core Curriculum in Geriatric Medicine*, 10th ed. New York, NY: American Geriatrics Society; 2019: http://geriatricscareonline.org.)

*ACE*, Angiotensin-converting enzyme; *NSAIDs*, nonsteroidal antiinflammatory drugs; *UI*, urinary incontinence.

cough again. Men should have a genital examination. A digital rectal examination can detect prostate nodules, rectal masses, and stool impaction, but does not provide reliable assessment of prostate size. A detailed neurologic examination is not necessary in the initial evaluation of UI, but one should be considered for patients with sudden onset of UI (especially urge), concomitant fecal incontinence, known neurologic disease (other than dementia), or new onset of neurologic symptoms. Sacral root integrity is assessed by including perineal sensation, resting and volitional tone of the anal sphincter, anal wink (visual or palpated anal contraction in response to a light scratch of the perineal skin lateral to the anus), and the bulbocavernosus reflex (anal contraction in response to a light squeeze of the clitoris or glans penis).

All patients should have a urinalysis, with reflex urine culture only if the patient has other symptoms of urinary tract infection (e.g., dysuria, fever) or if the UI is of new onset or new worsening. The primary purpose of urinalysis is to look for hematuria (and in diabetic patients, glycosuria, which can cause frequency).

There is no strong evidence to support routine PVR testing in the initial evaluation of persons with UI, including men because of the low prevalence (prior probability) of a significantly elevated PVR (Level of Evidence [LOE] = D).[30] Furthermore, there is no agreed-upon definition of an "abnormal" or "clinically significant" PVR. Patients for whom a PVR should be considered are those with complex neurologic disease, long-standing diabetes mellitus (especially if poorly controlled), women with marked pelvic organ prolapse, and patients with a high burden of anticholinergic medications (LOE = D). PVR can be measured by bladder scan or catheterization and should be done as soon after voiding as possible.

A team-based approach for incontinence screening and assessment might include medical assistants or nurses administrating UI screening, diagnostic and quality-of-life questionnaires, along with relevant cognitive and functional assessments, followed by physicians or advance practice provider reviewing medical conditions, medications, and conducting a physical examination.[31]

## Nocturia

Nocturia is a bothersome symptom that frequently coexists with UI. Although some patients have the same etiology for nocturia and UI (e.g., detrusor overactivity, bladder outlet obstruction), many patients have nocturia caused by other factors. These include disproportionate nocturnal urine excretion (nocturnal polyuria), a primary sleep disturbance (e.g., pain, depression, disruptive bed partner), or a combination.[32] Nocturnal polyuria is a common driver of nocturia in older persons. It is defined as greater than one-third of total 24-hour urine production occurring during hours of sleep.[32] Nocturnal polyuria can be assessed using a bladder (voiding) diary (Table 23.7). The differential causes of nocturnal polyuria include excess fluid intake (especially beverages with caffeine or alcohol), pedal edema (often associated with medications—see Table 23.5), congestive heart failure, and—importantly—sleep apnea.[33,34] Sleep apnea causes a nocturnal diuresis, as well as sleep disturbance, and should be considered in all patients with unexplained nocturnal polyuria, especially given its significant morbidity. Use of continuous positive airway pressure decreases nocturia[35] (see Chapter 31).

**ACTIVE SCREENING OF ALL OLDER PATIENTS**

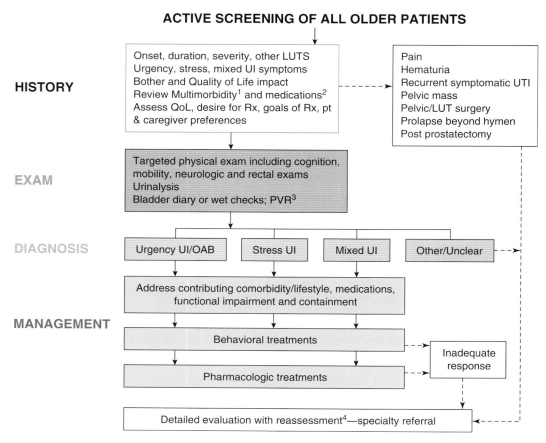

• **Figure 23.2** Evaluation and management of patients with urinary incontinence (UI).
[1]See Table 23.2.
[2]See Table 23.3.
[3]Postvoid residual (PVR) test is optional; considered for women with marked pelvic floor prolapse, longstanding diabetes, history of urinary retention or high PVR, recurrent urinary tract infections, medications that impair bladder emptying, chronic constipation, persistent or worsening UI on treatment with bladder antimuscarinics, or prior urodynamic study demonstrating detrusor underactivity and/or bladder outlet obstruction (grade C). If PVR is elevated (e.g., 200 mL), consider trial of alpha-blocker (men), treat constipation, decrease or eliminate anticholinergic medications and calcium channel blockers, and consider catheter drainage followed by voiding trial if PVR 300 mL.
[4]Detailed evaluation with reassessment could include the following: bladder diary and PVR, if not previously done; revisiting/testing for comorbidity (e.g., sleep apnea if nocturia with nocturnal polyuria is present); trial of alternative medication for urgency incontinence (another antimuscarinic or switch to beta-3 agonist, if not contraindicated); or addition of biofeedback for pelvic muscle exercise training.
*LUT,* Lower urinary tract; *LUTS,* lower urinary tract symptoms; *OAB,* overactive bladder; *PVR,* postvoiding residual; *Rx,* treatment; *UI,* urinary incontinence.
(Modified from DuBeau CE, Kuchel GA, Johnson T, et al. Incontinence in the frail elderly. In: Abrams P, Cardozo L, Khoury S, Wein A, editors. *Incontinence.* 4th ed. Paris: Health Publications; 2009:961–1025.)

## Management

### CASE

#### Anna Roberts (Part 3)

Pertinent findings on Mrs. Robert's examination are scant crackles at lung bases and moderate atrophic vaginitis. Patient Health Questionnaire-2 was 0, and STOP-BANG was 2. Her mobility is actually better now, since she completed her last course of physical therapy. Last month her hemoglobin $A_{1C}$ was 7.1, and urinalysis today is negative. She agreed to take furosemide, and you stopped amlodipine, increased lisinopril, and reminded her to use acetaminophen instead of NSAIDs for arthritis pain. You additionally recommend that she stop drinking coffee with dinner.

She returns a month later, at which time her weight has decreased 5 lbs, and edema is just trace. She is now getting up only once most nights.

However, her urge leakage has increased, and she is now using pads inside her pull ups and changing them twice a day.
1. How will you now treat her leakage symptoms?

Treatment of UI in older persons should proceed in a stepwise process, starting with addressing contributing comorbidity and medications, followed by lifestyle interventions, then behavioral treatment, pharmacologic treatment, and, if necessary, minimally invasive and surgical treatments (see Table 23.6). Management should focus on the most bothersome aspects of UI for an individual patient, and patient (and/or caregiver)—defined goals of care.[36] Complete cure (no leakage) is relatively uncommon and largely limited to persons with mild UI, women with stress UI treated surgically, or those with specific

## TABLE 23.6  Urinary Incontinence Treatments

| Intervention | Target Type of Incontinence |
|---|---|
| Lifestyle | All types |
| Behavioral | Urge, stress, mixed |
| Medications | Urge, urge-predom stress |
| Devices | Stress |
| Minimally invasive | Refractory urge, stress |
| Surgery | Stress |

contributing factors (e.g., medications, sleep apnea) when those are successfully treated or managed. However, many patients can expect improvement short of cure. For some patients, especially frail older adults, the goal may be (improved) contained incontinence, managed with protective garments.

## Lifestyle Interventions

Weight loss in moderately obese younger-old women remains the only evidence-based lifestyle intervention (LOE = A).[37] Other lifestyle interventions without an evidence base but nonetheless frequently recommended include avoiding excessive or inadequate fluid intake (the latter can lead to concentrated urine, which may be irritating), caffeinated beverages, and alcohol; minimizing evening fluid intake for nocturia; and quitting smoking for patients with stress UI. Afternoon administration of loop diuretics may decrease the volume of nocturnal polyuria and perhaps nocturia episodes (LOE = C), although it is not clear which patients are most likely to benefit.[32]

◆◆ **Behavioral therapy should be the first-line therapy for most older patients with UI.**

## Behavioral Therapies

Bladder training (BT) and pelvic muscle exercises (PMEs) are effective for urge, mixed, and stress UI (LOE = B),[38,39] including postprostatectomy UI (LOE = B).[40] BT and PME are often used

## TABLE 23.7  Using a Bladder Diary in the Evaluation of Nocturia

| Date | Time | Measured Amount of Urine (mL) | Approximate Amount of Leakage (mL) | Patient Comments | |
|---|---|---|---|---|---|
| 10/1 | 3:50 PM | 90 | | | Total 450 mL |
| | 6:05 PM | 90 | | | |
| | 8:15 PM | 120 | | | |
| | 10:20 PM | 150 | | | |
| 10/2 | 12:00 AM | 30 | | | Total 630 mL |
| | 2:15 AM | 150 | | | |
| | 3:40 AM | 120 | | | |
| | 5:00 AM | 120 | | | |
| | 6:05 AM | 240 | Maybe a drop | Almost had accident | |
| | 8:40 AM | 120 | | Coffee | Total 570 mL |
| | 12:50 PM | 120 | | | |
| | 6:00 PM | 120 | | | |
| | 9:20 PM | 210 | | Dribbled on way | |
| | 11:40 PM | 120 | | | Total 660 mL |
| | 2:00 AM | 150 | | | |
| | 4:50 AM | 180 | | | |
| | 6:20 AM | 180 | | | |

Adapted from Dubeau C. Urinary Incontinence. In: Harper GM, Lyons WL, Potter JF, eds. Geriatrics Review Syllabus: A Core Curriculum in Geriatric Medicine, 10th ed. New York, NY: American Geriatrics Society; 2019. http://geriatricscareonline.org
Bladder diary of an older woman with symptoms of 4-5 nightly episodes of nocturia, urgency with less than daily urge UI, and who denies daytime frequency.
Key points:
- Her nocturnal urine output (in red type, including all voids from bedtime up to and including first morning void) is 630–660 mL, or just over 50% of her 24-hour urine output on 10/2 (630 ÷ [630 + 570]).
- She meets diagnostic criteria for nocturnal polyuria (nocturnal excretion of >30% of total 24-hour urine output).
- Thus, despite the presence of daytime urgency and rare urgency UI, the cause of her nocturia is nocturnal polyuria. Evaluation and treatment should focus on causes of the polyuria.

## TABLE 23.8  Treatments for Incontinence

| COMPARATIVE EFFECTIVENESS | | |
|---|---|---|
| **Stress Incontinence** | | |
| | Odds Ratio (OR) (95% Confidence Interval [CI]) | Level of Evidence |
| Behavioral therapy more effective to achieve cure than no treatment | 3.1 (95% CI, 2.2–4.4) | High |
| Combination behavioral therapy and hormones more effective than no treatment | 4.4 (95% CI, 1.4–13.8) | Moderate |
| Behavioral therapy more effective than α-agonists (moderate strength of evidence) | 4.6 (95% CI, 1.4–15.8) | Moderate |
| Combination hormones and behavioral therapy more effective than α-agonists | 9.4 (95% CI, 1.2–73.6) | Moderate |
| No significant difference between periurethral bulking agents and no treatment | | Low |
| **Urge incontinence** | | |
| Behavioral therapy more effective than placebo or no treatment | 3.1 (95% CI, 2.2–4.4) | High |
| Anticholinergics more effective than placebo or no treatment[a] | 2.0 (95% CI, 1.3–2.9) | High |
| Combination behavioral and anticholinergics more effective than placebo or no treatment | 2.4 (95% CI, 0.8–7.0) | Moderate |
| Behavioral therapy significantly more likely to achieve cure than anticholinergics | 1.6 (95% CI, 1.0–2.4) | High |
| Onabotulinum toxin A (BTX) more effective than sham or no treatment | 5.7 (95% CI, 2.8–11.4) | High |
| Neuromodulation more effective than sham or no treatment | 3.3 (95% CI, 2.1–5.3) | High |

(From Kelleher C, Hakimi Z, Zur R, et al. Efficacy and tolerability of mirabegron compared with antimuscarinic monotherapy or combination therapies for overactive bladder: a systematic review and network meta-analysis. *Eur Urol.* 2018; 74: 324-333.)
[a]Mirabegron was not included in this review. A separate systematic review, which was industry-sponsored, found that mirabegron 50 mg was as effective as antimuscarinic therapy.

in combination (Table 23.8), because pelvic floor contraction can help with urgency suppression and forestalling voiding.[41] Recent metaanalyses suggest that behavioral therapies may be more effective than medications.[42]

Bladder training uses two principles: frequent voluntary voiding to keep bladder volume low, and urgency suppression using central nervous system and pelvic mechanisms (see online materials). The initial toileting frequency can be every 2 hours or based on the smallest voiding interval on a bladder diary. When urgency occurs, patients should stand still or sit down, do several pelvic muscle contractions, and concentrate on making the urgency decrease by taking a deep breath and letting it out slowly, and/or visualizing the urge as a wave that peaks and then falls. Once patients feel more in control, they should walk to a bathroom and void. After 2 days without leakage, the time between scheduled voids is increased by 30 to 60 minutes, and the process is continued until the person is dry (or has reached his or her symptom and function goal) when voiding every 4 hours. Successful bladder training usually takes several weeks, and patients need reassurance to proceed despite any initial failure.

PMEs strengthen the muscular components of urethral support. They require patient instruction and motivation, although simple instruction booklets alone have had moderate benefit.

To perform PME,[41] the patient (1) performs an isolated pelvic muscle contraction, without contracting buttocks, abdomen, or thighs (this can be checked during a bimanual examination in women), and holds it for 6 to 8 seconds (initially, only shorter durations may be possible); (2) repeats the contraction 8 to 12 times (one set), relaxing the pelvis between each contraction; (3) completes three sets of contractions starting three to four times a week, and continuing for at least 15 to 20 weeks. As patients progress, they should try to

increase the intensity and duration of the contraction, perform PMEs in various positions (sitting, standing, walking), and alternate fast and slower contractions. Many experts believe biofeedback can improve bladder retraining and PME teaching and outcomes, but marginal benefit is unproven. Medicare covers biofeedback for patients who do not improve after 4 weeks of conventional instruction.

For patients with dementia, the only behavioral treatment with proven efficacy is prompted voiding.[43,44] A caregiver monitors the patient and encourages him or her to report any need to void, then prompts the patient to toilet on a regular schedule during the day (usually every 2–3 hours), then leads the patient to the bathroom and gives the patient positive feedback when he or she voids. Patients most likely to improve with a 3-day trial have moderate voiding frequency (four or fewer during the day [12 h]) and are able to accept and follow the prompt to toilet at least 75% of the time.[44] If there is no decrease in UI after a 3-day trial, staff should stop prompted voiding and do check and change. Toileting routines without prompting, such as habit training (based on a patient's usual voiding schedule) and scheduled voiding (using a set schedule), are not effective and should be avoided.

## Pharmacologic Therapy

For patients with urge UI or mixed UI who fail or do not achieve their desired outcome with behavioral therapy, the next step is medications. Currently, there are no US Food and Drug Administration–approved medications for stress UI; duloxetine is effective in reducing stress UI (LOE = A)[42] but is not approved for this indication in the United States. Oral estrogen, alone or in combination with a progestin, increases stress UI in women (LOE = A).[45] Vaginal topical estrogen (cream, vaginal tablet, or

**TABLE 23.9   Pharmacologic Treatment for Urgency Urinary Incontinence**

| Indication(s) | Agent | Comments |
|---|---|---|
| Urgency UI OAB Urgency predominant—stress UI | All agents | With baseline average UI episodes/day of 1.6 to 5.3, mean reduction in episodes/day with placebo 1.08 (95% CI, 0.86—1.30); vs. IR formulations 1.46 (1.28, 1.64), and ER formulations 1.78 (1.61, 1.94). Head-to-head comparison trials of agents of limited quality |
| Antimuscarinics | Oxybutynin Immediate release (IR) 2.5—5 mg three to four times daily Extended release (ER, Ditropan XL) 5—20 mg once daily Topical patch (Oxytrol) 3.9-mg patch applied twice weekly Topical gel (Gelnique) 3% (84 mg, pump) and 10% (100 mg, sachet) once daily | Highest rate of dry mouth with immediate release, lowest with topical forms Application site rash in ~15% with patch |
|  | Tolterodine IR (Detrol) 1—2 mg one tab twice daily ER (Detrol LA) 2—4 mg once daily |  |
|  | Fesoterodine (Toviaz) 4—8 mg once daily | Prodrug of tolterodine |
|  | Darifenacin (Enablex) 7.5—15 mg once daily | Constipation |
|  | Solifenacin (VESIcare) 5—10 mg once daily |  |
|  | Trospium IR (Sanctura) 20 mg once to twice daily ER (Sanctura XR) 60 mg daily | Must be given on empty stomach |
|  | β-3 agonist |  |
| Urgency UI OAB | Mirabegron (Myrbetriq) 25—50 mg once daily | ADEs include hypertension; use with caution in patients with hypertension. Use with caution with metoprolol and digoxin |

*ADEs*, Adverse drug effects; *OAB*, overactive bladder; *UI*, urinary incontinence.

slow-release ring) (LOE = B)[46] is helpful for uncomfortable vaginal atrophy and may decrease recurrent urinary tract infections.

Antimuscarinic drugs and the beta-3 agonist mirabegron are moderately effective for urge UI, OAB, urgency-predominant mixed UI, and urgency associated with benign prostatic hyperplasia (BPH) (Table 23.9).[43,47] Both types of agents work by decreasing the basal excretion of acetylcholine from the urothelium, thereby increasing bladder capacity; they do not decrease or ablate uninhibited bladder contractions.[48] Routine monitoring of PVR is not necessary with drug treatment of urge UI (LOE = D) and it is unclear at what volume it is safe to administer antimuscarinics (LOE = D). Patients complaining of worsening UI while taking antimuscarinics should have a PVR checked. However, trials of antimuscarinics in men with BPH-associated lower urinary tract symptoms show no increased risk of retention with baseline PVR < 200 mL (albeit all coadministered with an alpha-blocker).

❖ **Discuss the potential risks of bladder antimuscarinics with patients, as well as possible other treatments before prescribing them.**

### Antimuscarinics

Antimuscarinics with established efficacy are oxybutynin, tolterodine, fesoterodine, trospium, darifenacin, and solifenacin (see Table 23.9). Based on systematic reviews,[17,42] these six antimuscarinic agents have generally similar efficacy in reducing urge UI frequency but differ in adverse events, metabolism, drug interactions, and dosing requirements.[48,49] Head-to-head trials are limited and are all industry supported. The only medication tested in a randomized controlled trial in vulnerable older adults is fesoterodine.[50]

Enthusiasm for antimuscarinics is increasingly tempered by concerns for immediate and long-term cognitive impairment.[51] This has led to specific recommendations for providers to counsel all patients on the associated risks, prescribe the lowest effective dose, and consider alternative medications in patients at risk.[52] Bladder antimuscarinics are included in the 2019 Beers Criteria Revision as potentially inappropriate;[53] however, they are not on the Center for Medicare and Medicaid Services 2019 High-Risk Medications list.[54] The situation is further complicated because the risk, incidence, type, and magnitude of cognitive changes from individual bladder antimuscarinics are not well characterized. No antimuscarinic is "safer" for all patients or those with dementia, nor has it been shown that the cognitive risk outweighs the potential treatment benefit (LOE = D).

The 2019 American Urological Association—Society for Female Urology and Urodynamics guidelines for treatment for OAB provide important considerations for drug treatment (Box 23.1). Antimuscarinics should not be used in combination with cholinesterase inhibitors because of lack of efficacy and risk of increased functional impairment (LOE = B).[49] Chronic

## • BOX 23.1 American Urological Association 2019 Guideline for Treatment of Overactive Bladder (OAB)

Clinicians should offer oral antimuscarinics or oral $\beta_3$-adrenoceptor agonists as second-line therapy. Standard (Level of Evidence [LOE] = B).

If an immediate release (IR) and an extended release (ER) formulation are available, then ER formulations should preferentially be prescribed over IR formulations because of lower rates of dry mouth. Standard (LOE = B).

Transdermal (TDS) oxybutynin (patch or gel) may be offered. Recommendation (LOE = C).

If a patient experiences inadequate symptom control and/or unacceptable adverse drug events with one antimuscarinic medication, then a dose modification or a different antimuscarinic medication or a $\beta_3$-adrenoceptor agonist may be tried. Clinical Principle.

Clinicians may consider combination therapy with an antimuscarinic and $\beta_3$-adrenoceptor agonist for patients refractory to monotherapy with either antimuscarinics or $\beta_3$-adrenoceptor agonists. Option (LOE = B).

Clinicians should not use antimuscarinics in patients with narrow-angle glaucoma unless approved by the treating ophthalmologist and should use antimuscarinics with extreme caution in patients with impaired gastric emptying or a history of urinary retention. Clinical Principle.

Clinicians should manage constipation and dry mouth before abandoning effective antimuscarinic therapy. Management may include bowel management, fluid management, dose modification, or alternative antimuscarinics. Clinical Principle.

Clinicians must use caution in prescribing antimuscarinics in patients who are using other medications with anticholinergic properties. Expert Opinion.

Clinicians should use caution in prescribing antimuscarinics or $\beta_3$-adrenoceptor agonists in the frail OAB patient. Clinical Principle.

Patients who are refractory to behavioral and pharmacologic therapy should be evaluated by an appropriate specialist if they desire additional therapy. Expert Opinion.

antimuscarinic use increases the risk of caries and tooth loss, and patients should have regular dental care.

All antimuscarinics, except trospium, are metabolized by cytochrome P-450 pathways and can interact with drugs that induce CYP2D6 (e.g., fluoxetine) or are metabolized by CYP3A4 (e.g., erythromycin, ketoconazole). Fesoterodine is a prodrug that is metabolized to tolterodine by nonspecific peripheral esterases. Trospium is renally cleared and should be given once daily in patients with renal insufficiency; it should be taken on an empty stomach.

◆◆ **The decision to use one antimuscarinic over another depends on avoidance of adverse drug effects (ADEs), drug–drug and drug–disease interactions, dosing frequency, titration range, and cost.**

Given that the six antimuscarinic agents have similar efficacy in reducing UI, the decision to use one antimuscarinic over another depends on avoidance of ADEs for which a patient may be most at risk along with other geriatric prescribing factors, including possible drug–drug and drug–disease interactions, dosing frequency, titration range, and cost. A lack of response to one agent does not preclude response to another.

### Beta-3 Agonists

Currently, mirabegron (Myrbetriq 25–50 mg once daily) is the only beta-3 receptor agonist approved in the United States for treatment of urge UI (LOE = B for efficacy).[55] It is the agent of choice for patients taking cholinesterase inhibitors, and, with the concerns about the antimuscarinic agents, is preferred for patients with cognitive impairment. Mirabegron can increase blood pressure; persons with hypertension should have periodic blood pressure checks while on mirabegron, and mirabegron should not be used in patients with severe uncontrolled hypertension. Only the lowest dose should be used in patients with severe renal or moderate hepatic insufficiency. Mirabegron should be used with caution in patients on anticholinergic medications. Mirabegron is a CYP2D6 inhibitor and if used with drugs metabolized by CYP2D6 (especially those with narrow therapeutic window [e.g., metoprolol]), close monitoring is needed and dose reduction of these drugs may be necessary. Mirabegron can raise serum digoxin levels.

### Desmopressin

This synthetic analog of antidiuretic hormone is used to treat younger patients with bothersome nocturia associated with nocturnal polyuria. However, desmopressin should not be used to treat nocturia in older, especially frailer, patients because of the risk of hyponatremia (LOE = A).[56]

### Miscellaneous Agents

There is insufficient evidence for the efficacy of propantheline, dicyclomine, imipramine, hyoscyamine, calcium-channel blockers, nonsteroidal antiinflammatory drugs, and flavoxate (LOE = C).[19] Furthermore, several of these agents are highly anticholinergic and are potentially inappropriate medications for older persons.[53]

## Minimally Invasive Procedures

There are several treatment options for patients with urgency UI refractory to behavioral and pharmacologic therapy (Table 23.10).[61,62,65]

## Surgery

Surgery is the gold standard treatment with the highest cure rates for stress UI in women. The most commonly used procedures are colposuspension (Burch operation) and slings (synthetic mesh, or autologous or cadaveric fascia, placed at the proximal or midurethra). Older women can have comparable outcomes to younger women, and age alone should not be a contraindication to surgery.[57] Periurethral injection of Coaptite is an alternative for women with sphincter insufficiency (rather than impaired urethral support); efficacy is relatively short term (6–12 months) and requires repeated injections.

### CASE 1

#### Discussion

Ms. Roberts describes urgency (of note, she has no impaired mobility contributing to UI), with daily urgency-associated UI and nocturia. She denied leakage with coughing and activity; thus she does not have stress UI. UI is having a major impact on her, leading to worsening of her heart failure because of skipping diuretic doses. She also has the out-of-pocket expense of adult diapers.

Several comorbid conditions can contribute to her urge UI. The most common urologic dysfunction in persons with diabetes is urge UI. Her diabetes is well controlled, and therefore it is unlikely that osmotic diuresis contributes to daytime and nighttime frequency. Heart failure and associated peripheral edema may be a cause of nocturia. Amlodipine could be contributing to peripheral edema as well. Another potential cause of nocturnal polyuria to consider is sleep apnea.

| TABLE 23.10 | Minimally Invasive Treatment for Refractory Urge Urinary Incontinence | | | |
|---|---|---|---|
| **Treatment** | **Method** | **Efficacy/Level of Evidence** | **Comments** |
| Botulinum toxin | Injection in detrusor during cystoscopy | Can reduce UI with a slightly higher cure compared with antimuscarinics, although with a greater risk of urinary retention (Level of Evidence = B)[63,64] | Patients must be willing to do self-catheterization because of the risk of urinary retention<br>Optimal dosing for specific patient groups such as older women is uncertain |
| Sacral nerve modulation | Percutaneous implantation of a trial electrode at the S3 sacral root, which is connected to an external stimulator. Patients responding to the trial have a permanent lead with a pacemaker-like energy source implanted | | Anticipated newer MRI-compatible models will end need to explant stimulators before imaging |
| Percutaneous tibial nerve stimulation[66] | | Very small trials only[66] | Patients unlikely to see efficacy before 6 weeks of treatment<br>Limited coverage by insurance |

*MRI,* Magnetic resonance imaging; *UI,* urinary incontinence.

Ms. Roberts's examination is normal except for an exacerbation of heart failure.

In terms of management of her UI, you explain to Ms. Roberts the association between heart failure and nocturia, and the importance of taking her diuretic, and prescribe compression stockings to reduce the edema. You also explain bladder training and give the patient a handout to follow.

When the patient returns to see you, her weight is down, and her pretibial edema is only a trace. She reports that she is getting up only twice a night now, but is still tired, and she is still leaking about once a day. She is willing to try an antimuscarinic, so you check her formulary, and select a preferred agent, which you start at low dose. You ask her to return in another month to review her progress, tolerance of the new medication, and adherence to the behavioral measures.

## Summary

UI is common but never normal in older patients, and all older persons should be routinely screened. Etiology is usually multifactorial, including multimorbidity, functional impairment, and medications, and behavioral therapies are effective for a variety of patients, especially when targeted to patients' functional and cognitive status. A combination of behavioral and drug therapy is more efficacious than either alone. Surgical treatment remains an effective option for older women with stress UI.

**Web Resources**

General: Each of these sites provides evidence-based guidelines and resources for providers to use in guiding patients.
International Continence Society; includes links to other continence organizations and resources: www.ics.org.
American Urological Association: www.auanet.org.
American Urogynecologic Association: www.augs.org.
Patient advocacy
National Association for Continence: www.nafc.org.
Simon Foundation for Continence: www.simonfoundation.org.

## Key References

17. Landefeld CS, Bowers BJ, Feld AD, et al. National Institutes of Health state-of-the-science conference statement: Prevention of fecal and urinary incontinence in adults. *Ann Intern Med.* 2008;148:449–458.
14. Holroyd-Leduc JM, Tannenbaum C, Thorpe KE, Straus SE. What type of urinary incontinence does this woman have? *JAMA.* 2008;299:1446–1456.
33. Gulur DM, Mevcha AM, Drake MJ. Nocturia as a manifestation of systemic disease. *BJU Int.* 2011;107 (5):702–713.
36. Fonda D, Abrams P. Cure sometimes, help always—a "continence paradigm" for all ages and conditions. *Neurourol Urodyn.* 2006;25(3):290–292.
38. Shamliyan T, Wyman J, Kane RL. Benefits and harms of pharmacologic treatment for urinary incontinence in women: a systematic review. *Ann Intern Med.* 2012;156 (12):861–874.

**References available online at** expertconsult.com.

# 24

# Constipation and Fecal Incontinence

ALAYNE D. MARKLAND

## OUTLINE

*Additional online-only material indicated by icon.*

## OBJECTIVES

*Upon completion of this chapter, the reader will be able to:*

- Define the various symptoms of constipation and fecal incontinence (FI), along with other associated bowel symptoms.
- Recognize types and subtypes of constipation and FI.
- List common medical conditions and medications associated with constipation and FI.

- Describe the clinical evaluation for older adults with constipation and FI, understanding when referral for further evaluation may be needed.
- Identify evidence-based nonpharmacologic and pharmacologic treatments for constipation and FI among older adults.

## CASE

### Angela McDonald (Part 1)

Angela McDonald, a 76-year-old woman with a 15-year history of constipation symptoms, presents to your office with new bowel complaints. She consistently has had one to two bowel movements a week for the last several years and often feels as though she has incomplete evacuation. Most of her stools are very hard and are rarely smooth in contour. She reports no blood in her stool, no pain with defecation, and no change in the caliber of her stools. Her weight and appetite have been stable.

Over the last 6 to 8 months, she admits to having weekly fecal incontinence (FI) episodes where she notes leakage of mushy stool consistency without any prior warning. She takes a stool softener on most days and

occasionally uses Milk of Magnesia when she has not had a bowel movement in 6 to 7 days. She notices that the Milk of Magnesia is no longer providing as much relief for her symptoms. She has not started any new medications and has had no dietary changes. Her medical history includes hypertension, gastroesophageal reflux disease, and mild urinary incontinence. She is very bothered because her episodes of FI have caused her to start wearing pull-ups on most days (she previously wore mini-pads for her urinary incontinence).

1. What is the most likely cause of her bowel symptoms?
2. Do her current symptoms warrant further evaluation with a colonoscopy or other bowel imaging?
3. What additional tests are needed (if any) for her bowel symptoms?
4. Given her current bowel symptoms, what is the best initial treatment for her symptoms?

❖❖ Constipation and FI are common, underrecognized, and underreported conditions in older adults.

Constipation in the older adult is often caused by functional chronic constipation or secondary to other causes.

Less is known about specific subtypes of FI.

Specialized bowel evaluation testing can help differentiate causes of constipation and FI in cognitively intact older adults.

The first step in treating chronic constipation and FI is with lifestyle and dietary modifications.

Long-term use risks and benefits of secretagogues, including lubiprostone, linaclotide, and plecanatide, in older adults need more evidence.

Fecal impaction is a common cause of FI in older adults with chronic constipation.

## Prevalence, Impact, and Definitions of Constipation and Fecal Incontinence

Constipation and FI can be classified as functional bowel disorders.[1] Functional bowel disorders are usually chronic ($>3-6$ months in duration at the time of presentation) and are attributable to the middle and lower gastrointestinal system. Constipation and FI are symptom-based diagnoses that may have multiple etiologies. Often, symptoms of constipation and FI occur simultaneously. Management will be discussed separately for constipation and FI, with a section on fecal impaction, which can present with symptoms of constipation and FI.

Constipation is a common complaint in older adults and affects an estimated 40% of people age $>65$ years.[2,3] In addition to age, risk factors for constipation include female gender, physical inactivity, low education and income, polypharmacy, comorbidity, and depression. In older adults who have poor dietary intake, constipation may be more common. Laxatives are used daily by 10% to 18% of community-dwelling older adults and 74% of nursing home residents.[4] Constipation has a major impact on wellbeing and healthcare costs. Nearly 85% of physician visits for constipation result in a prescription for laxatives, and more than $820 million is spent per year on over-the-counter (OTC) agents.

FI occurs in up to 15% of older women and men. FI is distressing, socially isolating, and possibly associated with an increased risk of dependency in activities of daily living, morbidity, and mortality. Many older individuals with FI do not volunteer the problem to their healthcare provider, and providers do not routinely enquire about the symptom. The condition can affect home-dwelling patients, with FI being cited as a reason for requesting nursing home placement by their caregivers. Because frail, older adults frequently have coexisting urinary symptoms (most often urinary incontinence) and other bowel symptoms (constipation), evaluation and management of other urinary symptoms and FI should be done simultaneously (see Ch. 23).[5] Even when noted by healthcare professionals, FI is often managed with absorptive or containment products, especially in the long-term care setting where it is most prevalent.

FI can result from constipation with stool impaction and may be more common in certain frail, older populations. Up to 81% of residents in long-term care settings had symptoms of constipation and FI.[6] However, the true prevalence of impaction and FI in nursing home residents and home-care settings is not known. Since constipation with FI (see later and section on fecal impaction) is difficult to diagnose, treatments should target constipation.

## Symptoms and Definitions

Constipation is often associated with other abdominal complaints (pain, bloating, and gas), as well as decreased overall wellbeing. It may involve infrequent defecation, difficulty in passing stool, or incomplete evacuation of stool. Physicians often define constipation as infrequent passage of stool; however, patients often define it as straining to defecate or sensation of incomplete evacuation. For chronic constipation (CC) to be diagnosed, symptoms should be present for at least 12 weeks.

According to the Rome IV criteria, functional constipation is defined as any two or more of the following symptoms: straining, lumpy hard stools, sensation of incomplete evacuation, use of digital maneuvers to relieve symptoms, sensation of anorectal obstruction or blockage with 25% of bowel movements, and decrease in stool frequency (less than three bowel movements per week).[7] Two or more of these symptoms must be present for the last 3 consecutive months with the onset of any symptoms at least 6 months before making a diagnosis of constipation. In addition, loose stools should rarely be present without the use of laxatives, and symptoms should not meet criteria for irritable bowel syndrome.

Differentiating symptoms of chronic idiopathic constipation (CIC) from irritable bowel syndrome with constipation (IBS-C) and diarrhea (IBS-D) may not be as important in older adults because those age $\geq 50$ years are associated with lower rates of IBS. However, management can differ between the two diagnoses. IBS-C is defined by recurrent abdominal pain or discomfort for at least 3 days per month in the previous 3 months (onset of symptoms $\geq 6$ months before the diagnosis) that is associated with at least two of the following symptoms: improvement of pain or discomfort upon defecation, onset of symptoms associated with changes in frequency of stool, and the onset of symptoms associated with a change in the stool form or appearance.[8]

The International Continence Society provides a definition of FI that is the "involuntary loss of liquid or solid stool that is a social or hygienic problem." Flatal incontinence may also be a bothersome symptom but is usually excluded from the definition for FI.[9] Other bowel symptoms that may present with FI include rectal urgency, loss of stool with straining or Valsalva, seepage of stool after bowel movements, incomplete evacuation, and loss of stool without any sensory awareness.

## Primary and Secondary Causes of Constipation and Fecal Incontinence

Constipation and FI can be subgrouped as primary colorectal dysfunction or secondary to several etiologic factors (e.g., because of a medical diagnosis or use of medications). The etiology of constipation and FI in older patients is often multifactorial. Primary types of constipation are categorized into three broad subtypes: slow transit constipation, dyssynergic defecation, and IBS-C. If the earlier criteria are present and secondary factors are not present, CIC may be an underlying cause. These patients often do not have any physiologic or anatomic abnormality on evaluation and testing. The primary types of FI are more open to interpretation. The primary types for constipation and FI are listed in Table 24.1 with secondary causes listed in Box 24.1 .

Many prescription and nonprescription drugs impact stool consistency and cause hard or liquid/loose stools. Medications can slow transit time and contribute to a hard stool consistency (e.g., narcotics, anabolic steroids, anticonvulsants, anticholinergic agents, antihypertensive

| TABLE 24.1 | Primary Pathophysiologic Types of Chronic Constipation and Fecal Incontinence |
|---|---|
| **Type of Chronic Constipation** | **Characteristics** |
| 1. Slow transit | • Increased intestinal transit time<br>• Reduced colonic motility through myopathy or neuropathy<br>• Multiple etiologies—gut, cellular, and protein level responses |
| 2. Dyssynergic defecation | • Difficulty with or inability to expel stool from the anorectum<br>• May also have prolonged colonic transit time<br>• Abnormalities in pressure and expulsion seen on anorectal manometry and inability to evacuate barium with defecography<br>• Pathogenesis not well understood, especially in older adults |
| 3. IBS-C | • Transit and stool frequency may or may not have slow transit or dyssynergia, but may have visceral hypersensitivity<br>• Characterized by abdominal pain with altered bowel habits[a] |
| **Fecal Incontinence Type** | **Characteristics** |
| 1. Urgency FI | • Often occurs with a strong urgency sensation to have a bowel movement<br>• Liquid stool or diarrhea often associated with the inability to hold stool in the rectal vault[a] |
| 2. Passive FI | • Bowel leakage without the sensation of the need to defecate<br>• May not be able to differentiate passing gas from having a bowel movement<br>• May also involve seepage after a bowel movement |
| 3. Overflow FI | • More common in older adults with impaired mobility and functional impairments (i.e., long-term care residents)<br>• May also involve seepage or smaller amounts of stool loss around an impaction<br>• Associated with symptoms of constipation<br>• May need to treat constipation symptoms to improve FI |

*FI,* Fecal incontinence; *IBS-C,* irritable bowel syndrome with constipation.

[a]Presence of pain increases the likelihood of a diagnosis of IBS-C.

---

**• BOX 24.1 Secondary Causes of Chronic Constipation and Fecal Incontinence in Older Adults**

• Malignancy (including the treatments for malignancy—surgical bowel resection and radiation)
• Medications/polypharmacy (prescription and nonprescription drugs—including opioids)
• Endocrine/metabolic (diabetes mellitus, hyper- or hypothyroidism, hypercalcemia, hypokalemia)
• Neurologic disorders (Parkinson disease, diabetic autonomic neuropathy, spinal cord injury, dementia, stroke)
• Nutritional (malabsorption syndromes, food sensitivities, low fluid and fiber intake)
• Rheumatologic disorders (systemic sclerosis and other connective tissue disorders)
• Psychological disorders (depression, eating disorders, alcohol or substance abuse)
• Anatomic dysfunction (strictures, postsurgical abnormalities, anal fissures, megacolon, hemorrhoids, fistulas, rectal prolapse, occult obstetrical sphincter tears)
• Decreased mobility/sedentary lifestyle

agents, tricyclic antidepressants). Nonprescription agents implicated in increased transit time and hard stools include antihistamines, calcium and iron supplements, antidiarrheals, nonsteroidals, and some antacids.

Diarrhea-inducing medications include those that decrease transit time and cause loose stool consistency. Medications that induce diarrhea may be time limited (i.e., a side effect that improves with time or with limited use of the medication), change intestinal bacterial flora, or be caused by higher than normal serum concentration of the medication. Medications with associated time-limited diarrhea include metformin, high doses of proton-pump inhibitors, acetylcholinesterase inhibitors, selective serotonin reuptake inhibitors, colchicine, and chemotherapeutic agents. Antibiotics may also cause loose stools and diarrhea by changing intestinal bacterial flora. Toxic levels of drugs, such as digoxin, can cause loose stools. Nonprescription medications that cause loose stools include laxatives and some nonsteroidal antiinflammatory drugs. Tube feedings may also be associated with loose stool.

## History and Physical Examination

In most cases, patients with constipation and FI do not warrant extensive diagnostic evaluation.[10] Older patients with a change in bowel symptoms who meet criteria for the warning or alarm symptoms (hematochezia, positive fecal occult blood test, obstructive bowel symptoms, acute onset of constipation, severe persistent constipation that is unresponsive to treatment, weight loss $\geq 10$ lbs, a change is stool caliber, family history of colon cancer or inflammatory bowel disease) should consider the benefits and risks of evaluation with colonoscopy or other invasive testing. This should prompt shared decision making for evaluation with invasive testing in older adults with other chronic comorbid conditions.

Often the first step in management of constipation and FI is to exclude secondary causes through the initial history and physical examination. Healthcare providers should inquire about constipation and FI because many older patients do not seek treatment for their symptoms. Using appropriate patient-oriented terminology, such as *accidental bowel leakage*, when asking about bowel habits is important. A focused history on stool frequency and consistency, and other bowel symptoms, helps identify types of constipation and FI. Dietary intake may identify contributing factors (e.g., poor dietary intake of fiber or lactose intolerance). Symptoms such as persistent nausea, vomiting, and abdominal pain should broaden the differential and evaluation, especially for an intestinal obstruction.

Physical examination should include a rectal examination, palpating for hard stool, assessing for masses, anal fissures, sphincter tone, prostatic hypertrophy in men, hemorrhoids, push effort during attempted defecation, and posterior vaginal masses in women. Laboratory testing should include a complete blood count, serum calcium, thyroid function tests, and fecal occult blood testing. The American College of Gastroenterology guidelines state that inadequate evidence exists to perform routine laboratory tests in patients with chronic constipation without alarm symptoms or signs (such as sudden change in bowel habits, blood mixed in the stool, unexpected weight loss, or a strong family history of colon cancer). However, the laboratory tests can identify metabolic conditions that may be secondary causes of constipation. Thyroid-stimulating hormone, calcium, and glucose could be considered selectively, but most major gastrointestinal societies recommend a complete blood cell count as a screening test because the finding of iron deficiency with anemia would prompt further testing.[10] New onset iron-deficiency anemia in the setting of bowel symptoms may indicate need for further evaluation with colonoscopy. Evaluation for causes of loose stool or persistent diarrhea should evaluate for infection (including *Clostridium difficile* evaluation, fat malabsorption, and the presence of leukocytes). Other testing could involve serum tests for celiac disease.

---

**CASE**

**Case Studies (Part 2)**

While the patient has a long-standing history of chronic constipation symptoms, she does have a new onset (6–8 months) of worsening symptoms that are not responding to over-the-counter laxative therapy with Milk of Magnesia. The most likely explanation for her bowel symptoms may be overflow fecal incontinence with fecal impaction.

She also does not endorse having any "alarm" symptoms. Even though you may not need further evaluation with endoscopy, you may consider doing further evaluation for worsening constipation and possible fecal impaction with an abdominal radiograph. Often fecal impaction is not identified on a digital rectal examination.

Laboratory testing to consider could involve thyroid function tests, serum calcium, and electrolytes. She does not endorse having diarrhea or loose stool so stool studies may not be indicated.

The best initial treatment would be to treat her constipation symptoms. She may benefit from higher doses and more consistent laxative treatment with Polyethylene Glycol (Miralax), which can be titrated to an effect. She may also benefit from an enema or a stimulant suppository to help with her fecal impaction while treating her slow-transit problems with oral laxative treatments. She will also need to improve her overall bowel habits once her impaction has improved. Hopefully, with the treatment of the fecal impaction, she will no longer have the fecal incontinence symptoms.

## Imaging and Specialized Testing

Overall, limited evidence exists to support the role of imaging in the evaluation of constipation in older adults.[10] Abdominal radiographs may indicate significant stool retention in the colon and suggest the diagnosis of fecal impaction, megacolon, volvulus, or a mass lesion. Abdominal ultrasound could be ordered if acute or chronic cholecystitis symptoms are suspected as a potential cause for the change in bowel symptoms.

Referral for specialized testing with endoscopy for constipation and FI is rarely indicated unless alarm symptoms and signs are present. If indicated, colonoscopy may be needed to evaluate for colonic lesions, mass or obstruction, volvulus, megacolon, strictures, or for mucosal biopsy to detect microscopic colitis or inflammation.

Four types of specialized testing may help with the diagnosis and pathophysiology of constipation and FI symptoms. Although findings on specialized testing may suggest more specific treatments, few have been evaluated for cost effectiveness. These tests are usually performed in patients who do not respond to initial therapies, such as lifestyle and dietary modifications and laxatives.

1. Motility studies or colonic transit studies in patients with constipation can help differentiate pelvic floor dyssynergia as a contributing cause for constipation. A motility marker study involves ingesting radiopaque markers with subsequent abdominal radiograph to detect the markers in the right, left, or rectosigmoid colon. Transit time evaluation with radioactive tracers and wireless motility capsule technologies (that record data after ingestion) are also available.
2. Anorectal manometry measures internal and external anal sphincter pressure at rest and during contraction. Sensation and rectal capacity can also be evaluated with a rectal balloon. Balloon expulsion tests can be used with anorectal manometry to evaluate pelvic floor dyssynergia and other defecation disorders.
3. Two- or three-dimensional endoanal ultrasound evaluates structural defects in the external or internal anal sphincters. Often, scarring or thinning of the muscle layers can also be detected. Endoanal ultrasound is done to evaluate patients with FI.
4. Defecography evaluates the defecatory process after a barium paste is inserted rectally and the patient defecates under fluoroscopy. Defecography can assess rectal emptying or structural abnormalities in the pelvic floor, such as obstruction or the presence of a rectocele.

## Treatment of Constipation

Once secondary causes of constipation have been evaluated and addressed, management of CIC varies by type. Treatment and prevention of constipation includes patient education about bowel habits, dietary changes, and drug therapies.[2,10] Management of dyssynergic defecation involves biofeedback, relaxation exercises, and suppository programs. Patients with slow transit and dyssynergic defecation should receive treatment for the dyssynergia first before other measures.

### Nonpharmacologic Treatments

Nonpharmacologic treatment options or lifestyle modifications involve dietary modifications, exercise, and bowel habit training

- Establish a regular bowel pattern
- Exercise to increase bowel motility
- Adequate plain water and total fluid intake
- Avoid excess straining at stool
- Increase fiber intake slowly—5 g/day at 1-week intervals until the intake is 25–30 g/day
- Probiotics *(Lactobacillus)* are probably helpful but commercial products are not standardized
- Dyssynergic defecation is effectively treated with biofeedback

(Box 24.2). Lifestyle modifications are the first step in treatment of constipation (Level of Evidence [LOE] = C). Establishing a regular pattern of bowel movement is important and part of a conditioned reflex. Colonic motor activity is more active after waking and after a meal. Excessive straining should be avoided.

Dietary options include increasing fluid and fiber. Adequate fluid may be an important general health recommendation and may impact treatment of constipation, especially with fiber supplementation. Although recommendations for plain water intake vary in the literature, consensus recommendations support taking in 91 ounces of total fluid from all beverages and food.[1] Recommended fiber intake is 20 to 35 g/day, but most Americans consume 5 to 10 g/day. Increasing dietary fiber is recommended given the effect on increasing stool bulk. Information should be given on the fiber contained in common foods. Patients should increase fiber intake slowly—5 g/day at 1-week intervals until the recommended intake is attained. Patients should know that an immediate response is not expected, and that flatus and bloating may occur but are usually temporary. Increasing fiber intake gradually may reduce these unwanted side effects. Some providers suggest a mixture of dietary fiber and use of the natural cathartic effect of prune or pear juice. "Constipation recipes" mixing high-fiber cereal (bran) and prune or pear juice (1–2 tablespoons of the mixture daily) with a warm beverage or oatmeal can be beneficial.

Probiotics have also been tested for the treatment of constipation. *Lactobacillus* and *Bifidobacterium* are symbiotics flora in the large intestine that may promote colonic mucosal health. Low levels of both have been reported in individuals with chronic constipation. Although properly controlled trials are lacking, some prospective evidence reports efficacy of probiotics *(Lactobacillus)* on constipation in nursing home residents. Survival and viability of probiotic bacteria in a commercial form has not been standardized for these treatments.

Increased physical activity is associated with lower rates of constipation in older adults. Physical inactivity may also be associated with increased colonic transit time (harder stool consistency). Exercise should be encouraged in older adults, when appropriate.

Bowel habits and the use of bowel retraining are important initial steps, in addition to diet and exercise. Establishing and recognizing a regular bowel pattern is an important component for treatment. Recognizing the postprandial gastrocolic reflex or urgency sensation may need to be retaught to older adults who have ignored or no longer experience this sensation. Often, encouraging defecation shortly after the same daily meal and maintaining a schedule can be beneficial. Caregivers and care providers in a long-term care setting could be taught to use these bowel retraining techniques. Clinical trial evidence suggests that scheduling bowel movements as part of a multicomponent intervention may improve bowel frequency in cognitively impaired nursing home residents.

Biofeedback is an effective treatment for dyssynergic defecation, which is characterized by paradoxic contraction or failure to relax the pelvic floor muscles during defecation. In patients with dyssynergic defecation, biofeedback using coordinated therapy was consistently found to be more effective than continuous use of PEG, standard therapy (other types of stool softeners and laxatives), sham therapy (aimed at overall body relaxation), or the use of diazepam in four randomized controlled trials. However, trials are needed to determine the efficacy of biofeedback in older adults. Cognitive function is an important consideration when treating constipation with biofeedback in older adults.

Many people will have already tried fluids, fiber, and fitness, but often not in a sustained manner. Most Americans do not consume enough dietary fiber, and increasing the intake of fiber and fluids may be enough to help prevent constipation in healthy older adults. Consideration may also involve nutritional expertise, pelvic floor physical therapy or physiotherapy (when appropriate), and family/caregivers in making dietary and exercise changes for the treatment of constipation. Preventing and treating constipation with nonpharmacologic and pharmacologic treatments may be needed in specific situations—that is, in the postoperative period, during hospitalization or other environments when decreased mobility is anticipated, and when using opioid medications.

## Pharmacologic Treatments (Including OTC Preparations)

OTC medication categories for constipation are bulk-forming laxatives, stool softeners/emollients, osmotic laxatives, stimulant laxatives, and suppositories.[4] The main prescription categories include some additional osmotic laxatives, colonic secretagogues, opioid antagonists, and 5-hydroxytryptamine receptor subtype 4 (5-HT$_4$) receptor agonists.[10] Table 24.2 lists the pharmacologic treatments for constipation.

Bulking-forming laxatives expand with water to increase fecal mass and result in softer stools. Patients may need to try different types of fiber to achieve the desired outcome with minimum side effects. Some patients may better tolerate soluble and synthetic bulking agents than insoluble agents. Types of fiber include naturally occurring plant fiber, synthetic polysaccharides, and cellulose derivatives. Systematic review findings are inconsistent, with one review reporting that psyllium (plant fiber) increases stool frequency in patients with chronic constipation over other forms of fiber, whereas another review found evidence supporting efficacy and safety with calcium polycarbophil (synthetic fiber). Adequate hydration may be necessary for the desired outcome. Patients taking fiber need to increase fluid intake to 30 mL/kg of body weight daily to avoid worsening of constipation or creating impaction. Fiber may also inhibit the absorption of some drugs and should be taken 1 hour before or 2 hours after other medications. Like dietary fiber, bulk-forming agents should be increased over weekly periods to avoid side effects. Bulk-forming agents are considered first-line agents for constipation. However, many older adults may not be good candidates for use. Instances when bulk-forming agents may not be the first-line agent for older adults include patients taking high doses of narcotic medications, those with difficulty swallowing or dysphagia (because of the consistency of certain types of fiber when mixed with water), anyone with surgical

## TABLE 24.2  Evidence-Based Pharmacologic Management Options for Chronic Constipation

| Therapy | Recommendations |
| --- | --- |
| **Bulking agents** | |
| Psyllium | Grade A |
| Calcium polycarbophil | Grade B |
| Methylcellulose | Grade B |
| **Stool softeners/emollients** | |
| Docusate calcium/sodium | Grade B |
| Mineral oil (linked with aspiration in older adults) | Grade C |
| **Osmotic laxatives** | |
| Lactulose | Grade A |
| Sorbitol | Grade B |
| PEG (polyethylene glycol) | Grade A |
| Magnesium hydroxide | Grade C |
| **Stimulants** | |
| Senna | Grade A |
| Bisacodyl | Grade A |
| **Chloride channel activator** | |
| Lubiprostone | Grade[a] |
| **Guanylate cyclase-C receptor antagonists** | |
| Linaclotide | Grade A |
| Plecanatide | Grade A |
| **5-HT$_4$ (serotonin) agonists** | |
| Prucalopride | Grade A |

[a]Data exist for adults > 65 years of age without significant comorbid disorders.

resection of the majority of the colon, patients who have a suspected rectal mass or possible bowel obstruction, and older adults with limited mobility, as well as those who do not consume adequate amounts of fluid.

Stool softeners and emollients act by a deterrent effect on stool consistency. This class of medications is well tolerated and does not interfere with other medications. However, limited data exist on clinical efficacy. Mineral oil is also an emollient and may help lubricate the stool through the colon; however, older adults are at risk for aspiration and lipoid pneumonia. Stool softeners are often used when bulking agents do not work or are not preferred. Because of their mechanism of action as a deterrent, stool softeners can also be used in combination with bulking agents. Like bulking agents, stool softeners alone are not good treatments for older adults on narcotic medications who have constipation.

Osmotic laxatives promote secretion of water into the intestinal lumen by osmotic activity and the hyperosmolar nature of these medications. Low-dose PEG (17 g/day) increases stool frequency and is well tolerated in older adults. Higher dose PEG (34 g/day) may cause abdominal bloating, cramping, and flatulence. Lactulose increases stool frequency and reduces the need for other laxatives in older adults compared with placebo, but is less effective than low-dose PEG for constipation symptoms. Common use of PEG or magnesium hydroxide containing preparations (Milk of Magnesia)

in patients with congestive heart failure or chronic renal disease should be done with extreme caution as they can cause electrolyte imbalances, such as hypokalemia and diarrhea, further worsening fluid/electrolyte balances. Osmotic agents are useful when first-line bulking agents and/or stool softeners are not effective.

Stimulants such as senna and bisacodyl-containing compounds increase intestinal motility by increasing peristaltic contractions. Stimulants also decrease water absorption from the lumen by affecting electrolyte transport across the intestinal mucosa. One study showed that senna given with fiber was more efficacious for constipation than lactulose in older nursing home residents and had a similar side effect profile. There is little evidence to support the safety or harm of long-term use of stimulant laxatives.

Suppositories and enemas are commonly used when oral agents are not effective for relieving symptoms of constipation. Glycerin and bisacodyl suppositories may help with dyssynergic defecation. Enemas (tap water, soapsuds) should be used sparingly in older adults. Adverse effects of soapsuds enemas include rectal mucosal damage. Sodium phosphate enemas should not be used in older adults given evidence on complications with use, including hypotension and volume depletion, electrolyte abnormalities, renal failure, and prolonged QT interval.

### CASE

#### Angela McDonald (Part 3)

After using twice daily doses of PEG and rectal suppositories for the first 2 weeks after her initial visit, she had three to four bowel movements per week with a softer stool consistency and less complaints of incomplete emptying after a bowel movement. Although we do not have recommendations for plain water intake, consensus recommendations support taking in 91 ounces of total fluid from all beverages and food. Given this, she started drinking at least 40 to 50 ounces of plain water daily. Although she was pleased with her current treatment, she still had some accidental bowel leakage that occurred after having a bowel movement. She noticed her leakage was not preceded by any fecal urgency symptoms. This passive leakage of stool occurred two to three times per month. Although she was only wearing the pull-ups when outside the house, she still wore pads daily. She wanted to know what else she could do to help with her symptoms.
1. What could be causing her current symptoms?
2. What would you recommend for treatment for her problems with passive leakage after bowel movements?

## Colonic Secretagogues (Increase Intestinal Fluid Secretion)

### Chloride channel activators

Lubiprostone is a chloride channel activator that improves intestinal motility by increasing intestinal fluid secretion without altering serum electrolyte concentrations. Retrospective data from three pooled clinical trials of lubiprostone in older patients ($n = 57$) without significant comorbidities showed improvement in stool frequency and consistency, and decreased straining compared with placebo. Side effects include nausea, diarrhea, headache, abdominal distention, and abdominal pain but are generally well tolerated.

Guanylate cyclase C receptor antagonists. Linaclotide and plecanatide stimulate intestinal fluid secretion and transit. Two large phase 3 trials of linaclotide in patients with constipation showed the treated groups had significantly higher rates of three or more complete spontaneous bowel movements per week and an increase in one or more complete spontaneous bowel movements from baseline during 9 of 12 weeks compared with placebo. The most common adverse event was diarrhea, which led to discontinuation in 4% of patients. The long-term risks and benefits of linaclotide in constipation are unknown.

5-HT$_4$ (serotonin) agonists. 5-HT$_4$ receptors are found in the colon and mediate the release of other neurotransmitters that enhance motility by increasing intestinal contractions. Prucalopride is a selective high affinity 5HT$_4$ receptor agonist that has some sub-group data on efficacy in patients age $\geq$ 65 years.

Opioid antagonists. Alvimopan and methylnaltrexone are peripherally acting mu opioid receptor antagonists that may have some role in treatment of opiate-induced constipation and paralytic ileus. Data are lacking in older adults. These medications do not cross the blood-brain barrier, thus not affecting the analgesic properties of opioids.

## Treatment of Fecal Impaction

Constipation is an important factor in the development of fecal impaction in older adults, especially those who have limited mobility and those in long-term care settings.[11] Fecal impaction results from an individual's lack of ability to sense and respond to stool in the rectum.

To diagnose fecal impaction, a digital rectal examination is important, but may also not be the only evaluation necessary. Impacted stool may not have a hard consistency, and the key finding is a large amount of stool in the rectum. Fecal impaction can also occur in the proximal rectum or sigmoid colon, which would not be detected on digital rectal examination. If fecal impaction is suspected, obtaining an abdominal radiograph may help identify the area of impaction.

The management of fecal impaction involves disimpaction and colon evacuation, followed by a maintenance bowel regimen. Digital disimpaction can be used to fragment a large amount of feces in the rectum. Following digital disimpaction, a warm-water enema with mineral oil may be used to soften the impaction and assist with evacuating the impacted area. Very little evidence exists in guiding treatment of fecal impaction. However, if digital disimpaction and enemas fail, local anesthesia to relax the anal canal along with abdominal massage may be useful. In rare cases, colonoscopy with a snare to fragment fecal material in the distal colon may be needed. Abdominal tenderness or bleeding may indicate bowel perforation or ischemia, and surgery may be necessary.

## Treatment of Fecal Incontinence

Given the multiple causes and contributors to FI, the treatments often include combinations of dietary changes, behavioral interventions, biofeedback, pharmacologic treatments, perianal-injectable bulking agents, and sacral neuromodulation (surgical and nonsurgical).[12] Special consideration is also needed to manage incontinence-associated dermatitis.

### Dietary and Behavioral Interventions for Fecal Incontinence

Initial treatment for FI includes conservative measures (dietary modifications, bowel habit training, and pelvic floor muscle training with or without biofeedback and electrical stimulation), and pharmacologic treatments (constipating agents and/or stool bulking agents). Conservative therapies are often combined and improve mild FI by 50% to 95% depending on the modality used. Dietary modifications should focus on avoiding triggers for loose stool such

as lactose-containing products. Increasing dietary or supplementary fiber may improve loose stool and decrease diarrhea by bulking the stool. Solid stool may be easier to retain in the rectum. A small study comparing psyllium or gum-arabic with placebo improved rates of FI in individuals with diarrhea-predominant FI. Bowel habit training and scheduled toileting with or without laxatives to empty the rectum may help those with cognitive or mobility problems.

### Biofeedback

Biofeedback involves a trained provider who uses an instrument with visual or auditory feedback on the proper control of voluntary muscle contraction and relaxation of the external anal sphincter and recognition of anal sphincter sensation. Strength training, sensory training, and coordinated training (strength and sensory) occur in most biofeedback protocols for FI. The goal is improved external anal sphincter muscle contraction in response to rectal sensation or distention. Most centers use electromyographic or manometric biofeedback equipment. For success, patients who undergo biofeedback treatment need to have awareness of their defecation symptoms and be able to actively participate during the office-based treatments and a home exercise program. Older adults with cognitive problems and adults with spinal cord injury may not be good candidates for biofeedback.

Biofeedback has been compared with anal exercises/pelvic floor muscle exercises along with other conservative treatments. Two randomized controlled clinical trials for FI comparing educational advice alone, loperamide with advice, biofeedback alone, and the combination of loperamide and biofeedback showed that loperamide and biofeedback were no better than advice alone in improving FI frequency.[13,14] A few studies show no improvement in FI with a home electrical stimulation unit over a sham unit or office-based treatment.

### Pharmacologic Treatment

The most commonly used pharmacologic treatments involve antidiarrheal drugs for FI associated with loose stool consistency/diarrhea. Only three randomized crossover trials with adequate methodology have evaluated pharmacologic treatment of diarrhea-predominant FI in adults.[15] All had decreased frequency of FI episodes, volume, and improved consistency. More people reported adverse events, including constipation, abdominal pain, diarrhea, headache, and nausea. Given the anticholinergic properties of diphenoxylate plus atropine, this treatment should be avoided in older adults, and loperamide should be considered given similar efficacy. Treatment of constipation-associated FI with laxatives can be very effective, especially in long-term care settings, when used with other behavioral interventions (see section, Treatment of Constipation).

Occasionally, when antidiarrhea drugs are not effective for improving diarrhea-associated FI, a trial with cholestyramine is warranted. Cholestyramine is a bile salt—binding medication used to lower cholesterol and can reduce diarrhea associated with the production of excess bile acid salts. Limited data exist on the use of this medication specifically for FI, especially among older adults.

### CASE

#### Case Study (Part 4)

The cause of her symptoms is likely long-standing constipation that increased compliance of the rectal wall and decrease the ability to have the same urgency sensation prior to bowel evacuation. However, she is having more leakage after having a bowel movement. This could indicate a rectal emptying problem. Problems with rectal emptying could occur from a having a vaginal posterior compartment defect (vaginal rectocele), problems with loose or unformed stool consistency, or weakened rectal sphincter muscles.

In addition to focusing on bowel habits with recognizing and responding to fecal urge, you may also consider decreasing the dose of polyethylene glycol to once every day or every other day. If the problem resulted from a posterior vaginal compartment defect or problems with stool consistency, you might consider increasing her total fiber content. Dietary fiber and supplementary fiber along with the polyethylene glycol, could improve stool consistency in a motivated patient who is also drinking plenty of fluids. Biofeedback and a home rectal sphincter-muscle exercise program would help increase rectal sphincter tone and to improve rectal sensation.

## Injectable Agents

When conservative measures for FI fail, minimally invasive injectable agents may be considered. An office-based procedure involves the perianal injection of dextranomer microspheres and hyaluronic acid. Initial data showed a reduction in FI episodes, and long-term data are needed.[16] Studies involving other injectable agents into the perianal area have not shown improvement in FI episodes.

## Sacral Neuromodulation

Percutaneous tibial nerve stimulation (PTNS) and a surgically implanted device involve the treatment of FI by "stimulating" the nerves that help control defecation. PTNS involves an office-based procedure to indirectly stimulate the sacral nerves through the posterior tibial nerve. A small, acupuncture-sized needle is inserted into the medial aspect of the lower extremity and attached to a stimulation device. Often, 12 weeks of treatment are needed to see improvement in symptoms. Data from adequately powered randomized controlled trials for PTNS treatment for FI did find improvements in FI symptoms except among participants with more urge-predominant FI symptoms.[17] After using PTNS or if PTNS is not an option, patients may consider a surgically implanted neuromodulation device.[18] These devices stimulate the sacral nerves (at S3) and improve symptoms compared with conservative measures.

## Other Surgical Approaches

Other surgical therapies include anal sphincter repairs, artificial bowel sphincter, and colostomy. Overlapping sphincteroplasty can be used to repair a torn anal sphincter, which most commonly results from an obstetric injury and can be an occult finding in older women. Although short-term benefits may occur in younger women, little is known about sphincter repairs in older women. Overall, longer term data on outcomes are needed. Use of artificial bowel sphincter has significant associated morbidity, and colostomy is essentially used as a salvage procedure.

## Treatment of Incontinence-Associated Dermatitis

Contact of fecal material with skin on the perineum can cause contact dermatitis, fungal infection, and pressure ulcers. Treatment of skin problems is dependent on correct classification and recognition. Incontinence-associated dermatitis in the perineal area occurs from wetness and moisture exposure, and with the use of pads and other forms of containment. Skin barrier cream is recommended to help prevent and occasionally treat erythema and maceration that can occur from FI.[19] Several moisture barrier/skin protectant creams/pastes are available for OTC use and often include zinc oxide and dimethicone.

## Summary

Constipation and FI are common bowel symptoms that older patients experience. Older adults often resort to self-treatment, and the impact of the symptoms is underrecognized by healthcare providers. Evaluation of potential causes and contributing factors is important. Evaluation with colonoscopy or other endoscopic procedures is not warranted unless alarm symptoms are present. Treatments often depend on the underlying cause of the constipation or FI. Conservative therapies are considered the initial treatment before using more invasive therapies, including medications and surgery.

### Web Resources

The Rome Foundation: http://romecriteria.org/

National Institutes of Health, NIDDK patient information website: http://digestive.niddk.nih.gov/ddiseases/pubs/constipation/ http://www.digestive.niddk.nih.gov/ddiseases/pubs/fecalincontinence/

National Institutes of Health, NIA patient information website: http://www.nia.nih.gov/health/publication/concerned-about-constipation

National Foundation for Continence (FI): http://www.nafc.org/index.php?page = fecal-incontinence

International Foundation for Functional Gastrointestinal Disorders: http://www.iffgd.org/

## Key References

1. Mearin F, Lacy BE, Chang L, et al. Bowel disorders. *Gastroenterology*. 2016;150(6):1393–1407.e5
2. Emmanuel A, Mattace-Raso F, Neri MC, Petersen KU, Rey E, Rogers J. Constipation in older people: a consensus statement. *Int J Clin Pract*. 2017;71–79.
7. Simren M, Palsson OS, Whitehead WE. Update on Rome IV criteria for colorectal disorders: implications for clinical practice. *Curr Gastroenterol Rep*. 2017;19:15.
10. Wald A. Constipation: advances in diagnosis and treatment. *JAMA*. 2016;315:185–191.
12. Norton C, Thomas L, Hill J, Guideline Development Group. Management of faecal incontinence in adults: summary of NICE guidance. *BMJ*. 2007;334(7608):1370–1371.

# 25

# Hearing Impairment

JESSIE JENKINS AND WILLIAM LYONS

## OBJECTIVES

*Upon completion of this chapter, the reader will be able to:*

- Describe the psychosocial and functional consequences of hearing loss.
- Identify common features of presbycusis.
- List the appropriate indications for audiology and otolaryngology referrals.

- Understand benefits and limitations of common treatments of hearing loss.

## Prevalence and Impact

Hearing impairment is a common cause of disability among older adults and is increasingly recognized as a pressing public health concern. In the United States, bilateral hearing loss increases geometrically with age, impacting roughly one-quarter of patients age 60 to 69 years, half of patients age 70 to 79 years, and over three-quarters of patients over the age of 80 years.[1] The prevalence is expected to double by 2060.[2] Untreated hearing loss impairs conversational abilities, predisposing to social isolation, depression, and impaired provider-patient communication.[3,4] It is also linked to a wide range of adverse health outcomes including falls, disability, hospitalization, and increased healthcare costs.[3,5–7] For all these reasons clinicians caring for older patients should set aside time during patient encounters to identify and manage hearing impairment.

> **After 80 years of age, three-quarters of patients have some degree of hearing loss.**

The increasingly recognized association between hearing loss and cognitive impairment (Level of evidence [LOE] = B) has garnered this ailment newfound attention among researchers.[3,8–12] The Lancet Commission on Dementia Prevention, Intervention, and Care identified hearing impairment as the largest potentially modifiable risk factor for dementia, ranked above smoking, depression, inactivity, social isolation, and hypertension. Modeling suggests that 9% of dementia cases could theoretically be prevented by complete elimination of hearing loss.[13] Lin et al. estimate the decline in cognition associated with mild hearing impairment as equivalent (gauged by measures of executive function and psychomotor processing) to 7 years of aging.[11] Although randomized controlled trials will be needed to determine whether treatment of hearing loss improves cognitive outcomes, extrapolation from research involving older cochlear implant recipients provides some support.[14] One recent longitudinal study[9] suggests hearing aid use may slow progression of cognitive decline, but most interventional studies investigating the effects of hearing aids on cognitive endpoints have been small and of limited quality, yielding mixed results.[10]

❖❖ **Hearing loss is associated with adverse outcomes, including social isolation, depression, and cognitive impairment.**

## Normal Anatomy and Physiology

The peripheral auditory system is divided into three regions; the outer ear, middle ear, and inner ear (Fig. 25.1). The outer ear consists of the pinna and auditory canal, which capture and funnel environmental noises inward to the tympanic membrane, causing it to vibrate. These vibrations set the trio of tiny ossicular bones within the middle ear into motion. The mechanical energy is in turn transferred to the inner ear via the oval window. The inner ear houses intricate components of both the auditory system (cochlea) and the vestibular system (semicircular canals). The cochlea is a fluid-filled, snail-shaped structure that contains the sensory apparatus of the ear (organ of Corti). Vibrations relayed from the middle ear travel through the cochlea, displacing the hair cells of the organ of Corti. The movement of the hair cells ultimately generates electrical signals that are carried centrally via the auditory nerve for further processing and interpretation.

## Risk Factors and Pathophysiology

Common risk factors for hearing loss include older age, male sex, and lighter complexion. Low educational attainment and toxic noise exposure are risk factors for high-frequency hearing loss. Vascular risk factors are frequently but inconsistently linked with hearing loss.[15] Importantly, genetic factors account for up to one-half of variation in hearing ability in later life.[16] Aging affects all auditory structures. Examples include degeneration of ossicular joints, metabolic changes in the cochlea, dulling of the tympanic membrane, and thickening of the cerumen.[17] These changes result in variable clinical consequences; although common, hearing loss is not an inevitable consequence of aging.

Presbycusis is sensorineural hearing loss that results from the cumulative, age-related degeneration of the auditory system and is the most common cause of late-life hearing loss.[18] It is symmetric and insidious, affecting high-frequency tones first. Because consonants use high-frequency sounds that give definition to speech, the brain is left to translate imperfectly encoded signals. Patients with presbycusis commonly complain, "I can hear you, but I can't understand you."

Complaints of "mumbled" speech can be heightened by imperfect listening conditions; the paradigm for a difficult listening environment is a cocktail party. Under these circumstances, the brain devotes increasing resources to comprehension. Any level of cognitive impairment diminishes the listener's ability to compensate and results in central auditory processing disorder.[19] This manifests as impaired comprehension out of proportion to objective deficits found on audiometry.

---

**CASE**

**Jim Wanek (Part 1)**

Jim Wanek is a 73-year-old Caucasian male who comes to your clinic today on his wife's urging. They have been married 45 years, and she has noticed some changes recently. He has difficulty following the plotlines of his favorite westerns and tends to fall asleep with the TV blaring. She is having to repeat herself frequently during conversations, and occasionally Jim's responses do not make sense. Their children have commented that he seems less engaged with the grandchildren at family gatherings and wonder if he could be depressed. He is a retired machinist and enjoys woodworking in his spare time. He has never smoked and drinks alcohol

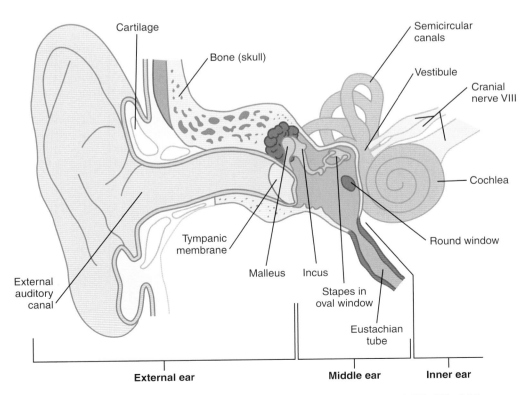

• **Figure 25.1** Anatomy of the ear. (From Baker Holly J, Sataloff Robert T. *Physician Assistant Clinics*. 2018;3(2): 223–245.)

infrequently. His past medical history includes osteoarthritis, hypertension, and allergic rhinitis. His medications include amlodipine, loratadine, and acetaminophen as needed.

1. What are Mr. Wanek's risk factors for hearing loss?
2. What office-based screening tests for hearing impairment are available?

❖ **The whispered voice test has good sensitivity and specificity for hearing loss. This functional test is a practical choice for screening geriatric patients in the primary care setting.**

## Screening

The US Preventative Services Task Force currently concludes that there is insufficient evidence to recommend screening for hearing loss in asymptotic older adults, although this recommendation is under review at the time of this writing.[20] Nonetheless, assessing for hearing impairment is a required element of the Medicare annual wellness visit. It is also an essential component of comprehensive geriatric assessment, especially when cognitive concerns or depressive symptoms are prominent. In this context, complaints of verbal repetitiveness, nonsensical responses, or socially isolative behaviors can be presenting symptoms of hearing impairment.

Simple screening approaches are preferred in the primary care setting. Single question screens, such as "Do you feel that you have any difficulty hearing?" or "Has anyone told you that you have difficulty hearing?" perform comparably to extensive questionnaires and should prompt further evaluation after an affirmative response. If there is concern that a patient is unable to reliably report symptoms, the whispered voice test is a logical alternative. To perform the whispered voice test, the examiner stands to the side of patient, with a fully extended arm covering the opposite ear. After fully exhaling to ensure consistent low volume, the examiner whispers a series of three letters and numbers for the patient to repeat. If the listener accurately repeats all three, the screen is considered negative. If the response is inaccurate, the examiner whispers a new combination of three letters and numbers. The screen is considered positive if the listener is unable to repeat a minimum three of the six offered letter/number combinations.[21]

An otoscope with a pure tone generator is another validated tool used to screen for hearing loss at specified frequencies (in Hz) and sound intensities (in decibels). The cost of this device is several hundred dollars. Test characteristics vary based on setting, frequency, and decibel level, but are not clearly superior to single question and whispered voice tests. Smartphone apps provide consumers with a highly sensitive screening option, although specificity varies significantly based on testing conditions.[22] See Table 25.1 for characteristics of office-based screening tests for hearing loss.

## Differential Diagnosis and Assessment

Once hearing loss is suspected, the primary care clinician should complete a history and physical examination focused on identifying readily treatable conditions and triaging appropriate referral. It is important to clarify the onset, laterality, and time course, and to inquire about associated symptoms, including tinnitus, otalgia, and otorrhea. The clinician should ask about recent viral illness or uncontrolled environmental allergies. The prior otologic history, including ear surgery, instrumentation, head trauma, and noise exposure, should be established. The drug list should be reviewed for ototoxic medications, including antibiotics, such as aminoglycosides and tetracyclines or chemotherapeutic agents, such as cisplatin. High-dose aspirin and intravenous loop diuretics may cause hearing loss, although the effects are reversible with drug discontinuation.[18]

The purpose of the otoscopic examination is to assess for obstruction, infection, effusion, or perforation. A brief neurologic examination to assess for coexisting cranial nerve deficits is also helpful. The Weber and Rinne tests, which have traditionally been used to differentiate conductive from sensorineural hearing loss, have variable test performance characteristics, and are heavily influenced by operator technique.[23] Tuning fork tests are therefore not well suited for decision making or diagnosis in the typical primary care setting.

The presence of any of the signs or symptoms delineated in Box 25.1 should prompt referral to an otolaryngologist. In the absence of these features, patients with suspected hearing loss should be referred to an audiologist. An audiologist is a healthcare professional with doctoral level training in diagnosis and treatment of both hearing disorders and vestibular disease. Pure tone audiometry, the gold standard for diagnosing and characterizing hearing loss, is the central component of the audiologist's evaluation. Audiometry measures the minimum sound intensity at which a patient can perceive a pure tone at various frequencies. A comparison between bone and air conduction thresholds provides important diagnostic classification. The results are plotted on an audiogram. Audiologic assessment may also include word recognition, acoustic reflexes, and tympanometry.[24] These tests provide additional detail that can help diagnose conditions, including otosclerosis and middle ear effusion.

**TABLE 25.1**   **Performance Characteristics of Screening Maneuvers for Hearing Loss of More Than 25 or 30 DB**

| | Sensitivity | Specificity | Median PLR | Median NLR |
|---|---|---|---|---|
| Single question | 0.67 | 0.80 | 3.0 | 0.40 |
| Questionnaire (HHIE-S) threshold >8 | 0.58 | .82 | 3.5 | 0.52 |
| Whispered voice | 0.95 | 0.82 | 5.1 | 0.03 |

(From Chou R, Dana T. *Screening for Hearing Loss in Adults Ages 50 Years and Older: A Review of the Evidence for the U.S. Preventive Services Task Force.* Rockville (MD): 2011; Agency for Healthcare Research and Quality.)

*NLR,* Negative likelihood ratio; *PLR,* positive likelihood ratio.

## • BOX 25.1  Indications for Otolaryngology Referral

1. Hearing loss with a positive history of ear infections, noise exposure, familial hearing loss, tuberculosis, syphilis, HIV, Ménière disease, autoimmune disorder, ototoxic medication use, otosclerosis, von Recklinghausen neurofibromatosis, Paget disease of bone, ear, or head trauma related to onset
2. History of pain, active drainage, or bleeding from an ear
3. Sudden onset or rapidly progressive hearing loss (<72 hours)[a]
4. Acute, chronic, or recurrent episodes of dizziness
5. Evidence of congenital or traumatic deformity of the ear
6. Visualization of blood, pus, cerumen plug, foreign body, or other material in the ear canal
7. An unexplained conductive hearing loss or abnormal tympanogram
8. Unilateral or asymmetric hearing loss (a difference of >15 dB pure tone average between ears); or bilateral hearing loss >30 dB
9. Unilateral or pulsatile tinnitus
10. Unilateral or asymmetrically poor speech discrimination scores (a difference of >15% between ears); or bilateral speech discrimination scores <80%

[a] Requires urgent Ear, Nose and Throat referral. Treatment with high dose systemic or intratympanic steroids if confirmed.

(From Position Statement: Red Flags-Warning of Ear Disease. https://www.entnet.org/?q = node/912)

| TABLE 25.2 | Differential Diagnosis of Hearing Loss | |
|---|---|
| **Conductive** | **Sensorineural** |
| Cerumen impaction | Presbycusis |
| Foreign-body impaction | Noise exposure |
| Otitis externa | Ototoxic medication |
| Perforated tympanic membrane | Inner ear infection (viral cochleitis or meningitis) |
| Otitis media | Autoimmune |
| Eustachian tube dysfunction | Tumor (acoustic neuroma) |
| Otosclerosis | Ménière disease |
| Cholesteoma | Diabetes mellitus |
| Tumor (SCC) | Gene mutation |
| Disarticulation of ossicular chain because of trauma | Cerebrovascular accident |
| | Multiple sclerosis |
| | Otosyphyllis |

◆◆ **Most hearing loss detected and evaluated during primary care visits is appropriately referred to an audiologist.**

Hearing loss is broadly categorized as conductive (CHL), sensorineural (SNHL), or mixed. See Table 25.2 for specific etiologies within these categories. Conductive loss results from abnormality of the outer or middle ear that impedes transfer of sound energy to the inner ear. It accounts for approximately 10% of cases in the geriatric population.[25] Although less common, CHL is important to recognize because medical or surgical treatments for conductive hearing loss are frequently curative.

Cerumen impaction is a commonly encountered and easily remedied cause of CHL. If cerumen is symptomatic or preventing adequate visualization of the tympanic membrane, it should be removed via manual extraction, application of softening agents, or a combination of both methods. Note that commercial cerumenolytics are not superior to warm water for this purpose and may

cause irritation with prolonged use. If impaction is refractory to these efforts, specialist referral is warranted.[26]

Sensorineural hearing loss results from dysfunction of the cochlea and/or auditory nerve. Cochlear hair cells are particularly sensitive to damage by noise, drugs, and aging, and as they do not regenerate, resulting deficits are permanent. Death of hair cells can be further compounded by degeneration of associated spiral ganglion neurons, whose axons form part of the eighth cranial nerve.[18]

◆◆ **Audiologists received doctoral level training in ear disorders, whereas hearing aid dispensers received 6 to 24 months of apprenticeship to learn audiometry and hearing aid fitting.**

## CASE

### Jim Wanek (Part 2)

During the appointment, you notice Mr. Wanek has a hard time understanding you, and he agrees that hearing has been problematic. He admits to avoiding social gatherings because he struggles to participate in conversation. He denies ottorhea and otalgia. He endorses mild, nonpulsatile tinnitus bilaterally that is only noticeable in quiet environments. Routine otoscopic examination reveals nonobstructive cerumen. Tympanic membranes are clear with normal landmarks. He has been hesitant to seek treatment as he knows several friends who were not satisfied with their hearing aids despite paying thousands of dollars. After discussing your recommendations, however, he agrees to audiology referral for a full hearing assessment.
1. What are appropriate indications for audiology and otolaryngology referral?
2. What are the expected benefits of treating hearing loss with optimum amplification?

## Management

Although enhanced understanding of the pathophysiology of degenerative hearing loss has motivated several ongoing therapeutic trials, there is currently no cure for SNHL. The goal of treatment therefore is to restore effective communication and minimize disability. This is accomplished through a combination of communication strategies (outlined in Box 25.2), amplification technology, and assistive listening devices.

## Hearing Aids

Amplification with hearing aids remains the cornerstone of management of SNHL. Audiologists identify candidates for amplification. In most patients with clinically significant hearing loss, hearing aids significantly improve hearing-related quality of life, listening, communication, and social participation (LOE = B). Hearing aids may also provide a benefit in overall quality of life and depression, although evidence is mixed.[27-29]

Hearing aids are classified as medical devices and regulated by the US Food and Drug Administration (FDA). Historically, sales have been restricted to licensed professionals, including audiologists and hearing aid dispensers. Unlike audiologists, the licensing requirements for hearing aid dispensers vary by state, and typically consist of a 6- to 24-month apprenticeship after high school. Dispensers are commonly employed by a hearing aid manufacturer and may rely on industry-provided rather than peer-reviewed sources for their education. Regardless of place of purchase, the cost of hearing aids is routinely bundled with services, such as postfitting

- Acknowledge hearing loss and ask the listener if he or she has tips to facilitate conversation
- Eliminate background noise
- Consider use of a personal amplification device
- Facilitate lip reading with appropriate lighting and use of corrective lenses
- Face the patient directly at a distance of approximately 2 feet
- Maintain the same register as conversational speech; shouting shifts the voice into a higher frequency range
- Speak slowly but naturally; overenunciating distorts speech and hinders lip reading
- Use written instructions, visual aids, and message boards
- Verify comprehension using teach-back method

adjustments, cleaning, repair, warranty, semiannual checks, reprogramming, and accessories. The hearing aids themselves account for only 30% to 40% of the total charges.[19] Consumers should request specifics of included services, as well as itemized prices in writing. There is usually a money-back trial period, and consumers should inquire about the terms of return.

Hearing aids are available in a wide range of designs and come equipped with a variety of customizable features (Fig. 25.2). Once an audiologist determines that a patient is a good candidate for hearing aids, an aid is selected based on the individual's degree of hearing loss, dexterity, lifestyle, and budget. Hearing aids are broadly categorized by shape, with options ranging from traditional behind-the-ear to tiny completely-in-the-canal models (see Fig. 25.2). Whereas inexperienced users may gravitate to smaller aids for cosmetic reasons, notable drawbacks include less amplification power, fewer features, and small batteries that both hold less charge and pose a challenge for patients with limited dexterity. Audiologists recommend bilateral hearing aids for most patients, which results in a higher out-of-pocket cost. Research to support this practice is lacking, although bilateral aids may improve sound

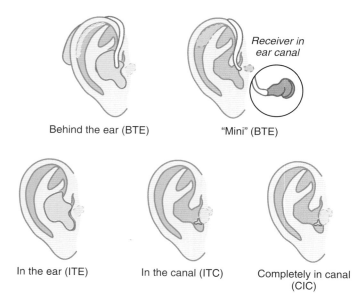

**Behind the ear (BTE)**       **"Mini" (BTE)**       *Receiver in ear canal*

**In the ear (ITE)**    **In the canal (ITC)**    **Completely in canal (CIC)**

• **Figure 25.2** Examples of traditional hearing aids. (From Baker Holly J, Sataloff Robert T. *Physician Assistant Clinics.* 2018;3(2): 223–245.)

localization and speech intelligibility in noisy environments.[24,30] Premium features also contribute to cost but do not necessarily translate into improved outcomes.[31]

Hearing aids can be well tolerated by many patients with dementia who enjoy the benefits of improved hearing-related quality of life.[32] To prevent loss, nylon line can be tied to a small metal loop on the device, with the other end pinned to clothing. Caregivers should be trained in hearing aid maintenance. In nursing facilities, staff should be educated in the hearing needs of residents, and hearing aid maintenance should be specifically delegated in the daily workflow.[33]

## Aural Rehabilitation

Aural rehabilitation refers to a holistic approach to hearing care, including sensory management through personalized amplification, instruction in the use of technology, perceptual training to improve speech understanding, and counseling on how to cope emotionally and practically with any remaining disability.[34] This education is delivered by audiologists in individual or group sessions for new hearing aid users. Although some aspects of aural rehabilitation may be bundled with hearing aid purchase, these services are not covered by most third-party payers.

Management of expectations is a key component of hearing rehabilitation. Hearing aids augment abnormal hearing but do not restore normal hearing. Patients should allow time to acclimate to the devices and should expect to return to place of purchase several times for troubleshooting and fine-tuning. Crowded environments can be especially difficult to navigate for new hearing aid users and often represent a significant source of dissatisfaction. The limiting obstacle to device efficacy in these settings is signal-to-noise ratio. Modern hearing aids attempt to optimize this through use of directional microphones, programming to augment frequencies associated with human voice, and complex digital algorithms designed to recognize and selectively amplify speech.

## Improving Access to Hearing Healthcare

Despite their known benefits, hearing aid utilization remains low. Just under 15% of adults with hearing loss over the age 50 years own hearing aids, although adoption increases with age and severity of impairment.[35] Several barriers to effective treatment exist. Many people view hearing loss as an inevitable and insignificant part of aging. For others, the insidious onset of hearing loss prevents them from recognizing their deficits. Cosmetic concerns and perceived stigma dissuade many. Cost remains the most commonly cited reason for not obtaining recommended aids. Unlike national health plans in other developed countries, Medicare does not cover hearing aids or aural rehabilitation. In the current model of payment, the average price for a pair of hearing aids with bundled professional services is $4700.[36] Some 28 states provide Medicaid coverage for hearing healthcare.[37] Some patients may find coverage through Veterans Affairs benefits or Medicare Advantage plans, although a majority of patients pay out of pocket.

❖ **Only about 15% of adults with hearing loss over the age 50 years own hearing aids.**

For a variety of reasons, hearing aid technology has not enjoyed the same reductions in price or rapid innovation cycles that are standard in electronic consumer technology. Potential explanations for the sustained price inflation include lack of competition, lack of price transparency, and excessive regulation. Only six hearing aid manufacturers account for 90% of the global market share for hearing aids in 2019.[38] Large-volume purchasers, such as the US Department of Veterans Affairs or the UK National Health Service, leverage their negotiating power to purchase midtier aids for approximately $400 per pair.[39]

With increasing recognition that hearing loss represents a serious public health concern for the aging population, consumer advocacy and governmental agencies are pressing for industry reform and increased access to affordable treatment. In response, Congress passed a law in 2017 directing the FDA to create a new regulatory class for hearing aids available for direct-to-consumer sale. The standards for over-the-counter (OTC) hearing aids are in development at the time of this writing. In general, this category of aids will be designed for mild to moderate hearing loss and will not require examination, audiometry, or involvement of licensed sales personnel. Opponents of direct-to-consumer hearing aids worry that some patients with hearing loss caused by serious medical conditions will delay seeking appropriate evaluation while self-treating with these devices. Another concern is that patients cannot know the severity of their hearing loss without formal testing, which may result in inadequate self-treatment of severe hearing loss. Advocates point to low incidence of medically significant causes of hearing loss and also draw analogies to OTC reading glasses. Consumers are trusted to recognize problematic eye concerns and to seek care if OTC magnification is insufficient.

⁍⁍ **The FDA is developing standards for OTC hearing aids, a step that is expected to substantially reduce cost and improve access for people with mild to moderate hearing loss.**

Increasing access to aural rehabilitation presents another promising domain of health policy change. There is evidence that patients who access hearing healthcare incur significantly lower overall healthcare costs, although the mechanism of this relationship is not well understood.[40]

## Personal Sound Amplification Products

Personal sound amplification products (PSAPs) comprise a category of wearable consumer technology designed to amplify sounds in specific situations, such as attending a lecture in a crowded space. To avoid FDA regulation, they cannot be marketed for daily use or as a treatment of hearing loss. It remains to be seen how PSAPs will differ from the FDA regulated, direct-to-consumer hearing aids. PSAPs are highly heterogeneous in terms of performance and cost, retailing anywhere from $30 to $400. Entry-level devices (i.e., less than $50) may overamplify low-frequency sounds and environmental noises. Users of budget devices may also be hindered by poor listening comfort and even reduced comprehension compared with using no device. Some popular devices incorporate advanced technology and perform comparably in head-to-head comparison with standard hearing aids.[41,42] Many devices require use of a smart-phone app for adjustments, but only a growing minority of older patients are facile with this technology. Overall, although these devices represent a good option for technologically-savvy, self-motivated, and cost-conscious persons, many older patients require hands-on support and education as they integrate this technology into their daily lives. These patients may be best served through involvement of professional audiology services.[43]

## Hearing Assistive Technology

Hearing assistive devices are products that help individuals with hearing loss safely function in specific situations where hearing aids alone would be insufficient. Closed captioning, vibrotactile alarms, video doorbells, and specialized telephones all fall into this category. Hearing aid adjuncts, such as remote microphones ("spouse mics" worn on a conversations partner's lapel) can optimize signal-to-noise ratio. Bluetooth equipped devices can sync with many personal electronic devices.

Personal amplification devices, best known by the popular brand name Pocketalker, can drastically improve communication with patients who cannot tolerate or do not have access to hearing aids. These devices consist of earphones for the listener, a microphone to be placed near the speaker, and a battery pack with volume control. This is an essential piece of equipment for any clinical setting serving older patients.

The Americans with Disability Act requires public places where communication is integral to the assembly space (i.e., churches, lecture halls) to incorporate assistive listening systems. This is accomplished through FM, infrared, or induction-loop technology. Listeners use headphones to selectively amplify the featured speaker, helping to overcome poor acoustics. Patients who use telecoil-equipped hearing aids can link to induction loop systems and forgo headphones.

### CASE

#### Jim Wanek (Part 3)

Mr. Wanek underwent audiometry, which revealed bilaterally symmetrical, mild to moderate, high-frequency sensorineural hearing loss. On speech discrimination testing, he recognized 87% of monosyllabic word listing in his right ear and 90% in his left ear with 40-dB amplification above his pure-tone thresholds. At normal conversational level, his word recognition score dropped to 70%. The audiologist felt he would benefit from hearing aids. Mr. Wanek's primary motivation in treating his hearing loss was to improve communication with his grandkids. He was also hopeful that the hearing aids would be compatible with his television and smartphone. The audiologist ultimately recommended a behind-the-ear hearing aid. Mr. Wanek experienced improved word recognition with use of the aid in the office but had a hard time getting used to it in noisy settings. He enrolled in a group aural rehabilitation course where he enjoyed learning tips and tricks from the audiologist and other patients on how to adjust to life with a hearing aid.

1. How can hearing assistive technology improve communication in difficult listening situations?
2. What treatment options are available for patients with severe hearing loss insufficiently treated with hearing aids?

## Surgical Treatments for Hearing Loss

Although less common, conductive hearing loss is important to recognize as medical or surgical treatment is first line and may be curative. Intervention is specific to etiology, and may include simple (e.g., cerumen removal) or more involved (e.g., stapedectomy for otosclerosis, or cholesteatoma removal) procedures.

Osseointegrated devices are an alternative for patients who cannot use standard aids because of anatomic defects, allergic reactions, or chronic infections of the external ear. Osseointegrated devices contain a titanium rod, which is surgically implanted in the skull and transmits sound directly through bone. The sound processor attaches directly or magnetically to the rod. Active middle ear implants are another option for patients with mild or moderate SNHL who cannot tolerate traditional hearing aids because of medical or cosmetic reasons. Components can be partially or fully implanted under the skin and function by directly stimulating the ossicles. Specifics vary by brand; patients should be aware of costs and reoperation rates.

For patients with severe to profound SNHL that is inadequately managed by traditional hearing aids, cochlear implants may restore functional hearing (LOE = A). The devices are placed in the outpatient setting. One component is an electrode array that is surgically implanted into the cochlea. A second component is the external speech processor, which converts sounds into electrical impulses; these, in turn, are transmitted to the electrodes, bypassing damaged hair cells and directly stimulating fibers of the spiral ganglion. Candidates must be highly motivated and agreeable to extensive aural rehabilitation after implantation. They also must be medically fit for general anesthesia. Unlike hearing aids, cochlear implantation is covered by Medicare. Recipients are eligible for a speech processor upgrade every 5 years to take advantage of technical updates.[17]

Cochlear implants are safe and effective in the geriatric population. Octogenarians and nonagenarians may expect favorable outcomes, with improvements in speech comprehension, social participation, and quality of life that are comparable with those of younger recipients. Although overall morbidity remains low, the very older adults experience a slightly higher rate of anesthetic complications.[44] As with hearing aids, management of expectations is important. Because a cochlear implant uses a limited number of electrodes (typically 12–22) to stimulate a reduced number of spiral ganglion cells, the pattern of nerve activity is crude compared with the complex resolution and high fidelity of the natural ear. Sounds may first be observed by patients to have a robotic quality, but that becomes smoother over time. Unfortunately, cochlear implants remain poor at restoring perception of harmonic pitch, speaker identity, or emotional content of speech.[45,46]

---

## CASE

### Discussion

Mr. Wanek's increasing social isolation is likely a result of his hearing impairment. Presbycusis predominantly affects perception of high pitches, making communication with grandchildren in group settings particularly challenging. When his hearing deficits persisted after treatment of the cerumen impaction, he was appropriately referred to an audiologist for comprehensive hearing healthcare. Mr. Wanek's case also illustrates the time and effort required to fully adapt to hearing aid use and the vital role aural rehabilitation plays in this process.

## Summary

Accurate and reliable hearing screening tools exist to identify persons for whom hearing specialist referral is warranted. Clinicians can improve the outlook for hearing-impaired persons by recognizing the serious consequences of hearing loss, assessing routinely for hearing loss, and counseling patients about the benefits of hearing health services. Hearing aids significantly improve the quality of life of patients with sensorineural hearing loss.

### Web Resources

CapTel captioning service is provided as part of a federally-funded program, regulated by the FCC, that is designed specifically to help individuals with hearing loss access the telephone: https://www.captel.com.

AARP Consumer Guide to Hearing Aids is a comprehensive educational packet for patients considering hearing aid purchase; it will be due for an update when OTC aids reach the market: https://assets.aarp.org/www.aarp.org_/articles/health/docs/hearing_guide.pdf.

US Food and Drug Administration—Protecting and Promoting Your Health: Medical Devices (Hearing Aids). Provides consumers a brief overview on hearing aids, hearing aids and cellphones, assistive listening devices, and surgical treatments for hearing loss; watch for updates on OTC aids: https://www.fda.gov/medical-devices/consumer-products/hearing-aids.

## Key References

9. Maharani A, Dawes P, Nazroo J, Tampubolon G, Pendleton N. Longitudinal relationship between hearing aid use and cognitive function in older Americans. *J Am Geriatr Soc*. 2018;66(6):1130–1136.

21. Strawbridge WJ, Wallhagen MI. Simple tests compare well with a hand-held audiometer for hearing loss screening in primary care. *J Am Geriatr Soc*. 2017;65(10):2282–2284.

43. Mamo SK, Reed NS, Nieman CL, Oh ES, Lin FR. Personal sound amplifiers for adults with hearing loss. *Am J Med*. 2016;129(3):245–250.

46. Sprinzl GM, Riechelmann H. Current trends in treating hearing loss in elderly people: a review of the technology and treatment options - a mini-review. *Gerontology*. 2010;56(3):351–358.

***References available online at* expertconsult.com.**

# 26

# Visual Impairment and Eye Problems

NATALIE A. MANLEY AND DEEPTA A. GHATE

## OUTLINE

*Additional online-only material indicated by icon.*

## OBJECTIVES

*Upon completion of this chapter, the reader will be able to:*

- Describe normal and abnormal changes of the eye associated with aging.
- Describe the functional and health impact of visual impairment on older people.
- Describe signs of eye emergencies.

- List the primary causes of blindness and vision loss in the older adult population.
- List common eye side effects of systemic medications and systemic effects of ophthalmologic medications.
- Describe diagnosis and management of common eye problems.

## Introduction

This chapter highlights what primary care providers (PCPs) should know to diagnose and manage common geriatric eye concerns; to provide primary prevention of vision loss; to refer to and communicate with eye consultants; and to recognize eye emergencies, ophthalmologic side effects of systemic medications, and systemic side effects of eye medications. A PCP can guide patients through the treatment options from specialists given the context of the patient's health. Lastly, the PCP should be knowledgeable when managing eye disorders when goals of care are purely for comfort. A PCP ensures that the patient's functional priorities are at the forefront of care. Lastly, for a nursing home or hospice provider, and when much of patient care occurs non face to face, it is important to know how to manage eye concerns over the phone.

---

### CASE 1

#### Mable Rose (Part 1)

Mrs. Rose is an 84-year-old female with insulin-dependent type 2 diabetes mellitus (DM) with peripheral neuropathy, Parkinson disease, hypertension, and seasonal allergies. You are seeing her at her assisted living facility in December. She had cataract surgery 5 years ago and sees ophthalmology for diabetic retinopathy (DR). She takes furosemide, carbidopa-levodopa, sertraline, lisinopril, metoprolol, aspirin, loratadine, and long-acting insulin. Her allergic symptoms occur in the spring. Lately, staff note that her eyes are a little red. The patient reports feeling like she has something stuck in her eyes, but denies eye pain or change in vision. Her visual acuity (VA) is 20/50 in the right eye and 20/40 in the left eye. Pupils are equal round and reactive; conjunctiva are injected bilaterally. There is no foreign body under the eyelids; fundus is normal; eyes are watery. She has dry, flaky skin on her scalp, forehead, and nasolabial folds.
1. What is the likely cause(s) of her red eyes? And what orders will you provide today?
2. Which medications and diagnoses could be contributing to her eye complaints?
3. How soon should she see an eye provider?

---

### ▶ Anatomic Landmarks of the Eye

Figs. 26.1–26.4 review anatomic landmarks; Table 26.1 defines ophthalmology abbreviations.

### Recommended Eye Examination Skills for the Primary Care Provider

Eye/vision concerns[1] should prompt an examination (see www.aao.org/basicvideo). Visual acuity (VA) is the vital sign

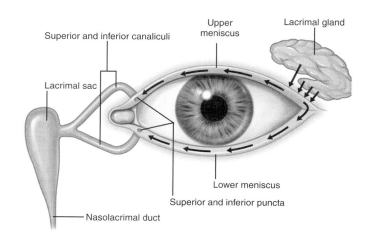

• **Figure 26.2** Anatomy of the lacrimal apparatus. (From Kellerman RD, Rakel DP. *Conn's Current Therapy* 2019. Elsevier; 2019: Figure 1, pages 475–477.)

for the eye. After assessing VA, check fields and inspect eyelids, surrounding tissues, conjunctiva, sclera, cornea and iris, extraocular movements, and pupils for direct and consensual responses. By ophthalmoscope, assess the anterior chamber, the lens for clarity, and the fundus (including the disc, vessels, and macula).

### Physiologic Changes With Age[1,2]

The primary change with aging is hardening of the crystalline lens. As the lens hardens, it loses ability to change shape (loss of accommodation), leading to presbyopia (decreased ability to focus on near objects).[1,2] Presbyopia becomes clinically apparent in a person's fourth decade and is corrected by bifocal lenses.[1,2] Other changes with age include decreased pupillary size, decreased ability to adjust pupil size to light, and lens opacification by cataracts. This leads to less light reaching the retina, and by the age of

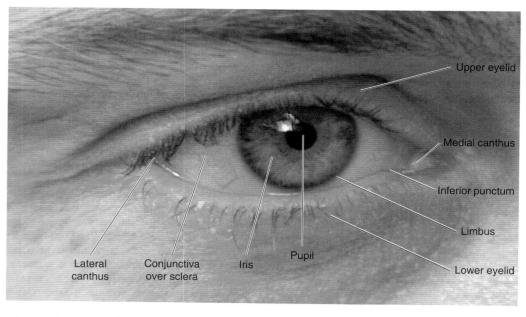

• **Figure 26.1** External eye anatomy. (From Swartz MH. *Textbook of Physical Diagnosis*, 7e. Saunders-Elsevier; 2014: Figure 7.1.)

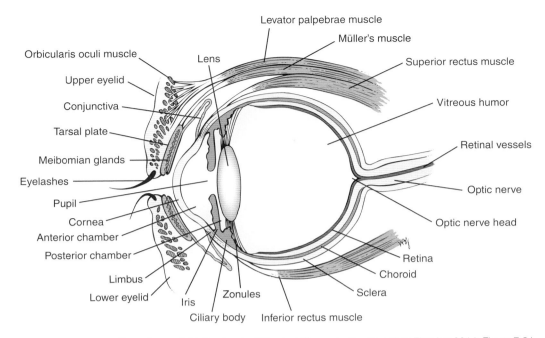

- **Figure 26.3** Cross-sectional anatomy. (From Swartz MH. *Textbook of Physical Diagnosis*, 7e. Saunders-Elsevier; 2014: Figure 7.2.)

60 years the retina receives two-thirds less light than at age 20 years.[2] Also, it takes longer for eyes to adjust to changes in light (e.g., going from indoors to outdoors). Cataracts cause sensitivity to glare from bright lights (e.g., automobile headlights).

## Common Age-Related Eye Problems

Age-related changes in the eye and periorbital tissues that may lead to pathology in older adults are listed in Table 26.2 (available online).

## The Geriatric Red Eye

A red eye is hyperemia or injection of superficially visible vessels of the conjunctiva, episclera, or sclera.[1] Most people with red eye do not have a vision threatening process. However, it is important to know symptoms and signs (red flags) of vision threatening conditions. Box 23.1 lists red flags for serious eye conditions. If any are present, the patient should see an eye provider on the same day. Box 23.2 (available online) is a physical examination guide for evaluating the red eye. Table 26.3 (available online) describes common diagnoses and treatments of benign red eye.

### CASE 1

#### Discussion

Mrs. Rose suffers from dry eye and also has a component of seborrheic blepharitis (dry, flaky skin over eyebrows and nasolabial folds). Treatment focuses on eye lubrication with drops and/or ointments, and with antidandruff therapy for seborrheic dermatitis. Her risk factors for dry eyes include age, female sex, neuropathy, polypharmacy, and Parkinson disease. Medications associated with dry eye include her diuretic, beta-blocker, antihistamine, and antidepressant.[3–5] Not all of these medications should be stopped, rather they should be reconsidered for risk and benefit. For her, loratadine can be discontinued given that it is not her allergy season. She should see ophthalmology if initial therapies are not helpful or if she develops red flag symptoms.

◆◆ **Patients who cannot effectively communicate should be assumed to have eye pain, when assessing a red eye.**

## Dry Eye Disease

### Prevalence and Impact

Dry eye disease (DED) or keratoconjunctivitis sicca, is a common geriatric eye complaint in primary care. Its prevalence increases with age and affects more women than men. Aside from dryness, patients complain of eye discomfort, burning, stinging, grittiness, tearing, ocular fatigue, or a foreign body sensation.[3,4,5] DED is associated with poor sleep, depression, anxiety, and stress. Quality of life scores associated with moderate and severe dry eye are similar to angina or hip fracture.[3]

◆◆ **The most important treatment for dry eye is identifying exacerbating factors and minimizing contributing medications.**

## Risk Factors and Pathophysiology

DED "is a multifactorial disease of the tears and ocular surface causing discomfort, visual disturbance, and tear film instability and may damage the ocular surface."[6] It can be episodic or chronic. Nonmodifiable risk factors include female sex, Sjögren syndrome, and age. Modifiable factors include dry environment, medications, blepharitis, smoking, alcohol use, long-term contact lens use, LASIK surgery, pollution, activities with decreased blinking (computer use), and topical ocular medications. Other causes include poorly fitting sleep apnea masks, decreased blink from Parkinson disease, peripheral neuropathy, sleep deprivation, lid abnormalities (ectropion—outward turning of the lid margin, and lagophthalmos—incomplete lid closure during sleep), and thyroid disease.[3] Sleep deprivation decreases tear secretion and osmolality, and worsens tear film breakup time. The symptoms of dry eye can worsen in sleep, creating a positive feedback loop. DED is also associated with depression, anxiety, and stress in a reciprocating manner.[7]

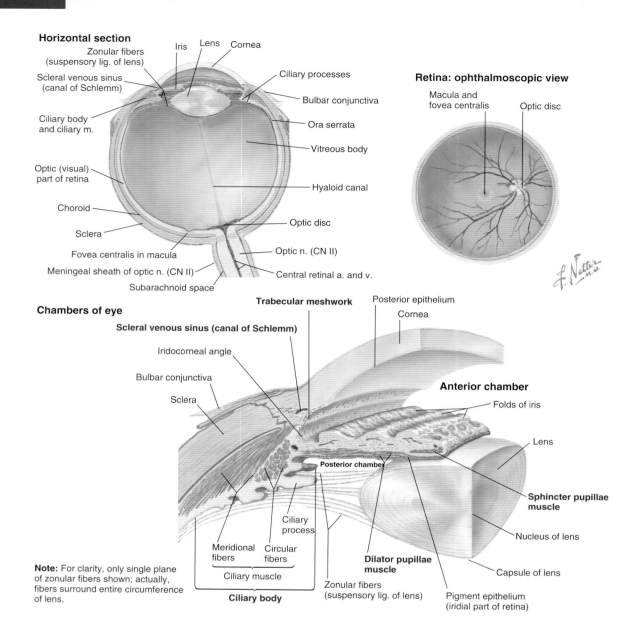

• **Figure 26.4** Retinal anatomy. (From Hansen JT. *Netter's Clinical Anatomy*, 4e. Elsevier; 2019: Figure 8.22.)

## Differential Diagnosis and Assessment

When diagnosing DED, look for any anatomic changes (e.g., ectropion, lagophthalmos), which may require surgery, and for other causative factors. Consider possible Sjögren syndrome by asking about dry mouth and examining parotid glands for enlargement.[3]

## Management

Interventions address exacerbating factors and minimize medications that contribute to DED. Hot compresses, artificial tears, and nighttime lubricating ointments are the mainstay of treatment. Use of artificial tears with preservatives more than three to four times a day will worsen DED, whereas preservative-free tears can be used as often as needed. Over-the-counter (OTC) "antiredness"

eye drops with naphazoline or pheniramine worsen DED if used for more than 3 to 4 days. Optimize sleep, mood, and Parkinson disease treatment when present. Refer to an eye provider when symptoms are not well controlled.

## Vision Loss in the Older Adult Population

### CASE 2

#### Larry Jones (Part 1)

Mr. Jones is a 65-year-old male who presents to clinic for his "Welcome to Medicare Preventative Visit." He has hypertension and diet-controlled type 2 DM. He smokes one pack of cigarettes/day and works as an accountant. He reports his parents are alive and well but that his mother goes to a low

| TABLE 26.1 | Common Ophthalmologic Abbreviations |
|---|---|
| **Abbreviation** | **Definition** |
| VA, DVA, NVA | visual acuity; distance VA; near VA |
| sc | uncorrected |
| cc | with correction (e.g., glasses, contacts) |
| ph | pinhole |
| OD | oculus dexter = right eye |
| OS | oculus sinister = right eye |
| OU | oculus uterque = both eyes |
| DFE | dilated ocular fundus examination |
| IOP | intraocular pressure |
| NPC | near point of convergence |
| NRA; PRA | negative relative accommodation; positive relative accommodation |
| MRx | manifest refraction (first number = sphere; second number = cylinder and axis) |

vision clinic. He worries about losing vision like her because he sees the impact it has on her independence. He reports he is due to see his eye care provider. His vision changes have been gradual. He denies distortion of vision, eye pain, or headache. His only medication is lisinopril. His corrected vision is 20/100 OD and 20/50 OS.

1. How would you address his concern about risk for development of low vision?

## Prevalence and Impact of Vision Loss

Some 37 million Americans age >50 years and 25% age >80 years suffer from vision impairment.[8] Visual impairment creates risk for decreased quality of life, functional loss, depression, falls, and social isolation.[9] The common causes of vision loss in those age >65 years is uncorrected refractive error, cataracts, age-related macular degeneration (AMD), DR, and glaucoma. These eye diseases are often asymptomatic early on, and prevention and early detection may prevent functional decline. A comprehensive eye evaluation for a person age ≥65 years should occur every 1 to 2 years.[10] Those with risk factors for vision threatening eye diseases should be seen as recommended by their eye care specialist.[10] Most with DM need annual eye examinations and those at risk for glaucoma should have a comprehensive eye evaluation every 1 to 2 years.[10]

◆◆ **Visual impairment decreases quality of life, function, and mood; it increases risk of falls and social isolation.**[9]

## Differential Diagnosis and Assessment of Vision Loss, Including Acute Vision Loss

The questions to consider when a patient reports vision loss include: What is the severity? Is it unilateral or bilateral? Is it acute or chronic/gradual? Is the eye painful? If vision loss is acute, severe, or painful, then urgent referral to an eye provider is needed. Full discussion of evaluation of acute vision loss is beyond the scope of this chapter; however, a few conditions associated with older age will be briefly described. A patient with bilateral painless sudden vision loss needs immediate neuroimaging to detect stroke within the treatment window for thrombolytics. Unilateral painless vision loss requires urgent examination by an ophthalmologist, for central retinal artery occlusion and management with thrombolytics and assessment for stroke. Painful vision loss needs urgent referral to rule out infectious or other causes.

◆◆ **Acute, painless vision loss should be emergently evaluated for possible stroke.**

## Chronic Vision Loss

### Refractive Error

One study found that 62% of low vision and 4% of blindness was caused by refractive error.[11] Older adults are at risk for uncorrected refractive error because of financial constraints, transportation, cognition, and communication issues.[12] One nursing home study found that refractive correction led to immediate improvements in reading, psychological distress, activities and hobbies, and social interaction.[11,13] The pinhole test is a rapid method to detect refractive error.

## Age-Related Macular Degeneration

### Prevalence and Impact and Risk Factors and Pathophysiology

AMD is a leading cause of severe, irreversible vision impairment in developed countries.[14] In AMD the sharp, "straight ahead" vision needed to see fine details is decreased by destruction of the macula.[15] This causes decreased ability to read, drive, recognize faces, and see colors.[15] Vision loss begins centrally and extends peripherally. Nonneovascular AMD (dry) causes 80% of cases, whereas neovascular (wet) AMD causes almost 90% of severe vision loss in AMD.[14]

Nonmodifiable risk factors for AMD include age, European decent, genetics, and female sex.[14,15] A primary modifiable risk factor for progression to late AMD is smoking.[14,15] The pathognomonic sign of AMD is drusen (yellow deposits on the macula from death of retinal cells). Neovascularization causes wet AMD, when vascular endothelial growth factor (VEGF) drives angiogenesis and increases vascular permeability and inflammation damaging photoreceptors and the retinal pigment epithelium.[15]

### Differential Diagnosis and Assessment[15]

AMD has early, intermediate, and late/advanced stages. The stages drive treatment and are based on changes on examination by an eye care specialist. Early AMD is often asymptomatic and is identified during dilated eye exams. Late AMD causes irreversible vision loss. Outcome is strongly associated with the acuity at the start of treatment, making early detection important.

Progression from early or intermediate AMD to late AMD can occur in a matter of days, causes loss of far and near vision, sudden visual distortion (e.g., straight lines or edges appear wavy), central vision loss, and change in color vision. Patients should be encouraged to do home monitoring with an Amsler grid and to immediately alert their eye care provider of changes.

**TABLE 26.2** Pathologic Anatomic Eye Changes That Commonly Occur With Aging

EXTERNAL CHANGES

| Anatomic Change | Consequence | Diagnosis | Image | Treatment by Ophthalmologist |
|---|---|---|---|---|
| Loss of skin elasticity | Brow sags over the superior orbital rim and can block vision | Brow ptosis | Image credit: Dr. Rao Chanduri-Truhlsen Eye Institute | Surgery if severe enough to restrict peripheral vision |
| Levator aponeurosis stretches or partially detaches from the superior tarsal plate | Upper eyelid moves down (closer to the visual axis) and can block vision | Ptosis | Image credit: Dr. Rao Chanduri-Truhlsen Eye Institute | Surgery if severe enough to restrict peripheral vision |
| Lower eyelid suspensor ligaments become lax | Eyelid margin rotates toward the cornea causing eyelashes to rub against the eye (trichiasis) | Entropion | Image credit: Dr. Rao Chanduri-Truhlsen Eye Institute | Surgery if tearing is bothersome or if there is any trichiasis |
| Lower eyelid suspensor ligaments become lax | Eyelid margin falls away from the globe leading to risk for dry eye | Ectropion | Image credit: Dr. Rao Chanduri-Truhlsen Eye Institute | Lubricating eye drops; surgery |
| Interruption of the normal eyelid architecture | Predisposition to dysfunction of the lacrimal pump drainage mechanism causes chronic tearing | Epiphora (tearing) | Image credit: Dr. Rao Chanduri-Truhlsen Eye Institute | Treat the cause |
| Lashes misdirected | Lashes rub the eye | Trichiasis | Kanski JJ, Bowling, B. *Kanski's Clinical Opthalmology*, 8e. Elsevier; 2016: Figure 1.32C. | Surgery, electrolysis of eyelashes |

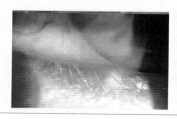

## TABLE 26.2   Pathologic Anatomic Eye Changes That Commonly Occur With Aging—cont'd

| | | | | |
|---|---|---|---|---|
| Conjunctiva loses accessory lacrimal glands and goblet cells | Dry eye | Dry eye syndrome | | Lubrication |
| Seventh nerve palsy, larger eyeball (proptosis because of thyroid eye disease or other reasons), lower lid ectropion | Inability to close eyelid completely over eye | Lagophthalmos | Craig JP, Downie LE. *Tears and Contact Lenses*. In: Phillips AJ, Speedwell L, eds. Contact Lenses. 6e. Elsevier; 2019: Figure 5.15. 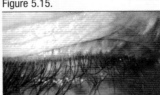 | Lubrication (if cornea is protected by the Bell reflex) or surgery |

**SELECTED INTRAOCULAR CHANGES**

| | | | | |
|---|---|---|---|---|
| Crystalline lens continues to grow with advancing age | Crowding of the anterior chamber angle with predisposition to glaucoma because of the shape of iris insertion into the sclera | Angle closure glaucoma (especially in the farsighted patient with shallow anterior chamber) | Sachsenweger, R. *Illustrated Handbook of Ophthalmology*. Elsevier; 2014: Figure 101. https://play.google.com/books/reader? id = hC7IAgAAQBAJ&printsec = frontcover&pg = GBS. PA67.w.7.1.15.0.2 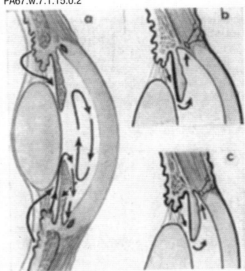 (a) Aqueous drainage with convection current in anterior chamber; (b) open anterior chamber angle; (c) narrow anterior chamber angle | Laser, medication, surgery |
| Slowed filtration of aqueous fluid through the trabecular meshwork | Progressive increase in intraocular pressure | Open angle glaucoma | Sachsenweger, R. *Illustrated Handbook of Ophthalmology*. Elsevier; 2014: Figures 110b, 110c. 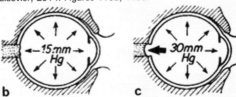 Glaucomatous cupping: effect of increased pressure | See glaucoma section, medication, lasers, surgery |

*(Continued)*

| TABLE 26.2 | Pathologic Anatomic Eye Changes That Commonly Occur With Aging—cont'd | | | |
|---|---|---|---|---|
| Vitreous humor develops pockets of liquefied vitreous in the previously homogeneous gel | Vitreous collapses inward and falls away from its attachments to the retina and optic disc | Posterior vitreous detachment (PVD) can cause retinal traction, tears, and detachment | Sachsenweger, R. *Illustrated Handbook of Ophthalmology.* Elsevier; 2014: Figure 120c. 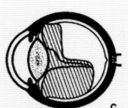 Posterior vitreous detachment causing retinal detachment. | Reassurance, laser if retinal holes found on examination |

❖ **People age ≥ 65 years without risk factors need a complete eye examination every 1 to 2 years.**

## Management

According the 2019 American Academy of Ophthalmology Preferred Practice Pattern for AMD, "Antioxidant vitamin and mineral supplementation as per the Age-Related Eye Disease Study (AREDS2) should be considered in patients with intermediate or advanced AMD."[14] The AREDS2 vitamins contain vitamins C and E, lutein, zeaxanthin, zinc oxide, and cupric oxide. There is no evidence supporting use of supplements for patients with less than intermediate AMD and no evidence of value for family members without signs of AMD[14] (Level of evidence [LOE] = A).

First-line treatment for wet AMD is intravitreal injection with anti-VEGF agents (aflibercept, bevacizumab, and ranibizumab) (LOE = A).[14,15] Adherence to monthly injections is difficult. In 2019 brolukizamab received approval; it requires fewer injections and has equal outcomes.[16]

**CASE 2**

**Discussion**

You have Mr. Jones see ophthalmology. He is at risk for AMD because of age, family history, and smoking and also for cataracts and DR. You advise him to stop smoking.

## Cataracts

### Prevalence and Impact[1]

Cataracts affect nearly 22 million Americans age ≥ 40 years, and all people age ≥ 70 years have some degree of cataract. Cataracts are only clinically relevant if they impact activities of daily living (ADLs). It is the primary cause of reduced vision in the United States, not correctable with glasses. Cataracts reduce illumination and contrast sensitivity, increase glare, and degrade color vision. These changes impact the patient's ability to perform ADLs and instrumental ADLs and decrease quality of life. Among Medicare beneficiaries, cataracts are the most common reason for eye examinations, and at 1.35 million/year, cataract surgery is the most frequently performed surgery costing $3.5 billion/year.

| TABLE 26.3 | Common Causes of Red Eye That Can Be Treated by the Primary Care Practitioner | |
|---|---|---|
| **Condition** | **Signs and Symptoms** | **Treatment** |
| Blepharitis and other dry eye syndromes | Red eye, no red flags, flaky deposits on eyelashes, worse on waking up | Warm compresses (tap water on clean washcloth) for 3–5 min BID. Eyelid margin scrubs (2 drops baby shampoo in 2 ounces of water) BID if eyelids seem oily. Lubricating drops BID or TID preferably preservative free |
| Subconjunctival hemorrhage | Very localized redness, completely asymptomatic | No treatment necessary. Monitor for any changes or worsening. |
| Stye and chalazion | Lump in eyelid Painful, red, and indurated (stye), painless, freely mobile, solid (chalazion) | Stye—Warm compresses or oral antibiotics, watch for signs of preseptal or orbital cellulitis (severe pain, worsening swelling, conjunctival congestion, any change in vision or pupil examination and pain on eye movements), which necessitates emergency room referral. Chalazion—Warm compresses to the affected eyelid BID to QID. If no improvement after 4–8 weeks, refer to ophthalmologist |
| Conjunctivitis | Conjunctival congestion, discharge, foreign body sensation, no red flags | Send swab of discharge. Very difficult to determine viral vs. bacterial conjunctivitis—topical antibiotics if bacterial. Supportive treatment includes cool compresses and artificial tears prn. Hand hygiene and avoid touching eyes or sharing towels, avoid communal activities, as long as discharge is present |
| Allergic conjunctivitis | Conjunctival congestion, discharge, foreign body sensation, no red flags | Lasts for longer than a week, challenging to distinguish from infectious conjunctivitis without a slit lamp examination. Supportive treatment includes cool compresses and artificial tears, topical antihistamines (includes ketotifen BID or olopatadine daily). Ophthalmology referral if no improvement |

(From Allen RC, Harper RA, eds. *Basic Ophthalmology: Essentials for Medical Students*. 10th ed. San Francisco, CA: American Academy of Ophthalmology; 2016; Jacobs D, ed. *Overview of the Red Eye*. Waltham, MA: UpToDate; 2019. Post TW, ed. UpToDate. Accessed September 30, 2019.)
*BID*, Twice a day; *QID*, four times a day; *TID*, three times a day.

## Risk Factors and Pathophysiology[17]

Risk factors for cataract include age, eye trauma, inflammation, metabolic or nutritional defects, smoking, alcohol consumption, ultraviolet radiation, and steroid use.

## Differential Diagnosis and Assessment

Cataracts are diagnosed with a slit lamp biomicroscope through a dilated pupil. Patients may describe blurring and reduced vision, or "second sight" when cataracts create a denser nucleus and patients no longer need glasses. Patients may also describe starbursts around lights, difficulty with night driving, and yellowed or brownish hue discoloration.

## Management

The treatment of cataracts is surgical. Extracapsular cataract extraction with posterior chamber intraocular lens implantation is standard. No medications prevent or abolish cataracts. The criterion for surgery is functional visual impairment and not a specific VA or maturity.[1] According to Shekhawat et al., "second eye cataract surgery improves visual function and quality of life well beyond levels achieved after first eye cataract surgery alone."[18] Visually impairing cataracts are associated with falls and first-eye cataract surgery appears to reduce falls.[19] Depth perception is affected with changes in the power of eye glasses after the surgery and falls may increase.[19] Special attention should be paid to patients until they adapt to the new refraction.[19] Cataract surgery is associated with improved cognition and reduced visual hallucinations.[20,21]

## Glaucoma

### Prevalence and Impact

Primary open angle glaucoma (POAG) is the second most common cause of legal blindness in the United States and the leading cause in Black persons.[22] POAG destroys peripheral vision first and central vision in late stages. Limited field of view makes mobility and driving difficult and increases fall risk. Glaucoma is also associated with depression and decreased quality of life.[23]

### Risk Factors and Pathophysiology[24]

Open angle glaucoma (open anterior chamber) causes progressive and asymptomatic optic neuropathy and visual field loss. Despite the open anterior chamber, there is reduced aqueous outflow.[22] Intraocular pressure (IOP) increases damaging optic nerve fibers. The most important risk factor for glaucoma is high IOP. Other risk factors include age, enlarged optic nerve cup, sub-Saharan African ethnicity, family history, high myopia, and male sex. Older age, hyperopia (far sightedness), female sex, and East Asian ethnic origin are risk factors for angle closure glaucoma. IOP is relative, some patients have low-pressure glaucoma and optic nerve damage at pressures < 21 mmHg, and others have ocular hypertension with no nerve damage at pressures > 21 mmHg. Low socioeconomic status is a risk for late detection of glaucoma and for progression because of healthcare access and therapy adherence issues.

## Differential Diagnosis and Assessment[24]

Half of patients with glaucoma are undiagnosed. Because damage to the optic nerve fibers can occur at normal IOP, these measurements have low sensitivity. The most reliable and sensitive method for detection is direct visualization of the optic nerve head and retinal nerve fiber layer. IOP measurement is vital for monitoring treatment and progression of disease. Visual field tests are most sensitive in later stage disease as a diagnostic and tracking tool.[22]

## Management[24]

Treatment for POAG is reduction of IOP with topical medications, but laser trabeculoplasty and surgery are increasing in use. Patients and caregivers using eye drops should know to gently occlude the lower lacrimal duct or to close the eyes after instilling the drops to reduce systemic absorption. Table 26.4 (available online) lists therapies.

Management of acute angle closure glaucoma is urgent. First-line therapy is lowering IOP using topical medications followed by immediate or urgent laser iridotomy.

## Diabetic Retinopathy

### Prevalence and Impact

Up to one-third of people with DM have retinopathy and one-third of those have vision threatening disease. It is the most common cause of preventable blindness in working aged adults and is associated with increased risk for the macrovascular complications of DM, such as heart attack and stroke.

## Risk Factors and Pathophysiology

Pathophysiology includes inflammation and oxidative stress. Risk factors for development and progression of DR are uncontrolled hyperglycemia, duration of hyperglycemia, hypertension, ethnicity (Black, Hispanic, South Asian), dyslipidemia, and cataract surgery.[25] DR has two stages. Nonproliferative DR is the early stage and is often asymptomatic. The more severe stage, proliferative DR, is characterized by neovascularization of the retina that can lead to vitreous hemorrhage or tractional retinal detachment. The primary cause of moderate vision loss in patients with DR is macular edema that occurs at any stage of DR. Symptoms include visual distortion and decreased VA.[26]

## Differential Diagnosis and Assessment

Patients with DM should be screened regularly by an eye specialist. Diagnosis of diabetic eye disease is made using slit lamp biomicroscopy and indirect ophthalmoscopy.

## Management

Treatment is management of the microvascular complications using anti-VEGF intravitreal therapy and laser treatment for diabetic macular edema and proliferative retinopathy. Other treatments include intravitreal antiinflammatories, steroids, interleukin-6 inhibitors, and integrilin.

### TABLE 26.4 Glaucoma Therapies

| Topical Drug | Examples | Mechanism of Action | Side Effects |
|---|---|---|---|
| Prostaglandin analogues (first line) | Latanoprost, bimatoprost, travoprost | ↑ Uveoscleral outflow | Eyelash lengthening<br>Loss of orbital fat<br>Iris darkening<br>Periocular skin pigmentation<br>Ocular allergy<br>No systemic side effects |
| β-adrenergic blockers (second line) | Timolol, betaxolol | ↓ Aqueous humor production | Bradycardia<br>Arrhythmias<br>Decreased blood pressure<br>Decreased libido<br>Bronchial spasm<br>Ocular allergy |
| Carbonic anhydrase inhibitors | Dorzolamide, brinzolamide | ↓ Aqueous humor production | Ocular allergy |
| α-adrenergic agonists | Brimonidine, apraclonidine | ↓ Aqueous humor production and ↑ uveoscleral outflow | Ocular allergy |
| Miotics | Pilocarpine | ↑ Transtrabecular outflow | Brow ache, limitation of vision especially with cataracts<br>Ocular allergy<br>Involuntary pupillary restriction but no major systemic side effects |
| ρ-kinase inhibitor | Netardusil | ↑ Transtrabecular outflow, possibly | Ocular allergy, corneal deposits |

(From Jonas JB, Aung T, Bourne RR, Bron AM, Ritch R, Panda-Jonas S. Glaucoma. *Lancet.* 2017;390(10108):2183–2193.)

| TABLE 26.5 | Visual Acuities Required for Common Daily Tasks |
| --- | --- |
| 20/20 | Physiologic vision |
| 20/30–20/100 | Driver's license, varies by state |
| 20/50 | Newspaper print |
| 20/70 | Large-print *Reader's Digest* |
| 20/100 | Check writing |
| 20/200 | Legal blindness |
| 20/400 | Paper currency |

(From Cioffi GA, Liebmann JM. Diseases of the visual system. In: Goldman L, Schafer AI. *Goldman-Cecil Medicine*. 26th ed. Philadelphia, PA: Elsevier; 2019 [table 395.1].)

## Low Vision

Consider patients with corrected VA < 20/40, contrast sensitivity loss, scotoma, or visual field loss for low vision rehabilitation.[27] Resources include low vision centers, state-based services for the visually impaired, online training, low vision websites, and support groups. These provide information on and access to adaptive equipment (magnifiers, electronic readers) and home modification. Table 26.5 (available online) shows functional loss at different visual acuities.

## Nursing Home, Homecare, and Hospice Eye and Vision Care

People in nursing homes have a higher prevalence of vision loss than their community peers, often because of refractive error or cataract. Poor vision is associated with reduced ADLs, falls, and mood and behavior changes. Visual loss causing functional decline is often missed. Treating refractive error leads to improved quality of life and depression scores.[13,28,29] Screening for vision loss should be done at admission, annually, and as needed (LOE = A).[30]

When patients have advanced dementia or are at the end of life, consider the burden of glaucoma drops or intraocular injections; burdens may outweigh benefits. Patients with dementia may have distress and agitation when eye drops are instilled. In this situation, discussing risks versus benefits of the drops is appropriate. Also consider corneal donation at end of life.[31] Phone management of acute vision change is facilitated by nurse training tools from paltc.org to determine if patients can be managed at the facility or need emergent transfer.

**At the end of life, discuss benefits and burden of glaucoma drops.**

## Summary

A principle of geriatric care is to identify functional impairment and maximize residual function. Vision care for the older adult population is no exception. VA is different than visual function. Older adults with good acuity may have degradation in visual function from environmental factors. Office performance should be correlated with how the patient functions at home. Identifying and treating refractive errors, AMD, cataracts, glaucoma, and DR improves function and quality of life. When vision cannot be corrected to 20/40 after disease treatment, use optical and nonoptical ways to enhance visual function.

Great website with videos of eye examination examples: www.aao.org/basicvideo
Lighthouse International: www.lighthouse.org.
The American Academy of Ophthalmology: www.aao.org
Vision Aware: for independent living with vision loss: https://www.visionaware.org/
Online interactive tool to experience the effects of eye diseases: https://simulator.seenow.org/

### Web Resources

The Eyes Have It. Great website with many pictures of eye diseases: http://kellogg.umich.edu/theeyeshaveit/

## Key References

1. Allen RC, Harper RA, eds. *Basic Ophthalmology: Essentials for Medical Students*. 10th ed. San Francisco, CA: American Academy of Ophthalmology; 2016.
4. Gayton JL. Etiology, prevalence, and treatment of dry eye disease. *Clin Ophthalmol*. 2009;3:405–412.
8. Pelletier AL, Rojas-Roldan L, Coffin J. Vision loss in older adults. *Am Fam Physician*. 2016;94(3):219–226.
24. Jonas JB, Aung T, Bourne RR, Bron AM, Ritch R, Panda-Jonas S. Glaucoma. *Lancet*. 2017;390(10108):2183–2193.
25. Cheung N, Mitchell P, Wong TY. Diabetic retinopathy. *Lancet*. 2010;376(9735):124–136.

**References available online at** expertconsult.com.

# 27

# Persistent Pain

ELLEN FLAHERTY AND MICHAELA PREISS

## OBJECTIVES

*Upon completion of this chapter, the reader will be able to:*

- Define persistent pain and discuss its impact on older adults.
- Discuss the pathophysiology of persistent pain.
- Describe age-related changes that influence the presentation and treatment of persistent pain.
- Take an accurate pain history and use assessment tools to quantitate and monitor pain syndromes.

- Choose appropriate pharmacologic treatments to manage persistent pain, including opioids.
- Apply nonpharmacologic approaches to the treatment of pain.

## Prevalence and Impact

Pain, although nearly universally experienced, is poorly understood. Pain is complicated, and its perception can be affected by a multitude of factors, including culture and past experience. Acute pain, prompted by an event like injury or illness, is generally simpler to manage and relief can often be achieved once the cause of the pain is treated. Acute pain also often presents with tachycardia, diaphoresis, and elevated blood pressure.

In contrast, ongoing or persistent pain cannot usually be linked to a specific event. This is common among older adults. There are misconceptions that this type of pain has no clear pathologic basis[1] and terms like "chronic pain" have negative associations—because of this, "persistent pain" is now the preferred terminology.

Persistent pain is commonly encountered in a geriatric practice and pain remains undertreated in nursing homes especially in certain subpopulations, including cognitively impaired and older

residents.[2] It is estimated that 25% to 50% of the older adult population may have persistent pain.[3] Some 65% of nursing home residents report having inadequately treated pain.[1] However, a recent study[4] looked at the long-term persistence of musculoskeletal pain. Over a 6-year period, approximately 20% had no musculoskeletal pain, one-third had persistent pain, one-third had intermittent pain, and one-sixth had pain in each of the 6 years. However, half of those with pain during 1 of the years had no pain during any of the other 5 years. This could imply that pain, although common, may be a more dynamic symptom than previously thought.

Persistent pain has a significant negative impact on patient's lives (Box 27.1). Sleep disturbances, feelings of loneliness, depression, and social isolation are all more common in those with persistent pain. There is a reduced ability to carry out the patient's social roles in their family or place of work. In addition, persistent pain often limits physical activity, worsening patients' physical conditioning and increasing their risk of cognitive difficulties and related

## • BOX 27.1 Impact of Persistent Pain

- Sleep disturbance
- Worsening physical conditioning
- Loneliness
- Loss of productivity
- Financial loss
- Loss of social support
- Potential of drug abuse/misuse

functional consequences.[5] A 2015 study showed persistent pain is also associated with poorer self-rated health and mobility, arthrosis, and rheumatoid arthritis when compared with persons without persistent pain. However, the study found only 15% of the persons with persistent pain were using any analgesics on a regular basis and one of every five was not taking any analgesics.[6]

In the United States, the annual cost of pain is estimated to be between $560 and $635 billion, not including costs associated with lost tax revenue or productivity. Medicare covers about $65.3 billion of this total, which equates to 14% of their budget. Concurrently, costs associated with disability top $300 billion per year. Persistent pain caused by arthritis and back/spine pain are cited as the top two causes of disability.[7]

❖❖ **Some 14% of the Medicare budget is consumed by pain treatment.**

## Pathophysiology

It is sometimes helpful from a clinical standpoint to classify persistent pain in pathophysiologic terms.[3] Nociceptive pain comes about from stimulation of peripheral pain receptors and may be from tissue or joint inflammation or degeneration, continuing injury, or skin or internal organ noxious stimulation. Inflammatory or degenerative arthritis, myofascial pain syndromes, or ischemia are examples of such pain. Pain with this etiology responds to usual analgesic medications and nonpharmacologic strategies. Neuropathic pain results from abnormal nerve stimulation, which involves peripheral or cranial nerves. Examples include diabetic or idiopathic peripheral neuropathy, trigeminal neuralgia, or phantom pain. Pain of this etiology is often more difficult to treat and may not respond completely to any treatment. Medications used include certain antidepressants or anticonvulsants. Another category is pain of mixed or uncertain etiology. Examples include recurrent headaches, vasculitis, somatization, or conversion reactions. Treatment of this category is difficult and should be individualized for each patient.

There is a difference in pain perception and tolerance when comparing the older adults with younger people. Myelinated and unmyelinated nerve fibers are decreased in density in older adults with prolonged latencies noted in peripheral sensory nerves. This slows transduction and transmission of the pain signals.[8] There is a lower density of descending pain inhibiting nerve fibers in the older adult population. In addition, there is a slower recovery from hyperalgesic states,[9] and once pain is established these changes may make it more likely that persistent pain develops after a noxious insult.

Most studies indicate that there is an increase in pain threshold with aging.[3] There is also an age-related decrease in the willingness to endure strong pain. From a clinical standpoint, such changes may be evident in the different pain presentations that the older adults have with either an acute myocardial infarction or a ruptured appendix.

❖❖ Neuropathic pain refers to pain originating from abnormal peripheral or cranial nerve stimulation. Nociceptive pain refers to pain originating from stimulation of peripheral pain receptors.

## CASE 1
### Cecelia Anderson (Part 1)

Cecelia Anderson is a 79-year-old who comes to your office with increasingly severe low back pain. She has had low back pain for at least 5 years, which has intermittently interfered with her ability to do housework and leave her house. However, the pain worsened after she stepped down hard off a curb 1 week ago. There has been no radiation of pain to buttocks or legs over the years.
1. What is the pathophysiology of her pain?
2. How does the etiology of the pain influence therapy?
3. What do you expect to find on examination?

## CASE 2
### James Walker (Part 1)

James Walker is a 76-year-old who had an episode of shingles 4 months ago involving the right T7 dermatome. The rash cleared rapidly but severe pain persisted in the prior area of rash. He got only minimal relief with acetaminophen or ibuprofen. You had previously given him hydrocodone, which gave slightly more pain relief.
1. What is the pathophysiology of his pain?
2. How does the etiology of the pain influence therapy?
3. What do you expect to find on examination?

## Pain Assessment

Accurate assessment of pain is necessary to successfully manage the patient. This typically can include taking medical and pain histories, a physical examination with special attention to the painful areas, and using appropriate pain scales. Patients should routinely be evaluated for persistent pain (Level of Evidence [LOE] = B).

When taking a pain history, it is important that the clinician convey to the patient that the pain complaint is acknowledged and believed. It is also important that the patient know that pain is not a normal part of aging and should not hesitate to discuss and describe the pain. The patient should be asked about a timeline of the pain, acerbating and alleviating factors, and previous treatments. Descriptors of pain, such as sharp, burning, aching, radiating, or tightness should be sought (LOE = D). Pain that awakens the patient from sleep may be particularly worrisome. How the pain affects the patient's everyday life should be assessed. The physical examination should pay particular attention to the painful areas and how function of those areas is affected (LOE = D). Areas of tenderness, inflammation, or tenderness should be sought. Weakness or limitation of motion, numbness, paresthesia, or change in reflexes is important. Simply observing the patient's gait can give information as to how the pain influences the patient's activities of daily living. The "get up and go" test can help quantify the patient's disability from the pain.

❖❖ **The patient must realize that the complaint of pain is taken seriously.**

## CASE 1

### Cecelia Anderson (Part 2)

On physical examination, Mrs. Anderson ambulates slowly with obvious pain. She has diffuse tenderness and spasm throughout the lumbar spine. There is more pronounced tenderness over the L3 spinous process. Her sensation and muscle strength of her lower extremities are normal. Her deep tendon reflexes are also normal. You suspect that Mrs. Anderson has a lumbar compression fracture superimposed on degenerative disc disease and osteoarthritis involving the lumbar spine. This would be considered to be nociceptive pain with no evidence of significant neuropathic involvement. The severity of her pain should be evaluated. Most likely she will require opioid therapy for her acute fracture. Once the acute pain has improved, her persistent, ongoing low back pain will need further evaluation.
1. What further imaging or testing would you now recommend?
2. What other conditions relevant to each patient should be addressed?

## CASE 2

### James Walker (Part 2)

On physical examination, Mr. Walker appears to be in pain and somewhat depressed. He has hyperalgesia involving the right T7 dermatome. There is no spine tenderness and his range of motion of the spine is normal. On further discussion with him, he admits that the constant nature of the pain has made him irritable and depressed.
1. What further imaging or testing would you now recommend?
2. What other conditions relevant to each patient should be addressed?

## Pain Quantitation

There are many tools to assess pain in the older adult population, both cognitively intact and cognitively impaired.[10] The most reliable way to evaluate the severity of pain of a cognitively intact patient is simply to ask the patient to estimate the pain.[3] For those with mild to moderate dementia, reliable pain scales are available for use (Fig. 27.1). Patients with advanced dementia are more difficult to evaluate, but clues from the patient's behavior or actions may be helpful.[11,12] Grimacing, grunting, or constant movement may be clues to uncontrolled pain. The mental status of the patient often deteriorates with persistent pain.

As the pain intensity should be measured serially, keeping a pain log is useful. This should include the pain intensity, how activity affects the pain, results of medication or nonpharmacologic treatments, and how pain is affecting daily life. Also, with each office visit, the pain should be quantified and changes noted (LOE = D) (see Fig. 27.1).

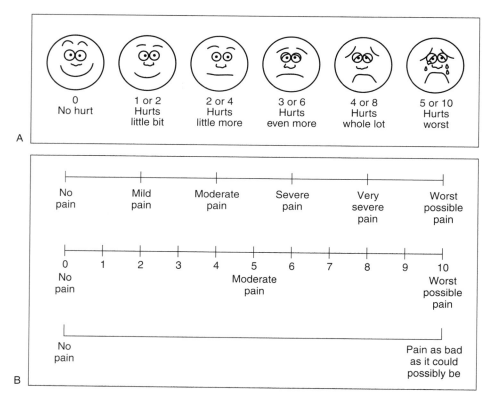

• **Figure 27.1** Pain intensity scales used in older patients. A, Faces scale. Ask the patient to "put an X by the face that best matches the severity of your pain right now." (From Hockenberry MJ, Wilson D, Rodgers CC: Wong's essentials of pediatric nursing, ed 10, St. Louis, 2017, Elsevier.) B, Visual analog scales. Ask the patient to "circle the number that best represents the intensity or severity of your pain right now." (Modified from Carr DB, Jacox AK, Cahpman CR, et al. Acute pain management: operative or medical procedures and trauma: clinical practice guideline. AHCPR publication 92-0032. Rockville, MD: US Public Health Service, Agency for Health Care Policy and Research, February 1992 and Jacox A, Carr DB, Payne R, et al. Management of Cancer Pain. Clinical Practice Guideline No. 9. AHCPR Publication No. 94-0592. Rockville, MD. Agency for Health Care Policy and Research, U.S. Department of Health and Human Services, Public Health Service, March 1994. With permission.)

## CASE 1

### Cecelia Anderson (Part 3)

A plain film of Mrs. Anderson's lumbar spine shows a moderate compression fracture of L3. Associated with this are facet arthritis and spurring of the lumbar vertebral bodies. As she rates her pain before her fracture on most days 6 out of 10 and currently an 8 out of 10, you recommend hydrocodone therapy. As she had a compression fracture without major trauma, a dual-energy x-ray absorptiometry (DEXA) scan was done, which revealed a T score of −2.9 over her lumbar spine. For further evaluation, a vitamin D level revealed a level of 20. Calcium, vitamin D, and bisphosphonates were recommended to prevent further fractures and pain. To address her ongoing back pain, physical therapy would be helpful after the acute pain of the fracture has improved.

1. What follow-up would you recommend?

## CASE 2

### James Walker (Part 3)

By history, Mr. Walker has postherpetic neuralgia and further imaging is not indicated. However, because of a self-reported possible depression, a Geriatric Depression Scale was administered. This showed a score of 8 out of 15 (>5 suggests depression). You discuss with him the possibility of using gabapentin for his neuralgia. Rather than using an oral medication, he asks about using lidocaine patches, which you prescribe. You also recommend discussing his depression with a counselor. He also agrees to try a selective serotonin reuptake inhibitor (SSRI) antidepressant. You had discussed with him the possibility of using duloxetine for both depression and possibly helping with the neuralgia, but the cost of the medication was prohibitive.

1. What follow-up would you recommend?

## Pharmacologic Treatment

Nearly all patients with persistent pain will require pharmacologic therapy, either constantly or intermittently. As with the treatment of any geriatric patient, the adage of starting low and slowly titrating upward on the dose applies. The drug that seems most effective and has the fewest side effects for the patient should be used, keeping in mind all the other comorbidities the patient may have. Also the type of pain the patient may have, either nociceptive or neuropathic, will dictate the type of medication used.

## Nonsteroidal Antiinflammatory Drugs

Nonsteroidal antiinflammatory drugs (NSAIDs) are a broad class of drugs (Table 27.1). Their main mechanism is to inhibit cyclooxygenase, which alters the transformation of arachidonic acid into prostaglandins, prostacyclins, and thromboxanes.

The primary use of NSAIDs is for inflammatory pain. They are more effective than acetaminophen for inflammatory pain, such as rheumatoid arthritis and are relatively effective in the short-term treatment of osteoarthritis and low back pain.[13–16]

NSAIDs are associated with gastrointestinal (GI), renal, and cardiovascular toxicity in older adults, even more than in younger patients.[17] GI toxicity is less in nonacetylated NSAIDs, such as salsalate when compared with aspirin, but the likelihood of GI toxicity is never zero.[18–20]

Renal toxicity and hyperkalemia may be significant side effects of NSAIDs. This is more often seen in the older adult population, those with congestive heart failure, hypertension, dehydration, preexisting mild renal dysfunction, and patients taking angiotensin-converting enzyme inhibitors or diuretics. Fluid retention is also seen and may be severe enough to worsen congestive heart failure. If some of these clinical signs are noted in the absence of prescription NSAID use, the patient should be queried about the use of over-the-counter NSAID use. With the numerous potential side

## TABLE 27.1 Information on Commonly Used Nonsteroidal Antiinflammatory Drugs

| Drug | Route | Aging Effect | Precautions and Recommendations | Cost |
|---|---|---|---|---|
| Aspirin | PO, PR | GFR decreases, which results in decreased excretion | Evaluate risks and benefits<br>Mostly used for cardiovascular protection | Generic |
| Ibuprofen | PO | Severity of GI toxicity increases with age and frequency | Treat acute or chronic inflammatory pain | Generic |
| Salsalate | PO | GI toxicity | GI toxicity lower than ASA | Generic |
| Naproxen | PO | COX-2 inhibitor, less GI toxicity; increases bleeding time | Moderate to severe inflammatory pain<br>Low risk of cardiovascular events | Generic |
| Diclofenac | PO | | Because of COX-2 selectivity has increased cardiovascular risk | Generic |
| Indomethacin | PO | More GI and central nervous system side effects | Not first-line drug for mild to moderate pain | Generic |
| Ketorolac | IM, PO | High GI toxicity and renal toxicity | Not recommended for long-term use | Generic |
| Nabumetone | PO | GI toxicity | Long half-life, low antiplatelet activity | 750 mg 60 tabs $68.99 |
| Celecoxib | PO | Selective COX-2 inhibitor | Fewer GI side effects | Generic |

*ASA*, Acetylsalicylic acid (aspirin); *COX-2*, cyclooxygenase 2; *GFR*, glomerular filtration rate; *GI*, gastrointestinal; *IM*, intramuscular; *PO*, by mouth; *PR*, per rectum.

effects of NSAIDs, they should be used rarely and with caution for long-term use (LOE = B).

## Acetaminophen

Acetaminophen is considered to be the initial drug of choice for management of mild to moderate persistent pain (LOE = A). Although it is an effective, safe medication for musculoskeletal pain, such as osteoarthritis and low back pain,[21,22] it is not as effective for chronic inflammatory conditions, such as rheumatoid arthritis.[23] It is not associated with significant GI bleeding, adverse renal effects, or cardiac toxicity. The suggested maximum daily dosing is 3 g/24 h but should be used with caution in those with significant renal or hepatic disease and in those with alcohol abuse. Side effects are minimal and may include transient elevation of alanine transferase, which does not translate into liver failure or dysfunction when maximum recommended dose is avoided. Chronic high-dose usage for many years may cause renal toxicity, but it is rare. When patients are prescribed drugs that combine acetaminophen, such as those with codeine, it is important to monitor the total daily amount of acetaminophen the patient is taking.

## Topical Agents

Topical agents may be useful for management of neuropathic pain or localized osteoarthritic pain. They are generally well tolerated with few significant systemic side effects. Care should be taken to apply them only to intact skin.

The 5% lidocaine patch is most useful for neuropathic pain, especially postherpetic neuropathy or diabetic neuropathy (LOE = B). There is little controlled data for other types of pain. Up to three patches should be applied to the painful area for up to 12 hours daily. Capsaicin cream may be used for neuropathic or nonneuropathic pain (LOE = B). It is an inhibitor of substance P, which is a mediator of inflammation. Patients should be warned that they may notice a burning sensation at the site of application, which may take several weeks of use to dissipate. Topical NSAIDs

(diclofenac and salicylate) are useful for localized nonneuropathic pain, particularly osteoarthritis. It is safe and effective, especially when used short term.[24,25] There is some systemic absorption so renal function should still be monitored (Tables 27.1 and 27.2).

## Opioids

Clinicians should carefully monitor and document opioid usage in older adults for drug-to-drug interactions, impact on cognition, and aberrant usage patterns.

Beyond individual factors, the current national concerns about opioid-related deaths have greatly influenced the terrain of pain management. Opioids (including prescription opioids, heroin, and fentanyl) resulted in more than 42,000 fatalities in 2016, more than any year on record. Of all opioid overdose deaths, 40% involve a prescription opioid.[36]

Continuous pain, especially cancer pain, should generally be treated with medications in long-acting or sustained-release formulations after total opioid requirements have been estimated by an initial trial of a short-acting agent. Fast-onset medications with short half-lives may be added to the long-acting regimen to cover episodes of breakthrough pain. Typically, a patient is offered approximately 5% to 15% of the total daily dose every 2 to 4 hours orally for breakthrough pain. In general, different opioids provide similar analgesic efficacy. Cost and route of delivery can help guide the choice of medication.

Long-term use of opioid analgesics often increases the risk of adverse events for the older adult population and should be avoided. Central nervous system (CNS) side effects, such as altered mental status, sedation, depression, delirium, and respiratory depression commonly occur, especially soon after initiation of the medication. GI side effects, such as constipation and nausea, are common. Constipation does not improve with continued use as CNS effects often will. It is worthwhile to anticipate this side effect and begin a bowel regimen consisting of physical activity, increased fluids and osmotic, or stimulant laxatives. Bulk building agents are usually ineffective in these cases. Methylnaltrexone injections, a selective peripheral mu-opioid antagonist, is available for severely ill patients with significant opioid induced constipation.

| TABLE 27.2 | Topical Agents | | | | |
|---|---|---|---|---|---|
| **Name** | **Route** | **Aging Effect** | **Precaution** | **Comparison** | **Cost** |
| Acetaminophen | Oral | Transient elevation of alanine aminotransferase | In hepatic insufficiency and alcohol abuse patient | No effects of GI bleeding, adverse renal effects, cardiac toxicity as of NSAIDS<br>Greater safety than NSAIDS so recommended as first-line therapy.[26]<br>NSAIDS better for short-term pain-OA,[27,28] low back pain[29,30] Acetaminophen less effective for chronic inflammatory pain than NSAIDS[26] | OTC, 100 tablets for $17.99 |
| Lidocaine 5% patch | Topical | Nontoxic with safe range of 4 patches in 24 h | Skin irritation | Limited for neuropathic pain Absence of toxicity, no drug interactions Contraindicated in advanced liver disease | Rx, $220.99 for a 30-patch box |
| Topical capsaicin cream | Topical | | Burning sensation of skin | Some benefit in reduction of neuropathic and nonneuropathic pain[31,32] | OTC |
| Topical NSAIDs | Topical | Reported toxicity is low when used in recommended doses.[33] Not fully understood | Check renal and hepatic function periodically | Effective and safe over short term (<4 weeks). Shown some efficacy in few studies of persistent pain management[34,35] | Rx, 30 patches of 1.3% for $189.99 |

*GI*, Gastrointestinal; *IM*, intramuscular; *NSAIDs*, nonsteroidal antiinflammatory drugs; *OA*, osteoarthritis; *OTC*, over the counter.

## TABLE 27.3  Short-Acting Opioids

| Drug | Route Available | Aging Effect | Precautions and Recommendation |
|---|---|---|---|
| Morphine | PO, SL, IV, SQ, PR | Active metabolite accumulation in renal insufficiency<br>More sensitive | Caution with low renal function<br>Anticipate and treat constipation |
| Hydromorphone | PO, SL, IV, SQ, PR | Active metabolite accumulation in renal insufficiency<br>More sensitive | Caution with low renal function<br>Anticipate and treat constipation |
| Oxycodone | PO, SL, PR | Active metabolite accumulation in renal insufficiency<br>More sensitive | Caution with low renal function<br>Anticipate and treat constipation |
| Hydrocodone | PO | | Usually comes with combination with other medication. Caution |
| Fentanyl | PO, SL, intranasal, IV, SQ, PR | Can be twice as sensitive as other age group | Anticipate and treat constipation |
| Codeine | PO | Active metabolite accumulation in renal insufficiency | Monitor for nausea, anorexia<br>Anticipate and treat constipation |
| Tramadol | PO | Active metabolite accumulation in renal insufficiency | Monitor for nausea, dizziness. Use with caution in patients with history of seizure disorders |

*IV,* Intravenous; *PO,* by mouth; *PR,* per rectum; *SL,* sublingual; *SQ,* subcutaneous.

After the patient's pain is stabilized, consideration could be given to the use of the longer acting opioids. These are available as a patch or in timed released oral form. The dose should be titrated depending on both the amount of short-acting pain medication required by the patient for relief and the effectiveness of the long-acting medication.

### Short-Acting Opioids

Commonly used and available short-acting opioids, along with precautions and changes expected in aging, are listed in Table 27.3.

### Long-Acting Opioids

Commonly used and available long-acting opioids, along with precautions and changes expected in aging, are listed in Table 27.4.

## Drug Misuse and Addiction

Prescription opioid misuse and diversion have been a great burden for the primary care provider and healthcare system as a whole. Careful initial assessment for the risk of such behavior is critical and there have been tools, such as the Opioid Risk Tool,[37] to screen high-risk patients. Addiction is the behavior characterized as impaired control over drug use, compulsive use, continued use despite harm, and craving for higher doses of the medication.[38] It is worthwhile for the patient to sign a contract with the clinician promising to not divert opioid medications. If there is any doubt, the patient could undergo periodic urine drug screens to ascertain if opioid metabolites are present.

## Adjunctive Therapy

Many topical agents, antidepressants, and anticonvulsants can be used as adjunctive therapy. Adjunctive therapy is usually used in combination with other analgesic strategies, but can be used to decrease the use of analgesics that may have major side effects. Because of its ability to alter and attenuate the perception of pain, this should be considered for neuropathic pain.

## Anticonvulsants

Anticonvulsant doses should always "start low and go slow"—increasing gradually depending on the patient's tolerance of the drug. Gabapentin

## TABLE 27.4  Long-Acting Opioids

| Drug | Route Available | Aging Effect | Precautions and Recommendation |
|---|---|---|---|
| Sustained release morphine | PO | Active metabolite accumulation in renal insufficiency | Escalate dose slowly because of possible drug accumulation (MS Contin, Kadian)<br>Use immediate-release opioid for breakthrough pain |
| Sustained release oxycodone | PO | Active metabolite accumulation in renal insufficiency | Start at lower dose |
| Hydromorphone extended release | PO | | Use after stabilized dose with short-acting medication |
| Fentanyl patch | Transdermal | Absorption may be variable, especially with thin subcutaneous fat | The lower-dose patch and after stabilized dose with short-acting medication are recommended. |

*PO,* By mouth.

- Tricyclic antidepressants
- Serotonin-norepinephrine reuptake inhibitor antidepressants
- Anticonvulsants
- Corticosteroids
- Muscle relaxants

and pregabalin are the most commonly used anticonvulsants today and can help manage persistent neuropathic pain. Others, like topiramate and lamotrigine, can be useful if other medication options are unsuccessful, but their evidence is limited. Carbamazepine may help treat trigeminal neuralgia, but should be used with caution as it can have bone marrow side effects and more drug-to-drug interactions.

## Antidepressants

Evidence shows tricyclic antidepressants (TCAs) can effectively control pain.[39] However, they should only be used in geriatric patients who cannot tolerate other treatment modalities, as they are associated with a significant risk of anticholinergic and cardiovascular adverse events. Selective norepinephrine reuptake inhibitor antidepressants such as duloxetine or venlafaxin are generally tolerated better than TCAs and can effectively address neuropathic pain. SSRIs can help manage depression but otherwise have limited use when it comes to pain management.

## Other Medications

Intermittent joint injections or trigger point injections with local anesthetics or corticosteroids and epidural steroid injections for refractory back pain (requires referral to pain management specialists) may relieve pain for weeks or more.

Baclofen, a muscle relaxant, can be used to treat muscle spasms that occur after a stroke. Notable side effects include weakness, fatigue, and confusion.

Corticosteroids may successfully work as an adjunctive therapy for some inflammatory conditions (Box 27.2). Notable side effects from chronic use include osteoporosis, glucose intolerance, or cataracts.

## Methadone

Methadone has received more attention for use in the management of persistent pain. However, it has unique pharmacodynamic and pharmacokinetic properties. It has a highly variable half-life with the potential for significant drug accumulation with resultant CNS depression. Use of this drug should be done only in carefully selected patients educated in its use and by clinicians experienced in dealing with its potential side effects.

## Cannabis

Cannabis is increasingly available for the treatment of chronic pain, yet its efficacy remains uncertain. There is low-strength evidence from 27 chronic pain trials that cannabis alleviates neuropathic pain but insufficient evidence in other pain populations.[40]

## Nonpharmacologic Strategies

The nonpharmacologic treatment of pain, either as a standalone treatment or in combination with medicine, is supported by substantial

data. Key to this strategy is patient education (LOE = A), to teach the patient more about the pain and what outcomes can reasonably be expected from nonpharmacologic treatments.

Many of these nonpharmacologic treatments can happen in a patient's home, including stretching, heat and cold therapy, and exercise. Physical or occupational therapists can be extremely helpful in teaching patients how to tailor these treatments to their specific type of pain and adjust their daily activities to work around their pain and conserve energy. Exercise programs can also be beneficial. These regimens can stave off physical deconditioning while encouraging social interaction (LOE = A).

Patients may be inclined to seek out alternative therapies such as acupuncture, homeopathy, or naturopathy. The efficacy of these treatments is generally not backed by controlled studies, but patients may report pain relief after participating. In this case, clinicians should not disparage the treatments but should ensure that they are not harmful and that the patient is not discontinuing other, evidence-based therapies (LOE = D).

Psychological interventions for the treatment of chronic pain in older adults have small benefits, including reducing pain and catastrophizing beliefs and improving pain self-efficacy for managing pain. These results are stronger when delivered using group-based approaches. Research is needed to develop and test strategies that enhance the efficacy of psychological approaches and sustainability of treatment effects among older adults with persistent pain.[41]

### CASE 1

#### Discussion

When seen 3 weeks later, Mrs. Anderson states her acute pain has improved to a level of 6 of 10. You recommend trying to decrease the use of hydrocodone and to start using acetaminophen on a regular basis up to 4 g daily. Physical therapy and regular exercise was recommended for her ongoing lumbar spine pain. In 2 years, you recommend repeating the DEXA scan for evaluation of her osteoporosis.

Mrs. Anderson is an example of a patient with persistent pain who has an acute injury complicating her pain. Once the acute pain has improved, the persistent pain still needs to be dealt with. This can be done with a combination of modalities. Medications from different classes of pain medications, physical and/or occupational therapy, antidepressants, counseling, or various treatments from complementary and alternative medicine may be used solely or in combination. For nociceptive pain, exercise and muscle strengthening can be very helpful once acute pain or pain exacerbations have improved.

### CASE 2

#### Discussion

When seen 3 weeks later, Mr. Walker reports some relief of his neuropathic pain, but still rates it at a 6. He agrees to try gabapentin. When seen again 3 weeks later his pain is down to a 4 and he agrees to continue the gabapentin and titrate the dose according to his pain level. In addition, talking with the counselor has helped him to better deal with his pain. He feels his mood has elevated with the use of the antidepressant.

Mr. Walker is an example of a patient with persistent pain because of his neuropathic pain. Although opioids, NSAIDs, or acetaminophen may occasionally be helpful, other classes of medications, such as anticonvulsants or antidepressants, may be more beneficial. Also, as patients with neuropathic pain often do not get complete pain relief from medications, nonpharmacologic therapy such as counseling may be helpful.

## Summary

Persistent pain is very common and sometimes challenging because of multiple complex issues related to aging changes and management options. However, persistent pain can be controlled by careful assessment of the etiology of the pain, selection of analgesics, their route of administration, dose and frequency, or other management options with careful monitoring of their effects and side effects. Reassessment for adjusting medication should be frequent enough to minimize the risk of potential side effects with various managements.

The clinician should understand that many aspects of the patient's life, such as interpersonal relationships, emotional health, and enjoyment of life are affected. Nonpharmacologic therapies such as physical and occupational therapy, counseling, complementary and alternative treatments can be used in certain patients. It should be emphasized that exercise is important for both general wellbeing and for strengthening of specific muscle groups related to the painful area.

Optimized use of recommendation from the American Geriatrics Society guidelines for persistent pain, as well as various assessment and screening tools, are also the key for successful pain management and improving the quality of life of patients and their family/caregivers.

## Acknowledgment

The author and editors would like to acknowledge the authors of this chapter from the sixth edition of this book—Jerome J. Epplin, Masaya Higuchi, Nisha Gajendra, and Soumya Nadella. They contributed the majority of the outstanding content.

## Key References

9. Hadjistavropoulos T, Herr K, Turk DC, et al. An interdisciplinary expert consensus statement on assessment of pain in older persons. *Clin J Pain*. 2007;23(1):S1—S43.
10. Herr K, Coyne P, McCaffery M, Manworren R, Merkel S. Pain assessment in the patient unable to self-report: position statement with clinical practice recommendations. *Pain Manag Nurs*. 2011;12(4):230—250.
14. Towheed TE, Maxwell L, Judd MG, et al. Acetaminophen for osteoarthritis. *Cochrane Database Syst Rev*. 2006; CD004257.
21. Chou R, Huffman LH. Medications for acute and chronic low back pain: a review of the evidence for an American Pain Society/American College of Physicians clinical practice guideline. *Ann Intern Med*. 2007;147:505—514.
41. Niknejad B, Bolier R, Henderson Jr CR, et al. Association between psychological interventions and chronic pain outcomes in older adults: a systematic review and meta-analysis. *JAMA Intern Med*. 2018;178(6):830—839.

**References available online at** expertconsult.com.

# 28

# Malnutrition and Feeding Problems

ROSE ANN DIMARIA-GHALILI AND MARTHA C. COATES

## OUTLINE

*Additional online-only material indicated by icon.*

## OBJECTIVES

*Upon completion of this chapter, the reader will be able to:*

- Understand the prevalence and impact of malnutrition (undernutrition) and feeding problems in older adults.
- Identify the risk factors for poor nutritional status in older adults.
- Describe the pathophysiology of malnutrition and feeding problems in older adults.

- List the differential diagnosis for malnutrition and feeding problems in older adults.
- Identify screening tools, approaches to assessment, and interdisciplinary management options to address malnutrition and feeding problems in older adults.

---

### CASE

#### Mr. Clarke (Part 1)

Mr. Clarke is an 87-year-old man who lives alone in an apartment. He has a past medical history of hypertension, hyperlipidemia, and macular degeneration (MD). He is fairly independent and ambulates without an assistive device. He recently stopped driving because of his MD.
1. What aspects of Mr. Clarke's life put him at risk for malnutrition?
2. Is malnutrition in the ambulatory setting common?

---

## Prevalence and Impact

Malnutrition generally refers to any nutrient imbalance, and older adults "who lack adequate calories, protein, or other nutrients needed for tissue maintenance and repair experience undernutrition."[1] This discussion on malnutrition in older adults focuses on undernutrition. Prevalence rates vary because of the different criteria used to characterize malnutrition across studies. The most recent malnutrition national estimates for hospitalized malnutrition are from the 2016 Healthcare Costs and Utilization Projects National Inpatient Sample.[2] Malnutrition was identified using the International Classification of Diseases, 10th Revision, clinical modification diagnosis codes for postsurgical nonabsorption, nutritional neglect, cachexia, protein-calorie malnutrition, weight loss or failure to thrive, and underweight.[2] Malnutrition was identified in 8% (or 2.2 million) of the 27.6 million total nonmaternal and non-neonatal stays.[2] Malnutrition was highest in older adults with the rates of protein-calorie malnutrition reported at 3754 per 100,000 for those age $\geq 85$ years, and rate of 1487 per 100,000 for those age 65 to 84 years.[2] Prevalence rates in nursing homes are reported between 1.5% and 67%.[3] Much less is known about the rate of malnutrition in community-dwelling older adults in the United States. One study reported 56.3% of community-dwelling older adults at risk for malnutrition and 5.9% were malnourished.[4]

Malnutrition is associated with negative health outcomes. The estimated annual cost attributed to disease-associated malnutrition in older adults in the United States is $51.3 billion.[5] Older adults with malnutrition have increased lengths of hospital stay,[2] more frequent hospital readmissions,[2] increased falls and physical disability, and increased mortality.[6]

◆◆ **The estimated annual cost attributed to disease-associated malnutrition in older adults in the United States is $51.3 billion.**

◆◆ **Older adults with malnutrition have increased lengths of hospital stay,[2] more frequent hospital readmissions,[2] increased falls and physical disability, and increased mortality.[6]**

Although sarcopenia, frailty, and malnutrition are distinct clinical entities, there are notable relationships. Sarcopenia (decreased muscle mass for age, sex, and race) increases with age, and approximately 7% of men and 11% of women over the age of 80 years are reported to have sarcopenia.[7] Older adults with sarcopenia have a decline in physical activity, functionality, and performance.[8] Approximately 25% of people over age 85 years have frailty (age-associated decline in reserve and function across multiple physiological systems[9]) and this clinical entity increases vulnerability to stress and adverse clinical outcomes.[8] Unintentional weight loss is a common characteristic of malnutrition and is associated with a loss of lean mass, which can contribute to sarcopenia and functional decline,[10,11] frailty,[12] hospital readmission,[13] falls,[14] and death.[15,16]

---

**CASE**

### Mr. Clarke (Part 2)

During a routine office visit Mr. Clarke complains of fatigue, poor appetite, poor sleep, and a weight loss of 10 lb over 2 months. He admits to feeling depressed since losing his wife 3 months ago. He also misses the independence of driving. Physical examination shows dry mucous membranes, generalized loss of subcutaneous fat, and decreased handgrip strength bilaterally.

Labs show a prealbumin of 14 mg/dL, albumin of 2.4 g/dL, hemoglobin of 12 g/dL, and a thyroid-stimulating hormone of 5.5 mU/L.
1. What factors are contributing to Mr. Clarke's weight loss?
2. What are your differential diagnoses?
3. What does his physical examination and laboratory work tell you?

---

## Risk Factors and Pathophysiology

Older adults are at risk for malnutrition (undernutrition) across the care continuum because of physiologic, psychological, social, economic, and environmental factors (Fig. 28.1). Often these risk factors contribute to alterations in nutritional requirements or the quality or quantity of food consumed with resultant unintentional weight loss.

## Age-Related Changes

Aging per say does not cause malnutrition, but age-related changes can impact the dietary quality and amount of food consumed, contributing factors to unintentional weight loss.[17] Some 20% of older adults are edentulous.[18] Alterations in oral health can impact the ability to lubricate, masticate, and/or swallow food, which can impact dietary intake. Xerostomia (dry mouth) can be caused by decreased saliva production usually because of medications.[19]

Older adults are more likely to experience chemosensory changes (impaired sense of smell and taste),[20] which can result in poor appetite.[17,19] Changes to gastric muscular tone and decreased motility can slow gastric emptying resulting in constipation and early satiety.[19,21] After age 50 years about 1% to 2% of muscle mass is lost per year,[7] and there is a redistribution of fat around the internal organs.[22] Because lean body mass contains metabolically active tissue, it burns more calories. As lean body mass decreases, so does the number of calories required.[22] Anthropometric measures may become altered because of shortening of the spine and changes in skin thickness, turgor, and elasticity.[22] Approximately 15% to 30% of older adults have anorexia of aging,[19] a physiologic reduction in appetite and food intake seen with advancing age.[23] Decrease in smell and taste perception, hormonal changes in gut mediators, and altered secretion pattern of ghrelin play a role in the early satiation and decreased appetite associated with anorexia of aging.[21]

◆◆ **Aging per say does not cause malnutrition, but age-related changes can impact the dietary quality and amount of food consumed, contributing factors to unintentional weight loss.[17]**

## Psychosocial and Environmental Risk Factors

Older adults who are recently widowed, lonely, or depressed may lose the desire to eat, have a diminished appetite, and thus lose weight.[17] Persons with Alzheimer disease (AD) will experience weight loss across the stages of the disease because of neuropathologic alterations that impact feeding behavior and memory, disturbed appetite signaling, volitional swallowing, and alterations in taste and smell.[24] Poverty and food insecurity increase risk of malnutrition; 1 in 11 older adults struggle with food insecurity.[25] Older adults with limited income or those with food insecurity may restrict the number of meals eaten each day or purchase food that is inexpensive and less nutritious.[22] Environmental factors, including housing, transportation, and accessibility to local resources, also play an important role in food access. Older adults with mobility limitations who live in apartments without elevators or ramps might not be able to carry groceries. The ability to shop for food can be impeded by lack of accessible public transportation especially for those older adults who do not drive.[17] Community-dwelling older adults who are malnourished are less likely to use the Internet and more likely to live alone, live below the poverty level, report difficulty with housing costs, receive food stamps, and use transportation and housing services.[4]

◆◆ **Poverty and food insecurity increase risk of malnutrition; 1 in 11 older adults struggle with food insecurity.[25]**

## Chronic and Comorbid Conditions

Chronic diseases (cancer, diabetes, congestive heart failure, dementia, chronic obstructive pulmonary disease, stroke, end-stage renal failure, human immunodeficiency virus, alcoholism, gastrointestinal [GI] disorders, and rheumatoid arthritis[26,27]) are more common in older adults and contribute to involuntary weight loss because of decreased appetite, restrictive diets, dysphagia, or concomitant limitations in activities of daily living (ADLs), which limit the ability to shop, cook, or feed oneself.[17] Inflammation associated with acute and chronic disease states can diminish physiologic reserve, placing them at risk for unintentional weight loss.[17] Medications (prescribed, over-the-counter, vitamins, and herbal

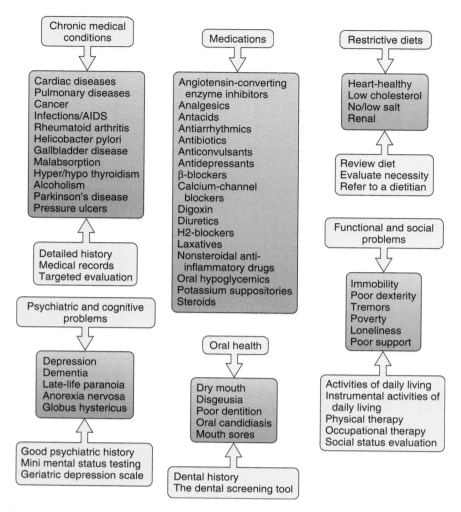

• **Figure 28.1** Risk factors for undernutrition illustrated by clinical approach. (Modified from Omran ML, Salem P. Diagnosing undernutrition. *Clin Geriatr Med.* 2002;18:719–736.)

supplements) used to manage chronic conditions can have unto-ward side effects that may affect appetite and dietary intake. These include changes in taste and smell, xerostomia, GI discomfort, slow gastric motility, early satiety, thirst, anorexia, and weight loss or gain.[17,27]

## Feeding and Swallowing Problems

Older adults with visual impairments and limitations in basic and instrumental ADLs caused by acute or chronic conditions may have difficulties shopping, cooking, or preparing meals; manipulating food; and feeding oneself.[17,19] These limitations impact the quality and quantity of food consumed. Individuals with dentition and oral health issues may have difficulty chewing food, which can impact dietary intake and quality. Loss of appetite, forgetting to eat, and reduced food intake are often experienced by individuals with cognitive impairment.[18,28]

Dysphagia, a risk factor for malnutrition, is difficulty in swallowing and chewing, with impairment of the various stages of swallowing and associated muscle weakness.[29] Dysphagia affects 7% to 13% of people over the age of 65 years[30] and is a known complication of many disorders seen in older adults (stroke, neurologic disorders, dementia, cancers, and respiratory disorders).[28,29]

Xerostomia is a common finding in older adults and also contributes to swallowing issues.[30] Signs and symptoms of dysphagia include self-reported difficulties with swallowing (coughing, choking, or sensations of food/drink sticking in the throat), pocketing of food in mouth, coughing, changes in voice quality (wet or hoarse voice), persistent throat clearing, upper airway sounds, and changes in breathing patterns.[29]

## Malnutrition

Malnutrition in older adults is usually linked to an inadequate intake of proteins and/or low intake of energy (protein-calorie malnutrition).[7,31] Marasmus, kwashiorkor, and mixed-marasmus kwashiorkor are terms traditionally used to define malnutrition (undernutrition) in children during famine and were applied to describe and diagnose disease-related malnutrition in adults, including older adults. An International Consensus Guideline committee acknowledged the negative impact of inflammation on nutrition status because of breakdown of skeletal muscle and proposed etiology-based diagnosis for starvation and disease-related malnutrition in adults.[32] In the United States, the Academy of Nutrition and Dietetics and the American Society for Parenteral and Enteral Nutrition collaborated to define three broad categories of malnutrition, which encompasses the etiology of malnutrition and the influence of illness and inflammation on nutritional state.[1] Starvation-related malnutrition (pure starvation or anorexia nervosa) is caused by energy deficit, without any underlying inflammation.[1] Chronic disease-related malnutrition is characterized by mild to moderate inflammation in the setting of chronic disease (disease or condition lasting $\geq 3$ months).[1] Acute disease or injury-related malnutrition is characterized by severe inflammation in the setting of acute illness (e.g., severe sepsis or trauma).[1]

---

## CASE

### Mr. Clarke (Part 3)

Mr. Clarke complains that food does not taste good. He also has trouble getting food now that he does not drive. His son takes him to the store once a week and he eats mostly soups and frozen dinners. He is worried about using the stove because of his vision loss.
1. What are some strategies to improve his intake?
2. What are some suggestions from the community that can improve his access to food?

---

## Differential Diagnosis and Assessment

### Nutrition Screening and Assessment

An interdisciplinary approach to address the nutritional needs of older adults includes screening for nutrition risk, conducting a nutrition assessment, initiating nutrition interventions, monitoring and evaluating responses to interventions, and diagnosing malnutrition when appropriate.[33] Nutrition screening is the first step in identifying an older adult who is malnourished or at risk for malnutrition to determine if a detailed nutrition assessment is indicated.[34,35] There are 21 different nutrition screening and assessment tools for use with older adults; however, the reliability, validity, specificity, and sensitivity of many of these tools are not well established. The Mini-Nutrition Assessment (MNA) short-form (SF)[37] (www.mna-elderly.com) and DETERMINE checklist[38] are two evidence-based screening tools recommended for use in older adults. The MNA-SF (developed from the full MNA)[34,35] consists of six questions on food intake, weight loss, mobility, psychological stress or acute disease, presence of dementia or depression, and body mass index (BMI). Calf-circumference can be used in place of BMI. The MNA-SF has a sensitivity of 89%, specificity of 82%, and a strong positive predictive value.[39] The MNA-SF can be administered by a clinician or the Self-MNA®[40] can be completed by an older individual. The DETERMINE checklist (Table 28.1) was developed by the Nutrition Screening Initiative and designed to be self-administered. Although the DETERMINE is an evidence-based nutrition risk screen, it has a high positive screen rate[41] and is most appropriate for use in community-dwelling older adults in the primary care setting. Screening for depression[28] and food insecurity[42] should also be integrated at regular intervals as depression and food insecurity are linked to weight loss and malnutrition in older adults.

❧❧ **Nutrition screening is the first step in identifying an older adult who is malnourished or at risk for malnutrition to determine if a detailed nutrition assessment is indicated.**[34,35]

## TABLE 28.1 Determine Your Nutritional Health

| Questions | Yes Points |
|---|---|
| I have an illness or condition that made me change the kind and/or amount of food I eat | 2 |
| I eat fewer than two meals a day | 3 |
| I eat few fruits or vegetables or milk products | 2 |
| I have three or more drinks of beer, liquor, or wine almost every day | 2 |
| I have tooth or mouth problems that make it hard for me to eat | 2 |
| I don't always have enough money to buy the food I need | 4 |
| I eat alone most of the time | 1 |
| I take three or more different prescribed or over-the-counter drugs a day | 1 |
| Without wanting to, I have lost or gained 10 pounds in the last 6 months | 2 |
| I am not always physically able to shop, cook, and/or feed myself | 2 |
| Total score: | |

Interpretation of scores:
0–2: Good. Recheck nutritional score in 6 months
3–5: You are at moderate nutrition risk. Recheck in 3 months
6 or more: You are at high nutritional risk. Review with healthcare provider.

An in-depth nutrition assessment (best performed by a registered dietitian or certified nutrition support clinician) should be performed when individuals screen positive. Components of a nutrition assessment are highlighted in Box 28.1. Loss of subcutaneous fat (orbital, triceps over rib cage), muscle loss (wasting of the temples, clavicles, shoulders, interosseous muscles, scapula, and calf), and fluid accumulation (extremities, vulvar/scrotal edema, or ascites) are physical signs suggestive of malnutrition.[1] Height and weight should be measured because self-report may not be reliable. Knee-height and demi-span measurements can be substituted for standing height in individuals who have difficulty standing erect.[22] Weight is an important vital sign in older adults. A weight loss (intentional or unintentional) of 5% of usual body weight in 6 to 12 months is clinically relevant and should be further evaluated (Fig. 28.2).[43] Clinical signs of inflammation should also be assessed (fever, tachycardia, hyperglycemia) as well as a functional assessment (handgrip strength to document physical decline).[1] Evaluation of prescription and over-the-counter medications for impact on nutrition status should be performed.[28]

Malnutrition can be diagnosed when two of six criteria are present: insufficient energy intake, weight loss, loss of muscle mass, loss of subcutaneous fat, localized or generalized fluid

---

### • BOX 28.1 Components of a Nutrition Assessment

**Anthropometric Measurements**
- Body mass index
- Usual adult weight
- Recent weight changes
- Skinfold measurements

**Biochemical Analysis**
- Complete blood count
- Protein status
- C-reactive protein
- Lipid profile
- Electrolytes
- Blood urea nitrogen/creatinine

**Clinical Evaluation**
- Physical examination
- Chronic conditions
- Current health status
- Oral health and dentition
- Medication use and polypharmacy

**Dietary History and Current Intake**
- Food preferences and food habits
- Cultural or religious habits
- Meal frequency
- Lack of control over food selection and choices
- Fluid intake
- Alcohol intake
- Special diet
- Vitamin/mineral/botanical supplement use
- Current intake compared with current nutritional needs
- Chewing and/or swallowing problems
- Functional limitations that impair independence with eating
- Cognitive changes affecting appetite and ability to feed self
- Physiologic changes that affect the desire to eat

---

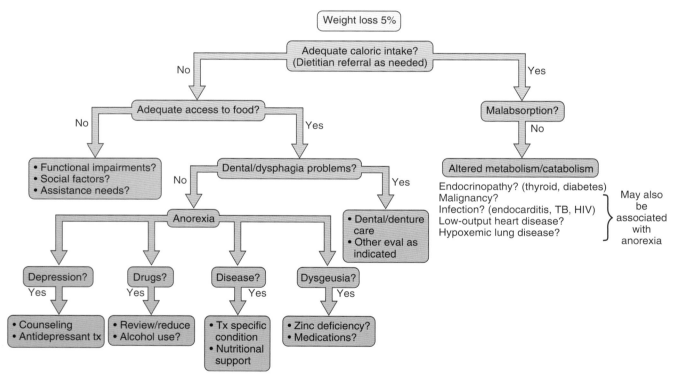

• **Figure 28.2** Weight loss algorithm. (Modified from Wallace JL, Schwartz RS. Involuntary weight loss in elderly outpatients-recognition, etiologies, and treatment. *Clin Geriatr Med*. 1997;13:717–33.)

---

accumulation, and diminished functional status by handgrip strength.[1] Biochemical indicators are no longer used to identify malnutrition. Albumin and prealbumin were often used to evaluate visceral protein status. In the setting of inflammation, these proteins are depressed and acute phase proteins, such as C-reactive protein (CRP), are produced. Low albumin or prealbumin may instead indicate illness and inflammation rather than nutritional status. Experts recommend interpreting albumin levels based on CRP. If CRP is normal and albumin is low, then the low albumin may suggest low protein status.[44]

TABLE 28.2   **Multidisciplinary Nutrition Interventions[a]**

| Intervention | Strategies |
|---|---|
| Encourage interprofessional collaboration | 1. Collaborate with nurse to develop a plan to assess and monitor nutrition risk factors, implement and evaluate nutrition interventions, and identify further issues related to feeding and eating[22] (Level of evidence [LOE] = D[b])<br>2. Collaborate with dietitian for comprehensive nutrition assessment and nutrition interventions[22] (LOE = D)<br>3. Consult with pharmacist to review medications for drug-nutrient interactions[22] (LOE = D)<br>4. Consult with social worker for referral to community-based resources for meal programs, food delivery, and financial resources[22] (LOE = D)<br>5. Consult with occupational therapist for adaptive eating equipment, positioning devices, and environmental modifications[22] (LOE = D)<br>6. Consult with speech therapist if dysphagia is suspected[8] (LOE = C)<br>7. Consult with physical therapist for exercise to support physical function and muscle mass[8] (LOE = C)<br>8. Consult with dental professional for oral health issues related to eating[8] (LOE = C) |
| Alleviate dry mouth | 1. Avoid caffeine, alcohol, tobacco, dry, bulky, spicy, salty or highly acidic foods[22] (LOE = D)<br>2. Sugarless hard candy or chewing gum to stimulate saliva if individual does not have dementia or dysphagia[22] (LOE = D)<br>3. Keep lips moist with petroleum jelly[22] (LOE = D)<br>4. Take frequent sips of water[22] (LOE = D) |
| Maintain adequate nutritional intake | 1. Daily requirements for healthy older adults include: 30 kcal/kg of body weight; 1.0 g/kg of protein per day[8] (LOE = C)<br>2. Requirements may differ depending on degree of malnutrition and physiologic stress[8] (LOE = C ) |
| Improve oral intake | 1. Avoid restrictive diets in individuals 75 years of age and older[8] (LOE = C)<br>2. Assess ability to eat and assist in feeding[45] (LOE = D)<br>3. Food fortification, such as adding eggs, oils or creams to food; or protein powders and maltodextrin to increase protein/energy density of meal[8] (LOE = C)<br>4. Engage in mealtime rounds to determine how much food is consumed and whether assistance is needed[45] (LOE = D)<br>5. Encourage family members to visit at mealtimes[22] (LOE = D)<br>6. Ask family members to bring favorite foods from home when appropriate[22] (LOE = D)<br>7. Honor patient food preferences[22] (LOE = D)<br>8. Suggest small frequent meals with adequate nutrients to help patients regain or maintain weight[22] (LOE = D)<br>9. Provide nutritious snacks[8] (LOE = C)<br>10. Mouth care and placement of dentures before food is served[45] (LOE = D) |
| Promote texture-modified diets | 1. Texture-modified diets are appropriate when individuals have chewing or swallowing problems. The type of diet depends on the extent of impairment of chewing and swallowing[8] (LOE = C )<br>2. Texture-modified diets include foods that are soft and bite-sized, minced and moist, pureed, or liquidized[29] (LOE = D)<br>3. Serve pureed or chopped foods in a visually appealing way[8] (LOE = C)<br>4. Dysphagia diets may also include drinks that are thickened with commercial thickeners[29] (LOE = D)<br>5. Consult with the speech therapist for specific safe swallow strategies such as chin tuck posture, effortful swallow, pacing or size of food, and drink mouthfuls[29] (LOE = D) |
| Provide oral supplements | 1. Supplements should not replace meals but should be provided between meals and not within the hour preceding a meal and at bedtime[46] (LOE = D)<br>2. Monitor the intake of the prescribed supplement[8] (LOE = C) |
| Provide specialized nutritional support | 1. Start specialized nutritional support (total parenteral nutrition or tube feeding) when a patient cannot, should not, or will not eat adequately and if the benefits of nutrition outweigh the associated risks[47,48] (LOE = D)<br>2. Before initiation of specialized nutrition support, review advanced directives regarding the use of artificial nutrition and hydration[47,48] (LOE = D) |
| Monitor for refeeding syndrome | 1. Carefully monitor and assess during the first week of aggressive nutritional repletion[49] (LOE = D)<br>2. Assess and correct hypophosphatemia, hypokalemia, hypomagnesemia, hyperglycemia, and hypoglycemia[49] (LOE = D)<br>3. Assess fluid status with daily weights and strict intake and output[49] (LOE = D)<br>4. Assess for congestive heart failure in patients with respiratory or cardiac difficulties[49] (LOE = D) |
| Create nil per mouth (NPO) orders | 1. Schedule older adults for tests or procedures early in the day to decrease the length of time they are not allowed to eat and drink[22] (LOE = D)<br>2. If testing late in the day is inevitable, order an early breakfast[22] (LOE = D)<br>3. Refer to the 2017 American Society of Anesthesiologists guideline recommending length of time patients should be kept NPO for elective surgical procedures[50] (LOE = C) |
| Consider mealtime and environmental aspects in dementia | 1. Arrange plate to facilitate self-feeding[51] (LOE = C)<br>2. Simplify meal presentation; serve one food at a time[51] (LOE = C)<br>3. Use verbal cueing and prompting to encourage self-feeding[51] (LOE = C)<br>4. Demonstrate eating motions so the person can imitate[51] (LOE = C)<br>5. Watch for cues that indicate the individual is being rushed or having trouble swallowing[51] (LOE = C) |

*(Continued)*

| TABLE 28.2 | Multidisciplinary Nutrition Interventions[a]—cont'd |
|---|---|
| **Intervention** | **Strategies** |
| | 6. Check for pocketing of food[51] (LOE = C) |
| | 7. Reduce distractions during mealtimes (eliminate noise, plain tablecloth or placemat)[51] (LOE = C) |
| | 8. Consult with occupational therapist for adaptive eating equipment[51] (LOE = C) |
| | 9. Use finger foods when individual is no longer able to use utensils[51] (LOE = C) |

[a]Modified in part from DiMaria-Ghalili, RA. Nutrition in the Older Adult. In: Boltz M, et al. *Evidence-based Geriatric Nursing Protocols for Best Practice*, 6th Edition. New York: Springer Publishing Company, 2020.

[b]Level of evidence modified from Sackett DL, Straus SE, Richardson WS, et al. Evidence-Based Medicine 2d Edition. Edinburg: Churchill Livingstone, 2000. A: supported by one or more high-quality RCT in an appropriate population; without contradictory evidence from other clinical trials. B: supported by one or more high quality nonrandomized cohort studies or low-quality RCTs. C: supported by one or more case series and/or poor-quality cohort and/or case-control studies. D: Supported by expert opinion and/or extrapolation from studies in other populations and/or settings.

## CASE

### Mr. Clarke (Part 4)

Mr. Clarke is now in the hospital with pneumonia. He is weak and now requires oxygen. He is assisted with meal setup but not with feeding. He is frequently found asleep during mealtime. The nursing staff states he eats 25% of his meals. He states he is too tired to eat.
1. What are Mr. Clarke's nutritional needs now that he is hospitalized?
2. What interventions can be put in place to increase his intake during his hospitalization?

## Management

### Nutrition Interventions

Many conditions and risk factors contribute to the development of malnutrition in older adults. Management should focus on treating the underlying cause when possible.[8] Evidence-based interdisciplinary nutrition interventions for older adults who are at risk for malnutrition or who are malnourished are outlined in Table 28.2. These interventions focus on strategies to engage in interprofessional collaboration, alleviate dry mouth, maintain and improve adequate nutritional intake, and implement nutritional support in the acute care, skilled care, or home setting. The approach presented here focuses on

increasing macronutrient (protein, carbohydrate, and fat) intake. However, providers should remember to monitor for signs of micronutrient imbalances because of impaired absorption, and supplement vitamin $B_{12}$, calcium, and iron when needed.[8] Several drugs have been tested for the stimulation of appetite in older adults with anorexia, but to date there is inadequate evidence to routinely incorporate in clinical practice.[28] Primary care physicians and nurse practitioners should also educate family caregivers on how to implement the most appropriate nutrition interventions for their loved ones.

## CASE DISCUSSION

Mr. Clarke is a common example of a community-dwelling older adult living in social isolation and experiencing malnutrition. He has multiple chronic medical problems that compound the normal aspects of aging that lead to malnutrition. Impaired access to food, limited transportation, and the loss of his wife have worsened his malnutrition risk. Mr. Clarke's malnutrition risk deteriorates when he is hospitalized for pneumonia, which puts his body in a hyperinflammatory state requiring increased nutritional needs. He will require supplementation and assistance with meals, including feeding assistance, to improve his intake while he is in the hospital. When Mr. Clarke discharges home, he will need continued nutritional support and assistance. Social services, home care, and community-based food assistance should be used along with close monitoring from his healthcare provider to ensure adequate nutritional status.

## Summary

Older adults are at risk for malnutrition (undernutrition) across the care continuum because of physiologic, psychological, social, economic, and environmental factors. A diagnosis of malnutrition is associated with increased healthcare costs and negative health outcomes. Early recognition and treatment of malnutrition can impact overall quality of life and health outcomes. Management of malnutrition is best accomplished through an interdisciplinary approach, which includes nutrition screening, assessment, and

implementation of nutrition interventions that take into consideration patient preferences.

### Web Resources
Nestle Nutrition Insititue: www.mna-elderly.com/
American Society for Parenteral and Enteral Nutrition (ASPEN): www.nutritioncare.org/Guidelines_and_Clinical_Resources/Malnutrition_Solution_Center/
Defeat Malnutrition Today: www.defeatmalnutrition.today/

## Key References

**8.** Volkert D, Beck AM, Cederholm T, et al. ESPEN Guideline on clinical nutrition and hydration in geriatrics. *Clin Nutr.* 2019;38(1):10–47.

**17.** DiMaria-Ghalili RA. Integrating nutrition in the comprehensive geriatric assessment. *Nutr Clin Pract.* 2014;29(4):420–427.

*References available online at* expertconsult.com.

# 29
# Frailty

REBECCA S. CROW AND PETER ABADIR

## OUTLINE

*Additional online-only material indicated by icon.*

## OBJECTIVES

*Upon completion of this chapter, the reader will be able to:*

- Describe the two major frailty paradigms and understand their similarities and differences.
- Describe the adverse outcomes associated with progression along the frailty spectrum.
- Understand frailty's all-encompassing effects on multiple subspecialty domains and organ systems.

- Review the interventions that have been studied to prevent progression and the limitations currently in terms of implementation into day-to-day practice.

## CASE

### Mrs. Jane S. (Part 1)

Jane S. is an 83-year-old female with significant past medical history of hypertension, hyperlipidemia, osteoporosis, mild dementia, atrial fibrillation, and frequent falls who lives at an independent living senior community. She is here to establish care and to discuss some acute concerns. Her daughter has brought her in a wheelchair because of distance from the parking garage. Jane has stopped driving; she says she is afraid she is "not as quick" as she used to be. Her daughter has taken over her finances because bills had a tendency to go unpaid. Otherwise Jane is independent in her activities of daily living (ADLs) and walks with a cane around her home and walker in the community. Her life space is her home, which she leaves only occasionally to go to a doctor's appointment or errand with her daughter. Over the last few months she has started to notice more swelling in her ankles and more shortness of breath when she goes to get the mail. You have to assist her onto the examination table and note on physical examination 2+ pitting edema in both her lower extremities and a 3+ holosystolic murmur at the left sternal border. Her vitals are otherwise stable and she is in no acute distress.

1. What are some clinical etiologies you are proposing as the possible reason for Mrs. S.'s progressive symptoms?
2. What concerns do you have about her overall health in addressing the etiology of her concern?

## Frailty: What Is This Geriatric Syndrome?

Approximately 10% of adults age >65 years and between 25% and 50% age >85 years are considered frail, making this a widely prevalent geriatric syndrome.[1] Lifestyle choices individuals make over a lifetime contribute to aging in either a positive or a negative way. Aging is individualized; all people age but not all who age are frail, which makes frailty a geriatric syndrome and not normal aging. Aging is the natural progressive loss of physiologic integrity, which leads to impaired function and increased vulnerability,[2] whereas frailty can be defined as homeostenosis or a decreased capacity to maintain homeostasis in times of acute stress.[3] A good

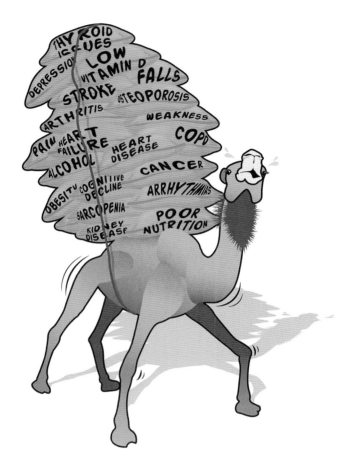

• **Figure 29.1** The famous proverb "the straw that broke the camel's back" serves as a good parallel to frailty in its imagery of diminished physiologic reserve weakened intrinsic capacity for handling acute, seemingly innocent stressors. (From Phil Davies [graphic artist] 2019.)

literary comparison can be found with the idiom "the straw that broke the camel's back." This initial 19th-century proverb refers to the growing burden of increasing weight added to the back of a camel who, despite the large weight, is able to stand upright until a small piece of straw is added and unexpectantly is the tipping point, leading to his collapse. With frail individuals, an otherwise trivial medical insult or physiologic change can have a domino effect of complications leading to systemic collapse because of the diminished physiologic reserve and resilience (Fig. 29.1). Frailty is felt to be somewhat reversible and responsive to interventions to alter its trajectory or possibly slow its progression.

## Nature Versus Nurture

The path to frailty varies from that of normal aging, but when do these two states divide and what are the influences? On a cellular level, homeostenosis seen with frailty is likely because of oxidative damage, chronic inflammation, mitochondrial exhaustion, and hormonal imbalance that is continuously asked of these individual's aging cells.[4] Chronic inflammation has been associated with upregulation of inflammatory markers interleukin 6, tumor necrosis factor alpha, and C-reactive protein.[5–7] Chronic inflammation over time leads to a catabolic neurohormonal state, muscle protein breakdown, and impaired immune system leaving an individual with a reduced ability to rebound from stress or disease.[8]

Environment and lifestyle also plays a strong role in the division from normal aging seen with frailty. A lifetime of obesity, inactivity, multiple chronic disease states, alcohol, and smoking further contribute to a decreased physiologic reserve state and decline in cognitive, cardiopulmonary, nutritional, neuroendocrine, muscular, and immune function.[2,8] Another strongly influential factor hypothesized is the concept of sarcopenia. Sarcopenia is defined as abnormally low lean muscle mass with low strength and function. It develops from low protein intake, chronic inflammation, disuse atrophy, and endocrine dysregulation.[9] With sarcopenia there are two systematic failures occurring. First, there is a reduced intake (anorexia), which lowers weight and inactivity (because of fatigue, low energy, fear of falling, etc.); secondly, the low muscle mass that results perpetuates further weakness and fatigue.

It has been demonstrated that those with lower education and lower income, as well as those with poorer health, have a higher risk of developing frailty status.[10] One study looked at the association of childhood and adult socioeconomic conditions and their impact on frailty progression. Here they showed that the more disadvantaged in childhood, the higher the odds of prefrail and frail state; however, this was mitigated if the adult conditions (education, occupation, low income) were improved.[11] This suggests that socioeconomic circumstances over a lifetime influence the development of frailty. All of these dynamic factors interplay to contribute to this complicated, all-encompassing syndrome.

## How We Define It?

Although there are over 51 current frailty scales available by one systematic review, there are currently two dominant paradigms to conceptualize frailty: a phenotype model (physical frailty) and a deficit accumulation model (frailty index).[12]

Fried and colleagues used the Cardiovascular Health Study to first define a frailty phenotype often termed "physical frailty."[1] The phenotype model defines frailty as a distinct clinical syndrome of five domains based on a biologic framework that is manifested outwardly with these signs and symptoms: unintentional weight loss (10 lbs in past year), self-reported exhaustion, weakness (grip strength), slow walking speed, and low physical activity.[1] In this model, frailty is defined by three or more of these factors, prefrailty by one or two and robust status by having none. The phenotype model views frailty as more of a "predisability" syndrome with decreased reserve from a cumulative decline and dysregulation across multiple physiologic domains.[1,13] Of all components of this phenotype, gait speed has been the most prominent element associated with disability and survival.[14]

The frailty index proposed and validated by Rockwood and colleagues take a different view on frailty, defining it by an accumulation of health and functional issues that serves more as an indication of reduced health state and requires more of a hands-on comprehensive clinical assessment.[13] The cumulative deficit model defines frailty by 70 items that evaluate six core domains: ADLs, physical performance or sarcopenia, cognitive function, neurologic signs, cardiopulmonary function, severity of present comorbidities. Rockwood developed the frailty index (total number of positive criteria expressed as a ratio of total deficits >70 denominator) and the clinical frailty scale (the abridged 7-point assessment tool) to conceptualize frailty as more of a multidimensional assessment of overall fitness and frailty.[15,16]

Although both these prominent scales are widely accepted and used in clinical research, they do function to identify separate groups of individuals by their definitions. A comparison study of

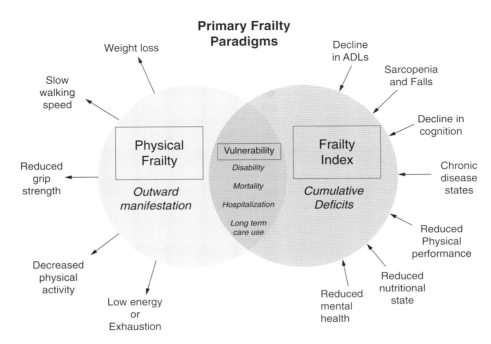

**Primary Frailty Paradigms**

- Weight loss
- Slow walking speed
- Reduced grip strength
- Decreased physical activity
- Low energy or Exhaustion

Physical Frailty

*Outward manifestation*

Vulnerability
*Disability*
*Mortality*
*Hospitalization*
*Long term care use*

Frailty Index

*Cumulative Deficits*

- Decline in ADLs
- Sarcopenia and Falls
- Decline in cognition
- Chronic disease states
- Reduced Physical performance
- Reduced nutritional state
- Reduced mental health

• **Figure 29.2** This Venn diagram is a representation of the two major frailty paradigms. Phenotypical or physical frailty is more defined by external manifestations whereas the frailty index views frailty more as an accumulation of deficits. Both share the commonality of increased vulnerability in this population. *ADLs*; Activities of daily living.

730 older adults showed the phenotype model identified 7% of individuals as frail whereas the frailty index defined 8.3%. However, there was only 12% agreement in who was deemed frail showing whereas both clinically valid, they are not to be considered interchangeable (Fig. 29.2).[17]

Other well-known scales available include the FRAIL scale, which defines frailty by five components: fatigue, resistance, ambulation, more than five illnesses, and 5% weight loss.[18] The Edmonton frail scale evaluates nine domains: cognition, general health status, functional independence, social support, medication usage, nutrition, mood, continence, and functional performance.[19] Other frailty assessment tools, such as the trauma-specific frailty index and gait speed, have been used in clinical subspecialties to define frailty.[20,21] Grip strength has been thought of as a quick single assessment tool for physical frailty; however, in one study it alone was not predictive of mortality at 2 years.[22] Although there are multiple scales out there, none have emerged to be the prominent tool for use both in research and medical literature. A scale to define frailty quickly, efficiently, and accurately in clinical day-to-day operations is still being evaluated.

## The Bad and the Ugly of Frailty

Frail patients tend to be older females with more comorbidities and they tend to have more disability a month after hospitalization at rates seven times their robust counterparts.[23–25] Numerous studies have shown that frailty has an association with inpatient hospital mortality[26] in addition to twice the risk of overall mortality, loss of ADLs, increasing physical limitation, as well as falls and fractures.[27] The same review showed frailty had an eightfold increased risk of hospitalization. A systematic review and meta-analysis demonstrated that frailty and prefrailty are both associated with increased rates of nursing home placement.[25] Although wound healing is slower even in a healthy octogenarian,

the disruption in homeostatic equilibrium seen with frailty is speculated to hinder the complicated process of wound healing in these individuals.[28] Improving quality of life whereas reducing early mortality, long-term care placement, and hospitalization are some of the pillars of quality geriatric care making frailty a valuable identification tool for these high-risk patients.

## Prefrailty: A Valuable Tool in Itself

Prefrailty is associated with a higher likelihood of reversibility than frailty, which argues for earlier recognition of this intermediate stage. Prefrailty in those with coexisting cognitive impairment has been associated with twice the prevalence of functional disability, reduced quality of life, along with increased mortality.[29,30] Prefrailty also appears to be an independent predictor of cardiovascular disease, cardiovascular-related mortality, as well as overall mortality.[30,31] A study looking at the transition along the frailty spectrum showed that participants who entered the study prefrail had a 78.4% chance of remaining prefrail or transitioning to robust over 36 months.[32] Those starting prefrail had higher rates of transitioning back to robust in the first 36 months and mortality was greater for those remaining prefrail over this 54-month period. This demonstrates that value in recognizing prefrailty and intervening early, which not only reduces mortality associated with the progression to frail status but also the morality risk in remaining prefrail as well. Prefrail status serves as a unique stage along the frailty spectrum that continues to gain interest in the research field.[33]

## Cognitive Frailty and Mental Health

Many criticisms about some current frailty measurements include the lack of cognitive screening and the influence of cognitive decline on outcomes that are not accounted for by standard metrics. A concept of "cognitive frailty" has been proposed and is defined as a presence of both physical frailty and cognitive impairment without the diagnosis of dementia (Mini-Mental State Examination [MMSE] score <26),[29] however the definition has yet to meet full consensus. Those who were cognitively frail had 13 times the rate of functional disability, 27 times increased incidence of low quality of life, and 5 times the risk of death.[29] In this study, 1.8% of the population were both physically frail and cognitively impaired. Frailty is also associated with a formal dementia diagnosis as it has been shown to be a significant predictor of Alzheimer disease, vascular dementia, and all dementias among community-dwelling older people.[34] Frailty and cognition function show many similar diagnostic overlaps and trajectories, as one study demonstrated that slow gait speed or a low hand grip strength could be predictive of 10-year cognitive decline,[35] suggesting these as a potential useful isolated metrics for both frailty and cognitive decline.

Frailty also has a relationship with other mental health disorders such as anxiety and depression. Frail older adults have increased odds of depression whereas those with depression also had increased odds of being frail suggesting a potential biway relationship.[36] The same relationship can be seen with anxiety with increasing levels of anxiety as one progresses along the frailty spectrum.[37] Having depression or anxiety coexisting with frailty leads to more accelerated cognitive impairment, especially in speech and executive function.[37,38] Anxiety, depression, cognitive decline, and frailty are all intertwined making it more of a chicken-or-egg hypothesis. The coexistence of frailty and mood disorders leads to a poorer sense of overall wellbeing, reduced physical performance, and reduced sense of communal contribution. What we do know now is that mental health and cognitive health play a larger role in frailty than previously acknowledged.

## Frailty's Use in Surgical Preoperative Care

Current established surgical risk tools, such as the American Society of Anesthesiologist Estimation of Physiologic Ability and Surgical Stress score[39] are designed to predict mortality and determine preoperative health before an operation. They focus on general demographics such as age and chronic comorbidities, along with the generalities of the procedure itself but poorly assess for vulnerability and trajectory seen with frail older adults. Frailty has been shown to be an independent risk factor for negative surgical outcomes and has strong association with adverse complications, prolonged hospitalization, need for postsurgical rehabilitation, as well as mortality.[8]

Because frailty identifies individuals with decreased physiologic reserve, this metric is a great tool to be used for surgical preoperative evaluation before engaging more aggressive treatment modalities. There are some barriers around integrating this into surgical preoperative care, which is thought to be caused by a lack of knowledge of providers and their understanding of frailty's effect on surgical outcomes.[40] However, more research is starting to demonstrate the benefits of this implementation in surgical practice. Transcatheter aortic valve implantation is a cardiac surgery for those with aortic stenosis felt too high risk for a major open heart procedure. In a systematic review, frailty assessment was able to identify those at highest risk for poor outcomes from this procedure above standard assessment tools.[41]

Frailty is not an isolated entity in itself as more research has demonstrated its utility in clinical outcomes in multiple organ systems further strengthening its value and scope of use (Table 29.1).

## Intrinsic Capacity and Resilience

Although frailty is dynamic, its operationalization is static in that its definition does not have the capacity to evaluate the body's response to past or present stressors and how this influences outcomes. Despite clinician's best efforts at prognostication, there are always cases where the outcome is unexpected: a frail patient who unexpectedly does very well with medical adversity or the robust patient who does not recover to the expected degree of his baseline status. From this arose the concepts of intrinsic capacity and physical resilience. Intrinsic capacity is the all-encompassing physical and mental capacity an individual has and serves as an indicator of healthy aging.[72] Resilience is the ability to resist functional decline and recover following an acute stressor (surgery, illness, or disease).[73] If the spectrum of robust to frailty status reflects the physiologic potential an individual has to recover from a stressor, then resilience refers to the actualization of that potential.[74]

With resilience testing, an individual undergoes a stress to evoke a dynamic recovery allowing for a true evaluation of reserve and resiliency. Proposed tools for this evaluation would be pre- and posttest assessment (i.e., looking at ADL or depression scores before and after elective surgery) or a stimulus response (i.e., evaluating heart rate around exercise testing) or the concept of microrecoveries (i.e., self-report of daily overall health suspecting that those with less variance would have more resiliency).[75] Some criticism is these evaluations is that they sway toward single organ system evaluation as currently there is no "whole body" resilience test currently available.

## Trajectories and Projections

Frailty is not thought to be a stagnant or unilateral downward process but much more dynamic with up to one-third of older adults making at least one transition (improvement or decline) over a 4.4-year period.[30] Higher rates of progression to frailty were seen if participants were older, female sex, obese, or had cardiovascular disease, osteoarthritis, history of smoking, vision impairment, ADLs dependence, reduced physical performance, polypharmacy, or hyperuricemia. Interestingly in this study, moderate alcohol intake, living alone, higher education, and being overweight had decreased frailty progression rates. Another study looking at transition rates found that 57.6% of participants had at least one transition along the frailty spectrum in the 54-month follow-up.[32] Also, the transition to greater frailty was 43.3% versus 23% to less frailty. Rates of transition from frail to robust were negligible, and the longer participants were classified as frail, the greater their chance of remaining frail and the higher their mortality. These findings suggest recognizing this diagnosis and implementing effective intervention strategies are more likely to lead to improvement or slow a decline known to have harmful or negative outcomes.

## Intervention Strategies

Few studies have looked at interventional therapies to reduce or improve frailty. Evidence has shown that aerobic and resistance exercises can improve aspects of frailty.[25] A large study, the Lifestyle Interventions and Independence for Elders Pilot Study, completed over 12 months, examined older adults at risk for disability and demonstrated that 150 min/week of activity plus balance training led to faster walking speed, but studies showing maintenance of these benefits over time are lacking.[76]

**TABLE 29.1    Known Association of Organ System Disease States With Frailty**

| System    Specific Disease State | Specific Association With Frailty |
|---|---|
| **Hematology** | |
| Acute myeloid leukemia, myelodysplasia, lymphoma, and myeloma | • Poor therapeutic response, increased toxicity from drug treatments, and worse survival rates[42–45]<br>• Frailty screening being used to assess patient's physiologic age to determine appropriate treatment |
| **Nephrology** | |
| Chronic kidney disease | • Risk increases as kidney disease progresses with the highest rates of association in those with end-stage renal disease[46,47]<br>• Coexistence has been shown to further increase falls, fractures, hospitalization, and mortality then either entity alone[48]<br>• In patients on hemodialysis, worsening frailty correlates with increased inflammation and hospitalization[49] |
| **Pulmonology** | |
| Chronic obstructive pulmonary disease | • Independent risk factor for 90-day hospital readmission for those admitted for acute COPD exacerbation<br>• Associated with more lung disease exacerbations, all-cause hospitalization, declines in functional status, and all-cause mortality<br>• Have a 42% higher odds of developing respiratory impairment<br>• Respiratory impairment led to a 58% higher risk of being prefrailty and frailty than those without impairment[50,51] |
| Lung transplant | • Associated with worse exercise capacity in lung transplant patients[52] |
| Interstitial lung disease | • Dyspnea severity more related to concurrent frailty than pulmonary function test severity[53]<br>• Frailty association with outcomes in this population is yet to be evaluated[53] |
| **Critical Illness** | |
| | • Frail survival tripled when comparing the 1990s to 2000s[54]<br>• More likely to be left with severe disability, longer hospital stays, and increased mortality at hospital discharge and 1-year postdischarge from critical illness admission[16,51,55]<br>• Highest need for palliative care assessment[56] |
| **Cardiology** | |
| Coronary artery disease | • Expedited onset cardiovascular disease and two- to threefold increase in cardiovascular mortality[31,57]<br>• Low energy expenditure, exhaustion, and slow gait speed predictive of new cardiovascular events[30] |
| Rhythm disorders | • 25% of patient evaluated for pacemakers<br>• Higher association with atrioventricular[58]<br>• Association with atrial fibrillation is still unknown[59] |
| Congestive heart failure | • 50% relationship with congestive heart failure across all age groups suggesting this association is not unique to the aging population[60] |
| **Endocrinology** | |
| Cortisol | • Association with elevated diurnal cortisol concentrations likely because of failure of homoeostatic control[61,62] |
| Testosterone | • Effect of treatment with testosterone and high caloric supplementation on frailty rates in undernourished older adults showed no improvement[63]<br>• Treatment may improve lean mass in frail and nonfrail men,[64] its benefit over risks are unknown |
| Growth hormone | • Associated with lower IGF-1 levels[65] |
| Thyroid disease | • Association with thyroid disease is still unknown<br>• Higher TSH levels in men and lower TSH levels in women seemed to correlated with increased risk of frailty[66] |
| Obesity | • Metabolic syndrome has not been shown to be associated[7]<br>• Associated with a <21 kcal/kg/day and a low protein diet whereas high dietary antioxidant capacity presents a lower risk[67]<br>• Lower serum albumin levels[68]<br>• Lower vitamin D levels than their robust counterparts making them higher risk for osteoporosis and fractures[6] |
| **Urology** | |
| Urinary incontinence | • Associated with urinary incontinence and increased mortality in these patients after hospital discharge[69] |
| Prostate disease | • Higher mortality, ICU complication and length of stay rates following radical cystectomy, transurethral resection of prostate among other urology procedures[70]<br>• Unknown association with benign prostate hypertrophy[71] |

*COPD*, Chronic obstructive pulmonary disease; *ICU*, intensive care unit; *IGF*, insulin-like growth factor; *TSH*, thyroid stimulating hormone

A review of current literature demonstrated that the most successful interventions included physical activity plus or minus nutrition and memory training and prehabilitation (which this study defined as physical therapy plus exercise plus home modifications).[77] The adherence rates in these studies was around 70%. However, although reduction in frailty may have been significant, several studies did not show improvement in ADL or reduced fall rates demonstrating we are not there yet in terms of effective, maintainable intervention techniques. Future studies are aiming to look not only at reducing frailty rates but improvement in its downstream sequela and adverse events, which is really where we will see improved outcomes in this vulnerable subset of the aging population.

---

## CASE

### Mrs. Jane S (Part 2)

You obtain an echocardiogram, which demonstrates severe high-grade aortic stenosis with an ejection fraction of 55%. She seeks the opinion of cardiac surgery and interventional cardiology who believe her to be a poor surgical candidate. It is recommended that she pursue a transcatheter aortic valve implantation. This decision was made based on her comorbidities, clinical condition, EuroSCORE, and STS score. Mrs. S. and her daughter return to your office to discuss concern of having this intervention and if it is the right choice for her since her memory and function have been getting worse (MMSE 19/30 and Timed up and Go [TUG] 18 seconds at visit). Mrs. S. says she is really content with her life, still really enjoys gardening and playing with her grandchildren, and wonders if she will live to see the benefit of having this intervention.

---

## CASE

### Discussion

One study showed that a multidimensional geriatric assessment, including frailty index calculation, may improve 1-year mortality prediction following transcatheter aortic valve replacement above commonly used evaluation scores used for cardiac procedures. The TUG was the highest single predictive test within the frailty index. Those deemed the most frail had a 50% mortality rate at 1 year, which demonstrates frailty a strong predictor for outcomes and further values goals of care and a realistic pursuit of aggressive interventions.[78] Ms. S. has components of dementia and meets criteria for phenotypic frailty. In this study 10% of patients like Mrs. S. had mortality at 1 year. Frailty is a valuable additional component to the discussion on outcomes after valve replacement. Like so much in geriatrics, there is no right or wrong answer. Reviewing the facts regarding the procedure, proposed realistic outcome, and risk with patient and her daughter will allow for the best decision for this patient considering her values and goals of care.

❖❖ Frailty is a complicated geriatric syndrome because there is no single disease or one organ system involved but serves as a power predictor of clinical outcome.

❖❖ The two main theories of frailty define it as a biologically driven syndrome versus a collection of diseases and comorbidities. There is no consensus as to the best way to define frailty at this time.

❖❖ The devil is in the details in caring for frail individuals. Frail patients are less forgiving to minor medical insults making medications, environment, and potential intervention decisions very impactful on their trajectory.

❖❖ Frailty is more accurate in predicting functional decline than age alone.

❖❖ Those defined as prefrail may have the highest benefit from intervention and improvement in long-term outcomes.

❖❖ Frailty can serve as a valuable marker of poor surgical outcomes over and above other prediction models in current use.

## Summary

Frailty is a dynamic syndrome defined by a decreased capacity to maintain homeostasis in times of stress leading to increased vulnerability. The two main paradigms to define frailty are by a phenotypic model and by a deficit accumulation model; however, they only have a 12% agreement rate in defining an individual as frail. Recognizing frailty early could lead to reduction in some of the known negative downstream effects, such as increased hospitalization, long-term care use, and mortality; however, successful intervention techniques are still being studied.

The concepts of intrinsic capacity and resilience have emerged to extend the continuum of frailty to define "healthy aging." Frailty still has many barriers to its use, including a lack of consensus of its definition, its lack of connection to meaningful prevention or treatment strategies, and current time-consuming screening tools for identification.[79] However, its growing use in the preoperative state demonstrates its growing value in the medical community as a means of advancing quality geriatric clinical care.

## Key References

1. Fried LP, Tangen CM, Walston J, et al. Frailty in older adults: evidence for a phenotype. *J Gerontol A Biol Sci Med Sci.* 2001;56(3):M146—M156.
16. Rockwood K, Song X, MacKnight C, et al. A global clinical measure of fitness and frailty in elderly people. *CMAJ.* 2005;173(5):489—495.
25. Kojima G. Frailty as a predictor of nursing home placement among community-dwelling older adults: a systematic review and meta-analysis. *J Geriatr Phys Ther.* 2018;41(1):42—48.
76. Cesari M, Vellas B, Hsu FC, et al. A physical activity intervention to treat the frailty syndrome in older persons-results from the LIFE-P study. *J Gerontol A Biol Sci Med Sci.* 2015;70(2):216—222.

**References available online at** expertconsult.com.

# 30

# Pressure Injuries

MONICA A. STOUT, E. FOY WHITE-CHU, AND AIMÉE D. GARCIA

## OUTLINE

## OBJECTIVES

*Upon completion of this chapter, the reader will be able to:*

- Define the stages of pressure injuries.
- Identify the risk factors that place a patient at risk for pressure injury development.
- Recognize and implement appropriate pressure redistribution strategies for the prevention of pressure injuries.
- Develop and implement a care plan for pressure injury management.

---

### CASE 1

#### Kevin Maloney (Part 1)

Kevin Maloney, an 89-year-old man, comes to the emergency room with altered mental status. He lives alone in his own home and his children check on him daily. The daughter reports that he has become incontinent over the last few days, and that she found many wet undergarments throughout the house. When she went to see him today, she found him confused and lying on the floor in his room. She saw no evidence of trauma, and the patient stated he "was tired and lay down on the floor." She is not sure how long he was there. On evaluation, the patient is oriented to name only. His vital signs are as follows: temperature 99.1° F, blood pressure 125/82 mmHg, respiration rate 18 breaths/min, pulse 82 beats per minute.

On physical examination, Mr. Maloney is found to have skin breakdown on the left buttock. The wound measures 6 cm × 5 cm × 0.1 cm. The wound bed is in the dermis, and is pink without necrotic tissue visible. It appears to have minimal serous drainage and no odor.
1. What stage would you document for Mr. Maloney's pressure injury?
2. What treatment recommendations would you make, and why?

---

### CASE 2

#### Meryl Curry (Part 1)

You are seeing Meryl Curry, a 75-year-old woman who resides in an assisted living facility, for an initial evaluation. She has diabetes, hypertension, chronic obstructive pulmonary disease (COPD), and a history of stroke with left-sided hemiparesis. She is on 2 L per minute of home oxygen for her COPD. She is incontinent of bladder and wears protective undergarments. She is continent of bowel and is able to toilet herself. Mrs. Curry recently lost her husband and has been depressed. She does not like to leave her apartment and sits in an easy chair most of the day. Since the loss of her husband, her appetite has diminished. The patient has had two admissions in the past 6 months for COPD exacerbation. She is a thin, frail-appearing woman with a flat affect.

On physical examination, the patient has very pronounced bony prominences. She is found to have skin breakdown on the sacral/buttocks area measuring 8 cm × 9 cm, which is covered with 100% necrotic tissue. There is erythema surrounding the site and foul-smelling drainage.
1. What stage would you document for Mrs. Curry's pressure injury?
2. What treatment recommendations would you make, and why?

## Epidemiology and Differential Diagnosis

With an aging population and a trend to provide more healthcare services in the home, primary care providers (PCPs) are providing more care for patients with pressure injuries. Incidence rates of pressure injuries vary widely. In previous studies, pressure injuries were noted to occur most frequently in acute care settings, with incidence rates as high as 38% in older persons. Efforts had reduced these rates considerably, but more recent data show that these rates are now trending back up, both in hospitals and long-term care settings.[1,2]

The PCP, when taking care of a patient with a pressure injury, must be mindful of the litigious nature surrounding this geriatric syndrome. Over 17,000 lawsuits related to pressure injuries occur every year.[3] Pressure injuries are often seen by family and patients as a sign of neglect. Careful assessment, documentation, and multi-disciplinary care planning are therefore important both to educate patients and to optimize healing and prevent litigation.[4]

Pressure injuries are not only devastating to the patient, but also have great impact on the healthcare system. A retrospective analysis of the Medicare 5% limited data set (for calendar year 2014) found that pressure ulcers were the second most expensive wounds—as much as $21,060 spending per beneficiary whether as a primary or secondary diagnosis.[5] Annual costs as high as $129,000 have been estimated for the treatment of stage 4 pressure injuries.[6]

As of October 2008, the Centers for Medicare and Medicaid Services have stopped reimbursing acute care facilities for treatment of stage 3 or higher pressure injuries that developed in-house. In 2011 the National Quality Forum considered recommending an expansion of this legislation to include postacute and long-term care, but this has not yet occurred.[7] This legislation was based on the belief that pressure injuries are largely preventable. Although these efforts to improve quality are to be applauded, it continues to be unclear how this decision will impact pressure injury prevention and treatment, especially considering the 2017 data showing a 6% increase in hospital-acquired pressure injuries.[2]

Pressure injuries develop when pressure forces exceed capillary blood flow, causing ischemia, and subsequent tissue necrosis occurs. Bony prominences, such as the coccyx, sacrum, heels, hips, and elbows, are most susceptible. Depending on the overall health and mobility of the patient, and on the hardness of the surface on which the patient is sitting or lying, tissue ischemia and necrosis can occur in as little time as 2 hours. Pressure injuries can also occur wherever skin is damaged by excessive friction or shear and moisture. Pressure injuries are the only wound type that should be staged (i.e., venous leg ulcers and other wound types are not staged).

⬥⬥ **When an open ulcer is seen on a geriatric patient, the clinician needs to consider not just pressure injury but other potential sources of skin breakdown.**

When an open ulcer is seen on a geriatric patient, pressure injury should be at the top of the differential diagnosis. However, there are multiple other causes of skin breakdown. Table 30.1 reviews the differential diagnoses of ulcerations that are commonly misdiagnosed as pressure injuries. Of these, several merit note:
- Moisture-associated skin damage (MASD) and abrasions are the most common misdiagnosis. Although MASD and friction put the patient at risk of pressure injuries, a discrete ulceration needs to form to differentiate pressure injury from these conditions.[8]

- A diabetic foot or arterial foot ulcer can be difficult to distinguish from a pressure injury; however, it is important therapeutically to determine the primary underlying cause. In the case of a diabetic foot ulcer, this would be neuropathy. For an arterial foot ulcer, the cause would be poor arterial flow, with weak or absent pulses a corroborating sign.
- Skin changes at life's end because of hypoperfusion of the skin and underlying tissues—also known as skin failure—is another increasingly recognized syndrome.[9,10] Thus far it has been challenging to diagnose this condition as distinct from pressure injuries.

The National Pressure Ulcer Advisory Panel states that some pressure injuries are unavoidable. The panel also recognizes pressure injuries as being separate from skin failure, but that the two diagnoses can coexist. For patients who have an illness that has caused poor tissue perfusion and thus low tissue tolerance to any pressure, the provider should consider documenting the pressure injury as "unavoidable" and that skin failure may be occurring.[11]

## Risk Factors and Prevention

⬥⬥ **Prevention efforts in every care setting should be used to limit the development of pressure injuries.**

Aggressive, 24-hour-a-day prevention efforts in every care setting are critical to limit the development of pressure injuries. The first step is to be aware of the factors that place patients at high risk. Risk factors are numerous and can be separated between intrinsic and extrinsic risk factors (Table 30.2).
- Intrinsic factors are those that alter skin integrity. They include limited mobility; medical comorbidities such as diabetes, COPD, congestive heart failure, or other medical conditions affecting perfusion and oxygenation, malignancy, and renal dysfunction; poor nutrition; and aging skin changes.
- Extrinsic factors are those external factors that can damage the skin. They include pressure, friction, shear, and moisture.

### Clinical Tools to Estimate Pressure Injury Risk

For pressure injuries, there are two validated and widely used risk assessment tools for the inpatient and long-term care setting: the Braden scale and the Norton scale.[12] Neither has undergone randomized trials to look at their impact on pressure injury incidence.[13] Risk assessment is required for inpatient and postacute or long-term care settings. The frequency varies between settings, and should also be done whenever the patient's condition changes. The score provided by the tool should be considered supplemental to clinical judgment. For those patients on Hospice, the Hospice Pressure Ulcer Risk Assessment (HoRT) scale has been validated.[14]

The more commonly used scale, the Braden scale, has six domains: sensory perception, moisture, activity, mobility, nutrition, and friction/shear. The first five domains are rated on a scale from 1 to 4, with 1 being worst and 4 being best; friction/shear is rated from 1 (problematic) to 3 (not a problem). The maximum score is 23. Typically, patients are considered at risk of pressure injury development if their Braden score is ≤ 18. Therefore scores ≤ 18 should trigger inpatient and postacute/long-term care nursing and other support staff to put in place more aggressive preventive measures, such as frequent turning, a specialized mattress, and perhaps a nutrition consult.

| TABLE 30.1 | Differential Diagnosis of Pressure Injuries | |
| --- | --- | --- |
| Diagnosis | Typical Location | Characteristics |
| Moisture-associated skin damage (also known as incontinence-associated dermatitis) | Perineum—sacrum, coccyx, gluteal folds, groin folds | Moisture must be present<br>Indistinct edges<br>No necrosis<br>Typically diffuse superficial excoriation, possible fungal appearance |
| Old pilonidal cyst excision | Gluteal cleft—inferior to coccyx | There is a history of pilonidal cyst excision or a scar is visible |
| Diabetic foot ulcer | Heel, plantar surface, toes | Neuropathy must be present |
| Arterial insufficiency—related foot ulcer | Heel, toes | Nonpalpable pulses |
| Venous insufficiency—related ulcer | On the lower extremity below the knee | Superficial ulcerations with ragged edges<br>Associated hemosiderin deposition noted on extremity |
| Edema/blisters | Anywhere on the body | Superficial ulcerations<br>Tend to be clean<br>Usually round |
| Abrasion/friction | Anywhere on body | Skin flap present or abraded/excoriated skin surface |
| Malignancy | Anywhere on body | Will not heal despite offloading and local wound care |
| Herpes simplex or zoster | Anywhere on body | Both simplex and zoster have punched out appearance<br>Tend to start out as blister or painful lesions<br>Zoster is dermatomal |
| Abscess | Anywhere on body | Starts as blister or localized swelling that will drain on its own |
| Skin failure | Anywhere on body, but commonly over a bony prominence | Skin changes at end of life; usually occurs concurrent with failure of other organ systems |

Individual item scores are important in planning care. For instance, a patient may score high in nutrition and have no sensory impairments but also be very immobile with poor activity and friction/shear forces at work. By looking at the items that engender risk, the provider can target interventions to the most important risk factors for that individual patient. However, when a patient has scored as "increased risk" every risk factor identified by the scale should have an action plan prepared and implemented.

## Preventive Measures

Some 70% of pressure injuries occur from the waist down. The main areas to examine when considering a patient's potential for skin breakdown are the sacrum, the trochanters, and the heels. If the patient is often in a seated position, the coccyx and ischial tuberosities become a site for greater risk of breakdown.

Once at-risk patients are identified, the healthcare provider can effectively put preventive interventions into practice. These include the following:

- *Maximizing treatment of the patient's medical conditions.* This is the first step. All medical conditions that could affect healing and skin integrity should be optimized. The provider and patient should make every effort to optimize diabetes control, blood pressure, and respiratory status depending on patients' comorbidities and life expectancies. A review of medications may find ones that cause easy bruising or skin tears, such as

warfarin or prednisone. If so, the provider should inquire as to whether they can be stopped, in consultation with the patient and other providers, and in consideration of the goals of care.

- *Nutrition consultation.* This should be considered early in the course of prevention, especially if there is concern that the patient's nutritional level is compromised. A systematic review found that many randomized controlled trials were poorly designed when addressing nutritional supplementation as a preventive measure for pressure injuries. The review concluded that a nutrition consultation is reasonable for patients at risk.[15]
- *Frequent repositioning.* If the individual is bedbound or chairbound, the patient and his or her caregivers should be educated about effective offloading strategies. A patient who spends most of the day in a wheelchair, recliner, or gerichair needs to be repositioned every hour. This can be easily done by reclining the chair, tilting the legs, or simply having the patient stand for about 30 seconds and then sit back down again.[16] A recent multisite randomized clinical trial found that there was no difference in pressure injury incidence for those frail older adults turned every 2, 3, or 4 hours in long-term care.[17] The recommendation remains to frequently reposition every 2 to 4 hours, depending on the goals of care. The exception would be a dying patient who has significant discomfort with frequent repositioning; that person should be kept comfortable even at the expense of skin integrity.

| TABLE 30.2 | Risk Factors for Pressure Injuries | |
|---|---|---|
| | **Factor** | **Examples** |
| Intrinsic factors (factors within the body) | Limited mobility | Delirium |
| | | Sepsis/critical illness |
| | | End-stage dementia |
| | | CVA with hemiplegia |
| | | Para-/quadriplegia |
| | | Severe osteoarthrosis |
| | | Spinal stenosis |
| | Sensory loss that reduces signaling to brain to reposition oneself | Hemi-/para-/quadriplegia |
| | | Diabetes mellitus with neuropathy |
| | Comorbid illness that reduces tissue oxygenation or immune response to injury | Diabetes mellitus |
| | | Coronary artery disease |
| | | Congestive heart failure |
| | | Peripheral arterial disease |
| | | Chronic obstructive pulmonary disease |
| | | Chronic kidney disease stage IV/ESRD with dialysis |
| | | Autoimmune disease |
| | | Malignancy |
| | | Urinary or fecal incontinence |
| | Body type | Underweight or obese |
| | | Older age |
| Extrinsic factors (factors in the immediate environment that affect the body) | Pressure | Standard mattress |
| | | Wheelchair that is too small or too large |
| | | Wheelchair seating |
| | Friction and shear forces | Rubbing heels in bed |
| | | Drag with repositioning |
| | | Aggressive hygiene cleansing |
| | | Head of bed greater than 30 degrees (body slides down in bed) |
| | | Reclining a wheelchair |
| | Moisture | Incontinence |
| | | Diaphoresis caused by pyrexia, autonomic instability, or ambient temperature |
| Both intrinsic and extrinsic factors | Inadequate nutrition | Hypercatabolic state (malignancy, infection, critical illness) |
| | | Low protein |
| | Supplemental nutrition | Patients on total parental nutrition (TPN) or gastrointestinal tube feeds |

*CVA*, Cerebrovascular accident; *ESRD*, end-stage renal disease.

- *Management of incontinence.* Urinary, and especially fecal, incontinence alters the pH balance of the skin surface, thereby increasing the risk of breakdown and pressure injury formation. Incontinence is best managed through toileting programs and, if needed, containment systems.

## Pressure Redistribution Systems

Pressure redistribution surfaces are a mainstay of prevention and treatment for pressure injuries. Unfortunately, insurance plans will pay for these devices only when a pressure injury is present. Many hospitals and healthcare facilities have purchased pressure redistribution surfaces on their own as part of their prevention protocols, however, in spite of the lack of insurance coverage.

◆◆ **Despite the use of a pressure redistribution system, patients will still need to be turned and repositioned if they cannot do so themselves.**

There are numerous different surfaces, ranging from gel mattress and overlays to low-air-loss and air-fluidized mattress systems. Clinicians will need to become familiar with the types of mattresses and features available within their healthcare system or refer the patient to a wound care specialist to obtain the appropriate device. Only a few high-quality randomized controlled trials have been done, however, and the question remains unanswered as to whether powered versus nonpowered mattresses are best for prevention or treatment.[15,18]

The other element of pressure redistribution is seating cushions because patients who spend many hours in a wheelchair, gerichair, Broda chair, or a regular chair at home are at risk for skin breakdown. The provider needs to take a thorough history and ask about decreasing mobility, especially in older patients with worsening musculoskeletal disorders, cardiac/pulmonary disorders, or dementia. The patient should have a cushion to prevent skin breakdown at the coccyx and ischial tuberosities. Again, there are many varieties of pressure redistribution cushions, and referral to a physical therapist or physiatrist for determination of the most appropriate type is warranted.

# Evaluation, Staging, and Documentation of Pressure Injuries

## Assessment and Documentation

There are a multitude of assessment frameworks available for wounds in general and pressure injuries in particular. Before assessing the pressure injury, the provider must thoroughly cleanse the wound of any excess drainage or wound care product. The key components to each assessment and documentation should include the following:

- Measurement—Traditional measurement is done with a paper ruler to measure length and width, along with a cotton-tipped applicator to measure the depth of the wound bed. However, this may result in poor inter- and intrarater reliability. There are various software programs available for measuring the wound bed based on digital imaging alone or in conjunction with projected laser beams, but budgetary constraints may preclude PCPs from using these systems.
- Appearance—Describe the wound location accurately. Location can be key to what is causing the pressure. For instance, sitting tends to cause ischial and coccyx pressure injuries, whereas lying down causes heel and sacrum pressure injuries. Pressure injuries on the earlobes tend to be from oxygen tubing or glasses. The provider should describe the borders (surrounding erythema or maceration) and the edge (well demarcated, or erosive/evolving, undermining). Undermining may be evidence of shear/friction forces. Describe the wound bed and percentage of presence of necrotic slough (wet, stringy tissue), necrotic eschar (dry yellow/brown/black tissue), or granulation tissue. Does the wound bed bleed easily, meaning it is friable? Is there scant, moderate, or heavy drainage, as evidenced by the dressing? What color is the drainage? And is there odor—this is an important patient concern that should be addressed, because odor and drainage may be indication for patient isolation.
- Photo documentation—This is becoming increasingly popular, and family members may also document wounds with cellular or other portable devices. If you choose to photograph pressure injuries in your clinic or facility, consultation with nursing and risk management representatives is important to develop a policy regarding written consent (if considered necessary), record-keeping, and storage.[19]

When documenting the incidence of a pressure injury, the physician must also document whether the patient is in the midst of severe illness or has significant comorbidities that would reduce the tissue tolerance to any pressure.[20] Determining the exact cause of the pressure injury is important in formulating a care plan. If the cause cannot be reversed, then the wound will not heal.

**❖❖ Patients' medical status will impact their risk for development of a wound, as well as their ability to heal.**

In addition, the clinician should estimate if the underlying causal process is reversible. This is done by carefully reviewing the care plan in collaboration with the family and direct care providers. For example, if a patient with end-stage Alzheimer disease has progressed to where he or she is no longer eating or drinking,

then despite all repositioning efforts the skin may still break down. These wounds may not have the potential to heal, and this should be clearly stated to the family and documented. The primary goal should be one of comfort and infection prevention, if possible.

## Staging

The most widely used staging system for pressure injuries is the one created by the National Pressure Ulcer Advisory Panel (NPUAP).[16] The stages are based on the degree of tissue damage (Fig. 30.1).

- **Stage 1**: Nonblanchable erythema of intact skin. The key to this definition is that the skin is intact. If there is any break in the surface of the skin, it is no longer stage 1. A physical examination of high-risk patients must include a tactile assessment of the skin because the stage 1 pressure injury may be tender and indurated. Special attention must be paid to dark-skinned individuals. In darker pigmented patients, the presence of nonblanchable erythema may not be as prominent, but the patient may have skin areas that are warmer, cooler, tender, firm, or boggy, indicating an area of stage 1 damage
- **Stage 2**: Partial-thickness skin loss with exposed dermis. May also present as an intact or open/ruptured serum-filled blister. A stage 2 pressure injury is superficial, and the wound bed is viable, pink or red, and moist. There is no granulation tissue, slough, or eschar within the wound bed. If a blister is present, it is filled with clear fluid. If the blister is filled with blood, it is not a stage 2. A wound is also not identified as a stage 2 if the site is a skin tear, tape burn, moisture-associated skin damage, or excoriation.
- **Stage 3**: Full-thickness skin loss. Subcutaneous fat may be visible but bone, tendon, or muscle is not exposed. Slough may be present but does not obscure the depth of tissue loss. May include undermining and tunneling. The depth of a stage 3 pressure injury will vary by the anatomic location. On the nose or ankle, where there is little subcutaneous tissue, a stage 3 may be very shallow. In an area, such as the buttock, a stage 3 may be very deep but still be in the subcutaneous tissue.
- **Stage 4**: Full thickness skin and tissue loss. Exposed or directly palpable fascia, muscle, tendon, ligament, cartilage, or bone are present. Slough or eschar may be present on some parts of the wound bed. Often includes tunneling and undermining.
- **Unstageable**: Obscured full-thickness skin and tissue loss. The extent of tissue damage cannot be confirmed, as the wound bed is covered by slough (yellow, tan, gray, green, or brown) and/or eschar (tan, brown, or black). The depth is unknown, however, if the necrotic tissue is removed, a stage 3 or 4 pressure injury will be exposed. This appearance often occurs after a deep tissue injury has evolved or if a pressure injury has progressed in the setting of continued pressure, friction/shear, and moisture forces.
- **Deep tissue injury**: Persistent nonblanchable deep red, maroon, or purple discoloration. Localized area of discolored intact skin or blood-filled blister resulting from damage of underlying soft tissue from pressure and/or shear. Sometimes with offloading these lesions will disappear. However, the provider must be aware that the wound could progress in a matter of days to weeks to full-thickness skin and tissue loss.

- **Figure 30.1** Staging of pressure ulcers. **A**, Normal skin, showing layers. **B**, Stage 1—redness without a break in the skin. **C**, Stage 2—superficial, confined to skin (can include dermis). **D**, Stage 3—penetrating into the subdermal tissues. **E**, Stage 4—down to the bone. **F**, Photograph of an unstageable pressure injury—one whose base is covered by necrotic material. (From National Pressure Ulcer Advisory Panel; photographs copyright Drs. Garcia and White-Chu. With permission.)

The provider should prepare family and support staff of this possibility, emphasizing that although the damage may have been done, efforts regarding offloading and care for the individual can be put into place.

An important aspect of pressure injury staging is that once a pressure injury is staged at a higher level of skin damage, the wound cannot then be backstaged. For example, if a wound is found to be involving muscle and tendon, it is a stage 4. If a month later, with good treatment, the wound is covered in granulation tissue, it is still a healing stage 4. Once closed, it is a healed stage 4.

Appropriate staging of the pressure injury is important, not only for care of the patient, but because reimbursement for many support surfaces and modalities is dependent on the staging of the pressure injury. There is also the issue of litigation. Appropriate documentation of wounds is an important piece in preventing and defending lawsuits associated with pressure injuries. Depending on the severity of the wound and whether infection is present, the wound can be reassessed every 2 to 4 weeks.

---

**CASE 1**

**Discussion**

In Mr. Maloney's case, the pressure ulcer would be a stage 2 pressure injury.

---

**CASE 2**

**Discussion**

In Mrs. Curry's case, the wound would be considered unstageable.

---

## Treatment Strategies

For wounds where the underlying cause is reversible and thus healable, treatment strategies need to be put in place quickly and effectively that will promote healing and prevent further progress of skin damage. Note that what the physician does with the wound locally is not nearly as important as reversing underlying conditions that are causing or worsening the wound. These include, as has been noted previously, managing underlying medical conditions, optimizing nutrition, and controlling fecal and urinary incontinence.

As also noted previously, comorbid conditions, such as uncontrolled diabetes mellitus, hypertension, congestive heart failure, malignancy, and inflammatory disorders, will put greater demands on the body and affect the functioning of cell lines critical to wound healing. The clinician should therefore make every effort to optimize each condition. These factors also will have impact on the clinician's estimate of the wound's prognosis for healing.

Nutrition is critical. Many geriatric patients are nutritionally compromised for multiple reasons, including dentition, anorexia-inducing medications, depression, lack of access to tasty and nutritious food, or other underlying comorbidities. A nutrition consult, where available, should be done early in the course of treatment to maximize protein and fluid intake. The NPUAP recommends intake of 30 to 35 kcal/kg body weight daily for adults at risk of a pressure injury or who currently have a pressure injury who are assessed as being at risk of malnutrition. They also recommend high-calorie, high-protein nutritional supplements if the nutritional requirements cannot be achieved with dietary intake alone.[16] Another multicenter randomized controlled blinded trial looked at providing supplementation with an enriched formula of arginine, zinc, and antioxidants versus supplementation alone to those patients in long-term care with stage 2 or higher pressure injuries. The study found that there was a significant reduction in pressure injury area over the 8-week course.[21] This study needs to be reproduced but raises the question of additional supplementation over and above the standard calorie and protein recommendations.

Management of incontinence is important to keep fecal and urinary contamination to a minimum. In an outpatient setting, a Foley catheter or fecal containment system is not optimal because of patient discomfort and risk of infection. However, if the healthcare team is unable to manage the incontinence and it is leading to skin breakdown, temporary use of these devices is sometimes needed. If the level of skin breakdown is advanced (stage $\geq 3$), and the provider is unable to contain fecal contamination, consideration may need to be given to a diverting colostomy until the patient is healed.

### Pressure Offloading

As previously stated, turning and repositioning of patients who cannot reposition themselves is essential for alleviating pressure. Small shifts in weight and use of positioning devices, such as pillows, can be very effective in offloading a bony prominence. The most appropriate pressure redistribution system(s) for the patient should be implemented promptly, taking into consideration comfort and cost (Table 30.3). It is important to note that despite the use of a pressure redistribution system, patients will still need to be turned and repositioned if they cannot do so themselves.

### Necrotic Tissue

Necrotic tissue in the wound must be debrided. This tissue contains a high bacterial load and can lead to further breakdown of the surrounding tissue. Debridement methods include mechanical debridement, sharp debridement, enzymatic debridement, biologic debridement, and autolytic debridement; Table 30.4 summarizes key aspects of each method. Conservative debridement, meaning debridement of only the necrotic tissue and not to the point of causing bleeding tissue, is indicated in almost every wound regardless of its potential to heal. The debridement reduces the bacterial burden in the wound and fosters granulation tissue formation. A large retrospective analysis of over 150,000 patients in wound centers found that more frequent sharp debridements led to swifter healing.[22] Theories include reduction of bacterial burden or biofilm removal as to why the wounds heal faster.

Depending on the clinical environment and the extent of tissue necrosis, referral to a surgeon may be necessary for debridement. Factors that may affect the need for surgical referral include the following: the physician's comfort level with debridement, the patient's pain level, the extent of necrosis, the underlying goals of care (i.e., cure vs. comfort care), the patient's ability to tolerate a surgical procedure, and use of anticoagulants.

### Provision of Moist Wound Healing

Once the wound is cleared of necrotic tissue, the goal of therapy is to achieve moisture balance and moist wound healing. If the wound has a lot of drainage, a dressing should be chosen that absorbs drainage, such as an alginate or foam. If the wound bed is dry, a dressing, such as a film, hydrocolloid, or hydrogel can be used. The choice of dressing will depend on the care setting and the wound characteristics. There are more than 2000 wound care products on the market. Collaborating with nursing staff can help the PCP to determine the best local wound care dressing.

### Diagnosing and Managing Infection

Infection continues to be a challenge in the care of patients with open wounds. There are different levels of bacterial invasion into wounds, and the majority of wounds do not require the use of

**TABLE 30.3 Support Surface Recommendations for Pressure Injury Prevention and Treatment**

| Type | Indications[a] | How it Works | Cost | Level of Evidence[b] |
|---|---|---|---|---|
| Nonpowered specialized mattress or overlay (filled with gel, foam, or combination) | Prevention to stage 2 | Redistributes pressure at bony prominences | $–$$ Medicare Group 1 support surface | Prevention—A (better than standard mattress) Treatment—Has not been studied against standard mattress |
| Low-air-loss mattress or overlay | Stage 3 or higher | Air sacs allow warmed air to pass through | $$$$ Static air mattress: Medicare Group 1 support surface Powered air mattress: Medicare Group 2 support surface | Prevention—B (no better than nonpowered specialized) Treatment—B (no better than nonpowered specialized overlay) |
| Alternating pressurized mattress | Stage 3 or higher | Alternates between high and low pressures, thus reducing time at high pressure | $$$$ Medicare Group 2 support surface | Prevention—B (no better than nonpowered specialized) Treatment—A (no better than nonpowered specialized overlay) |
| Air-fluidized mattress | Stage 3 or higher | Silicone-coated beads liquefy when air passes through them | $$$$$ Medicare Group 3 support surface | Prevention—B (no better than nonpowered specialized) Treatment—B (better when compared to alternating pressured mattress covered with foam) |
| Rotating bed | Critical illness | Bed rotates lateral for pulmonary toileting; not intended to replace turning and repositioning | $$$$$ | Prevention—X (no better than standard hospital or ICU beds) Treatment—D (expert opinion) |
| Specialized wheelchair cushion (foam, gel, air, or combination) | Prevention to stage 4 | Redistributes pressure at bony prominences | $–$$$ | Prevention—A (if combination gel/foam) Treatment—D (expert opinion) |

*ICU*, Intensive care unit.

[a]The National Pressure Ulcer Advisory Panel guidelines and other guidelines do not recommend a particular support surface for a particular stage of pressure ulcer. The indications listed here are regarding typical use of these surfaces.

[b]A = supported by one or more high-quality randomized controlled trials (RCTs); B = supported by one or more high quality nonrandomized cohort studies or low-quality RCTs; C = supported by one or more case series and/or poor-quality cohort and/or case-control studies; D = supported by expert opinion and/or extrapolation from studies in other populations or settings; X = evidence supports the treatment being ineffective or harmful.

**TABLE 30.4 Methods of Debridement for Pressure Injuries**

| Type of Debridement | Examples | Advantages | Disadvantages |
|---|---|---|---|
| Sharp debridement | • Scalpel, scissor, curette | • Fast<br>• Selective | • Requires expertise<br>• Level of comfort of practitioner<br>• Availability of equipment<br>• Painful |
| Autolytic debridement | • Manuka honey<br>• Hydrocolloid<br>• Hydrogel<br>• Film | • Painless<br>• Does not require expertise | • Slower acting |
| Enzymatic debridement | • Collagenase | • Selective<br>• Does not require expertise | • Slow acting<br>• Availability<br>• Cost |
| Mechanical debridement | • Wet-to-dry<br>• Pulsatile lavage<br>• Whirlpool | • Easily accessible<br>• Does not require expertise (except pulsatile lavage) | • Nonselective<br>• Painful<br>• Infection control problems can occur |
| Biologic debridement | • Maggot therapy | • Very selective | • "Ick" factor<br>• Often unavailable |

systemic antibiotics. The levels of bacteria in the wound can be classified as follows:

- *Colonization.* All wounds are colonized because bacteria live on our skin and in the environment. Colonization describes a bacterial level that is not affecting wound healing. Topical antiseptics or antimicrobials can effectively decrease bacterial load in the wound bed, and should be used whenever the clinician suspects that colonization is preventing healing. Systemic antibiotics are not indicated.
- *Superficial infection.* The bacteria are now at a concentration that is negatively impacting wound healing. The wound may appear clean but is not progressing toward healing. There may be increased drainage or odor. Aggressive local care (debridement and topical antimicrobials) is indicated. There are multiple dressings that can be used, including cadexomer iodine, Manuka honey, or ionized silver products. Dressings such as Dakin's, clorpactin, or betadine can be used for a very short time to decrease bacterial load in the wound bed, but long-term use of these products can impair wound healing.
- Cellulitis. Bacteria have now invaded the soft tissue and are causing the classic signs and symptoms of soft tissue infection, which may include erythema, pain, increased drainage, odor, fever, or elevated white count. For these patients, systemic antibiotics plus aggressive topical treatment are indicated.

## Summary

Pressure injuries are primarily caused by pressure, but poor nutrition and devices such as tubing and catheters also play a role. Most injuries occur beneath the waist and are associated with prolonged time in bed or chair. Treatment depends on stage and location, but includes pressure relief, local agents to promote healing, and debridement (enyzmatic or sharp). Remember that the "hole" is part of the "whole" patient and that pressure injury prevention and treatment requires a comprehensive, interdisciplinary approach.

### Web Resources

National Pressure Ulcer Advisory Panel website with photos, staging guide and pressure injury white papers, position statements, as well as a searchable database on pressure injury—related research: www.npuap.org.

Association for the Advancement of Wound Care's pressure injury prevention and treatment quick reference guide: http://aawconline.org/wp-content/uploads/2011/09/AAWCPU-Qwik-Ref-Final-23Sep11.pdf.

This National Database of Nursing Quality Indicators website has modules on pressure injury education. It was developed for nurses but is a great resource for all clinicians: https://www.nursingquality.org/NDNQIPressureUlcerTraining/default.aspx.

## Key References

11. Black JM, Edsberg LE, Baharestani MM, et al. Pressure ulcers: avoidable or unavoidable? Results of the National Pressure Ulcer Advisory Panel Consensus Conference. *Ostomy Wound Manage.* 2011;52:24—37.
13. Moore ZE, Cowman S. Risk assessment tools for the prevention of pressure ulcers. *Cochrane Database Syst Rev.* 2008;CD006471.
15. Reddy M, Gill S, Rochon P. Preventing pressure ulcers: a systematic review. *JAMA.* 2006;974—984.
16. National Pressure Ulcer Advisory Panel, European Pressure Ulcer Advisory Panel and Pan Pacific Pressure Injury Alliance. In: Emily H, ed. *Prevention and Treatment of Pressure Ulcers: Quick Reference Guide.* Osborne Park, Western Australia: Cambridge Media; 2014.
18. McInnes E, Bell-Syer SEM, Dumville JC, et al. Support surfaces for pressure ulcer prevention. *Cochrane Database Syst Rev.* 2008;4:CD001735.

**References available online at** expertconsult.com.

# 31

# Sleep Disorders in Older Individuals

STEPHEN J. BONASERA

## OUTLINE

*Additional online-only material indicated by icon.*

## OBJECTIVES

*Upon completion of this chapter, the reader will be able to:*

- Describe the molecular, cellular, anatomic, and physiologic aspects of sleep, and to describe the diagnostic criteria, pathophysiology, and treatment rationale for various sleep disorders.
- Differentiate different sleep disorders (e.g., circadian rhythm disorders vs. sleep-related breathing disorders vs. sleep-related movement disorders vs. parasomnias vs. primary insomnias vs. hypersomnias) by biologic and clinical characteristics.

- Identify aspects of history, validated questionnaire assessment tools, physical examination findings, and appropriate laboratory and physiologic testing required for diagnosis of sleep disorders.
- Know current, evidence-supported treatment options for patients with sleep disorders.
- Recognize public health consequences of sleep disorders.

## Introduction

Sleep is a highly familiar behavior that occurs in a wide range of multicellular organisms that have neurons. However, why organisms need to sleep, as well as the underlying neuronal organization that produces sleep, remains poorly understood.[1,2] Current research suggests that sleep fulfills many functions critical for life. These functions include immune defense against pathogens,[3,4] energy conservation,[5,6] restoration of brain energy stores,[7] maintenance of appropriate brain water volume and osmotic pressure[8] ("glymphatic" function), reversing cognitive and behavioral performance impairments that occur with prolonged periods of wakefulness,[9] and supporting neuronal synaptic plasticity and learning.[10] Maintaining appropriate sleep function is thus an important component of supporting healthy patient lifestyles.

## Older Adults Experience a High Incidence and Prevalence of Sleep Complaints

### CASE 1

**A 67-year-old woman**

A patient is a 67-year-old woman who reports a 3-month history of very vivid dreams. Her partner reports frequent vocalizations and significant leg and arm movements during sleep. For example, on one occasion, she poured a full pitcher of water over her partner's head while he slept; upon awakening, she reported a dream where she was watering a window box outside of their home. The patient was in otherwise excellent health, only requiring levothyroxine 0.1 mg qd for a longstanding diagnosis of hypothyroidism. She maintained a highly active lifestyle and often went on hiking excursions in the mountains surrounding her home.

## CASE 2

### A 77-year-old male

Patient is a 77-year-old retired veteran who comes for evaluation of difficulty falling asleep. He tries to maintain regular bed and rise times, and he avoids daytime naps and caffeine after 3 PM. He rarely uses alcohol and currently smokes about five cigarettes a day. He tells you that almost immediately after he lays down in bed to sleep, he begins to experience a difficult-to-describe, "almost burning" sensation in both of his legs from midcalf to his foot, with a concomitant urge to move his legs. This sensation almost immediately resolves when he gets out of bed and "stretches his legs." He alternates between laying down (and experiencing these sensations) and getting up for hours before the discomfort has faded enough for him to sleep. Because of these sensations, he usually sleeps while seated on the couch, and rarely uses the bed. His symptoms are not as bothersome during the day compared with night.

## CASE 3

### An 81-year-old male

Patient is an 81-year-old retired veteran referred for home-based primary care. His medical history is significant for severe chronic obstructive pulmonary disease (COPD) requiring baseline 3 to 4 L/min $O_2$ by nasal cannula, posttraumatic stress disorder, low back pain, hypertension, depression, and mild cognitive impairment. He requires significant assistance for all housework and some stand-by help when bathing, but continues to drive and do his own shopping. He tells clinic staff upon enrollment that he usually slept in his reclining chair at night, but did not sleep well and did not feel refreshed upon awakening in the morning. His caregivers reported that he often took daytime naps and snored loudly. He had deferred using continuous positive airway pressure (CPAP) in the past, telling his then primary care physician that he could not fall asleep while wearing the mask. His medications include albuterol, tiotropium, budesonide/formoterol, nortriptyline, clonazepam, baby aspirin, lisinopril, and metoprolol.

For each of the three cases described earlier:

1. What clues from the history indicate the presence of a specific underlying sleep disorder?
2. What are key points to be gathered from additional history, examination, and diagnostic testing?

Older adults often complain of poor sleep. Specific issues include insomnia (difficulty initiating and/or maintaining sleep), early morning awakenings, not feeling rested after sleep, daytime sleepiness, restless legs, periodic limb movements, snoring, and apneas. Some of these symptoms, such as periodic limb movements, snoring, and apneas, may be more apparent to the sleep partner than the patient. Many of these sleep complaints directly arise from chronic disease burden, including obesity, depression, pain, arthritis, stroke, diabetes, and cardiopulmonary disease.[11,12] Insomnia complaints in healthy older adults (with rigorous exclusion of individuals with chronic health disorders) range between 1% and 3%.[13] Recent estimates of insomnia prevalence in White and Black community-dwelling adults age $\geq$ 55 years were 36% and 12% in men, respectively, and 54% and 19% in women,

respectively.[14,15] Overall, insomnia prevalence is higher in older women compared with men.[16] In a 3-year longitudinal study of insomnia in older adults, 54% of persons with sleep complaints reported symptom remission; however, 27% of these individuals relapsed during the study period.[17] The incidence of sleep complaints in older adults previously reporting no sleep issues has been estimated at 5% to 15% per year.[11,18] Of note, 35% of persons reporting insomnia have a family history positive for insomnia, highlighting the genetic risks for illnesses contributing to both primary and secondary insomnia.[19] By itself, insomnia does not appear to influence overall mortality[20,21]; rather, it reflects mortality risks from underlying chronic conditions.[22–24] However, review of extant literature suggests that insomnia decreases health-related quality of life (HRQoL) in older individuals and that insomnia treatment can improve HRQoL.[25] In summary, these epidemiologic studies suggest that sleep problems are common in older adults (and particularly in older women), decrease quality of life, but do not increase the risk of mortality beyond the baseline risk(s) of the chronic illnesses that contribute to sleep problems.

## Sleep Stages and Their Temporal Ordering

At the simplest level, sleep can be defined as a reversible state of individual unresponsiveness to internal and external environmental stimuli. This state of unresponsiveness can itself be further classified into two distinct states: rapid eye movement (REM) and non-REM (NREM) sleep. NREM sleep is identified by electroencephalogram (EEG), and characteristically shows synchronized wave activity, sleep spindles, K-complexes, and high-voltage slow waves. Persons in NREM sleep do not display significant mental activity, and when awakened do not report dreams. NREM sleep is further classified into four stages (stage I through stage IV), reflecting progressively higher stimulus thresholds required for awakening.

By contrast, REM sleep is characterized by the occurrence of namesake rapid eye movement, as well as muscle atonia, periodic muscle twitching, and slight respiratory irregularities. In contradistinction to NREM sleep, the EEGs of individuals in REM sleep are highly desynchronized and resemble EEG tracings from awake individuals. Persons waking from REM sleep frequently report experiencing dreams.

Sleeping individuals progress through these cycles in a predictable manner (Fig. 31.1). An individual going to sleep progresses from wakefulness to stage I NREM sleep. Over the next 70 to 80 minutes, the EEG will progressively exhibit features of stage II NREM sleep, stage III NREM sleep, and stage IV NREM sleep. The first bout of REM sleep usually occurs 80 to 90 min from the start of stage I NREM sleep, and is relatively short in duration (5–10 min). For the remainder of the sleep period, individuals cycle between periods of NREM and REM sleep, with REM sleep accounting for a greater percentage of time as the sleep period progresses.

## Aging and Quantitative Measures of Sleep

The National Sleep Foundation has published guidelines for the appropriate amount of sleep for individuals of different age.[26] These guidelines state that adults age $\geq$ 65 years are recommended to have between 7 and 8 hours of sleep per day, and they are advised against having either less than 5 or more than 9 hours of sleep per day. Published metaanalyses of sleep parameters across the age spectrum[27] suggest that total sleep time, sleep latency,

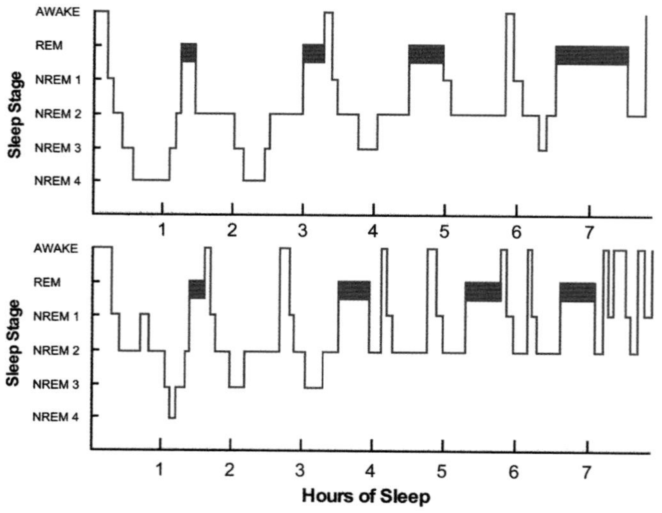

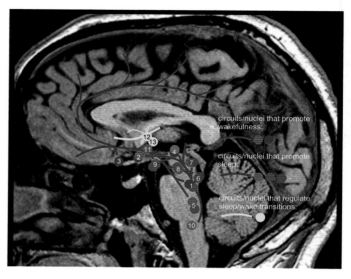

• **Figure 31.1** Exemplar hypnograms demonstrating sleep stage transitions in a young *(top)* and older *(bottom)* adult. Note that total duration of deepest sleep and rapid eye movement (REM) phase sleep decrease with aging, whereas total number of nighttime awakenings increase with age. Sleep fragmentation is an expected concomitant of aging.

• **Figure 31.2** Neuroanatomy of central nervous system (CNS) circuits promoting wakefulness and sleep. *Red lines* depict connectivity within CNS regions promoting wakefulness. *Red circles* depict critical components of this wakefulness circuit. *Maroon circles* depict regions that sculpt wakefulness behavior. *Blue lines* depict connectivity within CNS regions promoting sleep. *Violet circles* depict nuclei that promote sleep. *Purple circles* depict nuclei that broadly inhibit regions that promote wakefulness. *Blue circles* depict nuclei that locally inhibit neurons that promote wakefulness. *Yellow circles* depict nuclei forming the lateral hypothalamic "switch" that regulates transitions between wakefulness and sleep. Numbered nuclei/regions as follows: 1. parabrachial, pedunculopontine nuclei. 2. supramammillary nucleus. 3. basal forebrain. 4. periaqueductal grey matter. 5. locus ceruleus. 6. pedunculopontine nucleus. 7. lateraldorsal tegmental nucleus. 8. dorsal raphé nucleus. 9. tuberomammillary nucleus. 10. parafacial zone. 11. ventrolateral, median preoptic nuclei. 12. orexinergic neurons. 13. melanin-concentrating hormone neurons. Saper CB, Fuller PM. Wake-sleep circuitry: an overview. *Current opinion in neurobiology.* 2017;44:186−192.

duration of stage I to IV NREM sleep, percentage of REM sleep, and REM latency remain stable in older adults (albeit significantly different from younger adults). Older adults may have longer latencies to stage IV NREM sleep as well as less overall stage IV NREM sleep.

## Cellular and Neurophysiologic Clocks

The need to synchronize metabolism and behaviors to circadian cycles that predictably vary with season of the year has led to the evolution of multiple cellular clocks containing a wide variety of molecular components. In fact, recent studies suggest that critical biologic processes, including cellular ribonucleic acid (RNA) transcription, protein expression, and protein clearance, all vary on a circadian basis.[28−30] Circadian rhythms are sculpted by molecular mechanisms capable of timekeeping[31−33] and entraining the intrinsic period to light[34] and food availability cues.[35] Aging has distinctive effects on the human circadian clock, including an overall attenuation of circadian rhythmicity, altered intrinsic circadian periodicity, and blunted circadian entrainment through light and food cues.[36−39] These age-associated changes in circadian rhythmicity impact sleep function and may elevate the risks of metabolic syndrome,[40] inflammation,[41] and cancer.[42]

## CNS Anatomic and Neurophysiologic Substrates for Sleep

To understand how different pathologies might affect human sleep function, it is important to review the anatomy and physiology of brain systems involved in sleep production. Electrical activity resembling sleep can be observed in even relatively small neuronal ensembles.[43] However, human sleep behavior arises from the activity of multiple separate but interconnected brain regions spanning the basal forebrain to medulla (Fig. 31.2). Furthermore, these areas

can be broadly classified as systems that promote arousal and wakefulness, systems that promote sleep, and systems that control wake-to-sleep transitions.

Basal forebrain gammaaminobutyric acid (GABA)ergic neurons (defined by parvalbumin expression) are significant drivers of high-frequency cortical EEG activity closely associated with an awake state.[44] These basal forebrain neurons respond to internal environmental conditions, including hypoxia, hypercapnia, visceral stimuli, and pain.[45,46] In a parallel manner, GABAergic neurons and glutamatergic nuclei from multiple brain regions participate in maintenance of sleep and transitions between various sleep stages, including REM sleep. In the lateral hypothalamus, discrete populations of neurons expressing either orexin (aka hypocretin) or melanin-concentrating hormone (MCH) form a "switch" that controls transitions from wakefulness to sleep, or vice versa.[47−50]

As the earlier brief descriptions suggest, sleep regulation is a highly complex process requiring multiple central nervous system (CNS) regions spanning the basal forebrain, midbrain, pons, and medulla. Neurons that organize sleeping behaviors use multiple neurotransmitter systems, including glutamate, GABA, acetylcholine, histamine, galanin, orexin, and MCH. It is thus not surprising that sleep is exquisitely sensitive to lesions that may impact these CNS areas, or drugs whose actions may activate or inhibit the aforementioned neurotransmitter systems.

# Clinical Evaluation of Sleep Disorders in Older Adults

## CASE 1

### A 67-year-old woman

On examination, she has normal vital signs, is right-handed, and has an otherwise unremarkable physical examination. Laboratory studies, including a complete blood count, basic metabolic panel, and thyroid stimulating hormone (TSH), were all within established limits.

## CASE 2

### A 77-year-old male

On examination, the patient had normal vital signs and an unremarkable physical examination. Laboratory studies, including a complete blood count, basic metabolic panel, and
   TSH, were all within established limits. Serum ferritin was 18 ng/mL; hematocrit was 40%.

## CASE 3

### An 81-year-old male

On examination, the patient was a thin, frail-appearing gentleman noted to have bilateral temporal wasting. His vital signs included a blood pressure of 172/91 mmHg, pulse 78 beats per minute, respiratory rate 24 breaths/min saturating at 93% on $O_2$ 4 L/min by nasal cannula. Walking him about 50 feet around his home led to immediate desaturation on pulse oximetry to 85%. Chest auscultation demonstrated a marked decrease in air movement throughout all lung fields, with soft, monophonic wheezes present after exercise. He had 1 + pitting edema at both ankles. Metabolic panel revealed Na 139, K 3.2, Cl 99, $HCO_3^-$ 33, blood urea nitrogen (BUN) 22, creatinine 0.8. Posteroanterior (PA) and lateral chest x-rays revealed hyperinflation with prominence of lung apices and sharp diaphragmatic boundaries.
   For each of the three cases described earlier:
1. How does the information provided help in diagnosing the sleep disorder?
2. Would you order a polysomnogram in these patients? Why or why not?
3. What is the next step in helping treat the underlying disorder?

Evaluation of persons with sleep disorders entails obtaining a detailed and relevant history, physical exam, and relevant laboratory data. History should be obtained from the patient and sleep partner, and focus on sleep complaints (e.g., difficulty initiating/maintaining sleep, early-morning awakening, not feeling rested, restless legs, periodic limb movements, snoring, apneas), sleep hygiene (per Box 31.1), daytime impact (presence of daytime sleepiness, fatigue, exhaustion, poor energy, irritability, poor concentration, poor work performance), changes in sleep function (if present), and patient goals/preferences. Review of systems should focus on sleep complaints, as well as psychiatric comorbidities that may manifest as a sleep disruption (e.g., bipolar affective disorder) as well as medical conditions that may contribute to insomnia (Box 31.2). Medication review is critical, and focused on both medications known to disrupt sleep function (Box 31.3) and alcohol, caffeinated beverages, and similar "energy" drinks. Social history should focus

### • BOX 31.1    Recommended Sleep Hygiene Habits and Practices

Engage in at least 20 min per day of low-intensity exercise
Exposure yourself to natural light during the day, preferably in the afternoon
Limit screen time on television, computer, phone, etc.
Keep a regular bedtime, and follow a bedtime routine
Make sure the bedroom is dark, cool, and free of disturbing sounds
The bed is for sleeping and sex
Get out of bed if you can't fall asleep
Avoid caffeine, nicotine, and other stimulants after dinner
Limit fluid intake after 6:00 PM if you have to awaken more than twice a night to urinate
Avoid foods that may be disruptive before sleep
Avoid naps. If you do nap, keep total daily nap duration to less than 30 min per day

### • BOX 31.2    Medical Conditions That May Contribute to Insomnia

Neurologic: neurodegenerative disease (Alzheimer disease, Parkinson disease, frontotemporal dementia, etc.), cerebrovascular disease and stroke, demyelinating disease, neuropathy, chronic pain, chronic headache syndrome, traumatic brain injury, elevated intracranial pressure, seizure disorder
Cardiovascular: congestive heart failure, angina, supraventricular arrhythmias
Pulmonary: obstructive lung disease, restrictive lung disease, parenchymal disease
GI: peptic ulcer disease, GERD, inflammatory bowel disease, motility disorders, diverticulitis, biliary tract stones/disease
Endocrine: hyperthyroidism, hypothyroidism, hypercortisolism, hypocortisolism, h/o operative or radiation treatment to the pituitary gland, diabetes
GU: BPH, urinary incontinence, cystitis, polyuria
Musculoskeletal: degenerative arthritis, autoimmune arthritis (rheumatoid, ankylosing spondylitis, psoriatic), fibromyalgia
ENT: rhinitis, sinusitis, bruxism, periodontal disease.

*BPH*, Benign prostatic hypertrophy; *GERD*, gastroesophageal reflux disease; *ENT*, ear, nose and throat; *GI*, gastrointestinal; *GU*, genitourinary.

on the presence of new acute stressors impacting the patient's life, such as new jobs, relationships, bereavement, or financial strains. Use of illicit drugs, including marijuana, cocaine, amphetamine, sedatives, or opiates, must also be assessed (Box 31.3).

The American Academy of Sleep Medicine recommends that in addition to performing the aforementioned historical assessment, that clinicians administer a validated questionnaire quantifying the specific sleep disorder. Currently there are instruments designed to measure insomnia (Insomnia Severity Index [ISI][51]), daytime sleepiness (Epworth Sleepiness Scale [ESS][52]), sleep quality (Pittsburgh Sleep Quality Index [PSQI][53–55]), sleep apnea (STOP-BANG[56,57]), and restless legs syndrome (International Restless Legs Scale [IRLS][58]). The American Thoracic Society maintains a curated website[59] with descriptions of these and additional tools for evaluating sleep disturbances. The American Academy of Sleep Medicine also maintains a central site for practice guidelines regarding sleep disorders.[60]

Patients undergoing evaluation for sleep disorders should also document their sleep symptoms in a sleep log for at least 14 days. An exemplar sleep log can be found at the National Sleep Foundation website.[61] Physical examination should focus on general body habitus, vital signs, and findings associated with airway

• BOX 31.3    Medications/Medication Classes That May Be Problematic in Patients With Sleep Disorders

Selective serotonin reuptake inhibitors (fluoxetine, paroxetine, sertraline, citalopram, escitalopram, vortioxetine)
Dopamine agonists (pramipexole, ropinirole, levodopa)
Sympathomimetics (methylphenidate, Adderall)
Cholinesterase inhibitors (donepezil, rivastigmine, galantamine)
Antihypertensives (alpha blockers, beta blockers, ACE inhibitors/ARBs, clonidine)
Beta agonists
Theophylline
Diuretics (both loop and thiazide type)
Antihistamines (both first and second generation)
Steroids
Statins (particularly if there is muscle involvement)
Chondroitin/glucosamine (particularly if there is GI intolerance)

*ACE*, Angiotensin-converting enzyme; *ARBs*, angiotensin-receptor blocker; *GI*, gastrointestinal.

patency, including evaluation of the nasal turbinates and septum, sinuses, jaw, oropharynx (including low lying soft palate, enlarged tonsils, Mallampati Class III or IV airway anatomy, enlarged tongue, retrognathia, micrognathia, and/or a steep mandibular angle), and neck ($>$ 17-inch collar size associated with increased risk of obstructive sleep apnea [OSA]). Laboratory assessment of sleep disorders should exclude metabolic abnormalities, measure thyroid function, and assess hemoglobin/hematocrit. For patients with vascular disease, magnetic resonance imaging (MRI) of the brain to evaluate white matter integrity and identify potential completed cerebrovascular accidents (particularly along the neuraxis spanning the basal forebrain to medulla) may be indicated.

Monitored polysomnography, where patient sleep function is observed overnight in a facility, remains the gold standard for assessment of many sleep disorders, particularly when a need to assess airway patency and airflow during sleep arises (Fig. 31.3). Before undergoing monitored polysomnography, patients are asked to continue their regular medications but otherwise avoid naps, strenuous exercise, or stimulants on the day of their sleep study. Polysomnography continuously monitors brain electrical activity (EEG), extraocular movements (electrooculogram), chin and leg muscle activity (electromyogram [EMG]), nasal and oral airflow, pulse oximetry, abdominal/chest movements, and cardiac activity (electrocardiogram). A segment of a polysomnogram displaying an episode of OSA is provided as Fig. 31.4. Criteria are well established to identify obstructive apnea, hypopnea, mixed apnea, central apnea, respiratory-effort related arousals, Cheyne-Stokes respiration, sleep-related hypoventilation, periodic limb movements, EEG arousals, and bruxism from the earlier data streams.[62] In certain situations (availability of appropriately trained personnel, including a board-certified sleep specialist, patient with high pretest probability of OSA, or patient unable to undergo monitored polysomnography), a home polysomnography evaluation may be sufficient to confirm the diagnosis of OSA at lower cost. Guidelines for portable sleep monitoring studies have been published.[63] Portable sleep studies are not indicated for individuals who may have confounding sleep disorders (such as central apneas), situations (such as in diagnosis of REM behavioral disorder) where NREM must be differentiated from REM sleep, nor screening of asymptomatic patients.

For some patients with excessive daytime sleepiness, specialized workup, including multiple sleep latency test (MSLT) and maintenance of wakefulness test (MWT) may be appropriate.[64] Diagnosis of circadian rhythm disorders and primary insomnias may be facilitated by actigraphy, a technique whereby subjects use sensors (worn around the wrist, ankle, or belt) containing a small triaxial accelerometer to measure subject resting and movement at high temporal precision ($\leq$1-minute resolution) for 1 week or longer periods of observation. Patients requiring these assessments are appropriately referred to specialists for further evaluation.

## Sleep Disorders of Older Adults

### Human Circadian Rhythm Sleep Disorders

As previously discussed, human circadian rhythm arises from intrinsic cellular molecular clock activity further shaped by CNS regions that sculpt the frequency and stability of transitions from inactive to active states, and vice versa. Diagnosis of human circadian rhythm sleep disorders requires obtaining an appropriate history and physical examination (including sleep diary), as well as at least 1 week of actigraphy assessment,[65] and assessment of endogenous physiologic circadian rhythms, including those of temperature and melatonin.[66] Clinicians also need to rule out potential confounding factors, including poor sleep hygiene, social or environmental factors, and relevant psychiatric disorders (including anxiety, depression, substance abuse, and psychotic disorders) (Box 31.4).

### Delayed Sleep-Wake Phase Disorder (International Classification of Diseases [ICD]-10 Code G47.21)

Persons with delayed sleep-wake phase disorder (DSWPD) are often described as "night owls." Typically, individuals have normal sleep patterns, but (depending upon severity) may fall asleep sometime between 1:00 and 6:00 AM and awaken from sleep between 10:00 AM and 2:00 PM. Whereas DSWPD is relatively common in younger adults, its prevalence in older adults ranges between 0.2% and 1.7%.[67] Investigators suspect that individuals with DSWPD have a specific mutation in genes that form the cellular circadian clock; however, at this time no specific gene products have been identified. DSWPD is often associated with depression,[68] with more significant circadian misalignment associated with poorer antidepressant response.[69] Exposure to bright natural spectrum light (2000−2500 lux) between 7 AM and 9 AM, as well as avoidance of bright light in the evening, will usually promote earlier sleep and wake times in persons with DSWPD.[70]

### Advanced Sleep-Wake Phase Disorder (ICD-10 Code G47.22)

Persons with advanced sleep-wake disorder (ASWPD) are often described as "morning larks." These individuals also have normal sleep patterns, but they develop significant sleepiness in late afternoon/early evening hours with awakening and full alertness in early-morning hours when most individuals are at their nadir of alertness. The prevalence of ASWPD in young to middle-aged adults ranges between 0.25% and 7%,[71] and increases in older adults because of age-related blunting of internal circadian rhythms and alterations in anatomy/physiology (such as cataracts[72]) that decrease responsiveness to environmental time cues. Of note, ASWPD is associated with polymorphisms in cellular circadian clock genes, including *PER1*, *PER2*, *PER3*, and *CSNK1D*. Bright light therapy (2000−2500 lux) administered for 1 to 3 hours when the patient begins experiencing sleepiness is the mainstay therapy.[73]

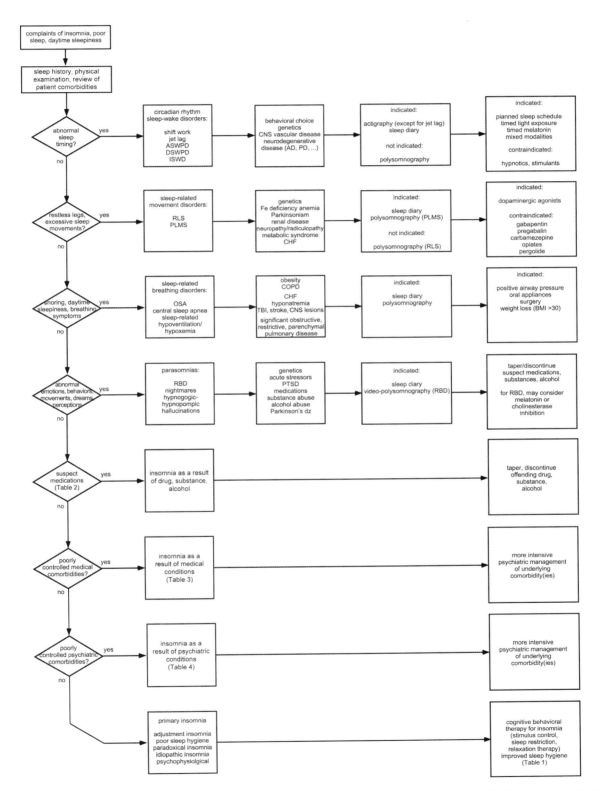

• **Figure 31.3** Flowchart for diagnosis, workup, and management of sleep disorders not characterized by hypersomnia. The first column depicts the flowchart that differentiates among specific sleep disorders, the second column delineates the specific family of sleep disorders associated with the target symptom, the third column notes risk factors associated with the chosen family of sleep disorders, the fourth column notes specific diagnostic modalities that may be required beyond a standard history/physical examination/lab studies, and the fifth column notes specific treatment indications and contraindications.

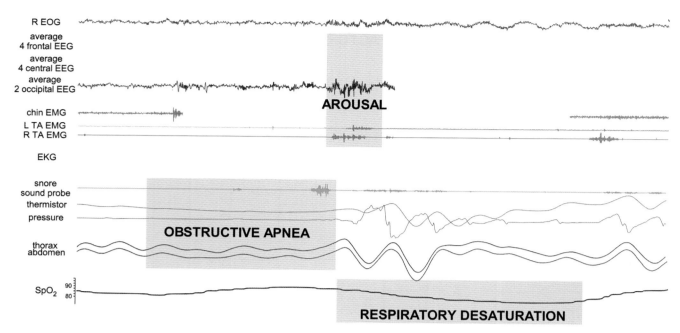

- **Figure 31.4** Polysomnography tracing from patient demonstrating an episode of obstructive sleep apnea. Traces depict (from top to bottom) extraocular movements (red), averages of frontal, central, and occipital electroencephalogram (*EEG*), 3 traces (*brown*), electromyograms for chin and left/right tibialis anterior, 3 traces (*orange*), electrocardiogram (*black*), snoring sound probe (*green*), thermistor and pressure transducer, 2 traces (*violet*), thorax and abdomen movement, 2 traces (*blue*), and SpO2 (*black*). Epochs demonstrating occurrence of airway obstruction, EEG arousal, and oxygen desaturation annotated on graph. *EKG, electrocardiogram; EOG, electrooculogram.*

---

**• BOX 31.4** **Psychiatric Conditions That May Contribute to Insomnia**

Substance-related and addictive disorders
  — Alcohol
  — Opioid
  — Sedative, hypnotic, anxiolytic
  — Stimulant
  — Caffeine
Anxiety disorders
Depressive disorders
Bipolar and related disorders
Obsessive-compulsive and related disorders
Trauma and stressor-related disorders (particularly posttraumatic stress disorder)
Somatic symptom and related disorders

---

## Irregular Sleep-Wake Disorder (ICD-10 Code G47.23)

Persons with irregular sleep-wake disorder (ISWD) have sleep characterized by naps of differing lengths occurring at irregular intervals throughout both day and night. This disorder is often comorbid with dementia from significant neurodegenerative and/or vascular brain disease, and its severity appears to track that of the underlying dementia.[74] Persons with ISWD often receive less exposure to important stimuli that entrain circadian rhythms, including bright light and physical activity.[75] Intrinsic 24-hour rhythms of body temperature may also be blunted or absent in persons with ISWD.[76] ISWD is often observed in residents of long-term care facilities, including assisted living and skilled nursing homes. Treatment is best focused on a multimodal program,

including activities to maintain alertness and wakefulness during the day, exposure to morning bright light, lowering the night-time soundscape volume, and evening fluid restriction to address nocturia. Programs focusing on these issues have been demonstrated to decrease nighttime wakefulness,[77–79] and by contrast, pharmacotherapy trials using melatonin were not found to be efficacious.[80]

◆◆ **Irregular sleep-wake phase disorder is highly prevalent in persons with dementia or stroke and those living in nursing home settings.**

◆◆ **Standard of care for irregular sleep-wake phase disorder includes increasing morning bright light, providing ample daytime opportunities for activity, and limiting night time fluids.**

◆◆ **Current evidence does not support pharmacotherapy as an appropriate treatment or adjunct for irregular sleep-wake phase disorder.**

## Other Circadian Rhythm Sleep Disorders

Jet lag is commonly associated with daytime fatigue, excessive sleepiness, insomnia, and early wakening. These symptoms usually occur after crossing two or more time zones (particularly eastbound), with more frequent travel, and older age. Steps to limit these symptoms include adjusting individual waking and sleeping hours to those of the destination over the days preceding the trip, bright light exposure (in early morning hours when traveling eastward; in evening hours when traveling westward), appropriate rest at the trip start, and providing ample opportunity to adjust to destination time schedule after arrival. Shift work disorder may impact older adults remaining in the workforce.[81] Finally, African sleeping sickness caused by *Trypanosoma brucei* may be considered in individuals with history of travel to sub-Saharan bush country.[82]

## Sleep-Related Breathing Disorders

Sleep-related breathing disorders (SRBDs) are among the most common sleep disorders encountered in older populations.[83] SRBDs may occur either as a result of peripheral (sleep-related problems in airway anatomy) or central (sleep-related dysfunction of respiratory pattern generation or respiratory neuronal output) causes. Regardless of cause, SRBDs lead to decreased ventilation during sleep. When severe enough, this decreased ventilation causes oxygen desaturation, leading to EEG changes associated with sleep-to-wake changes. SRBDs thus interfere with obtaining appropriate duration NREM and REM sleep on a nightly basis. Critically, SRBDs when untreated become significant risk factors for serious chronic comorbidities, including hypertension,[84] stroke,[85] insulin resistance,[86] heart failure,[87] major depression,[88] and cognitive impairment,[89,90] as well as motor vehicle accidents[91] and perceived occupational difficulties.[92]

### Obstructive Sleep Apnea (ICD-10 Code G47.33)

OSA is characterized by recurrent and reversible obstruction of the pharyngeal airway during sleep. With sleep onset, tone decreases in muscles that dilate the upper airway, causing a decrease in pharyngeal lumen area. Decreases in the diameter of the airway "pipe" in the setting of constant airflow lead to increased upper airway resistance. Persons who are awake compensate for increased upper airway resistance by increasing respiratory effort; however, persons who are asleep may not perceive changes in airway resistance.[93] Thus transitions from the awake to asleep state are often accompanied by airway narrowing or closure and consequent hypoventilation.

OSA is common in adults over 55 years of age, with a 24% prevalence of apnea/hypopnea index (AHI) of 5 or more and a 62% prevalence of respiratory disturbance index (RDI) of 10 or more[94] (see later for definitions of AHI and RDI). OSA is more common in men than women,[95] with incidence increasing as a function of age[96] and obesity. Regarding obesity, a weight gain of 10 kg over a 5-year period increased OSA risk by 5.2-fold in men and 2.5-fold in women[97]; furthermore, 43% of persons with body mass index (BMI) of $\geq 28$ kg/m$^2$ had comorbid OSA,[98] whereas > 85% of persons with a mean BMI of 52 kg/m$^2$ had comorbid OSA.[99] OSA further appears to have a strong hereditable component.[100,101]

Polysomnography is the gold standard for OSA testing and diagnosis. In this test, cessation of airflow for $\geq 10$ seconds with EMG-demonstrated myographic activity constitutes an obstructive apnea. A 30% reduction in airway flow over 10 seconds accompanied by a 4% or higher desaturation by pulse oximetry constitutes a hypopnea (an alternative criterion is a 50% reduction in airway flow over 10 seconds accompanied by either a $\geq 3\%$ desaturation or an arousal). A series of breaths with progressively increasing effort leading to an arousal constitutes a respiratory event—related arousal (RERA). Polysomnography studies are scored by determining the AHI, which is the sum of the total number of apneas and hypopneas, divided by total hours of sleep. Mild, moderate, and severe OSA are characterized by AHIs of 5 to 14, 15 to 29, and 30 or more, respectively.

Positive airway pressure (PAP) remains the standard treatment for OSA.[102] Current data support initiation of either continuous positive airway pressure (CPAP) or automatic positive airway pressure (APAP); the major difference between these two modalities is

that APAP may adjust pressures over time to compensate for acute or chronic changes in airway anatomy (medications, changes in body weight, etc.). Best practice suggests that patients should receive appropriate education before initiation of PAP. Components of these programs should include information educating patients regarding OSA and its health risks, and providing practical "troubleshooting" advice for overcoming common problems people first encounter when starting CPAP (wrong style/size mask, poor mask fit, finding comfortable position to sleep, dry nose/mouth, etc.). Machines capable of producing modified pressure PAP may also be better tolerated by patients. CPAP pressure should be at least 4 cm H$_2$O but not exceed 15 cm H$_2$O, with goal pressure set to avoid apneas.[103] Secondary goals include avoiding hypopneas and RERAs. Over 38 randomized controlled trials evaluating PAP versus no treatment show that PAP reduces daytime sleepiness in patients with OSA.[104] CPAP adherence also decreases risk of severe medical conditions associated with OSA, including congestive heart failure, coronary artery disease, cardiac arrhythmia (for review of CPAP and cardiac disease[105]), stroke,[85] and insulin resistance.[106] CPAP treatment of OSA also lowers the risk of fatal motor vehicle accidents. Factors that need to be addressed to maximize CPAP adherence include scrupulous attention to mask fit and comfort, air humidification, avoidance of air leaks,[107] and minimization of aerophagia.[108] For persons who are obese, weight loss to a BMI of 25 kg/m$^2$ or lower may ultimately obviate the need for PAP. Response to PAP must be evaluated by polysomnography (second night of a 2-day study or the last half of a split-night study).

For patients who are absolutely unable to tolerate PAP treatment, and for persons with mild disease, an oral appliance to maintain airway patency may provide good outcomes.[109] These appliances should be dispensed by a dentist, customized for each patient, and capable of titrating the amount of stenting. Again, treatment effects should be evaluated by polysomnography. Patients with extremely severe OSA, OSA with incomplete or poor response to PAP, persons who are unable to tolerate PAP or oral appliances, may be referred for surgical evaluation and potential management of their airways.[110] Current procedures include maxomandibular advancement (MMA), laser-assisted uvulopalatoplasty (LAUP), uvulopalatopharyngoplasty (UPPP), radiofrequency ablation (RFA), pharyngeal implants, implanted hypoglossal nerve stimulators, and tracheostomy. Patients must be thoroughly educated on surgical success rates, complications, alternatives, and likelihood of achieving personal goals before proceeding to surgery.

⧫⧫ **OSA is the most common sleep disturbance of older adults. A diagnosis is confirmed by polysomnography where the sum of apneas and hypopneas (called the AHI) is greater than 5 per hour.**

⧫⧫ **Nighttime PAP, usually provided by CPAP, is the definitive therapy for OSA.**

Central sleep apneas occur with failure of either the central pontine respiratory pattern generator to generate neural activity required to drive respiratory motoneurons or failure of the respiratory motoneurons to adequately drive respiratory muscle activity to perform ventilation.

Systemic diseases that impair the respiratory pattern generator include congestive heart failure, impaired left ventricular systolic function, ischemic stroke, hyponatremia, toxic metabolic encephalopathy, traumatic brain injury, and brain tumors. Persons with these conditions may demonstrate Cheyne-Stokes breathing, a 60- to 90-second cycle of accelerating and then decelerating respiratory rates separated by a prolonged apnea. The pathophysiology of Cheyne-Stokes respiration has been well studied (for recent review[111]). In addition to their acute actions suppressing respiratory drive, chronic use of opiates alters respiratory pattern generator sensitivity to hypoxemia and hypercapnia. Obesity-hypoventilation syndrome (OHS, also known as [aka] Pickwick syndrome) is present in individuals with BMI $> 30$ kg/m$^2$ and elevated arterial $CO_2$ tension ($P_ACO_2$ $>45$ mmHg) during wakefulness without other known causes of hypoventilation. In patients with either OHS or opiate-induced sleep hypoventilation, hypercapnia, and hypoxemia all worsen during sleep, leading to morning headaches and daytime hypersomnolence. Finally, an uncommon cause of respiratory pattern generator dysfunction is congenital central hypoventilation syndrome (aka Ondine's curse), a rare genetic etiology usually diagnosed during childhood (albeit less penetrant cases may present during adulthood).

By contrast, persons with impaired respiratory motor control have functional respiratory pattern generators but are unable to appropriately activate the respiratory musculature. These problems encompass neuromuscular disorders affecting motor neurons (amyotrophic lateral sclerosis [ALS], postpolio syndrome), motor axons (Guillan-Barré syndrome), the neuromuscular junction (myasthenia gravis, Eaton-Lambert syndrome), muscle physiology (myopathies, mitochondrial dysfunction, muscle dystrophies), and muscle anatomy (chest wall syndromes, kyphoscoliosis, ankylosing spondylitis, other processes pulling muscles into nonfunctional regions of their length/tension curves).

Although not as common as OSA, central sleep apnea prevalence is around 1% by polysomnography in middle-aged and older adults.[112] Central sleep apnea is also more common in men compared with women,[113] as well as individuals with congestive heart failure,[114] atrial fibrillation,[115] end-stage renal disease,[116,117] and cerebrovascular disease.[118,119] Some uncommon problems, including acromegaly, low cervical tetraplegia, and primary mitochondrial diseases, are also associated with increased incidence of central sleep apnea.

Polysomnography is also the gold standard test for diagnosis of central sleep apnea. Patients with mild to moderate central sleep apnea will first benefit from medical optimization of underlying chronic cardiac, renal, or neurovascular comorbidities. In patients with preserved cardiac ejection fraction, persons with moderate-to-severe central sleep apnea may benefit from PAP titrated for an AHI $< 5$. However, the role of PAP to treat patients with central sleep apnea and impaired cardiac ejection fraction at this time is controversial.[120] The SERVE-HF trial, which randomized 1325 patients with moderate-to-severe central sleep apnea and ejection fraction $< 45\%$ to either PAP + medical or medical therapy alone, showed that PAP could significantly lower the AHI in patients with central sleep apnea and impaired systolic function. However, individuals in the treatment group also had significantly higher all-cause mortality and cardiovascular mortality compared with the control group.

## Sleep-Related Hypoventilation/Sleep-Related Hypoxemia (ICD-10 Code G47.36, Also G47.34)

Many individuals who have respiratory disease are able to maintain appropriate ventilation and oxygenation while awake, but develop increased $P_ACO_2$ and decreased oxygenation consistent with hypoventilation and hypoxemia while asleep. Sleep-related hypoventilation and sleep-related hypoxemia are long-recognized problems for persons with obstructive airway disorders, restrictive lung disorders, and lung parenchymal disease. Airway obstruction includes common problems, such as COPD, asthma, and cystic fibrosis. Studies suggest that the severity of the sleep disorder in these patients tends to track the severity of airway obstruction.[121] Furthermore, patients with COPD frequently have an OSA comorbidity (and vice versa). In synergy, these two problems lead to more prominent nocturnal oxygen desaturations, worsening nocturnal hypercapnia, and elevated risk of acute respiratory failure.[122,123] Overnight supplemental oxygen is the mainstay of therapy for persons with severe obstructive airway disease, with demonstrated mortality improvement in two of six trials examining supplemental $O_2$ in persons with mild, moderate, and severe COPD.[124] Restrictive lung disorders encompass a broad category of pathologies that lead to dysfunction of the respiratory musculature, and the "bellows" anatomy of the lungs. Neural causes include ALS, postpolio syndrome, spinal cord injury, phrenic nerve injury, Guillan-Barré syndrome, myasthenia gravis, and Eaton-Lambert syndrome; muscular causes include toxic/metabolic myopathies, Charcot-Marie-Tooth syndrome, and muscular dystrophies. Alterations of chest wall anatomy, including those caused by kyphoscoliosis, ankylosing spondylitis, and morbid obesity, similarly alter lung bellows function. For all of these cases, sleep-related hypoventilation/hypoxemia is primarily because of inadequate ventilatory efforts during sleep, and may be addressed by noninvasive ventilation, including CPAP or bilevel PAP. *Lung parenchymal disorders* include interstitial lung disorders caused by inhaled particulate matter (pneumoconioses), pulmonary hypertension, and hemoglobinopathies (particularly sickle cell disease). Management of the underlying disease is the best approach to avoiding sleep hypoventilation/hypoxemia in these patients; persons with sickle cell disease may also benefit from supplemental $O_2$ at night, an intervention demonstrated to decrease sickle cell crises. Testing for sleep-related hypoventilation/sleep-related hypoxemia may include overnight oximetry, measurement of arterial $pCO_2$, and polysomnography. Positive findings include $SpO_2$ $< 88\%$ for at least 5 minutes, more than five combined apnea/hypopnea/respiratory–related arousal events per hour, five or more central apneas per hour, and $pCO_2$ $> 45$ mmHg or $> 10$ mmHg change in $pCO_2$ while sleeping.

## Sleep-Related Movement Disorders

Sleep-related movement disorders, and particularly restless legs syndrome (RLS), are common sleep disorders of older adults. Evaluation includes a history and physical examination as described, with disease quantification using one or more specially developed questionnaires,[125] including the Hening Telephone Diagnostic Interview (HTDI),[126] the Cambridge-Hopkins diagnostic questionnaire for RLS (CH-RLSq),[127] and the RLS Diagnostic Index (RLS-DI).[128] Diagnosis of periodic limb movement disorder (PLMD) is also facilitated by polysomnography and with or without actigraphy. Serum ferritin measurements are also appropriate.

### Restless Legs Syndrome (ICD-10 Code G25.81)

RLS is a chronic disorder characterized by a strong urge to move one's legs, particularly when at rest. Essential diagnostic criteria for RLS include (1) an urge to move the legs, usually accompanied or caused by uncomfortable and unpleasant leg sensations; (2) an urge to move or unpleasant leg sensations beginning or worsening during periods of rest or inactivity, such as lying or sitting; (3) the urge to move or unpleasant leg sensations that are partially or totally relieved by movement, such as walking or stretching, at least as long as the activity occurs; and (4) the urge to move or unpleasant leg sensations that are worse in the evening or night compared with the day or only occur in the evening or night.[129]

RLS is a relatively common disorder with estimated prevalence ranging between 7.1% and 23% in adults age >40 years.[130] In most studies, RLS prevalence is higher in women compared with men. RLS/aging interactions are unclear. RLS also demonstrates a strong autosomal dominant pattern of hereditability,[131] with high concordance rates in monozygotic twins compared with dizygotic twins,[132] as well as identification of multiple candidate genes serving as RLS risk factors, including *PTPRD*, *BTBD9*, and *MEIS1*.[131] Persons with genetic causes of RLS tend to present in their third decade of life. By contrast, RLS in older adults is associated with medical comorbidities, including parkinsonianism, neuropathies and radiculopathies, heart failure, metabolic syndrome, end-stage renal disease, and iron deficiency with low serum ferritin.[133,134]

At this time, there is an appropriate body of evidence to begin treatment of RLS with the dopaminergic agonists pramiprexole or ropinirole as first-line agents, and carbidopa/levodopa as a second-line agent.[135] Side effects are characteristic of increased brain dopaminergic activity and include impulse control disorders, such as pathologic gambling, compulsive shopping or eating, and hypersexuality.[136] Patients receiving long-term carbidopa/levodopa therapy typically (up to 85%) experience augmentation, a poorly understood complication where RLS symptoms worsen in severity, and may be felt in the upper extremities. Augmentation is more uncommon (2%−35%) in persons receiving dopaminergic agonists. RLS symptoms may also recur late at night or early in the morning. This "rebound" reflects decreasing duration of drug effect, particularly when using shorter-acting medications. Effective measures to counter rebound include using sustained release drug formulations or switching to agents that bind $\alpha_2\delta$-subunits of voltage-gated calcium channels (such as gabapentin or pregabalin). In patients with iron deficiency, iron supplementation (to achieve serum ferritin >75 ng/mL) may improve RLS symptoms after 11 weeks of treatment and obviate the need for dopaminergic therapy.[137,138] IRLS scores decreased from 24 to 7 in RLS subjects receiving intravenous iron sucrose, whereas subjects receiving the saline control had a decrease in IRLS score from 26 to 17.[139] A smaller study did not demonstrate similar benefits at an earlier, 2-week time point.[140] Patients receiving oral iron,[141] injectable ferric carboxymaltose,[142,143] and low-molecular-weight intravenous iron dextran[144] also showed sustained improvement in RLS symptoms.

⧫ **A diagnosis of restless leg disorder is based totally on patient history.**

⧫ **Current evidence states that dopaminergic agonists, such as pramiprexole or ropinirole, have greatest efficacy at diminishing restless leg symptoms.**

### Periodic Limb Movement Disorder (ICD-10 Code G47.61)

PLMD is an uncommon disorder characterized by the occurrence of repetitive limb movements, particularly at the toes, ankles, knees, and hips, that occur during sleep. These movements are slower than myoclonic jerks and tend to be separated by intervals of 20 to 40 seconds. PLMD may or may not result in arousals; persons with PLMD and arousals may report daytime sleepiness because of sleep fragmentation. Most limb movements in sleep are associated with either RLS (with patient consciously evoking limb movement to minimize discomfort), REM sleep behavioral disorder, or narcolepsy. Secondary causes of PLMD may include iron deficiency, type II diabetes, spinal cord disorders, anemia, poor renal function, and specific medications (antipsychotics, dopaminergic agonists, and first-generation tricyclic antidepressants).

Polysomnography remains the main diagnostic tool for evaluating PLMD. The periodic limb movements index (PLMI) is determined by dividing the total number of periodic limb movements observed during the sleep study by total sleep duration and is used to gauge intensity of symptoms as follows: mild = 5 to 24, moderate = 25 to 49, severe ≥ 50). Formal diagnoses of PLMD should be made by a certified sleep medicine specialist. Benzodiazepine, and in particular clonazepam, treatment is first-line therapy for PLMD. Some patients also may have improvement with dopaminergic agonists, including pramiprexole, carbidopa/levodopa, and ropinirole.

## Parasomnias

Parasomnias describe abnormal or unpleasant motor, verbal, or behavioral events occurring during sleep or at sleep-wake/wake-sleep transitions. In some individuals, these parasomnias may be so poorly tolerated that they lead to significant sleep fragmentation, poor quality of life, and stress. Persons awaking after a NREM parasomnia usually will be disoriented, confused, and not remember their actions or report a dream. By contrast, persons awakening after a REM parasomnia usually have high alertness and vividly recall dream content. Most of the parasomnias, including sleepwalking, confusional arousals, sleep terrors, sleep-related eating, and sleep-related sex, are more common in children or young adults, and tend to have resolved in persons age >50 years. Parasomnias may run in families; in particular, individuals with human leukocyte antigen (HLA) DQ B1*05:01 and HLA DQ B1*04 genotypes have an elevated risk for parasomnia.[145]

### REM Sleep Behavior Disorder (ICD-10 Code G47.52)

REM behavior disorder (RBD) parasomnias are relatively common in older adult populations, with an estimated prevalence of 1.06% in persons age ≥60 years.[146,147] Incidence is higher in males compared with females. RBD is characterized by both a subtle shift in dream content and dream enactment. First, persons with RBD more frequently experience dreams with greater violent content. Loss of REM-mediated motor suppression leads persons to perform many of the actions occurring in these dreams, including kicking, punching, yelling, and jumping. RBD is often identified by the sleep partner, who may be at risk for inadvertent injury. Given the strong association between RBD and REM sleep, patients tend to report RBD symptoms more commonly during the last half of a sleeping bout. Diagnosis may be facilitated by use of polysomnography coupled with video recording. Risk factors for RBD commonly include Parkinson disease (the onset of which RBD may predate by up to a decade), as well as pontine stroke, subarachnoid hemorrhage, multiple sclerosis, and narcolepsy. RBD is also a diagnostic component of Lewy body dementia (LBD), and its occurrence may predate more canonic symptoms, including rigidity, visuospatial deficits, and fluctuations of consciousness.[148] Rapid discontinuation of sedative hypnotic, selective serotonin reuptake inhibitors (SSRIs), tricyclic antidepressants, monoamine oxidase inhibitors, and cholinergic medications may also act as an RBD trigger. The estimated prevalence of RBD in persons with Parkinson disease ranges between 37% and 63%.[149,150] Current recommendations for RBD treatment include clonazepam for younger adults. However, the increase in fall risk makes this medication highly problematic in older adults. Rather, at this time data support use of either melatonin 3 to 12 mg qh or, in those with LBD, cholinesterase inhibition at higher doses (donepezil 10 mg; rivastigmine 4.5−6 mg bid).

◆◆ **Current evidence suggests that for older adults, the best treatment options for RBD include melatonin or, in those with LBD, cholinesterase inhibition.**

◆◆ **RBD may precede development of Parkinson disease or LBD by 5 to 10 years.**

### Other Parasomnias

Many medications are well associated with vivid dreams and nightmares, including cholinesterase inhibitors, SSRI antidepressants, levodopa, sedative/hypnotics, antihistamines (both first and second generation), stimulants, steroids, and beta-blockers. Patients may report the onset of visual or auditory hallucinations immediately before falling asleep (hypnogogic) or immediately upon awakening (hypnopompic). The hallucinations reported may vary greatly, from poorly formed visual shapes to well-defined objects; from indistinct sounds to conversation to musical phrases, and even cutaneous sensations. Individuals usually learn that these hallucinations are benign processes. Persons with new onset sleep-related hallucinations may require workup for narcolepsy.

### Primary Insomnias

Primary insomnias (Table 31.1) are long-term sleep complaints that cannot be attributed to circadian rhythm disturbances, sleep-related breathing disorders, sleep-related movement disorders, parasomnias, or pathology within CNS sleep substrates.

Prevalence estimates for primary insomnias vary depending upon whether investigators use the International Classification of Sleep Disorders (ICSD)-2, ICD-10, or *Diagnostic and Statistical Manual* (DSM)-V criteria for definition.[151] Regardless of definition used, insomnia risk increases in women, older adults, and persons with depression. Insomnia accompanied by daytime impairment or distress occurs in about 10% of older adults.[152] Clinical workup of the insomnias includes a history and physical examination, 2 weeks of a sleep diary, and a comprehensive review of sleep habits. Actigraphy may confirm paradoxic, psychophysiologic, and idiopathic insomnia.

Efforts to treat primary insomnia in older adults should include education, appropriate sleep hygiene practices (components of which are provided in Box 31.1), and referral for cognitive behavioral therapy for insomnia (CBTI) that may include components such as sleep restriction, stimulus control, cognitive therapy, and relaxation training.[162,163] CBTI encompasses four to eight sessions where clinicians characterize the patient's insomnia, educate patients to successfully complete a sleep diary, and use data from the sleep diary to individually tailor the different CBTI components. For example, the sleep diary is critical to limiting the number of hours a patient spends in bed to total sleep time (sleep restriction). Combined with stimulus controls (e.g., going to bed only when sleepy, limiting time in bed to sleeping and sex, leaving the bed if sleep is not achieved within a 15-min duration, keeping a constant wake time), cognitive therapy (challenging unrealistic beliefs regarding sleep, helping patients flexibly manage attitudes regarding sleep), and relaxation therapy, CBTI acts to normalize sleep-wake cycles, decrease stresses associated with insomnia, and provide patients with realistic, attainable goals for sleep. Current evidence suggests that CBTI is effective at reducing insomnia symptoms, improving patient quality of life, and improving patient sleep satisfaction.[164] CBTI may also have a role in facilitating older adults' transition away from chronic hypnotic medication use.[165]

◆◆ **Best outcomes for patients with sleep disorders occur when practitioners use therapy aimed at the specific sleep disorder**

| TABLE 31.1 | Primary Insomnias | | |
|---|---|---|---|
| Insomnia Type | ICD 10 Code | Brief Description | |
| Paradoxic insomnia | F51.03 | Chronic, severe insomnia, including long latency to sleep, but do not have functional or cognitive impairments consistent with their reported sleep loss. May be responsible for between 16% and 50% of all primary insomnia complaints.[153,154] Heightened awareness of surroundings while trying to sleep, exaggerated sleep onset latencies, underestimated sleep efficiencies. Normal sleep latency and normal NREM and REM sleep organization and duration. Treatment includes reassurance, education, cognitive behavioral therapy focusing on relaxation.[155] | |
| Adjustment insomnia | F51.02 | Acute condition lasting few days to a few months. May accompany affective stressors or changes in environmental conditions. By definition self-limited, and resolves with resolution of the underlying stressor or adaptation to the new environmental condition. | |
| Psychophysiologic insomnia | F51.04 | Common, learned habit that causes significant emotional distress.[156] Individuals experience increased anxiety at bedtime, and augmented anxiety with the passing of time in bed before sleep onset. More common in women than men, and may occur in families as a learned behavior rather than genetic predisposition. CBTI has been demonstrated to improve subjective[157] and objective[158] sleep quality. | |
| Idiopathic insomnia | F51.01 | Do not have paradoxic, adjustment, or psychophysiologic insomnia features, and who have appropriate sleep hygiene. First occurs during early childhood, and has few remissions throughout the life course. May result from either underactive CNS substrates to promoting sleep or overactive CNS substrates supporting wakefulness. | |

*CBTI,* Cognitive behavioral therapy for insomnia; *CNS,* central nervous system; *NREM,* nonrapid eye movement; *REM,* rapid eye movement.

## TABLE 31.2    Hypersomnias

| Hypersomnia Type | ICD 10 Code | Brief Description |
|---|---|---|
| Narcolepsy | G47.41 | See text |
| Idiopathic hypersomnia | G47.11, G47.12 | Uncommon disorder characterized by persons who have normal to increased nighttime sleep and multiple 1- to 2-hour-long episodes of NREM sleep during the day.[159] Daytime NREM sleep distinguishes this disorder from narcolepsy, where daytime REM sleep episodes occur. This disorder usually presents in individuals before age 30 years, often has a familial component, and may lead to devastating impacts on social and occupational function. |
| Recurrent hypersomnia | G47.13 | A rare, poorly understood syndrome. Persons display marked hypersomnia (often sleeping >20 h/day) with episodes ranging from a few days to a few weeks in duration.[160] Males are affected more than females. Usual presentation in teens, but has been reported in older adults. Hypersomnic episodes are interspersed among periods of normal function. When accompanied by food binging, sexual disinhibition, and other behavioral changes it is termed *Kleine-Levin syndrome.* Recurrent hypersomnia is thought to be the result of currently uncharacterized reversible changes in hypothalamic function. |
| Insufficient sleep syndrome | F51.12 | Under various social pressures, individuals may not appreciate that they are voluntarily sleep depriving themselves on a daily basis.[161] In this situation, persons rapidly accumulate a significant sleep deficit, manifested by daytime sleepiness. Adherence to better sleep hygiene is the definitive therapy. |

*NREM,* Nonrapid eye movement; *REM,* rapid eye movement.

(e.g., light therapy for persons with circadian rhythm disorders, or PAP for persons with SRBDs) AND optimize management of comorbid medical problems and issues with sleep hygiene.

◆◆ A brief (<1 week) course of hypnotic medications may rarely be appropriate for treatment of a limited sleep disorder, such as that arising from adjustment insomnia, but these medications are NOT appropriate long-term treatment options given increased risk of cognitive impairment and falls.

### Hypersomnias

Hypersomnia describes conditions where an individual is unable to appropriately sustain alertness during circadian epochs of wakefulness and activity (Table 31.2). Patients may describe daytime sleepiness, difficulty remaining alert, and lapses into drowsiness and sleep. Most individuals have experienced moderate sleepiness during periods of expected wakefulness and activity (and appreciate that individuals can increase their own alertness by performing an activity that is highly alerting, such as exercise). However, severe daytime sleepiness, characterized by a routine overwhelming need to sleep, frequent naps (that do not provide relief from sleepiness), and/or amnesia, indicate a significant problem, particularly if these occur during activities such as driving. The prevalence of hypersomnia in the general population ranges between 4% and 6%,[166] and represents between 15% and 30% of all sleep disorder complaints.[167] Appropriate questionnaire instruments focused on hypersomnia include the Functional Outcomes of Sleep Questionnaire, which is available in a 30- or 10-question version.[168,169] This questionnaire aims to quantify the impact of excessive daytime sleepiness on a person's daily functional status. The Stanford Sleepiness Scale[170] quantifies individual self-report of sleepiness during the day, whereas the ESS[52] examines how likely an individual is to fall asleep across a variety of different situations (average sleep propensity). Polysomnography should be performed to rule out common causes of daytime sleepiness from sleep-disordered breathing. Diagnosis may also be facilitated by MSLT and MWT. Laboratory studies should exclude anemia and hypothyroidism.

### Narcolepsy (ICD-10 Code G47.41)

Narcolepsy is an acquired sleep disorder characterized by excessive daytime sleepiness, hypnagogic hallucinations, sleep paralysis, disturbed nighttime sleep, and memory problems. Some individuals with narcolepsy experience sleep attacks, where symptoms are triggered by sudden or strong emotions. Sleep attacks are pathognomonic of narcolepsy with catalepsy. Narcolepsy is often accompanied by a number of significant medical problems. Narcoleptic patients are often obese, despite eating fewer calories on a daily basis compared with matched controls.[171–173] Weight loss plans for these individuals should thus focus on increasing caloric expenditure. Narcolepsy is also a risk factor for type II diabetes,[174] autonomic disturbances,[175] and potential susceptibility for risky behaviors.[176] Diagnosis of narcolepsy is confirmed with demonstration of at least two very short (<8 min) REM sleep onset latencies (time from alertness to polysomnographic demonstration of REM sleep) occurring during a MSLT. All individuals with narcolepsy benefit from heightened adherence to good sleep hygiene practices. Intravenous gamma globulin therapy administered at the start of symptoms may lessen catalepsy frequency.[177] Current evidence supports treating narcolepsy-evoked daytime sleepiness with the weak dopamine reuptake inhibitor modafinil, or amphetamine-related compounds, such as methylphenidate and Adderall. Limited available data suggest that side effect profiles for these medications are similar in older compared with younger adults; however, age-related differences in drug absorption, hepatic and renal clearance justify lower drug dosages and closer drug monitoring in older individuals.

## Pharmacotherapy Considerations

A number of newer agents show some promise in terms of efficacy and tolerability among older adults.[178] Recent trials have demonstrated effectiveness of low-dose doxepin (6–12 mg) in older adults with refractory insomnia and without significant comorbidity and with careful monitoring for anticholinergic side effects. Alternatively, evidence exists for safe and effective use of Ramelteon, a melatonin receptor agonist, among older adults. Finally, suvorexant, a dual orexin receptor antagonist (DORA), is approved for use for insomnia and has shown moderate effectiveness and tolerability among older adults in clinical trials. Little evidence exists to support other medications commonly prescribed for sleep in older adults, including trazodone or mirtazapine. All these agents should be used in consultation with a sleep specialist and while addressing medical and psychiatric comorbidities and initiating trials of CBTI. Newer generation Z-drugs have been advertised as effective and safe medications to promote sleep in adults. However, recent research suggests that these medications have similar and significant risks to older adults regarding adverse outcomes in driving safety,[181,182] falls and fractures,[183,184] cognition,[185,186] sedation,[187,188] and physiologic dependence.[189,190] Furthermore, under the best of conditions these medications have only produced slight improvements in subjective and polysomnographic sleep latency.[191] Unfortunately, provider prescribing patterns suggest that these medications continue to be overused.[192–194]

It is difficult to overstate the limited clinical indications for pharmacotherapy regarding sleep disorders, and conversely, the marked inappropriate overprescription of hypnotic medications, particularly benzodiazepines and other sedative hypnotics (often called the "Z-drugs"), including zolpidem, eszopiclone, and zaleplon. Benzodiazepines have a particularly high-risk profile in older adults: falls, fractures, cognitive impairment, sedation, and physiologic dependence. These medications have thus been considered potentially inappropriate medications since the first Beers recommendations examining medication safety in nursing home residents[179]; this recommendation has been further expanded to broadly cover all older adults.[180] As mentioned, even apprehensive patients may be transitioned off of benzodiazepines with CBTI and slow dosage tapering.

## Public Health Considerations

Over the past decade, a consensus has developed that sleep health and sleep disorders are a significant public health concern.[195] Inattention to appropriate sleep guidelines historically has significantly impacted the public, ranging from increased medical errors occurring during hospital night shifts,[196] to some of the more significant industrial disasters of the 20th century, including nuclear accidents at Three Mile Island and Chernobyl, the grounding of the Exxon Valdez, and the chemical release disaster at Bhopal Union Carbide. To address these public health dimensions, the US Centers for Disease Control and Prevention has created a Sleep and Sleep Disorders Team[197] to create and examine relevant policy. Curriculum focusing on essentials of sleep medicine should be required for all health practitioners who will be assessing or managing patients, either during the professional school or residency training phases of their career. Electronic medical records should have appropriate standardized templates for relevant sleep history, sleep questionnaire tools, polysomnography, and actigraphy data. Furthermore, physicians, nurse practitioners, physician assistants, allied health staff, and other healthcare providers should educate the public where and when possible regarding the importance of sleep and the need to treat sleep-related disorders. Health practitioners should push back against the culture of glorifying sleep deprivation as a badge of dedication to task. Recognition of the importance of sleep may also accelerate the changing of many hospital practices that currently lead to poor patient sleep hygiene.

## CASE 1

### Discussion

This patient's history strongly suggests REM behavioral disorder. Diagnostic hints included the nature of her movements (which were not repetitive or jerking in nature), her reports of dreaming that "matched" her nighttime behaviors, and her clear cognition when awakened during these events. Her only medication, levothyroxine, was not thought to be contributing to her symptoms. Because she had a low threshold for tolerating medication-related side effects, and her sleeping partner had grown accustomed to her nighttime movements, she elected against pharmacotherapy. About 3 years after this presentation she began noticing gradual difficulty with right-sided motor movements, particularly involving handwriting and fine finger tasks (such as crafting). Neurologic examination at this time revealed no evidence of tremor, but elevated, asymmetric truncal muscle tone (R > L), and more difficulty with right-sided movement accuracy and speed. Neuropsychologic examination revealed some slowing of executive function, particularly in performance of the Stroop test. MRI revealed subtle L-sided premotor cortex and superior parietal lobule atrophy. Unfortunately, her clinical presentation was consistent with corticobasalganglionic degeneration, a poorly understood parkinsonian-like syndrome.

## CASE 2

### Discussion

This gentleman voices all four of the IRLS criteria for RLS: he has pain characteristic of RLS that makes him want to move his legs, his pain is particularly prominent at rest, is worse at night compared with day, and is relieved by leg movement. We also note his low serum ferritin. He was first treated with oral iron supplementation (ferrous sulfate 325 mg per day) with a goal of increasing ferritin to a level above 75; on this regimen he noted that his symptoms improved but did not fully resolve. After 3 months of iron therapy, in discussion with his primary care provider he elected to begin ropinirole therapy over a 7-week titration schedule finishing at a total dose of 4 mg per day. With these therapies, his RLS symptoms have diminished to the extent that he feels it only minimally intrudes in his day-to-day life.

## CASE 3

### Discussion

With some difficulty, the patient was transported to the local Veterans Administration hospital for overnight polysomnography, which revealed an AHI of 75.2, with occurrence of both obstructive and central apneas. He was observed to have 6.4 hours of sleep over 8 hours of observation, of which he spent 43% of time with $SpO_2$ < 88% despite continuous oxygen by nasal cannula. Given his severe sleep apnea, respiratory therapy worked closely with the patient to provide a mask with appropriate fit that he could tolerate overnight. Repeat polysomnography with patient receiving both CPAP (10 mmHg) and supplemental $O_2$ (3 L/min) reduced his AHI to 17, and decreased time spent with $SpO_2$ < 88% to only 4% of observation. The veteran was unable to tolerate higher CPAP pressures and did not have the financial resources to purchase an APAP device. On follow-up after 3 months of appropriate CPAP adherence (at least 4 hours per night), the patient reported a significant increase in his daytime level of alertness, less napping, greater overall energy, better memory, and sharper thinking.

## Summary

As this chapter makes clear, sleep disorders are common in older adults. Primary care providers are thus tasked with determining which of their patients have sleep disorders and following up on these findings with history, examination, and study data to make a definitive diagnosis. For many common sleep problems, effective treatments, including timed bright light administration, PAP, CBTI, and pharmacotherapies, can provide patients with better sleep, while lowering the risk of common and serious comorbidities.

## Acknowledgments

The author thanks Kathryn S. Hentzen, Pharm.D., BCACP, BCGP and John J. Harrington, M.D. for review of Table 31.2 and provision of data for Fig. 31.4, respectively.

Dr. Heflin would like to acknowledge the contributions of authors from the prior edition of the diabetes mellitus chapter to this updated version. This includes Imaad Razzaque, John E. Morley, Konrad C. Nau, and Heather B. Congdon.

## Key References

102. Morgenthaler TI, Kapen S, Lee-Chiong T, et al. Practice parameters for the medical therapy of obstructive sleep apnea. *Sleep*. 2006;29(8):1031−1035.
135. Aurora RN, Kristo DA, Bista SR, et al. The treatment of restless legs syndrome and periodic limb movement disorder in adults—an update for 2012: practice parameters with an evidence-based systematic review and meta-analyses: an American Academy of Sleep Medicine Clinical Practice Guideline. *Sleep*. 2012;35(8):1039−1062.
147. Schenck CH, Mahowald MW. REM sleep behavior disorder: clinical, developmental, and neuroscience perspectives 16 years after its formal identification in SLEEP. *Sleep*. 2002;25(2):120−138.
163. Irish LA, Kline CE, Gunn HE, Buysse DJ, Hall MH. The role of sleep hygiene in promoting public health: a review of empirical evidence. *Sleep Med Rev*. 2015;22:23−36.
178. Sys J, Van Cleynenbreugel S, Deschodt M, Van der Linden L, Tournoy J. Efficacy and safety of non-benzodiazepine and non-Z-drug hypnotic medication for insomnia in older people: a systematic literature review. *European Journal of Clinical Pharmacology*. 2020;76(3): 363−381.

**References available online at** expertconsult.com.

# 32

# Sexual Health

THOMAS MULLIGAN

## OUTLINE

*Additional online-only material indicated by icon.*

## OBJECTIVES

*Upon completion of this chapter, the reader will be able to:*

- Be aware of the prevalence and pathophysiology of sexual dysfunction.
- Understand how to evaluate a patient with sexual dysfunction.
- Be knowledgeable of the treatment strategies for sexual dysfunction.

---

Our understanding of sexual function and dysfunction in older men has increased greatly in recent years. There is less available information on the sexuality of older women. Nevertheless, we now have a better understanding of the pathophysiology of age-associated sexual dysfunction and various effective treatments.

### CASE 1

#### Clifford Johnson (Part 1)

Clifford Johnson is a 68-year-old man and a new patient in your practice. During his initial visit, he mentions that he will soon be remarrying and is concerned that he will not be able to have sex with his new wife. His first wife died of breast cancer 5 years ago. He has not engaged in sexual activity since her death, except for occasional masturbation. He reports strong interest in sex since meeting his fiancé about 9 months ago. However, he fears his erections are not adequate to complete intercourse. Medications include hydrochlorothiazide 25 mg daily for hypertension, atorvastatin 10 mg daily for hyperlipidemia, and amitriptyline 50 mg daily for prolonged bereavement.

How can you discern if Mr. Johnson is sexually functional and what is the most likely etiology if he is dysfunctional?

## Male Sexuality: Age-Associated Changes

As men age, their sexual function changes. The frequency of intercourse and the prevalence of any sexual activity decrease. Young married men report intercourse three to four times per week, whereas only 7% of men aged 60 to 69 and 2% of those age ≥70 years report this same frequency (Level of Evidence [LOE] = A).[1,2] However, sexual interest often persists despite decreased activity. Factors contributing to a man's decreased sexual activity include poor health, decreased partner availability, decreased libido, and erectile dysfunction (ED). Although aging is associated with changes in sexual behavior and response (e.g., refractory period between erections is longer),[3] erectile failure is not a part of healthy aging but rather is caused by age-associated disease (e.g., peripheral arterial disease) or treatment (e.g., radical prostatectomy for prostate cancer) (LOE = B).[4]

**Normal age-associated changes lead to decreased sexual interest and ability; however, complete loss of sexual function is not a part of healthy aging.**

## Erectile Physiology and Dysfunction

In brief, testosterone, mental health, and an attractive partner stimulate libido. Fantasy, as well as visual, tactile, or other erotic stimuli trigger neural impulses from the brain or spinal cord to the penis. Neural impulses cause release of neurotransmitters (e.g., nitric oxide, cyclic guanosine monophosphate), which induce arterial vasodilation. Increasing arterial inflow dilates the corpora cavernosa, which impedes venous outflow. As the intrapenile (i.e., intracavernosal) pressure equilibrates to mean arterial pressure, the penis becomes rigid as blood is trapped in the penis.

ED, the inability to maintain an erection adequate for sexual intercourse, is the most common sexual problem of older men. The prevalence of ED increases with age; by 70 years of age, 67% of men have ED.[5] The common causes of ED in older men are outlined in Table 32.1.

The most common cause (30%–50%) of ED in older men is vascular disease (LOE = A).[6] Risk of vascular ED increases with traditional vascular risk factors (e.g., diabetes mellitus,[7] hypertension, hyperlipidemia, and smoking).[8,9] Obstruction from atherosclerotic arterial disease impedes the intracavernosal blood flow and pressure needed to achieve a rigid erection. Venous leakage[10] leading to vascular ED can result from Peyronie disease, arteriovenous fistula, or trauma-induced communication between the glans and the corpora. In anxious men who have excessive adrenergic-constrictor tone and in men with injured parasympathetic dilator nerves, ED can result from insufficient relaxation of trabecular smooth muscle.

❖ **Neurovascular problems are the most common causes of ED.**

The second most common cause of ED in older men is neurologic (17%–37%).[10] Disorders that affect the parasympathetic sacral spinal cord or the peripheral efferent fibers to the penis impair penile smooth muscle relaxation and prevent the vasodilation necessary for erection. In patients with prostate cancer, all forms of (curative) treatment frequently cause neurogenic erectile failure (brachytherapy or external radiation, 50%; radical prostatectomy with nerve sparing, 45%–80%) (LOE = B).[4] Common health problems such as diabetes mellitus and stroke can cause autonomic dysfunction,[11] and surgical procedures such as prostatectomy, cystectomy, and proctocolectomy commonly disrupt the autonomic nerve supply to the penis, resulting in postoperative ED.

Many medications are associated with ED.[12] Medications with anticholinergic effects, such as antidepressants (e.g., amitriptyline,), antipsychotics, and antihistamines, can cause ED by blocking parasympathetic-mediated vasodilation and trabecular smooth muscle relaxation. Almost all antihypertensive agents have been associated with ED; of these, clonidine and thiazide diuretics have higher incidence rates,[13,14] whereas angiotensin-converting enzyme (ACE) inhibitors and angiotensin-receptor blockers have lower incidence rates (LOE = B).[15,16] Numerous over-the-counter (OTC) medications can cause ED. Cimetidine acts as an antiandrogen[17] and increases prolactin secretion; thus it has been associated with loss of libido and erectile failure. Ranitidine can also increase prolactin secretion, although less commonly than does cimetidine.

The prevalence of psychogenic ED correlates inversely with age. Common causes[18] of psychogenic ED include performance anxiety, fear of sexually transmitted diseases, and "widower syndrome,"[19] in which the man involved in a new relationship feels guilt as a defense against subconscious unfaithfulness to his deceased spouse. A patient suffering only from "widower syndrome" should be able to achieve rigid erections with masturbation.

Hypogonadism, hypothyroidism, and hyperprolactinemia have been associated with ED. However, less than 5% of ED is caused by endocrine abnormalities.[20] Thus endocrine evaluation of men with ED but intact libido is of limited value (LOE = B). Even men with castrate levels of testosterone can attain erections in response to vigorous direct penile stimulation. It may be that erection from direct penile stimulation is less androgen dependent, whereas erection from fantasy is more androgen dependent. Thus testosterone plays a large role in libido and a smaller role in ED.[21]

**TABLE 32.1   Causes of Sexual Dysfunction in Older Men**

| Causes (in Order of Prevalence) | Characteristics |
|---|---|
| Vascular disease | Gradual onset<br>Vascular risk factors: diabetes mellitus, hypertension, hyperlipidemia, tobacco use |
| Neurologic disease (e.g., radiation therapy, spinal cord injury, autonomic dysfunction, surgical procedures) | Gradual onset (unless postsurgical)<br>Neurologic risk factors: diabetes mellitus; history of pelvic injury, surgery, or irradiation; spinal injury or surgery; Parkinson disease; multiple sclerosis; alcoholism<br>Loss of bulbocavernosus reflex |
| Medications (e.g., anticholinergics, antihypertensives, cimetidine, antidepressants) | Sudden onset<br>Lack of sleep-associated erections or lack of erections with masturbation<br>Temporal association with a new medication |
| Psychogenic (e.g., relationship conflicts, performance anxiety, childhood sexual abuse, fear of sexually transmitted diseases, "widower syndrome") | Sudden onset<br>Sleep-associated erections or erections with masturbation are preserved |
| Hypogonadism | Gradual onset<br>Decreased libido more than erectile dysfunction<br>Small testes, gynecomastia<br>Low serum testosterone concentration |
| Endocrine (e.g., hypothyroidism, hyperthyroidism, hyperprolactinemia) | Rare, <5% of cases of erectile dysfunction |

Therefore if a man has complaints of low libido (more likely the man's spouse urged him to seek evaluation for this problem), assessment of serum testosterone is warranted. Ideally, blood should be obtained in the morning to account for circadian rhythm and the result carefully interpreted. For example, a serum total testosterone concentration less than 200 ng/dL in a symptomatic man strongly suggests hypogonadism that will likely respond to treatment. A serum total testosterone concentration between 200 and 300 ng/dL in a symptomatic man likely also represents hypogonadism, but response to treatment is less predictable.

## Evaluation of Erectile Dysfunction

Sexual history should clarify whether the problem consists of decreased libido, inadequate erections, or orgasmic failure. The onset and duration of ED, the presence or absence of sleep-associated erections, and the associated decline in libido are clues to the likely cause.

Sudden onset (in the absence of pelvic surgery) suggests psychogenic or drug-induced ED. A psychogenic cause is likely if there is a sudden onset but retention of sleep-associated erections or if erections with masturbation are intact (LOE = A).[22] If sudden-onset erectile failure is accompanied by lack of sleep-associated erections and lack of erection with masturbation, temporal association with new medication should be investigated. A gradual onset of ED associated with loss of libido suggests hypogonadism. Gradual onset associated with intact libido (the most common presentation) suggests vascular, neurogenic, or other organic causes.

Medical history is directed at discerning those factors likely to be contributing to ED. Vascular risk factors include diabetes mellitus, hypertension, coronary artery disease, peripheral arterial disease, hyperlipidemia, and smoking. Neurogenic risk factors include diabetes mellitus; history of pelvic injury, surgery, or radiation; and spinal injury or surgery. A complete medication review, including OTC medications, is essential. Finally, the history should assess the patient's relationship with the sexual partner, the partner's health and attitude toward sex, economic or social stresses, living situation, alcohol use, and affective disorders.

On physical examination, attention should be paid to signs of vascular, neurologic, or endocrine diseases. A femoral bruit and diminished (or absent) pedal pulses suggest an arterial etiology. Palpation of penile plaques (i.e., Peyronie disease) suggests venous etiology. Orthostatic hypotension and loss of the bulbocavernosus reflex suggest neurologic etiology. Small testes and gynecomastia suggest hypogonadism or hyperprolactinemia.

### CASE 1

#### Clifford Johnson (Part 2)

On further questioning of Mr. Johnson, you determine that his libido and orgasmic function are intact but he has lost sleep-associated erections and is not able to get a rigid erection with masturbation. On examination you note a unilateral femoral bruit with good pedal pulses. He assures you he has no claudication.
What diagnostic testing should you perform?

Laboratory evaluations should target relevant comorbid conditions, such as diabetes mellitus and vascular disease or disorders suggested by the physical examination. The measurement of serum testosterone should be considered, especially in men with low libido.

An at-home therapeutic trial of a phosphodiesterase inhibitor (sildenafil or vardenafil) is considered first-line evaluation and treatment.[23] The initial dose should be low (sildenafil 25–50 mg or vardenafil 5–10 mg) in men suspected of having neurogenic ED. A poor response suggests vasculogenic ED. Further therapeutic trial with sildenafil at 100 mg or vardenafil at 20 mg may prove to be effective.

More extensive diagnostic testing is not commonly used. The penile-brachial pressure index[24] can be helpful in assessing arteriogenic ED. This index measures the loss of systolic pressure between the arm and the penis. When measured before and after exercise, it can be used to assess pelvic steal syndrome, which is the loss of erection associated with initiation of active pelvic thrusting, presumably because of the transfer of blood flow from the penis to the pelvic musculature. More invasive and expensive tests, such as Doppler ultrasound to assess penile arterial function, dynamic infusion cavernosometry to assess venous leakage syndrome, and penile arteriography are generally reserved for research or penile vascular surgery candidates.

### CASE 1

#### Clifford Johnson (Part 3)

Now that you know your patient's ED is likely caused by a combination of "widower syndrome," medication adverse effects, and possible mild vascular disease, what treatments are likely to help him regain adequate erectile function?

## Treatment of Erectile Dysfunction

Multiple effective therapeutic options are available for the treatment of ED.[25] Treatment should be individualized and based on etiology, personal preference, partner issues, and cost (Table 32.2). Oral therapy for ED with sildenafil, vardenafil, tadalafil, or avanafil has revolutionized treatment of male sexual dysfunction. Sildenafil is a phosphodiesterase inhibitor that potentiates the penile response to sexual stimulation. It improves the rigidity and duration of erection. It is taken 1 hour before sexual activity and has little effect until sexual stimulation occurs. Vardenafil is a more potent and specific phosphodiesterase inhibitor. A lower effective dose and better adverse-event profile (no effect on color vision) make vardenafil a reasonable option. Tadalafil is a longer-acting phosphodiesterase inhibitor with an adverse-event profile similar to that of vardenafil but with the added potential problem of muscle pain. Avanafil (approved in 2016) has a more rapid onset of action; it is taken 30 minutes before sexual activity. All four of these agents are contraindicated for concomitant use with nitrate medications, because the combination can produce fatal hypotension. In addition, combined use of α-blockers with phosphodiesterase inhibitors should be done with caution, starting with the lowest dose; hypotension may occur with higher doses. All phosphodiesterase inhibitors result in sufficient penile rigidity for an approximately 50% success rate. Because of the longer duration of action of tadalafil, men tend to select it when given the choice (LOE = B).[25] Daily dosing regimens have gained US Food and Drug Administration (FDA) approval for select phosphodiesterase inhibitors. The higher cost of daily dosing and the rapid onset of as-needed dosing suggest that as-needed dosing would be preferable for most patients.

Vacuum tumescence devices are another option. This consists of a plastic cylinder with an open end into which the penis is inserted. A vacuum device attached to the cylinder creates negative pressure

**TABLE 32.2   Treatment Options for Erectile Dysfunction**

| Treatment | Route/ Administration | Applicable Conditions | Onset | Duration of Action | Dosage | Selected Adverse Events |
|---|---|---|---|---|---|---|
| Sildenafil | Oral | N, A?, V? | 60 min | 4 h | 25–100 mg | Headache, flushing, rhinitis, dyspepsia, transient color blindness; contraindicated with nitrate use and α-blockers |
| Vardenafil | Oral | N, A?, V? | 45 min | 4 h | 5–20 mg | Headache, flushing, rhinitis, dyspepsia; contraindicated with nitrate use and α-blockers |
| Tadalafil | Oral | N, A?, V? | 45–60 min | 24–36 h | 5–20 mg | Headache, dyspepsia, flushing, rhinitis; contraindicated with nitrate use and α-blockers |
| Avanafil | Oral | N, A?, V? | 30 min | | 100 mg | Headache, flushing, prolonged erection; contraindicated with nitrate use and α-blockers |
| Vacuum device | External | P, N, V, A? | <5 min | 30 min | — | Petechiae, bruising, painful ejaculation |
| Papaverine | Intracavernosal | N, A?, V? | 10 min | 30–60 min | 15–60 mg | Prolonged erection, fibrosis, ecchymosis |
| Alprostadil | Intracavernosal | N, A?, V? | 10 min | 40–60 min | 5–20 mcg | Prolonged erection, pain, fibrosis |
| Phentolamine | Intracavernosal | N, A?, V? | 10 min | 30–60 min | 0.5–1 mg | Prolonged erection, fibrosis, headache, facial flushing |
| Medicated urethral system for erection (MUSE) | Intraurethral | N, A?, V? | 10–15 min | 60–80 min | 250–1000 mcg | Penile pain or burning, hypotension |
| Penile prosthesis | Surgical | N, A, V | | Replacement in 5–10 years | — | Infection, erosion, mechanical failure |
| Sex therapy | Counseling | P | Weeks | Years | Weekly | Anxiety |

*A,* Arteriogenic; *N,* neurogenic; *P,* psychogenic; *V,* venogenic.

causing blood to flow into the penis to produce penile rigidity. A penile constriction ring placed at the base of the penis then traps the blood in the corpora cavernosa to maintain an erection. The vacuum device is effective for psychogenic, neurogenic, and venogenic ED, but it requires a lot of manual dexterity. Local pain, swelling, bruising, and painful ejaculation are adverse events. It is important to remove the constriction ring after 30 minutes.

◆◆ **Type-5 phosphodiesterase inhibitors are now first-line therapy for ED. Combined use of α-blockers with phosphodiesterase inhibitors should be done with caution, starting with the lowest dose; hypotension may occur with higher doses.**

Intracavernous injection of drugs, such as papaverine, phentolamine, and alprostadil, is effective in producing erections (LOE = A)[26] but used much less frequently since oral therapy has become available. Alprostadil, the only agent approved by the FDA for intracavernosal injection, produces erections that last 40 to 60 minutes. Intracavernosal therapy should be reserved for patients in whom oral therapy with a phosphodiesterase inhibitor is not effective. Alprostadil can also be administered intraurethrally using a medicated urethral system for erection. This system contains a small pellet of alprostadil that is placed within the urethra and is rapidly absorbed through the urethral mucosa to produce an erection within

10 to 15 minutes. Possible adverse events are penile pain, urethral burning, and a throbbing sensation in the perineum.

Testosterone supplementation increases libido and can improve ED in men with hypogonadism (LOE = B). In patients with convincing symptoms of low libido, check morning fasting total testosterone level. For diagnosis of hypogonadism, levels should be less than 200 ng/dL.

Testosterone replacement is available as an intramuscular injection (testosterone enanthate or cypionate) or transdermal patch and gel. Follow serum levels during replacement and dose testosterone to achieve a level in the midrange of normal, about 450 ng/dL. Possible adverse events associated with testosterone include polycythemia, prostate enlargement, and fluid retention. It is important to obtain a baseline prostate-specific antigen level before beginning therapy. If prostate-specific antigen or hematocrit increases with testosterone therapy, it usually does so within the first 6 months. Therefore these levels should be checked every 3 months during the first year of therapy.

Surgical implantation of a penile prosthesis is an option, but is rarely done since the introduction of alprostadil and, more recently, phosphodiesterase inhibitors. Nevertheless, long-term patient satisfaction with penile prosthesis is actually higher than with oral therapy (LOE = B).[27] Penile revascularization surgery has limited success.

Men with psychogenic ED should be referred to a mental health or other professional specializing in treatment of sexual disorders for further evaluation and treatment.

---

**CASE 1**

**Discussion**

You refer Mr. Johnson to a counselor for his "widower syndrome." You also taper and stop amitriptyline (started after his wife's death) to decrease the anticholinergic burden, and change his antihypertensive from hydrochlorothiazide to lisinopril. The patient reports a return of erectile rigidity with masturbation. To provide additional assurance for his honeymoon, you offer a prescription for sildenafil 50 mg to be taken by mouth 1 hour before sexual activity if he finds that he needs it.

---

## Female Sexuality: Age-Associated Changes

Approximately 40% of adult women report some form of sexual dissatisfaction and nearly 15% report that this problem causes personal or interpersonal distress. Sexual dysfunction includes lack of interest in sex, impaired arousal, inability to reach orgasm, and/or pain with sexual activity. As women age and go through menopause, there is typically decreased sexual interest, responsiveness, and intercourse frequency.[28,29] And, there is an increase in urogenital symptoms, such as difficulty with lubrication (44%), inability to climax (38%), lack of pleasure during sex (25%), and pain during intercourse (12%).[30]

---

**CASE 2**

**Gloria Dean (Part 1)**

Gloria Dean, a 70-year-old woman, is seen in your office for an annual examination. During your review of systems, she admits to a lack of sexual interest. For several years, intercourse has been painful and she has been unable to achieve orgasm. Past medical history includes hypertension, hyperlipidemia, seasonal allergies, overactive bladder, and recurrent urinary tract infections. She takes lisinopril, simvastatin, cetirizine, and solifenacin. She is not on hormone replacement therapy. She had a hysterectomy with oophorectomy at age 39 years.
1. Are there additional elements in the history that will be helpful in making a diagnosis?
2. What other steps will be essential in identifying the etiology of Mrs. Dean's problem?

---

## Evaluation and Treatment

❖❖ **Many older women have sexual dysfunction but do not report it to their primary care provider unless asked.**

The urogenital symptoms associated with postmenopausal estrogen deficiency were previously referred to as vulvovaginal atrophy but now as the genitourinary syndrome of menopause (GSM). GSM includes genital dryness, burning, and irritation associated with diminished lubrication, as well as pain on penetration. With each subsequent encounter, the woman with GSM may anticipate pain, causing inadequate arousal with decreased lubrication. Other causes of painful penetration (dyspareunia) include vaginal infection, cystitis, Bartholin cyst, uterine or vaginal prolapse, endometriosis, dermatoses (lichen simplex chronicus,

lichen sclerosus, lichen planus), excessive penile thrusting, and pelvic floor hypertonus (previously known as vaginismus).[31] Vulvar or pelvic tumors are less common causes of dyspareunia, but important problems in themselves, the treatment of which may produce sexual dysfunction.[32]

Vaginal gels or moisturizers are first-line therapy for GSM (LOE = A)[35] as recommended by the North American Menopausal Society. In Europe, topical estrogen therapy is still considered first-line therapy for symptoms of GSM,[33,34] but estrogen therapy has little direct effect on libido or sexual satisfaction (LOE = B).[35] Libido is thought to depend more on physical, mental, and relational health than on simply estrogen or testosterone.[36]

❖❖ **Therapy for GSM is first vaginal moisturizers; topical estrogen may be used for severe or persistent symptoms.**

Many common medical conditions seen in older women may affect sexuality. Women with diabetes mellitus report decreased libido and lubrication and longer time to reach orgasm.[37] Rheumatic diseases affect sexuality via functional disability. After mastectomy for breast cancer, 20% to 40% of women[38] experience sexual dysfunction, possibly because of disruption of body image, marital and family problems, spousal reaction, adjuvant therapy, or the psychological impact of a breast cancer diagnosis. Several drugs can adversely affect sexual function, including antidepressants (especially selective serotonin reuptake inhibitors), antipsychotics, antiestrogens, antiandrogens, and anticholinergic drugs.[39] Psychosocial factors also have an important role in sexual dysfunction. Women live longer than men. Consequently, older women often spend the last years of their lives alone. Widowhood has a major influence on the frequency of sexual activity for women. Finally, lack of privacy can be a problem when an older couple lives with their children or in a nursing home.[40,41] Therefore medications, relationship issues,[42] the partner's health, and mood disorders[53] are all important in the evaluation of women with sexual dysfunction, as they are in men.

---

**CASE 2**

**Gloria Dean (Part 2)**

On further questioning Mrs. Dean describes pain on initial penetration. Pelvic examination shows no vulvar lesions, the vaginal mucosa is thin and friable with visible veins, and a poorly distensible vaginal vault. Pressure at the introitus reproduces her pain.
What are your next steps in evaluation and treatment?

---

The history is the most important part of the evaluation. Clinicians should ask about dyspareunia, lack of vaginal lubrication, and previous negative experiences, such as rape, child abuse, or domestic violence. Asking if dyspareunia occurs with initial penetration or if it occurs with deep thrusting helps to locate the pain as superficial or deep. For example, deep dyspareunia is a cardinal symptom of endometriosis. Medications should be carefully reviewed for those potentially interfering with sexual function (Table 32.3), including the commonly prescribed antidepressants.[43]

A woman with dyspareunia should undergo a pelvic examination that includes inspection of the external genitalia for atrophy and vulvar dermatoses. After providing a careful explanation, attempt to localize the source of pain. Apply gentle pressure against the inner thighs and then the external genitalia, including the

## TABLE 32.3  Drugs Associated With Sexual Dysfunction in Men and Women

| Therapeutic Class | Agent | Effect | Notes |
|---|---|---|---|
| Acid suppressants | Cimetidine, ranitidine, famotidine | ED<br>Loss of libido | Gynecomastia, which is rarely reported with some proton pump inhibitors |
| Anticonvulsants | Carbamazepine, phenytoin, phenobarbital, primidone | ED<br>Reduced libido | Increase metabolism of androgen |
| Anticholinergics | | Vaginal dryness | |
| Antidepressants | SSRIs | Reduced libido<br>Delayed orgasm | Sildenafil may reduce this side effect in both men and women |
| Antihistamines | | Vaginal dryness | |
| | Lithium | ED | |
| Antihypertensives | Spironolactone, centrally acting sympatholytics (e.g., clonidine) | ED<br>Reduced libido | Any antihypertensive can reduce genital blood flow |
| Antipsychotics | | Orgasmic dysfunction | More common with first generation (e.g., haloperidol) than second generation (e.g., quetiapine) |
| Aromatase inhibitors | | Vaginal dryness<br>Arousal issues | |
| Lipid-lowering agents | Fibrates<br>Statins | ED<br>Gynecomastia | |
| Opioids | All | Reduced libido<br>Anorgasmia | Reduced testosterone |
| Other | Alcohol | Reduced libido | At high doses |
| | Digoxin | Gynecomastia | |
| | Metoclopramide | Hyperprolactinemia | |

*ED*, Erectile disfunction; *SSRIs*, selective serotonin reuptake inhibitors.

vulvar vestibule, in a systematic fashion in an attempt to replicate the pain. Also examine pelvic floor muscles for tenderness; the uterus and cervix, ovaries, bladder, and rectum for pathology; and note the general elasticity of the vaginal tissue.

Therapy follows identified pathology. Vulvar dermatoses generally should be biopsied to distinguish malignant or premalignant lesions from benign conditions. Benign conditions (e.g., lichen sclerosis) respond to topical steroids. Tender pelvic floor muscles are a sign of high-tone pelvic floor dysfunction (pelvic floor hypertonus) and patients should be referred to physical therapists specializing in pelvic floor muscle dysfunction. Unfortunately, these specialists are not easy to find outside of major metropolitan areas.

Decreased lubrication, vaginal discomfort, itching, and dyspareunia caused by atrophic vaginitis respond equally well to vaginal gels and lubricants (e.g., Astroglide, K-Y Jelly, Replens) as to topical estrogen therapy (LOE = A) at least in perimenopausal women (mean age 61 years).[34] Vaginal lubricants are also first-line treatment for women with hormone-sensitive cancers. Importantly, local stimulation through regular intercourse helps maintain a healthy vaginal mucosa. Longer foreplay allows more time for vaginal lubrication.

Topical estrogen therapy may still have a role in women more remotely menopausal, those who fail simple lubricant therapy, and those with recurrent urinary tract infection. Improvement of symptoms can be expected within 2 to 4 weeks. The vaginal ring (replaced every 90 days) delivers low-dose estradiol locally with lower systemic absorption and risk of adverse events than conjugated estrogen cream. The estradiol ring may be preferred over topical estrogen creams because of ease of use. When creams are prescribed, they should be at a minimum dose to avoid systemic effects. Typically, patients are instructed to apply a dime-size amount to the vaginal introitus daily for 2 weeks, then 2 to 3 times per week. Topical estrogens also reduce the risk of recurrent urinary tract infection.

Alternative therapy for moderate to severe dyspareunia include the selective estrogen receptor modulator ospemifene. This daily oral agent is recommended for short-term use only; in women with a uterus, concomitant progestin treatment should be considered. Contraindications include stroke, myocardial infarction, deep vein thrombosis, pulmonary embolism, estrogen-dependent neoplasia, and genital bleeding. Also for moderate to severe dyspareunia prasterone (Intrarosa) in an intravaginal preparation likely acts through its estradiol and testosterone metabolites.

Decreased libido without identifiable cause may respond to flibanserin, the first FDA-approved medication for female sexual dysfunction. Studies were conducted in premenopausal women only; applicability to postmenopausal women is uncertain. Flibanserin is a centrally acting serotonergic agent, and daily use results in small increases in sexual desire and sexual activity. However, daily use and frequent side effects (somnolence, dizziness) limit its utility.

Bupropion may be a better option for women with sexual dysfunction who strongly desire pharmacologic intervention. Although not

FDA approved for female sexual dysfunction, the mechanism of action is similar to flibanserin, the side-effect profile is well known, long-term safety data are available, and a low-cost generic is available.

A third option for low libido is bremelanotide, a melanocortin receptor agonist, recently approved by the FDA for use in premenopausal women. However, it must be injected subcutaneously about 45 minutes before anticipated sexual activity and frequently causes nausea (40%) and/or headache (11%).

Decreased libido may respond to testosterone, but no androgen preparation is approved by the FDA for hypoactive sexual desire disorder in women. Several placebo-controlled, randomized trials showed that a low-dose testosterone patch delivering 300 mcg used twice weekly or daily improves sexual desire in women with natural or surgical menopause and on systemic estrogens (LOE = A).[44,45] Androgenic adverse events such as acne and hirsutism were uncommon. Although the testosterone patch seems effective, there are only limited data on the long-term safety of the testosterone patch in women.

Phosphodiesterase-5 inhibitors have no proven benefit in treatment of disorders of sexual arousal in women (LOE = A),[46,47] although they are effective for women with antidepressant-associated sexual dysfunction (LOE = A).[48] Finally, older women should receive education about male sexual aging in addition to female sexual aging. Otherwise, an older woman might mistakenly attribute her partner's diminished erection and need for more genital stimulation to her own inability to arouse her partner. Other psychological issues, including depression,[49] history of sexual abuse, and relationship problems, should be addressed and treated with antidepressants, psychotherapy, and marital therapy, as necessary (LOE = C).[50–52]

There is no evidence to support the use of herbal supplements in female sexual dysfunction.

---

**CASE 2**

**Discussion**

After the examination, you discuss with Mrs. Dean the potential benefits and safety of either water-soluble lubricants or low-dose vaginal estrogen. For this patient, estrogens may provide the additional benefit of reduced risk for recurrent urinary tract infections. You also provide written information to educate her and her spouse about aging and sexuality. She agrees to begin a gel lubricant and to return in 2 months to have you assess her progress.

## Summary

Normal aging is associated with decreased sexual interest and ability; however, complete sexual dysfunction is not normal and often has treatable causes in both men and women. Knowledge of those causes combined with a careful history and focused examination often provides a diagnosis that directs treatment without additional testing.

### Web Resources

The Mayo Clinic website provides good and detailed information. (Many websites are biased or inaccurate; the reader is advised to use a critical eye and look for websites from reputable sources.) www.mayoclinic.com/health/erectile-dysfunction/DS00162.

The National Institute on Aging offers a patient handout to help patients understand the normal and common pathologic changes in sexual function with age. www.nia.nih.gov/health/publication/sexuality-later-life.

## Key References

1. Alemozaffar M, Regan MM, Cooperberg MR, et al. Prediction of erectile function following treatment for prostate cancer. *JAMA.* 2011;306(11):1205–1214.

10. Mobley DF, Khera M, Baum N. Recent advances in the treatment of erectile dysfunction. *Postgrad Med J.* 2017;93:679–685.

23. Lee M. Focus on phosphodiesterase inhibitors for the treatment of erectile dysfunction in older men. *Clin Ther.* 2011;33(11):1590–1608.

29. Walsh KE, Berman JR. Sexual dysfunction in the older woman: an overview of the current understanding and management. *Drugs Aging.* 2004;21(10):655–675.

33. Mitchell CM, Reed SD, Diem S, et al. Efficacy of vaginal estradiol or vaginal moisturizer vs placebo for treating postmenopausal vulvovaginal symptoms: a randomized clinical trial. *JAMA Intern Med.* 2018;178(5):681–690.

**References available online at** expertconsult.com.

# 33

# Elder Mistreatment

MENGTING LI, E-SHIEN CHANG, MELISSA A SIMON, AND XINQI DONG

## OUTLINE

## OBJECTIVES

*Upon completion of this chapter, the reader will be able to:*

- Be aware of signs of elder mistreatment to improve geriatric primary care.
- Recognize the prevalence, risk/protective factors, and consequences of elder mistreatment.
- Be equipped with tool sets and strategies to implement screening, detections, and assessment for elder mistreatment.

- Identify different intervention strategies for managing and preventing elder mistreatment.
- Sensitize healthcare professionals to the fact that elder mistreatment might be a long-term issue and discuss related issues to follow up with elder mistreatment victims or perpetrators.

## Prevalence

Elder mistreatment is a growing public health concern. A widely accepted definition of elder mistreatment proposed by the US National Research Council[1] defines elder mistreatment as: "a) intentional actions that cause harm or create a serious risk of harm to a vulnerable elder by a caregiver or other persons who stands in a trust relationship, or b) failure by a caregiver to satisfy the elder's basic needs or to protect the elder from harm." Within this overarching framework, the following five subtypes of mistreatment are generally recognized by researchers, health practitioners, and legal statutes: physical mistreatment (i.e., act of intent of injury or pain), psychological mistreatment (i.e., verbal act resulting in anguish), sexual mistreatment (i.e., unwanted sexual violation), financial exploitation (i.e., fraudulent or otherwise unauthorized use of money or properties), and caregiver neglect (i.e., caregivers' failure to provide essential care).[2,3]

Self-neglect is considered as a separate entity as opposed to elder mistreatment perpetrated by others. The relationship between self-neglect and other forms of elder mistreatment is unclear. There is no consensus on the definition of self-neglect. The National Center on Elder Abuse defines self-neglect as failure to perform self-care tasks such that it threatens one's own health or safety.[4] Recent studies have attempted to characterize self-neglect as a geriatric syndrome. Self-neglect encompasses five different phonotypes: hoarding, personal hygiene, house in need of repair, unsanitary conditions, and inadequate utility.[5] In the United States self-neglect is the most common form of elder mistreatment reported to Adult Protective Services (APS).[6]

Best estimates to date suggested that global prevalence of elder mistreatment in the community setting was to be 15.7%, or approximately 141 million community-dwelling adults worldwide in 2015. A recent review of 18 studies reported overall prevalence rates using a 1-year period of 14.3% of global older persons experiencing mistreatment.[7] In the United States in 2008, 10% of adults age $\geq 60$ years experienced some form of mistreatment. The prevalence varies depending on subtypes of mistreatment: 4.6% for emotional mistreatment, 1.6% for physical mistreatment, 5.1% for potential caregiver neglect, and 5.2% for financial exploitation.[8]

❖ **Self-neglect is the most common form of elder mistreatment reported to APS.**

Evidence also suggests that racial/ethnic minority older adults are disproportionally affected by elder mistreatment. Population-based surveys and cohort studies have shown that Black older adults experienced higher rates of financial exploitation, psychological mistreatment, and elder self-neglect than their Caucasian counterparts, after controlling for all relevant covariates.[9,10] In a convenience sample of older Hispanic immigrants residing in Los Angeles, researchers estimated that 40.4% had experienced elder mistreatment in the previous year.[11] In another population-based study of older Chinese Americans, 15% reported elder mistreatment,[2] a rate also higher than nationally representative prevalence studies. Based on these population facts, it has been estimated that a busy primary care clinician will likely encounter at least one victim of elder mistreatment each week during routine practice.[12] As growing numbers of baby boomers age, so too will the absolute number of cases of elder mistreatment.

## Impact

The adverse health consequences of elder mistreatment are many. Elder mistreatment can often create a cascade of adverse effects with important practice and policy implications.[1] Elder mistreatment may result in adverse outcomes categorized by impaired physical health, increased psychosocial distress, financial costs to both individuals and societies, increased healthcare use, and premature mortality.[13-16]

Using different survey methodology, samples, and measures in various older populations, studies have consistently shown the relationships between elder mistreatment and its adverse impact on older adults' psychological and social wellbeing.[13,17,18] Depressive symptoms, anxiety, and posttraumatic disorders are some of the most prevalent psychological consequences.[16,19] Recent findings from the National Elder Mistreatment Study in the United States showed a strong prospective relationship between elder mistreatment and negative emotional health 8 years later.[18] Moreover, the same nationally representative study has shown that mental health problems resulting from past elder mistreatment may increase future risks of revictimization. Disruptions in social and family relationships may also occur as a consequence of elder mistreatment, which could take a toll on older adults' psychological wellbeing.[20]

❖ **A busy primary care clinician will likely encounter at least one victim of elder mistreatment each week during routine practice.**

Elder mistreatment also imposes significant financial costs to individuals, families, as well as society. Victims of financial exploitation, for example, may experience financial loss during a stage of life when it is particularly challenging to recover. Although underreported, the annual financial loss by victims of elder financial abuse is estimated to be at least $2.6 billion.[21]

Elder mistreatment is also associated with greater health service use, including increased emergency department use, increased hospitalization rates, 30-day readmission rates, and increased rates of institutionalization.[22,23] Furthermore, studies have consistently

found that older adults who experienced elder mistreatment were more likely to die prematurely compared to their abuse-free counterparts.[24,25]

### CASE 1

#### Mr. B

Mr. B is a 76-year-old Black older adult who resides in rural Tennessee. His 45-year-old niece has been living with him in exchange for his care. In recent visit, Mr. B persistently complains about increasing intensity and frequency of pain. You are puzzled by these complaints because the methadone you have prescribed should be controlling the pain. You finally ask a family member to bring in all of Mr. B's medications so that you could check for drug/drug interactions. Examination of the methadone tablets reveals that someone has switched most of the methadone with over-the-counter potassium tablets. Your questioning finds that Mr. B's niece was previously addicted with drugs and that she was responsible for his medication preparations each day. His family members suspect that she has been using drugs again, but are reluctant to probe too deeply because there was no one else to care for Mr. B.

1. What might you notice during these visits that could lead you to suspect possibility of elder mistreatment?
2. What other factors might you consider important in evaluating risks of elder mistreatment?
3. What issues would you discuss with Mr. B, his niece, and his family?

## Risk Factors

The ecologic model for categorizing risk factors for elder mistreatment includes the levels of the individual (victim and perpetrator), relationships, community, and society[1] (Table 33.1).

Older adults' functional dependence or disability has been found to be associated with greater risk of elder mistreatment, including psychological and physical mistreatment, and financial exploitation.[26] Older adults' cognitive impairment also significantly predicted elder mistreatment.[27] For instance, in a community-dwelling cohort of 2812 older adults in the United States, researchers found that both present cognitive impairment and the onset of new cognitive impairment were potent predictors of elder mistreatment.[27]

Despite recent systematic reviews that have reported inconsistent associations between sociodemographic and socioeconomic characteristics and elder mistreatment,[19] recent evidence from the United States and Canada suggests that racial/ethnic minority groups may be more likely to experience elder mistreatment compared with their counterparts. Compared with White persons,

**TABLE 33.1 Potential Risk Factors for Elder Mistreatment**

| Victim | Community |
|---|---|
| Poor health | Low levels of social support |
| Functional dependence | Low levels of social embeddedness |
| Cognitive impairment | Society |
| Substance abuse | Low socioeconomic status |
| Mental illness | Racial/ethnic minorities |
| Financial dependency | |

Black older adults were shown to be more likely to experience financial exploitation and psychological mistreatment.[9,26,28] For instance, in a community-dwelling cohort of 4156 cognitively intact older persons in New York State, researchers found that Black American race/ethnicity was associated with a 3.8-fold increased risk of past-year financial exploitation, relative to other groups of race/ethnicity.[28]

Recent research has only recently addressed perpetrator risk factors. Most population-based studies of perpetrator characteristics have collected data from older adults' self-reports, as opposed to perpetrators' own reports. Some common risk factors among perpetrators included poor mental health,[29] substance and alcohol abuse,[30] and abuser dependency.[31] Shared living arrangement also emerged as a strong risk factor, specifically for physical mistreatment and financial exploitation.[28]

On a community level, lower levels of social support and social embeddedness in social networks also significantly increase older adults' risk of elder mistreatment.[8] In a review of 49 studies, a low level of social support was a risk factor in four general population studies, with higher levels of social support reducing the risk of elder abuse. In four other studies of older adults requiring assistance with activities of daily living (ADLs), low social support increased the risk of abuse. There were mixed results with respect to living arrangements—living with others correlated with overall abuse (in four general population studies and one study of elders with dementia) but not financial abuse.[29]

## Detection

Older adults are two to three times more likely to visit a healthcare professional than younger individuals.[32] Identification of elder mistreatment can be achieved in healthcare settings, such as primary care, dental clinics, home health settings, emergency departments, and long-term care settings.[33] The American Medical Association (AMA) recommends that all older adults receive elder mistreatment screening.[34] The 2004 Survey of APS showed that only 1.4% of cases reported to APS came from primary care clinicians.[6] In contrast, in the context of child abuse, clinicians have continued to play a major role in the detection, intervention, research, reporting, and development of creative model programs. In 2013 the US Preventive Services Task Force concluded that current evidence was insufficient to assess the balance between benefits and harms of elder mistreatment screening among all older or vulnerable adults (physically or mentally impaired).[35]

To detect mistreatment in healthcare settings, healthcare professionals could incorporate routine questions related to elder mistreatment into their daily practice.[36] Even in cases of suspected cognitive impairment, it is reasonable to ask older adults about mistreatment, as they may still have the capacity to detect mistreatment during the early years of cognitive decline. If the patient has a significant degree of dementia and is unable to answer questions about mistreatment, the healthcare professional should seek out an appropriate respondent who is not likely to be a perpetrator.[32] Every clinical setting could have a protocol for the detection and assessment of elder mistreatment, which includes basic demographic questions on family composition and socioeconomic status, and questions related to overall wellbeing and elder mistreatment.[37]

There is no gold standard for elder mistreatment screening. However, several screening tools are designed to facilitate the detection of elder mistreatment (Table 33.2). The Hwalek-Sengstock Elder Abuse Screening Test (H-S/EAST), Vulnerability to Abuse Screening Scale (VASS), and Elder Abuse Suspicion Index (EASI) were developed for use in clinical practice. The H-S/EAST initially pooled and distilled more than 1000 items into a six-item instrument to measure violation of personal rights or direct abuse and potentially abusive situations.[38] The VASS measures vulnerability, dependence, dejection, and coercion. The EASI is

## TABLE 33.2  Brief Screening Measures for Elder Mistreatment

| Hwalek-Sengstock Elder Abuse Screening Test (H-S/EAST) | Vulnerability to Abuse Screening Scale (VASS) | Elder Abuse Suspicion Index (EASI) |
|---|---|---|
| 1. Has anyone close to you tried to hurt or harm you recently? | 1. Are you afraid of anyone in your family? | 1. Have you relied on people for any of the following: bathing, dressing, shopping, banking, or meals? |
| 2. Do you feel uncomfortable with anyone in your family? | 2. Has anyone close to you tried to hurt or harm you recently? | 2. Has anyone prevented you from getting food, clothes, medication, glasses, hearing aids, or medical care or from being with people you wanted to be with? |
| 3. Does anyone tell you that you give them too much trouble? | 3. Has anyone close to you called you names or put you down or made you feel bad recently? | 3. Have you been upset because someone talked to you in a way that made you feel shamed or threatened? |
| 4. Has anyone forced you to do things you did not want to do? | 4. Do you have enough privacy at home? | 4. Has anyone tried to force you to sign papers or to use your money against your will? |
| 5. Do you feel that nobody wants you around? | 5. Do you trust most of the people in your family? | 5. Has anyone made you afraid, touched you in ways that you did not want, or hurt you physically? |
| 6. Who makes decisions about your life—like how you should live or where you should live? | 6. Can you take your own medication and get around by yourself? | 6a. Doctor: Elder abuse may be associated with findings, such as poor eye contact, withdrawn nature, malnourishment, hygiene issues, cuts, bruises, inappropriate clothing, or medication compliance issues. Did you notice any of these today or in the last 12 months? |
| | 7. Are you sad or lonely often? | 6b. Doctor: Aside from you and the patient, is anyone else in this room during this questioning? |
| | 8. Do you feel that nobody wants you around? | |
| | 9. Do you feel uncomfortable with anyone in your family? | |
| | 10. Does someone in your family make you stay in bed or tell you that you are sick when you know you are not? | |
| | 11. Has anyone forced you to do things you did not want to do? | |
| | 12. Has anyone taken things that belong to you without your okay? | |

efficient to complete in the emergency department, and takes less than 2 minutes to administer.[39,40] A positive screen for elder mistreatment does not confirm that elder mistreatment is occurring, but does indicate that further information should be gathered.

❖ **Every clinical setting should have a protocol for the detection and assessment of elder mistreatment.**

## Reporting Procedures

The priority of the healthcare professional when mistreatment is detected or suspected is to ensure the safety of the victim. The second is to report the case to the appropriate state agency, such as APS, department of aging, or ombudsman, in accordance with state laws that govern elder mistreatment. States vary in reporting laws and procedures. Elder mistreatment prevention programs, including APS programs, are available nationwide to investigate and intervene when allegations of mistreatment are reported. According to the APS Survey, all states with the exception of New York currently have mandatory report laws for medical, behavioral health services, and social service providers to report reasonable suspicions of elder mistreatment cases.[41] The Eldercare Locator (https://eldercare.acl.gov/Public/Resources/LearnMoreAbout/Elder_Rights.aspx#Abuse, or 1-800-677-1116) can be used to identify the appropriate local elder mistreatment reporting agency and contact information. The additional resources for reporting or managing elder mistreatment are listed in Table 33.3.

When reporting suspected cases of elder mistreatment to a local agency, healthcare professionals do not need to prove that mistreatment is occurring. Some state laws specify that once authorities have been alerted to even the suspicion of elder mistreatment, an agent of the state will make an on-site investigation to corroborate the report. The information provided by healthcare professionals would be helpful for the investigation, such as the name, address, and contact information of the victim, the forms of mistreatment, and information about why this is a suspected elder mistreatment case. Some questions might be asked during the contact, such as "Are there any known medical problems (including confusion or memory loss)?"and "What kinds of family or social supports are there?" and "Have you seen or heard incidents of yelling, hitting, or other abusive behavior?" The local agency will also collect information on the contact information of the reporter, but most states will take the report even if the reporters do not identify themselves. The APS workers receiving reports may not disclose the identity of a reporter to the alleged perpetrators or victim.[33]

The healthcare professionals' legal obligations may vary depending on whether the patient resides at home or in an institution. In cases of mistreatment in the home, the healthcare professionals simultaneously may request a variety of other services, including respite care, a visiting nurse service, and a social work evaluation.

❖ **When reporting suspected cases of elder mistreatment to a local agency, healthcare professionals do not need to prove that mistreatment is occurring.**

| TABLE 33.3 | Resources for Healthcare Professionals |
|---|---|
| **System and Program** | **The Purpose of the Program and How It Works** |
| State Elder Abuse Helplines and Hotlines | If you suspect elder abuse, neglect, or exploitation, call your state's elder abuse hotline or reporting number. The website for the hotline information for each state: https://www.elderabusecenter.org/default.cfm_p_statehotlines.html. |
| Adult Protective Services (APS) | APS strives to ensure the safety and wellbeing of older adults who are in danger of being mistreated or neglected, are unable to take care of themselves or protect themselves from harm, and have no one to assist them. Adult protection interventions include: (1) receiving reports of elder abuse, neglect, and/or exploitation; (2) investigating these reports; (3) assessing victim's risk; (4) assessing victim's capacity to understand his/her risk and ability to give informed consent; (5) developing case plan; (6) arranging for emergency shelter, medical care, legal assistance, and supportive services; (7) service monitoring; and (8) evaluation. |
| Law Enforcement | The US Department of Justice Office of Community Oriented Policing Services has developed resources to help law enforcement officers respond effectively to cases involving elder abuse and is promoting many others developed by the Elder Justice Initiative and the Office of Justice Programs. |
| Long-Term Care Ombudsman Program | Every state has a long-term care ombudsman program, as established by the Older Americans Act in 1978. The long-term care ombudsman program works to resolve problems related to the health, safety, welfare, and rights of individuals who live in long-term care facilities, such as nursing homes, board and care and assisted living facilities, and other residential care communities. This program assists residents and their families in all states by providing a voice for those unable to speak for themselves. |
| State Survey Agencies | State survey agencies receive and investigate allegations against nurse aides regarding abuse, neglect, or misappropriation of property. When state survey agencies substantiate a finding of abuse in nursing homes, state survey agencies must report the substantiated finding to law enforcement and, if appropriate, the State's Medicaid Fraud Control Unit. |
| Medicaid Fraud Control Units (MFCUs) | MFCUs investigate and prosecute Medicaid provider fraud, as well as patient abuse or neglect in healthcare facilities and board and care facilities. MFCUs operate in 50 states, the District of Columbia, Puerto Rico, and the US Virgin Islands. |
| Nurse Aide Registry | A registry maintained by the state lists the names of nurse aides who have been found guilty of mistreatment. Nursing homes are required to check with the nurse aide registry before hiring staff |

## CASE 2

### Wanda

A 50-year-old man brings his mother, Wanda, to the doctor because she "had fallen down the stairs." Wanda has ADL impairments and lives with her son. Wanda looks frightened during the doctor visit. The primary care physician notes bilateral black eyes and bruises on her left arm and shoulder. When the attending physician asks about the origins of the bruises, Wanda attributes them to "clumsiness" on her part. The physician notifies APS. At the home visit, the agency's representative finds Wanda's bed covered with urine and feces. Wanda is referred to the interdisciplinary assessment and intervention team and is hospitalized. Wanda becomes agitated easily and will not let anyone approach her. The team institutes a comprehensive plan for her. After 1 month, Wanda's sleep improves, and she has better socialization with healthcare professionals and peers. She is moved to a long-term facility.

1. How would you detect elder mistreatment?
2. Who could be part of the interdisciplinary geriatric assessment and intervention team?
3. What interventions might the interdisciplinary team implement to help Wanda?

## Assessment

The purpose of the assessment process is to evaluate the person and situation of victim and perpetrator to determine need for assistance, immediacy of need, available resources to assist, and identified priorities for receipt of assistance.[42] Assessment interviews are best approached recognizing and respecting privacy, pacing, planning, pitch, and punctuality.[43] Awareness of some general principles in the initial stages, such as not blaming the victim, is likely to result in a better outcome. In-home assessment could be an effective way to detect self-neglect in older adults.

According to the AMA guidelines, healthcare professionals should consider safety, access (barriers limiting or preventing further assessment), cognitive status, emotional status (e.g., depression, shame, guilt, anxiety, fear, and/or anger), health and functional status, social and financial resources, and frequency, severity, and intent for elder mistreatment during the assessment (Table 33.4).[37]

## Intervention

There are different ways to categorize interventions for elder mistreatment.[44] Primary prevention includes interventions aimed at preventing the occurrence of elder mistreatment. Secondary interventions are actions aimed to prevent the recurrence of elder mistreatment. One model has been the development of shelters within existing long-term care facilities.[45] Tertiary intervention includes actions to manage the consequences after the occurrence of elder mistreatment.

There are short-term and long-term outcomes associated with intervention programs. Short-term outcomes include participant-, victim- or perpetrator-related outcomes, such as increased knowledge, attitudes and skills, and identification of mistreatment. Long-term outcomes include lower rates of elder mistreatment reporting or a reduction in the recurrence of elder mistreatment.

Culture may influence intervention strategies. Limited English language ability adds to the burden of help-seeking among minorities. The lack of English proficiency is also associated with limited access to healthcare and social services. Further, they may need to rely on a bilingual person to seek help when facing elder mistreatment. Multilingual translation services are needed in clinical practice to reduce the difficulty of identifying and reporting elder mistreatment among racial/ethnic minority groups.[46,47]

When elder mistreatment is suspected, the first step is a conversation with the older adult in a safe environment without the presence of caregivers. This conversation should lead to answers to several key questions that will help to determine the next steps in helping the older person (Box 33.1).

One of the most important developments in addressing elder mistreatment in recent years has been the use of multidisciplinary teams in hospitals and communities.[48,49] Multidisciplinary teams are created as an addition to existing APS to respond more efficiently and comprehensively to cases of elder mistreatment. These expanded services include forensic centers, vulnerable adult or financial abuse specialist teams, elder abuse prosecution units, and prevention teams that raise awareness of elder mistreatment.[50,51] Specialists in adult medicine, social work, nursing, psychiatry, the law, and law enforcement form a team that can help the primary care clinician to develop and implement an appropriate intervention plan.

⬥⬥ **When elder mistreatment is suspected, the first step is a conversation with the older adult in a safe environment without the presence of caregivers.**

| TABLE 33.4 | Primary Care Clinician Assessment of Elder Mistreatment | |
|---|---|
| **Observations** | **Physical Examination** |
| Caregiver dominates interview | Weight loss |
| Caregiver is overwhelmed | Dehydration |
| Older adult is inappropriately dressed | Abrasions/hematomas/burns |
| Older adult appears fearful | Pressure ulcers |
| History | Fractures |
| History of injuries with unclear cause | Rectal/vaginal bleeding |
| Delay in seeking care | Signs of sexually transmitted disease |
| Frequent emergency room visits | |
| Poor adherence to treatment | |

### • BOX 33.1 Elder Mistreatment: Guide to the Primary Care Clinicians Decision Making

- Is the older adult safe in the current setting; or does the person need to be moved to a safer location?
- Does the older adult have the decision-making ability to make informed decisions?
- If needed, what local services are available to assist the older adult?
- Should the case be reported to the local APS team?
- Does the caregiver/perpetrator need counseling or medical services?

## Programs to Increase Detection Rate for Prevention of Elder Mistreatment

There are programs that attempt to increase the elder mistreatment detection rate, such as home visits, home-based geriatric assessments, helplines, training for healthcare and social workers, and guidelines and protocols for screening. One study compared non-physician community mental health providers who used a new integrated system of clinical assessment with other providers who performed usual care, and found community mental health providers in the intervention group were more likely to screen for elder mistreatment.[52] Existing studies have not confirmed the effectiveness of these outreach programs in improving the outcomes for older adults at risk for abuse.

## Educational Interventions

Elder mistreatment educational programs are conducted for the older adults and caregivers, and professionals to increase awareness, improve attitudes, and build skills for prevention and management. Most educational interventions focus primarily on healthcare professionals. A few educational programs focus on both victims and perpetrators and attempt to improve their relationships. There is some limited evidence to suggest that educational interventions improve knowledge and attitudes toward elder mistreatment among healthcare professionals. There is no evidence to confirm educational interventions sufficiently prevent elder mistreatment, reduce recurrent elder mistreatment, or other related outcomes.[53]

## Program to Reduce Factors Influencing Elder Mistreatment

As discussed, risk factors, such as physical impairment of the patient, caregiver burden, detached family relations, and restricted social networks, increase the likelihood of mistreatment.[54–59] A large number of interventions aim to reduce risk factors for elder mistreatment, with some interventions that target perpetrators and others that focus on victims.

The programs targeted at perpetrators included legal assistance, psychiatric intervention, providing homemaker services for over-burdened caregivers, social support groups for caregivers, referrals to drug or alcohol rehabilitation for addicted perpetrators, and counseling that may involve conflict resolution skills.[37] Caregiver burnout is known to be a robust risk factor for elder mistreatment, and caregiver-based interventions reported different outcomes between family caregivers and paid caregivers. Studies targeting family caregivers found the treatment effect was not significant,[60,61] whereas studies focused on paid caregivers reported significant treatment effect.[62,63]

Programs for victims consist of APS, emergency shelters, temporary residential services, and relocation to long-term care settings. Victims are most likely to accept and benefit from concrete services (e.g., medical care and homemaking), or empowerment strategies (e.g., support groups and advocates).[64] The most common services for self-neglecting older adults were information and referral, supportive health care, case management, home health care, mental health services, home-delivered meals, and counseling.[65] More evidences is needed to identify the effective services

for victims and under what circumstances they are most likely to be helpful.

Victims are at times unwilling to accept voluntary services or lack capacity to consent.[66] The AMA guidelines suggest the following approaches: If victims have capacity, healthcare professionals could educate patients on elder mistreatment, including information about the forms of mistreatment, the older adults' right to be free from mistreatment, how to access local resources (e.g., providing emergency numbers and appropriate referrals), and develop a safety plan and a follow-up plan. If victims lack capacity, healthcare professionals could discuss with APS on financial management assistance, conservatorship, or guardianship.

## Follow-Up

Follow-up in elder mistreatment cases can have different purposes. Among the most important are evaluation of intervention effectiveness, reassessment of need, and situation monitoring to prevent the recurrence of elder mistreatment. In every instance, follow-up suggests the establishment of an ongoing relationship between victim (or perpetrator) and healthcare professionals.[42] Elder mistreatment often requires long-term or intermittent intervention before resolution.

### CASE 1

#### Discussion

Elder mistreatment is widespread in our society, and yet remains underrecognized by healthcare professionals. Caregiver neglect is one of the most prevalent forms of mistreatment. Clinicians in primary care are well placed to effectively prevent, recognize, and respond to mistreatment because they are likely to have frequent contact with older adults. When talking with Mr. B, it is important to find what supports he is receiving to assist with his current health needs. You could refer him to formal and informal services as needed, including respite care, day care, caregiver support, or information about medication management. You may also want to discuss options regarding Mr. B's living situation, such as seeking additional support from other family members, or having his niece evicted. Older persons considering such actions would also need your ongoing support to implement their decisions.

### CASE 2

#### Discussion

Separate interviews must be conducted with Wanda and her son because denial is often present. You can ask Wanda about the quality of her relationship with her son and the conditions of the home. During the interview, you should avoid blaming Wanda. When interviewing her son, you can offer empathy for the burdensome tasks of caregiving. The conversation should be documented. In the interdisciplinary assessment and intervention team, specialists in medicine, social work, nursing, psychiatry, and other fields offer suggestions to develop an appropriate intervention plan. For example, clinicians address the injuries. The social worker identifies strengths to empower the victim, and conduct psychological interventions to reduce the stress, anxiety, and depression. These specialists have referral information on social services in the community for Wanda and her son.

## Summary

Elder mistreatment is recognized worldwide as a serious public health problem. It is associated with adverse health and wellbeing. Healthcare professionals play an important role in the management of elder mistreatment, including detection, reporting, assessment, intervention, and follow-up. Healthcare professionals could work with social, legal, and other related professionals to reduce elder mistreatment.

**Web Resources**

https://eldercare.acl.gov/Public/Resources/LearnMoreAbout/ Elder_Rights.aspx#Abuse

## Key References

**37.** Aravanis SC, Adelman RD, Breckman R, et al. Diagnostic and Treatment Guidelines on Elder Abuse and Neglect. American Medical Association, 1992. Available at: http://tvfields.com/OtherLinks/AMAReport.pdf. Accessed 15.08.20.

**41.** Administration for Community Living. National Voluntary Consensus Guidelines for State Adult Protective Services Systems. Office of Elder Justice and Adult Protective Services, U.S. Department of Health and Human Services, 2019. Available at: https://acl.gov/sites/default/files/programs/2019-03/Proposed%20Updates%20to%20the%20APS%20Guidelines_All%20Content.pdf. Accessed 15.08.20.

**48.** Dong X, ed. *Elder Abuse: Research, Practice and Policy.* Springer International Publishing; New York, NY; 2017.

***References available online at*** expertconsult.com.

# 34

# Substance Use in Older Adults

SUSAN W. LEHMANN, MICHAEL FINGERHOOD, AND MATTHEW K. MCNABNEY

## OUTLINE

## OBJECTIVES

*Upon completion of this chapter, the reader will be able to:*

- Describe current trends in substance use among older adults.
- Identify the two most commonly abused substances among older adults.
- Discuss three differences between the presentation of substance use in older adults compared with younger adults.
- Identify five signs of problematic substance use in older adults.

- Describe the National Institute on Alcohol Abuse and Alcoholism drinking guidelines for older adults.
- Discuss three ways that marijuana can have deleterious impact on mental and cognitive health for older adults.
- Describe strategies for successful treatment of substance use disorders in older adults.

## Introduction

Concern about substance use disorders has grown in recent years. Although images and news stories frequently focus on rising rates of substance use among young and middle-age adults, rates of substance use are increasing among older adults as well. Historically, rates of substance use disorders have been significantly lower among older adults compared with younger adults. However, it is estimated that by 2020, rates of substance use among adults age ≥ 50 years in the United States will have increased to 5.7 million, up from 2.8 million in 2006.[1] A driving force behind this change involves changing demographics, most notably the aging of the population cohort known as the baby boomer generation. This is the very large cohort of individuals who were born between 1946 and 1964 and includes about 75 million individuals. The leading edge of this cohort turned 65 years in 2011. Whereas 12% of the US population was age ≥ 65 years in 2010, that number is expected to rise to about 21% of the population by 2030.[2] Rates of substance use have been higher among individuals of the baby boomer cohort, and they have continued to have higher rates of substance use than previous generations as they age.[1]

Although substance use poses harm to individuals at all ages, older adults are especially vulnerable to harmful effects of substances. Physiologic changes in hepatic metabolism with aging can affect the pharmacokinetics of both alcohol and other substances. Comorbid health conditions, whose incidence increases with age, such as diabetes, cardiovascular disease, and chronic pain conditions, as well as multiple prescription medications can interact with substance use and increase the risk of falls, confusion, cognitive impairment, and drug-drug interactions.[3,4] Yet, screening for substance use among older adults frequently does not occur in primary care settings, and detecting harmful use can be more challenging in the older adult as will be discussed later.

## Epidemiologic Trends and Illicit Substance Use

Evidence for increasing patterns of substance use among older adults comes from a number of large-scale studies. The Treatment Episode Data Set (TEDS) is a public use data surveillance system, maintained by the Substance Abuse and Mental Health Services Administration (SAMHSA) Center for Behavioral Health Statistics. All public and private substance abuse facilities that receive public funds are required to report information about admissions for substance use into this database. In 2012 the TEDS data system reported that 14,230 adults age $\geq 65$ years were admitted to substance abuse treatment programs. Most of these admissions were for treatment of alcohol use disorders, and most individuals were self-referred or referred by the criminal justice system.[5] Between 2000 and 2012, the proportion of admissions for substance use treatment for adults age $\geq 55$ years increased from 3.4% to 7.0%. Whereas the majority of admissions were for alcohol as the primary substance of abuse, there was an increasing trend for admissions for other substances, including cocaine/crack, marijuana, heroin, nonprescription methadone, and other opiates and synthetics. There was also an increase in admissions where more than one problem substance was reported.[6]

#### ❖❖ Rates of substance use are increasing among older adults.

The National Epidemiologic Survey on Alcohol and Related Conditions (NESARC) collected data on substance use in three separate waves: in 2001 to 2002, 2004 to 2005, and 2012 to 2013. In each wave, trained interviewers conducted semistructured interviews. A recent study used data from the NESARC to look at changes in lifetime prevalence of heroin use and heroin use disorder from 2001 to 2003 through 2012 to 2013. This study found that among 79,000 respondents, lifetime prevalence of both heroin use and heroin use disorder increased significantly during this time among all three age groups surveyed (18–29, 30–44, and $\geq 45$ years), although rates were significantly higher among younger, compared with older, age groups.[7]

The National Survey on Drug Use and Health (NSDUH) is an annual survey of the civilian, noninstitutionalized population that uses self-report questionnaires to obtain measures of drug use and health in the United States. Combining data from 2003 to 2012 from the NSDUH, Choi et al. reported that 4.3% of adults age 50 to 64 years and 1.7% of adults age $\geq 65$ years had alcohol use disorder and 8.7% of those age 50 to 64 years and 1.8% of those age $\geq 65$ years had any illicit drug use. Specifically, 5.9% of those age 50 to 64 years and 0.9% of those age $\geq 65$ years reported marijuana use.[8] The NSDUH found a significant increase from past surveys in cocaine use disorder in persons over age 50 years.[9] Findings from the NSDUH also indicate that among adults age $\geq 50$ years with a past-year history of substance use disorder, 11.5% have a comorbid mental illness. Of those individuals with comorbid mental health problems, only 59% of people age 50 to 64 years and 45% of those age $\geq 65$ years reported past-year mental health treatment.[10] These finding underscore the importance of screening for dual diagnosis of both substance use and mental disorders among older adults.

## Screening and Detection of Substance Use Disorders

Substance use and substance use disorders are often "hidden problems" among older adults, especially in primary care settings. There are a number of factors contributing to underdetection of substance use problems, including lack of time by providers during primary care visits, lack of age-appropriate screening tools to detect substance use, and lack of national guidelines for assessing older adults. Signs and symptoms of substance use can overlap with signs and symptoms of other health conditions, complicating recognition. As well, ageist attitudes toward older adults, both by clinicians and by family, may inhibit providers from probing for substance use problems. Healthcare providers may incorrectly assume that an older adult is unlikely to have a problem with substance because of age or may feel it is disrespectful to ask an older patient about substance use.

#### ❖❖ Older adults and their families may not appreciate deleterious consequences of long-term patterns of substance use or drinking.

Older adults themselves may underreport the quantity or frequency of their substance use, which hampers detecting problematic use. Both older adults and their family members may not appreciate that the older individual is drinking or using substances at a level that can cause harm. This is particularly true of older adults who have had long-time patterns of drinking or substance use. In addition, deleterious effects of alcohol and other substances on older adults can come from ingesting lower amounts of substances than for younger adults. Signs of problematic substance use include sleep disturbances, mood swings, unexplained falls, impaired coordination, memory impairment, and motor vehicle accidents.[11]

In recognizing and detecting problematic substance use, the *Diagnostic and Statistical Manual of Mental Disorders, Fifth Edition* (DSM-5) criteria are often less helpful for older adults. Although older adults are likely, as younger adults are, to develop cravings, to spend excessive time obtaining and using substances, and may continue use despite negative consequences, there are differences between older and younger substance users. Older adults are more likely to experience impairment from the same level of substance use they engaged in when younger and without evidence of physiologic tolerance. Withdrawal symptoms can be more subtle and might manifest as confusion or unexplained falls. Older adults with problematic substance use may live alone and may be retired, making it unlikely that impaired role function will be a signal of harmful substance use.[11]

The Center for Substance Abuse Treatment recommends screening for alcohol disorders and substance use as part of routine medical visits for all individuals aged $\geq 60$ years[12]; yet, the likelihood that a primary care provider has a discussion about alcohol use with a patient declines with age.[13] In 2003 SAMHSA launched SBIRT (Screening, Brief Intervention and Referral for Treatment), and it has become the recommended approach to detecting substance use disorders in all ages.[14] SBIRT involves a stepped approach to the patient, based on the individual's response to screening assessment. Although it has yet to be implemented on a national scale, a recent study reported on the successful application of the SBIRT approach to screening and intervention with older adults in Florida. Between 2006 and 2011, 85,000 older adults were screened for alcohol, illicit drug use, and medication misuse at 75 sites. The sites where screening took place included health fairs in addition to emergency departments (EDs), community mental health centers, and home nursing visits. A simple two-question screen was used to assess for problematic substance use: (1) Have you tried to cut down on drugs or medication? (2) Have you used drugs or medication more than you intended? This widespread screening process detected 8100 older adults who were at risk. The most common problems were alcohol and medication misuse. At 6-month follow-up, there was a significant reduction in substance use. This study showed that, although resource-intensive, applying the SBIRT approach to an older population was feasible and effective.[15]

Detection of problematic drinking starts with having a high level of suspicion based on the patient's presentation, history, and/or information from family or other informants. Probing for alcohol use in the course of an interview or appointment in a respectful and nonjudgmental way may reveal problematic drinking. There are three common screening tools used in the assessment for problematic alcohol use. The Michigan Alcoholism Screening Test has two geriatric versions (MAST-G and SMAST-G). The MAST-G has 24 items and the SMAST-G has 10 items. More than five "yes" answers are indicative of a problem with alcohol use.[16] The Alcohol Use Disorders Identification Test is a widely used instrument that was developed by the World Health Organization.[17] It does not have a geriatric version, but may be useful in office settings. It has 10 items and, typically, a score of 8 on a scale of 0 to 40 is considered indicative of hazardous drinking. For older adults, clinicians may want to consider using a lower cutoff score of 5. The CAGE (cut-annoyed-guilty-eye) questionnaire is a popular screening tool to assess for problematic drinking because of the simplicity of its four questions, prompted by the acronym.[18] It is not as reliable in detecting problematic use in older adults because it does not probe for binge drinking.[19]

## Alcohol Use

About two-thirds of older adults with problematic alcohol use have early onset alcohol use disorder that began when they were adolescents or young adults. Among the one-third of older adults with late onset problematic alcohol use, stressful life events, such as spousal loss, retirement, and medical disability or pain conditions are more likely to have been triggers for harmful use.[20] Using data from the NSDUH from 2008 to 2012, Choi et al. found that 4.3% of adults age 50 to 64 years and 1.7% of those age $\geq 65$ years had alcohol abuse or dependence. Although these rates were relatively low, rates of current alcohol use were high. Indeed, 87.8% of adults 50 to 64 years and 56.4% of adults age $\geq 65$ years reported current alcohol use in 2014.[8] Even more concerning, binge drinking, defined as having five drinks or more on the same occasion at least 1 day in the past 30 days, was endorsed by 14% of adults age 60 to 64 years and 9% of adults age $\geq 65$ years. Breslow et al. used data from the National Health Interview Surveys from 1997 to 2014 and found that during this time, the prevalence of both current drinking and binge drinking increased among adults age $\geq 60$ years, and were greatest among adults belonging to the baby boomer cohort.[21]

According to the National Institute on Alcohol Abuse and Alcoholism guidelines, adults age $\geq 65$ years should not consume more than seven drinks in a week and should not consume more than three drinks on a given day.[22] Yet, these guidelines are not widely known by older adults and often not known by their healthcare clinicians. The guidelines reflect the fact that older adults are more vulnerable to potential harms from drinking because of age-related changes in physiology and metabolism. As part of normal aging, there is a decrease in lean muscle mass and decrease in total body water, as well as diminished efficiency of liver enzymes that metabolize alcohol. As a result, older adults experience increased effective concentration of alcohol with high and longer lasting blood alcohol levels than younger adults for the same amount of consumption. In addition, older adults are more likely to have comorbid medical conditions and are more likely to be taking multiple prescription medications that can negatively interact with alcohol, amplifying risk for harm with drinking.

Chronic excessive alcohol use is known to contribute to regional brain atrophy. Knowing that normal aging is also associated with brain volume decline, Sullivan et al. used quantitative magnetic resonance imaging of 222 subjects with alcohol use disorder, age 25 to 75 years, compared with age-matched controls to examine the possible additive effects of drinking on brain volume. They found that subjects with alcohol use disorder had increased volume deficits and accelerated age-dependent cortical volume decline, even for subjects with late-onset alcohol use disorder.[23] Volume loss was most pronounced in frontal cortex. This is especially concerning as deficits were seen in the region of the brain most responsible for decision making, problem solving, and planning of executive functioning.

For all older patients with problematic drinking, a personalized approach to intervention must be done. Clinicians will want to provide information about the harmful effects of drinking and recommendations to cut down or stop. Motivational interviewing techniques, which were developed to promote behavior change among people with alcohol use disorder, are also effective in older adults. The goal is to use nonjudgmental language to encourage the patient to commit to changing behavior. For older adults, a strong motivation for behavior may be preservation of cognitive functioning and memory. All older adults who are advised to abstain from alcohol should be assessed for development of alcohol withdrawal. This can be done in the home, with family members or friends present to provide support. In older adults, development of withdrawal may not occur until 2 to 4 days after stopping drinking. Severity and duration of withdrawal increase with age, and confusion may be the predominant symptom rather than tremor or tachycardia.[24] Individuals with a history of severe withdrawal should be monitored and treated in the hospital. Benzodiazepines are the standard in the treatment of alcohol withdrawal, with dosing symptom-triggered.[25,26] There are no guidelines for the treatment of alcohol withdrawal that are specific to older adults.

Maintaining alcohol abstinence is an active process. Support groups such as Alcoholics Anonymous can be very helpful, but finding a group with similar peers is often challenging. Family involvement is crucial in the process of changing drinking behavior. Often the patient's spouse may also be drinking at a high level and will need behavior change counseling as well. Treatment plans should include undoing isolation and creating a social support system. Joining a senior center can be impactful toward maintain sobriety, fostering the development of new social contacts and interests.

---

### CASE 1

Alice Danforth is 72 year-old retired college professor. She lives with husband of 42 years. They live in retirement community where there are other people of similar age and social experiences. She has high cholesterol and hypertension as well as mild cognitive impairment (MCI). She reports noticing that she has trouble retrieving names, which frustrates her and worries her husband. When you are meeting with her, you probe more deeply into her substance use history and she reports 2–3 glasses of red wine most evenings and sometimes more at social gatherings in the community (which are fairly frequent). She also reports marijuana use 2–3 times per month. In reflection, her problems with memory do seem most apparent in the evenings.

1. What are some concerns you might have for someone like Ms. Danforth?

---

Less commonly, pharmacologic management is added to help minimize risk for relapse. As with the treatment of alcohol withdrawal, there are no guidelines for pharmacologic management specifically to decrease risk of relapse in older adults. Pharmacologic agents used to treat younger adults are also available to treat older adults. In general, naltrexone is considered first-line therapy and may be helpful in diminishing craving for alcohol. The usual dose range for naltrexone is 25 to 50 mg daily. Clinicians need to be mindful that it can be hepatotoxic, and that patients cannot also be receiving treatment with opioid medications because naltrexone blocks opioid receptors. Acamprosate is of limited effectiveness. Adherence is difficult as it is dosed three times daily and diarrhea is a very common side effect, limiting acamprosate's use. Disulfiram should be prescribed cautiously, if at all, for older patients because of its potential for adverse effects.

❖❖ **Alcohol and marijuana are the two most commonly abused substances by older adults.**

## Marijuana Use

There is increasing interest in marijuana, including products that have its components such as cannabidiol (CBD) and tetrahydrocannabinol (THC), which is considered the psychoactive alcohol, and marijuana use is increasing among older individuals. Between 2002 and 2003 and 2012 and 2013, the prevalence of marijuana use increased from 1.6% to 5.9% among adults age 45 to 64 years and 0% to 1.3% among adults age $\geq 65$ years.[27,28] Among adults age $\geq 50$ years, many users of marijuana have done so since their teen years and so marijuana use may be long term. The majority of older marijuana users perceive no risk or only slight risk from frequent use (defined as three times/week or more). This group of substance users have not received much research attention.

At the same time, there is growing societal interest in "medical marijuana." Although marijuana remains illegal from a federal standpoint, many states have taken steps to provide a legal pathway for adults to obtain marijuana for medicinal purposes from licensed dispensaries. Older adults are often drawn to these products as well. At the time of this writing, however, there are only three cannabis-derived products on the market that have approval from the US Food and Drug Administration (FDA). These include Epidiolex, which has FDA approval for the treatment of two severe forms of epilepsy, Marinol (dronabinol), which has FDA approval to treat anorexia and severe weight loss in acquired immunodeficiency syndrome patients, and Cesamet (nabilone), which has FDA approval for severe nausea and vomiting because of chemotherapy. Of these, Epidiolex is the only one that has a purified form of CBD. The other two medications are synthetically derived compounds that are similar to THC. All other cannabis-derived products are part of an unregulated industry, with wide variability in potencies, additives, and contaminants. A concern for clinicians who may be asked by their older patients about whether a "medical marijuana" product may be beneficial for them is that products that do not have FDA approval may still make unproven medical claims yet lack good clinical trials to support their use.

❖❖ **Older adults are likely to experience harm from lower levels of substance use than for younger adults and may be impaired from ingesting the same amount of a substance taken when they were younger.**

Although older adults frequently see marijuana as a "safer" alternative to alcohol or other illicit drugs, or prescription medications, there is evidence the marijuana use can lead to adverse health effects. In all ages, short-term use is associated with impaired short-term memory, impaired judgment and coordination, and impaired driving. There is evidence that high doses can precipitate paranoia and psychosis. Longer-term use can lead to addiction, as well as cognitive impairment and diminished motivation.[29] Growing evidence implicates marijuana as having a deleterious effect on still-developing brains of adolescents. Little is known about its effects on aging brains, or brains of older adults with cognitive disorders, which may be more vulnerable to adverse consequences. Certainly more research is needed in this area, given its high level of interest in the public and its underexamined potential for medical use. It is important for all clinicians to maintain a nonjudgmental stance with their older patients in eliciting history about marijuana use to provide the best guidance in helping patients make healthy decisions.

## Prescription Drug Misuse

Prescription drug misuse is defined as the intentional or unintentional use of a prescribed medication that does not conform to prescribed directions. It can include taking more of a medication than directed or taking a medication for purposes other than the one for which it was prescribed, such as using a prescription pain medication to elevate mood. The Drug Abuse Warning Network (DAWN) was a nationally representative public health surveillance system that existed from the 1970s until 2011. The DAWN system monitored drug-related ED visits to the hospital in which a drug or drugs were felt to have directly caused the visit, or in which drugs were felt to be a contributing factor to the ED visit. In 2011, which was the last year the DAWN program existed, the most common type of drug misuse leading to an ED visit for adults age $\geq 65$ years was for prescription and nonprescription pain relievers, especially narcotic pain medications.[30] Of note, the SAMHSA is reestablishing the DAWN program in 2019, with the goal of improving monitoring of the substance use crisis, especially for opioid medications.

---

**CASE 2**

Jon Rankowski is retired electrician who is 77 years old. He has been widowed for the past 4 years. He is fairly healthy with the exception of bilateral knee arthritis and chronic lower back pain. He does not like to see specialists and would not consider surgery even if recommended. He does not really have a primary care provider, but does occasionally see the geriatrician his wife was seeing before she died (she had a stroke 2 years earlier). He has noticed more problems with his back pain in the last year and he received a prescription for oxycodone in the past 6 months, which he has refilled regularly. The geriatrician is sympathetic to his situation but concerned that he now has a secondary problem related to the oxycodone use. Although never very "social", he reports not leaving the house except to go shopping with his daughter every two weeks. She is concerned about his growing apathy.

1. What would you say to the daughter and how might you engage in conversations about this with Mr. Rankowski?

---

Opioids have not only contributed to ED visits for older adults, but their use and misuse have also caused an increase in mortality. A study of over 184,000 cases of intentional misuse of prescription opioid medications reported to US poison control centers found that between 2006 and 2013, there was a linear increasing trend in mortality among adults age $\geq 60$ years. In addition, there was a significant linear increase in rates of opioid misuse with suicidal intent among older adults.[31]

During the early 2000s, opioid medications were increasingly prescribed in both medical office appointments and to patients in EDs. Data from the National Ambulatory Medical Care Study found that between 1995 and 2010, the number of medical office visits in which opioid medications were prescribed increased from 5 million to 26 million. The greatest increases in office visits with opioid prescriptions occurred among adults age $\geq 65$ years and among adults age 36 to 64.[32] Not surprisingly, opioid prescriptions were commonly part of medical office visits in which pain was the primary reason for the appointment. The National Hospital Ambulatory Medical Care Survey similarly found that between 2005 and 2015, there was a notable decrease in opioid prescribing to adult patients in EDs who were younger than age 64 years. However, rates of prescription of opioid medication to patients age ≥ 65 years who were seen in EDs remained the same.[33]

### ❖❖ Older adults benefit from screening, brief intervention, and treatment of substance use disorders.

In addition to opioid medications, older adults are frequently prescribed benzodiazepines. Data from the DAWN program indicates that between 2005 and 2011, ED visits involving benzodiazepines alone or in combination with opioids or alcohol were higher for baby boomer adults aged 45 to 64 years than for younger or older adults.[30] Even more concerning, long-term benzodiazepine use is common among older adults, and is higher among adults age 65 to 80 years than for younger adults. Indeed, the rate of benzodiazepine use increases with age, with higher rates seen among older women than among older men.[34] Maust et al., using data from the National Ambulatory Medical Care Survey, found that only 16% of medical office visits in which benzodiazepines were prescribed had any mental health diagnosis.[35] This finding suggests that benzodiazepines may be often prescribed for long-term use without clear mental health indication of need.

Benzodiazepines have been listed on the American Geriatrics Society (AGS) Beers list for potentially inappropriate medication use in older adults for many years. In 2015 the AGS Beers Criteria Update Expert Panel updated the Beers Criteria to include opioid medications.[36] Although data on prescription medication substance misuse among older adults is limited, it is clear that older adults are vulnerable to a number of harms from both benzodiazepine and opioid use.[37] These include increased risk for falls, fractures, and traffic accidents, as well as risk for addiction or intoxication. It is important for clinicians to develop plans with their older patients regarding deprescribing both opioid medications and benzodiazepines.

### ❖❖ Treatment most often works best in a cohort of peers and undoing isolation is essential.

## Summary

Alcohol use disorder, prescription drug misuse, and illicit drug use are all increasing in later life. Of these, alcohol is the most commonly used substance. But marijuana use is high, and is growing among older adults, many of whom view it as a safe alternative to other forms of standard medical treatment. Prescription misuse of opioids and benzodiazepines are also high among older adults, with risk of fatal outcomes. Opioid use disorder and related overdose deaths are being reported in increasing numbers in older

---

**CASE 3**

Jerry Carmichael is a 66 year old man who lives with his sister. He worked several years as a cement finisher and bricklayer. Past medical history includes diabetes, hypertension and a history of stroke. He has history of alcohol and heroin use (past 20 years). He is now in a methadone treatment program and is committed to long-term recovery.

1. How do you think about methadone treatment programs and older adults?

## Illicit Substance Use

The opioid overdose epidemic has impacted older adults as well. Clinicians should not abruptly stop prescribed opioids for pain in older adults as withdrawal symptoms can potentially lead to the use of illicit opioids and resultant overdose. Older adults being prescribed opioids for chronic pain should receive individualized care with careful decision making to continue or taper opioids. Older adults using illicit opioids should be considered for medication treatment with buprenorphine or methadone. Both medications are effective, but there are little data for them specific to older adults. Buprenorphine has no significant drug interactions, whereas drug interactions must be considered for methadone. Buprenorphine treatment can be integrated with primary care, whereas methadone treatment requires referral to a specialized methadone program. However, methadone treatment programs that specifically tailor treatment for older adults are rare. Older individuals in methadone treatment for opioid use disorder are more likely to have chronic medical problems and comorbid psychiatric disorders, such as major depressive disorder, generalized anxiety disorder, and posttraumatic stress disorder.[38,39] Cocaine use raises particular concern in older adults who already have higher risk for cardiovascular disease. There is no evidence for any pharmacologic treatment for cocaine withdrawal nor cocaine use disorder. General substance use disorder treatment modalities discussed previously are indicated.

adults. These conditions are often overlooked by healthcare providers and can be difficult to detect as patients and families are frequently not aware of deleterious substance use. Screening for substance use must be incorporated into all primary care settings. Future work is needed to develop appropriate screening tools designed for older adults. Research is also needed to identify best practices for treatment specific to older adults.

## Key References

36. American Geriatrics Society Beers Criteria Update Expert Panel. American Geriatrics Society 2019 Updated AGS Beers Criteria for potentially inappropriate medication use in older adults. *J Am Geriatr Soc*. 2019;67:674–694.
3. Cousins G, Galvin R, Flood M, et al. Potential for alcohol and drug interactions in older adults: evidence from the Irish longitudinal study on ageing. *BMC Geriatr*. 2014;14:57.
11. Lehmann SW, Fingerhood M. Substance use disorders in later life. *N Engl J Med*. 2018;379:2351–2360.

35. Maust DT, Kales HC, Wiechers IR, Blow FC, Olfson M. No end in sight: benzodiazepine use in older adults in the United States. *JAGS*. 2016;64:2546–2553.
31. West NA, Severtson SG, Green JL, Dart RC. Trends in abuse and misuse of prescription opioids among older adults. *Drug Alcohol Depend*. 2015;149:117–121.

***References available online at** expertconsult.com.

# 35

# Driving

ALICE K. POMIDOR AND SANDRA M. WINTER

## OUTLINE

*Additional online-only material indicated by icon.*

## OBJECTIVES

*Upon completion of this chapter, the reader will be able to:*

- Recognize important risk factors for driving disability in older adults.
- Describe strategies for fitness-to-drive risk screening, management, and referral.
- Identify strategies for risk reduction and counseling of older adult drivers and their caregivers.
- Discuss legal and ethical issues involved in reporting impaired drivers.

Driving has become an instrumental activity of daily living (IADL) for virtually all of us. Changes normally seen with age and the medical comorbidities that commonly occur can make driving difficult, thus reducing human contact, social interaction, access to nutrition and health care, and impairing independence and the enjoyment of life. Primary prevention of loss of driving ability, secondary detection, and treatment of impaired driving skills, and tertiary management of lost driving capacity, are essential if driving capacity and safety are to be maintained. Achievement of these goals can be challenging and time consuming in healthcare settings. Driving is a skill, and its loss is a social problem that does not fit typical healthcare paradigms. It can seem difficult to assess this skill in the office, especially when we all have significant time constraints. Legal and ethical questions may also deter some healthcare professionals from addressing driving. However, early intervention can prevent fatalities, injuries, unnecessary disability, and potentially the premature loss of driving skills and privileges, with concurrent serious adverse effects on the quality of life.

❖❖ **Driving is a learned skill and a privilege—it is not a right!**

---

### CASE 1

**Vera Hodges (Part 1)**

Vera Hodges, age 74 years, comes into your office for her annual health maintenance visit. The nurse screens her IADL; Mrs. Hodges reports, "I'm having difficulty driving, especially if I go to the city and get caught in afternoon traffic. I want to be safe when driving but I'm not sure what to do." She also reports being blinded from oncoming headlights and having trouble clearly seeing familiar landmarks at night.

1. Are Mrs. Hodges' safety concerns and actions regarding driving justified?

---

## Prevalence and Impact

The number of people older than 65 years is projected to increase to 88 million by 2050[1-3] and more than 80% of this group is licensed to drive.[4] Motor vehicle accidents are the second leading cause of death from unintended injury in those older than age 65 years.[5-7] Older drivers hospitalized after crashes have significantly higher mortality rates and longer hospital stays and are less likely to be discharged directly home.[8] The crash risk of older adults is similar to that of those aged $\leq 24$ years, although this is mostly because of the higher risk, urban nature of their lower average number of miles traveled (referred to as low-mileage bias).[9–11] Adults age $>70$ years make an average of 3.0 trips per day, with an average of 6400 miles a year, whereas adults in their 40s take a mean of 4.5 trips a day and average more than 15,000 miles a year.[12] Older women are at higher risk of crash-related injury and fatality compared with older men; such incidents most often occur during moving violations (e.g., missing signs and signals, crossing lines while passing, and making left-hand turns). Accidents of older drivers are usually lower speed and multivehicular, reflecting city traffic.[13] However, a larger proportion of older compared with younger adults have safe driving habits, including seat-belt use, and avoiding night driving, rush hour, bad weather, and unfamiliar areas; they also tend not to drive while under the influence of alcohol or other intoxicants.[14]

---

### CASE 1

#### Vera Hodges (Part 2)

Mrs. Hodges has had no changes in her basic ADLs, but reports changes in her routines for other ADLs, including doing more of her driving in the morning. She obtained stronger reading glasses recently but is considering an eye doctor appointment because of difficulty, including seeing when driving at night. Her chronic conditions include diabetes, osteoarthritis especially in her neck and hands, and seasonal allergies. She takes glipizide to control her blood sugar, and acetaminophen with diphenhydramine to help with allergy-related headaches and arthritis pain, and calcium with vitamin D daily.

1. What findings do you expect on vision testing?
2. Does Mrs. Hodges have other risk factors for future driving disability and injury?

---

## Risk Factors and Pathophysiology

### Physical Function

Impaired vision is the most clearly identified function placing older drivers at increased risk for accidents, particularly severe visual field loss and restricted useful field of view (UFOV).[15] Visual field loss may be present in 18% to 30% of adults age $\geq 70$ years as a result of glaucoma, macular degeneration, or retinopathy.[16] A UFOV test takes visual processing speed and cognitive skills (such as divided visual attention) into account, by measuring the speed of response to two vehicles simultaneously displayed on a monitor. Drivers in whom visual processing speed is impaired have an increased risk of motor vehicle collision of 2.2 times that of drivers without such impairment.[11] Static visual acuity does not predict crash involvement, although it is the most commonly used measure of vision, and the standards for passing assessment by departments of motor vehicles varies from state to state. Diminished static visual acuity may decrease driving performance when $<20/40$, particularly because of difficulty reading signage or interior control panels.[13] Glare and contrast sensitivity impairment from cataract disease, present in two-thirds of adults in their 70s, strongly affects driving performance and is reversible with treatment.[15,17]

The American Geriatrics Society's (AGS) *Clinician's Guide to Assessing and Counseling Older Drivers*, 4th Edition, is published under a collaborative agreement with the National Highway Traffic Safety Administration (NHTSA)[18] with the goal of helping healthcare providers to evaluate the ability of their older patients to operate motor vehicles safely and to prevent motor vehicle accidents and injury. Motor and sensory function measures recommended in this edition, earlier evaluated for their association with driving outcomes and falls, include the Rapid Pace Walk, the Get Up and Go test, and range of motion (ROM). Motor strength testing was not found to correlate with behind-the-wheel testing, most likely because of the availability of power controls and adaptive equipment in recent years. However, impaired ROM (especially the neck) and inability to walk 10 feet and back in $<9$ seconds did correlate with impaired driving skills.[19,20]

❖ **Impaired ROM of the neck and inability to walk 10 feet and back in $<9$ seconds are both associated with impaired driving.**

---

### CASE 1

#### Discussion

On examination, Mrs. Hodges's visual acuity has worsened from 20/70 last year to 20/100 at this visit and you see significant cataracts. She is unable to reach both hands behind her head, to touch her chin to her shoulders, or to fully close her hands. Her height has decreased by 0.5 inch over the past year. After further discussion, and a review of her blood sugar diary, you discuss making two medication changes. First, you suggest her allergy symptoms may be well controlled with less drowsiness on loratadine. Because she has been tracking low blood sugar levels in the afternoon, you decrease her glipizide dose. After referral to physical therapy (PT), her ROM improves substantially and she reports less arthritis pain. An occupational therapy (OT) consult is ordered to help her regain her desired afternoon activities and to ascertain whether a comprehensive driving evaluation with a certified driving rehabilitation specialist (CDRS) is warranted. After evaluation by an OT, a decision is made not to pursue a comprehensive driving evaluation at this time. In OT, Mrs. Hodges learns about two resources. She attends CarFit, a community event sponsored by the American Occupational Therapy Association in conjunction with the American Association of Retired Persons (AARP) and the American Automobile Association (AAA). At the event, she receives guidance from trained persons on how to best adjust seat and mirror, which improve her driving comfort. Also based on the CDRS recommendation, Mrs. Hodges explored the consumer website MyCarDoesWhat.org, which overviews the array of new car technologies, such as in-vehicle information systems and advanced driver assistance systems—both designed to support driving performance and improve safety. Mrs. Hodges decides to purchase a car with blind spot detection and collision avoidance to help increase her comfort and reduce risks associated with city driving. She has a few sessions of behind-the-wheel training scheduled with the CDRS to learn how to use her car's advanced safety features. She is advised to avoid busy times of day and school bus times. At her next follow-up, Mrs. Hodges reports that the medication changes, PT and OT, and successful cataract surgery have restored her driving confidence and her ability to go places in the evening.

---

### Cognitive Function

Cognitive skill is essential for safe driving. The primary concern in clinical care is which cognitive abilities can be easily and reliably evaluated and how to know which disabilities predict on-the-road driving impairment and crash risk.

Neuropsychologic testing scores that reflect actual performance and are not adjusted for age or demographics are good predictors of driving impairment and risk because the hazards that are inherent in the road and traffic do not adjust to the driver.[21] Speed and precision of visuospatial processing and attention, such as measured by the UFOV and by copying complex drawings, are key cognitive functions. The Trails Making Test—B (Trails B) evaluates processing speed, visual and motor function integration, symbol recognition and sequencing, and the ability to focus on two thought processes at once.[22] Memory loss appears to be an indicator of underlying neurologic illnesses impairing multiple cognitive domains, rather than an independent predictor of driving ability. Some patients with significant memory problems can perform most aspects of driving well.[23] This is consistent with the characteristically much later loss of procedural memory relative to the early loss of event memory in dementia of the Alzheimer type. Executive decision making is a critical function for planning and choosing what actions to perform, but this skill is not age dependent, and variability is high within age groups.[24]

◆◆ **Memory loss has less impact on driving skill than one might think; in Alzheimer disease, event memory is lost early and procedural memory is reduced much later in the illness.**

The Mini-Mental State Examination (MMSE)[25] is a frequently administered cognitive screening tool to investigate cognitive impairment of older adults and of their ability to drive. However, the MMSE was not designed to assess driving skills. It focuses on orientation, language, and memory, and omits the other domains of cognitive functioning important for driving competence. As such, the MMSE does not consistently predict future crashes or traffic violations.[26] The Porteus Maze, Snellgrove Maze Task, Clock Drawing, Trail-Making Test Parts A or B (TMT-A, B), UFOV, and Neuropsychological Assessment Battery tests do correlate significantly with on-road driving performance.[27] Of these, the Clock Drawing test and TMT-B as described in the AGS's Clinician's Guide are easily administered in the office or emergency room settings and are sensitive, identifying 92% of those who failed the behind-the-wheel test, although specificity is low at 50%.[23,27] The UFOV is commercially available. The Montreal cognitive assessment (MoCA) combines features of the MMSE, Clock Drawing, and Trails B, as well as testing abstract ability and verbal fluency (which tests retrieval speed). The MoCA has higher sensitivity than the MMSE for detection of early cognitive impairment, and in older adults with cognitive impairment referred for driving evaluation. Each 1-point decrease in the MOCA score correlates with an increased likelihood of 1.36 in failing the road test. Also a score of ≤ 18 may predict impaired driving safety.[28–31]

When following the disease course over time of a chronically progressive neurodegenerative disease, such as Alzheimer or Parkinson disease, the rate of disease progression is highly variable. It is important that any ongoing evaluation strategy for disease-related cognitive function include measures of the functional impact on driving.[21]

◆◆ **The MoCA is more sensitive in milder cognitive impairment than the MMSE and includes visuospatial skills, abstraction, and retrieval speed; a score of 18 may predict impaired driving safety.**

---

### CASE 2

#### Henry Dowd (Part 1)

Henry Dowd is a 78-year-old man who comes to your office for his quarterly checkup. His clinical problems include obesity, hypertension, low back pain, peripheral neuropathy (referred to his legs from the lower back), atrial fibrillation, and mild depression. Mr. Dowd's wife mentions recent concern about his driving. He looks distressed by this, but agrees, sharing that his daughter, who lives nearby, said she no longer feels comfortable with him taking the grandkids home from school. Mr. Dowd says "most of the time I feel fine" but reports having a few "dizzy" spells in the past few months, one of which led to a close call when he turned in front of an oncoming driver. On further discussion, his wife reports she has been providing more help with his daily medication management because he was forgetting doses. She also says they are doing more things together, including shopping and banking, because Henry was getting stressed and sometimes failing to complete errands. He is upset about the recent changes, but states that he has never had an accident in over 60 years of driving and cannot imagine giving up driving.

1. What driving skills appear to be already impaired in Mr. Dowd, and what risk factors does he have that add to his driving disability and chance of injury?
2. What information would be useful to him and his family?

---

## Medical Conditions and Medications

Conditions prevalent in older adults include neuropathy, dementia, polypharmacy, alcohol abuse, sleep apnea, and heart failure.[32,33] Older adults taking multiple medications or who use unsafe substances were 1.43 times more likely to be involved in an accident than those taking none, and those taking three or more potentially driving-impairing medications were 1.87 times at risk of a crash.[34] In a trauma population, those on two or more actively central nervous—acting medications had 7.99 times the risk of an accident (Box 35.1).[35]

Several organizations have recently reviewed the available evidence about medical conditions and driving fitness. The Federal Motor Carriers Safety Administration (FMCSA) has an ongoing series of comprehensive reviews of the crash risk associated with a variety of disorders.[36] These focus on commercial drivers, whereas NHTSA and AGS recommendations focus on drivers of private vehicles.[18] The AGS Clinician's Guide has reference tables of medical conditions, functional deficits, and medications that may impair driving skills, and also the associated consensus recommendations. All three organizations have developed medical report forms that reflect the medical conditions of greatest concern with respect to driving (Box 35.2).

---

### ● BOX 35.1  Classes of Medication That Should Be Avoided or Minimized in Older Drivers

- Anticholinergics
- Anticonvulsants
- Antidepressants
- Antiemetics
- Antihistamines
- Antiparkinsonian agents
- Antipsychotics
- Benzodiazepines and nonbenzodiazepine hypnotics
- Muscle relaxants
- Narcotic analgesics

(From Marrotoli R, Gray S. Medical conditions, functional deficits and medications that may affect driving safety. In: Pomidor A, ed. *Clinician's Guide to Assessing and Counseling Older Drivers*. 4th ed. New York: The American Geriatrics Society; 2019.)

**• BOX 35.2** Conditions With an Increased Relative Crash Risk

- Slight to moderate (odds ratio 1.2–2.0): cardiovascular disease, cerebrovascular disease, traumatic brain injury, depression, diabetes mellitus, musculoskeletal disorders, vision disorders
- Moderately high (odds ratio 2–5 or higher): alcohol abuse and dependence, dementia, epilepsy, schizophrenia, obstructive sleep apnea

(From Marshall SC. The role of reduced fitness to drive due to medical impairments in explaining crashes involving older drivers. *Traffic Inj Prev.* 2008;9(4):291–298; and U.S. Department of Transportation. How medical conditions impact driving (report). Available at https://www.fmcsa.dot.gov/regulations/medical/reports-how-medical-conditions-impact-driving)

The FMCSA advises physicians to consider the following: (1) the nature and severity of the condition (e.g., loss of strength), (2) the degree of limitation caused (e.g., ROM), (3) the likelihood of progression, and (4) the likelihood of sudden incapacitation occurring.[36,37]

## CASE 2

### Henry Dowd (Part 2)

Mr. Dowd's medications include apixaban, metoprolol, amiodarone, tizanidine, citalopram, and gabapentin daily. He reports no shortness of breath with exertion and moderate limitations in his ability to ambulate because of low back and leg pain. He reports no difficulty with his basic ADLs but agrees with his wife that some more complicated daily tasks such as medication management have become "confusing." During his "dizzy" spells, he reports lightheadedness and palpitations and says it occurs most often in the morning when he stands up, about an hour after he takes his medications. He has never passed out and denies any changes in his vision during the episodes. His vision was corrected by his ophthalmologist 4 months ago. On questioning, Mr. Dowd describes still feeling tired when he wakes up in the morning, occasionally drifting off during the day, especially when watching TV. He reports he has stopped driving on high-speed roads because he does not like the busy traffic, and that he keeps his trips close to home—"just the usual places, you know"—because of the combination of pain and fatigue. He has stopped attending exercise classes at the senior center, which is now "too much bother." Your physical examination reveals orthostatic changes in heart rate and blood pressure that reproduce his sensation of dizziness and palpitations. Other routine physical examination findings are unchanged from his baseline. Clock drawing is normal, but the rest of the visuospatial section of the MoCA, as well as the attention and delayed recall sections, are impaired, with an overall score of 24 of 30. He is able to walk 10 feet and back in 15 seconds.

1. What should be done to help reduce Mr. Dowd's driving disability and/or compensate for his decreased skills?
2. Should he continue to drive?

## CASE 2

### Discussion

Mr. Dowd has problems in several areas, and several types of intervention —including driving rehabilitation—should be considered. His lightheadedness is of particular concern, as well as some risky medications (two with orthostatic effects), and there is worsening depression. Slower reaction time when braking, mild cognitive impairment, and poor judgment on a left-hand turn reflect cognitive/neurologic impairment, which may be the first signals of neurologic illnesses, such as dementia, Parkinson disease,

**• BOX 35.3** How the Clinician Can Reduce Driving Risk

1. Identify medical conditions and/or functional deficits producing driving disability.
2. Treat those conditions to maximally restore functional ability and prevent functional decline, including referral to subspecialists and occupational therapy.
3. If a medication is probably producing impairment, reduce the dose if possible, substitute a different therapy, or discontinue the medication.
4. Counsel the patient about the risks to driving safety and document the discussion in the medical record.
5. Recommend driving restrictions or driving cessation and alternative transportation.
6. Refer to a driver rehabilitation specialist if available for driving evaluation and rehabilitation.

neuropathy related to his low back pain, or medication central nervous system side effects.

In view of his multiple risks, he should be (1) counseled not to drive for now, (2) referred to a driving rehabilitation specialist if possible, and (3) assisted with finding alternative transportation until he is able to complete an assessment and treatment targeted at these concerns. If he does not accept these recommendations, he must be counseled regarding the safety risks of continued driving and about restrictions that might reduce the risk (Box 35.3).

## CASE 2

### Henry Dowd (Part 3)

Mr. Dowd works through several adjustments to his medications over the next 6 months. He is able to see a driving rehabilitation specialist, resulting in improved driving performance as evaluated by on-the-road testing and by resolution of most of his previous areas of concern.

After an uneventful 18 months of routine care, he is brought by his daughter to see you for follow-up after an emergency room visit for involvement in a crash, where witnesses reported that he drifted into a neighboring lane and was rear-ended at moderately high speed by a following vehicle. "My neck is so sore from that fender-bender" he says. "The emergency room said that I had to come in and see you if the pain did not go away after a few days." Mr. Dowd denies all other complaints except mild right-sided chest pain, only with movement. His daughter states that he had another incident 2 months ago, which she only just found out about by finding on his mail table the traffic ticket for running a red light. Although he was not given any restriction by the emergency room, his wife and daughter would not let him drive today because of concerns about his driving safety. On physical examination he appears upset but generally cooperative. Physical findings are unremarkable except for blood pressure of 200/90 mmHg, irregular heart rate (104 beats per minute), and right-sided chest wall tenderness. He is able to perform his 10-feet walk and return without difficulty but blames his slower time of 20 seconds on soreness from the accident. His score on the MoCA has declined to 20 of 30. Questioned at the end of the visit, he is uncertain about why he is here in your office today.

1. Why has Mr. Dowd's driving ability changed? Is it possible to restore and/or compensate for his driving disability? Should he continue to drive?

## Dementia and Driving

Cognitive impairment that progresses to dementia is an especially challenging issue for driving disability evaluation and management. A diagnosis of early Alzheimer disease (AD) or other type of dementia does not necessarily preclude safe driving, but it is always a risk factor.

Driving impairment in adults with AD has been correlated with neuroimaging changes in regional cortical function. Neuropsychologic tests of visuospatial ability, executive function, and attention, such as clock drawing and TMT-B that assess corresponding frontal and right hemisphere resources, are more accurate predictors of driving competence than global measures of cognition. However, types of dementia other than AD, such as frontotemporal, Lewy body disorder, and vascular dementias, may create different patterns of cognitive deficits.[38]

Several professional societies and consensus groups (e.g., American Academy of Neurology, American Association for Geriatric Psychiatry, AGS, the Alzheimer's Association, and the Canadian Consensus Conference on Dementia) have published guidance for clinicians regarding how to detect drivers with dementia and when to remove them from active driving for their own safety, as well as that of other road users. However, although there is broad consensus that moderately severe dementia precludes safe driving, there is an insufficient evidence base and consensus about managing those with early, mild dementia who are minimally or mildly dependent on others for assistance with their other daily living activities.[39,40] Pooled data from two longitudinal studies involving 134 drivers with dementia showed that 88% of drivers with very mild dementia (Clinical Dementia Rating [CDR] scale score = 0.5) and 69% of drivers with mild dementia (CDR = 1.0) were still able to pass a formal road test. In one study, 77% of early driving terminations at 18 months (sooner than the mean of 2 years found in the study) were caused either by hazardous driving (55% were related to road test failure and 2% were related to motor vehicle accident) or family decisions based on the progression of dementia symptoms (20%). The median time to discontinuance of driving for those with very mild dementia was 2 years after dementia diagnosis, and for those with mild dementia the mean discontinuance was 1 year.[40,41] Even if the perceptual motor skills are unimpaired, such drivers often lack insight into their limitations or make poor judgments about their capacity to manage complex or challenging situations.[42] It is therefore both desirable and reasonable to follow such patients every 6 months to reassess their ability to drive safely.

## Diagnosis and Assessment

Medical evaluation of fitness to drive must be thorough enough to detect undiagnosed conditions that could affect driving, yet also must screen for specific driving skills. Multiple assessment algorithms have been developed. Box 35.4 summarizes aspects of assessment commonly recommended.

Interprofessional collaboration can assist older adults as they go through the driver assessment process and potentially transition out of driving as their main form of transportation. The *AGS Clinician's Guide for Assessing and Counseling Older Drivers*[18] provides guidance relevant to physicians, nurses, social workers, pharmacists, occupational therapists, and neuropsychologists and is accessible, comprehensive, and straightforward. The AGS Guide includes the Plan for Older Driver Safety (PODS) decision algorithm (Fig. 35.1), a collection of office-based assessment instruments called the Clinical Assessment of Driving Related Skills. Also included are reference tables for medical conditions, state regulations and counseling/transportation resources, billing information, and a companion smartphone application. It is freely available online in its 2019 format and has companion patient

education materials.[43] The PODS decision algorithm suggests roles for clinicians and provides guidance for specialty referrals, such as to a CDRS, an individual with the training and skills to perform a comprehensive driving assessment comprised of clinical tests and an on-road driving evaluation.

## Management

A general approach to risk reduction and counseling is summarized in Box 35.5.

**⁕⁕ Connecting the patient and caregiver to community transportation resources (if available!) through your local Area on Aging or equivalent resource is key to success.**

---

**• BOX 35.4  Driving Risk Assessment Areas**

- Questionnaire about driving habits and events plus traditional medical history
- Visual screen: acuity, fields, contrast sensitivity, processing speed
- Cognitive screen: MoCA (best) or SLUMS or MMSE plus visuospatial and executive function tests (e.g., clock draw, mazes, complex drawing, or TMT-A or B)
- Psychological screen: depression scale (e.g., GDS, others)
- Functional assessment: ADLs, IADLs, and AADLs
- Musculoskeletal screen: timed walk and range of motion of neck, shoulder, legs
- Sleep history: sleep habits, Epworth scale (see Ch. 31)
- Alcohol and drug use: CAGE, urine testing, etc. (see Ch. 34)
- Medications (prescribed and OTC) that could impair

*AADLs*, Advanced activities of daily living; *ADLs*, activities of daily living; *CAGE*, cut down, annoyed by criticism, guilty about drinking, eye-opener drinks (a test for alcoholism); *GDS*, Geriatric Depression Scale; *IADLs*, instrumental activities of daily living; *MMSE*, Mini-Mental State Examination; *MoCA*, Montreal Cognitive Assessment; *OTC*, over the counter; *SLUMS*, St. Louis University Mental Status; *TMT*, Trail-Making Test.

---

**CASE 2**

**Henry Dowd (Part 4)**

Mr. Dowd says that if he cannot drive, he will "just be a burden" to his wife and daughter, both of whom work. On discussion, he agrees to refrain now from driving while he finishes PT for neck and back pain following his crash and when taking pain medication. You support him in maintaining this decision by writing a prescription stating that he agrees not to drive for 6 weeks because of his acute injury, and both of you sign it. Your copy remains at the office, his family posts a copy where his keys hang at home, and in the car. During his therapy, you review his medical conditions and treatment to ascertain whether there are any contributing factors that may have led to the accident, refer to an ophthalmologist for comprehensive vision testing, and arrange for consultation with the local Area on Aging office to learn about alternative transportation.

At the end of the 6 weeks of therapy, Mr. Dowd says he and his wife spoke with a transportation coordinator at the senior center. Mr. Dowd's wife and daughter both learned how to use a smartphone application to arrange rides with a transportation network company or TNC (e.g., Uber, Lyft) to arrange rides for Mr. Dowd when they are working. Mr. Dowd reports success in arranging transportation and learned that if he gives up his license and car, the monthly savings will more than pay for TNC type rides. He especially likes that he can go places when he wants to without extra burden on his wife or daughter.

1. What are the potential risks for Mr. Dowd when he stops driving? What would you have done if he had not agreed to stop driving?

**Plan for Older Drivers' Safety (PODS)**

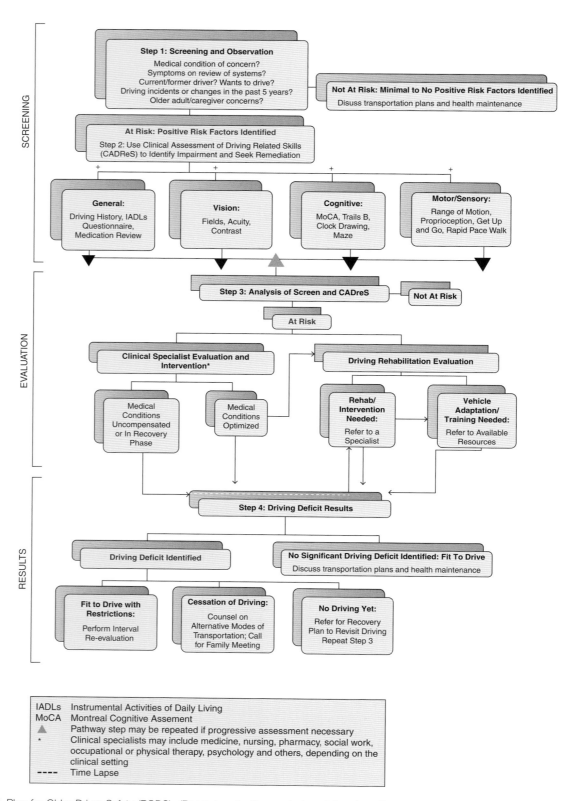

• **Figure 35.1** Plan for Older Driver Safety (PODS). (Reproduced with permission of American Geriatrics Society. Pomidor A, ed. *Clinician's Guide to Assessing and Counseling Older Drivers.* 4th ed. New York; The American Geriatrics Society: 2019.)

---

**• BOX 35.5   Risk Reduction and Counseling Strategies for the Older Driver**

- Seek treatment for reversible conditions/functional deficits
- Eliminate potential problem medications when possible
- Proper safety belt use
- Avoid severe weather conditions
- Avoid driving if sleep-deprived or acutely ill
- No driving with alcohol or when impairing meds could still be present
- No distractions: radio or music, cell phone use, eating and drinking
- One quiet adult passenger at most and no unrestrained children or uncaged animals
- Minimize night driving
- Avoid high-speed roads
- Avoid long, high mileage drives (or have a codriver)
- Plan your route: avoid left turns and overtaking; avoid school bus times
- Encourage driving refresher courses
- Use alternative transportation; buses, trains, and planes are safer per mile for long trips
- Refer to occupational therapist or driving rehabilitation specialist for formal evaluation and for rehabilitation after an immobilizing illness of any kind
- Know your state's mandatory reporting laws and other legal requirements
- If all else fails, recruit caregivers to assist: confiscate or grind keys down, park car out of sight, discontinue insurance, disable or sell car, report to local motor vehicle authority for potential license withdrawal

---

## Legal and Ethical Issues

Older adult drivers in the United States have "driving life expectancies" of approximately 11 years at age 70 years, so most older adults drive until their early 80s and will then probably need alternative transportation for an additional 5 to 10 years of life. Latino older drivers are an exception to this, with far fewer drivers overall in this age group and those who do drive stopping sooner with apparently poor health status.[44]

For many people, driving symbolizes freedom, independence, and having control. Driving refresher and training programs aimed at promoting the adoption of safe driving practices and strategies are popular approaches to the safe mobility of older drivers. Although their effectiveness on crash risk and driver performance are not well validated, they are regarded as an essential component of any strategy, particularly those that focus on improving awareness and behavior.[45] Overall, driving retirement is an expected but still highly stressful transition associated with depression, social isolation, and reduced access to services.[46,47]

Many physicians do not feel comfortable when having to confront a patient regarding his or her driving retirement and potentially reporting the patient for legal intervention by the state.

Furthermore in the United States, policies vary from state to state, with 33 states having laws and policies specifically relating to driver licensing for older adults and reporting. An overview of the state-by-state licensure policies by the Insurance Institute of Highway Safety is accessible online. In Canada, about 75% of physicians surveyed feel that reporting a patient as an unsafe driver places them in a conflict of interest and negatively impacts both the patient and the physician–patient relationship, and 72.4% agreed that physicians should be legally responsible for reporting unsafe drivers.[48] In the United States, a survey of vision care providers in Michigan found that when a change in driving status is deemed necessary, more than half recommend their patients modify their driving rather than stop driving altogether. More than half of these vision care providers were concerned that reporting would negatively influence the health of the provider–patient relationship, and more than 40% considered that reporting unsafe drivers breached physician–patient confidentiality. Because the main victim (should injury or death occur) is the driver, and because the death of innocent bystanders is unacceptable in a civilized nation, it is reassuring that most physicians believe the risks posed to the patient, his or her passengers, and the public by failing to report outweigh such negative consequences.[49]

Older drivers can have symptoms incompatible with safe driving that could occur at any age, such as syncope or presyncope, vertigo, arthritic or irrecoverable injuries, narcolepsy or the sleep attacks of undiagnosed sleep apnea, seizures, or transient ischemic attacks. If the patient does not mention driving, the clinician should take the initiative in patients with these symptoms and advise against driving. If the problem is persistent, patients will need to be advised to seek alternative transportation.

◆◆ **Always consider driving safety and do something about it if your patient or others are at risk. Hospitalized patients and patients treated in the emergency room should routinely be advised about driving (or not) before discharge, especially when they are taking newly prescribed sedative or narcotic medications.**

◆◆ **Even when a patient's symptoms or treatment appear to clearly preclude driving it should not be assumed that the patient is aware and understands the risks.**

Clinicians should counsel the patient and discuss a future plan regarding when to resume driving or how to arrange driving rehabilitation. Mandated reporting varies from state to state; these requirements are available through the Insurance Information Institute[44] or may be found in the AGS' Clinician's Guide. Only a handful of states have any type of required reporting of vision or dementia changes.[50] However, Maryland and Florida are exceptions and are pursuing driving safety for their older residents, with the stated mission of the Florida Safe Mobility for Life Coalition being to "improve the safety, access and mobility of older adults and to reduce their crash, fatality and injury rates."[51]

## Summary

Primary prevention of loss of driving ability, secondary detection and treatment of impaired driving skills, and tertiary management of lost driving capacity are all essential. The main medical factors affecting an older adult's ability to drive safely are age-related loss of physical and cognitive functions, increased prevalence of medical conditions, and use of multiple medications. Driving retirement can be a highly stressful transition associated with depression, social isolation, and reduced access to services. Licensure requirements, such as vision standards and frequency of in-person reexamination and mandated reporting, vary from state to state.

Clinicians should (1) identify medical conditions and/or functional deficits producing driving disability; (2) treat those conditions to maximally restore functional ability and prevent functional decline, including referral to subspecialists and OT; (3) reduce or discontinue potentially driving-impairing medications or substitute a different therapy (nonmedication, e.g., physical therapy);

(4) counsel the patient about the risks to driving safety and document the discussion in the medical record; (5) recommend driving restrictions or driving cessation and alternative transportation; and (6) refer to a driver rehabilitation specialist if available for driving evaluation and rehabilitation.

## Web Resources

AARP, AAA, and the American Occupational Therapy Association. Overview of the Car-Fit program: https://www.car-fit.org/

American Geriatrics Society Health in Aging Foundation Driving Safety for Older Adults: https://www.healthinaging.org/driving-safety

American Geriatrics Society & A Pomidor, ed. *Clinician's Guide to Assessing and Counseling Older Drivers*, 4th Edition. New York: The American Geriatrics Society; 2019. https://geriatricscareonline.org/ProductAbstract/clinicians-guide-to-assessing-and-counseling-older-drivers-4th-edition/B047

American Occupational Therapy Association. Resource page on Driving and Community Mobility: https://www.aota.org/Practice/Productive-Aging/Driving.aspx

Association for Driver Rehabilitation Specialists. A searchable listing of Driver Rehabilitation Specialists and Certified Driver Rehabilitation Specialists: http://www.driver-ed.org

Eldercare Locator, including transportation resources: https://eldercare.acl.gov/Public/Index.aspx/Eldercare.NET/Public/Index.aspx

Florida's Safe Mobility for Life Coalition: http://safemobilityfl.com/

Insurance Institute for Highway Safety and Highway Loss Data Institute. State licensure requirements and statistics on older drivers: https://www.iihs.org/topics/older-drivers

National Highway Traffic Safety Administration. The Effects of Medical Conditions on Driving Performance: A Literature Review and Synthesis: https://www.nhtsa.gov/sites/nhtsa.dot.gov/files/documents/13394-mediconlitreview-073018-v3-tag.pdf

National Highway Traffic Safety Administration. Older Drivers information page: https://www.nhtsa.gov/road-safety/older-drivers

National Safety Council. A guide to new car safety features: https://mycardoeswhat.org/

University of Florida. Free online driver screening tool for proxy rater (someone familiar with the person's driving) to determine category of driving risk: http://fitnesstodrive.phhp.ufl.edu/us/

## Key References

1. Pomidor A, ed. *Clinician's Guide to Assessing and Counseling Older Drivers*. 4th ed. New York, NY: The American Geriatrics Society; 2019.

23. Dickerson AE, Brown D, Ridenour C. Assessment tools predicting fitness to drive in older adults: a systematic review. *Am J Occup Ther*. 2014;68:670−680.

35. Lococo K, Staplin L, Schultz M. *The Effects of Medical Conditions on Driving Performance: A Literature Review and Synthesis* (Report No. DOT HS 812 526). Washington, DC: National Highway Traffic Safety Administration; 2018.

**References available online at** expertconsult.com.

# Selected Clinical Problems of the Organ Systems

*Whenever a man's friends begin to compliment him about looking young, you may be sure that they think he is growing old.*

**WASHINGTON IRVING, 1783–1859, US writer, in Bracebridge Hall**

*There are people who are beautiful in dilapidation, like old houses that were hideous when new.*

**LOGAN PEARSALL SMITH, 1865–1946 English writer US-born in Afterthoughts**

*When grace is joined with wrinkles, it is adorable. There is an unspeakable dawn in happy old age.*

**VICTOR HUGO, 1802–1865 French author in Les Misérables**

*The wise, for cure, on exercise depend.*

*God never made his work for man to mend!*

**JOHN DRYDEN, 1631–1700, English poet**

*No spring, nor summer beauty hath such grace, As I have seen in one autumnal face.*

**JOHN DONNE, 1572?–1631 English poet in Elegy "The Autumnal" 1635**

*To keep the heart unwrinkled, to be hopeful, kindly, cheerful, reverent — that is to triumph over old age.*

**THOMAS BAILEY ALDRICH 1836–1907 US poet, novelist, playwright in "Leaves from a Notebook", Ponkapog Papers 1903**

*Better is a poor and a wise child than an old and foolish king, who will no more be admonished.*

**THE BIBLE, Ecclesiastes 4:13**

*It is the common vice of all, in old age, to be too intent upon our interests.*

**TERENCE 195?–159 Roman playwright in The Brothers, 160 BC**

*I never accept lengthy film roles nowadays, because I am always so afraid I will die in the middle of shooting and cause such awful problems.*

**SIR JOHN GIELGUD, 1904–2000, in The Independent, *March 26, 1994***

*I think your whole life shows in your face and you should be proud of that.*

**LAUREN BACALL, 1924–2014, US film actress, remark in 1988**

*To live effectively, with a real purpose and not merely to exist, you must be active, interested, involved — both physically and mentally.*

**LAWRENCE J. FRANKEL, 1904–2004, exercise in old age pioneer, in Be Alive as Long as You Live**

*To get back my youth I would do anything in the world, except take exercise, get up early or be respectable.*

**OSCAR WILDE 1854–1900, in The Picture of Dorian Gray**

*I was so much older then, I'm younger than that now.*

**BOB DYLAN, b 1941, in My Back Pages**

*I grow old . . . I grow old . . . I shall wear the bottoms of my trousers rolled.*

**T. S. ELIOT, 1888–1965, U.S.- born British poet, in The Love Song of J. Alfred Prufrock**

*An old man loved is winter with flowers*

**German Proverb**

*Some old women and men grow bitter with age. The more their teeth drop out, the more biting they get!*

**GEORGE DENNISON PRENTICE 1802–1870 US editor and newspaperman in Prenticiana *1860***

*I wasted time, and now doth time waste me*

**WILLIAM SHAKESPEARE, 1564–1616, in Richard II *5.5.49***

*Last scene of all,*

*That ends this strange eventful history,*

*Is second childishness and mere oblivion;*

*Sans teeth, sans eyes, sans taste, sans everything.*

**WILLIAM SHAKESPEARE, 1564–1616, in As You Like It, II, 7**

# 36

# Hypertension

MARGARET R. HELTON

## OUTLINE

## OBJECTIVES

*Upon completion of this chapter, the reader will be able to:*

- Define hypertension and its pathophysiologic impact on the cardiovascular system.
- Discuss the evidence that treating hypertension is beneficial to the older adult population.

- Discuss the different types of hypertension.
- Discuss the treatment approach, including adjusting therapy in specific clinical conditions common in older people.

## Prevalence and Impact

Hypertension is one of the most common medical conditions in older adults. The percentage of adults with hypertension rises steadily and progressively as people age (Fig. 36.1).[1] Data on postmenopausal women in the Women's Health Initiative study identified prevalence rates of 27% for women 50 to 59 years of age, 41% for women 60 to 69 years of age, and 53% for women 70 to 79 years of age.[2]

In the United States, Black persons are more likely to have hypertension than White persons, a trend that continues as people age.[3] The prevalence of hypertension in Black persons in the United States is among the highest in the world and likely caused by a complex pathophysiology involving interaction of genetic, biologic, and social factors.[4] Hypertension explains the around 50% increased stroke risk among Black persons compared with White persons.[5] Native Americans and Asians generally have rates of hypertension similar to Whites, whereas Hispanic persons generally have lower rates.[1]

### Adverse Outcomes

Population data consistently show that people with hypertension have a higher rate of all cardiovascular events, including myocardial infarctions

(MI), stroke, peripheral arterial disease, and heart failure, and that risk of cardiovascular disease associated with hypertension increases markedly with age.[6] Hypertension is also linked to functional issues that affect quality of life, such as erectile dysfunction,[7] renal function,[8] and vascular dementia.[9] Hypertension is a risk factor for both Alzheimer disease (AD) and vascular dementia, because of cumulative damage to cerebral blood vessels and possible promotion of brain pathology.[10]

These adverse outcomes lead to increased death rates. The death rate associated with hypertension continues to increase, reflecting increasing numbers of older Americans and their higher prevalence of hypertension.

❖ **Hypertension is common in older adults and associated with increased cardiovascular morbidity and mortality.**

### Low Rates of Successful Treatment

Despite the prevalence of hypertension and evidence of its serious impact on health and mortality, the rate of successful treatment remains low in all ages. Among persons age ≥ 60 years, 77% of those with hypertension are aware of it, 71% are treated, although only 30% actually have their high blood pressure (BP) under control.[1]

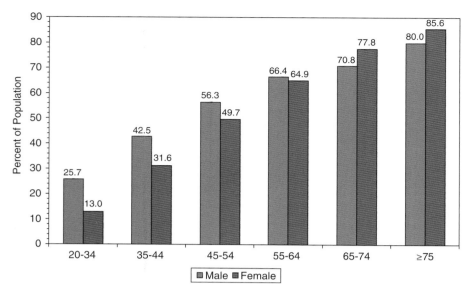

• **Figure 36.1** Prevalence of high blood pressure in adults age 20 years and over by sex and age. Based on NHANES 2013–2016. Hypertension is defined in terms of NHANES blood pressure measurements and health interviews. A person was considered to have hypertension if he or she had systolic blood pressure ≥ 130 mmHg or diastolic blood pressure ≥ 80 mmHg, if he or she said "yes" to taking antihypertensive medication, or if the person was told on 2 occasions that he or she had hypertension. *NHANES*, National Health and Nutrition Examination Survey. (From National Heart, Lung, and Blood Institute; National Institutes of Health; U.S. Department of Health and Human Services.)

These rates are higher than those of younger adults. Hypertensive control rates are lower for Black persons, Asian Americans, and Hispanic Americans, compared with White persons.[11] The good news is that the percentage of hypertensive adults in all racial subgroups who achieved BP control has steadily increased over the past 20 years.

## Rationale for Treatment

The benefits of treating hypertension in older individuals were established in the 1990s when large trials showed that treatment significantly lowered the rate of strokes and cardiovascular disease by 30% to 40% (Table 36.1).[12–16] These trials firmly established the benefits for individuals in their 60s and 70s, but concern remained regarding treatment in individuals age > 80 years until the Hypertension in the Very Elderly Trial (HYVET) was published in 2008.[17] In this older age group, treatment was associated with a 39% reduction in the rate of death by stroke, 23% reduction in rate of death from cardiovascular diseases, 64% reduction in rate of heart failure, and 21% reduction in the rate of death by any cause.

❖❖ **BP treatment and control can lower the risk of cardiovascular events and mortality in all age groups, including older adults.**

### CASE 1

#### Alice McAllister (Part 1)

Ms. McAllister is an 82-year-old White woman who lives in an assisted living facility. She moved to the area 3 years ago to be near her adult daughter. She has macular degeneration, breast cancer for which she underwent lumpectomy and radiation 10 years ago (and has remained disease-free), and arthritis in her knees, which requires her to use a rolling walker. Her only medication is a vitamin recommended by her eye doctor. Today her BP is 165/85 mmHg. In reviewing your last three visits with her, you notice

that those BPs were 152/82 mmHg, 158/86 mmHg, and 160/80 mmHg. She feels well and has no new complaints.
1. Does Ms. McAllister need medication?

### CASE 2

#### James Wilson (Part 1)

Mr. Wilson is a 77-year-old Black man with a long history of hypertension. He had a heart attack 4 years ago after which he received a stent in his left anterior descending artery and continues to be medically managed with metoprolol 25 mg twice daily, aspirin 81 mg daily, and clopidogrel 75 mg daily. He had a stroke last year, which left him with mild left hand weakness. He reports feeling shorter of breath and tired over the past months. His BP is 150/100 mmHg.
1. What information would be helpful in Mr. Wilson's history and examination?

## Risk Factors and Pathophysiology

Effective treatment of hypertension in older individuals requires an understanding of the pathophysiology that leads to increased BP. Some of these changes occur with normal aging but are also influenced by lifestyle factors.

Arterial BP consists of a forward wave generated by the heart and reflective waves returning to the heart from peripheral sites. In young people, the artery is distensible, so the pressure wave travels slowly and is reflected back in diastole. Aging is associated with a progressive increase in stiffness of the large vessels.[20] With this arterial stiffening, the waves move faster and reflect back to the proximal aorta during systole, augmenting the systolic pressure

## TABLE 36.1  Large Randomized, Blinded, Placebo-Controlled Trials of Pharmacologic Hypertension Treatment in the Older Adult Population

| | HYVET | SHEP | STOP HTN | MRC | Syst-Eur | Syst-China | STONE | EWPHE |
|---|---|---|---|---|---|---|---|---|
| No. of patients | 3845 | 4736 | 1627 | 4396 | 4695 | 2394 | 1632 | 840 |
| Mean age (years) | 84 | 72 | 76 | 70 | 70 | 66 | 66 (women) 67 (men) | 72 |
| Type of hypertension | Systolic | Systolic | Systolic and/ or diastolic | Systolic and/ or diastolic | Systolic | Systolic | Systolic and/ or diastolic | Systolic and/ or diastolic |
| Treatment regimen | Thiazide diuretic ± ACE inhibitor | Thiazide diuretic ± β-blocker, reserpine | Thiazide diuretic ± β-blocker | Thiazide diuretic ± ACE inhibitor | Calcium channel blocker ± ACE inhibitor, thiazide diuretic | Calcium channel blocker ± ACE inhibitor, diuretic | Calcium channel blocker | Diuretic ± methyldopa |
| **Relative Risk Reduction of:** | | | | | | | | |
| Stroke | 30% | 36%[a] | 47%[a] | 25%[ab] | 42%[a] | 38%[a] | — | 36% |
| Coronary artery disease | | 27%[a] | 13% | 19%[b] | 30% | — | — | 20% |
| Congestive heart failure | 64%[a] | 49%[a] | 51%[a] | Not reported | 29% | — | — | 22% |
| Other significant reductions | Coronary artery disease mortality | Coronary artery disease mortality | Major cardiovascular events Total mortality | | Vascular dementia | Cardiovascular mortality | Cardiovascular events | Fatal coronary events Cardiovascular mortality |

ACE, Angiotensin-converting enzyme; EWPHE, European Working Party on High Blood Pressure in the Elderly[19]; HYVET, Hypertension in the Very Elderly Trial[17]; MRC, Medical Research Council[16]; SHEP, Systolic Hypertension in the Elderly Program[12]; STONE, Shanghai Trial of Nifedipine in the Elderly[18]; STOP-HTN, Swedish Trial in Old Patients with Hypertension[13]; Syst-China, Systolic Hypertension in China Trial[15]; Syst-Eur, Systolic Hypertension in Europe Trial[14].

[a]Statistically significantly at P < .05.

[b]This reduction was only noted in the thiazide arm.

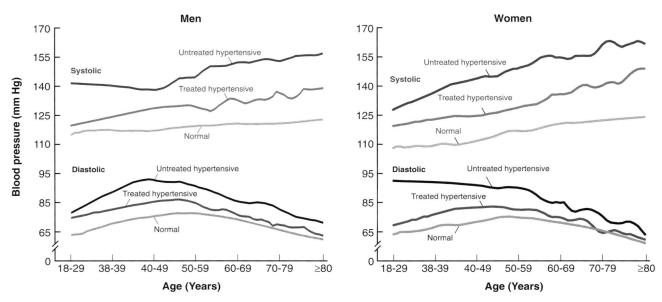

• **Figure 36.2** Mean systolic and diastolic pressure for men and women, by age and hypertension status. (From James PA, Oparil S, Carter BL, et al. 2014 Evidence based guidelines for the management of high blood pressure in adults: report from the panel members appointed to the eighth Joint national Committee (JNC 8). *JAMA* 2014;311:507–520.)

(SBP) and lowering the diastolic pressure (DBP), making isolated systolic hypertension the predominant problem in older adults (Fig. 36.2).[21] These changes lead to a widening pulse pressure (the difference between SBP and DBP) as people age, which is a better predictor of heart disease than either SBP or DBP.[22,23]

With age, blood vessels become less responsive to the vasodilatory effects of β-adrenergic stimulation,[24] changes that also contribute to hypertension. Plasma renin activity declines with age, probably because of age-associated nephrosclerosis, and plays less of a critical role in hypertension than the previously described vascular changes.[25] The decline in the aldosterone level leads to a greater risk of hyperkalemia in older individuals, especially when associated with the overall age-associated decline in renal function.

Lifestyle significantly influences BP. Smoking, excessive alcohol intake, and obesity have a complex and deleterious interplay with hypertension, all synergistically negative in the impact on health.

## Diagnosis and Assessment

### Definitions and Criteria

#### Hypertension

The Joint National Committee (JNC) on the Prevention, Detection, Evaluation, and Treatment of High Blood Pressure has long set the evidence-based standards for diagnosing and managing hypertension. The focus of its most recent release in 2014 (JNC 8) was on treatment thresholds, goals, and medications, rather than definitions, and for the first time drew a distinction based on age. Although they continue to advise that adults < 60 years of age start pharmacologic treatment at SBP 140 mmHg (or higher) or DBP 90 mmHg (or higher), they were more permissive in their guidelines for adults age > 60 years, advising that treatment be initiated at SBP 150 mmHg or higher with the same threshold of 90 mmHg or higher for DBP.[26]

Subsequent to the JNC 8 report, the American College of Cardiology (ACC) and the American Heart Association (AHA) released an updated clinical practice guideline on high BP, which suggested lower thresholds for treatment that did not vary by age. They suggested continuing the practice of categorizing BP as normal, elevated, or stage 1 or 2 hypertension (Table 36.2).[27]

#### Essential Hypertension

Most people with high BP have essential hypertension, which is defined as a rise in BP of unknown cause. It is likely because of an interaction between environmental and genetic factors and tends to coexist with other cardiovascular risk factors, such as aging, obesity, physical inactivity, insulin resistance, diabetes, and hyperlipidemia.[28] The term *essential* dates to the time when it was thought that an increase in BP was a necessary and appropriate response to guarantee adequate perfusion of organs.

#### Secondary Hypertension

Hypertension because of a secondary cause is uncommon in older adults but can be considered if there is a sudden rise in BP or a lack of response to three-drug therapy. Obesity-related hypertension is a distinctive form of hypertension with a complex pathophysiology.[29] This will have significant impact as the obesity epidemic persists as people age. Another cause of secondary hypertension in older people is renal disease although it is often hard to tell if the renal disease is causing the hypertension or vice versa. Renal artery stenosis because of atherosclerotic disease should be suspected if there is an acute kidney failure (a rise in serum creatinine of ≥ 0.5−1 mg/dL) after starting an angiotensin-converting enzyme (ACE) inhibitor or angiotensin receptor blocker (ARB) or with severely worsening hypertension.[30] The renal arteries can be evaluated with imaging; however, medical management is recommended for adults with atherosclerotic renal artery disease because it is as effective as revascularization with similar rates of BP control

## TABLE 36.2  Categories of Blood Pressure in Adults

| BP Category | SBP | | DBP |
|---|---|---|---|
| Normal | <120 mmHg | and | <80 mmHg |
| Elevated | 120–129 mmHg | and | <80 mmHg |
| Hypertension | | | |
| Stage 1 | 130–139 mmHg | or | 80–89 mmHg |
| Stage 2 | ≥140 mmHg | or | ≥90 mmHg |

(From Whelton PK, Carey RM, Aronow WS, et al. 2017 ACC/AHA/AAPA/ABC/ACPM/AGS/APhA/ASH/ASPC/NMA/PCNA Guideline for the prevention, detection, evaluation, and management of high blood pressure in adults: a report of the American College of Cardiology/American Heart Association Task Force on Clinical Practice Guidelines. *J Am Coll Cardiol.* 2018;71:e127–e248.)
*DBP,* Diastolic blood pressure; *SBP,* systolic blood pressure.

and cardiovascular deaths and without the risks associated with surgery.[27,31] Thus diagnosing renal artery stenosis may be of little value in most older adults.

Thyroid disease can cause hypertension and can occur in middle or older age. Thyroid-stimulating hormone is a sensitive measurement for diagnosis. Parathyroid disease can also increase BP and can be evaluated by measuring calcium and parathyroid hormone levels.

Hypertension because of medications should be considered. Nonsteroidal antiinflammatory drugs (NSAIDs), steroids, and decongestants can increase BP.

### Resistant Hypertension

Patients whose BP remains above goals despite treatment with three or more antihypertensive medications at optimal doses, including a diuretic, or those who require four or more antihypertensive medications for control, are considered to have resistant hypertension.[27] The most common cause is nonadherence to the prescribed medications.

### Pseudohypertension

In rare cases, peripheral arteries may be so stiff and rigid that measuring BP with the arm cuff may lead to an overestimate of the arterial pressure because of incomplete compression of the brachial artery.[32] This should be considered in patients whose hypertension does not respond to treatment or who have postural symptoms with treatment.

### Markedly Elevated Blood Pressures

Severe asymptomatic hypertension is defined as SBP 180 mmHg (or higher) or DBP 110 mmHg (or higher) without symptoms of acute target organ injury, although they may have symptoms, such as headache, nausea, palpitations, and shortness of breath. These patients are at minimal increased risk in the short term and can be managed in the outpatient setting with adjustment of medications over weeks.[33] Hypertensive emergencies have the same parameters but manifest with acute target organ damage, such as aortic dissection, acute renal failure, acute coronary syndrome, pulmonary edema, or stroke, requiring parenteral drug treatment in a hospital.[27]

### Blood Pressure Measurement

A diagnosis of hypertension should be based on two or more BP readings obtained on two or more separate occasions.[27] The principles of BP measurement have changed little since Korotkoff introduced the procedure 100 years ago. Mercury sphygmomanometers remain the gold standard, but their use is being phased out in many countries because of environmental and health concerns. Electronic, or digital, devices are safe and convenient and base readings on oscillometric measurements when the device is placed at the upper arm or wrist. They do not require auscultation so can be used in noisy environments but may not be accurate in patients with arrhythmias.

Proper technique starts with an appropriately sized cuff, with the cuff inflatable bladder length at 75% to 100% of the upper arm circumference. The cuff bladder width should be 37.5% to 50% of the patient's arm circumference (a length to width ratio of 2:1). The cuff should cover 80% of the area from the elbow to the shoulder.[34] Too small a cuff may produce an artificially elevated SBP. The patient should be quietly seated for at least 5 minutes with no caffeine, smoking, or exercise in the preceding 30 minutes. The patient's arm is supported or resting on a table at the level of the heart and the cuff inflated until the brachial artery is occluded and then slowly deflated at a rate of 2 mmHg per second. When blood starts to flow in the artery, a pounding sound is heard with the provider's stethoscope or detected by the digital device (first Korotkoff sound), indicating the SBP. With further release of the cuff pressure, eventually no sound is heard or detected, indicating the DBP.

Inappropriately low SBP readings in older individuals can occur because of an auscultatory gap, which is the interval of pressure where the Korotkoff sounds that indicate systolic pressure fade away and reappear at a lower pressure point. This gap is related to arterial stiffness and is associated with an increased risk of cardiovascular disease, especially carotid atherosclerosis.[35] The true systolic pressure can be obtained by palpating the radial artery pulse, which is recommended whenever a manual BP is taken and is usually around 10 mmHg lower than the pressure heard with auscultation. Or the gap can be avoided by making sure the BP cuff is always inflated to about 30 mmHg higher than that needed to occlude the brachial artery.

Office measurement of BP may not accurately reflect a patient's baseline BP with differences between ambulatory and in-office BP as much as 19/11 mmHg, which is enough to affect treatment decisions and inaccurately estimate risk as both ambulatory and home BP monitoring are stronger predictors of all-cause and cardiovascular mortality than BP measurements taken in the clinic.[36] The BP in the office may be elevated because of patient anxiety ("white coat hypertension"), a phenomenon that is even more common in older adults.[37] Conversely, office BP measurement may systematically fail to identify patients with BPs that are usually higher than that measured in the office because of a masking effect. For accurate diagnosis and monitoring, out-of-office BP monitoring is recommended using an ambulatory BP monitor or, as a practical alternative, home monitoring with a validated oscillatory device (Level of evidence [LOE] = A).[35]

---

### CASE 1

**Alice McAllister (Part 2)**

On physical examination, Ms. McAllister weighs 116 lbs. and is 5'2" in height. You decide to start her on chlorthalidone 25 mg daily.
1. What laboratory and other investigations are appropriate?

---

### CASE 2

**James Wilson (Part 2)**

Further history reveals that Mr. Wilson was a one-pack a day smoker for 50 years but successfully stopped after his heart attack. On physical examination, he has moderate arteriovenous nicking in the fundi. He has normal carotid upstrokes. On chest examination he has bibasilar rales and a soft systolic murmur over the aortic outflow area. He has 1 + peripheral edema and diminished pulses in his feet.
1. What laboratory and other investigations are appropriate?

---

### Medical History

The evaluation of the patient with hypertension should assess for other cardiovascular risk factors that affect prognosis and treatment. The history should include duration of the condition, previous treatments, weight gain, diet, physical activity, alcohol use, lifestyle changes, and family history.

### Physical Examination

Physical examination should assess for end-organ damage and includes evaluation of optic fundi (arteriolar narrowing, hemorrhage), heart (murmur, displaced apical impulse, arrhythmia), and peripheral circulation (abdominal pulsation or bruit, carotid bruit, peripheral pulses, jugular venous distention). The thyroid gland should be palpated, and the lungs auscultated. Neurologic examination should look for any deficit that might indicate previous stroke. Memory testing is often indicated in older adults if there are concerns regarding cognition.

### Laboratory Tests

Laboratory studies assess for target organ damage and other cardiovascular risk factors and include fasting blood sugar, complete blood count, lipid profile, creatinine, sodium, potassium, calcium, thyroid-stimulating hormone, and urinalysis. An electrocardiogram (ECG) will identify left ventricular hypertrophy or signs of previous cardiac events.

## Management

### Goals of Treatment

The guidelines and goals for the treatment of hypertension vary (Table 36.3). The JNC 8 advises that in the general population of adults age ≥ 60 years, pharmacologic treatment should be initiated when the SBP is 150 mmHg (or higher) or when the DBP is 90 mmHg (or higher). The target SBP is < 150 mmHg and DBP < 90 mmHg. These goals and targets are permissive compared with those of adults < 60 years of age for whom the SBP treatment threshold is 140 mmHg with the same DBP threshold of 90 mmHg. A corollary recommendation states that if treatment results in SBP < 140 mmHg and treatment is not associated with adverse effects on health or quality of life, treatment does not need to be adjusted.

Subsequent to the JNC 8 recommendation, the ACC and the AHA released a new guideline that removed the age-related permissiveness regarding BP definition and treatment thresholds, and recommended treating adults age ≥ 65 years with an average SBP of > 130 mmHg to a goal of < 130 mmHg.[27]

The ACA/AHA guidelines were informed by updated results reported in 2016 of the Systolic Blood Pressure Intervention Trial (SPRINT).[38] This paper described the outcomes for a prespecified subgroup of adults age ≥ 75 years with hypertension. In this trial of > 9000 patients with SBP 130 mmHg (or higher), the intensive target of < 120 mmHg was associated with a 33% relative risk reduction in the composite outcomes of fatal and nonfatal cardiovascular outcomes (absolute risk reduction [ARR] of 1.26%/year; number needed to treat [NNT] 27 over 3 years). The rate of serious adverse events was similar between the two groups.

The generalizability of SPRINT has been debated and remains controversial. These more aggressive guidelines would classify 48% of the US adult population as hypertensive. The American Academy of Family Physicians and the American College of Physicians do not endorse these more aggressive treatment recommendations and continue to endorse the evidence-based guidelines from JNC 8.[39] Clinical judgment, patient preference, comorbidities, and life expectancy are factors to consider when weighing the

---

| TABLE 36.3 | Practice Guidelines for Treatment of Hypertension in Older Adults | | |
|---|---|---|---|
| Guideline Entity | | BP Threshold for Treatment (mmHg) | BP Goal (mmHg) |
| Eighth Joint National Committee (JNC 8) for the general population of adults age > 60 years[26] | | SBP > 150 or DBP > 90 | SBP < 150 and DBP < 90 |
| ACC/AHA Task Force on Clinical Practice Guidelines for noninstitutionalized, ambulatory, community-living adults age ≥ 65 years[27] | | > 130/80 | < 130 (SBP) |

*ACC*, American College of Cardiology; *AHA*, American Heart Association; *DBP*, diastolic blood pressure; *SBP*, systolic blood pressure.

risks and benefits of treatment for hypertension in older adults. Adults with ischemic heart disease or heart failure, including adults age > 75 years, should be treated to attain a BP of < 130/80 mmHg (class 1 recommendation).[27,40]

**How aggressive to be in treating hypertension in older adults requires considerable clinical judgment.**

---

### CASE 1

### Alice McAllister (Part 3)

Her blood work, including renal function and electrolytes, was initially normal, but 3 months after starting the chlorthalidone, Ms. McAllister appears in the clinic with her daughter who expresses concerns that she seems more confused. Blood work reveals a sodium of 128 mmol/L with a creatinine of 0.66 mg/dL.
1. What are the next steps?

---

### CASE 2

### James Wilson (Part 3)

An ECG on Mr. Wilson shows an old anteroseptal MI, diffuse nonspecific ST and T wave changes, and left ventricular enlargement. You order a chest x-ray because of the crackles on his lung examination. It shows moderate cardiomegaly, fluid in the fissures, and small bilateral pleural effusions. His BP is 152/88 mmHg.
1. What are the next steps?

---

## Nonpharmacologic Treatment

Given the cost, poor adherence, and unwanted side effects of many medications, it is important to emphasize lifestyle changes that can effectively reduce BP (Table 36.4). These lifestyle interventions can help with health problems and increase overall quality of life, although change is notoriously challenging for people.

### Weight Loss

In the United States, the prevalence of obesity is 40%, a rate that persists as people age.[41] How this epidemic will affect an aging population is complex, but it is certain that being overweight or obese complicates the aging process. The evidence that being overweight increases BP is overwhelming at all ages, including in older adults.[42] Although most studies showing the efficacy of weight loss in lowering BP involve middle-aged adults,[43] several were conducted in older persons and demonstrated that older persons can successfully achieve and maintain weight control and reduce BP.[44]

### Physical Activity

Multiple trials have reported that BP is reduced with physical exercise, including for older adults.[44] The benefits of exercise are abundant and include reduction in lipids and insulin resistance, improvement in mental health, and lower risk of falls, with an overall improvement in quality of life that benefits older adults, including those with chronic disease.

### Reduced Salt Intake

The relationship between dietary salt (sodium chloride) intake and BP is direct and progressive and it is recommended that salt intake be limited to 2.3 g per day.[45] The effects of salt restriction on BP reduction is most pronounced in Black persons, older persons, and people with hypertension, diabetes, or chronic kidney disease. Excess salt consumption is a worldwide problem across societies with inherent challenges because of high consumption of processed foods, and individual efforts to reduce added salt will be limited without a strategy to reduce salt in processed foods from food manufacturers and restaurants.[46,47] It is worth noting that these recommendations are still debated with some arguing against population-wide sodium restriction.[48]

### Dietary Approaches to Stop Hypertension Eating Plan

The Dietary Approaches to Stop Hypertension (DASH) eating plan has been shown to reduce BP. It emphasizes fruits, vegetables, low-fat dairy products, whole grains, poultry, fish, and nuts with reduced intake of fats, red meat, sweets, and sugar-containing beverages.[49,50] The diet is rich in potassium, phosphorus, and protein, so it is not recommended for persons with stage 3 or 4 chronic kidney disease.

---

**TABLE 36.4  Effects of Lifestyle Modifications on Blood Pressure**

| Lifestyle Modification | Specifics | Level of Evidence | Approximate Reduction in Systolic Blood Pressure |
|---|---|---|---|
| Weight loss | Maintain BMI <25 kg/m² | A | 5–20 mmHg per 10 kg weight loss |
| Physical activity | At least 30 minutes per day | A | ~5 mmHg |
| Reduce salt intake | Limit sodium to 2.4 g per day | A | ~5 mmHg |
| Heart-healthy diet, such as DASH | Low fat diet with fruits and vegetables | A | ~11 mmHg |
| Potassium supplementation | Preferably as part of dietary modification | A | ~4 mmHg |
| Stop smoking | | A | 1–6 mmHg |
| Moderation of alcohol consumption | Limit alcohol to ≤2 drinks/day for men and ≤1 drink/day for women | A | ~4 mmHg |

(Modified from Whelton PK, Carey RM, Aronow WS, et al. 2017 ACC/AHA/AAPA/ABC/ACPM/AGS/APhA/ASH/ASPC/NMA/PCNA Guideline for the Prevention, Detection, Evaluation, and Management of High Blood Pressure in Adults: A Report of the American College of Cardiology/American Heart Association Task Force on Clinical Practice Guidelines. *J Am Coll Cardiol.* 2018;71:e127–e248.)
*A,* Supported by one or more high quality randomized trials; *BMI,* body mass index, *DASH,* Dietary Approaches to Stop Hypertension.

## Potassium Intake

Multiple trials have documented an inverse relationship between potassium intake and BP, leading to a recommendation that individuals have a potassium intake of at least 4.7 g per day.[45,51] However, the concern for hyperkalemia leads to reluctance to recommend potassium intake and often limits the use of renin-angiotensin-aldosterone system blockers, especially in patients with heart failure and chronic kidney diseases.[52]

## Smoking

Significant progress has been made in reducing cigarette smoking by US adults with 14% of adults currently smoking cigarettes, a decline of 67% since 1965.[53] For adults age $\geq 65$ years, the rate of smoking is lower at 8%, likely because many smokers do not make it far into old age; 480,000 US adults die from cigarette smoking and secondhand smoke exposure each year.[54] Smoking works synergistically with hypertension to significantly increase the risk of coronary artery disease and stroke.[55,56] Smoking cessation lowers BP in older adults and should be strongly encouraged.[57] Smoking cessation significantly reduces the risk of cardiovascular disease within 5 years relative to current smokers; however, the risk remains significantly elevated for many years compared with never smokers.[58] Still, despite skepticism and fatalism among both clinicians and patients, when offered support for smoking cessation, older smokers quit smoking at rates comparable with those of younger smokers.[59] Multiple online resources are available, including some aimed at older adults (60plus.smokefree.gov) (see Ch. 5).

## Alcohol

Drinking alcohol, especially outside of meals, increases BP in all age groups. Alcohol and hypertension work synergistically to increase morbidity and mortality. Reducing alcohol intake lowers BP in a dose-dependent manner, and implementation of effective alcohol interventions in people who drink more than two drinks per day would reduce the disease burden from both alcohol overuse and hypertension.[60] Alcohol consumption should be limited to no more than two drinks per day for men and no more than one drink per day for women[27] (see Ch. 34).

## Caffeine

Coffee does seem to increase BP within hours of drinking, including in older adults, but the long-term clinical significance of this is not clear.[61,62]

❖ **Lifestyle interventions are important, but most older people with hypertension will require medications.**

## Pharmacologic Treatment

### Overview of Medications

For decades, JNC recommended diuretics as the first-choice treatment in hypertension. JNC 8 advises that diuretics are still a good first choice, but for the general population, ACE inhibitors, ARBs, and calcium channel blockers (CCB) are also appropriate choices for initial therapy (moderate recommendation: grade B).[26] For adults age $\geq 60$ years, diuretics and CCBs are more effective and should be selected as first-line pharmacotherapy. If the target BP is not reached within 1 month after initiating therapy, the dosage of the initial medication should be increased, or a second medication should be added. Reduction of end-organ disease from

hypertension depends on successful reduction of BP rather than on the choice of any specific medication.

An algorithm for treatment of hypertension in older adults is presented in Fig. 36.3.

Table 36.5 lists the most commonly used antihypertension drugs.

### CASE 1

#### Alice McAllister (Part 4)

At the last visit you changed Ms. McAllister's medication from chlorthalidone to amlodipine, but she called the nurse 4 weeks later, explaining that the amlodipine was making her lower legs swell. You instructed the nurse to have Ms. Johnson stop the amlodipine and begin lisinopril 5 mg daily. You see her in follow-up today and she reports that the lisinopril is making her "swimmy headed." You have her come into the office and her BP is 139/82 mmHg.
1. How will you address Ms. McAllister's concerns?

### CASE 2

#### James Wilson (Part 4)

Mr. Wilson has coronary artery disease, a previous stroke, probable peripheral vascular disease, and now signs of congestive heart failure. You realize he is at high risk for further cardiovascular events if his BP and other risk factors are not better controlled. You congratulate him on stopping smoking and advise that he reduce salt consumption and review with him the principles of the DASH eating plan, although he admits it does not sound very appealing to him.
1. What medications will you add to Mr. Wilson's regimen?

### Treatment in Specific Clinical Circumstances

**Uncomplicated Hypertension.** Diuretics and dihydropyridine CCBs are the recommended initial choices for older adults. ACE inhibitors or ARBs can be used, although are potentially less effective given that older adults have a less active renin-angiotensin system than younger individuals. Most older adults with hypertension need two or more drugs to effectively lower their BP. A second drug can be chosen from among the other classes suggested for initial therapy.

Beta-blockers are not recommended as first-line therapy for uncomplicated hypertension in adults age $\geq 60$ years. A metaanalysis of 13 randomized controlled trials reported an increased risk of stroke with beta-blockers compared with other antihypertensive agents in this older age group.[59] Their use is recommended in older patients with compelling indications because of concomitant conditions, such as certain arrhythmias, essential tremor, ischemic heart disease, angina, recent acute coronary syndrome, or heart failure with reduced ejection fraction.

❖ **Thiazide diuretics or CCBs are especially effective treatments in older adults.**

**Isolated Systolic Hypertension.** Arterial stiffness associated with aging causes SBP to rise and diastolic pressure to fall, and isolated systolic hypertension predominates. In the Systolic Hypertension

Targets are systolic blood pressure <150 mmHg and diastolic blood pressure <90 in adults ≥60 years of age

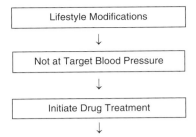

| Without Compelling Indications | |
| --- | --- |
| Non-Black persons | Black persons |
| Thiazide-type diuretic **or CCB or ACEI or** ARB, alone or in combination | Thiazide-type diuretic **or CCB** |

If SBP and DBP goals not met with the first medication, add a second medication from a different class. If still not met, add a third medication from another class. May maximize medication doses before adding another class. Avoid combined use of ACEI and ARB.

Reinforce medication and lifestyle adherence throughout.

Cease target SBP if DBP is reduced to <65 mmHg

| With Compelling Indications | |
| --- | --- |
| Comorbidity | Initial Therapy Options |
| IHD or high CVD risk | BB, ACEI or ARB |
| Post Myocardial Infarction | BB, ACEI or ARB, ALDO ANT |
| Angina Pectoris | BB, CCB |
| Heart Failure | BB, ACEI or ARB, ALDO ANT |
| Aortic Aneurysm | BB, ACEI or ARB, THIAZ, CCB |
| Diabetes | ACEI or ARB, CCB, THIAZ, BB |
| Recurrent stroke prevention or TIA | THIAZ, ACEI or ARB, CCB |
| Chronic kidney disease | ACEI or ARB |

• **Figure 36.3** Algorithm for treatment of hypertension in older adults. (Modified from James PA, Oparil S, Carter BL, et al. 2014 evidence-based guideline for the management of high blood pressure in adults: report from the panel members appointed to the Eighth Joint National Committee (JNC 8). *JAMA* 2014; 311:507–520.)

in the Elderly Program (SHEP), treatment with the diuretic chlorthalidone in patients with systolic pressure of ≥ 160 mmHg and diastolic pressure < 90 mmHg had impressive reductions in the incidence of stroke and heart disease.[12] Similarly positive results were demonstrated with a CCB.[63]

**Wide Pulse Pressure.** Widened pulse pressure whether pretreatment or treatment induced, is independently predictive of increased risk of stroke, heart failure, and other cardiovascular disease.[64,65] Data from large trials suggest that thiazide diuretics are more effective in reducing pulse pressure than ACE inhibitors or CCBs.[66,67]

**Resistant Hypertension.** The most common cause of inability to control BP despite three or four antihypertensive medications is nonadherence to the prescribed medications. Patients should have outpatient BP monitoring to exclude white coat effect. If elevated BP is established and adherence is confirmed, focus on lifestyle factors, such as obesity, physical inactivity, excessive alcohol intake, and diet. Medications that can elevate BP, such as NSAIDs, stimulants, or decongestants, should be eliminated. The possibility of a secondary cause of hypertension should be considered, although

this is less likely in older adults. Treatment strategies include maximizing diuretic therapy, adding a mineralocorticoid receptor agonist, agents from a category not yet tried, or loop diuretics in patients with chronic kidney disease.[27]

**Ischemic Heart Disease.** Recall that arterial stiffening with age causes the systolic pressure to increase and the diastolic pressure to decrease. Lowered diastolic pressure can impair coronary blood flow and predispose to myocardial ischemia, which explains why the relationship between diastolic pressure and cardiovascular risk is bimodal in older individuals, with diastolic pressures of > 90 mmHg associated with similar increased risk as that associated with diastolic pressures < 70 mmHg.[22,68] Studies on hypertension have repeatedly found a paradoxic increase in cardiovascular events with lower BP, known as the J-curve hypothesis. No J-curve effect was seen regarding the incidence of stroke, which may be caused by the fact that the heart is perfused mostly during diastole and is therefore more susceptible to reduction in diastolic pressure.[69] In the International Verapamil SR-Trandolapril Study (INVEST), the Hypertension Optimal Treatment, and A Coronary Disease Trial Investigating Outcome with Nifedipine studies, the risk of death and MI but not stroke rose progressively with low diastolic

## TABLE 36.5 Antihypertensive Drugs

| Drug Class | Mechanism of Action | Possible Adverse Effects |
|---|---|---|
| Thiazide-like diuretics<br>Chlorthalidone<br>Hydrochlorothiazide<br>Indapamide<br>Potassium-sparing diuretics<br>Triamterene<br>Spironolactone | Inhibit sodium and chloride reabsorption in the kidney, reducing intravascular volume and peripheral vascular resistance | Volume depletion hypotension, hyponatremia, hypokalemia, hypomagnesemia, hyperuricemia (gout), hyperglycemia, renal impairment |
| Angiotensin-converting enzyme inhibitors (ACE inhibitors)<br>Benazepril<br>Captopril<br>Fosinopril<br>Lisinopril<br>Ramipril | Inhibits ACE, interfering with conversion of angiotensin I to angiotensin II, reducing vasoconstriction | Hyperkalemia (with impaired renal function), cough, angioedema, rash, renal impairment, altered taste |
| Angiotensin II receptor blockers (ARB)<br>Candesartan<br>Irbesartan<br>Losartan<br>Valsartan | Antagonizes angiotensin II AT1 receptors, reducing vasoconstriction | Hyperkalemia, renal impairment<br>Do not use an ACE inhibitor and an ARB simultaneously |
| Beta-Blockers<br><br>Beta$_1$ Selective<br>Metoprolol<br><br>Dual acting<br>Carvedilol<br>Labetalol | Selectively antagonizes β-1 adrenergic receptors<br><br>Antagonizes α-1, β-1, and β-2 adrenergic receptors | Sinus bradycardia, heart block, fatigue, bronchospasm, hyperglycemia, confusion. Not recommended as first-line agents unless the patient has ischemic heart disease or heart failure |
| Calcium channel blockers—Nondihydropyridines<br>Diltiazem<br>Verapamil | Prolong AV node refractory period and have negative inotropic effect; less effective as vasodilators | Sinus bradycardia, heart block, heart failure, rash, GERD, constipation, gingival hyperplasia |
| Calcium channel blockers—Dihydropyridines<br>Amlodipine<br>Felodipine<br>Nicardipine<br>Nifedipine | Inhibit calcium influx, relaxing vascular smooth muscle and decreasing peripheral resistance causing vasodilation with little or no negative effect upon cardiac contractility or AV nodal conduction | Peripheral edema |
| Alpha-adrenergic agonists, centrally acting<br>Methyldopa<br>Clonidine | Stimulates α-2 adrenergic receptors centrally | Sedation, dry mouth, constipation. Avoid in older adults because of central nervous system adverse effects |
| Alpha$_1$ selective adrenergic antagonists, peripherally acting<br>Doxazosin<br>Prazosin<br>Terazosin | Antagonizes peripheral α-1 adrenergic receptors | Orthostatic hypotension. Consider in patients with benign prostatic hypertrophy |

*GERD*, Gastroesophageal reflux disease.

pressure readings in patients with ischemic heart disease and hypertension.[70-72]

With these precautions in mind, older adults with hypertension and stable angina and/or prior MI should be treated with a beta-blocker followed by a long-acting dihydropyridine CCB if hypertension or angina persists.[73] They should also be given an ACE inhibitor or an ARB, especially if left ventricular function is compromised (see Ch. 38).

**Heart Failure.** The most common cause of heart failure is ischemic heart disease, for which hypertension is a significant risk factor, so treatment is important in prevention. In patients who develop heart failure with reduced ejection fracture (HFrEF), or systolic heart failure, both preload and afterload should be reduced, and the recommended antihypertensive medications are ACE-I or ARB and beta-blocker (LOE = A).[74] They also benefit from aldosterone receptor antagonists. Nondihydropyridine CCBs should not be prescribed in adults with HFrEF.

Patients with heart failure with preserved ejection fraction (HFpEF), or diastolic heart failure (limited diastolic filling because of ventricular stiffness), should have their hypertension treated per clinical guidelines, but otherwise treatment recommendations are much less clear, compared with HFpEF. CCB, ACE inhibitors, ARBs, and diuretics may be used with monitoring for hypotension because of excessive preload or afterload reduction. These patients may benefit from aldosterone antagonists, so spironolactone can be considered[75] (see Ch. 38).

### Previous Stroke or Transient Ischemic Attack.
Older adults without a history of treatment for hypertension who have had an ischemic stroke or transient ischemic attack (TIA) and, after the first several days, have SBP 140 mmHg (or higher) or DBP 90 mmHg (or higher) should be treated with an antihypertensive (LOE = B).[76] For those patients previously treated for high BP, and who have SBP 140 mmHg (or higher) or DBP 90 mmHg (or higher) several days after the stroke or TIA, should have their treatment resumed, as this will prevent recurrent stroke or other vascular events (LOE = A). Any medication works, although diuretics and ACE inhibitors are generally recommended (LOE = A)[76,77] (see Ch. 40).

### Diabetes.
Patients with diabetes are already at significantly increased risk of cardiovascular events, and guidelines often suggest aggressive reduction in BP to < 130/80 mmHg.[27] However, the INVEST reported that tight control of systolic pressure was not associated with improved outcomes in older patients (mean age 62 years) with hypertension, diabetes, and coronary artery disease compared with usual control and could potentially be hazardous over the long term.[78] JNC 8 recommended a treatment goal of SBP < 140 mmHg and DBP < 90 mmHg in adults age ≥ 18 years[26] (see Ch. 41).

Like other conditions, the reduction of vascular complications in older adults with diabetes and hypertension depends more on reducing BP than on the type of drug used, and all first-line classes of antihypertensives (diuretics, ACE inhibitors or ARBs, and CCBs) are useful and effective (LOE = A).

### Chronic Renal Disease.
Hypertension can worsen the decline in renal function that accompanies aging, and both are independent risk factors for cardiovascular events and adverse outcomes. BP control itself is the most important goal in slowing progression of kidney failure. JNC 8 recommended treatment goals of SBP 140 mmHg (or lower) and DBP 90 mmHg (or lower) for adults with chronic kidney disease (LOE = D).[26]

ACE inhibitors or ARB therapy is reasonable and likely effective in slowing the progression of chronic kidney disease in patients with proteinuria (LOE = B).[27] However, the benefit of these medications in older adults is uncertain because most of these patients do not have proteinuria and most trials did not enroll patients over age 70 years.[79] If these agents are used, renal function and electrolytes should be monitored as ACE inhibitor or ARB therapy in older adults with kidney disease can cause a decline in the glomerular filtration rate and alterations in potassium levels.

### ◆◆ Comorbidities influence medication selection in the treatment of hypertension.

### Dementia.
The understanding of the relationship between hypertension and dementia is evolving. The HYVET, a double-blind, placebo-controlled trial of antihypertensive treatment in people age ≥ 80 years, did not show a significant reduction in the onset of dementia in treated patients; however, it did suggest that patients with a wider pulse pressure may possibly have an increased risk for dementia.[80,81] Other studies, such as SHEP and Syst-Eur, showed a modest trend toward reduction in dementia with treatment.[12,82]

Part of the challenge in generating hypotheses, clinical trials, and treatment guidelines is separating AD, which results from neurodegeneration, from vascular dementia, which is caused in part by hypertension. It is not always possible to tell which form of dementia the patient has, and many have both. The PROGRESS study showed that lowering BP reduced the rate of dementia and cognitive decline in patients with cerebrovascular disease.[83] The different pathophysiologic processes of the dementias cloud any hypotheses regarding treatment for hypertension.

Still, there is wide recognition of a complex association between midlife hypertension and later development of AD. There are emerging theories that the renin-angiotensin system, which plays an important role in BP regulation, may have alterations in patients with AD, which may contribute to the neuropathology in AD.[84] With an aging population and a rising incidence of these dreaded diseases, more research is urgently needed. Multiple trials are underway (see Ch. 18).

### Frail Elderly.
Data on patients > 85 years of age are limited, particularly those who are frail or have multiple comorbidities. Although the HYVET study provided clear evidence that BP lowering with antihypertensive medication reduced the risk of stroke, heart failure, and cardiovascular disease in the very elderly, subjects in this study were in relatively good physical health for their age and did not include frail and medically compromised patients. The use of medications in frail patients should be judicious with close follow-up.

### Benign Prostatic Hypertrophy.
Although they can be helpful in reducing lower urinary track symptoms because of benign prostatic hypertrophy (BPH), the use of alpha-adrenergic blockers should be limited in older adults. The Antihypertensive and Lipid-Lowering Treatment to Prevent Heart Attack Trial showed doxazosin was associated with 25% excess cardiovascular events compared with the diuretic chlorthalidone.[85] This led many to conclude that in men with both BPH and hypertension, the two conditions should be treated independently with the best available medications[86] (see Ch. 51).

### Erectile Dysfunction.
Phosphodiesterase-5 inhibitors both treat erectile dysfunction and have the primary effect of lowering BP.[87] Many antihypertensives affect erectile function, which can be mitigated with an alternative agent or with the use of a phosphodiesterase-5 inhibitor.[88]

### Osteoporosis.
The use of thiazide diuretic agents in older adults is associated with a reduction of approximately one-third in the risk of hip fracture.[89] This effect is likely caused by increased availability of calcium from both a reduction in urinary excretion of calcium and an increase in serum bicarbonate, which reduces acid-induced bone buffering[90] (see Ch. 43).

## CASE 1

### Discussion

After trying numerous medications over the past year, Ms. McAllister reluctantly agrees to take the lisinopril 5 mg after you encouraged her to do so, educating her on the risks of untreated hypertension. Although not the first choice in older adults, the ACE inhibitor is proving effective and, importantly, she is tolerating it, which was not the case with the recommended diuretic or CCB. Intolerance of medications and reluctance to take them is common in patients. Strategies to improve adherence include once daily dosing, patient registries in the electronic medical record with outreach efforts including team-based care, phone calls, and telehealth. Hypertension control is a common quality metric in new value-based payment systems.

Ms. McAllister's case illustrates a common scenario in hypertensive management in older adults. Medication adherence is challenging, and patients often stop medications because of real or perceived side effects. Time, patience, and a willingness to listen and work with older individuals builds trust, which can help increase adherence and therefore successful treatment.

❖❖ Strategies to improve medication compliance include education on potential side effects, once-daily dosing, avoiding expensive medications, and a plan for medication management such as a pill box or calendar, with use monitoring by a nurse, pharmacist, or family member.

## CASE 2

### Discussion

Mr. Wilson's symptoms of heart failure with reduced ejection fraction along with his suboptimally controlled hypertension lead you to add furosemide 20 mg daily to his treatment, while continuing the metoprolol. You suggest adding an ACE inhibitor (benazepril), which will help with both his systolic heart failure and his hypertension. You advise him that his kidney function and fluid status will need close monitoring, so you arrange to check his electrolytes and creatinine in a week.

## Summary

Hypertension, especially systolic hypertension, is prevalent in older adults and is associated with increased cardiovascular morbidity and mortality. These risks can be reduced with treatment. Lifestyle interventions are appropriate, but most older people will require pharmacologic management. Considerable clinical judgment is required regarding treatment decisions as comorbidities and intolerance of medications are common.

❖❖ There are several different guidelines ton the BP thresholds for treatment in older adults. Which guideline to follow is based on shared decision making, combining the clinical judgment of the provider with patient preference.

❖❖ Familiarly with the different classes of medications, and their side effects, and consideration of any comorbidities help in selection of pharmaceutical agents.

❖❖ Adherence to medications is a challenge and requires patient education, follow-up, listening, and shared decision making.

### Web Resources

A list of validated blood pressure measuring devices is available at www.dableducational.org

## Key References

26. James PA, Oparil S, Carter BL, et al. 2014 Evidence-based guideline for the management of high blood pressure in adults: report from the panel members appointed to the Eighth Joint National Committee (JNC 8). *JAMA*. 2014; 311(5):507−520.

27. Whelton PK, Carey RM, Aronow WS, et al. 2017 ACC/AHA/AAPA/ABC/ACPM/AGS/APhA/ASH/ASPC/NMA/PCNA Guideline for the prevention, detection, evaluation, and management of high blood pressure in adults: a report of the American College of Cardiology/American Heart Association Task Force on Clinical Practice Guidelines. *J Am Coll Cardiol*. 2018;71(19):e127−e248.

39. Qaseem A, Wilt TJ, Rich R, Humphrey LL, Frost J, Forciea MA. Pharmacologic treatment of hypertension in adults aged 60 years or older to higher versus lower blood pressure targets: a clinical practice guideline From the American College of Physicians and the American Academy of Family Physicians. *Ann Inter Med*. 2017;166(6):430−437.

*References available online at* expertconsult.com.

# 37

# Coronary Artery Disease and Atrial Fibrillation

S. MICHAEL GHARACHOLOU AND CHRISTINA BUNGO

## OUTLINE

## OBJECTIVES

*Upon completion of this chapter, the reader will be able to:*

- Understand the epidemiology, pathobiology, and risk factors for patients across the CAD spectrum (stable ischemic heart disease (SIHD) and acute coronary syndromes (ACS))
- Apply risk stratification to guide management decisions regarding risk reduction interventions
- Understand the distinction between risk stratification for unstable angina (UA)/non-ST elevation myocardial infarction (NSTEMI) and reperfusion for ST-elevation myocardial infarction (STEMI)

- Be able to understand the impact of age and geriatric multimorbidity in the care and clinical outcome of patients with SIHD and ACS
- Identify risk factors for the development of atrial fibrillation (AF)
- Develop strategies to decrease AF morbidity and mortality through anticoagulation, rate, and rhythm control

Coronary artery disease (CAD) affects nearly 17 million people in the United States, and incident coronary events, defined as myocardial infarction (MI) or CAD death, affects more than 700,000 Americans per year.[1] Although cardiovascular (CV)–related deaths have been on the decline, CAD remains the leading cause of

death (44%) when compared with other CV deaths, such as stroke (17%), hypertension (9%), or heart failure (9%).[1] Because the prevalence of CAD rises with advancing age, primary care providers are often diagnosing, managing, and treating older adults with suspected or known CAD. Among adults age 80 years and older, it has been estimated that 37% of men and 23% of women have CAD.[2] Costs, both direct and indirect, for patients with CAD are substantial, estimated at over $150 billion annually.[3] Much of the cost is related to hospitalization and use of invasive procedures, such as percutaneous coronary intervention (PCI). Among older adults, however, a significant portion of spending includes long-term care costs, such as home health, durable medical equipment, and short-term rehabilitation in skilled nursing facilities.[3] Indirect costs such as work absences (patients and caregivers), lower productivity, and potential adverse drug reactions nearly equate with direct costs.[4] As healthcare costs increase, Medicare and other government payers have initiated programs that seek to place priority on quality measures over traditional fee-for-service payment models for many CV conditions, including MI and heart failure (HF), though effects of such programs on outcomes remains unknown.[5]

## Pathobiology

Coronary arterial plaques form when interactions occur between leukocytes and the coronary endothelium, promoted by proinflammatory cytokines, and accelerated further by risk factors, such as elevated blood glucose, smoking, and hypertension.[6-8] CAD may cause narrowing of the arterial lumen resulting in coronary blood flow limitation and the clinical syndrome of stable angina (i.e., demand exceeds supply) or the plaque may develop erosion, fissuring, or rupture leading to an acute coronary syndrome (ACS), manifesting clinically as unstable angina (UA) or acute MI (non-ST elevation myocardial infarction [NSTEMI] or ST-elevation myocardial infarction [STEMI]). Studies have previously shown that vascular inflammation plays a pivotal role in the development of ACS,[9] and these plaques often have evidence of "high-risk" findings, such as complex atheroma or thrombus.[10]

❖ **Atherosclerosis is a systemic condition where patients develop atherosclerotic plaques in different vascular beds. Older age is a primary risk factor for development of atherosclerosis.**

### CASE 1

#### Eleanor Beasley (Part 1)

Eleanor Beasley is an 85-year-old married woman with hypertension and hyperlipidemia that you are seeing in follow-up. She always comes to her appointments with her husband who is generally healthy but has moderate cognitive impairment. Mrs. Beasley takes hydrochlorthiazide 25 mg daily and amlodipine 10 mg daily. She believes in a healthy diet and does not take lipid lowering therapy. Previously, you calculated her 10-year CAD risk using her blood pressure (BP) of 145/85 mmHg and most recent lipid profile (total cholesterol of 250 mg/dL, high-density lipoprotein [HDL] of 35 mg/dL, and low-density lipoprotein [LDL] of 160 mg/dL) and it was 2%. She has no concerns for you regarding her current visit and her examination is normal.
1. What interventions, if any, should be offered for her risk factors?
2. What psychosocial factors should be considered?

## Traditional Coronary Artery Disease Risk Factors and Risk Factor Modification

The premise of risk reduction is to lower the patients' risk for future CV events, such as MI, stroke, or death. Clinical recommendations must be tailored to the estimated CV risk, derived on the basis of clinical impressions, or calculated using risk models in patients without known disease. Clinical risk factors include smoking, hypertension, diabetes, hyperlipidemia, chronic renal disease, family history of CV disease, or peripheral artery disease. However, because diabetes has been considered a CAD risk equivalent, some risk scores omit diabetes in risk prediction models. Risk calculators use multivariable models to derive a risk estimate, though few of these incorporated older adults in the derivation cohort (Table 37.1). Older adults benefit from risk factor reduction strategies, such as smoking cessation, lipid management, BP control, diet and nutrition counseling, diabetes management, use of cardiac rehabilitation, and exercise instructions. In fact, given that age confers higher baseline CV risk, older adults have perhaps the most to gain from risk factor reduction strategies.

| TABLE 37.1 | Risk Estimators for Cardiovascular Events in Patients Without Known Coronary Artery Disease | | |
|---|---|---|---|
| Clinical Risk Estimator | Purpose of Risk Estimator | Limitations | Web or Mobile App Available |
| ASCVD Risk Estimator | 10-year risk of ASCVD event (CV death, MI, stroke) | Not validated for patients ≥ 80 years old, excludes family history | Yes |
| Framingham Risk Score | Estimates risk for CV death, MI, stable and unstable angina | Excludes family history | Yes |
| MESA Risk Score | 10-year risk for CV death, MI, cardiac arrest, coronary revascularization | Excludes family history | Yes |
| Reynolds CVD Risk Score | Estimate risk for CV death, MI, stroke, revascularization | Does not account for treatment of hypertension | Yes |
| Adult Treatment Panel (ATP) III | Estimate risk for death or MI | Excludes DM or family history | Yes |

*ASCVD*, Atherosclerotic cardiovascular disease; *CV*, cardiovascular; *DM*, diabetes mellitus; *MESA*, Multi-Ethnic Study of Atherosclerosis; *MI*, myocardial infarction.

## Smoking

The association between smoking and CAD has been clearly established over many decades of epidemiologic studies. Lower life expectancy and more life-years lost in smokers has been demonstrated in a large cohort of older adults with prior MI.[11] Patients who survive acute MI and are smokers are at risk for future coronary stent problems, such as stent thrombosis.[12] Pooled studies have shown that smoking cessation has been associated with a 36% relative risk reduction of death, with health benefits during the first few years of smoking abstinence.[13] A multifaceted approach combining physician counseling, pharmacotherapy, and behavioral or support therapy to smoking cessation may provide a greater likelihood of success.

## Hyperlipidemia

The relationship between elevated LDL cholesterol and CAD events has been demonstrated in patients with and without known CAD.[14,15] Long-term follow-up after acute MI has shown that elevated cholesterol is associated with increased risk for reinfarction and cardiac mortality.[15] Although HDL levels remain relatively constant with increasing age, LDL metabolism changes over time contributing to rising levels in both men and women.[16] Numerous randomized trials and metaanalyses have demonstrated that reduction of LDL cholesterol using an HMG-CoA reductase inhibitor (statin) is associated with lowering risk of MI, stroke, and death.[17,18] Secondary analysis of these data ascribes an equal or greater treatment effect in older adults,[19,20] who are often undertreated with lipid-lowering therapy as compared with younger patients.[21] Yet despite the proven benefit in older adults, side effects, such as myopathy, may limit use in a substantial portion of patients. Furthermore, the benefits of statin therapy are observed over time, which may not be congruent with the care plan of a frail older adult with reduced life expectancy. Individualization is key to implementing prevention strategies that provide net clinical benefit without complicating prescription practices and contributing to untoward effects.

## Hypertension

Hypertension is an established risk factor for cardiac events, namely stroke, HF, MI, and CV death, and accounts for significant disability-adjusted years missed. Older adults typically have increased arterial stiffness, reduced arterial compliance, and higher rates of systolic hypertension. Treatment benefits extend to older adult populations as was demonstrated in the Hypertension in the Very Elderly Trial (HYVET).[22] In HYVET, 3845 patients age ≥ 80 years were randomized to BP control with the diuretic indapamide and angiotensin-converting enzyme (ACE) inhibitor perindopril to achieve a target BP of 150/80 mmHg versus placebo. At 2 years, treatment was associated with significant reductions in rate of stroke (30% reduction), stroke mortality (39% reduction), HF (64% reduction), and CV-related death (23% reduction) when compared with placebo.[22] More recently, Systolic Blood Pressure Intervention Trial (SPRINT) tested the hypothesis that further reduction of target BP to systolic goal of ≤ 120 mmHg (intensive treatment) would be more beneficial in terms of reducing clinical events than the standard of ≤ 140 mmHg (standard treatment).[23] Intensive treatment was associated with a significantly lower rate of the composite outcome (MI, stroke, HF, or CV death) as compared with standard treatment (hazard ratio [HR], 0.75; 95%

confidence interval [CI], 0.60−0.90; $P=.003$). Of note, higher rates of syncope, acute kidney injury, and hypotension, but not injurious falls, were observed in the intensive treatment group. For older adults, the established benefit of BP reduction on clinical events should be balanced with the known risk of increased side effects from intensive lowering. The adage "start low, but go slow, but do go" certainly applies to BP management in older adults, particularly those with geriatric syndromes that include mobility difficulty, polypharmacy, or cognitive impairment.

## Diabetes Mellitus

Diabetes mellitus (DM) is strongly associated with atherosclerosis, and deaths in patients with DM are often accounted for by CAD. Although the totality of data suggest that intensive glycemic control leads to lower rates of CV events, it also increases risk for hypoglycemic events, such that DM management should be individualized for patient-specific factors. Lifestyle modifications are important components to DM management, as those interventions will also improve coexisting CV risk factors. In older adults without decompensated HF or significant renal failure (estimated glomerular filtration rate <45 mL/min), metformin is often initially prescribed in combination with lifestyle recommendations. In those patients with DM and CAD, the addition of novel agents including sodium-glucose cotransporter 2 (SGLT2) inhibitors and glucagon-like peptide-1 receptor agonists (GLP-1RAs) have shown reduction in adverse CV events and are recommended to be used in eligible patients.[24] Empagliflozin, an SGLT2 inhibitor, has been shown to reduce cardiac events, including HF-related hospitalization and cardiac-related mortality. Liraglutide, a GLP-1RA, has shown reduced cardiac events and is approved for this indication in patients with DM and CAD. An SGLT2 inhibitor may increase the risk for infections. The GLP-1RAs may be associated with transient nausea and vomiting.

## Diet and Exercise

It is recommended that patients with CAD adhere to a diet low in saturated fats, while increasing intake of fruits, vegetables, whole grains, nuts, legumes, and nontropical vegetable oils. Total caloric intake will vary depending on age and daily energy expenditure, including whether the dietary goal is weight loss, weight gain, or weight maintenance. A Mediterranean diet translated to benefits for reducing CV events in patients at high risk of CV events but without overt CAD.[25] Moderate intensity aerobic activity, primarily walking, should be performed most days per week.[26] Exercise may translate into improved quality of life, reduced burden of angina, improved psychosocial scores, and more optimal control of risk factors. Cardiac rehabilitation has established benefits for several important clinical outcomes, though data suggest it may be underused in older adults who perhaps have the most to gain from exercise training and risk factor modification.[27,28]

The current class I recommendations and associated level of evidence for risk factor modification from practice guidelines in patients with CAD[3] are listed in Box 37.1.

⇜ **Patients without known CAD should follow recommendations for primary prevention, which focuses on reducing CV risk through treatment of modifiable risk factors. Older adults are often at greater CV risk than younger patients, and thereby may derive even greater benefit from risk reduction strategies.**

**Hyperlipidemia**

1. Lifestyle modifications to include physical activity and weight management for all patients with CAD (LOE=B)
2. Diet should include reducing saturated fats, trans fats, and total cholesterol (LOE=B)
3. Consider moderate- to high-dose statin therapy in addition to lifestyle modifications if no contraindications or documented adverse effects (LOE=A)

**Hypertension**

- Lifestyle modifications to include weight management and dietary changes, aerobic physical activity, sodium reduction (LOE=B)
- Antihypertensive therapy should be started in addition to or after a trial of lifestyle modifications if patients have BP 140/90 mmHg or higher[a] (LOE=A)
- Specific antihypertensives should be based on patient characteristics to ultimately achieve an ideal BP goal (LOE=B)

**Physical Activity**

- Encourage 30 to 60 minutes of moderate-intensity aerobic activity, such as brisk walking, for at least 5 days per week. This should accompany increasing activity during daily lifestyle routines (LOE=B)
- Risk assessment with either a physical activity history and/or an exercise test is recommended (LOE=B)
- High-risk patients may benefit from supervised exercise programs, such as cardiac rehabilitation (LOE=A)

**Weight Management**

- Body mass index and/or waist circumference should be assessed at every visit and clinicians should encourage a healthy weight through balance of lifestyle modifications (physical activity, diet) (LOE=B)
- Initial goal of weight loss therapy should target body weight reduction by 5% to 10% of baseline (LOE=C)

**Smoking Cessation Counseling**

- Smoking cessation and avoidance of second-hand smoke should be encouraged for all patients with CAD. A stepwise strategy for smoking cessation using special programs and pharmacotherapy are recommended (LOE=B)

**Immunizations**

- An annual influenza vaccine is recommended for patients with CAD (LOE=B)

[a] Recommendations for the BP treatment threshold may change based on recent literature showing benefits of intensive BP control

*BP*, Blood pressure; *CAD*, coronary artery disease; *LOE*, level of evidence.

## Depression and Coronary Artery Disease

Psychosocial factors may underlie CV disease and screening for depressive symptoms with the Patient Health Questionnaire in patients with CAD has been recommended.[29] In a cohort of older adults with CAD undergoing PCI, one-fifth had depressive symptoms and moderate/high depressive symptom severity was associated with nearly twofold increased risk of mortality (HR, 1.90; 95% CI, 1.02–3.53; $p=.043$).[30] Improved quality of life in patients with CAD has steadily emerged as a laudable endpoint in clinical trials and a goal for patients with CAD. Despite its primary use in research, the Seattle Angina Questionnaire offers prognostic information while capturing disease-specific limitations in

function and quality of life.[31] In patients with angina, studies measuring health status and quality of life have shown the benefits of medical therapy and PCI, and also help clarify their mutual roles in patient management.

## Stable Ischemic Heart Disease

Patients with CAD are typically stratified as having either asymptomatic stable ischemic heart disease (SIHD) or symptomatic SIHD. In the former group, the patient may have been diagnosed with CAD based on results of diagnostic tests, such as a coronary artery calcium scan, or may have had an abnormal functional test (i.e., stress test) performed in the absence of any pretest symptoms, a practice that continues to occur though is generally discouraged.[32] Because these patients are asymptomatic, the treatment objective is to lower CV risk by aggressively treating risk factors. Pharmacotherapy for these patients often involves the use of low-dose aspirin and statin medications as an adjunct to behavioral and lifestyle modifications. Given that these patients do not report angina or anginal-equivalent symptoms, there is no role for the use of antianginal medications.

In patients with symptomatic SIHD, the fundamental goal is similar—to reduce risk for future CV events, and entails an aggressive approach to risk reduction. In addition, these patients complain of exertional symptoms related to obstructive CAD, which often warrants the addition of antianginal medications to existing risk-reduction strategies (Table 37.2). Many patients respond well to initiation and titration of medical therapy and symptom burden improves.

## Stress Testing

Clinicians may pursue additional testing to determine the presence or absence of ischemia. Exercise is the preferred method for stress testing in those patients able to do so given the prognostic information obtained from the functional aerobic capacity. Test accuracy is improved with addition of cardiac imaging, such as echocardiography or perfusion (nuclear or magnetic resonance) imaging. Most stress imaging studies have good test operating characteristics, with sensitivity and specificity ranges of 75% to 85%, and the selection of test type depends more often on clinical factors than superiority of one technique over another. For example, patients with underlying conduction abnormalities (i.e., left bundle branch block), preexisting regional wall motion abnormalities, or systolic dysfunction may achieve a more diagnostically useful examination with nuclear perfusion imaging than with stress echocardiography. Stress echocardiogram may be preferred to evaluate valvular disease or filling pressures with exercise, which can aid with diagnosis of nonischemic etiologies of cardiac symptoms. Pharmacologic stress is an alternative to exercise testing for patients unable to exercise or who cannot achieve an adequate workload or heart rate response with exercise. Pharmacologic agents used include dobutamine-atropine, adenosine, or dipyridamole. Test characteristics remain similar and selection of one agent over another depends on clinical factors. For example, dobutamine may exacerbate atrial fibrillation (AF) with rapid ventricular response in patients with this dysrhythmia. Adenosine or dipyridamole should be used with caution in patients with reactive airways disease or preexisting atrioventricular block. Although a negative (i.e., normal) stress test suggests low event rate (1%–2%) in the subsequent year, certain populations, such as diabetics or older comorbid adults, may have higher event rates. Although many providers view stress test results as either "positive (abnormal)" or "negative (normal)," it should be emphasized that

**TABLE 37.2    Pharmacotherapy for Patients With Asymptomatic or Symptomatic Stable Ischemic Heart Disease**

| Asymptomatic SIHD | Comments |
|---|---|
| **Antiplatelet** | |
| • Aspirin (Class I: LOE=A) | Although the optimal dose of aspirin has not been established, current recommendations for secondary prevention (i.e., known CAD) are for low dose (81 mg) once daily. Clopidogrel 75 mg once daily may be used as monotherapy for patients that are allergic to aspirin or who cannot take aspirin (Class I: LOE=B). |
| • HMG CoA reductase inhibitor (statin) (Class I: LOE=A) | Several generic statins are widely available. Intolerance (myopathy) to one agent may not necessarily translate to intolerance of another and is often dose-dependent. Reduction of LDL cholesterol proportional to estimated CV risk is recommended (i.e., aggressive LDL reduction for patients at high CV risk). |
| **Symptomatic SIHD** | |
| • Beta blocker (Class I: LOE=A) | Effective antianginals but also improve outcome in specific clinical settings (post-MI, low EF). Benefit for relief of ischemia may be additive when combined with oral nitrates. Caution in patients with preexisting bradyarrhythmia, advanced AV block, or sick sinus syndrome without permanent pacemaker. BB may worsen fatigue or mask signs of hypoglycemia. |
| • ACE-I or ARB (Class I: LOE=A) if patients have history of hypertension, DM, low EF, or CKD | Reduces risk for future clinical events, with treatment effect enhanced among high-risk subgroups (post MI, DM, or heart failure with low EF). |
| • Calcium channel blockers (Class I: LOE=B) | For angina not controlled with BBs or in patients not tolerating BBs, CCBs exert negative inotropic effect and smooth muscle relaxation. Short acting dihydropyridine CCBs may elicit reflex tachycardia and exacerbate anginal symptoms. Side effects may include edema, palpitations, and constipation. Metabolized through CYP3A4. |
| • Long-acting nitrates (Class I: LOE=B) | Usually used in combination with BBs and/or CCBs, long-acting nitrates relax vascular smooth muscle and are effective antianginals (lowers ventricular filling pressures, augments collateral coronary blood flow, and reduces myocardial wall tension). Long-acting nitrates are used when angina remains uncontrolled with BBs and/or CCBs. Typical side effects are related to the vasodilatory action of the drug (headache, hypotension, reflex tachycardia). |
| • Ranolazine (Class IIa: LOE=A) | Used in combination with BBs and long-acting nitrate, or in lieu of BBs in those patients intolerant of BBs. Ranolazine does not exert significant changes to heart rate or blood pressure. Mechanistically, it blocks the late sodium current and reduces cellular calcium overload. Caution with CCBs and simvastatin given CYP3A4 metabolism. |

*ACE-I*, Angiotensin-converting enzyme inhibitor; *ARB*, angiotensin-receptor blocker; *AV*, atrioventricular; *CAD*, coronary artery disease; *BB*, beta blocker; *CCB*, calcium channel blocker; *CKD*, chronic kidney disease; *CV*, cardiovascular; *DM*, diabetes mellitus; *EF*, ejection fraction; *LDL*, low-density lipoprotein; *LOE*, level of evidence; *MI*, myocardial infarction; *SIHD*, stable ischemic heart disease.

stress testing, and in particular exercise testing, helps the clinician with further estimation of CV risk, not merely to evaluate obstructive CAD.[32,33] Inherent in diagnostic tests are limitations of sensitivity and specificity, and this is certainly true of stress tests in patients with presumed or suspected CAD. Application of diagnostic tests, such as stress tests, without an estimate of pretest probability of disease, renders limited diagnostic information. For example, a "positive" exercise electrocardiogram (ECG) performed in a young, healthy patient without CV risk factors is 3 times more likely to be a false positive than it is to represent obstructive CAD. Use of these tests are enhanced when applied in a framework of estimating pretest probability of obstructive CAD (low, intermediate, or high) based on information obtained through symptom characteristics and readily available clinical characteristics (age, previous history, risk factors). These methods are based on Bayes theorem of conditional probability, which incorporates information regarding pretest disease prevalence into the operating characteristics (i.e., sensitivity and specificity) of diagnostic tests[34] (Box 37.2). Using a Bayesian approach to interpretation of diagnostic test results may help with reducing testing in patients at very low pretest probability of CAD and avoid pitfalls associated with false-negative and false-positive results, which have impact on patient anxiety

and wellbeing. Whether the results of the diagnostic test are likely to change clinical management remains fundamental to the decision-making process.

## Revascularization in Stable Ischemic Heart Disease

The decision to perform revascularization, either by PCI or coronary artery bypass grafting (CABG), should be patient centered and weigh the benefits and risks of each procedure (PCI or CABG) versus optimal medical therapy (OMT). In older adults, factors that merit consideration include recovery and rehabilitation, ability to comply with medical therapy, and patient preference. CABG may be better suited for patients with complex CAD and associated medical comorbidities, such as low left ventricular ejection fraction (LVEF) or DM.[35,36] PCI would be favored for less complex disease where dual antiplatelet therapy (aspirin + P2Y12 inhibitor) can be tolerated. Importantly, the primary role for revascularization in SIHD is to improve ischemic symptoms. Clinical trials comparing OMT versus PCI have demonstrated improvement in angina with

**Simplified Bayesian Approach to Estimating Pretest Probability of Coronary Artery Disease**

**Symptoms**

- Are symptoms (chest pressure, shortness of breath, arm/neck/jaw) related to physical exertion?
- Are symptoms relieved by rest or use of sublingual nitroglycerin?
- Are there historical or physical examination features that refine the pretest probability?
  - Supports or increases pretest likelihood of CAD: history of CAD, traditional CV risk factors (DM, PAD, stroke/TIA, hyperlipidemia, hypertension), abnormal resting ECG
  - Lowers the pretest likelihood of CAD: reproducible symptoms on physical examination (costochondritis, osteoarthritis), abnormal lung examination (consolidation, COPD), alternative diagnosis appears more likely

**Apply a pretest likelihood of obstructive CAD (prevalence)**

- Very low (<5%)
- Low (5%–10%)
- Medium (10%–80%)
- High (>80%)
  
  **Determine whether diagnostic testing, if applied, will change posttest probability (accuracy) or patient management**

*CAD*, Coronary artery disease; *COPD*, chronic obstructive lung disease; *CV*, cardiovascular; *DM*, diabetes mellitus; *ECG*, electrocardiogram; *PAD*, peripheral artery disease; *TIA*, transient ischemic attack.

PCI but without significant reduction in MI or death,[37] a finding that has been mirrored in several trials of revascularization for SIHD.[38] Therefore patients may derive symptomatic benefit with OMT as an initial strategy, reserving revascularization for those patients who remain symptomatic. Finally, patients with symptomatic SIHD benefit from referral to cardiac rehabilitation programs that, in addition to exercise training, provide important counseling regarding diet, risk factor modification, and coordination of care.[39]

❖ **Patients with symptomatic CAD should have risk reduction and addition of antianginal medications to improve their quality of life. For those patients who remain symptomatic on medical therapy, coronary revascularization with PCI or CABG may be considered.**

---

**CASE 1**

**Eleanor Beasley (Part 2)**

Your received a call from Mrs. Beasley's daughter that she has been experiencing increased fatigue, shortness of breath, and mild chest pressure on exertion over the past several months. She performs her usual daily routines without any significant symptoms. The prior week, she was taken to the local hospital at the insistence of her daughter where she had a stress test performed, which showed mild ischemia in the inferior wall. Her exercise ability on the test was very good (10.0 metabolic equivalents at 110% of her functional aerobic capacity) and her BP response during exercise was normal. There were no abnormal ECG findings during the study. The patient declined to be admitted and preferred to follow up with you in clinic. You agree to see them both and corroborate the history and test results. Her vital signs show BP of 155/90 mmHg and heart rate of 90 beats per minute. There is no interval change in the examination. Her ECG and relevant laboratories are normal. In reviewing her discharge medications, she was prescribed a sublingual nitroglycerin tablet to use on an as needed basis. No other medications were prescribed. You discuss with Mrs. Beasley and her

daughter that medical therapy with addition of antianginal medications may help improve her symptoms and quality of life. She is leery of having any invasive procedures performed because she needs to care for her husband.

1. What is her current diagnosis?
2. How should she be initially treated?
3. When would it be appropriate to consider invasive angiography with intent to revascularize?

---

## Acute Coronary Syndromes

### Unstable Angina/Non-ST Elevation Myocardial Infarction

Ischemic symptoms may result in ECG changes and/or elevation of cardiac biomarkers, such as high sensitivity troponin (hsTn). Unstable angina (UA) may be present when there are ischemic symptoms with or without ECG changes of ischemia and without elevation of troponin. Non-ST elevation myocardial infarction (NSTEMI) may be more likely to show ECG changes of ischemia but demonstrates confirmation of myocardial injury with a rise and/or fall of troponin. Both syndromes may show acute regional wall motion abnormalities on transthoracic echocardiography (TTE). Given similarities of UA/NSTEMI, they are often grouped together based on shared mechanism, triage strategies, and clinical management.[40] Although cardiac troponin is integral to a diagnosis of acute MI, both cardiac and noncardiac conditions may cause nonischemic myocardial injury that are distinct from acute MI (Box 37.3). The initial ECG may be normal; however, changes are often dynamic, therefore serial ECG tracings are recommended. Typical findings may include ST-segment depression or T-wave inversions, which may improve with institution of antiischemic

**Differential Diagnosis of Elevated Troponin Other Than Acute Coronary Syndrome**

**Noncardiac**

- Renal failure
- Pulmonary hypertension
- Pulmonary embolus
- Adverse drug reactions/toxicity
- Burns
- Sepsis
- Respiratory distress/failure
- Neurological injury (CNS bleed, stroke)
- Hypoxia
- Severe hypertension
- Severe hypotension (shock)
- Acute pancreatitis

**Cardiac Related**

- Heart failure
- Myocarditis, pericarditis
- Cardiomyopathies (hypertrophic, peripartum, stress, chemotherapy-related)
- Acute aortic syndromes (aortic dissection, intramural hematomas, penetrating ulcers)
- Arrhythmias
- Stimulants (methamphetamines, cocaine)
- Physiologic stress in setting of known CAD
- Post-PCI or postcardiac surgery

*CAD*, Coronary artery disease; *CNS*, central nervous system; *PCI*, percutaneous coronary intervention.

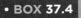

## BOX 37.4    Initial Medical Therapy in Patients With Unstable Angina/Non ST Elevation Myocardial Infarction

**Antithrombotic[a]**

- Aspirin
- Anticoagulation with unfractionated heparin or low-molecular-weight heparin
- P2Y12 inhibitor[b] (clopidogrel or ticagrelor)
- Discontinue any NSAIDs

**Nitrates**

- Sublingual nitroglycerin or IV nitroglycerin if pain recurs or significant hypertension

**Beta blockers**

- Oral beta blockers may be effective at relieving angina and should be started if there is no contraindication (acute heart failure, bradycardia, hypotension)

**Statin**

- Early (in-hospital) use of statin in patients with UA/NSTEMI has been associated with better outcomes and should be initiated at time of presentation

**ACE Inhibitor**

- In the absence of renal failure, clinical trials have shown improved outcomes for patients treated with an ACE inhibitor. It should be considered for patients that are hypertensive
- Supplemental oxygen is only necessary for patients that are hypoxic

[a] Attention to dosing of antithrombotic medications is essential in older adults as data suggests excess dosing is often performed and leads to worse outcomes.

[b] Owing to higher rates of bleeding, the P2Y12 inhibitor prasugrel is not recommended in older adults ≥ 75 years of age, patients with prior stroke or transient ischemic attack, or low body weight (< 60 kg) and is not administered before coronary angiography.

*ACE*, Angiotensin-converting enzyme; *NSAIDs*, nonsteroidal antiinflammatory drugs, *NSTEMI*, non-ST elevation myocardial infarction; *UA*, unstable angina.

medications. Treatment for initial stabilization of UA/NSTEMI is listed in Box 37.4. Rapid risk stratification is accomplished with cardiac troponin, with currently used high sensitivity (fifth generation) assays being preferred for clinical use (hsTn) as it can clarify an ACS diagnosis within a few hours of patient presentation. The typical approach is to evaluate the change in hsTn from initial presentation (time=0 hours) and at 2 hours postpresentation (time=2 hours). If NSTEMI is diagnosed, then appropriate management can be initiated. If the diagnosis is uncertain, hsTn testing at 6 hours postpresentation (time=6 hours) is recommended. Most emergency rooms and chest pain programs have algorithms regarding troponin testing and interpretation of results. Patients with elevated troponin are at increased risk by virtue of myocardial injury and most information regarding risk stratification of UA/NSTEMI patients can be obtained shortly after patient arrival to the emergency department.

## Early Invasive Versus Initial Conservative

After initial medical stabilization of UA/NSTEMI and risk assessment, a decision regarding referral for coronary angiography with an intent to revascularize (i.e., early invasive) versus medical management (i.e., initial conservative) can be made. High-risk features, such as hemodynamic abnormalities, ventricular arrhythmias, shock, or HF, warrant an early invasive strategy. Given that older age is heavily weighted in risk scores, older adults have potentially greater benefits for revascularization in ACS; however, they may also be at greater risk for adverse outcomes and complications. A secondary analysis of adults age ≥ 65 years with UA/NSTEMI from the TACTICS-TIMI (Treat Angina with Aggrastat and Determine Cost of Therapy with an Invasive or Conservative Strategy—Thrombolysis in Myocardial Infarction) 18 trial comparing early invasive versus initial conservative strategies demonstrated a lower risk of death or MI at 6 months with the early invasive strategy (8.8% vs. 13.6%; *P*=.018), translating to nearly 40% relative risk reduction.[41] These benefits were even greater when the cohort of patients age ≥ 75 years were studied, showing a 56% relative risk reduction in death or MI. In addition, data from clinical registries have also shown benefits among nonagenarians with NSTEMI that are treated in accordance with evidence-based recommendations.[42] Despite previous data showing benefits in patients treated with intravenous (IV) glycoprotein IIb/IIIa inhibitors for NSTEMI, more recent studies showed tendency for these agents to be excessively dosed in older adults, resulting in more bleeding, and less benefit when applied "upstream" to PCI. Geriatric comorbidities also factor in decision making regarding optimal treatment for patients with UA/NSTEMI. Previous studies have shown that geriatric comorbidities, such as frailty and cognitive impairment, are associated with worse outcome after acute MI,[43,44] and that functional limitations and loss of independence may often be observed in survivors.[45] A patient-centered approach focusing on expectations and goals from treatment of UA/NSTEMI should be undertaken. Despite aggressive care and revascularization in older adults with UA/NSTEMI, many patients remain at high risk for subsequent rehospitalization and mortality during follow-up.[46]

## ST Elevation Myocardial Infarction

Patients presenting with STEMI should be referred immediately for reperfusion therapy, either with administration of systemic fibrinolysis (thrombolysis) or primary PCI (emergency angiography and PCI). The type of reperfusion delivered is less important than the goal of providing any form of reperfusion to all eligible STEMI patients. All emergency departments in the United States that do not have primary PCI availability are recommended to develop processes of care to either administer fibrinolytics or to transfer STEMI patients to a facility capable of performing primary PCI.[47] Although there has been a gradual decrease in STEMI rates as compared with an increase in UA/NSTEMI, likely reflecting the demographic shift in CAD patients, STEMI still accounts for up to one-third of acute MI admissions and carries substantial morbidity and mortality.[47,48] Patients that present with concomitant HF, shock, anterior infarct, and mechanical or electrical complications are at particularly increased risk. In the APEX-AMI (Assessment of Pexelizumab in Acute Myocardial Infarction) study, age was the strongest independent predictor of 90-day mortality in STEMI patients referred for primary PCI (HR, 2.07 per 10-year increase in age; 95% CI, 1.84−2.33).[49] Older adults may also have higher risk features including presentation delay, HF, and more procedural complications.

Benefits of reperfusion wane as time from initial STEMI diagnosis increases. Although studies have compared the benefits of fibrinolysis versus primary PCI, primary PCI is generally preferred if it can be accomplished expeditiously because it is considered safer, has lower rate of reperfusion failure, and likely associated with better outcomes.[50,51] It may also be preferred in older adults that may carry higher bleeding risk from fibrinolysis.[52] After the acute recognition of STEMI, patient-centered discussion regarding risks and benefits of reperfusion should be undertaken. Among older adults, delays to reperfusion may involve delays in obtaining consent. Older adults have higher rates of cognitive and communication disorders that may impair capacity and require the involvement of family members in the decision-making process. Although STEMI presentations are emergency scenarios, treating providers must seek to provide a thorough understanding of potential risks among patients and families and to foster trusting relationships through a calm and supportive dialogue.

## Post-ST Elevation Myocardial Infarction Care

After STEMI reperfusion, patients are often continued on secondary prevention medications. These include dual-antiplatelet therapy (low-dose aspirin combined with a P2Y12 inhibitor), high-intensity statin, beta blocker, and an ACE inhibitor. These medications have been shown to improve clinical outcomes postacute MI and are combined with important behavioral modification counseling that are received as part of an integrated cardiac rehabilitation program. STEMI patients are at risk for subsequent CV events, therefore secondary prevention is a critical aspect of CAD management. Importantly, older adults may also be at greater risk for adverse drug reactions and side effects, especially if prescribed several new prescriptions post-MI. Pharmacy intervention with the goal of improving education, adherence, and recognition of adverse events should be considered before hospital discharge. This becomes important if patients are often coadministered higher risk medications, such as anticoagulants and antiarrhythmic drugs.

❖❖ **Patients with UA/NSTEMI should have risk stratification with a discussion regarding an early invasive strategy versus an initial conservative strategy. The dialogue allows for making patient-centered decisions with discussion of risks and benefits for the various strategies. Patients with STEMI should be referred for reperfusion (primary PCI or fibrinolysis). Providing prompt access to reperfusion for eligible patients is more important than the type of reperfusion ultimately recommended.**

---

### CASE 1

#### Eleanor Beasley (Part 3)

You are called by the emergency room physician for Mrs. Beasley. She presented via emergency medical services for chest pressure and dizziness. Her initial ECG in the ambulance showed ST segment depression in V2 through V4. Her symptoms and ECG abnormalities resolved after two sublingual nitroglycerin tablets. Her hsTn at time of presentation and at 2 hours was 24 ng/mL and 82 ng/mL, respectively, confirming that she has had acute myocardial injury. She is diagnosed with an ACS (NSTEMI) and started on unfractionated heparin and given clopidogrel 300 mg. She already takes an aspirin, statin, beta blocker, and ACE inhibitor. She consults with you regarding her treatment options. She tells you that her symptoms were very concerning, and she enjoys her quality of life. She would be willing to have revascularization if it would help her. You consult with her cardiologist and verify that she does not have major geriatric comorbidities that would preclude an early invasive strategy. The following morning, she undergoes angiography via radial arterial access and has successful PCI of a 90% stenosis in the proximal left anterior descending coronary artery with a drug-eluting stent. She had no other significant coronary lesions. She is discharged with good secondary prevention medications, cardiac rehabilitation consultation, and recommendations to continue clopidogrel for a minimum of 1 year.

1. Are Mrs. Beasley's presentation symptoms typical for older adults?
2. What would be the criteria for then changing to an invasive approach if Mrs. Beasley preferred an initial conservative (i.e., medical) strategy to manage her NSTEMI?
3. What are the advantages of radial access over femoral access?
4. How long should Mrs. Beasley take clopidogrel after PCI for NSTEMI?

## Risk-Treatment Paradox

Health disparities in the medical field are not uncommon and cardiovascular care is unfortunately no different. Older adults have more prevalent CAD and are at higher risk for adverse events than their younger counterparts. Despite guideline recommended benefits for medical treatment of CAD, there continues to remain evidence of therapeutic inertia for implementing best clinical practice in the older adult with CAD. Lower use of statins among eligible older patients has been previously described,[21] and similar findings for lower use of aspirin and ACE inhibitors has been reported.[53] Among Medicare beneficiaries hospitalized for acute MI, both substantial regional differences in use of cardiac catheterization and risk-avoidance for cardiac catheterization exist.[54] On the positive end, the treatment gap appears to be improving, and research has suggested that other factors, such as functional status and mood disorders, may account for some of the observed differences.[55,56] Risk assessment for patients with or without known CAD provides objective evidence for implementing best practice and tailoring patient risk to management strategies. Individualizing care, particularly in older patients with multiple comorbidities, remains a central tenant to care of patients with CAD as very few clinical trials in CAD enrolled older adults with geriatric syndromes exist.

## Geriatric Considerations in Coronary Artery Disease and Acute Coronary Syndrome

Beyond ageing, there has been increasing recognition of geriatric syndromes and their intertwined role in managing patients with CV disease. A movement away from a traditional "organ-system" based approach to a "patient-centered" framework for providing care to older adults with CAD has emerged given the complexities of patient management and interrelated conditions in older patients.[57] Enhancing communication between primary providers and geriatric specialists with other health providers helps bring attention to the patient-centered approach. Fig. 37.1 illustrates a contemporary characterization of factors relevant in the evaluation of older adults with CAD.[58] In an era of minimally invasive procedure for complex cardiac structural heart disease, the relevant role of frailty, nutritional deficiencies, cognitive impairment, impaired mobility, fracture history, and loss of independence have gained greater relevance during cardiovascular evaluations. Frailty is prevalent among hospitalized CAD patients[59] and is associated with worse outcomes after revascularization.[43] Characterized as a biologic vulnerability to physiologic stressors, frailty has a shared inflammatory basis in its etiology as CAD, and these factors may converge to development of frailty traits.[60]

Polypharmacy in older adults with geriatric syndromes and CAD increases their risk for adverse events, toxicities, and

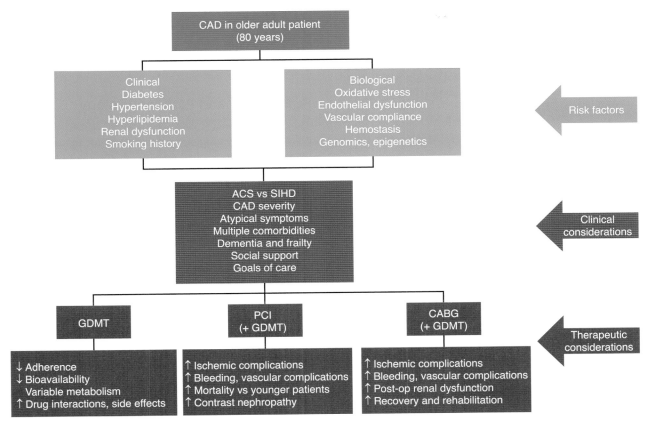

- **Figure 37.1** Risk factors, clinical influences, and treatment considerations in older patients with coronary artery disease (*CAD*). *ACS,* Acute coronary syndrome; *CABG,* coronary artery bypass grafting; *GDMT, Goal directed medical therapy; PCI,* percutaneous coronary intervention; *SIHD,* stable ischemic heart disease. (From Madhavan MV, Gersh BJ, Alexander KP, et al. Coronary artery disease in patients ≥80 years of age. *J Am Coll Cardiol.* 2018;71:2015-2040. With permission.)

drug-drug interactions. Deprescribing, defined as medication dose reduction or removal based on benefits versus harms assessment, as a strategy to align treatment with the overall care plan (goals, functional status, life expectancy)[61] is increasingly recognized as often overlooked in CAD patients. Refer to the section on polypharmacy and deprescribing for more information. Ongoing studies to evaluate deprescribing interventions of commonly used CV medications in older adults will help inform this area of practice.

## CASE 1

### Discussion

Part 1: Although the risk estimator identifies her as having low risk for future CAD or CV event, her risk factors are not optimally controlled. She may require the addition of a third antihypertensive medication to bring her closer to a goal of 120/80 mmHg. Dietary and lifestyle recommendations are reasonable for her hyperlipidemia, without necessarily instituting statin therapy. She should be advised on a Mediterranean-type or low-fat low-cholesterol diet and aerobic physical activity, such as walking. She should have continued follow-up to see if risk factors change over time. It should be acknowledged that she may also have psychosocial stressors related to care for a spouse with cognitive dysfunction. It has previously been shown that caregiver stress is associated with future adverse health outcomes. This may also impact her ability to manage her own chronic comorbidities and keep future health visit appointments.

Part 2: Her symptoms are suggestive of CAD and may be exacerbated by uncontrolled hypertension. She meets a diagnosis of symptomatic SIHD

and has documented ischemia by stress testing. Many patients, such as Mrs. Beasley, may decline invasive testing and prefer medical therapy for SIHD. Her exercise capacity and normal BP responses were also prognostically favorable. Her treatment should include low-dose antiplatelet therapy with aspirin 81 mg daily and statin. Her BP should be brought under better control, and this may be accomplished by introducing a beta blocker and/or an ACE-I. Ranolazine may be used to reduce anginal symptoms and does not significantly affect heart rate or BP. The decision regarding the need for angiography may be reserved for patients that have ongoing symptoms despite optimal medical therapy or have high burden of symptoms at baseline.

Part 3: Although older adults may present with atypical symptoms of myocardial ischemia (i.e., fatigue, dizziness, abdominal symptoms, back pain), typical symptoms, such as chest pain, still remain the most common. When an initial conservative strategy is pursued, the institution of antianginals and antithrombotics is used to medically treat UA/NSTEMI. If patients have rapid symptom resolution and hemodynamic stability, a predischarge stress test may be used to further risk stratify the burden of ischemia. Low-risk stress findings can be used to support ongoing conservative management. However, crossover to an invasive strategy would be recommended for patients with postinfarct angina (i.e., recurrent chest pain after initial index MI), dynamic ST-segment changes, HF, electrical instability, or high-risk findings on stress testing. An important downside for invasive procedures relates to bleeding at the arterial access site. Radial artery access, as compared with femoral artery access, has been associated with reduced risk of bleeding, fewer transfusions, and perhaps, because of this, better survival. Radial access also has been associated with less need for sedating or analgesic medications, earlier ambulation time, and lower risk for access site complications. It has been considered the default access site approach for ACS patients, given the heightened risk of bleeding related to concomitant antithrombotic medications. Current practice guidelines recommend clopidogrel and aspirin for a minimum of 1 year after PCI for patients treated during an ACS. The risk:benefit calculus for abbreviating or extending therapy should be individualized. Low-dose aspirin would be recommended indefinitely in the post-PCI patient, unless they are also being treated with a chronic anticoagulant (vitamin K antagonist or direct oral anticoagulant), such as for AF.

## Coronary Artery Disease Summary

Older adults have a high prevalence of CAD and important aspects for management center on implementing risk reduction strategies, such as diet and lifestyle modifications along with medical therapy. Age carries strong prognostic weight in all CAD risk models, therefore treatment benefit for certain therapies are likely to be greater in older adults as compared with younger patients. Given these observations, older adults should receive guideline recommended therapies for treatment of ACS, which often includes revascularization to reduce risk for recurrent MI and improve survival. However, this must be balanced with potentially increased risks for adverse events from therapeutic intervention, whether medical in nature or procedural. Primary care clinicians often partner with specialty providers and other members of the treatment team (cardiologist, pharmacist, therapist, dietitian) to align patient treatment with goals of the care plan. The multidisciplinary team approach often proves essential to providing patient-centered care, with recognition of geriatric comorbidities that often impact care of the patient with CAD.

## Atrial Fibrillation

### Prevalence and Impact

AF is the most common cardiac arrhythmia encountered in clinical practice. It is defined as a supraventricular arrhythmia characterized by unregulated, chaotic atrial electrical activity. AF is more prevalent with advancing age because of an accumulation of risk factors and age-related changes in the heart's conduction system. Approximately 12% of adults over age 75 years have AF.[62] AF is associated with increased morbidity and mortality. Individuals with AF are twice as likely as age- and gender-matched controls to be hospitalized annually.[63] Irregular contraction of the atria leads to turbulence and clot formation, particularly within the left atrial appendage, predisposing to a four- to fivefold increased risk of stroke.[64] In older adults, AF has been associated with cognitive decline, physical disability, and falls.[65]

---

### CASE 2

#### Rupert O'Donnell

Mr. O'Donnell is a 79-year-old male patient who presents to your clinic earlier than his scheduled appointment because of fatigue and dizziness. His past medical history includes hypertension, untreated sleep apnea, hypothyroidism, and diabetes. He lives with his spouse, who assists with bill-pay and manages his medicines. He is independent with his activities of daily living. He has had two falls in the previous 3 months and uses a cane for ambulation. In your office, his vital signs include: blood pressure 132/64 mmHg, heart rate 108 beats per minute, respiratory rate 15, O2 sat 98%. His examination reveals an irregularly irregular heart rhythm. The remainder

of his examination is unchanged from previous visits. An ECG shows new onset of AF, with heart rate 110 beats per minute.
1. What risk factors does your patient have for developing AF?
2. What are the most common presentations of AF?

---

## Risk Factors and Pathophysiology

There are a number of mechanisms by which AF occurs, from isolated electrophysiologic dysfunction to an accumulation of underlying factors. Age is an independent risk factor for the development of AF because of atrial fibrosis and structural remodeling. Box 37.5 lists risk factors for AF. Hypertension, diastolic dysfunction, and obstructive sleep apnea are risk factors that are increasingly prevalent in older populations. Similar to other disorders in geriatric medicine, transient factors, such as dehydration, stress, infection, and postoperative state, may precipitate the incidence of AF in a patient with underlying risk factors.[66]

## Presentation and Assessment

Presenting symptoms of AF include fatigue, palpitations, shortness of breath, and lightheadedness. Older patients may present with geriatric syndromes, such as falls, delirium, or syncope. AF can be persistent or fleeting and intermittent, termed paroxysmal. Physical examination will identify an irregularly irregular rhythm, but the diagnosis of AF requires an ECG or electrical monitoring. Lastly, patients may present emergently with tachycardia, HF, or

---

### • BOX 37.5 Risk Factors for the Development of Atrial Fibrillation

**Demographics**
Age
Male sex
European ancestry

**Diseases**
HTN
DM2
History of MI
Valvular heart disease
OSA
Obesity
Heart failure
Diastolic dysfunction
CAD
Parenchymal lung disease

**Lifestyle factors**
Alcohol use
Tobacco use
Long-term endurance exercise

**Transient factors**
Postoperative state
Cardiothoracic surgery
Pulmonary embolism
Hyperthyroidism

*AF,* Atrial fibrillation; *CAD,* coronary artery disease; *DM2,* type 2 diabetes; *HTN,* hypertension; *MI,* myocardial infarction; *OSA,* obstructive sleep apnea.

## TABLE 37.3   Diagnostic Testing for New Onset Atrial Fibrillation

| Laboratory testing | CBC, liver function, electrolytes, renal function, TSH, ± troponin |
|---|---|
| Radiography | Chest plain film |
| Cardiac studies | ECG, echocardiogram for structural heart disease and/or thrombus, stress testing, event monitor, EP studies |
| Noncardiac studies | Overnight oximetry, sleep study |

*CBC,* Complete blood count; *ECG,* electrocardiogram; *EP,* electrophysiology; *TSH,* thyroid stimulating hormone.

## TABLE 37.4   CHA$_2$DS$_2$-VASc Score and Associated Increased Annual Risk For Stroke

| | | |
|---|---|---|
| C | Congestive heart failure | 1 |
| H | Hypertension | 1 |
| A | Age >75 years | 1 |
| D | Diabetes | 1 |
| S | Stroke, TIA | 2 |
| V | Vascular disease | 1 |
| A | Age 65−74 years | 1 |
| Sc | Sex (female) | 1 |

| Total score | Annual risk of stroke |
|---|---|
| 0 | 0.2% |
| 1 | 0.6% |
| 2 | 2.2% |
| 3 | 3.2% |
| 4 | 4.8% |
| 5 | 7.2% |
| 6 | 9.7% |
| 7 | 11.2% |
| 8 | 10.8% |
| 9 | 12.2% |

*TIA,* Transient ischemic attack.

stroke. Once new onset AF is identified, an investigation for provoking factors is warranted through history, physical examination, laboratory testing, radiography, and/or advanced cardiac studies. Diagnostic testing, as directed by history and physical examination, is listed in Table 37.3.

### CASE 2

#### Rupert O'Donnell (Part 2)

Mr. O'Donnell is hemodynamically stable and willing to complete an outpatient workup, including labs and echocardiogram. He agrees to use his continuous positive airway pressure more frequently. He is already taking five medicines: amlodipine, lisinopril, levothyroxine, metformin, and atorvastatin. He is hesitant to start additional medications.
1. What treatments should be initiated during his visit?
2. What risks are associated with treatment?

## Management

The goal of AF treatment is to prevent long-term morbidity and mortality. Management strategies should be individualized for each patient, with a focus on (1) reduction of stroke risk, and (2) minimizing symptoms related to heart rate and rhythm. An anticoagulation strategy is necessary for patients with AF to decrease the risk of stroke. The risk of stroke is predicted by the CHADS2Vasc model, with increasing risk correlating with higher CHADS2Vasc score (Table 37.4) (Level of evidence [LOE] = B). The use of anticoagulants also carries risk, primarily because of increased major bleeding events, such as gastrointestinal or intracranial hemorrhage. In older adults, a comprehensive assessment of risks versus benefits is indicated at initiation of anticoagulation and frequently thereafter. Risk-prediction scores, such as HAS-BLED and HEMORR$_2$HAGES, have modest performance in predicting clinically relevant bleeding events.[67,68] In practice, the risk of hemorrhage is often overstated in comparison with the relatively greater risk of ischemic stroke in patients with frailty or falls, leading to underprescription of anticoagulation to those who may be most likely to benefit.[69] New left atrial appendage occlusion devices, such as the Watchman device™, can be used in patients with both high stroke and bleeding risks, to avoid complications of long-term anticoagulation.

The choice of anticoagulant also requires a comprehensive assessment. Patients are characterized as either valvular or nonvalvular AF. Valvular AF refers to patients with mechanical valves and/or moderate/severe mitral stenosis. This group of patients are recommended to use warfarin for anticoagulation (LOE = B).[70] Nonvalvular AF patients may be candidates for direct oral anticoagulant (DOAC) therapy, a newer class of medication that includes dabigatran, rivaroxaban, apixaban, and edoxaban. Renal and liver function must be assessed before initiation of a DOAC because the available agents have varying degrees of hepatic and renal clearance. Apixaban has a US Food and Drug Administration−approved dose adjustment for age, low body weight, and impaired renal function. The other agents may be dose-reduced for renal insufficiency, although use is prohibited in both severe renal and hepatic impairment. Benefits of DOACs over warfarin use include fewer drug and food interactions, decreased need for monitoring, and decreased mortality because of major bleeding. Cost of DOAC therapy exceeds warfarin substantially. When costs or contraindications prohibit the use of DOAC therapy, warfarin is recommended.

**In older adult patients, choosing an anticoagulant in AF to decrease risk of stroke requires an individualized comprehensive assessment of AF type, bleeding and stroke risk, renal and hepatic impairment, medication interactions, transportation, and cost.**

AF can manifest with tachycardia, termed rapid ventricular response (RVR), or bradycardia with slow ventricular response.

Management of heart rate can prevent morbidity from AF RVR, hypotension, and exacerbations of heart failure. Beta blockers and nondihydropiridine calcium-channel blockers (diltiazem and verapamil) are most frequently used for long-term rate control (LOE = B).[71] Less often, patients may be prescribed amiodarone or digoxin for rate control, although use is limited by adverse effects. AF with slow ventricular response may indicate the need for reduction in rate controlling medication in the older adult patient or may be an indication for a permanent pacemaker.

In patients whose heart rate and/or symptoms remain poorly controlled with rate-limiting agents alone, a rhythm control strategy, often using membrane-active antiarrhythmic medications, may be used. Antiarrhythmics, including amiodarone, flecainide, propafenone, sotalol, and dofetilide, are most frequently administered under the guidance of a cardiologist. However, it should be noted that antiarrhythmics do not improve mortality and can lead to increased hospitalizations and resource utilization.[71] A rhythm control strategy is indicated for patients who remain symptomatic with reduced quality of life while in AF. Electrical cardioversion is performed for highly symptomatic AF with or without an antiarrhythmic medication for patients in whom the clinical decision has been made to have them on a rhythm control strategy. Finally, an electrophysiologist can perform radiofrequency or cryoballoon ablation procedures, termed pulmonary vein isolation, in patients who fail the aforementioned drugs or therapies. The role of AF ablation is less established in older patients.[72]

---

**CASE 2**

### Discussion

You replace Mr. O'Donnell's amlodipine with carvedilol, which is successful in managing his heart rate and symptoms. You calculate his CHADS2Vasc as 4, indicating a moderate-high risk of stroke. He agrees to start anticoagulation. Additional recommendations are provided to decrease his risk of falls, including a trial of gait/balance therapy and use of grab bars in his home.

---

## Summary

AF is increasingly prevalent with older age and is associated with increased hospitalization, stroke, and functional decline. Diagnostic workup at presentation should focus on identifying correctable underlying factors. Appropriate management focuses on decreasing morbidity and mortality, generally through anticoagulation, rate, and rhythm control agents. The choice of medications in the older adult population must balance the risks of adverse effects with the benefits of therapy. In AF, a comprehensive geriatric assessment is beneficial to determine the safest choice of anticoagulation to prevent stroke while balancing risk of major hemorrhage from falls or gastrointestinal bleeding.

### Web Resources

Heart risk calculator of the American College of Cardiology/American Heart Association Atherosclerotic Cardiovascular Risk Calculator: www.cvriskcalculator.com.

American Heart Association sparctool.com. Stroke Prevention in Atrial Fibrillation Risk Tool: www.heart.org.

---

## Key References

### Coronary Artery Disease

3. Fihn SD, Gardin JM, Abrams J, et al. 2012 ACCF/AHA/ACP/AATS/PCNA/SCAI/STS guideline for the diagnosis and management of patients with stable ischemic heart disease. *Circulation.* 2012;126:e354−e471.
31. Spertus JA, Jones P, McDonell M, et al. Health status predicts long-term outcome in outpatients with coronary disease. *Circulation.* 2002;106:43−49.
37. Boden WE, O'Rourke RA, Teo KK, et al. Optimal medical therapy with or without PCI for stable coronary disease. *N Engl J Med.* 2007;356:1503−1516.
41. Bach RG, Cannon CP, Weintraub WS, et al. The effect of routine early invasive management on outcome for elderly patients with non-ST-segment elevation acute coronary syndromes. *Ann Intern Med.* 2004;141:186−195.
57. Forman DE, Rich MW, Alexander KP, et al. Cardiac care for older adults: time for a new paradigm. *J Am Coll Cardiol.* 2011;57:1801−1810.

### Atrial Fibrillation

64. Wolf PA, Abbott RD, Kannel WB. Atrial fibrillation: a major contributor to stroke in the elderly: the Framingham Study. *Arch Intern Med.* 1987;147:1561−1564.
71. January C, Wann J, Alpert J, et al. 2014 AHA/ACC/HRS guideline for the management of patients with atrial fibrillation. a report of the American College of Cardiology/American Heart Association Task Force on Practice Guidelines and the Heart Rhythm Society. *JACC.* 2014;64 (21):e1−76.
72. Calkins H, Kuck K, Cappato R, et al. 2012 HRS/EHRA/ECAS expert consensus statement on catheter and surgical ablation of atrial fibrillation: recommendations for patient selection, procedural techniques, patient management and follow-up, definitions, endpoints, and research trial design: a report of the Heart Rhythm Society (HRS) Task Force on Catheter and Surgical Ablation of Atrial Fibrillation. *Heart Rhythm.* 2012;9:632−696.

**References available online at** expertconsult.com.

# 38

# Heart Failure

BRITTANY M. DIXON AND MICHAEL W. RICH

## OBJECTIVES

*Upon completion of this chapter, the reader will be able to:*

- Understand the epidemiology and clinical features of heart failure (HF) in older adults.
- Recognize the differences between HF with reduced ejection fraction and HF with preserved ejection fraction.
- Understand the important role of guideline-directed medical therapy in the treatment of HF.

- Be familiar with the appropriate use of heart failure medications, including angiotensin-converting enzyme inhibitors, angiotensin receptor blockers, beta blockers, mineralocorticoid receptor antagonists, and newer classes of drugs.

## Introduction

Heart failure (HF) is a condition frequently encountered in the geriatric population and may present with atypical symptoms.

### CASE 1

#### Barry Jones (Part 1)

Barry Jones is a 78-year-old man who reports decreasing ability to take care of himself. Mr. Jones is now short of breath with minimal exertion and has difficulty sleeping at night. On examination, his heart rate is 105 beats per minute and blood pressure is 116/43 mmHg. He has moist rales bilaterally, jugular venous distention, and 2 + pedal edema. His heart rhythm is regular with both S3 and S4 gallops. Labs are notable for creatinine 1.2 mg/dL and N-terminal prohormone B-type natriuretic peptide (NT-proBNP) 2525 pg/dL.
1. What is the best way to assess volume status in this patient?
2. What further tests may be useful in confirming the diagnosis?

## Prevalence and Impact

HF is a growing epidemic worldwide and affects approximately 6.2 million adults in the United States.[1] HF incidence increases with age and approaches 10 per 1000 population after age 65 years. Furthermore, the prevalence among adults age $\geq 80$ years is 8.6% in men and 11.5% in women.[2] Despite advances in medical treatment, mortality among HF patients remains high, with 5-year survival rates of approximately 50%.[1] In addition, increasing age is one of the strongest predictors of less favorable prognosis.

HF also contributes to chronic disability in the older population. HF is the most common cause of hospitalization and rehospitalization among Medicare beneficiaries, accounting for 1 million admissions annually. More than 70% of HF hospitalizations involve persons older than age 65 years, and almost 20% of patients are readmitted within 30 days.

## Risk Factors and Pathophysiology

HF results from alterations to the myocardium with a broad list of potential causes, including ischemic heart disease, hypertension, infection, genetic mutations, alcohol/illicit drugs, cardiotoxic medications, and valvular disease. In addition, normal aging is associated with extensive changes in the cardiovascular system that reduce cardiovascular reserve and predispose to the development of HF (Table 38.1).

In the early stages of HF, the ventricle may undergo remodeling with increased ventricular volume and/or increased wall thickness to maintain cardiac output. However, this remodeling eventually fails to preserve cardiac output, especially during stress (e.g., myocardial infarction, pneumonia, major surgery), and may lead to clinical HF. HF also involves activation of several neurohormonal systems to augment cardiac output and regulate fluid balance, electrolytes, and blood pressure. Specifically, the renin-angiotensin-aldosterone system (RAAS) and adrenergic nervous system play a major role in HF and are the target of many pharmaceutical interventions.

Recent guidelines from the American College of Cardiology (ACC) and American Heart Association (AHA) define four stages of HF, which are distinct from the widely used New York Heart Association (NYHA) classification of symptoms. Stage A refers to patients who are "at high risk for HF but without structural heart disease or symptoms" and includes individuals with known risk factors for HF, such as hypertension, obesity, or coronary artery disease.[3] Stage B refers to patients who have "structural heart disease but without signs or symptoms of HF."[3] Stage B includes patients with asymptomatic left ventricular systolic or diastolic dysfunction, as well as patients with left ventricular hypertrophy or significant valvular heart disease in the absence of symptoms. Stage C is defined as "structural heart disease with prior or current symptoms of HF," whereas stage D refers to "refractory HF."[3] Although many patients with stage A or B HF eventually progress to clinical HF (stage C or D), other patients remain asymptomatic for prolonged periods of time, especially if risk factors, such as hypertension, are well controlled.

## Differential Diagnosis and Assessment

### General Principles

The assessment of suspected HF begins with a careful history and physical examination. Important components of the history that support a diagnosis of HF include dyspnea at rest or with exertion, decreased exercise tolerance, orthopnea, paroxysmal nocturnal dyspnea, and lower extremity edema or abdominal distension. The diagnosis of HF in older adults may be difficult because the symptoms are often atypical or difficult to elicit (Table 38.2). Geriatric patients may present with worsening fatigue, decreased functional capacity, altered sensorium (e.g., delirium/confusion), or gastrointestinal disturbances (anorexia, nausea, abdominal bloating). The most useful way to assess volume status is by estimating jugular venous pressure (JVP). Elevated JVP suggests intravascular volume overload. An S3 gallop reflects left ventricular volume overload and almost always indicates HF because of systolic dysfunction in older patients. An S4 gallop is caused by increased stiffness of the left ventricle and is often present in older adults with or without HF. Pulmonary rales are a hallmark of pulmonary edema but may also be caused by atelectasis or chronic lung disease in older patients. Lower extremity edema may also be sign of a HF, but may be caused by other causes such as medications (especially calcium channel blockers), venous insufficiency, or kidney disease in the geriatric population.

**⇔ The best way to assess volume status on physical examination is to estimate jugular venous pressure.**

Basic laboratory evaluation for suspected HF includes a chest x-ray, 12-lead electrocardiogram (ECG), and selected blood tests. The chest x-ray may show an enlarged heart (cardiomegaly), enlarged hila with indistinct margins (perivascular edema), engorged veins draining the upper lobes (cephalization of flow), or frank pulmonary edema with Kerley B lines and pleural effusions. The ECG may show left and/or right atrial enlargement, left ventricular hypertrophy, or evidence of acute ischemia or prior myocardial infarction. Routine blood tests should include a comprehensive metabolic panel and complete blood count. B-type natriuretic peptide (BNP) and NT-proBNP are high yield tests for evaluating HF but have some limitations in older patients. Individuals with low levels of BNP or NT-proBNP are unlikely to have acute HF as the cause of their symptoms. However, it is important to recognize that BNP and NT-proBNP increase with age, and that women have higher levels than men.[4] One study proposes the following thresholds for NT-proBNP values used to diagnose clinical HF: 450 or higher for age < 50 years, 900 or higher for age 50 to 74 years, and 1800 or higher for age ≥ 75 years.[5] In addition, BNP and

| TABLE 38.1 | Major Effects of Normal Aging on Cardiovascular Structure and Function |
|---|---|
| **Alteration** | **Impact** |
| Increased stiffness/decreased elasticity of large arteries | Increased impedance to LV ejection; gradual increase in systolic BP |
| Increased myocardial stiffness and impaired LV relaxation | Altered diastolic filling predisposing to HFpEF and atrial fibrillation |
| Impaired responsiveness to beta-adrenergic stimulation | Declines in peak HR (220-age), peak contractility, and peripheral vasodilation |
| Decreased sinus node function and degenerative changes in conduction system | Sick sinus syndrome, bradyarrhythmias, supraventricular and ventricular arrhythmias, conduction disturbances |
| Altered baroreceptor responsiveness | Predisposition to lightheadedness, falls, and syncope |
| Impaired endothelium-dependent vasodilation | Decline in peak coronary blood flow; predisposition to ischemia because of supply/demand mismatch |

*BP*, Blood pressure; *HFpEF*, heart failure with preserved ejection fraction; *HR*, heart rate; *LV*, left ventricular.

**TABLE 38.2 Classical and Atypical Manifestations of Heart Failure in Older Adults**

| Classical | Atypical (Noncerebral) | Atypical (Cerebral) |
|---|---|---|
| Shortness of breath with exertion | Abdominal discomfort or bloating | No history or poor/unreliable history |
| Orthopnea | Anorexia/weight loss | Confusion/delirium |
| Paroxysmal nocturnal dyspnea | Nausea | Decreased sensorium |
| Lower extremity swelling | Change in bowel habits | Lethargy |
| Decrease in exercise tolerance | Nocturia | Behavioral disturbances, (e.g., irritability) |
| Fatigue/low energy | Chest pain or discomfort | Falls |
| Cough | | Insomnia |
| Weight gain | | Syncope |
| Weakness | | Depression |

NT-proBNP are cleared by the kidneys and levels are influenced by renal function. This is important to consider when evaluating older patients, in whom renal function declines progressively with age, as it is common for BNP or NT-proBNP to be elevated in older patients with renal disease, even in the absence of overt HF. Cardiac troponins are useful to evaluate for ischemia as a cause of acute decompensated HF. Troponin levels are also affected by renal dysfunction and may be slightly elevated in older adults without active ischemia.

◆◆ **The diagnostic utility of BNP and pro-BNP may be affected by age, sex, and renal function.**

In most cases, a transthoracic echocardiogram (TTE) is recommended to evaluate left ventricular systolic and diastolic function, wall thickness and chamber sizes, valve function, and right ventricular function and pulmonary artery pressure. It may be appropriate to obtain additional diagnostic tests to investigate potential etiologies of HF (e.g., stress test to evaluate for ischemia; cardiac magnetic resonance scan to evaluate for cardiac amyloid). Consultation with a cardiology specialist should be considered in cases of diagnostic uncertainty.

## Precipitating Factors

Conditions that increase cardiovascular demand or interfere with compensatory mechanisms may precipitate HF symptoms (Box 38.1).

### CASE 1

**Barry Jones (Part 2)**

Upon further review of the medical record, you discover that Mr. Jones has a history of HF with reduced ejection fraction (HFrEF), coronary artery disease, and hypertension. He states that recently he has been drinking more water and that he frequently consumes canned vegetables and soup at home. Current medications include aspirin 81 mg daily, lisinopril 5 mg daily, carvedilol 3.125 mg twice daily, and furosemide 20 mg daily. He relates that he usually takes his medications as prescribed but that he ran

**• BOX 38.1 Common Precipitant of Heart Failure**

- Alcohol or illicit drugs (esp. cocaine, amphetamines)
- Anemia
- Arrhythmias (esp. atrial fibrillation/atrial flutter)
- Chronic obstructive pulmonary disease exacerbation
- Dietary or medication nonadherence[a]
- Drugs: cardiac depressants (e.g., antiarrhythmics, antineoplastics)
- Excess fluid intake (including intravenous fluids)
- Hypoxia
- Hyperthyroidism
- Infection (pneumonia, sepsis)
- Medication withdrawal (e.g., ACE inhibitors, digoxin, diuretics)
- Myocardial infarction/ischemia
- Pulmonary embolism
- Renal insufficiency
- Stress (e.g., major surgery, major life events)

[a] Most common precipitating cause outside hospital.
*ACE*, Angiotensin-converting enzyme.

out of his furosemide "a couple of weeks ago." His ECG reveals sinus tachycardia and no ischemic changes. A recent TTE demonstrated moderate left ventricular (LV) systolic dysfunction with ejection fraction (EF) 30% to 35%. You counsel him on a low-sodium diet, advise him to cut back on his fluid intake, and increase his furosemide dose.
1. What other medication changes should be considered at this time?
2. How should the patient be monitored in the future?

## Management of Heart Failure with Reduced Ejection Fraction

### Goals of Treatment

HF presents several challenges in both acute and long-term management. The goals of treatment are to alleviate symptoms, maximize functional status, improve quality of life, reduce the number of hospitalizations, and prolong survival. However, management of the older patient is often complicated by the presence of multiple medical comorbidities, geriatric syndromes (e.g., frailty, incontinence, cognitive impairment), and polypharmacy. Furthermore, aging is associated with altered pharmacokinetics and pharmacodynamics of most medications. Ultimately, treatment decisions should incorporate both evidence-based medicine and individual patient factors, including personal preferences and goals of care.

## Medications

Angiotensin-converting enzyme (ACE) inhibitors and angiotensin-receptor blockers (ARBs) improve both survival and quality of life in patients with reduced EF. Potential adverse effects include hypotension, worsening renal function, hyperkalemia, and angioedema. Cough may occur in up to 20% of patients using ACE inhibitors because of effects of increased bradykinin. Cough and angioedema occur much less frequently with ARBs. Doses should be low initially and progressively increased as tolerated while the clinician monitors the blood pressure, renal function, and electrolytes. In Black patients with advanced HF symptoms, the combination of hydralazine and nitrates provides additional benefit to use of an ACE inhibitor or ARB.[3]

❖ **HF medications should be started at low doses in geriatric patients and uptitrated slowly.**

Beta blockers are also beneficial in patients with reduced EF. Beta-receptor blocking agents improve LV function, increase survival, and reduce hospitalizations.[3] Beta blockers approved for treatment of HF in the United States include metoprolol succinate (sustained release), carvedilol, and bisoprolol. Contraindications to use of beta blockers include bradycardia, hypotension, severe lung disease and/or bronchospasm, and acute decompensated HF. Again, doses should be low initially and uptitrated slowly. A small minority may not be able to tolerate beta blockers because of side effects. In the geriatric population, beta blockers may negatively impact functional status. Therefore use of beta blockers in older adults should weigh the survival benefit against the potential decrease in quality of life.

Spironolactone and eplerenone are mineralocorticoid receptor antagonists (MRAs) that are beneficial in patients with reduced EF, especially those with EF under 35%.[3] Production of aldosterone, a potent sodium- and water-retaining steroid with additional actions that are deleterious to the heart and blood vessels, is upregulated in chronic HF but blocked by MRAs. Potential adverse effects include hypotension, hyperkalemia, worsening renal function, and gynecomastia. Eplerenone is a more selective MRA, and gynecomastia is less common with this agent. MRAs are contraindicated if creatinine >2.5 mg/dL or serum potassium >5.0 mEq/L. As with other HF medications, the initial dose should be low (12.5−25 mg daily) with appropriate monitoring of renal function and potassium.

Digoxin is no longer a first-line drug for treatment of HF but is recommended when patients remain symptomatic despite optimization of other treatments.[3] Digoxin has mild inotropic properties that improve symptoms and reduce hospitalizations, but digoxin has not been shown to reduce mortality. Potential adverse effects include arrhythmias (bradycardia, heart block, supraventricular, and ventricular arrhythmias), gastrointestinal symptoms, and neurologic effects. The dose of digoxin must be reduced when renal function is impaired and the therapeutic range for digoxin is 0.5 to 0.9 ng/mL.

In recent years, newer classes of drugs have become available for the treatment of chronic HF. Sacubitril-valsartan is a neprilysin inhibitor in combination with an ARB. Sacubitril-valsartan is now recommended as a first-line therapy for patients with reduced EF and is a reasonable alternative to ACE inhibitors or ARBs.[6] If a patient is already taking an ACE inhibitor or ARB, it is important to wait 36 hours for washout before initiating sacubitril-valsartan. A second medication that has become available in recent years is ivabradine. Ivabradine inhibits the "funny channel" of the sinoatrial node and is approved for use in HF patients with sinus rhythm and resting heart rates over 70 beats per minute despite maximally tolerated doses of beta blockers. Ivabradine reduces hospitalizations and HF-related deaths.[7] There are emerging data on use of sodium-glucose cotransporter-2 inhibitors for the treatment of HFrEF, including patients who do not have diabetes mellitus.[8] However, more data are needed on outcomes in geriatric populations.

Loop diuretics (furosemide, torsemide, bumetenide) are often necessary for treatment of HF symptoms but have not been shown to improve survival. The goal is gentle diuresis to relieve symptoms, avoiding hypotension and its consequences. Diuretics are often dosed incorrectly or discontinued prematurely because of concerns about rising creatinine. However, it is appropriate to initiate diuretic therapy in patients with elevated creatinine because of volume overload and acute cardiorenal syndrome (i.e., worsening renal function in the setting of worsening cardiac function, often related in part to passive congestion of the kidneys). Serum magnesium and potassium should be measured routinely and repleted if necessary. When the patient has suboptimal response to loop diuretics, metolazone or indapamide may be added. These agents should be given 30 minutes before administration of loop diuretics to potentiate their effects. Close monitoring of renal function and electrolytes (including sodium) is critical with use of these drugs.

❖ **Continue diuretics if worsening renal function because of volume overload!**

Optimal therapy for HF fosters polypharmacy, which may be particularly challenging for older adults who are often taking multiple medications for comorbid conditions. Effectively navigating polypharmacy requires shared decision making with delineation of the patient's goals of care, including the relative importance of length versus quality of life. As discussed earlier, ACE inhibitors, ARBs, beta blockers, MRAs, sacubitril-valsartan, ivabradine, and hydralazine/nitrates all improve survival in selected patients with HFrEF. Among these, ACE inhibitors/ARBs, MRAs, and especially sacubitril-valsartan have been associated with improved quality of life. Diuretics and digoxin alleviate symptoms but have not been shown to improve survival.

## Nonpharmaceutical Interventions

Lifestyle modifications play an important role in managing HF. In general, HF patients should adhere to a moderately low-sodium diet (<3 g/day) and avoid excessive fluid intake (i.e., no need for 8−10 glasses of water a day). Mild aerobic exercise, such as walking or cycling, increases functional capacity and quality of life.[9] Many HF patients benefit from formal cardiac rehabilitation programs once acute symptoms have been controlled. Education of patients and their families should be a cornerstone of every office visit and hospital interaction.

HF patients with reduced EFs (EF $\leq$ 35%) are at increased risk for sudden cardiac death (SCD) because of ventricular arrhythmias. Implantable cardioverter-defibrillators (ICDs) reduce SCD in high-risk patients with systolic dysfunction. However, the benefit of ICDs declines with age, and ICDs may introduce adverse effects (i.e., postprocedural complications, inappropriate shocks) that can impair quality of life.[10] The decision regarding ICD or cardiac resynchronization therapy in older patients should carefully weigh the benefits and risks using a shared decision-making process. Deactivation of the ICD may be appropriate in patients with worsening prognosis or in those pursuing palliative care, and older adults should be counseled on the option of future ICD deactivation as part of the initial shared decision-making process.

## End-Stage Heart Failure

HF is associated with a worse prognosis than most forms of cancer, and older age is a potent risk factor for reduced survival. End-of-life care should focus on shared decision making and use a multidisciplinary approach. LV assist devices (LVAD) are increasingly being used as "destination therapy" (i.e., final treatment with no plan to pursue heart transplantation) in older patients with highly symptomatic advanced HF and have been shown to improve quality of life and survival in selected patients at least up to age 80 years. However, most older patients are not candidates for advanced HF therapies, such as an LVAD or heart transplantation because of the effects of age, comorbidities, and limited life expectancy. A multidisciplinary team, including advanced HF specialists, can play an important role in evaluating a patient's candidacy for such therapies. Patients with refractory symptoms despite optimal medical therapy may benefit from palliative care or hospice.[11] Prognosis should be discussed openly, and completion of advanced directives regarding healthcare preferences should be encouraged.

### CASE 1

#### Discussion

Barry Jones presented with classic signs and symptoms of HF. He was found to have systolic dysfunction and should be started on appropriate medical therapies to improve symptoms, quality of life, and survival. Consideration of additional interventions should be predicated on disease trajectory, comorbid medical conditions, and personal preferences.

### CASE 2

#### Sally Lou (Part 1)

Sally Lou is an 82-year-old woman with hypertension, hyperlipidemia, and paroxysmal atrial fibrillation. She presents to your office complaining of worsening shortness of breath, nocturnal cough, and lower extremity swelling. Vital signs include blood pressure 150/80 mmHg, heart rate 92 beats per minute (regular), respiratory rate 16 breaths/min., and temperature 97° F. On examination, she has bilateral peripheral edema, elevated JVP, and bibasilar rales. ECG shows normal sinus rhythm and LV hypertrophy.
1. What factors may be contributing to her worsening symptoms?
2. What test(s) would you order next?

## Heart Failure with Preserved Ejection Fraction

HF with preserved EF (HFpEF), sometimes referred to as diastolic HF, increases with age, especially among women. Cardiac contractility is preserved but with increased filling pressures and abnormal relaxation, which causes (elevated pulmonary pressures and congestion, etc.). The clinical signs and symptoms of HFpEF are almost identical to those of systolic HF (an important difference is that an S3 gallop is uncommon in HFpEF). The prognosis of HFpEF is similar to that in HFrEF. The majority of data available for HF therapies are for patients with reduced LV systolic function (EF <40%). However, although there have now been numerous trials testing a multitude of pharmacologic agents for the treatment of HF with mildly reduced or preserved EF, none of these studies have demonstrated a beneficial effect on all-cause mortality.

### CASE 2

#### Sally Lou (Part 2)

You order an echocardiogram for Sally Lou to evaluate function and to determine if the HF is related predominantly to systolic or diastolic dysfunction. TTE reveals LVEF 67%, moderate diastolic dysfunction, normal pericardium, and no evidence of significant valvular disease.
1. How does treatment of HFpEF differ from that of HFrEF?
2. What is Ms. Lou's prognosis compared with a similar patient with reduced EF?

## Management of Heart Failure with Preserved Ejection Fraction

The first-line treatment for HFpEF is decreasing pulmonary congestion and venous pressures with diuretics. However, overdiuresis should be avoided because patients may rely on high filling pressures to maintain cardiac output and may be preload dependent. Adequate control of blood pressure is essential to managing HFpEF. Tachycardia or arrhythmias, such as atrial fibrillation, may worsen HFpEF owing to shortening of diastole. Patients with atrial fibrillation should have heart rates adequately controlled with beta blockers or calcium channel blockers. Alternatively, restoration to sinus rhythm may be desirable. Unlike systolic dysfunction, medications such as ACE inhibitors, ARBs, and beta blockers have not shown clear mortality benefit in patients with HFpEF. In the PARAGON-HF trial, sacubitril-valsartan did not reduce hospitalizations or mortality among patients with HFpEF but did improve some aspects of quality of life.[12] In the TOPCAT trial, spironolactone reduced hospitalizations in patients with HFpEF but had no effect on mortality.[13]

### CASE 2

#### Discussion

Sally Lou has HFpEF. This condition can present similarly to HFrEF and has a similar prognosis. The mainstay of therapy for HFpEF is control of volume status with diuretics and management of hypertension. In patients with persistent symptoms, the addition of spironolactone or sacubitril-valsartan is reasonable.

## Summary

HF is a growing medical problem worldwide and a common cause of hospitalizations, especially among older adults. HF diagnosis may be confirmed with a combination of history, physical examination, laboratory studies (especially BNP or NT-proBNP), and imaging tests (chest x-ray, TTE). Several classes of drugs have been shown to provide morbidity and mortality benefits for patients with HFrEF. These include ACE inhibitors and ARBs, beta blockers, MRAs, and neprilysin-ARB in combination. Other medications, such as diuretics, are helpful for controlling symptoms. With older adults, it is important to start with low doses and slowly uptitrate HF medications. Patients should be monitored for hypotension, renal dysfunction, or electrolyte abnormalities. Lifestyle modification is equally important. Patients should follow a reduced sodium diet and be encouraged to exercise. Device therapy may be appropriate in some patients but has limitations in the geriatric population. Management of refractory HF symptoms is best accomplished using a multidisciplinary team and shared decision making. To date, no interventions have been shown to improve survival in patients with HFpEF. Treatment of these patients includes optimizing volume status, controlling blood pressure, and lifestyle modifications as recommended for patients with HFrEF.

### Web Resources

American Heart Association (excellent source of materials for both practitioners and patients): www.americanheart.org

Cardio Smart (excellent source for patients from American College of Cardiology): https://www.cardiosmart.org/Heart-Conditions/Heart-Failure

Heart Failure Society of America (source materials for physicians and patients): www.hfsa.org

## Key References

3. Yancy CW, Jessup M, Bozkurt B, et al. 2013 ACCF/AHA guideline for the management of heart failure: a report of the American College of Cardiology Foundation/American Heart Association Task Force on Practice guidelines. *J Am Coll Cardiol.* 2013;62:e147–e239.

9. O'Connor CM, Whellan DJ, Lee KL, et al. Efficacy and safety of exercise training in patients with chronic heart failure: HF-ACTION randomized controlled trial. *JAMA.* 2009;301(14):1439–1450.

11. Rogers JG, Patel CB, Mentz RJ, et al. Palliative care in heart failure: the PAL-HF randomized controlled clinical trial. *J Am Coll Cardiol.* 2017;70(3):331–341.

***References available online at*** expertconsult.com**.**

# 39
# Peripheral Vascular Disease

JONATHAN R. THOMPSON AND JASON M. JOHANNING

## OBJECTIVES

*Upon completion of this chapter, the reader will be able to:*

- Describe the three most common types of peripheral vascular disease.
- Describe the current diagnostic strategy for workup of peripheral vascular disease.
- Describe the indications for treatment, including minimally invasive and open surgical options.

## Peripheral Vascular Disease

### CASE 1

#### James Fisher (Part 1)

James Fisher is a 73-year-old former maintenance worker who comes to your office with complaints of lower leg cramping with activity. He is obese with a long-standing history of type 2 diabetes mellitus treated and well controlled with oral medications. He is hypertensive despite being on two antihypertensive agents. He has some chronic kidney disease with a mildly reduced glomerular filtration rate.

1. What are the ideal diagnostic studies with which to confirm the presence of significant peripheral vascular disease?

Peripheral vascular disease (PVD) is primarily a disease of older adults. The average age of patients seeking treatment is approximately 70 years, with approximately 14.5% of patients age > 70 years having PVD.[12] Given the expected increase in our elderly population, the diagnosis and treatment of PVD will become a priority. A working knowledge of the most common sites of disease, the initial diagnostic tests, and options for treatment, as well as their outcomes, are necessary to provide optimal guidance for these patients.

A basic framework for diagnosis of vascular disease relies heavily on the vascular laboratory. The majority of structures involved in vascular disease, including retroperitoneal vascular structures, can initially be imaged using ultrasonography because of increasing resolution of and advances in hardware and software. In addition, in the periphery and supraclavicular region, vessel proximity to the skin level and the dynamic image acquisition often allow diagnosis and treatment without need for advanced imaging modalities. In fact, the vascular laboratory should be able to document the presence and extent of carotid, aortic, and lower extremity disease for the vast majority of patients, with advanced imaging (computed tomography [CT] and magnetic resonance imaging [MRI]) reserved for those patients in whom diagnosis is in question or for pretreatment planning. With regard to CT and MRI, these techniques also have increased in accuracy and clarity. Thus noninvasive imaging focusing heavily on CT angiography has replaced diagnostic angiography for detection of vascular disease, with angiography primarily reserved for confirmation of disease during planned endovascular intervention.

**❖ Noninvasive imaging has replaced diagnostic angiography for detection of vascular disease, with angiography primarily reserved for confirmation of disease during planned endovascular intervention.**

Similar to the increasing role of noninvasive imaging, there has been an increasing shift in vascular disease treatment to less invasive interventions. Vascular interventions for all patients can follow four different paths. All patients with vascular disease benefit both locally, at disease location, and systemically (i.e., presume coronary disease) with optimal medical management. This involved treatment with antiplatelet agents and cholesterol-lowering agents, primarily in the form of statin agents. In addition, we are beginning to understand the importance of aggressive blood pressure control and blood sugar control on outcomes in patients with vascular disease. Increasingly, patients are being treated in the lower extremities with solely minimally invasive percutaneous interventions (balloons, stents, atherectomy) requiring arterial access via catheters and guidewires. Although decreasing in usage, open surgical revascularization remains the gold standard against which all techniques are judged with regard to outcomes (patency and limb salvage). Lastly, a combination of open and percutaneous endovascular interventions can be combined to create a hybrid operation chosen to address complex vascular disease where outcomes are best served by a unique approach. The important point to remember is the patient at any time can be served by any of these techniques and therefore patient assessment, clinical judgment, and informed consent are paramount in choosing the appropriate intervention.

# Carotid Artery Disease

## Indications for Diagnostic Study

---

**CASE 2**

**Wayne Johnson (Part 1)**

Wayne Johnson is a 70-year-old retired custodian who has transient monocular blindness that he describes as a window shade covering his eye intermittently. He smokes one pack per day despite having coronary artery bypass grafting 10 years previously.

You discuss with Mr. Johnson next steps regarding diagnostic testing.

1. What are the options specific to the expected outcome for surgical treatment of carotid stenosis?

---

## Carotid Stenosis

Proper diagnosis, management, and treatment of carotid stenosis are important for reducing risk of ischemic stroke in older adult patients. Stroke is the third leading cause of death in the United States and results in significant disability. In general, 80% of strokes are ischemic and 20% hemorrhagic. Of the 80% of ischemic strokes, 20% to 30% are attributed to atheroembolic disease, resulting from stenosis of one carotid artery more than 50%. Focus has been placed on risk stratification for proper selection of appropriate treatment especially in the setting of a patient with carotid stenosis who is asymptomatic. Treatment will vary depending on

degree of stenosis and presence of symptoms and comorbid conditions that could potentially increase operative risks.

**❖ Of the 80% of ischemic strokes, 20% to 30% are attributed to atheroembolic disease resulting from stenosis of one carotid artery more than 50%.**

### History

A complete history is important to identify those patients at increased risk for carotid disease and stroke. It is important to determine if the patient is symptomatic or asymptomatic because this information, in combination with various imaging studies, will dictate what types of treatment are appropriate for patients with varying degrees of stenosis. Patients with prior or current cardiovascular disease may be at increased risk for concurrent carotid disease; therefore knowing a patient's cardiac history is critical. Neurologic symptoms, such as unilateral weakness, numbness or paresthesias, aphasia or dysarthria, history of transient ischemic attack (TIA), prior stroke, or amaurosis fugax (transient unilateral loss of vision) are all significant historical findings. Patients with TIA, stroke, or amaurosis fugax in the past 3 months are at greater risk for stroke and this warrants further workup for carotid disease. Symptoms not usually associated with carotid disease are vertigo, ataxia, diplopia, nausea, vomiting, decreased consciousness, and generalized weakness.

### Risk Factors

Risk factors for carotid disease are similar to those of atherosclerosis in other arterial beds and include smoking history, advanced age, male gender, and positive family history. Risk factors for stroke are multifactorial, but for patients with carotid disease, the most important are a history of neurologic symptoms, the degree of carotid stenosis, and plaque characteristics.

### Physical Examination

Complete physical examination is important to determine the possibility of carotid disease, as well as to assess the general health of patients who could potentially undergo a procedure. Focused physical examination includes auscultation of heart, palpation of distal pulses, a complete neurologic examination, including a cranial nerve examination, musculoskeletal examination for overall strength and symmetry, as well as examination of face for unilateral weakness or facial droop. Ocular examination can identify Hollenhorst plaques, but may not, and carotid auscultation for bruit is a classic finding, but its absence does not rule out potentially significant carotid disease.

## Optimal Diagnostic Study

Multiple radiologic studies can be used to assess the carotid arteries, including duplex ultrasonography (DUS), angiography with CT or MRI, and conventional digital angiography (DA). Each has utility in specific situations and these studies should not be used interchangeably. Imaging aids the clinician by providing information about the degree of stenosis and the plaque's morphology and location.

### Duplex Ultrasonography

Ultrasound (US) is an accurate, reliable, noninvasive imaging modality used to characterize carotid vascular disease. It is often the initial study to identify patients with disease. The degree of stenosis is determined by peak velocity through a narrowed lumen. DUS is also very useful for determining plaque morphology. This cost-effective study is operator dependent and can assess only the extracranial carotids but does allow for primary diagnosis of carotid stenosis.

## Computed Tomography

CT imaging without contrast is not sufficient to evaluate disease burden; thus contrasted CT angiography of the head and neck must be used for accurate imaging of the carotid arteries. This may preclude some patients with contrast allergy or preexisting renal disease from this imaging modality. When possible, it is a very effective imaging technique with high resolution and allows full examination of neck and cranial arteries. High calcium content in plaque can obscure contrast and thus occasionally makes identifying plaque morphology difficult. This modality, although noninvasive, does expose the patient to ionizing radiation and can be expensive.

## Magnetic Resonance Imaging

MRI is a good alternative to CT because contrast is not required for evaluation of arteries, but is required for concurrent soft tissue evaluation. Newer sequences, such as time-of-flight, may give the arterial enhancement needed without additional contrast. An MRI is noninvasive and allows for plaque morphology analysis, as well as examination of intracranial arteries. Magnetic resonance angiography can tend to overestimate the degree of stenosis. It is limited by cost and availability, and because it cannot be used with any implanted ferrous devices. Some centers now have protocols for MRI in patients with implantable defibrillators and pacemakers. MRI should not be used for first-line imaging.

## Digital Angiography

Conventional peripheral catheter-based digital subtraction angiography is considered the gold standard for carotid imaging. It provides excellent images that are easy to interpret. The degree of stenosis and location and morphology of plaque can all be assessed with this modality. It is most useful in patients with conflicting imaging before operation or at the time of stent-based interventions. Major limitations are cost, risk of stroke, systemic risks associated with a percutaneous intervention under mild sedation, and possibly poor vascular anatomy that could preclude a percutaneous study.

An area of continued study and debate involves the current recommendations for screening of asymptomatic patients. It is generally agreed that population screening examinations for asymptomatic patients are not cost effective. Highly selected patient populations may benefit from screening. This includes patients age >60 years with one or more risk factors, such as hypertension, coronary artery disease, current smoker, a first-degree relative with history of stroke, or if they may be undergoing a planned coronary artery bypass grafting procedure. Screening is not recommended for patients based solely on presence of an abdominal aortic aneurysm, presence of a carotid bruit, or prior head and neck radiotherapy.

❖ **Asymptomatic patients that may benefit from screening for coronary artery stenosis include those older than 60 years with one or more risk factors, such as hypertension, coronary artery disease, current smoker, a first-degree relative with history of stroke, or if they may be undergoing a planned coronary artery bypass grafting procedure**.

For postoperative patients, follow-up imaging recommendations include postoperative DUS within 30 days to assess status of the artery, as well as contralateral imaging to monitor any disease progression when there is >50% stenosis. Most surgeons will then follow the patient yearly with a repeat duplex. Specific timing for surveillance DUS is not established; however, with little risk associated and minimal cost, there is little concern about timing as long as it is done.

## Treatment

Once a diagnosis of carotid stenosis is made several factors are examined when considering optimal treatment. First is whether or not the patient's stenosis is symptomatic or asymptomatic. Second pertains to the degree of stenosis. Lastly, comorbidities, location of plaque, and patient preferences must be considered. In general, medical management is reserved for low-grade stenosis (<50%) in asymptomatic patients. Surgical correction of stenosis is performed for patients with symptomatic stenosis >50% or in asymptomatic patients with stenosis of 70% to 99%.

### Endovascular

Carotid artery stenting (CAS) via percutaneous approach has become an acceptable way to manage carotid stenosis. This approach allows for a less invasive technique for potentially poorer operative candidates. CAS also allows for angiography, angioplasty, and stent placement all with one procedure, but it does have limitations. Anatomic conditions of femoral vessels, the aorta, and the aortic arch must be appropriate. Furthermore, plaque characteristics such as long segment lesions may lead to multiple stents, and soft plaques can rupture, increasing perioperative stroke risk. CAS may be more beneficial in asymptomatic patients with >60% stenosis and for symptomatic patients with >50% stenosis with coronary artery disease (CAD) or prior head or neck radiation. CAS can reduce the number of perioperative myocardial infarctions, but it does have a higher risk of periprocedural stroke, including contralateral stroke risk because of aortic arch manipulation. Medicare will not reimburse for carotid stenting procedures in patients age >80 years given poor data to support use in octogenarians.

### Open Repair

Carotid endarterectomy (CEA) is the gold standard operative procedure for correction of carotid stenosis. In symptomatic patients with lesions >70% CEA has been shown to reduce stroke risk to 13% over 5 years from 28% when compared with medical management alone. CEA is generally preferred for patients with carotid stenosis because of the improved outcomes with reduction in overall stroke risk and risk of periprocedural death. The procedure requires excision between the plane of the inner and outer medial layers, resulting in removal of intima, plaque, and part of the media. A patch is sewn in place to close the carotid artery. CEA is preferred in patients with longer segment disease, or with stenosis >70%. Patients are monitored overnight in the hospital often in the intensive care unit and can be discharged the following day barring any complications or concerns.[1]

### Transcarotid Arterial Revascularization

A new approach to cerebral revascularization combines elements of open and endovascular surgery, a true hybrid procedure. Transcarotid arterial revascularization (TCAR) is indicated for patients with high-risk lesions. Such high-risk characteristics include age >75 years, poor physiologic status (including severe chronic obstructive pulmonary disease [COPD] and CAD), previous neck dissection, restenosis after carotid endarterectomy or carotid artery stenting, high lesion not accessible via standard open techniques, prior neck irradiation, contralateral occlusion, and cervical spine immobility. Results from trials, using very strict inclusion criteria, are promising and have the lowest reported stroke rate for any carotid intervention, 1.4%.[2]

## Medical

Medical management is important for all patients with carotid disease regardless of the degree of stenosis. Treatment is aimed at decreasing stroke risk and minimizing progression of stenosis. Treating underlying comorbid conditions is important. Hypertension, diabetes mellitus, and lipid abnormalities are all treatable conditions. Smoking nearly doubles stroke risk and cessation will markedly improve patients' risk. All patients with documented carotid disease should be on a high potency statin regardless of their cholesterol levels. Universal antiplatelet recommendations have not been adopted because there is no evidence suggesting antiplatelet agents other than aspirin have improved benefit in asymptomatic carotid stenosis patients. Antiplatelet agents are recommended for patients with non-cardioembolic ischemic stroke or TIA associated with carotid atherosclerosis. Aspirin is the most commonly used antiplatelet therapy and for symptomatic patients a combination of aspirin and clopidogrel are often used. For asymptomatic patients, combination of aspirin and clopidogrel offered no benefit in large trials.

## Outcomes

Complications associated with surgical repair include stroke, cranial nerve injury, hematoma, re-occlusion, and complications with anesthesia. As noted earlier, risk of myocardial infarction is higher in CEA patients, and perioperative stroke rates are higher in CAS. Morbidity and mortality can range from 1% to 2% to as high as 10%. Accepted 30-day stroke and death risk is about 3% or lower for patients with > 60% stenosis and who are expected preoperatively to live > 5 years.[3]

# Abdominal Aortic Aneurysm

## CASE 3

### James Roberts (Part 1)

James Roberts is a 75-year-old male who on workup for an unrelated disease was found to have a 6-cm asymptomatic abdominal aortic aneurysm (AAA). He was a previous smoker who quit 40 years ago. His past medical history includes hypertension and hypercholesterolemia.

Mr. Roberts is reluctant to think about surgery.

1. What information can you provide Mr. Roberts about the risk that his abdominal aortic aneurysm will rupture?

## Indications for Diagnostic Study

AAA is a degenerative disease of the aorta in which progressive remodeling of the arterial wall leads to progressive dilatation and possibly rupture. AAA is defined by increase in vessel diameter by > 50% compared with a normal-size vessel. The infrarenal aorta is considered aneurysmal when it is > 3.0 cm. AAA is a progressive disease that can result in a long indolent period or unexpected rupture, which is associated with high morbidity. It is most commonly seen in men age > 65 years. AAAs are often asymptomatic, but if they are symptomatic, patients will present with symptoms of abdominal pain radiating to the back or a pulsatile abdominal mass.

## History

A thorough history is helpful in determining a patient's risk for developing an AAA, as well as risks associated with complications; the history is also useful for identifying comorbidities that may affect surgical repair. Estimation of the patient's functional and cardiac status is critical to assess the patient's preoperative reserve and ability to tolerate surgical repair. The metabolic equivalent unit (MET) is a standard criterion for assessing a patient's activity level and is frequently used to assess a patient's preoperative status. A complete cardiac history is important because CAD is the leading cause of mortality after AAA repair. Poor cardiac status often leads to a delay in repair to allow for optimization of heart function. Other comorbidities that contribute to morbidity and mortality are COPD and diabetes mellitus.

## Risk Factors

Identifying patients at risk for an AAA is part of a complete history. Development of an AAA is associated with smoking, advanced age, CAD, atherosclerosis, high cholesterol, hypertension, first-degree relative affected, and male gender. Risk factors for expansion include advanced age, severe cardiac disease, prior stroke, and tobacco use. Independent risk factors for rupture of AAA include female gender, large initial diameter, low forced expiratory volume ($FEV_1$), current smoking, and elevated mean blood pressure. Patients with family history for inherited disorders such as Marfan syndrome, Ehlers–Danlos syndrome, and familial thoracic aortic aneurysm and dissection are also at increased risk for developing AAA at a younger age.

## Physical Examination

Complete physical examination is critical to assess overall patient function. Abdominal examination may or may not reveal a pulsatile mass in the midabdomen. This is highly dependent on patient body habitus and size of the AAA if present. AAAs between 3.0 and 3.9 cm are detected only 29% of the time, whereas an AAA > 5.0 cm can be detected 76% of the time. In addition to abdominal examination, femoral and popliteal pulses, peripheral pulses, and cardiac and pulmonary examinations should be performed at a minimum.[4]

## Optimal Diagnostic Study

Multiple radiologic studies can be used to assess AAA, including US, CT, and MRI. Each has utility in specific situations and should not be used interchangeably.

### Ultrasound

US is an inexpensive, noninvasive, and accessible means to detect an AAA. Sensitivity and specificity for detection are close to 100%. Limitations include operator skill level, variability from examiner to examiner, and nonvisualization resulting from bowel gas or body habitus. US is ideal for screening, but it is not good for preoperative anatomic assessment. When done in the same accredited vascular lab, diameter of the AAA can be reliably followed over time. The Society of Vascular Surgery (SVS) recommends using US, when able, for aneurysm screening and surveillance.[5]

### Computed Tomography

CT is an excellent means of imaging AAA and is generally more reproducible than US with more consistent measurements between examinations. CT also allows for examination of the entire aorta, intraabdominal/pelvic structures, and allows for three-dimensional reconstruction of vessels. Use of intravenous contrast allows for greater detail and information about the aneurysm, arterial calcification, and presence of thrombus. CT also provides excellent imaging of related anatomy, such as femoral, iliac, and renal vessels, which are important for preoperative planning when undergoing endovascular or open repair. CT has become more accessible yet still can be expensive and exposes the patient to radiation and contrast.

### Magnetic Resonance Imaging

MRI can be used to evaluate AAA; however, because of expense, time, and limited access, MRI should not be first-line imaging for AAA.

Current recommendations for screening based on the SVS guidelines is a one-time US screening for men or women ages 65 to 75 years with a history of tobacco use or with first-degree relatives who have a history of AAA.[5] Currently, Medicare offers US screening as part of its Welcome to Medicare physical examination to men who have smoked at least 100 cigarettes or to any patient with a family history.

No definitive recommendations have been established for surveillance if an AAA is detected. Current practice is to follow up at 12-month intervals for 3.5- to 4.4-cm AAAs and 6-month intervals for 4.5- to 5.4-cm AAAs. A 3- to 5-year follow-up is appropriate for 2.6- to 3.3-cm AAAs. All follow-up should include repeat imaging to accurately assess any change in AAA diameter. Should an AAA become symptomatic, imaging may be indicated sooner.

## Treatment

Treatment for AAA is specifically aimed at reducing a patient's risk of rupture. The new diagnosis of an aneurysm can often lead to anxiety in patients. Rupture rates for small aneurysms are exceedingly low. The 12-month risk of rupture based upon diameter is as follows: 3.0 to 3.9 cm, 0.3%; 4.0 to 4.9 cm, 0.5% to 1.5%; 5.0 to 5.9 cm, 1% to 11%; 6.0 to 6.9 cm, 11% to 22%; >7 cm, >30%. Therefore principles of treatment weigh the risk of rupture for a patient's AAA with the risk of morbidity and mortality associated with the surgical repair. Size is the major determining factor for risk of rupture, but rate of expansion can also be used. Aneurysms can be expected to grow between 0.1 and 0.4 cm per year; they rarely stay the same size. It is generally accepted that AAAs >5.5 cm for men and >5.0 cm for women have a high enough yearly risk for rupture that surgical intervention is indicated on an elective basis. Any AAA that enlarges 0.5 in 6 months or 1 cm in 12 months, regardless of size, is also an indication for surgical repair.[6]

### Endovascular Aneurysm Repair

First described in 1991, the endovascular aneurysm repair (EVAR) approach uses the femoral arteries as access points for catheters and wires, allowing for a graft to be placed intraluminally under fluoroscopy. This technique has numerous benefits over the traditional open approach. Benefits include no abdominal incision, less postoperative pain, shorter hospital stay, and lower 30-day mortality. These benefits allow for patients who could not tolerate an open procedure to have their AAA repaired, as well as quicker recovery for ideal surgical candidates. In spite of these perioperative benefits, numerous studies have not shown any improvement in quality of life or long-term morbidity and mortality. Endovascular repair is limited to patients with specific aneurysm characteristics and locations, and can also be limited by less favorable femoral and iliac artery anatomy. Control of ruptured AAAs can also be managed endovascularly with quick access and avoidance of a large incision that could possibly depressurize a rupture that has tamponaded in the retroperitoneum. Risks associated with EVAR include rupture, graft migration, endoleaks, perforation, infection, femoral artery aneurysm, hemorrhage, infection, and others.

### Open Aneurysm Repair

Open repair of an AAA requires either a transperitoneal or retroperitoneal approach, with midline laparotomy common. Open approach is generally used for patients who do not meet anatomic specifications for EVAR, or for those who require more complex repairs. This approach may also be indicated for redo procedures on the aorta. Once the aorta has been dissected from the retroperitoneum it can be clamped to stop blood flow into the aneurysm. The AAA is then opened and a graft is sewn intraluminally proximally and distally with the aneurysm sac closed over the newly placed graft. Patients are monitored in the intensive care unit postoperatively and generally do well both short and long term, although there is a higher 30-day morbidity and mortality when compared with EVAR. Risks associated with open repair include iatrogenic injury, bowel ischemia, hemorrhage, infection, hernia, and others.

### Medical

Optimal medical management is indicated for all patients with AAA. This includes smoking cessation, hypertension control, lipid control, diabetes management, diet and exercise lifestyle modifications, and regular follow-up with the primary care provider. New evidence also suggests that small asymptomatic AAAs may be amenable to medical therapy. Matrix metalloproteinases (MMPs) have been found to play a critical role in development of AAA. These enzymes can be inhibited with doxycycline; this property is independent from the drug's antimicrobial properties. Research has shown decreased rate of growth and even reversal of AAA size in some cases. Currently, no recommendation for use of doxycycline for management of small AAAs exists, but clinical trials are currently underway.[7]

### Outcomes

With proper diagnosis, surveillance, and medical management, patients can go years without needing surgical repair for their AAA. For those who do qualify for elective repair, discussion with patient and surgeon to address the best approach is critical. EVAR has more short-term perioperative benefits. However, the cost for fewer short-term complications is more complications over the long term and secondary interventions associated with graft durability. The reintervention rate at 6 years for EVAR patients was 29.6%, versus 18.1% for those who had had open repair. In a recent prospective trial, 6-year survival for EVAR was 68.9%, versus 69.9% for open repair.[8]

## Lower Extremity Arterial Disease

### Indications for Diagnostic Study

Lower extremity arterial disease is commonly referred to as peripheral arterial disease (PAD). It is clearly a disease of the older adult population, with studies documenting a 15% incidence in patients age >70 years. The presentation of PAD varies over a continuum. The most common presentation is that of claudication, or cramping of the lower extremity muscles. The cramping or aching occurs primarily in the calves, less often in the thighs and buttocks, and is relieved within 10 minutes of cessation of activity. Although claudication secondary to arterial disease may seem significant and can cause the patient significant distress, the rate of progression of disease to rest pain (severe ischemic pain caused by insufficient arterial inflow), gangrene, and subsequent amputation is low (10%) even in the absence of any intervention. Interventions should not be performed on vascular claudicants solely for the purpose to prevent limb loss.

## History

A focused history of ambulation is able to confirm the diagnosis of claudication in the majority of patients. The patient with true vasculogenic claudication will complain of pain with ambulation that starts after a known distance (often at presentation this will be on the order of two to three blocks, a distance that commonly interferes with activities of daily living). Upon cessation of activity and with simple standing, the pain will subside and the patient will be able to ambulate again a similar distance. This cycle in vasculogenic claudication can be repeated indefinitely. In the older adult patient, coexistent disease is common and must be distinguished. The two most common conditions are neurogenic claudication secondary to spinal stenosis and osteoarthritis of the hip or knee. Osteoarthritis is more easily differentiated from claudication as the pain of osteoarthritis generally localizes to the joint, improves with pain medications, and has a varying course of improvement and worsens throughout the day. Neurogenic claudication is the most difficult to differentiate from vasculogenic disease because of the frequency of spinal stenosis in the older adult population. The most common presenting symptom of neurogenic claudication is pain in the calves and posterior thigh and buttocks. In contrast to vasculogenic disease, neurogenic claudication has a variable distance to onset, often takes 15 minutes to several hours to relieve the pain, and claudication distance can be significantly increased with the use of an assistive device, such as a shopping cart on which the patient can lean and relieve the pressure on the nerves within the spinal canal. Unfortunately, often all three conditions in the older adult patient can coexist and then diagnosis of the primary limiting condition is of utmost concern to achieve an optimal outcome and maintain ambulatory independence.

## Risk Factors

Risk factors for PAD are similar to those of atherosclerosis in other peripheral arteries and include smoking history, advanced age, male gender, and positive family history.

## Physical Examination

Lower extremity examination and documentation includes inspection of the legs to assess for and document lesions consistent with arterial ischemia. Arterial lesions are primarily located on the toes or distal foot and tend to be painful because of loss of arterial flow. Loss of hair on the toes and distal ankles is also a common finding in patients with arterial compromise. Palpation of pulses in the femoral, popliteal, and tibial (dorsalis pedis and posterior tibial) allows a relatively quick determination of location of disease (loss of femoral pulses = aortoiliac disease; loss of popliteal pulses with preservation of femoral pulse = superficial femoral artery disease; loss of tibial pulses with preservation of popliteal pulse = tibial arterial disease of the lower leg).

## Optimal Diagnostic Study

Multiple radiologic studies can be used to assess the lower extremity arteries, including DUS, angiography with CT or MRI, and conventional DA. Each has utility in specific situations and should not be used interchangeably. Although these are noninvasive, simple Doppler analysis in the form of segmental arterial pressures and ankle brachial index (ABI) can be very useful in providing an adequate physiologic picture of the peripheral vasculature. ABIs should be the first test ordered in a patient to confirm the diagnosis of PAD suspected after the physical examination.

### Duplex Ultrasonography

US is an accurate, reliable, noninvasive imaging modality used to characterize lower extremity vascular disease. The degree of stenosis is determined by peak velocity through a narrowed lumen. DUS is also very useful for determining plaque morphology. It is operator dependent and can assess only the femoral vessels and below, not the iliac system. This is generally used for helping guide therapy and should not be the first test ordered.

### Computed Tomography

CT imaging alone is not sufficient to evaluate for lower extremity arterial disease; contrasted angiography must be used for accurate imaging of the lower extremities. This may preclude some patients with contrast allergy or preexisting renal disease from this imaging modality. When possible, CT angiography is a very effective imaging technique with high resolution and allows full examination of the aorta, iliac, and lower extremity arteries. High calcium content in plaque can obscure contrast and thus occasionally makes identifying plaque morphology difficult. This modality, while noninvasive, does expose the patient to ionizing radiation and can be expensive.

### Magnetic Resonance Imaging

MRI is a good alternative to CT because contrast is not required for evaluation of arteries (but contrast is required for concurrent soft tissue evaluation). MRI is noninvasive and allows for plaque morphology analysis, as well as examination of intraabdominal arteries. Magnetic resonance angiography can tend to overestimate the degree of stenosis. MRI is limited by cost and availability, and cannot be used in patients with any implanted ferrous devices. MRI should not be used for first-line imaging. Special sequences, such as time-of-flight, may allow for good analysis of stenotic segments without the use of contrasted agents.

### Digital Angiography

Conventional peripheral catheter-based DA is considered the gold standard for lower extremity imaging. It provides excellent images that are easy to interpret. The degree of stenosis and the location and morphology of plaque can all be assessed with this modality. DA is most useful in patients with conflicting imaging before operation. $CO_2$ can be used as a contrast agent to eliminate or significantly reduce the iodinated contrast requirements in patients with chronic kidney disease. A major advantage includes the ability to diagnose and often intervene in the same setting. Major limitations are cost, risk associated with a percutaneous intervention under mild sedation, and possibly poor vascular anatomy (calcified access vessels) that could preclude a percutaneous study.

Current recommendations for screening asymptomatic patients for lower extremity arterial disease are in constant debate. It is generally agreed upon that population screening examinations for asymptomatic patients are not cost effective. Highly selected patient populations may benefit from screening. This includes patients age > 70 years, current or former tobacco use, diabetics, those with an abnormal pulse exam, or presence of other established cardiovascular disease.[9]

## Treatment

Once a diagnosis of PAD is made, initial treatment should consist of medical management of the patient's atherosclerotic disease and a thorough assessment of the patient's cardiac status should be conducted; 90% of patients with PAD will have documented CAD based on angiographic evaluation with absence of overt symptoms secondary to lack of activity.

Medical management should consist of an antiplatelet agent in conjunction with a statin agent. Secondly, a walking program in which the patient is encouraged to walk 30 minutes at a time, preferably three times a week, should be initiated. With a walking regimen that is followed, patients can double or triple their maximal walking distance. Supervised exercise therapy is offered at many centers often in the same locations as cardiac and pulmonary rehabilitation programs. This has been approved by Medicare to treat intermittent claudication: 12 weeks, up to 36 sessions, are covered. Drugs, such as cilostazol (Pletal) may be prescribed, taking into account side effects and contraindications. If tolerated, there is evidence that these agents do improve ambulation in patients with claudication; however, the maximal gain in walking distance is somewhat limited compared with exercise therapy. Interventions to restore blood flow are indicated: (1) in patients with significant disease that limits ambulation thus resulting in subsequent lifestyle changes that are unacceptable, (2) in patients with pain at rest, or (3) in patients with gangrene and tissue loss.

❖❖ **Exercise consisting of a 30-minute walk three times a week can double or triple maximal walking distance in patients with lower extremity arterial disease and can have outcomes that are comparable to iliac angioplasty and stenting.**

### Endovascular

PAD treatment via the percutaneous approach has become the preferred initial treatment modality for those patients with both lifestyle-limiting claudication and rest pain/tissue loss. The approach is usually from the femoral arteries for both iliac and femoral/tibial lesions. Short focal stenosis responds very well to angioplasty and stenting, whereas long segment stenosis and occlusions are more challenging to treat and have a reduced patency rate. Although generally believed to be less durable than open surgical approaches, the endovascular approach provides a reduction in major complications compared with open surgery and can be repeated two to three times after the initial revascularization procedure while still maintaining the ability to perform open surgical bypass in the future.

### Open Repair

Open surgical bypass of occluded or stenotic segments still remains the gold standard against which percutaneous interventions are gauged. Bypass of iliac stenosis using aortobifemoral bypass or bypass of the occluded superficial femoral artery or proximal tibial arteries is the most commonly performed procedure to provide pulsatile flow to the distal leg in the setting of lesions or gangrene. The downside to open surgical revascularization is the definite risk of mortality and morbidity that accompanies these procedures despite the much more reliable provision of blood flow.

### Outcomes

Complications associated with percutaneous intervention include vessel thrombosis, embolization, dissection, and rupture. Although complications can be serious, they are worth tolerating because of the severity of PAD; acute complications of PAD can necessitate amputation and the patient should be made aware of the potential for limb loss. Outcomes for percutaneous intervention are improving, with patency rates of intervened segments approaching 80% at 2 years for iliac stents and 70% at 2 years for superficial femoral artery stents. Aortoiliac revascularization using aortobifemoral bypass has a 90% 5-year patency. Femoral popliteal and femoral tibial bypass have 70% to 80% and 60% to 70% 5-year patency, respectively. More important, limb salvage is > 90% in the majority of patients at 2 years and this is confirmed by large-scale data documenting a reduction in amputation rates in population-based studies.[10] A large trial sponsored by the National Institutes of Health, the BEST-CLI (Best Endovascular vs. Best Surgical Therapy in Patients With Critical Limb Ischemia) trial, recently completed enrollment. This study randomized patients with critical limb ischemia to endovascular or open revascularization. The anticipated results may help guide decision making regarding optimal revascularization strategy[11] in patients with tissue loss.

## Summary

Knowing how to diagnose and manage peripheral vascular disease is important for the geriatrician because there is a high incidence of the disease in the older adult population. A trend toward noninvasive diagnosis and minimally invasive approaches is noted. However, a treatment plan based on knowledge of current treatment paradigms with attention to provider- and patient-specific factors should be taken into consideration to achieve optimal treatment outcome.

## Key References

3. Ricotta JJ, AbuRahma A, Ascher E, et al. Updated society for vascular surgery guidelines for management of extracranial carotid disease. *J Vasc Surg.* 2011;54(3):e1−31.
4. Chaikof EL, Brewster DC, Dalman RL, et al. The care of patients with an abdominal aortic aneurysm: the society for vascular surgery practice guidelines. *J Vasc Surg.* 2009;50 (suppl 4):S2−49.
10. Silva MB, Choi L, Cheng CC. Peripheral arterial occlusive disease. In: Townsend C, Beauchamp RD, Evers BM, Mattox KL, eds. *Townsend: Sabiston Textbook of Surgery.* 19th ed. Philadelphia, PA: Elsevier Saunders; 2012: p. 1725−1784.

**References available online at** expertconsult.com.

# 40

# Stroke and Transient Ischemic Attack

MARCO A. GONZALEZ CASTELLON AND KARINA I. BISHOP

## OBJECTIVES

*Upon completion of this chapter, the reader will be able to:*

- Properly define stroke and transient ischemic attack.
- Identify stroke risk factors and appropriate management.
- Describe most common clinical presentations of stroke.
- Recommend appropriate acute stroke treatment, including intravenous thrombolysis, mechanical thrombectomy, and blood pressure management.

- Prescribe adequate secondary stroke prevention measures, including antiplatelet agents, anticoagulants, and lipid-lowering drugs.
- Identify long-term complications of stroke and management.

## Definition of Stroke

Stroke was defined for many years by the World Health Organization as "rapidly developing clinical signs of focal (or global) disturbance of cerebral function, lasting more than 24 hours or leading to death, with no apparent cause other than that of vascular origin." This includes cerebral infarction, intracerebral hemorrhage, and subarachnoid hemorrhage.[1] Recent advances in basic science, pathophysiology, and diagnostic imaging make this definition obsolete. In 2013 a new definition was proposed by the American Heart Association/American Stroke Association (AHA/ASA). Transient ischemic attack (TIA) is defined as a transient episode of neurologic dysfunction caused by focal brain, spinal cord, or retinal ischemia, without evidence of central nervous system (CNS) infarction.[2] Ischemic stroke is defined as an episode of neurologic dysfunction caused by focal CNS infarction.[3] CNS infarction is brain, spinal cord, or retinal cell death attributable to ischemia, based on (1) pathologic, imaging, or objective evidence of focal ischemic injury in a defined vascular distribution; or (2) clinical evidence of cerebral, spinal cord, or retinal focal ischemic injury based on symptoms persisting equal or more than 24 hours or until death, and other etiologies excluded.[3] Intracerebral hemorrhage is defined as a focal collection of blood within the brain parenchyma or ventricular system that is not caused by trauma.[3] Subarachnoid hemorrhage is the bleeding into the subarachnoid space (the space between the arachnoid membrane and the pia matter of the brain and the spinal cord).[3]

## Classification of Stroke

Stroke can be classified by phenotype or etiology. Phenotypic classification usually provides a summary of abnormal test findings without suggesting a possible etiology. Etiologic classification usually identifies the cause of stroke using clinical, imaging, and laboratory information. Identifying the cause of stroke is useful for appropriate management, prevention of secondary injury, and stroke recurrence.

In broad terms, stroke is classified as ischemic stroke, hemorrhagic stroke, or subarachnoid hemorrhage. In Western nations, ischemic stroke accounts for approximately 80% to 85% of all strokes, hemorrhagic stroke 15% to 20 %, and subarachnoid hemorrhage 0% to 5 % of all strokes.[4] In Asia, the distribution of stroke types is slightly different as hemorrhagic stroke has a higher incidence. In Asian nations, ischemic stroke accounts for approximately 65% to 70% of all strokes, hemorrhagic stroke 16% to 40%, and subarachnoid hemorrhage 1% to 8%.[5] Ischemic stroke can be further classified based on etiology. Possible etiologies for ischemic stroke include embolism from the heart, artery-to-artery embolism, and in-situ small vessel disease.[6] The most widely used classification for ischemic stroke is the one used for the Trial of Org 10172 in Acute Stroke Treatment (TOAST). The TOAST classification system includes five categories: (1) large-artery atherosclerosis, (2) cardioembolism, (3) small-artery occlusion (lacune), (4) stroke of other determined etiology, and (5) stroke of undetermined etiology (Box 40.1).[7] Large artery atherosclerosis refers to patients with clinical and imaging findings of either stenosis or occlusion of a major brain artery or branch cortical artery, presumably because of atherosclerosis.[7] Cardioembolism refers to patients with arterial occlusions presumably because of an embolus arising in the heart.[7] Small-artery occlusion refers to patients with occlusion of small penetrating branches in the deep hemispheric white matter and brainstem. These are usually ≤ 1.5 cm in diameter.[7,8] Acute stroke of other determined etiology pertains to patients with rare causes of stroke, including nonatherosclerotic vasculopathies (inflammatory, infectious, and genetic), hypercoagulable states, and hematologic disorders.[7] Stroke of undetermined etiology refers to events for which a cause cannot be determined because of an incomplete assessment or lack of conclusive diagnosis despite an extensive workup.[7] The TOAST classification has many drawbacks, including low reliability in minor strokes and overinflating strokes of undetermined source. Several modified classifications have been proposed, including the Stop Stroke Study-TOAST (SSS-TOAST) and the Causative Classification of Stroke System (CCS).[9] These classification were designed to improve the reliability of the TOAST scale. SSS-TOAST added three levels of evidence: evident, probable, and possible. These changes improved the classification reliability and reduced the undetermined group. Unfortunately, because of the level of complexity, this classification has not been widely accepted. The CCS uses a web-based system that consists of a questionnaire-style classification scheme for ischemic stroke. An automated algorithm reports the stroke subtype and a description of the classification rationale.[10] In 2009 the ASCO (atherosclerosis; small vessel disease; cardiac sources and other) classification was proposed by Amarenco et al.[11] This classification was updated in 2013 by adding dissection as a standalone etiology and renaming it ASCOD (atherosclerosis; small vessel disease; cardiac sources; other; and dissection).[12] ASCOD grades all diseases present in a given patient, captures the overlap between the diseases, and weighs the potentially causal relationship between every disease detected and the ischemic stroke. In the ASCOD classification, every patient is graded into the five predefined phenotypes. Each phenotype is graded from 0 to 3 depending on the level of causality and 9 if the workup has been insufficient to grade the disease.[12] A major advantage of the ASCOD grading system over the TOAST classification is the very low proportion of ischemic strokes in which no ASCOD evidence grades of 1, 2, or 3 can be identified.[13] Using ASCOD classification identifies all possible pathologies that should be addressed in patients with ischemic stroke.

## Impact of Stroke in the United States and the World

Each year in the United States approximately 795,000 people experience stroke. Approximately 610,000 are first stroke and 185,000 are recurrent attacks. On average, every 40 seconds someone in the United States has a stroke.[14] Approximately 7 million Americans over the age of 20 years self-report experiencing a stroke in their lives. The prevalence of stroke increases with advancing age in both men and women.[14] In 2016 stroke accounted for approximately one of every 19 deaths and was the fifth cause of death in the United States.

Worldwide there are approximately 11.6 million incident ischemic strokes and 5.3 million incident hemorrhagic strokes. Most of the burden of stroke is in low- and middle-income countries.[15] The incidence of stroke varies by country. The highest incidence of stroke, adjusted to World Health Organization World Population, is in Portugal, Russia, and Belarus.[16] Between 1990 and 2010, the incidence of stroke remained the same in low- and middle-income countries and decreased by 13% (95% confidence interval [CI], 6%–18%) in high-income countries creating significant disparities in stroke treatment and prognosis. In 2016, 5.5 million deaths worldwide were attributed to stroke. Worldwide, a total of 2.7 million individuals died of ischemic stroke and 2.8 million of hemorrhagic stroke.

❖❖ **Over the period from 2010 to 2050, the number of incident strokes is expected to more than double, with the majority of the increase among the older adult population (aged ≥ 75 years) and minority groups.[18]**

## Stroke in the Older Adult Population

Approximately 17% of all stroke patients are older adults ( > 85 years).[17] Over the period from 2010 to 2050, the number of incident strokes is expected to more than double, with the majority of the increase among the older adult population (aged ≥ 75 years) and minority groups.[18] Older adult patients have longer hospital stays with higher disability and mortality. They are also more likely to receive less evidence-based care and less likely to return to their original place of residence.[14] Most observational studies suggest that the benefits of intravenous thrombolysis[19] and mechanical thrombectomy[20] is reduced in the older adult population.

### CASE

### A 75-year-old woman (Part 1)

A 75-year-old previously independently living right-handed woman with a past medical history of essential hypertension, hyperlipidemia, and type 2 diabetes mellitus presents to the emergency room (ER) after developing right face, arm, and leg weakness associated with slurred speech and word finding difficulties. Her symptoms started approximately 1 hour before arriving to the ER. On examination, her blood pressure (BP) is 210/100 mmHg and her heart rate (HR) is 98 beats per minute. She has an irregularly irregular heart rhythm. She is awake, but unable to speak. Her eyes are deviated to the left and she has weakness involving the right side of her face, arm, and leg. Her arm is weaker than the leg.
1. What are her stroke risk factors?
2. What vascular distribution appears to be affected by her stroke?
3. What treatment options are available to this patient?

## Stroke Risk Factors

Stroke risk factors can be classified into nonmodifiable and modifiable risk factors. Nonmodifiable stroke risk factors include age, gender, race-ethnicity, genetics, and prior history of stroke or TIA. The incidence of stroke increases with age, with the incidence doubling for each decade after 55 years of age.[14] In general, more strokes occur in women than men likely because of longer life spans of women when compared with men.[14,21] With respect to racial differences, Black persons have twice the incidence of stroke and have higher mortality when compared with White persons.[22] Hispanic persons also have an increased risk of stroke. Genetic risk factors increase the risk of stroke through several single gene mutation syndromes. Examples include cerebral autosomal dominant arteriopathy with subcortical infarcts and leukoencephalopathy, cerebral autosomal recessive arteriopathy with subcortical infarcts and leukoencephalopathy, familial amyloid angiopathy, and collagen 4 mutations. Other single gene mutation syndromes can result in stroke as one of several possible manifestations of the disease. Examples include Fabry disease, Marfan syndrome, and mitochondrial encephalopathy with lactic acid and strokelike episodes. Lastly, some variants of genetic polymorphisms have been associated with stroke.[23]

Modifiable stroke risk factors include both medical conditions and lifestyle risk factors. For the most part, 10 modifiable risk factors are collectively associated with approximately 90% of the risk of stroke around the world.[24] Well-documented medical conditions associated with stroke include hypertension, diabetes mellitus, hyperlipidemia, and atrial fibrillation (AF). Risk factors in rank order have been summarized in Box 40.2. Hypertension is the most important modifiable stroke risk factor, with a direct

### • BOX 40.2 Modifiable Stroke Risk Factors (In Rank Order)

- Hypertension
- Diabetes mellitus
- Hyperlipidemia
- Atrial fibrillation
- Obstructive sleep apnea
- Tobacco use
- Alcohol use
- Physical inactivity

linear relationship between BP and stroke risk. Even among patients without a formal diagnosis of hypertension, stroke risk increases as BP increases.[23] Diabetes mellitus doubles the risk of stroke; even patients with prediabetes have an increased risk of stroke.[23] AF is a major risk factor for stroke with a fivefold risk increase. The percentage of strokes attributable to AF increases steeply from 1.5% at 50 to 59 years of age to 23.5% at 80 to 89 years of age.[14,23] The cumulative incidence of AF among patients with stroke of unknown etiology is approximately 30% by 3 years.[25] Left atrial enlargement is associated with AF and stroke. As such, left atrial size is significantly associated with an increased risk of stroke and death in both men and women[26] and is also an independent marker of recurrent cardioembolic or cryptogenic stroke in patients with prior stroke.[27] Although lipid abnormalities are a well-documented risk factor for coronary heart disease, observational studies have mostly found weak associations between them and ischemic stroke.[28] Obstructive sleep apnea (OSA) is a risk factor for incident stroke and is associated with worse outcomes on those patients with established diagnosis. OSA significantly increases the risk of stroke and death and is an independent risk factor for stroke.[29] Patients with prior diagnosis of OSA have a fivefold greater risk for worse functional outcomes and death within the first month after acute ischemic stroke.[30] Lifestyle stroke risk factors include tobacco use, alcohol consumption, and physical inactivity. Tobacco use is an important stroke risk factor. Smokers have approximately double the risk of stroke.[23] This increase in risk seems to be dose dependent, with higher risk in those with heavy tobacco use.[31] The association with stroke of other forms of tobacco is less clear. However, smokeless tobacco use is associated with an increased risk of cardiovascular disease incidence.[32] Alcohol consumption appears to have a J-shaped relationship with stroke risk. Light to moderate consumption is associated with a decreased risk of stroke and heavy consumption is associated with an increased risk of stroke.[23] Excess alcohol intake is clearly associated with hypertension and poor BP control in patients with hypertension.[33] Physical inactivity has been associated to a greater risk of stroke mainly in those age $\geq$ 80 years in a multiethnic prospective cohort study.[34]

## Ischemic Stroke

### Ischemic Stroke Clinical Presentation

Stroke symptoms usually present abruptly and are focal in nature. Most patients with stroke will present with signs and symptoms in a pattern consistent with cerebral dysfunction in a defined vascular territory. Most common stroke signs and symptoms include sudden unilateral weakness of the face, arm, and leg; sudden unilateral sensory loss; sudden speech difficulties (producing or understanding speech); sudden slurring of speech; sudden loss of vision or double vision; sudden loss of balance, vertigo, or clumsiness; and sudden onset of severe headache. Stroke symptoms are quite heterogeneous and trying to memorize all can be quite difficult. The most effective method for stroke recognition is to associate signs and symptoms with defined vascular territories. In broad terms, the stroke symptoms can be divided in anterior circulation syndromes (internal carotid artery, anterior cerebral artery, and middle cerebral artery [MCA]), posterior circulation syndromes (posterior cerebral artery, basilar artery, cerebellar arteries, and vertebral arteries), and lacunar stroke syndromes (deep small penetrating branches).[8,35] Most common clinical stroke syndromes are summarized on Table 40.1.

## TABLE 40.1  Stroke Syndromes

| Middle Cerebral Artery Stroke Syndromes[8] | Anterior Cerebral Artery Stroke Syndromes[8] |
|---|---|
| Contralateral gaze deviation<br>Contralateral homonymous hemianopsia<br>Contralateral hemiparesis involving face, arm and leg (arm > leg)<br>Left hemisphere stroke: patients will present with aphasia<br>Right hemisphere stroke: patients will present with dyspraxia and hemineglect | Cognitive changes, including confusion, disorientation and memory loss<br>Abulia or apathy<br>Euphoria or disinhibition<br>Contralateral hemiparesis (leg > arm)<br>Impaired bladder control |

| Posterior Circulation Stroke Syndromes (Includes Posterior Cerebral Artery, Basilar Artery, and Vertebral Arteries)[8] | Lacunar Stroke Syndromes[8] |
|---|---|
| Dizziness and vertigo<br>Nausea and vomiting<br>Double vision, nystagmus and dysconjugate gaze<br>Slurred speech, difficulty swallowing and hoarseness<br>Limb and truncal ataxia<br>Crossed signs (symptoms involving one side of the face and contralateral side of body)<br>Changes in consciousness, amnesia, and behavioral changes | Pure sensory stroke<br>Pure motor stroke<br>Sensory-motor stroke<br>Dysarthria-clumsy hand syndrome<br>Ataxia-hemiparesis |

Older adults often present with severe strokes (high National Institutes of Health stroke scale [NIHSS]) in the anterior circulation distribution. This phenomenon is most likely related to higher prevalence of cardioembolic stroke in this population.[36] Anterior circulation strokes are more common, in both younger and older adult patients, and usually present with weakness and language deficits. Posterior circulation strokes are rarer and can be more difficult to diagnose. Always be suspicious of a posterior circulation stroke in patients who present to the ER with sudden onset of vertigo, dizziness, loss of balance, difficulty swallowing, and eye movement abnormalities. Lacunar stroke usually presents with well-defined syndromes as summarized in Table 40.1.

## Ischemic Stroke Clinical Assessment

Acute ischemic stroke is a medical emergency that has highly effective treatment options. Patients presenting with acute ischemic stroke warrant an accurate and thorough examination done in a timely fashion. Current guidelines recommend complete assessment and treatment of acute ischemic stroke patients within 60 minutes of arrival to the ER.

Obtaining an accurate history is extremely important because most stroke treatment options are time sensitive. Establishing a clear time of symptom onset can be challenging, but along with imaging, is critical to decision making regarding treatment. Additional strategies to confirm times include talking to family members, checking patient and family member's phones/receipts, asking what was on the TV or radio, and so on. Once time of onset

has been determined, a thorough chronology of symptoms should be obtained. Stroke is usually sudden with maximum deficits at onset. Establishing chronology of symptoms is useful in differentiating stroke from common mimics, such as migraine, seizures, and conversion disorder.[37] Obtaining the patient's past medical history is important because some elements can render the patient ineligible for intravenous (IV) thrombolysis. Prior history of stroke (ischemic or hemorrhagic), recent surgery, bleeding disorders, and current use of anticoagulants should be obtained. Additional considerations when assessing an older adult patient for treatment with IV thrombolysis are the presence of cerebral microhemorrhages and cerebral amyloid angiopathy (CCA). Microhemorrhages are thought to be the result of small arterial rupture in the basal ganglia or subcortical white matter and are often asymptomatic.[38] These microhemorrhages have a prevalence of 4.7% to 6.4% in healthy adults with the average age of 60 years.[39,40] In hypertensive patients, the prevalence can be as high as 56%.[41] In older adults, cerebral microhemorrhages are associated with CAA. Sporadic CAA is caused by deposition of amyloid beta fibrils in cortical and leptomeningeal blood vessels.[42] Presence of cerebral microhemorrhages has been proposed as a possible risk factor for cerebral hemorrhage after IV thrombolysis. However, a recent metaanalysis of more than 800 patients showed a trend for higher symptomatic intracerebral hemorrhage risk after IV thrombolysis without reaching statistical significance.[43] A complete list of indications and contraindications for IV thrombolysis is available at the end of this chapter (Table 40.2).

The neurologic examination of a patient with acute ischemic stroke starts as soon as the patient enters the ER. Initial assessment includes observations of how the patient responds to the ambulance crew. Is the patient conscious? Is he/she following commands? Is his/her speech garbled or nonsense? Is he/she paralyzed/weak in the face or limbs? A quick survey examination should be done next. The examiner should look for gaze deviation, pupil size, facial weakness, motor tone, and spontaneous movements. Vital signs and capillary glucose should be checked as soon as the patient arrives. Once this initial survey has been completed, the patient should proceed to imaging. Once imaging has been completed, an NIHSS should be completed and documented. At times, older adults may have concurrent problems that may make it more difficult to interpret if symptoms are new—for example, a prior stroke, cognitive impairment, and Parkinson disease can all confound the evaluation.

The NIHSS is a highly reliable and valid screening assessment of patients with acute stroke. This scale has 11 items and measures stroke severity by assigning points depending on response to questions and physical examination findings. Scores vary from 0 to 42 with higher scores associated with more severe strokes. This scale can be completed in 6 to 7 minutes and can be administered consistently by nurses or physicians.[44] The NIHSS is not a perfect scale, it is biased in favor of dominant hemisphere strokes and underestimates posterior circulation stroke severity[35] but is an effective method of communicating stroke severity between providers. Training for correct application of the NIHSS is easy and can be done through various websites and live programs.

Laboratories should be obtained once the initial examination and imaging have been completed. Current guidelines require only a finger-stick glucose to be available before starting treatment with IV alteplase,[45,46] with the exception of patients taking warfarin who should have an international normalized ratio (INR) available before considering treatment. Obtaining other laboratories, including complete blood count (CBC), electrolytes, renal

| TABLE 40.2 | Eligibility Criteria for Intravenous Alteplase in Patients With Acute Ischemic Stroke |
|---|---|
| Eligibility criteria 0–3 hours | • Age ≥ 18 years<br>• Symptoms consistent with acute ischemic stroke<br>• There are no contraindication for treatment of patients with severe stroke symptoms<br>• Mild but disabling symptoms should be treated |
| Eligibility criteria 0–4.5 hours | • Age ≥ 18 years<br>• Symptoms consistent with acute ischemic stroke<br>• No contraindications for treatment in the 3–4.5 hour window |
| Contraindications | • Last known well >3 or 4.5 hours<br>• CT shows intracranial hemorrhage<br>• CT shows extensive area of cerebral infarction<br>• Prior history of ischemic stroke within 3 months<br>• Prior history of head trauma within 3 months<br>• Prior history of intracranial/spinal surgery in the last 3 months<br>• Prior history of intracranial hemorrhage<br>• Patients presenting with symptoms of subarachnoid hemorrhage (SAH)<br>• Patients with GI malignancy or recent hemorrhage (21 days)<br>• Patients with coagulopathy:<br>  ○ Platelets <100 000/mm$^3$<br>  ○ INR >1.7<br>  ○ aPTT >40 s<br>  ○ PT >15 s<br>• Received treatment dose of low-molecular-weight heparin (LMWH) within the last 24 hours<br>• Patients taking direct thrombin inhibitors or direct factor Xa inhibitors<br>  ○ Alteplase can be considered when appropriate laboratory tests are normal (aPTT, INR, platelet count, ecarin clotting time, direct factor Xa activity)<br>  ○ Patient has not received a dose for >48 h<br>• Patients with infective endocarditis<br>• Patients with aortic arch dissection<br>• Patients with intraaxial intracranial neoplasm |
| Contraindications in the 3–4.5 hour window | • For patients with >80 years, IV alteplase may be beneficial<br>• For patients with prior stroke and diabetes mellitus, IV alteplase may be a reasonable option<br>• For patients taking warfarin with an INR ≤ 1.7, IV alteplase appears safe and may be beneficial<br>• The benefit of IV alteplase in patients with very severe stroke symptoms (NIHSS >25) is uncertain |

(Modified from Powers W, Rabinstein A, Ackerson T, et al. 2018 Guidelines for the early management of patients with acute ischemic stroke: a guideline for healthcare professionals from the American Heart Association/American Stroke Association. *Stroke.* 2018;49:e46–e49.)

*aPTT,* Activated partial thromboplastin time; *CT,* computed tomography; *GI,* gastrointestinal; *INR,* international normalized ratio; *NIHSS,* National Institutes of Health stroke scale, *PT,* prothrombin time.

function, and troponins, are suggested in the acute stroke evaluation. Obtaining these laboratories should not delay treatment.[37]

The goal of brain imaging is to differentiate between a hemorrhagic and an ischemic stroke. In most cases, a noncontrast head computed tomography (CT) is sufficient to make a treatment decision. Current acute ischemic stroke treatment guidelines recommend obtaining brain imaging within 20 minutes of arrival to the hospital.[45,46] Obtaining advanced imaging (like an magnetic resonance imaging [MRI]) should not delay treatment; if these studies are needed, these should be obtained once treatment has been started.

## Acute Ischemic Stroke Management

Acute ischemic stroke is a medical emergency with specific treatment. Patients with suspected stroke must be assessed and treated promptly. For every minute without treatment, a stroke patient loses approximately 1.9 million neurons, 14 billion synapses, and 12 km of myelinated fibers.[47] Treatment success depends on rapid identification, diagnosis, and appropriate treatment. The treatment goal in stroke is revascularization either by chemical (thrombolysis) or mechanical (thrombectomy) methods. Current treatment options are summarized in Table 40.3. BP control

should be achieved before considering treatment. Target BP will depend on eligibility for thrombolysis and other therapies. A summary of BP goals and options for pharmacologic management can be found in Boxes 40.3 and 40.4.

Intravenous thrombolysis continues to be the mainstream treatment for acute ischemic stroke. Intravenous alteplase was approved by the US Food and Drug Administration (FDA) in 1995 after the National Institutes of Neurological Disorders and Stroke tissue plasminogen activator trial. Eligibility criteria for its use are summarized in Table 40.2. Patients treated with IV alteplase within 0 to 3 hours from symptom onset had a 30% increase in probable minimal to no symptoms at 90 days with a 6.4% risk of symptomatic intracranial hemorrhage.[48] Patients were treated with an alteplase dose of 0.9 mg/kg (maximum of 90 mg) over 60 minutes, with 10% of the dose given as a bolus over 1 minute.[45,46] Thrombolysis in patients older than 80 years of age has been found to be beneficial with similar complication rates and mortality.[49] The treatment window was extended in 1998 after the publication of the European Cooperative Acute Stroke Study III trial. This trial showed favorable outcomes in patients treated between 3 and 4.5 hours from symptom onset. This trial excluded patients age ≥ 80 years, patients with prior diabetes and stroke,

**TABLE 40.3 Treatment Options for Acute Ischemic Stroke**

| Time Window | Treatment Options |
|---|---|
| 0–3 hours | IV thrombolysis with alteplase<br>Mechanical thrombectomy (terminal ICA or M1 occlusion) |
| 3–4.5 hours | IV thrombolysis with alteplase (relative contraindications)<br>Mechanical thrombectomy (terminal ICA or M1 occlusion) |
| 4.5–6 hours | Mechanical thrombectomy (terminal ICA or M1 occlusion) |
| 6–24 hours | Mechanical thrombectomy (large vessel occlusion + favorable perfusion imaging)<br>a. 6–16 hours (DEFUSE 3 Criteria):<br>  i. Occlusion of terminal ICA or MCA - M1<br>  ii. Clinical imaging mismatch<br>    i Infarct core volume <70 mL<br>    ii Mismatch volume >15 mL<br>    iii Mismatch ratio (penumbra/core) >1.8<br>b. 16–24 hours (DAWN Criteria):<br>  i. Occlusion of terminal ICA or MCA - M1<br>  ii. Clinical imaging mismatch:<br>    a. ≥ 80 y.o., NIHSS ≥10 + core <21 mL<br>    b. < 80 y.o., NIHSS ≥10 + core <31 mL<br>    c. < 80 y.o., NIHSS ≥20 + core <51 mL |
| Wake-up stroke | • Age 18–80 years old<br>• Stroke symptoms at awakening or could not report symptom onset<br>• MRI brain including DWI, FLAIR, a sequence sensitive to hemorrhage, and time-of-flight magnetic resonance angiography of circle of Willis<br>• Patients are eligible for thrombolysis if:<br>  ○ Abnormal signal in DWI + no signal change in FLAIR |

*DWI,* Diffusion-weighted imaging; *FLAIR,* fluid-attenuated inversion recovery; *ICA,* internal carotid artery; *MCA,* middle cerebral artery; *MRI,* magnetic resonance imaging; *NIHSS,* National Institutes of Health stroke scale.

---

**• BOX 40.3 Blood Pressure Goals in Acute Ischemic Stroke**

• If not a candidate for thrombolysis: <220/120 mmHg
• If candidate for thrombolysis: <185/110 mmHg
• After thrombolysis: <180/105 mmHg
• After revascularization: <140/80 mmHg

---

**• BOX 40.4 Options for Treatment of Arterial Hypertension in Patients With Acute Ischemic Stroke Who are Candidates for Acute Reperfusion Therapy**

For patient eligible for acute reperfusion therapy to maintain blood pressure <185/100 mmHg

• Labetalol 10–20 mg intravenous (IV) over 1–2 minutes, may repeat 1 time
• Nicardipine 5 mg/h IV titrate up to 2.5 mg/h every 5 to 15 minutes, maximum 15 mg/h
• Clevidipine 1–2 mg/h IV, titrate by doubling the dose every 2–5 minutes
• Other agents (e.g., hydralazine, enalaprilat) may also be considered

(Modified from Powers W, Rabinstein A, Ackerson T, et al. 2018 Guidelines for the early management of patients with acute ischemic stroke: a guideline for healthcare professionals from the American Heart Association/American Stroke Association. *Stroke.* 2018;49:e46–e49.)

---

and patients taking warfarin independent of current INR.[50] Treatment of patients age ≥ 80 years in the extended window can be considered in a case-by-case approach given the lack of specific evidence. Current AHA/ASA guidelines state that treatment of the very old may offer the same benefits as in younger patients.[45,46]

**Treatment of patients age ≥ 80 years in the extended window can be considered in a case-by-case approach given the lack of specific evidence. Current AHA/ASA guidelines state that treatment of the very old may offer the same benefits as in younger patients.**[45,46] Rapid recognition and treatment of patients presenting with TIA symptoms is extremely important as it is an important risk factor for subsequent stroke. Several studies show a short-term elevated risk of stroke after an episode. This risk is particularly high in the first few days after a TIA with most studies finding stroke risk above 10% in the first 90 days after a TIA.[2]

For patients waking up with stroke without a large vessel occlusion, treatment with IV alteplase might be an option. The WAKE-UP trial showed improved functional outcomes in treated patients when compared with placebo (53.3% vs. 41.8%, odds ratio 1.61; P = .02). This evidence should be taken with caution as treated patients had higher hemorrhagic complications and their improvement was less than expected when compared with historical controls.[51] Recently, tenecteplase (TNK) has surged as a possible alternative to alteplase. TNK is a genetically modified variant of alteplase and is a newer generation fibrinolytic agent with several advantages over alteplase. TNK has a longer half-life allowing administration as a bolus rather than an infusion. Also prior trials suggest a lower incidence of hemorrhagic complications.[52] A formal meta-analysis of head-to-head trials in acute ischemic stroke patients demonstrated that TNK is noninferior when compared with alteplase. Different doses have been proposed for management of acute ischemic stroke, including 0.1 mg/kg, 0.25 mg/kg, and 0.4 mg/kg.[53] The 2018 Acute Stroke Management Guidelines by the AHA/ASA indicate that tenecteplase might be considered as a possible alternative to alteplase in patients with minor neurologic impairment and major intracranial occlusion.[45,46]

Mechanical thrombectomy: Patients presenting with a large vessel occlusion (terminal internal carotid artery or M1 portion of the MCA) treated with thrombolysis have low rates of recanalization (13%–50%),[54] therefore these patients should be treated with mechanical thrombectomy. In 2015 five randomized trials (MR CLEAN, SWIFT PRIME, EXTEND IA, ESCAPE, and REVASCAT) demonstrated that patients treated with IV thrombolysis and mechanical thrombectomy had significant better clinical outcomes when compared with those treated with intravenous thrombolysis only. This evidence led to the recommendation that all patients, with normal premorbid function, who present with a large vessel occlusion and could be treated within 6 hours of symptoms onset should be treated with mechanical thrombectomy.[55] Current guidelines recommend treating with mechanical thrombectomy all patients presenting between 6 and 16 hours from symptom onset with acute ischemic stroke and large vessel occlusion who meet either DAWN or DEFUSE 3 criteria.[45,46,56,57]

## Transient Ischemic Attack

TIA is defined as a transient episode of neurologic dysfunction caused by focal brain, spinal cord, or retinal ischemia, without evidence of CNS infarction.[2] Most patients with TIA will have symptoms for 15 to 20 minutes with complete recovery. Because of this characteristic, estimating the true incidence and prevalence of TIA is difficult. There is lack of TIA recognition among the general population, leading to significant underreporting and undertreatment. The TIA incidence in the United States has been estimated to be approximately 200,000 to 500,000 per year with a population prevalence of 2.3%.[58] Rapid recognition and treatment of patients presenting with TIA symptoms is extremely important because it is a notable risk factor for subsequent stroke. Several studies show a short-term elevated risk of stroke after an episode. This risk is particularly high in the first few days after a TIA with most studies finding stroke risk above 10% in the first 90 days after a TIA.[2] TIA is also associated with an elevated risk of cardiovascular events. In a large study, 2.6% of TIA patients were admitted to the hospital with cardiovascular events within 3 months.[59] Knowing these risks then is important to identify those patients who are most at risk. Multiple tools have been developed for this purpose. The ABCD2 score provides a robust prediction of the patient's risk. Patients are scored if they have the following factors: (1) age $\geq$ 60 years (1 point); (2) BP $\geq$ 140/90 mmHg on presentation (1 point); (3) clinical symptoms of focal weakness with the spell (2 points) or speech impairment without weakness (1 point); (4) duration of symptoms $\geq$ 60 minutes (2 points) or 10 to 59 minutes (1 point); and (5) diabetes (1 point). The 2-day risk of stroke is 1.0% with a score of 0 to 3, 4.1% with a score of 4 to 5, and 8.1% with 6 to 7.[60] Independent of risk, patients presenting with TIA should undergo expedited workup. Hospitalization should be considered in those patients with moderate to high risk to allow close observation and a rapid workup. Patients presenting with TIA symptoms should have neuroimaging within 24 hours of symptom onset. MRI, including diffusion weighted imaging, is the preferred brain diagnostic imaging. Blood vessel imaging, including intracranial and cervical vessels, is also recommended.[2] Given concerns about the association of TIA with heart disease and occult AF, patients presenting with TIA symptoms should have a baseline electrocardiogram (ECG) and further cardiac testing, including echocardiography, and long-term rhythm monitoring should be considered in patients with an unclear origin after imaging. Initial treatment of TIA will depend on the etiology of their symptoms, but, pending diagnosis, initial efforts should focus on control of risk factors associated with stroke and TIA.

### CASE

#### A 75-year-old woman (Part 2)

Our patient has stroke risk factors of essential hypertension, hyperlipidemia, and type 2 diabetes mellitus. She has evidence of new onset AF. Her history and neurologic examination is suggestive of an acute ischemic stroke, most likely because of the occlusion of the left MCA at the M1 segment. A noncontrast head CT was obtained showing no hemorrhage and no ischemic changes. Her symptoms started 1 hour before arrival to the ER. Therefore she is eligible for treatment with IV thrombolysis with alteplase and mechanical thrombectomy. Before treatment, her BP should be

controlled to $\leq$ 180/105 mmHg with labetalol, nicardipine, or clevidipine. Her treatment was successful with good reperfusion. She was admitted to the stroke unit for close observation and BP control. After a few days, she regained the ability to speak a few words and to move her right arm and leg against gravity. She was able to do 3 hours of therapy per day but still needed assistance for walking and activities of daily living. Family reports her prior expressed desire to live at home independently and would not like to live at a nursing home.

1. What would be the best next step in the recovery of this patient?
2. What should be done for secondary stroke prevention?

## Secondary Ischemic Stroke Prevention

BP control is the single most important treatable risk factor for stroke. Current AHA/ASA guidelines recommend initiation of BP treatment for those patients with established systolic BP 140 mmHg (or higher) and diastolic 90 mmHg (or higher).[61] For patients with prior history of hypertension, treatment should be resumed a few days after stroke. A BP goal of systolic $\leq$ 140 mmHg and diastolic $\leq$ 90 mmHg is reasonable.[61] The recent Secondary Prevention of Small Subcortical Strokes trial showed lowering BP below 130 mmHg 2 weeks after a lacunar stroke was associated with a nonstatistically significant lower risk of recurrent stroke.[62] Therefore for patients with a recent lacunar stroke, it might be reasonable to target a systolic BP (SBP) $\leq$ 130 mmHg.[61] Furthermore, a recent systematic review and metaregression analysis showed that both SBP and diastolic (DBP) reduction is linearly associated with the magnitude of risk reduction in recurrent cerebrovascular and cardiovascular events suggesting that a target of SBP $\leq$ 130 mmHg would be an effective secondary stroke prevention target for patients with cerebrovascular events.[63] In the course of titrating medications toward a lower BP in older patients, clinicians should very carefully monitor for adverse events related to overtreatment of BP, including orthostatic hypotension, falls, and kidney injury.

Almost all patients should be treated with an antiplatelet agent after their first stroke. Aspirin (50–100 mg daily), clopidogrel (75 mg daily), and the combination of aspirin-extended-release dipyridamole (25 mg/200 mg twice a day) are all acceptable options for preventing recurrent noncardioembolic ischemic stroke. Selection of antiplatelet agents will depend on the underlying stroke etiology. Patients with TIA and minor stroke will benefit from dual antiplatelet therapy (DAPT). Two recent trials (Clopidogrel in High-Risk Patients with Acute Nondisabling Cerebrovascular Events [CHANCE] and Platelet-Oriented Inhibition in New TIA and Minor ischemic Stroke [POINT]) showed a risk reduction of 28% to 33% of stroke recurrence when DAPT was started within 12 to 24 hours after stroke onset. The CHANCE trial continued DAPT for 21 days and the POINT trial treated patients with DAPT for 90 days. The optimal duration of DAPT is not well defined but should not be extended for $\geq$ 3 months.[64] Current AHA/ASA guidelines recommend consideration of DAPT within 24 hours of minor ischemic stroke or TIA and continuation for 21 days.[61] In patients with intracranial atherosclerosis, treatment with aspirin 325 mg is recommended over warfarin. In patients with severe intracranial atherosclerosis (70%–99%) addition of clopidogrel 75 mg daily for 90 days is reasonable.[61]

For patients with hyperlipidemia, the use of statins decreases the risk of stroke. The beneficial effect of statins is likely caused by antiatherothrombotic properties and as opposed to reduction in cholesterol. The Stroke Prevention by Aggressive Reduction in

Cholesterol Levels (SPARCL) trial showed that in patients with recent stroke or TIA and without coronary artery disease, addition of atorvastatin 80 mg daily was associated with recurrent stroke risk reduction.[65] For patients who tolerate them, high intensity statins are suggested for patients with TIA or ischemic stroke of atherosclerotic origin. Some advocate for the initial use of moderate- rather than high-intensity statins based on a concern for a greater likelihood of side effects and potential for drug interaction in the setting of polypharmacy. For older individuals who were not started on a high-intensity statin, consideration can be given to uptitrate to high-intensity statin within 3 months if they have tolerated the moderate dose. Other lipid lowering therapies like fibrates and diet have no significant impact on stroke incidence. In frail geriatric populations, shared decision making is important as the overall benefit from statin therapy in individuals with a limited life expectancy (<5 years). For patients who are intolerant of high-intensity statin therapy, alternatives are moderate- and low-intensity statin therapy. If patients are intolerant to these groups as well, the suggested treatment is another class of lipid lowering drug.

Anticoagulation and other measures for cardioembolic stroke: For secondary stroke prevention, virtually all patients with AF who have a history of stroke or TIA of cardioembolic origin should be treated with lifelong anticoagulation in the absence of contraindications. Warfarin, dabigatran, apixaban, rivaroxaban, and edoxaban are all acceptable options, but for older patients with adequate renal function, direct oral anticoagulants (DOACs) are preferred to warfarin. There is no preference for a specific DOAC, but dose adjustments should be made for weight or renal function appropriately.

For patients unable to take oral anticoagulants, the AHA/ASA guidelines recommend aspirin 325 mg daily. Adding clopidogrel to aspirin therapy might be a reasonable option.[61] It is important to mention that anticoagulation therapy is far superior to antiplatelet therapy with both options having a similar hemorrhagic risk to warfarin. For example, the ACTIVE W trial (warfarin vs. aspirin + clopidogrel) was stopped early because of clear superiority of warfarin over aspirin and clopidogrel. Patients in this trial had a higher hemorrhagic complication risk in the aspirin plus clopidogrel arm.[66]

An option for patients unable to tolerate anticoagulation is the placement of a left atrial appendage (LAA) occlusion devices. Currently, there are several LAA occlusion devices: the Watchman (Boston Scientific), Amplatzer Amulet (Abbot), WaveCrest (Coherex Medical), the ultrasept LAA closure device, the LAmbre LAA Closure system (Lifetech Scientific), and the Occlutech LAA occluder (Occlutech). Only the Watchman device has been approved by the FDA for stroke risk reduction in patients with nonvalvular AF (2015). A metaanalysis of the PROTECT AF and PREVAIL trials showed similar benefit as warfarin in the prevention of stroke, systemic embolism, and cardiovascular death. All-cause bleeding was similar between groups. Warfarin patients had higher bleeding rates when periprocedural hemorrhage was excluded.[67]

For patients with AF who require temporary interruption of oral anticoagulation and are at high risk for stroke (CHADS2 score of 5 or 6, stroke or TIA within 3 months, or rheumatic heart valve disease), bridging therapy with subcutaneous low-molecular-weight heparin is reasonable.[61] The risk of intracranial hemorrhage and mechanical falls that may lead to subdural hematomas is increased in older adult patients taking oral anticoagulants, but no specific guidelines exist on when to stop anticoagulation in older adults at risk of falling. Thus concern about increased risks of falls

with resultant intracranial hemorrhage leads to reduced use of oral anticoagulants in older adult patients. In our practice, we carefully assess the relative benefits and risks of oral anticoagulation in patients at risk of falling, and in most cases, we recommend continuing anticoagulation.

Diabetes, hyperlipidemia, and smoking cessation: Appropriate control of diabetes and hyperlipidemia are also important components of secondary stroke prevention. No randomized controlled trials of smoking cessation for stroke prevention exist; however, observational studies demonstrate that stroke risk declines steadily after cessation and is equivalent to nonsmokers 5 years after quitting. Finally, increasing evidence suggests that low physical activity and prolonged sitting increases the risk of cardiovascular disease, including stroke.

---

**CASE**

### A 75-year-old woman (Part 3)

Our patient left the hospital a few days after treatment. She was transferred to an acute rehabilitation facility where she underwent 3 hours of therapy per day. She had an excellent recovery. Three months after her stroke, she was able to speak in short sentences and was able to walk unassisted.

Her stroke risk factors include essential hypertension, hyperlipidemia, type 2 diabetes mellitus, and AF. For secondary stroke preventions she should start anticoagulation with warfarin or a NOAC (apixaban, dabigatran, rivaroxaban, or edoxaban), continue high-intensity statins, control her BP to a goal of ≤140/90 mmHg, and manage her diabetes. Her family endorses worsening memory and not wanting to leave her home. They also think her memory has worsened as she is leaving the stove on and missing steps when cooking a recipe.

1. What are common complications after a stroke?
2. What is the management of the late complications of stroke?

---

## Cerebrovascular Disease Complications

Stroke survivors are at risk of developing significant medical complications and have higher disability and mortality.[68] Complications of stroke include hemiparesis, dysphagia, poststroke fatigue, poststroke pain, poststroke seizures, sleep disorders, including OSA, spasticity, cognitive changes, and depression.

Falls present a particular hazard for older adults after stroke. This is particularly problematic in those who have hemiparesis. Hip fractures constitute almost half of all fractures after a stroke. The disuse of the affected limbs predisposes patients to bone resorption and "hemiosteoporosis." This and the inability to have a protective response like an outstretched arm are the reasons why most fractures after stroke occur on the paretic side. The impaired mobility caused by a stroke also predisposes patients to pressure ulcers and deep vein thrombosis.

Dysphagia, most often impairment in oropharyngeal function, is a major risk factor for developing aspiration pneumonia and is a common cause for weight loss in older adults after a stroke.

Poststroke fatigue is often misdiagnosed as poststroke depression and thought to be caused by disturbances in cortical excitability and inflammatory changes. There are no proven therapies available, but interventions like exercise and avoiding excessive alcohol and sedatives hypnotics, as well as treating pain and mood disorders, are encouraged.

Poststroke pain is a frequent but often neglected complication of stroke. Onset of pain can happen at any time with most patients developing symptoms 1 to 3 months after the stroke and can range from mild pain to debilitating limb pain and complex regional pain syndrome. Poststroke pain is usually described as aching, dull, burning pain. The pathophysiology of poststroke pain is not well described. Several factors, including history of depression, stroke severity, younger age, and smoking, have been associated with its development. Treatment of poststroke pain is challenging. Several medications have been found useful in the management of poststroke pain. Anticonvulsants and antidepressants are mainstream medications used in the management of poststroke pain. Gabapentin, pregabalin, carbamazepine, and lamotrigine are the most used medications. Other options include amitriptyline, fluvoxamine, venlafaxine, desvenlafaxine, and duloxetine.[69]

Interprofessional teamwork provides the most effective strategy for treatment and/or prevention of poststroke complications. Working with physical therapists, occupational therapists, speech therapists, pharmacists, social workers, dieticians, and nursing staff provides the best opportunity for recovery to the patient.

Poststroke seizures: Stroke is the most common underlying etiology of seizures in older patients. Approximately 45% of those with epilepsy above 65 years of age have a history of stroke.[69] Patients with hemorrhagic stroke, involvement of the cortical structures, severe neurologic deficits, family history of epilepsy, and younger age have an increased risk of poststroke seizures (Box 40.5).[70,71] Seizure appearance can be divided into early seizures and late seizures. Early seizures are those seizures that occur within 2 weeks after stroke. Early seizures are thought to be secondary to acute neuron injury, ion shifts, blood-brain barrier disruption, and release of excitotoxic neurotransmitters in the ischemic cascade.[72] Late-onset seizures are those that occur more than 2 weeks after stroke and are thought to be caused by membrane property changes, chronic inflammation, neurodegeneration, and altered synaptic plasticity that leads to hyperexcitability and increased synchronization of neuronal activity.[72] Poststroke seizures are associated with poor functional recovery and outcome. Clinically, patients present with focal seizures with or without impaired awareness (simple partial and complex partial seizures). Patient can have secondary generalization and can progress to convulsive status epilepticus. Prophylaxis with antiepileptic drugs (AED) is not recommended. Evidence in favor of the use of AEDs to prevent poststroke seizures is lacking and AED have significant side effects that worsen patient outcome.[73] Poststroke seizures have a high risk of recurrence and must be treated with an AED. The few randomized trials that have assessed treatment of poststroke seizures suggest that lamotrigine, levetiracetam, and gabapentin have similar efficacy. However, lamotrigine had fewer side effects. Two small trials assessing levetiracetam showed 80% seizure control with minimal side effects.[74]

Sleep disorders and OSA: Breathing disorders are both a novel risk factor for stroke and a complication after stroke. OSA has been associated with wake-up stroke[75] and brainstem strokes. After stroke, breathing disorders are very common. Patients can present with several breathing conditions, including OSA, central sleep apnea (CSA), and Cheyne-Stokes breathing (CSB). CSA and CSB are associated with cardiac dysfunction and disruption of the central autonomic networks.[76] CSA and CSB are worse in acute stroke patients and improve as they recover. After stroke, prevalence of OSA is high. Approximately 53% of patients will have an apnea-hypopnea index over 10/h 1 month after a stroke.[76] OSA is associated with poor poststroke BP control, worse neurologic recovery, and longer hospital stays.[76] Patients with OSA should be treated with continuous positive airway pressure once the diagnosis has been made. Treated patients have significant improvements in neurologic recovery, sleepiness, depression, and recurrent vascular events.[76]

Poststroke depression: Depressive symptoms complicating stroke recovery have been recognized for more than a 100 years. Patients with ischemic stroke are at increased risk of developing depression. Recent meta-analyses and systematic review report an incidence of depressive symptoms between 31% and 52% in the 5 years after stroke.[77,78] The association between stroke mechanism and location with subsequent development of depressive symptoms remains unclear. Left frontal lesions have been associated with development of depression[79]; however, this relationship has been challenged. Recent studies have found no significant association between stroke location and depression.[78] Stroke patients with depressive symptoms have higher mortality and disability.[80] Patients who develop depressive symptoms should be offered treatment. Several studies evaluating the efficacy of psychotherapy and pharmacotherapy show improvement of symptoms with either therapy or combination of both.[80] Pharmacologic treatment has not been only associated with improvement of depressive symptoms but also with benefits in stroke recovery. Treatment with selective serotonin reuptake inhibitors (SSRIs) (fluoxetine and citalopram) have been associated with improved motor recovery[81] and enhanced cognitive performance.[82] The decision to treat patients should be made with caution as antidepressant (SSRI) use has been associated with an increase in hemorrhagic complications and falls.[83]

Poststroke spasticity: Spasticity is a common complication of stroke. Approximately one-quarter of stroke survivors will develop spasticity[84] within the first 6 weeks and can appear at any time after stroke. It is defined as "a motor disorder characterized by a velocity dependent increase in tonic stretch reflexes (muscle tone) with exaggerated tendon jerks, resulting from hyperexcitability of the stretch reflex, as one component of the upper motor neuron syndrome."[85] In practice, spasticity will affect patient mobility and activities of daily living. Patients with spasticity will have increased pain and stiffness in the affected limb that negatively impacts recovery. Spasticity treatment is multidisciplinary and includes daily stretching exercises, physical therapy, occupational therapy, splinting and orthoses, as well as pharmacologic and surgical treatments. Pharmacologic treatments should be offered to patients in whom more conservative measures have not provided adequate relief from and those who develop and worsening motor function. Treatment options include oral and injectable medications. The most common treatment options include baclofen, benzodiazepines, gabapentin, tizanidine, and dantrolene. Most of these medications have significant adverse effects and therefore should be used with caution. Baclofen is the most common treatment used as a first-line agent. Baclofen is a gamma-aminobutyric acid (GABA) agonist that crossed the blood-brain barrier and binds to the GABA-b receptors in the spinal cord use. Patients with persistent symptoms despite treatment should be considered for treatment with botulinum toxin (BoNT). BoNT blocks

---

• **BOX 40.5** **Blood Pressure Goals in Hemorrhagic Stroke**

- For patients presenting with systolic blood pressure (SBP) between 150 and 220 mmHg and without contraindication to acute blood pressure treatment, lowering to SBP of 140 mmHg is safe.

(From Coupland C, Dhiman P, Morriss R, et al. Antidepressant use and risk of adverse outcomes in older people: population based cohort study. *BMJ.* 2011;343:d4551.)

acetylcholine release at neuromuscular junction reducing muscle contraction and is more selective and safer than some oral treatment. Treatment with BoNT should be a part of the multidisciplinary approach to patients with spasticity. Stroke patients treated with BoNT have improved mobility and autonomy.[86]

◆◆ **Poststroke complications in older adults include hemiparesis that predisposes to falls and pressure ulcers, dysphagia that predisposes to weight loss and apathy, and cognitive impairment that predisposes to mood disorders/dementia and urinary and fecal incontinence.**

## CASE

### Discussion

After several weeks of intensive rehabilitation, our patient was able to return to her apartment. She required supervision but was able to take care of herself. She was started on appropriate secondary stroke prevention, including anticoagulation, BP, and diabetes control.

## KEY POINTS

- All patients presenting with acute ischemic stroke should be considered for treatment with intravenous thrombolysis and mechanical thrombectomy (see Box 40.3).
- Intravenous thrombolysis can be administered up to 4.5 hours from symptom onset and mechanical thrombectomy can be performed, on selected patients, up to 24 hours after symptom onset.
- Identifying the stroke mechanism is important for the selection of appropriate secondary stroke prevention.
- Rehabilitation should be started as soon as possible to improve recovery.

## Summary

TIA and stroke are heterogeneous diseases with significant consequences if left untreated. Sudden onset of focal neurologic deficits is the core feature of ischemic stroke presentation. Initial assessment needs to be efficient and precise as rapid recognition and treatment is vital for optimal recovery. All patients, independent of age, presenting with acute stroke symptoms should be considered for treatment with intravenous thrombolysis and mechanical thrombectomy. Secondary stroke prevention will depend on accurate stroke etiology identification and management of risk factors. In the older adult population, monitoring for arrhythmias is important as AF is frequent stroke etiology. Evaluating mobility and swallowing function becomes a priority before discharge and selecting the appropriate venue for care after stroke can improve recovery. Management of long-term complications needs a multidisciplinary approach.

## Key References

2. Easton JD, Saver JL, Albers GW, et al. Definition and evaluation of transient ischemic attack. *Stroke*. 2009;40:2276−2293.
3. Sacco R, Kasner S, Broderick J, et al. An updated definition of stroke for the 21st century. A statement for healthcare professionals from the American Heart Association/American Stroke Association. *Stroke*. 2013;44:2064−2089.
45. Powers W, Rabinstein A, Ackerson T, et al. 2018 Guidelines for the early management of patients with acute ischemic stroke: a guideline for healthcare professionals from the American Heart Association/American Stroke Association. *Stroke*. 2018;49:e46−e49.
46. Powers W, Rabinstein A, Ackerson T, Adeoye O, et al. Guidelines for the early management of patients with acute ischemic stroke: 2019 update to the 2018 guidelines for the early management of acute ischemic stroke: a guideline for healthcare professionals from the American Heart Association/American Stroke Association. *Stroke*. 2019;50:e344−e418.
60. Kernan W, Ovbiagele B, Black H, et al. Guidelines for the prevention of stroke in patients with stroke and transient ischemic attack. *Stroke*. 2014;45:2160−2236.

**References available online at** expertconsult.com.

# 41
# Diabetes Mellitus

MITCHELL T. HEFLIN

## OUTLINE

*Additional online-only material indicated by icon.*

## OBJECTIVES

*Upon completion of this chapter, the reader will be able to:*

- Understand the changing epidemiology of adult diabetes mellitus (DM) and the impact it has on the older adult population.
- Identify the risk factors for DM in older persons.
- Understand the continuum of the disease process of DM and how this affects the diagnostic criteria.
- Identify appropriate goals for treatment based on status of health and function.

- Be able to assess the older adults with DM in a multisystem and multidisciplinary fashion, including the common geriatric syndromes.
- Describe management strategies, including indications and contraindications for pharmacologic and nonpharmacologic treatments of DM.

## CASE

### Maria Sanchez (Part 1)

Maria Sanchez is a 72-year-old Latinx woman who comes to your office with her daughter for hypertension follow-up and remarks that for 2 months she has had bilateral burning and numbness of her feet and that she has fallen recently at home without injury. Medications include hydrochlorothiazide 25 mg daily and metoprolol 50 mg twice a day. Her blood pressure is 160/88 mmHg, pulse 60 beats per minute, weight 173 lbs, and body mass index 30 kg/m$^2$; monofilament and light touch sensation is diminished in a stocking distribution, Achilles reflexes are $+1$ and dorsalis pedis pulses are $+1$, and the remainder of the examination is unremarkable. Fasting serum glucose is 130 mg/dL, blood urea nitrogen 19 mg/dL, creatinine 1.2 mg/dL, and electrolytes are normal.

1. Can you name at least four of Ms. Sanchez's risk factors for diabetes?
2. Can you make the diagnosis of diabetes at this time?
3. What additional laboratory tests would you order?

## Prevalence and Impact

One-quarter of adults in the United States age $> 65$ years have a diagnosis of diabetes mellitus (DM) and nearly half qualify as having prediabetes (Fig. 41.1).[1,2] The rising prevalence of obesity predicts that these numbers will continue to increase in the coming decades. DM is even more common among the frailest and most dependent patients with estimated rates of 25% to 34% among nursing home residents in the United States.[3] Males tend to have a higher prevalence than females, and Latinx and Black Americans have a higher prevalence than White Americans. Older adults diagnosed with diabetes have a similar spectrum of macrovascular and microvascular complications as their younger counterparts; however, the overall risk of cardiovascular disease is substantially higher. In addition to high rates of traditional complications of diabetes, older persons with the disease have more functional disability, mobility impairment, depression, falls, incontinence, and cognitive impairment.[4] The presence of these geriatric syndromes not only

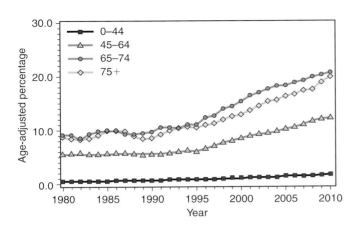

• **Figure 41.1** Increasing prevalence of diabetes.

<table>
<tr><td colspan="4">**TABLE 41.1**  **Diabetes in Old Age Compared With "Classical" Types 1 and 2**</td></tr>
</table>

| Age | Young | Old | Middle Aged |
|---|---|---|---|
| Body habitus | Thin | Thin or mild visceral obesity | Obese |
| Coma | Ketoacidotic | Mixed/lactic acidosis | Hyperosmolar |
| Glucose induced insulin release | Very low | Low | Increased but insufficient to overcome insulin resistance |
| Insulin mediated glucose disposal | Normal | Mild or decreased | Markedly decreased |
| Fasting hepatic glucose output | Increased | Normal | Increased |

reflects the effects of living with diabetes as a chronic disease, but also confounds older adults' ability to safely and independently manage the disease. Not surprisingly, substantial costs are incurred annually in care for older adults with diabetes related to management of the disease and its complications.[5]

The cumulative impact of diabetes has important effects on longer-term health outcomes and prognosis. Multiple studies have demonstrated that a diagnosis of diabetes may shorten life expectancy by a decade or more.[6,7] In addition, lifetime remaining is characterized by poor health status and disability. A British study of persons older than age 85 years found that only 32% of the remaining life of persons with diabetes was active, compared with 42% among those without diabetes.[8]

⁘ **Older adults with diabetes suffer from high rates of functional disability and geriatric syndromes, such as cognitive impairment and falls, that can confound their ability to manage the disease independently and safely.**

## Pathophysiology

The physiologic course of diabetes follows a predictable progression from the asymptomatic prediabetic state, with insulin resistance, through mild postprandial hyperglycemia and/or mild fasting hyperglycemia, to diagnosable type 2 diabetes.[9] Increased resistance to insulin-mediated glucose disposal and a decrease in noninsulin-mediated glucose uptake play a role in the development of DM in older persons.[10,11] The resistance to insulin-mediated glucose disposal is, in part, caused by triglyceride infiltration into muscle and mitochondrial defects in the muscle. In addition, independent of changes in body weight, older adults experience an increase in relative adiposity. This physiologic change, combined with a reduction in physical activity, can exacerbate other biologic changes to increase insulin resistance. Among older persons, a reduction in glucose-induced insulin release from beta cells in the pancreas further exacerbates glucose control. This reflects the impact of aging, comorbid conditions, inflammation, and possible genetic effects on beta cell function with time. Older persons have fewer abnormalities in fasting hepatic glucose output compared with middle-aged persons. The differences in how DM manifests in older persons compared with how it appears in "classical" manifestations are highlighted in Table 41.1.

Much debate also exists about the diagnosis and rates of type 1 versus type 2 diabetes in older adults.[9] Although the vast majority of DM in older adults is related to insulin resistance and classic features of type 2, type 1 diabetes with islet cell dysfunction occurs and may be difficult to distinguish. Older adults can have classic features of type 1 with rapid onset and dramatic presentation with weight loss and ketonuria, but also be gradual in onset and may not be recognized as such until it is found that they have a poor response to oral hypoglycemics. A separate category, latent autoimmune diabetes in adults (LADA), has been established and is characterized by immunologic features of type 1, including antibodies to glutamic acid decarboxylase, insulin, or islet cells. LADA is associated with other autoimmune conditions. Often, the only distinguishing feature of these patients from classic type 2 diabetes is the early need for insulin.

## Differential Diagnosis and Assessment

### Presenting Symptoms

DM can present atypically in older adults. Up to 30% of undiagnosed patients do not have the "3 Ps" (polyphagia, polydipsia, polyuria). The renal threshold for glucose increases with age because older persons often have a higher thirst threshold; thus glycosuria may not occur.[11] Instead of classic polydipsia, the presentation may be dehydration with altered thirst perception and delayed fluid supplementation. Polyuria can present as incontinence. More often, changes such as dry eyes, dry mouth, confusion, incontinence, or diabetic complications are the presenting symptoms.[12] Older patients may occasionally present with weight loss or hyperosmolar nonketotic coma. The common age-associated syndromes of persistent pain, urinary incontinence, cognitive impairment, depression, injurious falls, and polypharmacy are all increased and may constitute presenting symptoms in persons with diabetes.

### Confirming the Diagnosis and Initial Assessment

The laboratory diagnosis, similar to the pathophysiology, involves a continuum from prediabetes to the diabetic threshold

(Boxes 41.1 and 41.2). A fasting blood glucose (FBS) of 126 mg/dL or greater is still the preferred test to screen for prediabetes and diabetes.[13] Older persons should be screened for DM annually; however, up to 30% of older diabetics have an FBS of less than 126 mg/dL yet have a 2-hour oral glucose tolerance test (OGTT) of more than 200 mg/dL.[13] The vast majority of those who meet the OGTT criteria for diabetes, but not the FBS criteria, will have a hemoglobin (Hb)$A_{1C}$ less than 7.0%.

Assessment of older adults with diabetes should include a clinical history and examination conducted by a multidisciplinary, interprofessional team that ascertains overall health status and risk factors for complications, including concurrent geriatric syndromes that affect prognosis and management. Ideally, this includes evaluation for the following:

1. Macrovascular complications. Morbidity and mortality from vascular disease presents the greatest health risk for older adults with diabetes. This includes a history of coronary, carotid, and peripheral atherosclerosis either by diagnosis or symptoms. Patient interviews should focus on neurologic symptoms, syncope, chest pain—often atypical, exertional dyspnea or fatigue, and claudication. This includes measures of blood pressure in office and at home. A systolic blood pressure goal of 140 mm Hg or lower has been set for people with hypertension, as well as diabetes with some evidence supporting even lower targets for those who tolerate treatment. Blood pressure should also be measured when not at the physician's office because "white coat" hypertension occurs in 25% of patients. In addition, patients should have a fasting lipid profile, liver function, and a 12-lead electrocardiogram.

2. Microvascular complications. Although often diagnosed later in life, older adults still incur substantial long-term risk of the range of microvascular complications. This includes nephropathy as assessed routinely by urinalysis, urinary microalbumin, and serum creatinine to yield measures of creatinine clearance; retinopathy requiring an annual ophthalmologic visit for dilated retinal examination; glaucoma and cataracts should also be included in the screening; peripheral neuropathy with foot complications, such as undetected injury and ulcers should be assessed regularly, including a monofilament test and examination for posterior column disease.

3. Age-friendly care for patients with diabetes. Clinical assessments for older adults with diabetes should also reflect the elements of high-quality, person-centered care encompassed in the age-friendly care initiative.[14] In addition to the disease-specific complications, broader evaluations inclusive of the "4 Ms" (mentation, mobility, medications, and matters most) become particularly important in this most vulnerable population. This includes:

   - Memory and mood. Older diabetics develop cognitive impairment and mood disorders at a significantly higher rate than the unaffected population. In addition, comorbid cognitive and mood disorders confound the ability to manage diabetes safely and effectively. Case finding for mood and cognition should be considered annually.

   - Mobility and personal safety. A diagnosis of diabetes in older adults increases the risk of falls.[15] This risk, undoubtedly, relates to the myriad of concurrent problems with vision, peripheral nerve function, muscle strength, and the need for multiple medications. The risk is particularly pronounced among those taking insulin, likely related to overtreatment and hypoglycemia. In addition, screening for home safety, including driving ability, use of power tools, yard and housework, heat-generating appliances, and firearms, all are critically important. In addition, all diabetics need to have orthostatic blood pressure and heart rate measured at every visit. Persons who complain of dizziness or falling within 2 hours of a meal should be screened for postprandial hypotension, which is present in 20% of patients with diabetes.

   - Medications. Older adults with diabetes take more medications than those without the diagnosis.[16,17] This relates not only to the frequent use of medications to treat both hyperglycemia and macrovascular and microvascular complications, but the high prevalence of other comorbid conditions that require medications to manage—including arthritis and nerve conditions causing pain, mood disorders, sleep disruption, and vision problems.

   - Advance directives (i.e., what matters most). Given the high rates of comorbid conditions and a clear connection between diabetes and worse prognosis and shortened life expectancy, routine care should also include proactive advance care planning discussions.[18] Providers should identify expectations, goals, and preferences to include documentation of advance directives, including healthcare surrogates and specific directives included as part of a living will, code status and, when appropriate, use of specific orders for life-sustaining

---

### • BOX 41.1 Criteria For The Diagnosis of Diabetes[a]

$A_{1C}$ 6.5% or greater[b]

OR

FPG 126 mg/dL or greater (7.0 mmol/L or greater)[c]

OR

2-hour PG during OGTT 200 mg/dL or greater (11.1 mmol/L or greater)[d]

OR

Random PG 200 mg/dL or greater (11.1 mmol/L or greater)

OR

When classic symptoms of hyperglycemia or hyperglycemic crisis are present

[a]$A_{1C}$, FPG, or OGTT results should be confirmed by repeat testing unless unequivocal hyperglycemia is present.

[b]Must be done in a lab using an NGSP-certified method, standardized to the DCCT assay.

[c]Fasting = no caloric intake for at least 8 hrs.

[d]Test as WHO describes, with glucose load equivalent to 75 g anhydrous glucose dissolved in water.

*DCCT*, Diabetes control and complications trial; *FPG*, fasting plasma glucose; *OGTT*, oral glucose tolerance test; *PG*, plasma glucose; *NGSP*, National Glycohemoglobin Standardization Program; *WHO*, World Health Organization.
(From ADA. Standards of Medical Care in Diabetes—2013. Diabetes Care 2013;36:S11−66.)

---

### • BOX 41.2 Factors That Predispose Older Adult Patients with Type 2 Diabetes to Hypoglycemia

- Poor or erratic nutritional intake
- Changes in mental status that impair the perception or response to hypoglycemia
- Increased polypharmacy and noncompliance with medications
- Dependence or isolation that limits receipt of early treatment for hypoglycemia
- Impaired renal or hepatic metabolism
- Presence of comorbid conditions that can mask or lead to misdiagnosis of hypoglycemic symptoms (dementia, delirium, depression, sleep abnormalities, seizures, myocardial infarction, cerebrovascular accident)
- Presence of other endocrine disorders, such as adrenal insufficiency

treatments (medical orders on scope of treatment [MOST] or physician's orders for life-sustaining treatment [POLST]). Such discussions can avoid unwanted interventions and improve experience and quality of life near the end of life.

## CASE

### Discussion (Part 1)

Maria Sanchez has multiple risk factors for DM, including age > 65 years, Hispanic ethnicity, body mass index > 25 kg/m², hypertension, and use of a thiazide diuretic. Her physical examination and history are compatible with peripheral neuropathy, of which diabetes is a leading cause among older adults. Although a single fasting plasma glucose of 130 exceeds the 126 mg/dL threshold for diabetes, the World Health Organization and American Diabetes Association require two fasting plasma glucose levels equal to or exceeding 126 mg/dL to establish the diagnosis of DM. Additional laboratory tests to consider would be a lipid panel, HbA₁C, urinalysis, and urine microalbumin. Should the repeat FBS be less than 126 mg/dL, then a couple of glucose levels 2 hours after her largest meal should be obtained. A 2-hour value of ≥ 200 mg/dL would be sufficient to diagnose DM. Mrs. Sanchez also has a geriatric syndrome seen in diabetics, namely, persistent pain. Diabetics should be screened for pain, cognitive decline, depression, injurious falls, urinary incontinence, and polypharmacy. Diabetes is also a recognized risk factor for osteoporosis.

## CASE

### Maria Sanchez (Part 2)

A repeat FBS was 127 mg/dL, and her HbA₁C was 8.9; total cholesterol was 205 mg/dL, triglycerides 250 mg/dL, high-density lipoprotein (HDL) 34 mg/dL, low-density lipoprotein (LDL) 121 mg/dL, and urine microalbumin 40 mg/L.
1. What treatment goals should you establish for Mrs. Sanchez?
2. What changes would you make in her medications?

## Management

Management of diabetes in older adults accounts for a range of factors that inform the safety and effectiveness of various treatment options. These factors include (1) overall health status, (2) cognition and functional status, (3) social factors, and (4) personal preference. Measures of health status include the presence of multiple comorbid conditions that influence the complexity and cost of particular treatment regimens, as well as prognosis and life expectancy. Chronic illness and limited life expectancy may lead providers and patients to prioritize comfort and quality over tight control of blood glucose aimed at preventing long-term complications. Similarly, impairments in cognition and/or functional status may impede a person's ability to adhere to a prescribed regimen. In addition, social factors, such as health literacy, access to care, and cost, directly affect the practical implementation of a treatment regimen. Another factor that becomes particularly important in considering treatment goals in older adults is risk of adverse effects. Specifically, while lower blood glucose levels may reduce long-term risk of complications, they also substantially increase the risk of hypoglycemia, which, in the short run, may present a greater threat to health and independence. This balance of factors has led the American Diabetes Association to provide general recommendations about selecting treatment goals for older adults in terms of target HbA₁C levels.[19] Specifically, for those older adults with good health and function, a treatment goal of a HbA₁C < 7.5% provides the right balance of long-term risk reduction while minimizing the risk of hypoglycemia. For those with other confounding factors, including multiple comorbid conditions and impairments in cognition or function, a goal of 8% to 8.5% allows for simpler medication regimens and slightly higher daily blood glucose levels to avoid more complex monitoring and medication regimens and, importantly, to minimize risk of hypoglycemia. Finally, for those with limited life expectancy and severe functional impairments, treatment goals place a higher premium on safety and simplicity and allow for a HbA₁C goal up to 8.5%, a threshold intended to prevent or minimize the short-term complications of hyperglycemia. Table 41.2 provides a convenient view of these treatment goals. In the end, these goals should be highly individualized and require shared decision-making approaches with patients and caregivers.

Ultimately, safe and effective management of diabetes in the older adult requires a combination of nonpharmacologic and pharmacologic strategies that optimizes health and function and reduces the risk of complications, including geriatric syndromes. A comprehensive review of the management of diabetes is beyond

## TABLE 41.2  Treatment Goals for Blood Glucose and Blood Pressure Based on Health Status

| Health Status/Function | Implications for Survival | Suggested HbA₁C Goal | Fasting or Preprandial Glucose | Blood Pressure |
|---|---|---|---|---|
| Healthy with few if any coexisting chronic illnesses, intact cognitive and functional status | Longer remaining life expectancy | <7.5% | 90–130 mg/dL | <140/90 mmHg |
| Moderately complex health issues with multiple chronic illnesses or 2+ instrumental ADL impairments or mild-to-moderate cognitive impairment | Intermediate remaining life expectancy (potential for high treatment burden, hypoglycemia, falls, other adverse events) | <8.0% | 90–150 mg/dL | <140/90 mmHg |
| Very complex or poor health with LTC needs or end-stage chronic illnesses or moderate-to-severe cognitive impairment or 2+ ADL dependencies | Limited remaining life expectancy makes benefit uncertain | <8.5% | 100–180 mg/dL | <150/90 mmHg |

*ADL,* Activities of daily living; *HbA₁C,* hemoglobin A₁C; *LTC,* long-term care.

the scope of this chapter. General guidance in implementation and prioritization of various strategies and combination therapies is provided.

◆◆ **Among older adults, treatment goals for diabetes depend on a number of factors, including health status, functional ability, and life expectancy. Those with robust health and preserved cognitive and physical ability may have a $HbA_{1C}$ goal of $< 7.5\%$, whereas those with frail health and limited life expectancy may liberalize goals to a higher $A_{1C}$ to simplify care and avoid complications such as hypoglycemia.**

## Diabetes Education

All diabetics should receive formal education and counseling from an interprofessional team. Certified diabetic educators (CDEs) are nurses, pharmacists, or dietitians who have passed a comprehensive national examination and can instruct patients about nutrition, home glucose monitoring, recognition and prevention of hypoglycemia, and other complications. CDEs are central to the healthcare team; they gain insight into their patients' functional capacity and adherence. Similarly, initial management for older adults, as well as their caregivers, should include comprehensive diabetes self-management education, which is a covered benefit under Medicare Part B. Patients should be advised that home blood glucose self-monitoring, when appropriate, has been associated with improved glycemic control. Team members should review monitoring technique as functional ability may change over time. Education regarding medication use is vital; package inserts are often written in small print or on poor-quality paper. Language and health literacy may also be barriers to obtaining important information about medications.

## Lifestyle Interventions

### Diet

Medical nutrition therapy (MNT) must be individualized by body type and energy requirements. Carbohydrate intake remains key to glycemic control. Extremely low carbohydrate diets ($< 130$ g/day), however, are not recommended because carbohydrates are important for energy, water-soluble vitamins and minerals, and fiber. In fact, 45% to 65% of daily calories should be carbohydrates. Weight loss by diet should be only undertaken with caution in older persons because it has been shown to increase mortality rate in diabetics.[20]

### Exercise

Physical activity improves insulin sensitivity, glycemic control, and selected risk factors for cardiovascular disease (hypertension, dyslipidemia), and decreases the risk of coronary artery disease. Resistance exercise is particularly effective when coupled with aerobic exercise. Current recommendations for exercise in older adults encourage 150 minutes of moderate exercise per week. The addition of balance training and strengthening can further improve function and reduce falls.

## Pharmacologic Therapy

Medication and monitoring regimens that maximize compliance and account for treatment goals are recommended, started at the lowest dose, and titrated gradually to targets or side effects (Table 41.3). Newer medications offer a broader range of options that minimize risk of hypoglycemia, but may increase cost, complexity, and still have important side effects in older patients.

### Biguanides

The primary mechanism of action of biguanides is to decrease hepatic production and intestinal absorption of glucose while improving insulin sensitivity. Metformin is the first-line therapy of choice in older adults with type 2 DM. As monotherapy, metformin typically does not cause hypoglycemia or long-term weight gain. Common side effects include gastrointestinal discomfort, diarrhea, decreased appetite, and weight loss.[21] Metformin is contraindicated in any patient with an estimated glomerular filtration rate (eGFR) $< 30$ mL/min/1.73m$^2$ and should be held before the administration of iodinated contrast for imaging in patients with eGFR of 30 to 60 mL/min/1.73m$^2$. Metformin should also be avoided in situations of potential hypoxemic stress (cardiovascular collapse, respiratory failure, acute myocardial infarction, septicemia), impaired liver function, or congestive heart failure because of the rare but real risk of lactic acidosis.

### Sulfonylureas

Sulfonylureas enhance beta cell secretion of insulin from the pancreas causing a decrease in glucose output from the liver and an increase in insulin sensitivity in the periphery. These medications have traditionally served as first-line monotherapy but have likely been overused in the past. Although they are affordable and reasonably effective early in the disease, they carry a risk of hypoglycemia and their efficacy declines as beta cell function wanes with aging. Longer acting agents, such as glyburide and chlorpropamide, should be avoided because of the substantial risk of hypoglycemia. Shorter acting medications, such as glimepiride and glipizide, remain an affordable option with appropriate education regarding signs and symptoms of hypoglycemia.

### Thiazolidinediones

The thiazolidinediones, pioglitazone and rosiglitazone, lower glucose by improving target cell response to insulin, without increasing pancreatic insulin secretion; thus they are unlikely to cause hypoglycemia. Although this mechanism of action may be attractive for achieving glucose control with less risk in older adults, substantial concerns exist regarding a range of adverse effects. These include liver dysfunction, heart failure with fluid retention, and increase in bone loss and fracture rates. Given side effects and safer alternatives, this class has fallen out of favor for use in older diabetics.

### Meglitinides

Repaglinide and nateglinide are used less frequently in older adults because of the risk of hypoglycemia. They provide increased insulin secretion for improved postprandial control, but incur risk of hypoglycemia and weight gain given the mechanism of action. Although a plausible part of a combination regimen in younger diabetics, they should only be used with caution in older patients.

### Alpha-Glucosidase Inhibitors

Acarbose and miglitol can be used as an adjunct to diet and exercise or in combination pharmacotherapy. They reversibly inhibit intestinal alpha-glucosidases, resulting in delayed glucose absorption and lowering of postprandial hyperglycemia and increased

**TABLE 41.3    Choices of Pharmacotherapy in Diabetes Mellitus With Medications**

| Class/Medication | Pharmacologic Activity | Pros | Cons |
|---|---|---|---|
| Biguanide<br>• Metformin | Hepatic glucose production;<br>↑insulin-mediated uptake of glucose in muscles | No weight gain<br>Minimal hypoglycemia<br>Likely ↓in both microvascular and macrovascular events | Gastrointestinal side effects (diarrhea and abdominal discomfort)<br>Lactic acidosis<br>Contraindicated in renal insufficiency, liver, or cardiac failure |
| Sulfonylureas<br>• Glipizide<br>• Glimepiride<br>• Glyburide | ↑Insulin secretion from pancreatic beta cells | ↓ Microvascular events | Hypoglycemia (esp. with longer half-life: glyburide)<br>Weight gain<br>Skin rash (including photosensitivity) |
| Meglitinides<br>• Repaglinide<br>• Nateglinide | ↑Insulin secretion from pancreatic beta cells | ↓Postprandial glucose excursions<br>Dosing flexibility (before meals) | Hypoglycemia<br>Weight gain<br>Frequent dosing schedule |
| TZDs<br>• Pioglitazone<br>• Rosiglitazone | ↑Insulin sensitivity | Minimal hypoglycemia ↑HDL-C<br>↓Triglycerides (pioglitazone) | Weight gain<br>Edema/heart failure<br>Bone fractures<br>↑LDL-C (rosiglitazone)<br>Possible ↑MI |
| DPP-4 inhibitors<br>• Sitagliptin<br>• Saxagliptin<br>• Vildagliptin<br>• Linagliptin<br>• Alogliptin | ↑Insulin secretion (glucose-dependent) ↓Glucagon secretion (glucose-dependent) | Minimal hypoglycemia<br>Well tolerated<br>Once-daily dosing | Urticaria/angioedema<br>Possible increased risk of pancreatitis<br>?↑Heart failure hospitalization<br>High cost |
| GLP-1 receptor agonists<br>• Exenatide (Byetta) Exenatide extended release<br>• Liraglutide<br>• Dulaglutide<br>• Albiglutide<br>• Lixisenatide | ↑Insulin secretion (glucose-dependent) ↓Glucagon secretion (glucose-dependent)<br>Slows gastric emptying<br>↑Satiety | Minimal hypoglycemia Weight reduction ↓Postprandial glucose excursions | Gastrointestinal adverse effects (nausea, vomiting)<br>↑Heart rate<br>Acute pancreatitis<br>C-cell hyperplasia/ medullary thyroid tumors in animals |
| Glucosidase inhibitors<br>• Acarbose<br>• Miglitol | Slows intestinal carbohydrate digestion or absorption | Minimal hypoglycemia<br>↓Postprandial glucose excursions<br>Possible ↓CVD events | In general, modest A$_{1C}$ reduction<br>Flatulence and abdominal discomfort<br>Contraindicated in cirrhosis<br>Frequent dosing schedule (with meals) |
| SGLT-2 inhibitors<br>• Canagliflozin<br>• Empagliflozin<br>• Dapagliflozin | ↓Glucose reabsorption by the kidney<br>↑Urinary glucose excretion | Minimal hypoglycemia Weight reduction<br>↓Blood pressure<br>Effective at all stages of T2D<br>Once-daily dosing | Caution in patients with renal insufficiency<br>Genitourinary infections<br>Genital yeast infections<br>Polyuria<br>Hyperkalemia<br>Orthostatic hypotension<br>Pancreatitis |

*CVD*, Cardiovascular disease; *DPP-4*, dipeptidyl peptidase-4; *GLP-1*, glucagon-like peptide-1; *HDL-C*, high-density lipoprotein-C; *LDL-C*, low-density lipoprotein-C; *MI*, myocardial infarction; *SGLT-2*, sodium glucose transport-2; *T2D*, type 2 diabetes; *TZDs*, thiazolidinediones.

glucagon-like peptide 1 (GLP-1). Flatulence and diarrhea are common side effects and often prohibitive for use in older adults. Acarbose and miglitol are not recommended in chronic kidney disease and are contraindicated in diabetic ketoacidosis, cirrhosis, and many intestinal diseases.

## Glucagon-Like Peptide 1 Agents

GLP-1 is an intestinal hormone that stimulates the release of insulin as glucose rises in the postprandial period. As such, drugs that work via this mechanism are unlikely to cause hypoglycemia and

may be important adjuncts for achieving glucose control in older diabetics. Two medication classes act upon GLP-1. **GLP-1 agonists** require a daily injection to lower glucose. They also produce anorexia, gastrointestinal upset, and weight loss. As such, these drugs may not be appropriate for older persons, although they can be excellent for overweight middle-aged persons. Agents available include exenatide and liraglutide. Dipeptidyl peptidase IV (DPP-4) inhibitors block the breakdown of GLP-I. They can be used as monotherapy and do not produce hypoglycemia. The three drugs of this class available in the United States are sitagliptin, linagliptin, and saxagliptin. These drugs can cause a severe skin rash. In combination with angiotensin-converting enzyme (ACE) inhibitors they can produce angioedema. Mixed evidence exists regarding the potential for DPP-4 inhibitors to reduce the risk of cardiovascular events.

### Sodium Glucose Transport 2 Inhibitors

The sodium glucose transport 2 (SGLT-2) inhibitors are oral agents that increase urinary excretion of glucose and can be used once daily with less risk of hypoglycemia. This mechanism of action can result in a diuretic effect that can lower blood pressure and weight. They can, however, also result in orthostatic hypotension, as well as increased rates of both genital yeast and urinary tract infections. They should be used with caution in older adults with chronic kidney disease or other genitourinary conditions. Emerging evidence indicates that use of SGLT-2 inhibitors lowers risk of cardiovascular events.

### Insulin

Insulin is indicated for treatment of diabetes that has not responded to diet, exercise, and oral agents. Its use is sometimes required as the diabetic patient ages because of a progressive loss in beta cell function that mitigates the response to insulin secretagogues or GLP-1 based therapies. Of course, its use requires a higher level of cognitive and physical function to independently manage injections and to monitor for hypoglycemia. This includes adequate vision and dexterity to self-administer injections. As such, decisions to transition to insulin therapy can depend on the availability of adequate caregiver support. In most cases, adequate control can be achieved with low risk of hypoglycemia with long-acting basal insulin given once daily. Options include glargine 100 or detemir insulin, both of which have minimal peak and trough effects and some flexibility as to what time of day they may be given. Multiple daily dosing and, in particular, preprandial short-acting insulins must be used with more caution in older adults because of their higher risk of hypoglycemia. If a need for control of postprandial glucose spikes exists, a rapid-acting insulin, such as aspart or lispro, with shorter onset and duration of action are preferred.

### Combination Therapy and Deintensification

As the disease progresses, older diabetics may require the use of combinations of medications. Whereas the use of multiple agents with different mechanisms of action may be attractive for better control, these changes must be made with caution because of increased risk of hypoglycemia and other side effects. Specifically, if lifestyle interventions and metformin have not achieved adequate control, the addition of a sulfonylurea, DPP-4 inhibitor, or SGLT-2 inhibitor may be appropriate. The latter two have the advantage of a lower risk of hypoglycemia, but also incur greater expense. Alternatively, the addition of basal insulin is often an attractive option for the older adults with sufficient abilities or care resources. Particular caution should be taken in transitioning from a sulfonylurea to insulin with a clear plan for tapering and discontinuing the oral agent. As detailed earlier, treatment goals and, specifically, $HbA_{1C}$ targets change with age, ability, and life expectancy. Providers caring for older adults with diabetes should continually reassess these goals with patients and care teams and recognize opportunities for "deintensification" or deprescribing of pharmacologic regimens. Examples include changes in regimens that can occur during acute illness when glucose levels may increase with stress or from other prescribed medications, such as glucocorticoids. Hospital follow-up should include a careful review of both treatment goals and targets and recognition of opportunities to lower doses or discontinue medications added during hospitalization. Cognitive decline provides another example. As dementia worsens, attention should be given to simplifying drug regimens to ensure the patient and caregiver can safely manage their diabetes. This may involve adjusting expectations for glucose control and deprescribing medications to reduce complexity.

❖❖ **As a person with diabetes ages, providers need to continually reassess goals and consider approaches to deintensification of treatment regimens. This may be particularly important with the progression of other chronic diseases, such as dementia, or with changes in health status around acute episodes of illness**.

---

### CASE

#### Discussion (Part 2)

The additional laboratory studies indeed confirm your suspicion of DM and suggest hyperlipidemia and the presence of Mrs. Sanchez's diabetes for at least 2 to 3 months. Mutual goal setting would be desirable, and because she is otherwise healthy and presumably has good functional capacity, it would be reasonable to aim for blood pressures below 140/80 mmHg. Her elevated blood pressure should be confirmed on at least two home measurements, and she should have a blood pressure measured standing. A low-dose ACE inhibitor would be preferred because of her diabetes with microalbuminuria. You should stop her hydrochlorothiazide and beta-blocker, because this will reduce polypharmacy. The theoretical problems with exacerbation of glucose intolerance with thiazides and the masking of hypoglycemic symptoms with beta-blockers are rarely clinically significant. It is reasonable to set a goal of getting her $HbA_{1C}$ down to 7%, and for her total cholesterol to be below 200, triglycerides below 150, HDL above 45, and LDL below 120. We can wait a few months to see if exercise and improved glycemic control are able to bring the lipids to goal. Individualized MNT and diabetic education will be ordered, and self-glucose testing can be recommended. Should this prove ineffective after several months, then oral agents would be indicated. Metformin is a good choice because it is somewhat associated with weight loss and is proven to prevent macrovascular complications.

---

### CASE

#### Maria Sanchez (Part 3)

Twelve weeks later Mrs. Sanchez has substantial relief from her foot discomfort, and her blood pressure is 135/78 mmHg on a low-dose ACE inhibitor. Her $HbA_{1C}$ is 7.5 on metformin. Her FBS is in the 110 to 130 mg/dL range.

What other measures can you recommend to her to reduce the macrovascular complications of coronary artery disease?

---

## Long-Term Management Guidelines

Effective management of diabetes in older adults goes well beyond blood glucose control and requires vigilance in health optimization with respect to vascular risk and geriatric syndromes.

## Hypertension Management

Hypertension is associated with stroke, coronary artery disease, peripheral vascular disease, retinopathy, nephropathy, and potentially neuropathy. Blood pressure control in diabetes is very important. A goal of < 140/80 mmHg is recommended if tolerated; lowering below 130/80 mmHg may have additional benefit in those with elevated 10-year cardiovascular risk but has the potential to cause more adverse effects in older adults and those with chronic kidney disease.[5] Gradual reduction is preferred. Systolic pressure should initially be lowered by no more than 20 mmHg; if this is well tolerated, further reduction may be made. Patients with blood pressure > 160/100 mmHg should be offered pharmacologic and behavioral interventions within 1 month.[22] ACE inhibitors and angiotensin receptor blocking agents (ARBs) are preferred in diabetic hypertension because of their efficacy in lowering blood pressure and slowing the progression of proteinuria and nephropathy. Diabetes is not a barrier to the use of beta-blockers for cardioprotection in myocardial infarction or in hypertensive patients with diabetes and congestive heart failure. Little evidence exists to support withholding beta-blockers from diabetic patients because of metabolic concerns or fears of masking hypoglycemia. Because ACE inhibitors and ARBs are associated with renal impairment and hyperkalemia, renal function and serum potassium should be tested within 1 to 2 weeks of starting the drugs, once a year, and at dose increases.[18]

## Smoking

Smoking is the most important modifiable cause of premature death associated with macrovascular and microvascular complications. Twelve percent of patients older than age 65 years smoke.[23] Smoking cessation in the older adult population may drop the risk of macrovascular and microvascular complications to presmoking levels. All diabetic patients who smoke should be assessed for willingness and offered counseling and pharmacologic interventions as appropriate.[22]

## Eye Care

Diabetic retinopathy is the most frequent cause of new cases of blindness among adults age 20 to 74 years.[24,25] The incidence of retinopathy is associated with the quality of glycemic control over the past 6 years and elevated blood pressure; progression of retinopathy is linked to older age, male sex, and hyperglycemia. Early detection and treatment of diabetic retinopathy is paramount. Older patients with new-onset diabetes should have an initial screening, dilated-eye examination performed by an eye-care specialist, and a dilated-eye examination annually if they are at high risk for eye disease (e.g., those with symptoms of retinopathy, glaucoma, or cataracts; HbA$_{1C}$ > 8%; type 1 DM; or blood pressure > 140/80 mmHg). At lower risk, the dilated-eye examination can occur every 2 years.

## Nephropathy

Diabetic nephropathy is the leading cause of end-stage renal disease; it occurs in 20% to 40% of patients with diabetes. In the absence of previously demonstrated macroalbuminuria or microalbuminuria, an annual microalbumin screening test should be performed; it should also be done at the time of diagnosis of type 2 diabetes. Blood pressure and glucose control will slow the progression of nephropathy. ACE inhibitors delay the progression from microalbuminuria to macroalbuminuria and can slow the decline in the GFR in patients with macroalbuminuria.

## Neuropathies and Foot Care

Diabetic neuropathy is a microvascular complication of diabetes that can lead to foot ulcerations and even lower-limb amputation. Early recognition and management is key. Persons with diabetes for > 10 years, males, those with poor glycemic control, or those with cardiovascular, retinal, or renal complications incur the highest risk. Patients should be educated on proper foot care and have a comprehensive foot examination at least once a year, more frequently if problems are already present. Diabetics are at greater risk for vascular foot ulcers, pressure ulcers, and amputation. Diabetics need special attention to footwear and should be taught to protect their feet. A regular visit to the podiatrist to examine their feet and trim their toenails is important.

Painful peripheral neuropathy from diabetes affects up to 50% of older type 2 diabetic patients. Presentation is as an acute painful sensation, gradual onset numbness, or an asymptomatic foot ulcer. The monofilament pressure perception test, Achilles reflex, and 128-Hz tuning forks are tools useful in diagnosing peripheral neuropathy. Gabapentin and pregabalin are the two most widely used medications for neuropathic pain; gabapentin is often used at much higher daily doses than were initially recommended, but individual patients respond quite differently with respect to pain relief and side effects. Specifically, gabapentin is renally cleared and therefore doses need to be adjusted in patients with chronic kidney disease. Other medications (including adjunctive use of antidepressants) may add to their effectiveness. Podiatry consultation for footwear and physical therapy consultation (for gait training and possible nerve stimulation [e.g., with a transcutaneous nerve stimulator unit]) should also be offered.

Many persons with DM have autonomic neuropathy, which can be detected by examining the failure of the R-R interval to change during the Valsalva maneuver or by the squat test.[14] Persons with autonomic neuropathy often also have a prolonged QTc, and this combination results in a markedly increased risk of arrhythmias, syncope, and sudden death. Many of these diabetics need further investigation with an event monitor and may need insertion of an implantable loop recorder.

## Falls and Fracture

DM is a major cause of faints and falls in older persons.[20] Diabetes has a number of effects that potentially increase falls: gait abnormalities, vision problems, orthostatic hypotension, foot deformities, vestibular abnormalities, altered vibration sense, neuropathy, a decrease in ankle dorsiflexion and step length, muscle weakness, and hypoglycemia. Although patients with type 2 diabetes have greater bone mineral density than those without diabetes, the bone is porous and more fragile; this puts patients with type 2 diabetes at increased risk for developing fractures.[26]

## Cognition

Hyperinsulinemia and both hyperglycemia and hypoglycemia are directly related to declines in memory-related cognitive scores. The risk of Alzheimer dementia directly attributable to hyperinsulinemia or diabetes is as high as 39%.[27] Whether glycemic control decreases cognitive decline is speculative at present. Paradoxically, nasal insulin has been suggested as a treatment for dementia. Regardless, cognitive problems are critical to recognize given the implications for diabetes self-management.

## CASE

### Discussion (Part 3)

Mrs. Sanchez should be encouraged to exercise. She has made great progress. Her $A_{1c}$ has dropped from 8.8 to 7.5 with lifestyle modifications and a low-cost medicine. Overall morbidity and mortality will be prevented by achieving the blood pressure target, which has a greater impact on cardiovascular events than does glycemic control, and is a more powerful influence on microvascular complications. (She has achieved the target of

<140/80 mmHg.) Adding DPP-4 inhibitor (e.g., sitagliptin) or SLT-2 inhibitor would be a consideration in the future because it could improve her $HbA_{1c}$ without producing hypoglycemia.

In addition, ongoing education and reinforcement, recognizing that her skills and even cognition may change over time, with close follow-up with laboratory tests and actual observations of foot and other aspects of her overall care, are crucial to maintaining the current success of her management. You—the primary care provider—will need to actively follow up, with scheduled visits to maintain observation for proteinuria and renal function, orthostasis, falling (often unreported), blood pressure control, and regular eye examinations. Her family members and other caregivers need to know about her illnesses and the need for professional care, because she will need more help with time.

## Summary

Older persons have an increased incidence of diabetes and should be screened yearly for DM with a fasting venous plasma glucose level. Diabetes presents atypically in older individuals. Upon diagnosis of diabetes or prediabetes (formerly called impaired fasting glucose and impaired glucose tolerance), diabetic education, dietary education, exercise, and weight loss are appropriate interventions. Treatment goals for blood glucose in diabetes take into consideration health status, cognitive and physical function, and resources for care. In particular, the provider must work with the patient to balance the benefits of tighter glucose control on macrovascular and microvascular complications with the risk of adverse effects, particularly hypoglycemia. For healthy, high functioning older adults, a goal $HbA_{1C}$ may be < 7.5%, for those with multiple chronic conditions and functional impairment, 8% to 8.5%, and for those with limited life expectancy, ≥ 8.5%. Efforts to reduce diabetes-related mortality should focus on macrovascular complications, including heart disease and stroke. Older diabetics are at particular risk for the geriatric syndromes of persistent pain, urinary incontinence, cognitive impairment, depression, injurious falls, and polypharmacy, and they should be screened for these syndromes within 3 to 6 months of initial diagnosis and regularly thereafter. Older adults with diabetes benefit greatly from person-centered, age-friendly care focused on optimizing function and minimizing adverse events and provided by an interprofessional team that includes the primary care provider, diabetic educators, podiatrists, ophthalmologists, therapists, social workers, nutritionists, and pharmacists.

### Web Resources

Centers for Disease Control National Diabetes Education Program: www.cdc.gov/diabetes/ndep.
American Association of Diabetes Educators: www.diabeteseducator.org.
American Diabetes Association: www.diabetes.org.

## Key References

7. Kilvert A, Fox C. Diagnosis and management of diabetes in older people. *Pract Diabetes.* 2017;34(6):195–199.
9. Lee PG, Halter JB. The pathophysiology of hyperglycemia in older adults: clinical considerations. *Diabetes Care.* 2017; 40(4):444–452.
15. Yang Y, Hu X, Zhang Q, Zou R. Diabetes mellitus and risk of falls in older adults: a sys-tematic review and meta-analysis. *Age Ageing.* 2016;45(6):761–767.
16. Al-Musawe L, Martins AP, Raposo JF, Torre C. The association between polypharmacy and adverse health consequences in elderly type 2 diabetes mellitus patients; a systematic review and meta-analysis. *Diabetes Res Clin Pract.* 2019;155:107804.
19. American Diabetes Association. Older adults: standards of medical care in diabetes—2020. *Diabetes Care.* 43(suppl 1): S152–S162.

***References available online at*** expertconsult.com.

# 42

# Thyroid Disorders

GINA S. FERNANDEZ AND PETER R. DIMILIA

## OBJECTIVES

*Upon completion of this chapter, the reader will be able to:*

- Describe the presentations of hypothyroidism in an older adult population.
- Describe the presentations of hyperthyroidism in an older adult population.
- Define the euthyroid sick syndrome.

- Understand the risks and benefits of thyroid replacement therapy in an older adult population.

## Prevalence and Impact

### Prevalence

Limited data are available on exact prevalence of thyroid dysfunction in older adults.[1] Evidence of hyperthyroidism in older adults has a prevalence rate as high as 3%,[2] with more recent estimates around 1%.[1] Hypothyroidism, including subclinical hypothyroidism, has a prevalence rate of nearly 24% among adults age ≥ 65 years.[1] The reported prevalence of hypothyroidism is 3 times higher among women than men.[3] Abnormal thyroid-stimulating hormone (TSH) values are found in as many as 40% of acutely ill older adult patients.[4] It is important to note that there is a debate regarding clinical significance of elevations of TSH in the older adult population, particularly among the oldest old and acutely ill.[5] Controversy exists about issues as critical as whether having mild thyroid dysfunction may actually have an improved mortality among older persons.

❖ **Abnormal TSH does not mean thyroid disease**.

---

**CASE 1**

**Carol Weise (Part 1)**

Carol Weise is an 86-year-old new patient to your office who presents for a complete evaluation. Initial history is remarkable for mild cognitive impairment, dysthymia, fatigue, and decline in instrumental activity of daily living (IADL) function. Physical examination is remarkable for slowing of deep tendon responses, bradycardia, and slowing of mobility as assessed by the "get up and go" test.
1. What would be appropriate initial screening laboratory test(s)?

---

### Impact

Fluctuations in thyroid hormone function increases with age and some evidence exist that unstable thyroid function in older adults has been associated with increased mortality. Thyroid dysfunction can also lead to suboptimal function of multiple organs and systems. For instance, hypothyroidism may have significant impact on the high rate of mental illness, particularly depression, among older adult persons. Thyroid dysfunction is also significantly related to lipid abnormalities. Lipid levels should be checked in all patients with thyroid underactivity, and thyroid activity should be checked in all patients with elevated cholesterol levels.[5]

Thyroid disorders are more likely to go undiagnosed in patients age > 65 years than in younger populations as hypothyroid and hyperthyroid symptoms are common findings in numerous geriatric syndromes.[6] Hypothyroidism has been associated with a general slowing of mental and physical function, cold intolerance, weight gain, constipation, effects on blood pressure, and anemia. Hyperthyroidism is associated with irregular heart rhythms, congestive heart failure, weight loss, and muscular weakness.[6]

❖ **Thyroid dysfunction must be sought when evaluating depression (and other mental illness) in elders**.

## Risk Factors and Pathophysiology

A negative feedback mechanism exists between the pituitary hormone thyrotropin or TSH and thyroid hormones triiodothyronine (T3) and thyroxine (T4). This mechanism is affected by multiple factors including age. Some evidence suggests that TSH typically increases with age thus mild elevations may not truly relate to thyroid dysfunction, rather a function of normal aging.[7] With age the thyroid gland atrophies, fibrosis occurs, and there is accompanied lymphocytic infiltration, as well as increasing colloid nodular production. Production of T4 decreases with age; however, clearance is also reduced leading to unchanged T4 levels. T3 levels remain unchanged in healthy older subjects.[8] The body's decreased use of thyroid hormone is felt to be related to a decline in lean body mass, including the metabolically active muscle, skin, bone, and viscera.

---

### CASE 1

#### Carol Weise (Part 2)

Ms. Weise is screened for thyroid dysfunction with a serum TSH, and this reveals a TSH of 38 IU/L. This was confirmed by a low T4.
1. Is this patient a clear candidate for thyroid placement?
2. Is this patient likely to have other identifiable symptoms of hypothyroidism on further review?

---

## Hypothyroidism

In the older population, the prevalence of overt hypothyroidism has ranged between 0.2% and 5.7% and subclinical hypothyroidism between 1.5% and 12.5%.[7] Populations at high risk of thyroid dysfunction include people with high levels of radiation exposure, the older adult population, and people with Down syndrome.[9] People with diabetes are also felt to be at high risk of hypothyroid dysfunction.

The most common etiology of hypothyroidism in older adults is Hashimoto disease (a cell-mediated autoimmune inflammatory process with the presence potentially of four different types of thyroid-directed antibodies). It can also result from irradiation, surgical removal of the thyroid gland, and pituitary and hypothalamic disorders leading to TSH deficiencies. Other causes include iodine-induced hypothyroidism most commonly from the use of

medical agents, such amiodarone, potassium iodide, lithium, antithyroid drugs, or radio contrast agents.[5]

See "CASE 1 Discussion."

## Hyperthyroidism

Prevalence in the older adult patient of overt hyperthyroidism is 0.2% to 2%, which is similar to that in the general population.[1] In older adults, similar to the younger population, hyperthyroidism is most likely caused by Grave disease, an autoimmune disorder with antibody formation with TSH-like activity that binds to the TSH receptor and/or thyroid follicular cells. Multinodular goiter and uninodular active goiter are also more common in older adults than in young adults. Other etiologies include granulomatous or lymphocytic thyroiditis, in which there is leakage of thyroglobulin from the follicles. There are also iatrogenic sources of hyperthyroidism, including that induced by substances containing iodine or the use of amiodarone or from the overingestion of thyroid repletion agents.[2]

## Thyroid Nodules/Thyroid Cancer

Prevalence of thyroid nodules increases with age. Radiation is a risk factor for thyroid cancer. However, in the very old if that exposure was > 50 years ago, there is no indication of higher risk of cancer.[10] Papillary thyroid cancer is more common in older adults, as is anaplastic carcinoma, the most fatal histologic type of thyroid carcinoma. In 2020, thyroid cancer will represent an estimated 4.4% of all new cancer cases among women and 1.4% among men.[11]

## Differential Diagnosis and Assessment

---

### CASE 2

#### Grace Palmer

Grace Palmer is a 79-year-old woman evaluated in your office for mild dysthymia. She has a history of hypertension, glaucoma, and osteoarthritis. She has recently lost her husband of 56 years. As part of your evaluation, you check serum TSH, which is 9.7 IU/L. You order a T4 test, which is at the lower end of the normal range.
1. Is Ms. Palmer suffering from hypothyroidism?
2. Would Ms. Palmer benefit from thyroid replacement?

---

### CASE 2

#### Discussion

Ms. Palmer most likely is suffering from bereavement. The low-normal T4 and the relatively mild elevation of TSH are consistent with subclinical hypothyroidism, and many of these patients do not progress to clinical hypothyroidism. Exposing her to thyroid replacement may not be beneficial.

---

## Subclinical Hypothyroidism

The syndrome of subclinical hypothyroidism is a relevant differential from symptomatic hypothyroidism in the older adult population. Debate is currently ongoing regarding the benefits or possible risks of treating subclinical hypothyroidism. Subclinical hypothyroidism is defined by a normal serum-free T4 level combined with an elevation of the TSH level (commonly but arbitrarily defined as > 4.5 mIU/L).[9] The transition from subclinical to overt hypothyroidism is not inevitable and may only occur in 5% to 8% of the population with subclinical hypothyroidism on an annual basis.[12] However, a recent study indicated that compared with euthyroid participants, participants with subclinical thyroid dysfunction were 10- and 16-fold more likely to develop overt hypothyroidism and hyperthyroidism, respectively.[13] Levels of TSH above 10 mIU/L are considered to be clearly abnormal and typically needs treatment with levothyroxine. Those between 4.5 mIU/L and 10 mIU/L are considered to be of uncertain significance in the absence of any symptoms or signs of hypothyroidism and treatment with levothyroxine remains controversial.[9] One study has indicated potential detrimental effects of treatment of subclinical hypothyroidism by actually shortening survival.[14] Other studies have indicated a survival advantage in patients with higher TSH levels; studies indicate if TSH elevated and T4 in low normal T4 levels had better survival.[15] Further, recent randomized controlled trial evaluated levothyroxine treatment in older adults with subclinical hypothyroidism and found no consistent beneficial effect of treatment on thyroid-related symptoms after 12 months.[16]

## Hypothyroidism

There are a multitude of relatively nonspecific symptoms of hypothyroidism (Box 42.1). It is important to note that older adult patients have significantly fewer symptoms with hypothyroidism than do their younger counterparts. The complaints are often subtle, vague, and (if present) more likely to be misattributed to an age-biased view of normal aging or other comorbid conditions.[7] Clearly a high index of suspicion for hypothyroidism is indicated in evaluation of the geriatric patient.

## Screening of the Asymptomatic Patient

There are various recommendation guidelines for screening asymptomatic, well, older adults. The American Academy of Family Physicians and the American Association of Clinical Endocrinologists recommends to measure thyroid function periodically in all older

---

**• BOX 42.1  Symptoms of Hypothyroidism**

Probably less common in elders:
Fatigue
Weakness
Depression
Dry skin
Significantly less common in elders:
Weight gain
Cold intolerance
Muscle cramps
Parasthesias
   Libido
   Appetite
   Arthralgias
   Confusion
   Constipation
   Brittle nails
   Loss of hair
   Easy bruisability
   Low back discomfort

(Modified from Ingbar SH. The thyroid gland. In: Wilson JD, Foster DW. *Williams Textbook of Endocrinology.* 7th ed. Philadelphia: WB Saunders Company 1985:682–815.)

---

adults, especially women.[5] The American College of Physicians recommends screening women age > 50 years with one or more general symptoms that could be caused by thyroid disease.[17] The American Thyroid Association recommends screening in older adult patients and all patients with autoimmune disease or with a strong family history of thyroid disease. Further, the American Thyroid Association and American Association of Clinical Endocrinologists jointly recommend considering screening in asymptomatic older adults.[5] The Canadian Task Force on Periodic Health Examination recommends maintaining a high index of clinical suspicion for nonspecific symptoms presenting with hypothyroidism (Box 42.2), but recommends against screening for thyroid dysfunction in asymptomatic adults.[18] The US Preventive Services Task Force (USPSTF) did not find sufficient evidence to recommend screening in asymptomatic older adult women; however, they advise a high index of suspicion of low threshold for checking thyroid function in the at-risk population.[9] Care must be used in the screening of patients who are otherwise ill, as a substantial portion will have abnormal thyroid function in the absence of true thyroid disease owing to euthyroid sick syndrome.

Regarding screening for thyroid cancer, at this time there is no clearly defined screening mechanism that increases the benefit by providing early detection with significant differential treatment outcomes. Palpation of the thyroid gland remains part of good clinical practice and routine examination, although there is not high-quality evidence to conclude that regular neck palpation could have a major effect on the natural history of this infrequent cancer. According to the USPSTF, there is inadequate evidence to estimate the accuracy of neck palpation and use of thyroid ultrasound as a screening test for asymptomatic individuals. The task force hence recommends against screening for thyroid cancer in adults who do not have symptoms except in patients with a high risk of thyroid cancer, such as those who were exposed to radiation to the head or neck in the past.[19,20]

◆◆ **Ill patients may have the euthyroid sick syndrome: abnormal thyroid function, but *not* true thyroid disease.**

---

**• BOX 42.2  Clinical Conditions With Clear Indication for Thyroid Dysfunction Screening**

Depression
Down syndrome
Postpartum depression
Women with family history of autoimmune disease
Hyperlipidemia

---

**CASE 3**

**Andrew Taylor**

Andrew Taylor is a long-term patient of yours and presents for his routine physical and well-adult care update in the fall. In addition to requesting his flu vaccination, he reports the following nonspecific symptoms: slowed mentation, diarrhea, and weight loss. His daughter reports as well he has decreased appetite. On examination, he has a blood pressure of 142/86 mm Hg, pulse 88 beats per minute, respiratory 20 breaths/min, and temperature 37.0° C. Testing reveals a Mini-Mental State Examination of 22/30 and a global deterioration scale of 5/15. The physical examination is otherwise unremarkable. Your evaluation includes a TSH of 0.2 mIU/L and an elevated T4 on repeat examination; you suspect his thyroid gland may be enlarged without discrete nodule.
1. What further studies would you consider?
2. Are his clinical findings consistent with hyperthyroidism?

## Hyperthyroidism

Less than 35% of hyperthyroid patients age >65 years present with atypical symptoms.[10] Like younger patients, two-thirds present with symptoms of tachycardia, goiter, and eye symptomology. Older patients are more likely to present with relative tachycardia, weight loss, apathy, and fatigue as primary symptoms. Diarrhea and sweating are also far less common presenting symptoms in older individuals. Instead, older patients often have persistent constipation. Likewise, a sense of agitation or anxiety is less commonly reported in older persons. It has been reported that the tremor is as likely to appear in both age groups (Box 42.3).

---

**• BOX 42.3    Symptoms and Signs of Hyperthyroidism**

Tachycardia[a,b]
Fatigue[a]
Weight loss[a]
Tremor
Atrial fibrillation
Anorexia
Nervousness

[a] This triad presents in more than 50% (From Cavalieri RR. The effects of nonthyroid disease and drugs on thyroid function tests. *Med Clin North Am*. 1991;75(1):27–39.
[b] Clinical suspicion should be raised at heart rates 90 beats per minute or greater in older persons.

---

Older adult patients are likely to have both heart failure and the possibility of angina at time of presentation, and as many as 27% will present with atrial fibrillation.[2] Hyperthyroidism in older adults can be complicated by depression, myopathy, and osteoporosis. But the most dangerous complication is clearly thyroid storm. The elder person with thyroid storm may be at greater risk for death from the fever, tachycardia, nausea, vomiting, mental status changes, and heart complications. Assessment is still best done initially with the serum TSH.

**CASE 4**

**Matthew Dillon**

Matthew Dillon is a 74-year-old man who was recently admitted to the hospital for an acute right middle cerebral artery distribution cerebrovascular accident complicated by congestive heart failure and acute renal insufficiency. He was noted to have a slowing of cognition and was assessed with a TSH, as well as other tests for reversible causes of functional decline.
1. If the TSH is elevated, can you conclude Mr. Dillon has hypothyroidism?
2. How long would it be reasonable to wait after his episode of acute illness before reassessment of TSH?

## Nonthyroidal Illness Syndrome (Euthyroid Sick Syndrome)

Abnormalities in thyroid function tests can occur in the setting of critical illness. Many will have low concentration of T3 with normal to low concentrations of TSH and T4, an entity currently termed as nonthyroidal illness syndrome. Previously, these patients were believed to be euthyroid, hence the term "euthyroid sick syndrome." Current evidence, however, suggests that critically ill individuals may undergo a transient state of thyroid dysfunction characterized by a central suppression of the thyroid hormone that can affect adaption during periods of severe physiologic stress and survival.[21] It is uncertain if treatment of this entity is beneficial, and hypothyroidism should only be diagnosed in a patient with acute illness when there is an evaluation of T4 and suppression of TSH,[5] which does not normalize within 2 weeks after the resolution of the acute medical or psychiatric illness.

## Management

**CASE 1**

**Carol Weise (Part 3)**

Ms. Weise agreed to initiation or replacement therapy and has no significant coronary artery disease (CAD).
1. What would be a reasonable starting dose of L–T4?

**CASE 1**

**Discussion**

Ms. Weise has clinical hypothyroidism. TSH is the most appropriate screening test. As she has symptomatic hypothyroidism, she would benefit from replacement of thyroid hormone with low-dose Levo T4. Once clinically suspected, more symptoms/signs attributable to hypothyroidism are likely to be appreciated.

## Hypothyroidism

Overt hypothyroidism with symptoms is treated by careful repletion of thyroid hormone with synthetic thyroid. It is important to assess for the possibility of CAD. In situations of high risk for CAD and potential for long-standing hypothyroidism, a stress cardiac imaging study is appropriate before reinitiating a normal metabolic rate. As with other geriatric pharmacology, starting low and going slow is clearly appropriate. A starting dose of 12.5 to 25 mcg per day is appropriate. The dosage should be increased every 6 weeks. It is rare to require doses greater than 75 to 125 mcg per day in an older person. Treatment goal is to restore T4 to the normal range and TSH to the upper range of normal. These goals have to be tempered by coexisting cardiovascular disease. Over time, dosage may need to be decreased. Of particular note is the risk of overtreatment leading to osteoporosis in women.

▸▸ **With a high CAD risk and potentially long-standing hypothyroidism, do a stress test before treatment; and always "start low, go slow."**

## Subclinical Hypothyroidism

As previously described, it is currently debated as to whether or not treatment should be instituted for levels between 4.5 mIU/L and 10 mIU/L without clear evidence of symptoms. Most important is to analyze and monitor for the appearance of true clinical hypothyroidism or an elevation into more clearly defined ranges of TSH.

## Hyperthyroidism

Cases owing to diffusely overactive thyroid or hyperfunctioning nodule(s) are optimally treated with antithyroid medications propylthiouracil and methimazole. There is also a role for beta-blockade to improve symptomatic treatment, before the antithyroid medication restoring the patient to the euthyroid function. After a period of stabilization, radioactive iodine can be used for definitive treatment. After radioactive iodine treatment, the patient must be monitored for the appearance of hypothyroidism. In the case of possible underlying malignancies, surgical options may be entertained. In the case of inflammatory disease, the etiology of hyperthyroidism tends to spontaneously resolve over weeks to months but may require temporizing symptomatic treatment for relief. This is accomplished with a cautious use of beta-blockade. Of note in severe cases of inflammation, there may be a period of hypothyroidism after the acute event that may temporarily require thyroid replacement. Subclinical hyperthyroidism is estimated to occur in 0.8% to 2% of older individuals and is believed to uncommonly lead to full-blown hyperthyroidism.[2]

## Summary

Hypothyroidism, including subclinical hypothyroidism, has a prevalence rate of nearly 24% among adults age 65 and older. The reported prevalence of hypothyroidism is three times higher among women than men. The most common cause of hypothyroidism is previous Hashimoto's disease. Hyperthyroidism is less common in older adults and is most likely due to Graves' disease. Thyroid dysfunction can lead to suboptimal function of multiple organs and systems. Thyroid disorders are more likely to go undiagnosed in patients over the age of 65 than in younger populations as hypothyroid and hyperthyroid symptoms are common findings in numerous geriatric syndromes. Hypothyroidism has been associated with a general slowing of mental and physical function, cold intolerance, weight gain, constipation, effects on blood pressure, and anemia. Hyperthyroidism is associated with irregular heart rhythms, congestive heart failure, weight loss, and muscular weakness.

## Key References

2. Samuels MH. *Hyperthyroidism in Aging*. South Dartmouth, MA: MDText.com, Inc.; 2018.
4. Finucane P, Rudra T, Church H, et al. Thyroid function tests in elderly patients with and without an acute illness. *Age Ageing*. 1989;18(6):398−402.
5. Garber JR, Cobin RH, Gharib H, et al. Clinical practice guidelines for hypothyroidism in adults: cosponsored by the American Association of Clinical Endocrinologists and the American Thyroid Association. *Endocr Pract*. 2012;18(6):988−1028.
13. Roberts L, McCahon D, Johnson O, Haque MS, Parle J, Hobbs FR. Stability of thyroid function in older adults: the Birmingham Elderly Thyroid Study. *Br J Gen Pract*. 2018;68(675):e718−e726.
16. Stott DJ, Rodondi N, Kearney PM, et al. Thyroid hormone therapy for older adults with subclinical hypothyroidism. *N Engl J Med*. 2017;376(26):2534−2544.

**References available online at** expertconsult.com.

# 43

# Osteoporosis

RICHARD HSANG-YOUNG LEE AND WANDA COOK LAKEY

## OUTLINE

*Additional online-only material indicated by icon.*

## OBJECTIVES

*Upon completion of this chapter, the reader will be able to:*

- Estimate the risk of fracture among those with osteoporosis and those with previous fracture.
- Identify risk factors for osteoporosis and fracture, including medications and medical comorbidities.
- Identify individuals who should be evaluated/screened for osteoporosis and who should be treated with pharmacologic agents.

- Determine when calcium and vitamin D supplementation or other nonpharmacologic therapies are required.
- Describe the available pharmacologic treatments for osteoporosis, including contraindications and potential adverse effects.

---

## CASE

### Lily Stephens (Part 1)

Ms. Lily Stephens is a 66-year-old female with history of breast cancer, diabetes, hypertension, hyperlipidemia, and osteoarthritis who presents to your primary care office after she fell and sprained her wrist. She tripped over the curb while walking in the parking lot, braced her fall with her left hand, and felt an immediate pain after landing. She went to the emergency room nearby; fortunately, x-rays showed no bone fractures. She was placed in a splint, which she has been wearing for the past 2 weeks. The swelling has gone down, and the pain is getting better. However, she is concerned that next time she will break her wrist.

1. Does Ms. Stephens have any risk factors associated with osteoporosis and fractures?
2. What key questions should be obtained from her personal and family history?
3. Are there key physical examination findings that would suggest the presence of osteoporosis?

## Definition and Epidemiology

Osteoporosis is a systemic skeletal disease characterized by decreases in bone quality and bone mineral density (BMD) that result in decreased strength of the bones and the increased risk of bone fractures. Osteoporotic fractures typically occur with minimal or no trauma, most notably of the hip, spine, and wrist. However, in the absence of fracture, osteoporosis is often an asymptomatic condition. Because of this, the World Health Organization (WHO) developed diagnostic criteria for osteoporosis based on bone density measurement. In postmenopausal women and men age $> 50$ years, osteoporosis is defined as a T-score of $\leq 2.5$ standard deviations below the mean of a young reference group. Similarly, osteopenia in this group is defined as a T-score between $-1.0$ and $-2.5$. For the femoral neck and total hip regions, the International Society for Clinical Densitometry recommends using the young, female Caucasian reference group derived from the National Health and Nutrition Examination Study III cohort data, which are included on most commercial bone density machines.[1]

There are over 8.9 million fractures annually worldwide because of osteoporosis.[2,3] In the United States, the population with osteoporosis has been estimated to be 25 million persons, including 1 in 4 women and 1 in 20 men age > 65 years. There are approximately 300,000 hip fractures annually in the United States in older adults. More than 95% are caused by falls. The incidence of hip fractures is greater among women compared with men (78 vs. 56 per 100,000 at age 60 years).[4] Risks of major osteoporotic fractures and hip fractures are greatest among White persons compared with other racial and ethnic groups.[5]

Osteoporosis and osteoporotic fractures are associated with significant morbidity and mortality. Within 5 years of an initial fracture, 24% of women and 20% of men will sustain another fracture. Osteoporotic fractures lead to significant functional limitations, requirement for increased assistance with activities of daily living, and placement in skilled facilities. Estimates of the cost of osteoporosis and fractures in the United States are over $16 billion annually. Furthermore, the 5-year mortality among older adults after an incident fracture is 39% among women and 51% among men. After a hip fracture, older adults have a five- to eightfold increased risk for all-cause mortality during the first 3 months.[6] Although the incidence of hip fracture is greater in women, the excess mortality from hip fracture is significantly greater among men.

## Pathophysiology and Risk Factors

Peak bone mass is the maximum bone accrued by 18 to 25 years of age. The ability to reach peak bone mass is affected by multiple factors, including genetics, general health, nutrition, physical activity, medications, alcohol ingestion, and cigarette smoking.[7] Balanced remodeling maintains healthy bone by resorption of old bone via osteoclasts and formation of new bone by osteoblasts.[8] When bone remodeling becomes skewed toward accelerated bone removal without subsequent replacement of new bone, there is a reduction in the mass of the remaining bone. Aging, menopause, and hypogonadism are known risk factors for accelerated bone loss. Fracture risk increases when the microarchitecture of bone is altered and weakened from age-related bone loss or other risk factors (Fig. 43.1).

A number of conditions have been associated with low bone density and increased fracture risk. These include lifestyle, genetic factors, medical conditions, and medications (Table 43.1). Falls increase the risk of fractures. Multiple factors increase the risk of falls.[7,9] Environmental risk factors include poor lighting, tripping hazards, slippery environments, and lack of assistive devices in the bathroom. Sedating medications can impair cognition and coordination. Malnutrition and dehydration can cause loss of strength and imbalance. Additional medical risk factors for falls include age, poor vision, depression and anxiety, arrhythmias, urinary incontinence, and vitamin D [25(OH)D] insufficiency impairing muscle strength and function. Neurologic and musculoskeletal abnormalities also increase the risk of falls. These include diminished proprioception, deconditioning, poor balance, impaired transfer and mobility, sarcopenia, and kyphosis.

## Assessment and Differential Diagnosis

### History and Physical

A thorough history should be performed to identify and assess for risk factors for osteoporosis and fractures, such as a history of frequent falls. Self-reported height loss of > 3 cm has been found to have a positive likelihood ratio of 3.2 and negative likelihood ratio of 0.4.[10] Additional history should include family history of osteoporosis, metabolic bone disease, or low trauma fractures, especially in regard to history of parental hip fractures.[11] Medical history should include tobacco and alcohol use, as well as history of medication exposures, radiation therapy, and chronic medical conditions.[7] A dietary history should include intake of dairy products or calcium-containing foods, as well as dietary restrictions, such as lactose intolerance.

The physical examination should focus on factors related to risk of fracture. For example, height and objective signs of height loss should be assessed. Nearly two-thirds of radiographic vertebral fractures do not present clinically. Occult vertebral fractures are suggested with decreased rib-pelvis distance. A rib-pelvis distance of < 2 finger-breadths between the inferior margin of the ribs and the superior surface of the pelvis in the midaxillary line is associated with a positive likelihood ratio of 3.2 and negative likelihood ratio of 0.6.[10] Similarly, the inability to touch the occiput to the wall when standing with back and heels to the wall has been associated with a positive likelihood ratio of 4.6 and negative likelihood ratio of 0.5. Other factors in the physical examination associated with osteoporosis include weight < 51 kg, presence of kyphosis, and grip strength. Also it is important to assess for risk of falls in the clinical examination, including gait assessment and timed get-up-and-go.

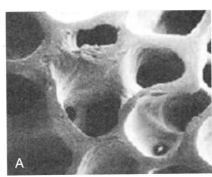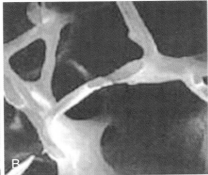

• **Figure 43.1** Micrographs of normal (A) versus osteoporotic (B) bone. (From National Osteoporosis Foundation. Physicians' guide to prevention and treatment of osteoporosis. http://www.nof.org.)

## TABLE 43.1 Risk Factors and Medications Associated With Osteoporosis and Fractures

**Lifestyle Factors**

| | | |
|---|---|---|
| Alcohol abuse | Frequent Falling | Immobilization |
| Smoking (active or passive) | Inadequate physical activity | Excessive thinness |
| Low calcium intake | Vitamin D insufficiency | |

**Hypogonadal States**

| | | |
|---|---|---|
| Hyperprolactinemia | Panhypopituitarism | Androgen insensitivity |
| Premature menopause | Mumps orchitis | Anorexia nervosa |

**Endocrine Disorders**

| | | |
|---|---|---|
| Hyperparathyroidism | Thyrotoxicosis | Diabetes mellitus |
| Adrenal insufficiency | Cushing syndrome | |

**Gastrointestinal Disorders**

| | | |
|---|---|---|
| Celiac disease | Inflammatory bowel disorder | Primary biliary cirrhosis |
| Gastric bypass | Malabsorption syndromes | Pancreatic insufficiency |

**Hematological Disorders**

| | | |
|---|---|---|
| Multiple myeloma | Thalassemia | Monoclonal gammopathies |
| Sickle cell disease | Leukemia and lymphomas | |

**Rheumatic Disorders**

| | | |
|---|---|---|
| Rheumatoid arthritis | Systemic lupus | Sarcoidosis |
| Ankylosing spondylitis | | |

**Neurologic Disorders**

| | | |
|---|---|---|
| Epilepsy | Multiple sclerosis | Stoke |
| Parkinson disease | Spinal cord injury | |

**Other Conditions**

| | | |
|---|---|---|
| AIDS/HIV | End-stage renal disease | Depression |
| Chronic obstructive lung disease | Posttransplant | Weight loss |
| Congestive heart failure | Hypercalciuria | |

**Medications**

| | | |
|---|---|---|
| Glucocorticoids | Anticonvulsants | Heparin |
| Aromatase inhibitors | Thiazolidinediones | Lithium |
| Depomedroxyprogesterone | Selective serotonin reuptake inhibitors | GnRH (gonadotropin-releasing hormone) agonists |

(Modified from Office of the Surgeon General (US) (2004) Bone health and osteoporosis: a report of the Surgeon General. Office of the Surgeon General (US), Rockville (MD). Available from: http://www.ncbi.nlm.nih.gov/books/NBK45513/. Accessed March 2014.)
*AIDS,* Acquired immunodeficiency syndrome; *HIV,* human immunodeficiency virus.

❖❖ Common examination findings of osteoporosis include height loss >4 cm, rib-pelvis distance <2 finger-breadths, and inability to touch the occiput to the wall when standing with heels to the wall.

### CASE

#### Lily Stephens (Part 2)

Ms. Stephens's mother had broken her hip in her 80s. Ms. Stephens was diagnosed with breast cancer 4 years ago and had a lumpectomy. She has been taking letrozole for the past 3 years to prevent breast cancer recurrence. She has had diabetes for about 12 years and takes metformin and glipizide. Her other medications include lisinopril, hydrochlorothiazide for hypertension, atorvastatin for cholesterol, and a low-dose aspirin daily. She exercises regularly, does not smoke, and drinks alcohol only occasionally. She reports only one fall this past December on icy pavement at her sister's house. She reports no height loss.

She is 5'4" and weighs 152 lbs. She walks without an assistive device. Her blood pressure is 132/88 mmHg, pulse is 89 beats per minute. She has some decreased sensation to monofilament on exam. Her gait is mildly antalgic but with a narrow base.

1. What are potential secondary causes of low BMD or osteoporosis that should be considered?
2. What laboratory tests and imaging modalities should be done to assess Ms. Stephens's current state of bone health?

## Laboratory and Radiologic Testing

Common laboratory tests performed during the evaluation of osteoporosis are found in Table 43.2. Laboratory testing is used to differentiate osteoporosis from other causes of low bone density or metabolic bone disease. An elevated serum calcium with elevated parathyroid hormone level may indicate primary hyperparathyroidism. An elevated alkaline phosphatase level with focal uptake on bone scan is consistent with Paget disease. A low 25-hydroxyvitamin D level may indicate osteomalacia. Measurement of bone turnover markers (BTM), such as urinary N-telopeptide (NTX) and procollagen type 1 N-terminal propetide (P1NP), may also be considered. These tests assess the bone remodeling process and may predict fracture risk and treatment response.[12,13] However, variability both in BTM levels intrinsically throughout the day and in test characteristics have limited their clinical utility (see further discussion later).

The National Osteoporosis Foundation (NOF) and International \Society of Clinical Densitometry (ISCD) recommend BMD screening for women age >65 years and for postmenopausal women age <65 years or women during the menopausal transition with clinical risk factors, such as low body weight, prior fracture, use of high-risk medications (e.g., corticosteroids), or conditions associated with bone loss (e.g., rheumatoid arthritis).[1,7] The ISCD also recommends BMD screening in men age >70 years and men age <70 years with clinical risk factors. Similarly, current recommendations from the US Preventative Services Task Force (USPSTF) suggest screening for osteoporosis among older women age 65 years and among postmenopausal women younger than 65 years who have significant fracture risk based on formal clinical risk assessment tools.[14] However, the USPSTF does not recommend screening in men.

## TABLE 43.2   Laboratories for Evaluation of Low Bone Density and Osteoporosis

| Laboratory Testing for Secondary Causes of Osteoporosis | |
| --- | --- |
| **Blood or Serum** | **Urine** |
| Complete blood count (CBC) | 24-hour urinary calcium, creatinine |
| Chemistry levels (calcium, renal function, phosphorus, and magnesium) | Bone turnover markers: NTX |
| Liver function tests | |
| Thyroid-stimulating hormone (TSH) ± free T4 | |
| 25-hydroxyvitamin D | |
| Parathyroid hormone (PTH) | |
| Bone turnover markers: CTX, P1NP, bone-specific alkaline phosphatase | |
| **Consider in selected patients** | |
| Serum protein electrophoresis (SPEP), serum immunofixation, serum-free light chains | Urine protein electrophoresis (UPEP) |
| Tissue transglutaminase antibodies (IgA and IgG) | Urinary free cortisol level |
| Iron and ferritin levels | Urinary histamine |
| Homocysteine | |
| Total testosterone and gonadotropin | |
| Prolactin | |
| Tryptase | |

(Modified from Cosman F, de Beur SJ, LeBoff MS, et al. Clinician's guide to prevention and treatment of osteoporosis. *Osteoporos Int.* 2014;25(10):2359–2381.)
*CTX,* Carboxy-terminal collagen crosslinks; *Ig,* immunoglobulin; *NTX,* urinary N-telopeptide.

Common clinical risk assessment tools for identifying individuals to screen include SCORE, ORAI, the fracture risk assessment tool (FRAX), and the osteoporosis self-assessment tool (OST).[15–18] The OST is an index calculated from a person's age and weight designed to identify those individuals at increased risk of fracture who would benefit from osteoporosis screening. The tool has been validated in multiple populations, including White women, men, Asian women, and Black persons. The most widely used fracture assessment tool is FRAX. Developed by WHO, FRAX is a computer-based algorithm that uses clinical risk factors to estimate 10-year fracture risk of major osteoporotic fractures and hip fractures. FRAX can be used with or without data from BMD assessment. In the Screening in the Community to Reduce Fractures in Older Women study, 12,483 women age 70 to 85 years living in the United Kingdom were randomized to screening based on calculated FRAX risk or usual care.[19] In the screening group, those with a 10-year probability of hip fracture greater than an established screening threshold based on age were referred to dual-energy x-ray absorptiometry (DXA) screening. Results of the study did not show a reduction in the primary outcome of incidence of all osteoporosis-related fractures (hazard ratio [HR] 0.94, 95% confidence interval [CI], 0.85–1.03, $P = .178$); however, screening did reduce the incidence of hip fractures (HR 0.72, CI 0.59–0.89, $P = .002$).

Because up to two-thirds of morphometric vertebral fractures do not present clinically, the ISCD recommends that x-rays of the spine or vertebral fracture assessment (VFA) be considered to exclude occult fractures.[20] VFA uses the same DXA technology for BMD assessment to image the thoracic and lumbar vertebrae. Alternatively, plain x-rays of the vertebrae should be performed to assess for occult fractures. Other radiologic testing to assess BMD includes quantitative ultrasound, quantitative computed tomography (CT), and high-resolution peripheral quantitative CT; however, these modalities have limited clinical use and are typically used for research purposes.

## Management

In the United States, the NOF recommends pharmacologic therapy in individuals who (1) have sustained a hip or vertebral fracture (clinical or morphometric), (2) have BMD T-scores $\leq -2.5$, or (3) have BMD T-scores between $-1.0$ and $-2.5$ and a 10-year probability of hip fracture $> 3\%$ or 10-year probability of major osteoporotic fracture $> 20\%$. Most fractures occur in those with osteopenia or BMD T-scores between $-1.0$ and $-2.5$. Therefore fracture risk assessment with FRAX has been recommended to further identify those individuals at increased fracture risk who should be treated for low bone density. FRAX has become the most widely used clinical algorithm for fracture risk estimation, although a number of limitations remain. The duration and dose of tobacco use and corticosteroid use are important determinants of fracture risk. However, the quantification of these risks are not included in the FRAX algorithm. Also FRAX incorporates BMD from the femoral neck using DXA. However, DXA assessment includes measurement at the lumbar spine and total hip, which are not included in the FRAX algorithm. Finally, there are a number of medical conditions that impact fracture risk independent of BMD that are not included in FRAX. These include type 2 diabetes mellitus and frequent falls. Other validated fracture risk calculators also exist. For example, the Garvan calculator uses data from the longitudinal study of the population in Dubbo in southern Australia. This calculator includes falls frequency, as well as number of prior fractures.

◆◆ **Management of osteoporosis depends on history of hip and/or vertebral fracture, T-score on bone density, and/or absolute fracture risk assessment.**

### CASE

#### Lily Stephens (Part 3)

Lily Stephens returns to clinic after completing her diagnostic evaluations. Her chemistry panel shows calcium 8.9 mg/dL with albumin 3.8 mg/dL. Her creatinine is 0.9 mg/dL. Her thyroid-stimulating hormone (TSH), parathyroid hormone (PTH), and alkaline phosphatase levels are within the normal range. Her 25(OH)D level is 19. DXA results: L-spine T = −2.2; total hip T = −1.9, femoral neck T = −2.0; 1/3-radius T-score = −2.0. She does not drink milk and does not like dairy foods because she develops gastrointestinal upset. She asks if she should make any changes to her diet or multivitamin.

1. Do guidelines support the addition of calcium and/or vitamin D supplements?
2. What nondairy items could she consume to increase her amount of dietary calcium?
3. Would a clinical risk assessment tool be useful to predict the future risk of a fracture?

## Nonpharmacologic Therapy

There are several nonpharmacologic therapies and interventions that can be used alone or in conjunction with US Food and Drug Administration (FDA)–approved osteoporosis drugs, including optimal nutrition, supplementation with calcium and vitamin D, exercise, and falls prevention. Maintaining adequate caloric intake with a balanced diet throughout an individual's lifetime is imperative to build and maintain healthy bone density. Ideally, dietary intake of calcium and vitamin D should meet the recommended daily intake to reach peak bone mass in young adults. Calcium-containing food items include dairy products, vegetables (broccoli, kale, collard greens), fruit (oranges, figs, raisins), grains, legumes, seafood (salmon, sardines, shrimp), poultry, and eggs. The Institute of Medicine (IOM) recommends 1000 mg of calcium per day for adult females 19 to 50 years of age, with an increase to 1200 mg per day for females 51 years of age or older because of the decrease in bone density related to menopause.[21] The IOM recommends adult males consume 1000 mg of calcium per day until 70 years of age, with an increase to 1200 mg after 70 years of age. Some metaanalyses have demonstrated a weak association between calcium supplementation and an increased risk in cardiovascular events, but this has not been a consistent finding.[22–24] For this reason, obtaining the recommended daily calcium intake from the diet when possible is advised.

Few food items are significant sources of vitamin D. These include fatty fish (salmon, tuna, mackerel), fish liver oils, cheese, beef liver, and egg yolks. Most dietary sources of vitamin D are from fortified foods. The IOM recommends a daily intake of vitamin D of 600 IU for males and females 19 to 70 years or age and 800 IU for males and females age > 70 years. For diets that do not meet the recommended daily intake of calcium and vitamin D, supplementation should be initiated. Consuming higher than recommended daily intakes of calcium and vitamin D can be associated with adverse effects, such as hypercalcemia, hypercalciuria, nephrolithiasis, and constipation.[25–27]

Calcium and vitamin D supplements are frequently used for primary prevention of osteoporosis or treatment for osteoporosis as adjunctive therapy to FDA-approved medications or standalone therapy. However, randomized-controlled trials and metaanalyses demonstrate inconsistent data on fracture reduction with calcium and vitamin D supplementation that may not be generalizable to the entire population.[25,28,29] The USPSTF has reviewed the use of calcium and vitamin D supplementation, alone or in combination, for primary prevention of fractures in community-dwelling, asymptomatic adults.[30] Because of insufficient data to analyze the risks and benefits, the USPSTF was unable to provide recommendations for calcium and vitamin D supplementation in men and premenopausal women. The data were also insufficient to evaluate the risks and benefits of daily vitamin D doses > 400 IU and calcium doses > 1000 mg in postmenopausal women. The USPSTF does not recommend daily vitamin D supplementation for postmenopausal women, as supported by a recent USPSTF metaanalysis of 11 RCTs that did not find a reduction in fractures associated with vitamin D supplementation or a combination of vitamin D and calcium supplementation in community-dwelling adults age ≥ 50 years.[31] However, there are important caveats to consider related to the USPSTF conclusions and recommendations. These do not apply to individuals in a nursing home or other care settings. In addition, the conclusions and recommendations are not applicable to individuals with a known diagnosis of osteoporosis or osteoporotic fractures, vitamin D deficiency, or an increased risk of falls. Despite the debate regarding whether calcium intake can prevent the accelerated bone loss associated with menopause, the IOM believes that avoiding inadequate calcium ingestion by following their recommended daily intake of calcium can avoid exacerbating the bone

loss. The Endocrine Society also supports calcium, preferably from dietary sources, and vitamin D in specific situations. The Endocrine Society recommends calcium and vitamin D for postmenopausal women with osteoporosis as adjunct therapies for individuals at an increased risk of fractures and as primary therapy for hip fracture prevention in individuals at an increased risk of fracture who are unable to tolerate FDA-approved osteoporosis drugs.

The US Surgeon General recommends regular physical activity equivalent to 150 minutes of moderate-intensity aerobic activity (brisk walking) or 75 minutes of vigorous-intensity activity or a combination of both per week for adults.[32] For older adults at risk for falls, balance training at least 3 times per week is also recommended. In older adults, a combination of weight-bearing aerobic and muscle-strengthening exercises can decrease the risk of falls. Improvements in balance, posture, muscle tone, and strength most likely contribute to the reduction in falls. In addition, exercise training programs have demonstrated modest improvements in bone density in both men and postmenopausal women.[33,34]

In addition to weight-bearing and muscle-strength training exercises, additional fall prevention measures may help reduce the risk of falls and subsequent fractures.[35] These include correction of visual impairments, maintenance of adequate nutrition and vitamin D levels, avoiding dehydration, removal of tripping hazards (loose rugs, cords), dose reduction or discontinuation of sedating medications, improved lighting, and addition of assistive devices in bathrooms. A home safety assessment by an occupational therapist may help identify additional individual risks for falls.

⬥⬥ **Essential nonpharmacologic elements of a fracture prevention plan include exercise, adequate intake of calcium and vitamin D, and falls prevention.**

## Pharmacologic Therapies

There are a number of osteoporosis drugs approved by the FDA for postmenopausal osteoporosis, male osteoporosis, and corticosteroid-induced osteoporosis (Table 43.3). These drugs are divided by their mechanism of action as anabolic or antiresorptive medications according to the principle cell type they affect (osteoblast vs. osteoclast).

### Antiresorptive Agents

The most widely prescribed medications for osteoporosis are the bisphosphonates. The oral bisphosphonates include alendronate, risedronate, and ibandronate. Bisphosphonates work by inhibiting osteoclastic activity and therefore slowing the remodeling process and thus increasing BMD. In the Fracture Intervention Trial, 2027 postmenopausal women with prevalent vertebral fracture and/or low BMD (approximately T-score < −2.0 at the femoral neck) were randomized to alendronate equivalent to 70 mg weekly or placebo.[36] In those treated with alendronate, there was a 55% relative risk reduction in clinical vertebral fractures with an absolute risk reduction of 2.7%. There was also a 51% reduction in hip fractures and 48% reduction in wrist fractures. Similarly, in the Vertebral Efficacy with Risedronate Trial of 2458 postmenopausal women with prevalent vertebral fracture, women treated with the equivalent of 35 mg weekly of risedronate had 59% reduction in new vertebral fracture and 39% reduction in nonvertebral fractures, compared with placebo.[37]

Zoledronic acid is an intravenous bisphosphonate given as a once yearly infusion. The HORIZON Pivotal Fracture trial included

**TABLE 43.3   US Food and Drug Administration-Approved Treatment for Osteoporosis**

| | Dose | Route | Frequency | Postmenopausal | Glucocorticoid-induced | Men | Fracture Risk Reduction | | | Renal Contraindication | Consider Drug Holiday | Level of Evidence |
|---|---|---|---|---|---|---|---|---|---|---|---|---|
| | | | | | | | Vertebral | Nonvertebral | Hip | | | |
| **ANTIRESORPTIVE AGENTS** | | | | | | | | | | | | |
| Alendronate | 70 mg | Oral | Weekly | ✓ | ✓ | ✓ | + | + | + | CrCl <35 | Yes | A |
| Risedronate | 35 mg | Oral | Weekly | ✓ | ✓ | ✓ | + | + | + | CrCl <30 | Yes | A |
| Ibandronate | 150 mg / 3 mg | Oral / IV | Monthly / Q 3 months | ✓ | | | + | | | CrCl <35 | Yes | A |
| Zoledronate | 5 mg | IV | Annually | ✓ | ✓ | ✓ | + | + | + | CrCl <35 | Yes | A |
| Denosumab | 60 mg | SubQ | Q 6 months | ✓ | ✓ | ✓ | + | + | + | None | No | A |
| **ANABOLIC AGENTS** | | | | | | | | | | | | |
| Teriparatide | 20 mcg | SubQ | Daily × 2 years | ✓ | ✓ | ✓ | + | + | | None | No | A |
| Abaloparatide | 80 mcg | SubQ | Daily × 2 years | ✓ | | | + | + | | None | No | A |
| Romosozumab | 210 mcg | SubQ | Monthly × 12 months | ✓ | | | + | | | None | No | A |
| **OTHER AGENTS** | | | | | | | | | | | | |
| Raloxifene | 60 mg | Oral | Daily | ✓ | | | + | | | None | No | A |
| Estrogen | Dosage varies | | | ✓ | | | + | + | + | None | No | A |
| Calcitonin | Not a preferred agent | | | ✓ | | | + | | | None | No | A |

postmenopausal women with BMD $< -2.5$ at the femoral neck or those with low BMD and prevalent vertebral fracture. Compared with placebo, those treated with 5 mg infusion once yearly had a 77% reduction in clinical vertebral fractures and 25% reduction in nonvertebral fractures. There was also a 41% reduction in hip fractures.[38] The HORIZON Recurrent Fracture trial studied older adults both men and women who had sustained a recent low-trauma hip fracture. Those treated with once yearly infusion had a 55% reduction in vertebral fracture and 29% reduction in nonvertebral fracture. There was also a 28% reduction in mortality.[39]

Alendronate is contraindicated in renal dysfunction with creatinine clearance $< 35$ mL/min. Risedronate is contraindicated at creatinine clearance $< 30$ mL/min. To avoid the side effect of esophageal irritation/inflammation, patients prescribed oral bisphosphonates should be instructed to take the medication on an empty stomach with a full glass (8 oz) of water, staying upright and waiting to eat or take other medications for 30 to 60 minutes. Additional common side effects of the oral bisphosphonates include other gastrointestinal (GI) complaints, such as gastritis and abdominal pain; myalgia and/or arthralgias, and hypocalcemia. Rarer adverse effects of bisphosphonates include osteonecrosis of the jaw (ONJ) and atypical femoral fractures (AFF), especially after prolonged use ($> 3-5$ years).[40] AFFs are located in the subtrochanteric region and diaphysis of the femur. They have been reported in patients taking bisphosphonates and other antiresorptive medications and may represent a stress or insufficiency fracture. In the task force report from the American Society for Bone and Mineral Research, the incidence of AFF was estimated at 3.2 to 50 cases per 100,000 person-years.[41]

Denosumab is a monoclonal antibody that binds to the receptor nuclear factor κB (RANK) ligand and thereby blocks the binding to RANK. This inhibits the development and activity of osteoclasts and decreases bone resorption. In the Fracture Reduction Evaluation of Denosumab in Osteoporosis Every 6 Months (FREEDOM) trial, postmenopausal women age 60 to 90 years with T-score $< -2.5$ but not $< -4.0$ at the lumbar spine or total hip were randomized to subcutaneous injection of denosumab 60 mg every 6 months or placebo.[42] Compared with those receiving placebo, those treated with denosumab had a 68% reduction in incident vertebral fracture and 20% reduction in nonvertebral fractures. There was a 40% reduction in hip fracture. Common adverse effects include myalgias and/or arthralgias, eczema, cellulitis, and urinary tract infections. Unlike the bisphosphonates, there is no contraindication of denosumab based on creatinine clearance[43]; however, denosumab should be used cautiously in patients with severely reduced renal function who are at risk for renal osteodystrophy.

## Anabolic Agents

Teriparatide is a recombinant PTH analog, consisting of the first 34 amino acids of the native protein. Teriparatide stimulates osteoblastic activity through the PTH receptor, increasing anabolic activity. In the Fracture Prevention trial, postmenopausal women were randomized to 20 mcg or 40 mcg of teriparatide daily subcutaneous injection or placebo.[44] Compared with placebo, the efficacy of the two teriparatide doses were comparable, with 65% to 69% reduction in new vertebral fractures and 53% to 54% reduction in nonvertebral fractures. The FDA approved teriparatide at 20 mcg daily injection dose with a black box warning noting a possible increased osteosarcoma risk in preclinical testing and limited total duration of treatment to 2 years. However, an increased incidence of osteosarcoma has not been detected in postmarketing surveillance of teriparatide use. Teriparatide should not be used in patients with Paget disease, history of osteosarcoma, or history of external beam radiation. Common adverse effects of teriparatide include transient hypercalcemia, orthostatic hypotension, dizziness, nausea, leg cramps, and arthralgias.

In contrast, abaloparatide is an analog of the PTH-related protein (PTHrp), having approximately 60% homology to the native PTHrp and PTH proteins. Abaloparatide was designed to selectively bind the PTH receptor in the anabolic conformation. The Abaloparatide Comparator Trial In Vertebral Endpoints (ACTIVE) study enrolled postmenopausal women with T-score at the femoral neck or lumbar spine $< -2.5$ but $> -5.0$.[45] Subjects also had to have radiologic evidence of vertebral fracture or history of low-trauma nonvertebral fracture. In this high-risk population, those treated with subcutaneous abaloparatide 80 mcg daily had an 86% reduction in incident vertebral fractures and 43% reduction in nonvertebral fractures, compared with placebo. The ACTIVE study also had an arm that received teriparatide at standard doses. Those randomized to teriparatide had an 80% reduction in vertebral fractures and 28% reduction in nonvertebral fractures. There were fewer hypercalcemia adverse events in the abaloparatide-treated group, compared with the teriparatide-treated group. Similar to teriparatide, abaloparatide has a black box warning regarding osteosarcoma. The FDA approved abaloparatide for a total of 2 years, inclusive of teriparatide use.

Romosozumab was approved by the FDA in 2019 for the treatment of osteoporosis in postmenopausal women at high risk for fracture. Romosozumab is a monoclonal antibody that binds and inhibits sclerostin. Sclerostin is a negative regulator of bone formation that is secreted by osteocytes, which works by inhibiting Wnt signaling, a stimulus for osteoblast development and function. In the Fracture Study in Postmenopausal Women with Osteoporosis, women age 55 to 90 years with a T-score of $-2.5$ to $-3.5$ at the femoral neck or total hip were randomized to 210 mg subcutaneous injection of romosozumab once monthly or placebo for 12 months, followed by open-label denosumab every 6 months.[46] Those treated with romosozumab had a 75% reduction in vertebral fracture; there was also a 25% reduction in nonvertebral fractures, although this was not statistically significant. Common adverse effects include injection-site reactions and arthralgias. Romosozumab has also been compared with alendronate in the head-to-head Active-Controlled Fracture Study in Postmenopausal Women with Osteoporosis at High Risk.[47] Compared with those treated with once-weekly alendronate, postmenopausal women with osteoporosis, who received once-monthly romosozumab for 12 months followed by alendronate, had a 48% reduction in incident vertebral fracture and 19% reduction in nonvertebral fractures. Injection-site reactions were common, and there was also an imbalance in serious cardiovascular events, including cardiac ischemia and stroke. The FDA approved romosozumab with a black box warning stating the potential increased risk for myocardial infarction, stroke, and cardiovascular death.

## CASE

### Lily Stephens (Part 4)

Based on her age, weight, height, parental hip fracture, and femoral neck T-score, Ms. Stephens's calculated fracture risk by FRAX was major osteoporotic = 20%, hip = 2.1%. She was started on alendronate 70 mg once weekly. Because she has limited dietary calcium intake, she

was instructed to increase calcium with vitamin D supplement to twice daily at mealtimes.
1. Would Ms. Stephens be a candidate for nonbisphosphonate therapies?
2. How should her response to alendronate be monitored during and after therapy?

## Monitoring

Monitoring response to therapy may be assessed by measuring changes in BMD with serial DXA, height measurements or, less frequently, with BTMs. Significant decreases in BMD on serial DXA measurements, insufficient changes in BTMs, or fracture while on therapy should prompt consideration for noncompliance, unidentified secondary causes for continued bone loss, or the need to change osteoporosis therapy.

Changes in BMD greater than the densitometer's least significant change (LSC) is considered significant. Increasing or stable BMD on serial DXA measurements is generally believed to indicate a good therapeutic response.[48] There is no consensus on the optimal timing to perform serial DXA measurements after initiating osteoporosis therapy. The Endocrine Society recommends reassessing BMD by DXA in postmenopausal women at high fracture risk with low BMD every 1 to 3 years after initiating therapy, whereas the American College of Physicians does not recommend serial DXA monitoring in women during the treatment period, and the ISCD recommends repeating BMD measurement 1 year after initiating or changing therapy. Longer intervals for reassessment have been proposed when the expected therapeutic effect has been achieved, whereas shorter intervals should occur if a concurrent condition may cause continued bone loss.[49,50]

Yearly height measurements should be performed throughout osteoporosis treatment. Vertebral imaging to assess for new vertebral fractures should be performed when a loss of 2 cm (0.8 inches) or more in height is observed. BTMs may be measured when there are concerns about nonadherence or therapy efficacy. The effect of antiresorptive therapy can be measured by bone resorption markers (serum carboxy-terminal collagen crosslinks [CTX] and NTX). The bone formation marker P1NP can be measured to determine the effect of anabolic bone agents. BTMs should be measured in the morning while in the fasting state to account for diurnal variations and food effects. Baseline BTMs should be compared with repeat markers 3 to 6 months after initiating therapy; however, the extent of changes in BTMs that constitutes a response is unclear. Nevertheless, bone resorption markers should decrease with antiresorptive therapies, whereas bone formation markers increase with anabolic bone therapies.

❖❖ **Monitoring of osteoporosis treatment includes measurement for changes in height, BMD, and fracture risk, as well as assessment for treatment compliance and side effects.**

The recommended duration of therapy for bisphosphonates varies according to the specific agent, patient preferences, and individual risk factors. Oral bisphosphonates should be continued up to 5 years. Intravenous bisphosphonates should be continued up to 3 years. An individual's fracture risk should be reassessed after 3 to 5 years of initial therapy. Prolonged bisphosphonate therapy > 5 years may increase the risk of ONJ and AFF. Temporary discontinuation of bisphosphonate therapy after several years may decrease the risk of AFF, as suggested by limited observation data.[51] The benefits of continuing bisphosphonate therapy beyond 3 to 5 years should be carefully weighed against potential risks. Long-term effects of bisphosphonates after 3 to 5 years in postmenopausal women were evaluated in two trials: the Fracture Intervention Trial Long-Term Extension (FLEX) and the extension to the HORIZON-Pivotal Fracture Trial.[52,53] The FLEX trial compared the effects of randomizing women who completed 5 years of alendronate with placebo or continuing alendronate for 10 years. Women who remained on alendronate for 10 years had a significant reduction in clinical vertebral fractures (relative risk, 0.45; 95% CI, 0.24–0.85) and less bone loss observed at all bone sites compared with those who discontinued alendronate after 5 years. Similarly, the HORIZON study extension compared the effects of randomizing women who completed 3 years of zoledronic acid with placebo or continuing zoledronic acid for 6 years. BMD decreased slightly at all sites in the placebo arm compared with women on zoledronic acid for 6 years, but did not decrease below pretreatment levels. There were no other significant differences in fracture reduction noted. Management guidelines incorporating data from the FLEX and HORIZON extension trials for long-term bisphosphonate treatment in postmenopausal women have been released by the Task Force of the American Society of Bone and Mineral Research and the Endocrine Society.[40,48] Extrapolation of the recommendations to men and glucocorticoid-induced osteoporosis may be reasonable.

A bisphosphonate drug holiday begins when a patient discontinues bisphosphonate use after 3 to 5 years of therapy. A drug holiday may last up to 5 years. At cessation of the bisphosphonate drug holiday, bisphosphonate therapy is generally restarted; however, individual risk factors should be reassessed to determine if bisphosphonate therapy is still the most appropriate treatment option. There is no operational consensus on how best to evaluate patients during a drug holiday to determine the optimal time to restart bisphosphonate therapy, thus most guidance originates from expert opinion. Monitoring during a bisphosphonate drug holiday may include one or a combination of the following every 2 to 4 years: serial DXA measurements, fracture risk evaluation, or BTMs. Restarting bisphosphonate therapy may be guided by multiple factors. Bisphosphonate therapy may be empirically restarted within 5 years of initiating a drug holiday. Alternatively, bisphosphonate therapy may be restarted after identifying significant increases in fracture risk, significant decreases in BMD on serial DXA measurements, or increases in serial bone turnover markers. The development of a new fragility fracture while on drug holiday should also prompt consideration for restarting bisphosphonate therapy. Prolongation of a bisphosphonate drug holiday beyond 5 years may be reasonable for individuals in whom there has been no significant increase in fracture risk factors and BMD stability has been observed on serial DXA measurements.

The recommended duration of treatment for nonbisphosphonate therapies must be carefully balanced with the detrimental effects on bone after discontinuation of these therapies. Unlike bisphosphonate therapy, there are no long-term residual bone effects of nonbisphosphonate therapies after discontinuation. Data from the FREEDOM extension trial support continued use of denosumab up to 10 years.[54] Discontinuation of long-term denosumab leads to rapid decreases in BMD and an increase in BTMs within the first year.[55,56] In addition, there have been reports of an increased risk of vertebral fractures immediately after the discontinuation of denosumab.[57] Therefore denosumab therapy should not be discontinued for a drug holiday, but either continued indefinitely or with follow-on osteoporosis therapy to maintain the BMD gains achieved with denosumab. Similarly, rapid loss in BMD gains occurs after discontinuation of anabolic agents, such as teriparatide and abaloparatide. Teriparatide and abaloparatide are approved by the FDA for a combined 2 years of use, and the sclerostin inhibitor romosozumab is FDA approved for 12 months. To prevent rapid decline in BMD gains after discontinuation of anabolic agents, follow-on therapy with an antiresorptive agent, such as zoledronic acid or denosumab, should be initiated. Continued increases in BMD were observed in all sites at 24 months using denosumab as follow-on therapy to 24 months of teriparatide in postmenopausal women.[58]

---

### CASE

#### Lily Stephens (Part 5)

Ms. Stephens returns for follow-up appointment 6 months later. After her last visit, she started alendronate on Sunday mornings. She describes taking the pill on an empty stomach, with a full glass of water. She remained upright for at least 60 minutes after taking the pill, finishing her daily routine. She would then take her other medications, as well as prepare breakfast. However, she would have stomach pains for the rest of the day and stopped taking the medicine after 2 weeks. Unfortunately, she fell 1 month later and suffered a right femoral neck fracture. She underwent open reduction and internal fixation of the fracture and was discharged to an acute rehabilitation facility. She spent 2 months at the facility and was able to return home with physical therapy services for another month. At her follow-up appointment with Orthopedics, she was given an infusion of zoledronic acid. She tolerated the infusion initially, but says she felt like she had the "flu" for a week afterwards. She is currently walking with a rolling walker but still able to cook meals for herself and independent with her activities of daily living.

1. Why was Ms. Stephens switched to zoledronic acid for her osteoporosis therapy?
2. What are the symptoms of an acute phase reaction after receiving zoledronic acid?

---

### CASE

#### Discussion

Ms. Lily Stephens has a number of risk factors for osteoporosis and fractures that were detailed during the history and physical examination. She has a family history of parental hip fracture. With her history of breast cancer, she was treated with an aromatase inhibitor, which may lead to secondary bone loss. She did not have radiation therapy for her breast cancer, so that teriparatide may still be a treatment option. She also has diabetes, so it is important to identify diabetic complications, such as peripheral neuropathy, as well as potential hypoglycemic events and risk of falls. She does not consume dairy in her diet, so additional calcium is needed either with alterations in her diet or through calcium supplements. Her laboratory evaluation reveals an inadequate 25-hydroxyvitamin D level, indicating that vitamin D supplementation should be started to target a level > 30 mg/dL.

Ms. Stephens has osteopenia by DXA, given her lumbar spine and hip T-scores, so calculating her fracture risk helps determine if treatment should be initiated. Given her FRAX risk of major osteoporotic fracture > 20%, the recommendation is to start alendronate therapy. Proper dosing of alendronate is important to achieve efficacy, and a DXA for BMD monitoring could be considered at 2 years of therapy. Unfortunately, she sustained a hip fracture in the interim and was transitioned to intravenous zoledronic acid, which has been shown in clinical trial to decrease secondary hip fractures. Adverse effects of zoledronic acid include arthralgias, myalgias, and low-grade fever after infusion, which may be mitigated with acetaminophen predose and as needed afterwards. Additional nonpharmacologic therapy should include assistance with ambulation, reduce risk of falls, and regular weight-bearing exercise.

---

## Summary

Osteoporosis is a common, systemic disease that results in increased risk of bone fractures and in significant morbidity and mortality among older adults. Multiple medications and medical conditions are risk factors for osteoporosis and fractures, including glucocorticoid use and frequent falls. DXA is the primary screening test, along with fracture risk assessment calculators, to estimate absolute risk and indicate if treatment is warranted. A number of pharmacologic treatments are available that differ in mechanism of action and adverse effects. Completion of anabolic therapy course should be followed by antiresorptive agent. A drug holiday should be considered after 3 to 5 years for bisphosphonate therapy, but not for denosumab.

### Web Resources

Guide to Calcium-rich Foods: http://www.nof.org/patients/treatment/calciumvitamin-d/a-guide-to-calcium-rich-foods/ https://www.iofbonehealth.org/osteoporosis

FRAX: Fracture Assessment Tool: https://www.sheffield.ac.uk/FRAX/

ASBMR Task Force Reports: https://www.asbmr.org/asbmr-task-force-reports

---

## Key References

7. Cosman F, de Beur SJ, LeBoff MS, et al. Clinician's guide to prevention and treatment of osteoporosis. *Osteoporos Int.* 2014;25(10):2359–2381.
13. McCloskey EV, Vasikaran S, Cooper C. Official positions for FRAX(R) clinical regarding biochemical markers from Joint Official Positions Development Conference of the International Society for Clinical Densitometry and International Osteoporosis Foundation on FRAX(R). *J Clin Densitom.* 2011;14(3):220–222.
35. Grossman DC, Curry SJ, Owens DK, et al. Interventions to prevent falls in community-dwelling older adults: US Preventive Services Task Force Recommendation Statement. *JAMA.* 2018;319(16):1696–1704.
40. Adler RA, El-Hajj Fuleihan G, Bauer DC, et al. Managing osteoporosis in patients on long-term bisphosphonate treatment: report of a Task Force of the American Society for Bone and Mineral Research. *J Bone Miner Res.* 2016;31(1):16–35.

**References available online at** expertconsult.com.

# 44

# Arthritis and Related Disorders

DEVYANI MISRA AND UNA E. MAKRIS

## OUTLINE

*Additional online-only material indicated by icon.*

## OBJECTIVES

*Upon completion of this chapter, the reader will be able to:*

- Understand the differential diagnosis of common rheumatic conditions affecting older adults.
- Recognize that arthritis in later life is different from that in younger populations and may be complicated by multimorbidity and polypharmacy.
- Describe the pharmacologic and nonpharmacologic modalities used to treat common musculoskeletal disorders in older adults.
- Become familiar with timing and indications for appropriate referral to rheumatology, physical/occupation therapy, and other services.

---

### CASE 1

#### Mrs. Montes (Part 1)

Mrs. Montes, a 78-year-old woman, comes to the office with long-standing intermittent knee pain that now has become persistent pain. Pain is exacerbated with standing and walking. She has tried 1 g of acetaminophen three times a day without relief. She also reports knee buckling and giving way. She uses a cane to help with ambulation. She describes morning stiffness lasting for 15 minutes. On examination, she is noted to have swelling in her right knee without warmth or erythema. She has varus deformity (bowing of both knees). She also has prominent Heberden and Bouchard nodes in both hands.

1.  What are the likely causes of Mrs. Montes's complaints?

### CASE 2

#### Mr. Smith (Part 1)

Mr. Smith is a 75-year-old gentleman who presents for 3 to 4 months of prolonged stiffness in the morning lasting for more than 2 to 3 hours. He reports joint pain in both shoulders, hands, and wrists and has swelling in the joints as well. He reports difficulty in turning the door knob and opening jars. He initially responded to over-the counter-ibuprofen but now nothing seems to be helping his pain. On physical examination, he has fusiform swelling and warmth in multiple proximal interphalangeal (PIPs) and metacarpophalangeal joints. Both wrists are swollen. He has reduced range of motion in wrists and shoulders.

1.  What are the likely causes of Mr. Smith's complaints?
2.  How is the treatment approach different for Mrs. Montes and Mr. Smith?
3.  What is the significance of Heberden and Bouchard nodes compared with fusiform swelling of the PIPs?

## Prevalence and Impact

Arthritis is gaining more attention as a common cause of both disability and years lived with functional impairments. Osteoarthritis (OA) is the most common joint disease among older adults, affecting 13.9% of US adults, or 26.9 million people (Table 44.1). Other rheumatic disorders prevalent among older adults are rheumatoid arthritis (RA; 1.5 million cases in the United States), gout (6.1 million cases), pseudogout (10,000–40,000 people age 65–85 years), polymyalgia rheumatica (PMR; approximately 450,000 cases, 90% of whom are age $\geq 60$ years), and giant-cell arteritis (GCA; 110,000 Americans, 90% of whom are >60 years).

## Risk Factors and Pathophysiology

### Osteoarthritis

Arguably advanced age is the most important risk factor for OA, although the exact aging-related causal mechanisms are not completely understood. Other risk factors for OA include obesity, female gender, trauma or joint injury, quadriceps muscle weakness, and possibly genetics. Cartilage loss is the hallmark pathology although synovial inflammation, osteophyte formation, and subchondral bone sclerosis are other intraarticular (IA) pathologic features.

### Rheumatoid Arthritis

The distribution of RA is bimodal, with a peak in the 30s and another in the 70s. Genetic predisposition, cigarette smoking, and periodontal disease are some of the known risk factors for RA. The phenotype of late-onset RA is different from young-onset RA in terms of joint distribution, prevalence of positive antibodies, and so on. The characteristic pathology in RA is synovial inflammation that extends to the cartilage (pannus formation) and can invade the adjacent bone, causing erosions.

### Gout and Pseudogout

Gout, an inflammatory reaction to monosodium urate (MSU) crystals deposited in the joint, is associated with hyperuricemia. Risk factors include advancing age, male gender, renal disease, and genetic predisposition. Risk factors for a gout flare include factors that either impair excretion of uric acid or increase production or both, and include alcohol use, diuretic use, and red meat/shellfish consumption. A similar inflammatory reaction occurs to calcium pyrophosphate dehydrate (CPPD) crystal deposition in joints, commonly known as *pseudogout*. Advanced age is the most important risk factor for CPPD, other risk factors include disorders of phosphate, magnesium, parathyroid and thyroid hormone, and hemochromatosis. Trauma, acute diseases, or surgery provoke CPPD attacks.

### Polymyalgia Rheumatica and Giant-Cell Arteritis

PMR and GCA are closely related conditions in that they are seen almost exclusively in older adults. The disease initiating triggering of the immune system in PMR is unknown. GCA is a chronic, systemic vasculitis that affects the elastic membranes of the aorta and its extracranial branches, particularly the external carotid artery with its superficial temporal division.

## Other Rheumatic Diseases

Late onset systemic lupus erythematosus (SLE), primary Sjögren and psoriatic arthritis, are also seen in older adults, although less frequently, and can vary in presentation and severity as compared with younger-onset disease (refer to Table 44.1). As primary care providers and geriatricians, it is important to have a low threshold to refer to specialists if there is a high index of suspicion for autoimmune disease or inflammatory arthritis.

## Differential Diagnosis and Assessment

The differential diagnosis and assessment for arthritic conditions in older adults is similar to that of younger individuals, although comorbidities and medical and social complexity sometimes delay diagnosis. Table 44.1 lists laboratory and x-ray studies to assist with differential diagnosis. A component of assessment is determining whether the symptoms with which the patient presents are atypical manifestations of typical diseases, as indicated in Table 44.2.

### Osteoarthritis

OA is the most common joint disease affecting older adults. It usually has an insidious onset and chronic course. It affects the DIP joints, causing characteristic Heberden nodes, and the proximal interphalangeal (PIP) joints, causing Bouchard nodes. In addition, there is frequent involvement of the hips, knees, back, and neck. The development of Heberden and Bouchard nodes may take several years; they may be painful and soft initially and later harden and calcify as pain subsides. Bowing (varus) or knock knees (valgus) indicate misalignment of the knees. OA of the knee is associated with thigh muscle weakness, functional limitation, disability, and poor quality of life. Two-thirds of patients age $\geq 65$ years and 90% of those age $\geq 90$ years have x-ray changes consistent with OA.[1,2] Laboratory studies reveal negative antinuclear antibodies (ANA) and rheumatoid factor (RF). The inflammatory marker, C-reactive protein (CRP), may be mildly elevated.[3] X-ray features include joint space narrowing, osteophytes, subchondral sclerosis, and cystic changes. Magnetic resonance imaging (MRI) shows correlated bone marrow lesions with meniscal derangement in symptomatic knees.[4] Synovial fluid assessments show generally noninflammatory fluid with total nucleated cell count $\leq 1000$ cells/mm.[3]

➤➤ **Osteoarthritis is the most common cause of arthritis, has an insidious onset, chronic course, minimal morning stiffness, and significant impact on quality of life and daily function.**

### Rheumatoid Arthritis

RA is also a chronic arthritis but has a more acute or subacute onset as compared to OA. Late-onset RA has different characteristics than young-onset RA.[5] For example, proximal joint involvement as presenting symptoms, equal gender distribution, less frequent RF positivity, and more aggressive disease course is more common in elderly-onset RA as compared with young-onset RA. X-ray features of RA include loss of articular space, multiple erosions, juxtaarticular osteopenia, and ulnar deviation.

➤➤ **RA has a more acute presentation in older than in younger individuals, with more involvement of proximal joints.**

**TABLE 44.1   Differential Diagnosis of Prevalent Rheumatic Disorders in the Older Adult Population**

| Disorder | Prevalence etc. | Impact on Mortality | Pathophysiology and Risk Factors | Clinical Comparison | Laboratory | X-rays | Management |
|---|---|---|---|---|---|---|---|
| Osteoarthritis (OA) | 13.9% of US adults or 26.9 million people | Prevalence of coronary artery disease (CAD) in patients with OA is 27% | Risk Factors: Age, obesity, female, genetics, quadriceps weakness, joint injury/instability, poor proprioception, heavy physical activity | Insidious and chronic in DIPs, PIPs, CMCs, hips, knees, back, and neck Heberden nodes (DIPs) and Bouchard nodes (PIPs) common | ANA (−), RF (−); ESR normal; CRP normal | Osteophytes, loss of articular space, subchondral sclerosis | See Table 44.3 |
| Late-Onset Rheumatoid Arthritis (>60 years) | Unknown sex distribution 1:1 | No data | HLA DR4 is present in RF (+) and less likely in RF (−) patients | More acute and infectious like Symptoms: >proximal Outcome: worse | ANA (±), RF (+) 32%–89%, ESR higher at onset | As YORA | See Table 44.4 Low-dose steroid |
| Gout in older people | 5.1 million: Most are men, onset in midlife. Late-onset gout is after age 60 years, sex distribution is 1:1. After age 80 years, women are almost all | Hyperuricemia may produce HTN | It is associated with diuretic use and renal disease. Other classical risk factors include obesity, hypertension, and heavy alcohol use (less common). Gout is an inflammatory response to MSU crystals | Elderly-onset gout is still acute but more polyarticular, more likely to involve small joints and develop tophi more rapidly and in unusual locations | ANA (−), RF (−), High serum uric acid, MSU (negative birefringent) on synovial fluid | Overhanging edge, with erosions Affects mainly the first MTP, but it is common in hands | NSAIDs, colchicine allopurinol, steroids PA or intraarticular. Diet low in red meats and seafood |
| Pseudogout in older people | Age 65–75 years; 10,000 to 15,000. Age >80 y: 40,000 per 100,000 | Unknown | Inflammation to CPPD crystals. With intraarticular chondrocalcinosis | Affects mainly older population, most commonly the knee Concomitant OA | Crystals positive birefringent in synovial fluid | Hands, pelvis, and knees mostly | NSAIDs, intraarticular steroids |
| Late-onset SLE (>50 years) | Female to male (6.9:1) Compared with younger onset SLE, more common in White persons | 5-year survival rate is comparable with younger onset SLE | Genetic factors, nongenetic, environmental, and lifestyle factors | Milder. Weight loss, muscle aches and pains, disturbances of cognition/ affect Arthritis and arthralgias of hands and wrists, rash, Raynaud, vague central nervous system symptoms | ANA (weakly +) (36% of healthy older people have nonspecific low titers ANA), Anti dsDNA, AntiSm, AntiRo/SSA (+), C3, C4 low ESR/ CRP high | Same as younger-onset SLE | Same as younger-onset SLE Careful with side effects |

*(Continued)*

**TABLE 44.1** Differential Diagnosis of Prevalent Rheumatic Disorders in the Older Adult Population—cont'd

| Disorder | Prevalence etc. | Impact on Mortality | Pathophysiology and Risk Factors | Clinical Comparison | Laboratory | X-rays | Management |
|---|---|---|---|---|---|---|---|
| Polymyalgia Rheumatica (PMR) | 600/100,000 90% are >60 years. 450,000 in US, mostly White persons | Overall life expectancy is essentially identical to the general population | Unknown. Synovitis with T-cell and macrophage infiltration | ≥1 month aching/ morning stiffness in ≥2 of 3 areas: shoulders /upper arms, hips/thighs, neck/torso | ESR/CRP high, RF (−), anti-CCP (−) | Negative | Steroids |
| Giant Cell Arteritis (GCA, temporal arteritis) | 200/100,000 Americans | 15%–20% with PMR also have GCA. 15% with GCA have visual loss | Related to PMR | Headache, jaw claudication, vision change, scalp tenderness, fever, weight loss, fatigue | ESR/CRP high Positive temporal artery biopsy (can be negative because of skip lesions) | Negative imaging, unless patient has a stroke | Steroids, ASA to prevent strokes |
| Idiopathic inflammatory myopathy (IIM), polymyositis (PM), dermatomyositis (DM), sporadic inclusion body myositis (S-IBM) | Unknown prevalence. S-IBM is the most common after age 50 years | Onset after age 50 y associated with increased mortality Frequency of malignancy in patients with PM-DM increases with age | Consider hypothyroidism, hyperthyroidism, osteomalacia, amyloid myopathy, drug-induced, corticosteroids, alcohol, colchicines, lipid lowering agents | Weakness of limb-girdle and anterior neck flexors, progressive over weeks to months | High: ESR/CRP, CK, aldolase, AST/ALT, LDH; + Anti-Jo antibodies (PM-DM) EMG/NCS often positive. Muscle biopsy is the gold standard | None | Steroids/ DMARDs. S-IBM often not responsive to Tx Response of older with PM-DM < younger adults |

*ANA*, antinuclear antibodies; *anti-CCP*, anticyclic citrullinated peptide; *APS antibodies*, lupus anticoagulant and anticardiolipin antibodies; *ALT*, alanine aminotransferase; *ASA*, acetylsalicylic acid; *AST*, aspartate aminotransferase; *CAD*, coronary artery disease; *CK*, creatinine kinase; *CMC*, carpometacarpal joints; *CPP*, anti-cyclic citrullinated peptide; *CPPD*, calcium pyrophosphate dehydrated; *CRP*, C-reactive protein; *dsDNA*, double-stranded deoxyribonucleic acid; *DIP*, distal interphalangeal joints; *EMG/NCS*, electromyogram/nerve conduction studies; *ESR*, erythrocyte sedimentation rate; *HLA*, human lymphocyte antigen; *HTN*, hypertension; *LDH*, lactate dehydrogenase; *MSU*, monosodium urate crystals; *NSAIDs*, nonsteroidal antiinflammatory drugs; *PIP*, proximal interphalangeal joints; *RF*, rheumatoid factor; *Sm*, Smith antibodies.

| TABLE 44.2 | Musculoskeletal Manifestations of Typical Diseases |
|---|---|
| Shoulder pain | Acute myocardial infarction, pneumonia, costochondral pain, intraabdominal bleeding, or perforation |
| TMJ pain | Acute myocardial infarction joint pain |
| Hip pain | Pancreatitis, psoas muscle abscess or hematoma, hip fracture, hernia |
| Back pain | Bone metastasis, osteomyelitis, tumor, or deep venous thrombosis |
| Myalgias | Rhabdomyolysis |

*TMJ,* Temporomandibular joint.

## Gout and Pseudogout

Gout is acute in both older and younger individuals, but intermittent, unlike OA or RA, which are chronic. It characteristically involves the first metatarsal phalangeal joint (MTP) but can affect any joint. ANA and RF are negative, and serum uric acid is elevated (except perhaps during an acute attack). MSU crystals are found in the synovial fluid and are needle-shaped crystals that are bright yellow when parallel to the axis or negatively birefringent on a polarizing microscope. MSU crystals are inside the neutrophils in active inflammation because of phagocytosis. X-ray studies may show erosions that are usually slightly removed from the joint, which is atrophic and hypertrophic, leading to erosions with an "overhanging edge."

Pseudogout presents as acute intermittent arthritis of the knee, wrist, hand, or any peripheral joint. It is also a cause of acute neck pain with characteristic crownlike calcifications around the odontoid process ("crowned dens") on radiograph of the cervical spine accompanied by acute neck pain, stiffness, fevers, and raised inflammatory markers. Pseudogout is common in patients with OA and is confirmed by the finding of CPPD crystals in the synovial fluid. Crystals are rod-check shaped and blue when parallel to the axis or positively birefringent on a polarizing microscope and x-rays show chondrocalcinosis primarily in the hands, wrists, pelvis, and knees.

◆◆ **Crystal arthritides present with acute intermittent inflammatory arthritis. Gout often affects the first MTP whereas pseudogout more commonly affects knees and wrists.**

## Polymyalgia Rheumatica and Giant-Cell Arteritis

PMR is a clinical diagnosis that presents with acute onset of achiness, pain, and morning stiffness in shoulders and upper arms, hips, thighs, neck, and torso. Characteristically, erythrocyte sedimentation rate (ESR) and CRP are elevated and RF, anticyclic citrullinated peptide (anti-CCP), and ANA antibodies are negative. There are no characteristic x-ray features. All patients suspected of having PMR should also be evaluated for possible GCA by asking about symptoms of headache, jaw claudication, visual disturbances, fever, weight loss, and fatigue. On examination, scalp arteries (e.g., a temporal artery) may be tender during scalp palpation. GCA has traditionally been diagnosed by biopsy of the temporal artery. The biopsy should be at least 1 cm in length and even then false negatives are common. More recently, imaging with ultrasound of the temporal arteries, computer tomography, or MRI angiography of large arteries (subclavian, axillary, or aorta) have shown diagnostic changes with good sensitivity and specificity for diagnosis.

GCA is a vasculitis of both cranial and large arteries. When the diagnosis is suspected, the patient requires urgent treatment to prevent sudden and painless vision loss related to involvement of the ophthalmic artery.

◆◆ **PMR presents as acute onset achiness or pain in the shoulder and hip girdles and elevated inflammatory markers. All patients with PMR should be evaluated for GCA.**

## Role of Arthrocentesis

Examination of joint fluid from arthrocentesis aids in the differential diagnosis of many arthritic conditions. Fluid is evaluated for cell count, crystals, and culture. Noninflammatory fluids have $\leq 1000$ white blood cells (WBC)/mm$^3$, whereas inflammatory fluids tend to have $\geq 2000$ WBC. Fluid with $\geq 100,000$ WBC indicates septic arthritis until proven otherwise. Carefully selecting the kind of needle for this procedure is important. For instance, ordinarily, an 18- to 21-gauge needle can be used safely in the knee. If the patient is anticoagulated, a 22- or 25-gauge needle minimizes risk of bleeding. There is no need to stop anticoagulation if the procedure is properly done. There should be an attempt to obtain clean, blood-free fluid for accurate analysis. As much fluid as possible should be drained with one needle-stick to minimize discomfort from the swollen joint.

◆◆ **Arthrocentesis and synovial fluid analysis (with cell count, crystals, and Gram stain/culture) is important to evaluate for an infection (septic joint) and distinguish between OA, crystal arthritis, and other inflammatory arthritides.**

## Imaging

There is poor correlation between joint symptoms and x-ray findings. Patients may have moderate to severe x-ray findings but remain asymptomatic and fully functional. In contrast, patients may have absent or mild x-ray findings with severe pain and functional impairment and disability, and in some conditions (e.g., PMR) there may be no findings on x-rays. Therefore imaging is not necessary to establish the diagnosis in most cases.[6] Most rheumatic conditions are based on thorough history and physical examination; laboratory data and imaging are used to confirm a clinical suspicion.

◆◆ **Severity of disease on imaging rarely correlates with clinical findings or response to therapy, especially in OA.**

## Management

### General Considerations

Appropriate management of an older adult with rheumatic diseases requires assessment of pain, functional status, and quality of life.[7] Further, it is important to diagnose appropriately early on, to maintain function and prevent deformity. Depending on the diagnosis and severity, early referrals to rheumatology, physical therapy (PT), occupational therapy (OT), physical medicine and rehabilitation, or pharmacy colleagues are central to managing arthritis in older adults. In addition, the choice of therapy will vary based on comorbidities, medications, and potential for drug-drug or drug-disease interactions. Special consideration in older adults includes the presence of frailty, cognitive impairment, and social support.[8] Older adults with rheumatic disorders are more likely to die from cardiovascular events and complications than from their musculoskeletal condition. Therefore it is critical for primary care to actively manage comorbid cardiovascular disease especially in patients with inflammatory arthritis and other autoimmune conditions.

The overall goals of management are to reduce pain, maximize function, and maintain independence in activities of daily living (ADLs) for as long as possible. Goals should be established early on and must be realistic given the patient's specific circumstances. Sometimes, it is not possible to be pain-free; however, it is often still possible to be functional, carry out ADLs, and enjoy hobbies. Reassessing progress to goals, tailoring expectations, and adapting to circumstances as they arise are important parts of clinic visit discussions at the initial and follow-up visits. Thus first-line management for all arthritis involves education, counseling, and establishing goals of care.

The interprofessional team is critical when caring for older adults with arthritis. PTs and OTs can train patients to compensate for lost function, gain strength and flexibility, and help select and use assistive devices. Social workers assist in finding and connecting patients to community resources, including transportation services to clinics or PT, and arrange for home-based care when needed. Pharmacists can assist with medication reconciliation and find ways to reduce costs and avoid interactions of prescribed medications.

❖❖ **Understanding the patient's goals is key to managing and monitoring arthritis in older adults. A multimodal approach with attention to optimizing pain management, improving functional status, and managing comorbidities is needed for management of arthritis in older adults.**

## Osteoarthritis

Treatment options for OA, with the level of evidence that supports those options, are detailed in Table 44.3.[9] Nonpharmacologic and behavioral interventions include weight loss (if patient is overweight or obese) and an exercise program.[10,11] Exercise and physical activity based interventions strengthen muscles around the

### TABLE 44.3 Treatment of Osteoarthritis

| Treatment Method | Evidence | Recommendation Level[a] |
|---|---|---|
| Weight loss (if patient is overweight or obese) | Effective and safe | LOE = D, Expert opinion |
| Exercise | Effective for pain and function, especially in supervised setting Effect depends on sustainability of land-based exercise program, so home exercise programs following physical therapy are suggested Discuss fall prevention, balance training and safety with graduated physical activity | Core part of treatment |
| Brace/splinting | May be effective | Limited evidence |
| Tai Chi, Yoga, Qi Gong | Variable efficacy, safe, limited by access | Limited evidence |
| Acupuncture | Variable efficacy, depends on individual offering the services Safe, limited by access | Limited evidence |
| Acetaminophen (APAP) (up to 4 g/day) | Efficacy for symptom relief is small compared to oral NSAIDs but better safety profile, daily cumulative dose <3–4 g | Limited evidence |
| Nonaspirin NSAIDs for OA of the hand, knee, and hip | Although efficacy is smaller, topical NSAIDs are preferred over oral NSAIDs because of the gastrointestinal, renal and cardiovascular adverse effects of oral NSAIDs. Use lowest effective dose for shortest duration. If duration of use >2 weeks suggest gastric mucosa protection. | LOE = D, High consensus, conditional |
| Intraarticular steroids | Moderate efficacy with improvement in pain and function in the short term | LOE = D, High consensus, conditional |
| Intraarticular viscosupplementation | Efficacy is small and clinically not meaningful. Potential for postinjection reactions (usually effusion) leading to ED visits | LOE = D, Low consensus, conditional |
| Glucosamine | Safe but not effective | LOE = D, Low consensus |
| Topical analgesics (capsaicin, lidocaine) | Safe but questionable efficacy | LOE = D, Low consensus |
| Opioids, including tramadol | Not effective and several adverse effects | LOE = D, Low consensus |

*ED*, Emergency department; *LOE*, level of evidence; *NSAIDs*, nonsteroidal antiinflammatory drugs, *OA*, Osteoarthritis.
Total knee arthroplasty and total hip replacement
Effective in select surgical candidate, best before severe functional impairments

[a]Based on OARSI treatment Guideline 2019 for non-surgical treatment of Osteoarthritis. The variability for the site of OA (knee, hip, and hand), lack of placebo controlled group (especially for studies on exercise) and small size of random control trials makes it complex.

joints affected by OA, maintain range of motion, relieve pain, and reduce instability.[12] PT and OT may recommend assistive devices for ambulation, such as canes and walker. Braces and splints may provide joint protection. Other behavioral interventions include cognitive behavioral therapy for chronic pain and acceptance commitment therapy.[13]

There are no disease modifying pharmacologic drugs available at this time. Hence, the treatment is primarily symptomatic. First-line pharmacotherapy is a trial of topical nonsteroidal anti-inflammatory drugs (NSAIDs) and oral acetaminophen, based on the safety profile even though evidence for efficacy in clinical trials is limited. Use of oral NSAIDS is discouraged because of cardiovascular, gastrointestinal, and renal toxicity. Cyclooxygeanse (COX)-2 inhibitors exhibit similar adverse risk profiles. Trials of non-NSAID topical therapies, including capsaicin, menthol, and lidocaine based cream/gel, have few adverse events because of limited systemic absorption. Opioids, including tramadol, have not shown efficacy in symptom or functional improvement, and are best avoided because of adverse effects, including falls, mental status changes, constipation, respiratory depression, and sometimes death.[14,15] IA steroids have shown moderate efficacy in improving pain in the short term (1−2 weeks) for knee OA but sustained benefit beyond 1 to 2 weeks is not consistent.[16] IA steroids are generally considered safe although a recent randomized clinical trial showed slightly greater risk of cartilage loss compared with placebo when steroid injections were repeated every 3 months over 2 years.[17] The efficacy of IA steroids in hand OA is not convincing. There is insufficient evidence for supplements (glucosamine, chondroitin, fish oil/omega-3 fatty acid) and visco-supplements (hyaluronic acid) for use in OA.[9]

Decision to refer for joint replacement is made on an individual basis based on comorbidities and functional status. If selected appropriately, joint replacements can improve pain and function for patients suffering from OA.

## Rheumatoid Arthritis

RA is treated initially with disease modifying antirheumatic drugs (DMARDs) as outlined in Table 44.4. Long-term glucocorticoid therapy is not disease modifying and is associated with many adverse effects and should not be considered first-line therapy for RA, although many patients are started on glucocorticoids before referral to rheumatology for symptomatic relief. If a patient is on steroids (e.g., prednisone $\geq 7.5$ mg orally daily) for $\geq 3$ months, the patient should be considered for osteoporosis prophylaxis.[18] Ideally, patients are tapered off steroids while using DMARD therapy and before development of long-term consequences from steroid use.

The goal for RA management is to diagnose early and treat to target, meaning treat the disease manifestation until remission is achieved. First-line therapy is typically triple therapy with DMARDs under care of a rheumatologist. Triple therapy often includes a combination of methotrexate, hydroxychloroquine, and leflunomide or sulfasalazine. Table 44.4 outlines specific cautions for starting and monitoring these medications. For example, hydroxychloroquine should be avoided in older adults with macular degeneration. If hydroxychloroquine is used, annual ophthalmologic evaluation to screen for retinal deposits is recommended. Routine toxicity monitoring with labs and adverse effects from methotrexate, sulfasalazine, and leflunomide are suggested every 8 to 12 weeks.[19] Triple therapy is noninferior to biologicals but for RA patient who do not achieve disease remission or have low disease

activity (depending on the patient's threshold to escalate therapy), biologicals are the next step, sometimes in combination with methotrexate or other nonbiological DMARDs.[20] Before initiating biological DMARDs, it is essential to evaluate for tuberculosis, hepatitis B, and hepatitis C because biologicals can reactivate these infections. Also before DMARDs, other vaccinations (pneumococcal, influenza, and varicella vaccinations) should be up to date. Of note, there is recent evidence that influenza vaccine has improved immunogenicity (and may be more effective) if methotrexate is held 2 weeks following administration of the vaccination.[21]

Older adults with RA should be evaluated for extraarticular manifestations that suggest more aggressive disease and worse prognosis: these include presence of rheumatoid nodules, interstitial lung disease, rheumatoid vasculitis, deformities, or erosions on imaging. Treat-to-target (disease remission) prevents deformities from developing and hopefully reduces the risk of extraarticular manifestations. Importantly, lower disease activity in RA is also associated with a decrease in cardiovascular events.[22]

◆◆ **Cardiovascular mortality is high in older adults with RA and other inflammatory arthritides. In addition to control of disease activity, it is critical to control cardiovascular risk factors.**

## Gout and Pseudogout

Gout is treated with a combination of lifestyle modification, uric acid lowering therapy, and acute abortive therapy. Uric acid lowering therapy is warranted if the patient has had two to three acute attacks, renal complications from hyperuricemia, or in the presence of tophi or erosive disease.[23] Gout patients should avoid excessive alcohol intake, as well as shellfish and organ meats. Treatment with xanthine oxidase inhibitors is suggested to reduce the serum uric acid level to $\leq 6$ mg/dL. Allopurinol is first-line uric acid lowering therapy and is well tolerated. Serious hypersensitivity reactions are rare. Further, allopurinol can be safely titrated up despite renal insufficiency, which is especially important in older adults. If a patient does not respond to or has a reaction to allopurinol, febuxostat can be trialed. However, a recent trial found higher all-cause mortality and cardiovascular death associated with febuxostat use compared to allopurinol, raising safety concerns, hence the first-line urate lowering treatment recommended is allopurinol.[24]

Prophylaxis is recommended during initiation of uric acid lowering therapy to prevent acute gout flares as uric acid levels fall to normal levels (this can take $>3−6$ months). Depending on comorbidities, prophylaxis can include colchicine (0.6 mg PO daily) or low dose steroids. Acute, abortive therapy includes IA steroid injection if one to two joints are involved. If more than two joints are involved, colchicine or a short course of steroid can be used. Indomethacin is not the recommended abortive therapy in older patients with gout.[25] Uric acid lowering therapy should not be stopped during acute flares. Rarely, for severe, refractory gout flares, interleukin (IL)-1 inhibitor (Anakinra) can be used.[26] Pseudogout is also treated with IA steroid injection if one to two joints are involved. Similar to gout therapy, both colchicine and steroids are used while NSAIDs are used with caution in older adults.

## Polymyalgia Rheumatica and Giant-Cell Arteritis

Steroids at different doses are used to treat PMR and GCA. The initial dose for PMR is prednisone 12.5 to 25 mg daily (or

**TABLE 44.4** Disease Modifying Drugs and Biologicals for Rheumatoid Arthritis

| Drugs | Usual Dose | Side Effects and Cautions |
|---|---|---|
| **DMARDS** | | |
| Methotrexate | 7.5–25 mg per week in a single dose orally or SQ. Start low and increase by 5 mg every 1 to 2 months until desired effects are achieved | Myelosuppression, hepatotoxicity, hepatic fibrosis, cirrhosis, pulmonary infiltrates or fibrosis, mouth sores (daily folic acid can prevent this), nausea, hair loss |
| Sulfasalazine (Azulfidine, Azulfidine EC) | 500–3000 mg per day in 2 to 4 divided doses orally | Myelosuppression, hepatotoxicity, nausea |
| Hydroxychloroquine sulfate (Plaquenil) | 200–400 mg per day in two divided doses orally Not to exceed 6.5 mg/kg of actual body weight | Retinal toxicity, rash |
| Leflunomide (Arava) | 10–20 mg per day in a single dose orally | Myelosuppression, hepatotoxicity, cirrhosis, diarrhea, hair loss |
| Azathioprine (Imuran) | 50–150 mg per day in 1 to 3 divided doses orally | Myelosuppression, hepatotoxicity, lymphoproliferative disorders, nausea, hair loss; check TPMT before initiation |
| **BIOLOGICALS** | | Must check Tspot and hepatitis B and C serology before starting all biologicals; discuss updating vaccinations before initiation |
| **TNF blockers:**<br>Adalimumab (Humira)<br>Etanercept (Enbrel)<br>Infliximab (Remicade)<br><br>Golimumab (Simponi)<br>Certolizumab (Cimzia) | 40 mg SQ once a week or every 2 weeks<br>25 mg SQ twice a week, or 50 mg SQ once a week<br>3–10 mg/kg IV. Given at 0, 2, 6 weeks then every 8 weeks (usually taken with methotrexate)<br>50 mg SQ once a month<br>400 mg SQ loading at 0, 2, 4 then 200 mg q 2 weeks vs 400 mg q 4 weeks | Increased risk of infections, tuberculosis, histoplasmosis or others;<br>Injection site or infusion reaction;<br>Congestive heart failure |
| **T-cell costimulation blocker:**<br>Abatacept (Orencia) | 500–1000 mg IV 0, 2, 4 weeks then every 4 weeks or 500–1000 mg IV one time, then 125 mg SQ weekly | Increased risk of infections; Injection site or infusion reaction; COPD exacerbation |
| **IL-6 blocker:**<br>Tocilizumab (Actemra) | 4–8 mg/kg IV every 4 weeks; 162 mg SQ once every other week or weekly | Increased risk of infections; Myelosuppression; Hepatotoxicity; Hyperlipidemia |
| **B-cell depletion:**<br>Rituximab | 1000 mg IV 0, 2 weeks and again when arthritis becomes active. On average every 6 months | Increased risk of infection; progressive multifocal leukoencephalopathy (PML); tumor lysis syndrome |
| **IL-1 blocker:**<br>Anakinra | 100 mg SQ daily, 100 mg SQ every other day in severe kidney disease | Increased risk of infections; Injection site reaction |

*COPD*, Chronic obstructive pulmonary disease; *IL*, interleukin; *TPMT*, thiopurine S-methyltransferase; *TNF*, tumor necrosis factor.

equivalent); the initial dose depends on patient's risk of relapse and other comorbidities (e.g., diabetes mellitus, congestive heart failure).[27] Higher risk of relapse has been associated with female sex, high ESR (> 40 mm/h), and peripheral inflammatory arthritis. Typically, PMR responds within 2 to 4 weeks at these doses of prednisone. The steroid taper begins once remission is achieved and is individualized to the patient based on symptom monitoring, ESR/CRP levels, and adverse effects from steroids. A taper may take 12 to 18 months with initial dose reduction within 4 to 8 weeks, followed by 1 mg/ month taper thereafter. Often, patients are started on osteoporosis prevention as prednisone doses can exceed 7.5 mg/d for ≥ 3 months. Steroid sparing medication are considered if patient experiences adverse effects from steroids or for relapse during the taper. Although effectiveness of methotrexate is not clear, studies have shown a decrease in the cumulative dose of steroids.

GCA is treated with higher doses of glucocorticoids, and treated early based on a convincing history and symptoms because a delay in treatment may result in sudden blindness. Typically, prednisone 1 mg/kg PO is given and maintained for 4 to 8 weeks or until symptomatic relief and normalization of the ESR and/or CRP. Intravenous glucocorticoids may be considered for initial treatment if a patient presents with transient or permanent vision loss, diplopia, transient ischemic attack, or stroke. Glucocorticoid treatment typically continues for 1 to 3 years as symptoms and inflammatory markers are monitored. Glucocorticoid therapy at doses that exceed prednisone 20 mg daily for ≥ 1 month warrants prophylaxis for osteoporosis and possibly for *Pneumocystis* pneumonia. Several trials show lower relapse rates and less overall steroid dosages with the addition of IL-6 blocker (tocilizumab), which is now approved for GCA. Few small studies show possibly reduced cumulative dose of steroids in the treatment of GCA with use of methotrexate but no evidence supports other steroid sparing agents (antitumor necrosis factor). Low-dose aspirin is used concurrently to decrease the risk of vision loss and cranial ischemic complications. The clinician should remain vigilant for development of aortic aneurysm even after immunosuppression has been discontinued.

◆◆ **Long-term use of steroids requires prophylaxis or treatment for osteoporosis; there are steroid sparing agents available to help reduce the total steroid dose needed.**

## CASE 1

### Discussion

Mrs. Montes's presentation is consistent with OA of the knees and hands. Mrs. Montes was anticoagulated with warfarin (Coumadin) so oral NSAIDs are contraindicated. However, she can use topical NSAIDS that are safe and moderately effective.[28] She should also be referred for PT given presence of quadriceps atrophy on examination and history of knee instability (buckling, giving way).[9] Referral to OT for hand exercises and possibly splinting is also suggested. Knee bracing may be helpful.[29] Encouraging the patient

to continue a home exercise program for both hand and knee OA will be important to sustain results. Because she has swelling in her knee, she should undergo synovial fluid aspiration of the knee to rule out concomitant CPPD, refer to rheumatology or orthopedics when needed. Aspiration of fluid and IA corticosteroid injection will also provide symptomatic relief.

## CASE 2

### Discussion

Mr. Smith's presentation is consistent with late-onset RA with inflammation in hands, wrists, and shoulders. The fusiform swelling of PIP joints indicates synovial inflammation compared to bony enlargement of the Heberden and Bouchard nodes typical of OA. Inflammatory markers and antibodies for RF and anti-CCP may be helpful in confirming the diagnosis. Early referral to rheumatology will help in initiating disease modifying treatment that is key in preventing joint damage and potentially other extraarticular manifestations. Given increased mortality associated with presence of RA, assessment of and optimization of cardiovascular risk factors are warranted.

## Summary

Early recognition of and diagnosis of rheumatic conditions in older adults is critical for appropriate referral to rheumatology and interdisciplinary management of arthritis and/or autoimmune disease. Education, physical activity/exercise/PT are all integral aspects of nonpharmacologic therapy and are particularly important in older adults to reduce unnecessary medications or surgery. Referral to rheumatology facilitates early DMARD and/or biologic therapy and follow-up for potential toxicity and to monitor disease activity. Comanagement between rheumatology and primary care is ideal for managing cardiovascular comorbidity, vaccinations, and polypharmacy in this vulnerable population. A coordinated approach to arthritis and autoimmune conditions will help older adults optimize social, mental, and physical function.

### Web Resources

National Institutes of Health's National Institute of Arthritis and Musculoskeletal Diseases: https://www.niams.nih.gov/health-topics/arthritis-and-rheumatic-diseases

Go4Life Campaign: promoting exercise and physical activity from National Institute of Aging: https://go4life.nia.nih.gov

Arthritis Foundation: https://www.arthritis.org

American College of Rheumatology: https://www.rheumatology.org

Centers for Disease Control and Prevention: https://www.cdc.gov/arthritis/

## Key References

7. Hootman JM, Helmick CG, Brady TJ. A public health approach to addressing arthritis in older adults: the most common cause of disability. *Am J Public Health.* 2012;102(3):426–433.

8. Makris UE, Abrams RC, Gurland B, Reid MC. Management of persistent pain in the older patient: a clinical review. *JAMA.* 2014;312(8):825–836.

9. Hochberg MC, Altman RD, April KT, et al. American College of Rheumatology 2012 recommendations for the use of nonpharmacologic and pharmacologic therapies in osteoarthritis of the hand, hip, and knee. *Arthritis Care Res.* 2012;64(4):465–474.

19. Singh JA, Saag KG, Bridges Jr SL, et al. 2015 American College of Rheumatology Guideline for the Treatment of Rheumatoid Arthritis. *Arthritis Care Res.* 2016;68(1):1–25.

23. Qaseem A, Harris RP, Forciea MA, Clinical Guidelines Committee of the American College of P. Management of acute and recurrent gout: a clinical practice guideline from the American College of Physicians. *Ann Intern Med.* 2017;166(1):58–68.

***References available online at* expertconsult.com.**

# 45
# Foot Problems

JEFFREY M. ROBBINS, ERIK MONSON, CARLY B. ROBBINS, AND ARTHUR E. HELFAND

## OUTLINE

## OBJECTIVES

*Upon completion of this chapter, the reader will be able to:*

- Recognize the primary clinical changes in the aging foot.
- Identify the primary systemic diseases associated with foot complications, ailments, conditions, and/or disorders.
- Understand the important principles and protocols of podogeriatric and chronic disease assessment of the aging foot and its related structures.

- Identify the essential complicating foot problems in the older adult.
- Recognize the importance of diabetic, avascular, and neurosensory-related foot problems in the aging patient.
- Understand the primary need to manage foot and related problems in the older patient to maintain quality of life.

## Primary Care Considerations in the Older Patient

Diseases and disorders of the foot and its related structures represent some of the most painful, distressing, and disabling afflictions associated with aging. They may alter the patient's quality of life, and may contribute to institutionalization. There are two important catalytic factors in the older individual's ability to remain a vital part of society; they are a keen mind and the ability to ambulate. Podiatric care is an essential service to foster mobility and independence among older persons and to protect their general health and a sense of wellbeing. The ability to remain ambulatory may be the only dividing line between institutionalization and remaining an active viable member of society.[1]

Foot and related pathologies in the older patient are a significant health concern, both from a standpoint of prevalence and incidence. The immobility that results from a focal foot problem or as the result of complications of a systemic disease, such as diabetes mellitus (DM), peripheral vascular diseases, (arterial and venous), sensory and motor neurologic disease, and degenerative joint changes, can have a significant negative impact on the patient's ability to maintain a quality of life as a useful member of society.[2]

There are many systemic and/or life changes not already mentioned that can directly contribute to high-risk foot problems. These include agitation, compulsive activities, increased foot perspiration, neurologic and sensory deficits, neurotic excoriation, changes in mental status, self-mutilation, chronic constipation and incontinence, weakened muscle and bone structure, impaired cardiovascular function, reduced interest and/or participation in social activities, decreased and/or loss of mobility, pododynia dysbasia, sleep problems, reduced interest and/or participation in social activities, and a reduction of independent and/or instrumental activities of daily living. Good foot care is essential for older adults who prize remaining independent.[3]

# Foot Deformities

The majority of foot deformities (bunions, hammertoes, pes cavus, pes planus, tailors bunion, etc.) in the older adult patient are treated conservatively. This treatment consists of footwear modifications, orthotics, padding, debridement of hyperkeratotic tissue, keratolytic medications, and so on. Oftentimes this treatment is successful and keeps the patient functioning and in less pain. When all conservative therapy has been exhausted and the patient has significant pain or ambulation restrictions that limit quality of life, then surgery would be the remaining option. Age itself should not be the final determining factor in considering surgery. The main consideration is whether or not the benefits/potential outcomes of the surgery outweigh the potential complications/risks. This decision should occur after a thorough discussion with the patient/family regarding the benefits of surgery versus the potential risks. If the benefits outweigh the risks, then surgery would certainly be an option despite the patient's age. Consider a 52-year-old patient with long-standing DM, neuropathy, renal transplant, coronary artery disease with two prior myocardial infarction versus an 83-year-old patient who is relative healthy with hypertension and hypercholesterolemia who both have a painful second-digit hammertoe that limits ambulation. Despite being 31 years older, the 83-year-old patient would have less risk of complications with the hammertoe correction surgery.

❖❖ **The immobility that results from a local foot problem or as the result of complications of a systemic disease such as DM, peripheral vascular diseases (arterial and venous), sensory and motor neuropathy and degenerative joint changes, and diseases identified in the Americans for Disabilities Act of 1990 can have a significant negative impact on the patient's ability to maintain quality of life as a useful member of society.**

## Changes in the Foot in Relation to Age

There are many factors that contribute to the development of foot problems in the older adult population, including the aging process itself and the presence of multiple chronic diseases. Other significant factors include the degree of ambulation, balance issues, the duration of prior hospitalization, limitation of activity, prior institutionalization, episodes of social segregation, emotional adjustments to disease, multiple medications for multiple chronic diseases, and the complications and residuals associated with other diseases. The management of foot problems in the geriatric patient requires a comprehensive team approach by those licensed to maximize the quality of care provided.

### Skin Changes

The skin of the foot is usually one of the first structures to demonstrate early change. There is usually a loss of hair below the knee and on the dorsum of the foot and toes.

Atrophy then follows with the skin appearing parchment-like and xerotic. Brownish pigmentations are common and related to the deposition of hemosiderin. Hyperkeratosis, when present, may result from keratin dysfunction, a response to repetitive pressure, atrophy of the subcutaneous soft tissue, and/or as space replacement as the body attempts to adjust to the changing stress placed on the foot.[4]

### Nail Changes

The toenails undergo degenerative trophic changes (onychopathy), thickening, and/or longitudinal ridging (onychorrhexis) related to

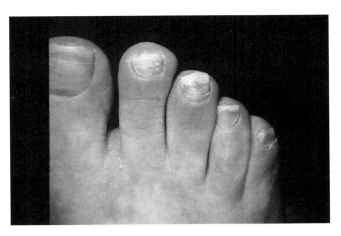

• **Figure 45.1** Marked ischemia and peripheral arterial disease related to diabetes mellitus.

repeated microtrauma, disease, and nutritional impairment. Deformities of the toenails become pronounced and complicated by xerotic changes in the periungual nail folds as onychophosis (hyperkeratosis) and tinea unguium (onychomycosis). These conditions are usually long-standing, chronic, and very common in the older adult population and, in the case of onychomycosis (Fig. 45.1), present a constant focus of infection.

❖❖ **Deformities of the toenails become pronounced and complicated by xerotic changes in the periungual nail folds as onychophosis (hyperkeratosis) and tinea unguium (onychomycosis). These conditions are usually long-standing, chronic, and very common in older adults and, in the case of onychomycosis, present a constant focus of infection.**

### Musculoskeletal Changes

There is a progressive loss of muscle mass and atrophy of tissue caused by disease. Decreased function and a lack of activity increases the susceptibility of the foot to injury; thus even minor trauma can result in a fracture and a marked limitation of activity.

---

**CASE 1**

**A 70-year old male**

A 70-year-old male with a history of mild congestive heart failure presents to your office. Pedal pulses are present and there are early clinical symptoms and signs of peripheral arterial disease (PAD). He has pain and a small hematoma on the dorsum of his left second toe. He indicates that he dropped a can on his foot, but that he was wearing a soft slipper. The toe has continued to hurt, especially when walking. Mild hammertoes were noted and the patient indicated that he has had arthritis for some time.
1. What would be your initial steps?

---

**CASE 1**

**Discussion**

Initial management would include radiographs to rule out a fracture. If there is a fracture in good position, immobilization by "buddy splinting" (with hypoallergenic tape with proper precautions to protect the web space from maceration) can be used to immobilize the toe with the possibility of a surgical shoe for ambulation. Without evidence of fracture, a "buddy splint" can still be used for a shorter period to splint the joint, followed by the use of a protective tube and/or surgical shoe. While there are palpable pedal pulses, there are also some signs of arterial disease. As such, special care when applying the "buddy splint" must be taken to minimize any constriction in the toes. Disruption of the vascular supply could precipitate necrotic changes distal to the trauma site so that reassessment and follow-up are important. The patient should be instructed to take special care when at home to minimize additional trauma by wearing the prescribed protective device(s).

## Podogeriatric Assessment

The initial evaluation of the older patient should include a comprehensive assessment and risk stratification process. A comprehensive podogeriatric and chronic disease assessment protocol (Helfand Index),[5] developed for the Pennsylvania Department of Health, enables practitioners to initiate a diagnostic and risk stratification procedure that includes multiple elements. The comprehensive assessment tool can be used to assess both pathology and risk factors. These elements include demographics, history of present illness, and past medical history. Current prescriptions and over-the-counter medications should be noted.[6]

The dermatologic evaluation should include but is not limited to the following: hyperkeratosis, bacterial infection, ulceration, cyanosis, xerosis, tinea pedis, verruca, hematoma, rubor, discoloration, and preulcerative changes.

The foot musculoskeletal evaluation includes but is not limited to osseous deformities, such as bunions and hammer toes, as well as muscle strength and range of motion.[7-9]

The peripheral vascular evaluation should include but is not limited to arterial and venous signs and symptoms: coldness, trophic changes, palpation of the dorsalis pedis and posterior tibial pulses, capillary refill time, the history of rest pain and/or claudication, edema, atrophy, varicosities, venous insufficiency, and presence of, or history of, venous/arterial ulcers, and prior amputation or partial amputation.

The neurologic evaluation should include but is not limited to pain assessment, Achilles, patellar and superficial plantar reflexes, vibratory sensation (pallesthesia), loss of protective sensation (with a 10-g monofilament), sharp and dull reaction, joint position (proprioception), burning, and balance assessment.[10]

**◆◆ The two main factors that predispose geriatric patients to problems are PAD and neuropathy. PAD makes it difficult for patients to heal any type of wound and neuropathy predisposes them to developing foot ulcers.**

## Diabetes and Foot Care

The older patient with diabetes presents a special problem in relation to foot health.[11] It has been projected that 50% to 75% of all amputations in the diabetic cohort can be prevented by early intervention where pathology is noted. This can be accomplished by improved foot care health education, and by periodic assessment before the onset of symptoms and pathology (secondary and tertiary prevention). The older adult patient with diabetes is subject to all of the problems related to the disease itself. These include vascular impairment, sensory and motor neuropathy, and

dermopathy. These factors are also complicated by the social restrictions related to these multiple pathologies.[12-14]

**◆◆ The older patient with diabetes presents a special problem in relation to foot health. It has been projected that 50% to 75% of all amputations in the diabetic can be prevented by early intervention where pathology is noted. This can be accomplished by improved health education, and by periodic evaluation before the onset of symptoms and pathology (secondary and tertiary prevention).**

The older patient with diabetes and neuropathy has insensitive feet that will usually exhibit some degree of paresthesia, sensory impairment to pain and temperature, motor weakness, diminished or lost Achilles and patellar reflexes, decreased vibratory sense, a loss of proprioception, xerotic changes, anhidrosis, neurotrophic arthropathy (Charcot), atrophy, neurotrophic ulcers, and the potential for a marked difference in size between two feet. Foot drop and a loss of position sense may be present. Arthropathy gives rise to deformity (Charcot), altered gait patterns, and a higher risk for ulceration and limb loss. There is a greater incidence of infection, necrosis, and gangrene.[15]

Vascular impairment may demonstrate pallor on elevation, dependent rubor, a loss or decrease in the posterior tibial and dorsalis pedis pulse, a decrease in the venous filling (capillary refill) time, coolness of the skin, and trophic changes. Numbness and tingling, as well as cramps and pain, can be demonstrated. There is usually a loss of the plantar metatarsal fat pad that predisposes the patient to ulceration in relation to the existing bony deformities of the foot and repetitive microtrauma.[15-17]

Hyperkeratotic lesions form in response to pressure and friction and form space replacements. They can provide a focus for ulceration because of increased pressure on the soft tissues with an associated localized avascularity from direct pressure and counter pressure. The mechanical changes caused by tendon contractures and claw toes (hammertoes) are a common cause of hyperkeratotic lesions. Ulcerations can form under hyperkeratotic lesions especially when there is a loss of protection sensation. When ulceration is present, the base is usually roofed by hyperkeratosis often preventing healing. Infection, necrosis, and gangrene are associated with infection with eventual occlusion and amputation.

Risk assessment models similar to one used in the Department of Veterans Affairs Prevention of Amputation in Veterans Everywhere (PAVE) Program can identify patients at risk for foot wound and amputations and those at high risk. It involves assessment for disease procurers, in this case peripheral vascular disease, loss of protection sensation, and foot deformities, and assigning a risk level to each patient. A management and referral algorithm is used to quickly refer those patients at high risk for care and schedule those at lower risk for ongoing surveillance. This is always coupled with foot care health education and follow-up on adherence of those behaviors.[18-20]

**◆◆ Hyperkeratotic lesions in the diabetic patient form as space replacements and provide a focus for ulceration because of increased pressure on the soft tissues with an associated localized avascularity from direct pressure and counterpressure.**

The most commonly demonstrated nail changes are noted but not limited to the following: onychomycosis (fungal), onychocryptosis (ingrown), diabetic onychopathy (nutritional and vascular changes), onychorrhexis (longitudinal striations), onycholysis

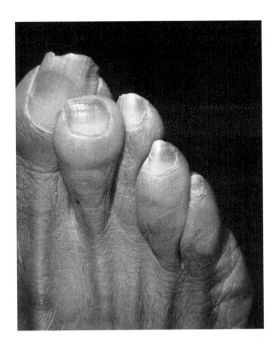

• **Figure 45.2** Hallux valgus, hammertoes, bowstring dorsal tendons, overriding second toe, onychodystrophy.

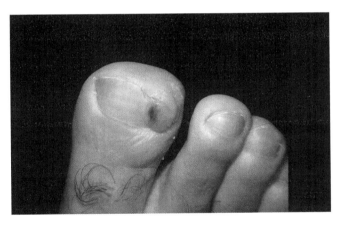

• **Figure 45.3** Infected ingrown toenail with periungual ulcerative granulation tissue, hallux.

(shedding from the distal portion), onychomadesis (shedding from the proximal portion; Fig. 45.2), subungual hemorrhage (bleeding in the nail bed), onychophosis (keratosis), onychauxis (thickening with hypertrophy), onychogryphosis (thickening with gross deformity), onychia (inflammation; Fig. 45.3), onychomycosis (fungal infection), subungual ulceration (ulceration in the nail bed), deformity, hypertrophy, incurvation or involution (onychodysplasia), subungual hemorrhage (nontraumatic), and autoavulsion.

Radiographic findings in the foot in older patients with diabetes usually demonstrate thin trabecular patterns, decalcification, joint position changes, osteophytic formation, osteolysis, deformities, and osteoporosis. Pruritus and cutaneous infections are more common in diabetes. Dehydration, trophic changes, anhidrosis, xerosis, and fissures are predisposing factors to calcaneal ulceration.[21–23]

**CASE 2**

**A 75-year-old female (Part 1)**

A 75-year-old female with a 12-year history of adult-onset (noninsulin-dependent) diabetes mellitus is adequately diet controlled, as reported by her endocrinologist. She reports noticing a dark spot under her left great toenail in recent months but with no pain. She has trophic changes and diminished pedal pulses. Doppler studies detect both pedal pulses. Testing with a monofilament demonstrates a loss of sensation to the forefoot. All toenails demonstrate onychorrhexis (thickening and/or longitudinal ridging), and xerosis of the skin was noted. No other significant clinical findings were noted.

1. What is the most important consideration in the differential diagnosis given the lack of pain?
   a. Subungual heloma (callus)
   b. Subungual ulceration
   c. Subungual hematoma
   d. Subungual exostosis/spur
   e. Subungual melanoma

**CASE 2**

**Discussion**

Initial management includes radiographs to rule out an exostosis or spur or other bony change. If the concern is related to a possible melanoma, biopsy should be completed with appropriate surgical referral. With a history of trauma, a subungual hematoma should be considered. Without trauma, a subungual diabetic ulcer should be considered. If there is an enlargement of the dorsal aspect of the tip of the distal phalanx on x-ray examination, a subungual heloma (callus) should be considered. Appropriate management depends on the diagnosis. A depth shoe or other protective padding can then be used to help reduce pressure. The patient should avoid walking barefoot and injuring the toe without knowing because of the neuropathy.

## Onychia

Onychia is an inflammation involving the posterior nail wall and nail bed. The onychial changes that occur in the older adult patient are the result of a new disease or are the residual of chronic disease, injury, and/or functional modification. It is usually precipitated by local trauma or pressure, a complication of systemic diseases, such as DM, and is an early sign of a developing infection. Mild erythema, swelling, and pain are the most prevalent findings. Treatment should be directed at removing all pressure from the area and the use of tepid saline compresses for 15 minutes, three times per day (note: do not soak feet). With systemic complications, systemic antibiotics should be instituted early along with radiographs and scans to detect bone change at its earliest sign. Lamb's wool, tube foam, or shoe modification should also be considered to reduce pressure to the toe and nail. If the onychia is not treated early, paronychia may develop with significant infection and abscess of the posterior nail wall. The infection progresses proximally and deeper structures may become involved. The potential for osteomyelitis is greater in the presence of DM and vascular insufficiency. Necrosis, gangrene, and the potential for amputation become reality. Management includes establishing drainage, culture and sensitivity, radiographs and scans as appropriate, the use of saline compresses, and appropriate systemic

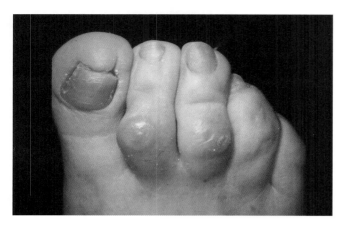

• **Figure 45.4** Hallux valgus, multiple hammertoes, heloma related to contractures and pressure, and onychodystrophy.

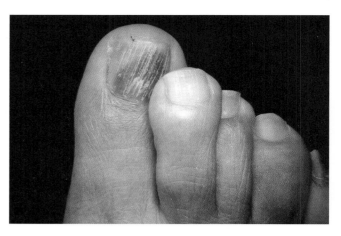

• **Figure 45.5** Subungual hematoma and onychorrhexis of hallux with onychomycosis, deformity of second toe with early onychia.

antibiotics and possible topical antibiotics with a dressing changes. Always advise against soaking the feet because it can lead to maceration of tissue. If patients prefer to soak, have them limit this to only a few minutes to avoid maceration. They should also test the water first to avoid burns. This is especially true for those patients with sensory neuropathy and the loss of protection sensation, as well as those with PAD as even 99o F temperatures have been known to cause tissue damage because of the inability of the body to dissipate heat. Early follow-up is essential because these conditions can result in significant problems in management.[24]

❖ **Treatment of onychia should be directed toward removing all pressure from the area and the use of tepid saline compresses for 15 minutes, three times per day, continuing surveillance, and appropriate antibiotics, as indicated. Note: Foot soaking is not recommended.**

Deformities of the toenails are the result of repeated microtrauma, degenerative changes, or disease. For example, the continued rubbing of the toenails over the years against the inferior toe box of the shoe is sufficient trauma to produce change. The initial thickening is termed onychauxis. Onychorrhexis with accentuation of normal ridging, trophic changes, and longitudinal striations are onychopathic when related to disease and/or nutritional etiology. When debridement is not completed on a periodic basis, the nail structure elongates, continues to thicken, and becomes deformed with shoe pressure. Onychogryphosis or "ram's horn nail," is usually complicated by fungal infection. The resultant disability can prevent older adults from wearing shoes. Pain is usually associated with shoe pressure and the deformity. In addition, a traumatic avulsion of the nail is more frequent with this condition. The exaggerated curvature (onychodysplasia; Fig. 45.4) may even penetrate the skin, with resultant infection and ulceration. Management should be directed toward periodic debridement of the onychial structures both in length and thickness, with as little trauma as possible. The degree of onycholysis (freeing of the nail from the anterior edge) and onychoschizia (splitting) helps determine the level of debridement. With the excess pressure of deformity, the nail grooves tend to become onychophosed (keratotic). When this occurs, debridement and the use of mild keratolytics and emollients, such as urea preparations, provide some measure of home care for the patient. With

onycholysis, subungual debris and keratosis develop, which increases discomfort and may generate pain. However, the patient may not complain of pain and discomfort because of neuropathy and care should be provided for the deformity. The loss of protective sensation in the form of sensory neuropathy may be present, which tends to defer care by the patient until a complicating condition occurs (Fig. 45.5).[25,26]

## Onychomycosis

The most common nonbacterial infection of the toenails is onychomycosis. It is a chronic and communicable disease with four clinical subtypes, including (1) distal subungual, (2) white superficial, (3) proximal subungual, or (4) total dystrophic. In the superficial variety, the changes appear on the superior surface of the toenail and generally do not invade the deeper structures. In distal, proximal, and total dystrophic manifestations, the nail bed, as well as the nail plate, are infected. There is usually some degree of onycholysis (freeing of the nail from the distal edge) and subungual keratosis. In the older adult population, because of the longstanding chronic nature of this condition, the posterior nail wall and eponychium demonstrate xerotic changes and hypertrophy, as does the nail plate. Candida is most common in patients with some form of chronic mucocutaneous manifestation.

❖ **The most common nonbacterial infection of the toenails is onychomycosis. It is a chronic and communicable disease, and clinically it may appear as distal subungual, white superficial, proximal subungual, total dystrophic, or candida (mold) onychomycosis.**

The older adult patient with this condition usually has the presenting symptom of chronic infection, involving one or more of the nail plates. The entire thickness of the nail plates is usually involved with resultant hypertrophy and deformity. Pain is usually not a significant factor because of the normal lessening of sensation in older adults but can be present when the deformity becomes excessive and is related to external pressure. Mycotic onychia; autoavulsion; subungual hemorrhage; a foul, musty odor; and degeneration of the nail plate are common findings. The most practical form of treatment in older adults is one of management. Because

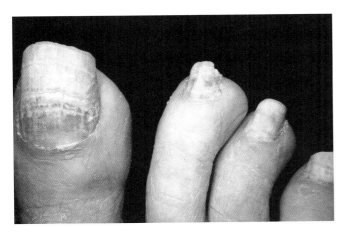

• **Figure 45.6** Onychauxis, onychomycosis, onychodystrophy, xerosis, and distal digital deformity.

of the chronicity of the condition and the fact that once the matrix of the nail is involved and hypertrophy and deformity occur, the residuals cannot be reversed. In addition, multiple drug use for systemic diseases and vascular impairment limits systemic management. Periodic debridement, the use of 35% to 50% urea to aid in debridement, and the use of a topical fungicide in an alcoholic base to permit penetration provide a conservative approach to management, which also reduces the risk of recurrent or chronic tinea pedis infection. Systemic antifungals can also be used as indicated but carry the risk of hepatotoxicity. Onychomycosis must be viewed as a chronic infectious disease, deserving management as any other chronic condition, such as hypertension and/or DM (Fig. 45.6).

## Ingrown Toenails (Onychocryptosis)

Ingrown toenails in older adults are usually the end result of deformity, improper care, and long-standing onychodysplasia. When the nail penetrates the skin, an abscess and then infection result. If not managed early, periungual granulation tissue may form, which complicates treatment. Deformity and involution also provide a complicating factor. In the early stage, a segment of the nail can easily be removed using a nail splitter (English or anvil type), then incision and drainage established to establish drainage, saline compresses used for 15 minutes three times a day, and antibiotics used as indicated. It should be noted that providing antibiotics without removing the offending portion of toenail will not resolve the problem. Measures should be taken to prevent the problem in the future. When granulation tissue is present, excision, fulguration, desiccation, or the use of caustics (such as silver nitrate [75%]) and astringents may be used to reduce the granulation tissue. In all cases, removal of the penetrating nail is primary. Partial excision of the nail plate and matrix can be completed using local anesthesia followed by chemical cautery of the matrix area with liquefied phenol or sodium hydroxide, for example. With this procedure, postoperative management may include isopropyl alcohol or saline compresses, topical steroid solutions, and/or a topical antibiotic, three times per day to healing. Surgical excision of the matrix without chemical cautery is also a valid option. Although removal of the ingrown portion of the nail is essential to clearing the infection, it should also be noted that the patient's vascular status should be evaluated before any caustic chemicals are applied.

With aging, we also find changes in the nail plate, which when viewed distally appears C-shaped. This abnormal curvature is incurvation or involution. When present, the pressure of the nail plate on the nail bed and folds produces onychophosis (hyperkeratosis in the nail folds) and discomfort, with complaints similar to an ingrown toenail. The condition may precipitate pressure ulcerations and infection. When this condition is severe, early and total removal of the nail plate and matrix should be considered to avoid complications as the patient ages.[28]

## Dryness and Xerosis

Dryness of the skin and xerosis are common problems in the older patient. They result from a lack of hydration and lubrication, and to some degree are part of the normal aging and degenerative process. There is usually some evidence of keratin dysfunction that can be associated with xerosis. Fissures develop as a result of dryness and when present on the heel, with associated stress, present a potential hazard for the development of infection and ulceration. Initial management includes the use of an emollient following hydration of the skin; urea and/or lactic acid preparations may be helpful to aid as a mild and safe keratolytic. A plastic or Styrofoam heel cup can be of assistance in minimizing trauma to the heel, thus reducing the potential for complications. Pruritus is a common complaint of older adults and is usually more severe in the colder weather. It is related to dryness, scaliness, decreased skin secretions, keratin dysfunction, and environmental changes of the skin that can be precipitated by the constant use of hot foot soaks. The patient will scratch with excoriations noted on examination. Chronic tinea, allergic, neurogenic, and/or emotional dermatoses should be considered as part of the differential diagnosis and treated accordingly. Management consists of hydration, lubrication, protection, topical steroids if indicated, and judicious use of antihistamines in minimal doses to control the itching, which is usually the primary complaint, unless medically contraindicated. If excoriations are infected, proper antibiotic therapy should be instituted. Foot soaks should be avoided.

◆◆ **Initial management of fissures that are a result of dryness on the heel includes the use of an emollient following hydration of the skin; urea and/or lactic acid preparations may be helpful to aid as a mild and safe keratolytic. A plastic or Styrofoam heel cup can be of assistance in minimizing trauma to the heel, thus reducing the potential for complications.**

## Tinea Pedis

Tinea pedis in the older adult population is many ways an extension of onychomycosis, which serves as a focus of infection. It is more common in warmer weather with the chronic keratotic type more common clinically in the older adult population. Poor foot hygiene in many older patients and the inability to see their feet may motivate patients to seek care only when the condition becomes clinically significant. Proper foot health education is also an important element of care. The variety of topical medications available can usually control this condition. Solutions and/or creams (water washable or miscible) should be used when the patient is unable to easily remove an ointment base. For those patients who have difficulty seeing or reaching their feet, a mirror on a stick and sponge on a still can aid in proper daily foot inspections and daily hygiene. These are readily available at local medical supply companies.

## Hyperkeratotic Lesions

Common complaints of most older adults are the many forms of hyperkeratotic lesions, such as tyloma (callus) and heloma (corn) and their varieties, which include hard, soft, vascular, neurofibrous, seed, and subungual. Intractable keratoma, eccrine poroma, porokeratosis, and verruca must be differentiated from these keratotic lesions, although each may present initially as a hyperkeratotic area. The biomechanic and pathomechanic factors that help create these problems are those associated with stress (i.e., compressive, tensile, and/or shearing). The loss of soft tissue as part of the aging process and atrophy of the plantar fat pad increase pain and limit ambulation. Contractures, gait changes, deformities, and the residuals of arthritis are all additional factors that need to be considered in management. The incompatibility of the foot type (inflare, straight, or outflare) to the shoe last is another factor to be considered. It is important to recognize that there is usually not one factor but a multiplicity of conditions, including skin tone and elasticity, which result in the development of keratotic lesions in the older adult population. Their management is not routine and the term *management* signifies a period of continuing care, as with any other chronic condition in the older adult population, to provide for ambulation and comfort.

The common sites for the development of hyperkeratotic lesions (calluses and corns) are generally over bony prominences (e.g., dorsal or distal digital, plantar metatarsal heads, marginal calcaneal, and with deformities such as hammertoes [Fig. 45.7], digital rotations, contractures, hallux valgus, bunion, and/or tailor's bunion). These deformities are precipitating factors to foot-to-shoe-last incompatibilities that produce excessive pressure and friction on segments of the foot. Management and treatment should be directed toward the functional needs of the patients and on their activity needs for daily living. Considerations include debridement, padding, emollients, shoe modifications, and shoe last changes, orthoses, and surgical management as indicated. Materials to provide soft tissue replacement, weight dispersion, and weight diffusion are also indicated. It is important to recognize that keratotic lesions of long standing represent a hyperplastic and hypertrophic pathology and that even when weight bearing is removed they tend to persist. In a sense, hyperkeratotic lesions are a form of body protection to pressure and friction and are symptoms of an abnormal state. If permitted to persist, enlarge, and condense, they become primary irritants. With pressure, such as weight bearing and ambulation, they produce local avascularity,

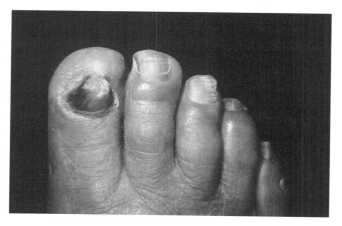

• **Figure 45.7** Onychodysplasia—incurvated hallux toenail, onychomycosis, multiple hammertoes.

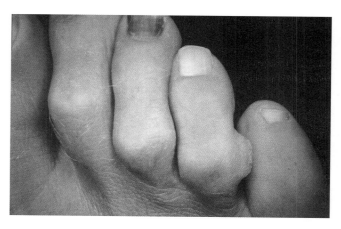

• **Figure 45.8** Multiple hammertoes with dorsal hypertrophy and heloma molle, fourth toe.

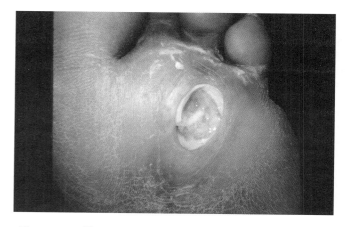

• **Figure 45.9** Plantar diabetic ulcer, metatarsal prolapse, anterior metatarsal fat pad displacement.

which can precipitate ulceration and their resultant sequelae. Pressure ulcers in the foot usually begin with subkeratotic hemorrhage (Figs. 45.8 and 45.9). Once debrided and managed properly, they usually heal but may be repetitive unless adequate measures are instituted to reduce the pressure to the localized areas of ulceration. Even with all measures, the problem may persist because of residual deformity and systemic diseases, such as DM. Thus management and monitoring are similar to any other chronic condition in the older adult population and can have a significant impact on the social elements of society, for without ambulation the older adult patient often needs to be institutionalized.[29,30]

❖ **The common sites for the development of hyperkeratotic lesions (calluses and corns) are generally over bony prominences (e.g., dorsal or distal digital, plantar metatarsal heads, marginal calcaneal, and with deformities such as hammertoes, digital rotations, contractures, hallux valgus, bunion, and/or tailor's bunion).**

## Foot Deformities

There are a variety of foot deformities that can be present in multiple combinations in the older adult population. These include but

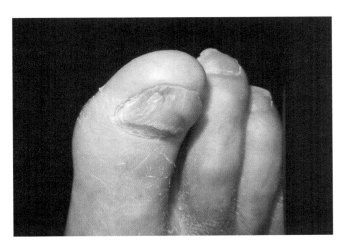

• **Figure 45.10** Onychomadesis, onychomycosis, hallux toenail.

are not limited to hallux valgus, hallux varus, splay foot, digiti flexus (hammertoe), digiti quinti varus, overlapping toes (Fig. 45.10), underriding toes, pes cavus, pes planus, pronation, hallux limitus, and hallux rigidus.

Biomechanical, pathomechanical, and stress-related pathologies create functional problems in relation to gait and obtaining adequate footwear. Examples include plantar fasciitis, spur formation, periostitis, decalcification, stress fractures, tendonitis, tenosynovitis, pes planus, pes cavus, hallux valgus, digiti flexus (hammertoes), rotational digital deformities, joint swelling, pain, limitation of motion, and painful and limited ambulatory function (pododynia dysbasia—ambulatory dysfunction). Treatment consists of both nonsurgical and surgical considerations. Age itself should not be the final determining factor in considering surgery. It is important to determine what can be planned to maintain a quality of life for the patient. Consideration should also be given to the patient's ability to adapt to change in relation to ambulation; to have an anatomically corrected joint and a patient who cannot ambulate without pain defeats the purpose of treating the older adult population.

Conservative modalities include shoe last changes, shoe modifications, orthoses (ankle and foot), digital braces, physical medicine, exercises, and mild analgesics for pain. Deformities can limit ambulation and the ability of the patient to maintain a good quality of life.

The deformities can produce inflammatory changes, such as periarthritis, bursitis, myositis, synovitis, neuritis, tendonitis, sesamoiditis, and plantar myofasciitis, for example, which should be managed medically, physically, and mechanically to keep the patient ambulatory and pain free.[31]

◆◆ **Conservative modalities to treat biomechanic and pathomechanic abnormalities include shoe last changes, shoe modifications, orthoses (ankle and foot), digital braces, physical medicine, exercises, and mild analgesics for pain.**

## Summary

Much of the ability to remain ambulatory in the period of aging is directly related to foot health. To maintain foot health, and thus ambulation, practitioners must think comprehensively, and recognize that team care must be an essential part of geriatrics and gerontology. Foot health education, such as programs developed by Feet First and If the Shoe Fits, are available to both patients and professionals, and should be used as a part of all geriatric patient education programs. With the high prevalence and incidence of foot problems in the older adult population, much of their quality of life will depend on their ability to remain mentally alert and ambulatory.[32]

## Key References

1. Banks A, Downey MS, Martin DE, Miller SJ. *McGlamry's Forefoot Surgery.* Philadelphia, PA: Lippincott, Williams & Wilkins; 2004.
11. Foster AVM. *Podiatric Assessment and Management of the Diabetic Foot.* Edinburgh, Scotland: Churchill-Livingstone-Elsevier; 2006.
15. Ham RJ, Sloane PD, Warshaw GA, et al. *Primary Care Geriatrics—A Case Based Approach.* 5th ed. Philadelphia, PA: Mosby/Elsevier; 2007.
24. Helfand AE. Clinical assessment of peripheral arterial occlusive risk factors in the diabetic foot. *Int J Clin Pract.* 2007;61(4):540–541.
28. Merriman LM, Turner W. *Assessment of the Lower Limb.* 2nd ed. New York, NY: Churchill Livingstone–Elsevier; 2002.
32. Yates B. *Merriman's Assessment of the Lower Limb.* 3rd ed. Edinburgh, Scotland: Churchill Livingstone–Elsevier; 2009.

**References available online at** expertconsult.com.

# 46

# Cancer

MIRIAM B. RODIN AND MATTHEW K. MCNABNEY

## OBJECTIVES

*Upon completion of this chapter, the reader will be able to:*

- Be aware of age-related differences in cancer biology that affect age-related decisions for the management of specific cancers.
- Summarize general principles of cancer management applied to the older adult population.
- Be prepared to apply geriatric principles to maintaining functional status of older adult cancer patients.

- Be familiar with disease-specific treatment guidelines for several common cancers in the older adult population.
- Apply current cancer prevention and cancer screening guidelines appropriately to the older adult population.
- Understand special issues in the care of cancer survivors.

## Cancer in the Older Adult Population

Cancer is the second leading cause of death and a major cause of morbidity for persons age 65 years and older. More than 50% of all new solid tumor diagnoses are made among people over 65 years of age.[1,2] In addition, there are now more than 11 million cancer survivors in the United States, 6.5 million of whom are of Medicare age.[3] Cancer control in older individuals includes early diagnosis, prevention, individualized treatment plans, supportive care, end-of-life care, and survivor care. The primary care physician (PCP) plays a key role in each stage of cancer care, and it is increasingly clear that patients benefit from having a multidisciplinary team.

Frequently, it is the PCP who first detects the cancer. It is important that geriatricians and other primary care providers have a good understanding of the risks and benefits of current therapies for various cancers to interpret specialist recommendations and assist patients and families to make realistic decisions, which are neither irrationally optimistic nor pessimistic. Furthermore, an informed PCP can often be the best advocate for a patient who is also encountering oncologists with overly optimistic or pessimistic biases with respect to older adults. Referral to an oncologist sometimes results in differing perspectives on treatment, so having the specialist and PCP involved and on the same page helps patients with difficult decisions and complex treatments.

## Jane Thompson (Part 1)

Jane Thompson, an 81-year-old woman, is brought to the hospital semicomatose by an ambulance. Two weeks earlier, she was reported by her daughter to be in excellent general health, with the exception of osteoarthritis. She was independent in her activities of daily living (ADLs) and in her instrumental ADLs (IADLs). She had lived alone for 12 years since the death of her husband. After fluid resuscitation in the emergency department and correction of her electrolytes on the inpatient service, the patient becomes responsive but is still confused. She is unable to tolerate oral fluids or food. An esophagogastroscopy shows gastric outlet obstruction by a mass. The biopsy reveals it is a diffuse large B-cell lymphoma (DLBCL). By computed tomography (CT) scan the tumor appears unresectable. You initiate intravenous total parenteral nutrition (TPN) and call an oncologist for consultation.

1. Who will make decisions regarding how aggressive Mrs. Thompson's medical care will be?
2. What options are available to provide nutritional support to Mrs. Thompson?
3. What cancer-directed treatment options are available to provide treatment for Mrs. Thompson's tumor?
4. Before this event, what was Mrs. Thompson's estimated remaining life expectancy?
5. If Mrs. Thompson is treated with standard chemotherapy, what is the likelihood of complete remission?
6. What is the likely duration of that remission?
7. What are her risk factors for severe treatment toxicity?
8. What can/should be done to control the risks of treatment?

## Cancer Biology and Aging

More than half of new diagnoses of the common solid tumors, including lung, breast, colon, prostate, and ovarian cancers, occur in those age 65 years and older. For most of these cancers, incidence increases with age at least to 85 years of age, after which the rate of increase levels off. However, the biological behavior of most common solid tumors changes with the age of the patient as a result of mechanisms shown in Table 46.1.[4]

Worse survival of older adults with cancer is partly because of differences in the cancer biology but also because of the choices made about their treatment. Examples of neoplasms of older people that

are less responsive to chemotherapy include osteosarcomas, glioblastomas, and several hematological and lymphatic malignancies. Acute myelogenous leukemia (AML) and Hodgkin and non-Hodgkin lymphomas have different genetics and different prognostic characteristics in the older adult population. Age itself should not determine the treatment of cancer. Some 67% of older persons with AML have a poor prognosis biology that is multidrug resistant, but 33% have a disease responsive to current chemotherapy. Although 80% of older women have an indolent form of breast cancer that is hormone sensitive, the remainder have aggressive disease that may benefit from adjuvant chemotherapy and radiotherapy.[8]

Recent advances in genetic analysis of tumor cells promise to improve chemotherapy targeting. For some malignancies, oncologists can predict which cancers will respond to available chemotherapy agents and those which will not. In the older adult population, this is especially useful because the decision to accept highly toxic treatment should be conditioned upon the probability of response. Examples of cancer cell markers effectively selected by newer targeted chemotherapy agents include the human epidermal growth factor receptor 2 (HER2/neu), which indicates responsiveness to trastuzumab; KRAS in colon cancer predicts sensitivity to cetuximab. Other genetic markers are BRAF and mTOR. Molecular profiling of tumors is rapidly emerging as an exciting modality, and testing has greatly grown in availability.[9]

In addition to tumor biology, aspects of host resistance may account for poorer survival in the older adult population. This includes both systemic responses and age-related differences in the tumor microenvironment. Immune senescence impairs surveillance for abnormal cells.[6] Microenvironmental factors such as angiogenesis and tissue growth factors differ with age, as do whole organism characteristics such as renal function and cardiovascular fitness. One well-studied example is the inflammatory response. For example, the concentration of interleukin (IL) 6 in the circulation increases with age. Some cancers also stimulate the inflammatory response. Chronic inflammation may play a role in tumor formation, for example in some gastrointestinal (GI) malignancies, such as colon cancer. Blunted T-cell and natural killer (NK) cell immune surveillance has been thought to undermine host response to neoplastic cells.[6,7] Clinical applications of these observations include the following: contrary to expectations, some cancers such as myeloid and lymphoid malignancies may become more aggressive with age. Some, such as non–small cell lung

**TABLE 46.1  Selected Age-Related Changes in Tumor Biology**

| Disease | Prognosis in Older Patients | Mechanism |
|---|---|---|
| Acute myelogenous leukemia | Worse | Increased multiple drug resistance; increased incidence of stem cell leukemia[5] |
| Large cell non-Hodgkin lymphoma | Worse | Increased circulating IL-6 stimulates lymphoid proliferation[6,7] |
| Breast cancer | Better | Increased expression of hormone receptors, well differentiated, slowly proliferating; reduced production of tumor growth factors by host |
| Non–small cell lung cancer | Better | Less chemotherapy responsive but more indolent for unknown reasons |
| Celomic ovarian cancer | Worse | Unknown |

(From Dendaluri N, Ershler WB. Aging biology and cancer. *Semin Oncol.* 2004;31:3580–3587; Irminger-Finger I. Science of cancer and aging. *J Clin Oncol.* 2007;25:1844–1851; Hornsby PJ. Senescence as an anticancer mechanism. *J Clin Oncol.* 2007;25:1852–1857.)

*IL-6,* Interleukin 6.

adenocarcinoma, estrogen/progesterone responsive positive breast cancers, and prostate adenocarcinomas, are more indolent because the microenvironment does not stimulate growth.

⬥⬥ **More than half of new diagnoses of the common solid tumors, including lung, breast, colon, prostate, and ovarian cancers, occur in those age 65 years and older.**

## Evidence-Based Treatment

Applying clinical trials findings to practice always involves comparing the trials population with the local clinical population. In cancer treatment, the clinical trials conducted by the cooperative groups rarely include patients older than age 70 years. One factor for the low inclusion rate is that older adults are rarely asked to participate even though they are typically just as willing as younger patients.[10] If clinical trials require considerable travel, older adult patients may be reluctant to drive or may lack a household driver.

Trials are also typically sponsored by the drug manufacturers who may set recruitment criteria that exclude the older adult population, specifically because of age, coexisting conditions, and burden of travel. Nonetheless, a few trial have included significant numbers of patients older than age 70 years; secondary analyses of cooperative group trial databases have attempted to pool or perform metaanalysis to extract age-related treatment data; and the National Cancer Institute–Medicare merged database has been productively explored for population-level experience.

The subgroup analyses of clinical trials of adjuvant chemotherapy for breast and colon cancers have shown equal benefit from equal treatment (among older and younger patients) in terms of standard oncology endpoints of tumor response and disease-free survival. However, population-based data demonstrate that older adult patients do worse than younger patients and receive less treatment even when adjusted for stage of disease and inferred performance status.[11] The reasons for differences between the clinical trial results and community results include referral bias of the most fit patients to the trial centers; better adherence to standards of cancer-directed care, including choice of agents, dose-density and toxicity monitoring at referral centers; and better quality of supportive and follow-up care through the trial centers.

At least two oncology professional societies have studied these data and offered recommendations for the treatment of specific cancers in older adult patients. The International Society of Geriatric Oncology (SIOG) and the National Comprehensive Cancer Network (NCCN) maintain updated treatment recommendations and online links to current literature for the older adults on their websites. The cooperative trials groups have shown heightened awareness of the need for age-representative trial design and enrollment, and more patient-centered rather than disease-centered outcomes.[12]

The overall goal is to avoid undertreating curable and controllable disease in consenting patients, and to avoid overtreating both indolent and poor-prognosis disease. Finding the "just right" approach requires experience, collaboration, and expertise. Principles for cancer treatment in older adults have been endorsed by SIOG and the NCCN (Box 46.1).

## Staging the Aging

Oncologists typically assess patients as fit or unfit for standard therapy (Fig. 46.1). If they feel a patient will not tolerate standard therapy, they may attempt dose-reduced therapy or treatment with a

---

> ● **BOX 46.1** **Principles of Cancer Treatment in Older Adults**
>
> - Treatment should be based on the extent and biology of the tumor, not the age of the patient.
> - Healthy older adults derive equal benefit from equal treatment for their cancers.
> - Vulnerable older adults require weighing the risks and benefits of treatment in terms of both risk and quality of life during treatment as the "down payment" for extension of life after active treatment. (Especially true when the goal of cancer treatment is not cure but an estimated likelihood of surviving 1, 2, or 5 years without symptomatic cancer progression or recurrence. If the likelihood of early recurrence is high relative to estimated remaining life expectancy, the calculus changes to time spent with poor quality of life caused by treatment vs. caused by cancer.)
> - Geriatric principles accurately identify fit, vulnerable, and frail patients, that is, staging the aging.
> - Standard geriatric assessments predict cancer treatment intolerance because they identify specific vulnerabilities that can be remediated to improve treatment tolerance.
> - Excellent supportive care, symptom management, and attention to maintaining functional status may improve treatment tolerance and prevent toxicity-related hospitalizations.
> - Elective cancer surgery poses no greater risk than noncancer surgery.
> - Many radiotherapy protocols are well tolerated by the older adult population. Newer technology has improved efficacy for selected cancers with reduced total body tissue exposures.
> - Treatment decisions should be guided by the patient's treatment goals.
>
> (From National Comprehensive Cancer Network.)

---

single agent as opposed to combination therapy. This approach is flawed because it is not evidence-based, and because for reasons previously explained, the evidence base is limited with regard to older patients. International data reveal that older adult patients receive less cancer-directed therapy, so the lessened toxicity is also accompanied by less efficacy.[13]

Global functional/fitness-for-treatment assessments do not explicitly identify the clinician's subjective biases. The most commonly used functional assessments in the United States are the Eastern Cooperative Group Performance Status and the Karnovsky Performance Status scales. Both are subjective but nonetheless have withstood the test of time and continue to be highly predictive of early mortality.[14] These scales are used to track treatment tolerance, not to predict it. They do not identify specific risk factors for treatment intolerance that may be remediable.

There are differences in practice style. Some oncologists choose to front load the treatment to give as much chemotherapy as possible before the patient needs a break. Some choose to test tolerance by lowering doses and spreading them out to lessen toxicity, but that also lessens tumor cell killing. Neither approach has clinical trial–based evidence. For example, in breast cancer, single agents, either alone or as a sequential regimen in metastatic disease, are better tolerated than combination therapies. The combination therapies produce better results in terms of tumor shrinkage, but survival does not seem to differ between the approaches. The current weight of opinion among oncologists specializing in treating older adults is to try to give standard protocols for which there is evidence if the patient is fit and willing.[15]

Over the past several years, there have been increasing numbers of studies in which geriatric screening tools are used to describe clinical samples of older adult cancer patients. As yet, there are limited data showing that geriatric screening tests incorporated into

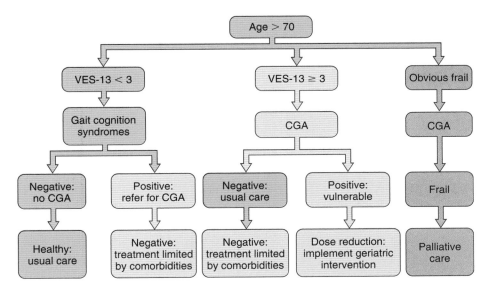

• **Figure 46.1** A decision tree for staging the aging. *CGA*, Comprehensive geriatric assessment; *VES*, Vulnerable Elders Survey. (From Rodin MB, Mohile SG. A practical approach to geriatric assessment in oncology. *J Clin Oncology [Rev.]* 2007;25(14):1936–1944; Mohile SG, Bylow K, Dale W, et al. A pilot study of the Vulnerable Elders Survey-13 as compared with comprehensive geriatric assessment for identifying disability in older prostate cancer patients receiving androgen ablation. *Cancer* 2007;109:802–810.)

cancer treatment affect decisions or outcomes.[16] However, there are a few preliminary studies, mainly from France, that may soon yield results.[16a,17] A source of resistance to routine geriatric assessment has been that oncologists are concerned that performing many screening tests will be too time consuming for their practices and that the screening tests will generate information that they cannot use.[18] Several studies have tested short screens to identify only those patients who should be comprehensively evaluated and to quantify the amount of time it takes to gather the data.[19–21]

The various components of a comprehensive geriatric assessment include functional status (ADLs and IADLs), cognitive screening, review of medications for potentially harmful or just unnecessary polypharmacy, nutritional status, vision and hearing, gait and fall risk assessment tools, depression, and delirium. There is no reason to choose one specific validated screening tool over another with which the clinician is familiar or has comparative data in the medical record for the patient. It is important to recognize that these tools were devised to determine intermediate- to long-term outcomes, including loss of independence (nursing home placement) and longevity over a range of several years.[22]

Remaining life expectancy (RLE) is a prognostic indicator, obviously not an absolute prediction of the future. For an older person with a long RLE, a new cancer diagnosis may shorten RLE.

The value of having an estimate is to draw a frame around the expected course of the disease within a realistic span of time (Table 46.2).[23] A highly treatable cancer may have a low probability of recurrence within the patient's RLE, even if it is not completely "cured." The mirror image of this assessment is whether the treatment poses a higher risk than the cancer or whether the cancer is likely to progress during the patient's RLE or not. Heuristically, is the patient's precancer life expectancy less than 5, 5 to 9, or 10 or more years? With successful treatment, what is the probability of symptomatic progression within 5 years? Is it less than 10%, less than 50%, less than 80%? Do the risks of standard treatment— including surgical risk, serious toxicity, or suffering or death—outweigh any theoretical benefit? Several studies have specifically examined the performance of common functional scales for chemotherapy tolerance.[24–27]

Low-risk asymptomatic cancers can be watched in frail patients; cancers that are likely to become symptomatic during a short time and that are responsive to low-toxicity therapy can be treated in frail patients. Treatment for high-risk tumors requiring highly toxic therapy should be offered only to the most fit patients where RLE will allow them to enjoy their survival. Extreme frailty is usually recognized without difficulty. Because oncologists generally see a selected group of reasonably healthy older patients,

| TABLE 46.2 | Remaining Life Expectancy in Years by Age (5 y), Sex, and Quartile (Lowest, Middle 2, Highest) | | | | | | | | | | | | | |
|---|---|---|---|---|---|---|---|---|---|---|---|---|---|---|
| | 70 Y | | | 75 Y | | | 80 Y | | | 85 Y | | | 90 Y | | |
| Sex | L | M | H | L | M | H | L | M | H | L | M | H | L | M | H |
| Men | 6.7 | 12.4 | 18.0 | 4.9 | 9.3 | 14.2 | 3.3 | 6.7 | 10.8 | 2.2 | 4.7 | 7.9 | 1.5 | 3.2 | 5.8 |
| Women | 9.5 | 15.7 | 21.3 | 6.8 | 11.9 | 17.0 | 4.6 | 8.6 | 13.0 | 2.9 | 5.9 | 7.9 | 1.8 | 3.9 | 6.8 |

(Modified from Walter LC, Covinsky KE. Cancer screening in elderly patients: a framework for individualized decision-making. *JAMA* 2001;285:2750–2756.)
*H,* High quartile of LE; *L,* low quartile of LE; *LE,* life expectancy; *M,* middle quartile of LE.

geriatricians' greatest contribution is in decision making for the apparently fit but "vulnerable" or "subclinical frail" patients.[20]

The NCCN recognizes that some form of geriatric assessment provides information essential to the treatment of persons age 70 years or older.[28] These guidelines also recognize the importance of caregiver support, out-of-pocket costs for people on fixed income, access to care, depression, malnutrition, and polypharmacy. Patients who are dependent in IADLs, especially in the use of transportation, ability to take medications, and money management, are at increased risk for complications.

It is important to lay out in a clear and systematic manner the likely course of the cancer if not treated or with best possible treatment and best expected outcome based on the cancer alone. Then the individual's life expectancy based on stable comorbidities and functional status needs to be measured against the likely duration of toxic therapy and duration of remission to be gained. Then it makes sense to let the patient weigh the balance and set his or her goals.[29,30]

❖ **Geriatric assessment provides information essential to the treatment of cancer in persons age 70 years or older.**

Recently, two important studies have shown a role for geriatric consultation. One trial involved randomizing advanced lung cancer patients to usual care or to proactive palliative care assessments. The palliative care group lived longer and terminated active treatment earlier.[31] In an observational study in the context of a clinical trial, advanced lung cancer patients who had previously documented IADL dependencies were 50% more likely, patients who could not walk a block outside their homes were 75% more likely, and patients who had a previous fall were 2.5 times more likely to experience serious chemotherapy toxicity.[24] Geriatricians have been careful to separate the patient's functional status from comorbidity burden. This separation appears to hold with cancer patients, because studies confirm that toxicities are independently predicted by functional variables and by summary comorbidity variables. Simply doing assessments will not change outcomes. However, the geriatric model of multidisciplinary continuity of care may improve outcomes as demonstrated in a multicenter Veterans Administration trial showing that among functionally impaired veterans randomized to geriatric outpatient care, those with cancer benefitted the most with respect to quality of life.[32] Adverse events beyond direct drug toxicity should be considered in future studies when additional outcomes can be built into the trial protocols.

Oncologists know the direct toxic effects of the agents they use, including nausea and vomiting; bone marrow suppression; and acute renal, neurological, cardiac, and pulmonary toxicities. With the introduction of new biological agents, the more common toxicities of the cytotoxic agents (e.g., mucositis, nausea and vomiting, neutropenia, neuropathy, and hair loss) are somewhat mitigated. Oncologists are also aware of subjective symptoms, such as depression and fatigue, but they have a relatively limited armamentarium for effective intervention. Furthermore, delirium is common on inpatient oncology units, but there are little data on low-grade delirium in oncology outpatients. Geriatric assessments and geriatric interventions may prove to be effective for maintaining functional status in older adult cancer patients.

Chemotherapy is largely an outpatient procedure, and oncology nurses are skilled in administering preventive protocols to reduce immediate nausea and vomiting, cutaneous itching and burning, and anxiety. However, older adult patients who experience less immediate chemotherapy induced nausea (CIN) are more subject to delayed toxicities, including nausea, bone marrow suppression, neutropenia, anorexia, fatigue, and diarrhea.[33] The impact of known late toxicities may be more serious in the older adult population because of preexisting vulnerabilities. At some institutions, out-of-town patients may be kept close by in dedicated housing near the hospital or admitted to skilled nursing facilities (SNFs) to carry them through chemotherapy. Thus, nursing homes need to be aware and prepared to manage predictable delayed toxicities. SNF-level care anticipates functional problems. An older adult patient at home, especially alone, who is suffering from fatigue, anorexia, or low-grade delirium may not be able to recognize, report, and self-manage toxicities. Recognizing mild mobility problems, mild cognitive impairment, or dementia is crucial for an older adult patient's ability to maintain nutrition and hydration, and avoid falls. Minor mobility problems may get worse as a result of orthostatic hypotension, fatigue, anorexia, and sleep dysfunction. Nausea, vomiting, diarrhea, anorexia, and mucositis require adequate supports in the home to manage medications, fluids, and toileting. Active supportive symptomatic management is crucial.

## General Principles of Cancer Management

Cancer treatment includes local and systemic treatment. Local treatment includes surgery and radiation therapy. Systemic treatment includes several classes of drugs: cytotoxic chemotherapy, hormonal therapy, biological therapy, and targeted therapy. Each treatment modality has predictable potential side effects.

### Local Therapy

Elective surgery for cancer is reasonably safe through the ninth decade of age.[35,36] The major differences in surgical mortality between younger and older individuals are seen in emergency surgery of the GI tract. Standard screening for cancer of the large bowel may substantially reduce the need for emergency surgery. Elective cancer surgery poses no greater risk than noncancer surgery. The usual perioperative risk stratification and monitoring for delirium and early nutritional support should be performed. Early mobilization and referral for rehabilitation should also be encouraged.

Surgical practice with respect to breast cancer has trended toward less extensive procedures. For example, in breast cancer, radical and modified radical mastectomies are now rarely performed. Lumpectomy with sentinel lymph node dissection has for many patients obviated the need for axillary dissection, given the low risk for extended axillary involvement (if less than three lymph nodes) and high morbidity (lymphedema, pain, shoulder weakness, and contractures.)

By contrast, surgical debulking of ovarian cancers is trending toward longer procedures to achieve more complete excisions. Improved radiation technology, such as cyberknife, may in some cases eliminate the need for surgical excision of isolated small tumors.[37]

Several studies attest to the safety of radiation therapy in older patients, even those age 80 years or older.[38] Radiation therapy can sometimes be used in lieu of surgery for curative purposes in selected patients and for palliation of pain and obstruction. The combination of chemotherapy and radiation for cancer of the larynx, esophagus, and small rectal tumors produces results comparable to surgery with the advantage of organ preservation.[39] Radiation and surgery remain effective strategies for curative prostate cancer therapy, but the best use of these interventions is actively under discussion.[40]

◆◆ **Studies attest to the safety of radiation therapy in older patients, even those age 80 years or older.**

## Systemic Therapy

Systemic therapy involves oral and intravenous agents of several classes (Box 46.2).

### Hormonal Therapy

The aromatase inhibitors (AIs) have proven more effective than the older selective estrogen receptor modulators (tamoxifen and toremifene) in the management of breast cancer. For the majority of practitioners, these compounds are now the initial treatment of choice, both in the adjuvant setting and in metastatic disease.[41] The AIs are active even in tumors that overexpress the HER2neu protein, for which selective estrogen receptor modulators (SERMs) are generally ineffective. The risk of endometrial cancer, thrombosis, and cataracts is lower with AIs compared with SERMs. Despite this advantage, AIs are known to increase osteoporosis, and that raises the risk for subsequent bone fractures. In addition, letrozole has been shown to increase the levels of circulating low-density lipoprotein and has been associated with an increased risk for

---

> ### • BOX 46.2  Classes of Systemic Antineoplastic Treatment
>
> **Hormonal Therapy**
> Selective estrogen receptor modulators (SERMs)
> Aromatase inhibitors
> Progestins
> Luteinizing hormone-releasing hormone (LHRH) analogs
> LHRH antagonists
> Estrogens
> Androgens
> Androgen antagonists
> Adrenal antagonists
> Corticosteroids
>
> **Biological Therapy**
> Interferons
> Interleukin 2
>
> **Tumor Vaccines (Mostly in Clinical Trials)**
> HPV is given for prevention of cervical cancer. Future uses include likely penile and possibly oropharyngeal cancers.
>
> **Cytotoxic Chemotherapy**
> Alkylating agents
> Antimetabolites
> Antibiotics
> Plant derivatives
>
> **Targeted Therapy**
> **Monoclonal antibodies**
> Immune destruction of the tumor
> Carriers of cytotoxic material inside the tumor
> Inhibitors of the action of tumor growth factors
>
> **Tyrosine kinase inhibitors**
> Farnesyl transferase inhibitors
> Angiogenesis inhibitors
>
> *HPV,* Human papillomavirus.

---

cardiovascular deaths in a European study. A bone density study before AI therapy should be done. With osteopenia or osteoporosis, it is prudent practice to also give bisphosphonates and replete vitamin D.[41]

A new SERM, fulvestrant, is a pure estrogen antagonist that has recently become available. Its activity may be comparable with that of AIs. This agent is administered by intramuscular injections. Poor adherence to oral antiestrogens has made this attractive in some circumstances. Progestins, whose activity is inferior to that of AIs, are used occasionally as third-line agents in metastatic breast cancer.

Gonadotropin-releasing hormone (GnRH) analogs cause medical castration and are currently preferred in the management of prostate cancer. Treatment with GnRH analogs may be given along with oral androgen antagonists (e.g., bicalutamide, flutamide) during the first 2 weeks of treatment to counteract the burst of testosterone after the first dose of analogs. As single agents, the androgen antagonists are inferior to luteinizing hormone-releasing hormone (LHRH) analog therapy. Adrenal suppressors, including aminoglutethimide and ketoconazole, at high doses have some activity as second- or third-line hormonal treatment of relapsed prostate cancer.[40]

### Cytotoxic Chemotherapy

Cytotoxic chemotherapy includes diverse groups of drugs that preferentially kill proliferating cells and spare resting-phase cells. The common toxicities of cytotoxic chemotherapy are listed in Table 46.3. Age is a risk factor for most of these complications because the reserves of progenitor cells are lower. The timing of the toxicities is related to the mechanisms of the drugs. For example, nausea may be an acute reaction to drug crossing the blood–brain barrier, or it may be delayed and a result of depression of GI motility. Mucosal injury and hair loss peak within the normal turnover cycle of rapidly dividing endothelial cells. Knowing the drugs and their toxicity profiles helps to anticipate potential problems.

A number of steps may ameliorate the toxicity of chemotherapy in older individuals:[42]

- Adjust the dose to the renal function. In particular for patients older than age 65 years, the dose of chemotherapy should be adjusted to the calculated glomerular filtration rate from a measured 24-hour urine sample.
- Reduce the dose to test tolerance with the intent that doses may be escalated in subsequent cycles if the drugs are tolerated. This strategy is ill advised in situations in which chemotherapy is administered for cure, because the full dose is based on clinical trials and improves the chances of achieving a cure.
- Older patients are more likely to experience severe bone marrow suppression, including anemia, thrombocytopenia, and neutropenia. Support with hematopoietic growth factors. NCCN and SIOG guidelines recommend routine preventative use of agents to prevent neutropenia.[28] Pegfilgrastim prevents neutropenic infections in approximately 50% of cases and has largely replaced granulocyte colony stimulating factor (G-CSF) because it can be administered once for each cycle of chemotherapy (with a minimum of 14 days between treatments), whereas G-CSF requires daily administrations for 7 to 10 days.
- Anemia may be caused by the cancer or by the treatment, and initially it was hoped that treating anemia aggressively would also relieve the burden of fatigue many cancer patients feel. Epoetin A and darbepoetin A will raise hemoglobin levels in

| TABLE 46.3 | Chemotherapy-Related Toxicity in Older Individuals | |
|---|---|
| **Type of Toxicity** | **Agents Involved** |
| Myelodepression | All agents, except vincristine, bleomycin, L-asparaginase, streptozotocin |
| Alopecia | Most agents except gemcitabine (oral fluorinated pyrimidine, 5-FU) |
| Mucositis (diarrhea) | Fluorinated pyrimidines, methotrexate, anthracyclines (doxorubicin, daunorubicin, idarubicin, epirubicin) |
| Cardiotoxicity | Anthracyclines (doxorubicin, daunorubicin, idarubicin, epirubicin), mitomycin C |
| Peripheral neurotoxicity | Alkaloids (vincristine, vinblastine, vinorelbine), cisplatin, podophyllotoxins (etoposide, teniposide), taxanes (Taxotere, paclitaxel) |
| Central neurotoxicity | All agents (delirium, "chemo brain," possibly dementia), high-dose cytarabine and 5-FU (cerebellar toxicity) |
| Anemia | Nearly all antineoplastics |
| Fatigue | Nearly all antineoplastics |
| Depression | Interferons |

(From Gonsalves W, Ganti AK. Targeted anti-cancer therapy in the elderly. *Crit Rev in Oncol-Hem.* 2001;78:227–242;e3.)
*5-FU,* 5-Fluorouracil.

approximately 75% of patients. Management of anemia during cytotoxic chemotherapy has two goals: prevention of functional decline caused by fatigue, and treatment of fatigue itself, if it is caused by profound anemia. Clinical trials have failed to support the goal of normalizing hemoglobin as effective treatment of cancer fatigue.[43] Current guidelines advise against using these agents either in patients being treated for cure or for patients in palliative care because of excess thrombotic events and the potential for stimulating tumor growth, especially with head and neck and non–small cell lung cancer.

• Cardiotoxicity occurs as early (reversible) congestive heart failure with trastuzumab and a late-onset restrictive form associated with anthracyclines. Anthracycline cardiotoxicity is not dose related; it occurs several years after completion of treatment and may contribute to congestive heart failure in long-term survivors. There appear to be individual susceptibilities, but these have not yet been identified, so many oncologists are reluctant to give anthracyclines to older adult patients who may already have cardiomyopathy. Cardioprotective strategies, including giving anthracyclines as continuous infusions rather than bolus, concomitant administration of doxorubicin and dexrazoxane (which prevents the formation of free radicals in the myocardium), and administration of pegylated liposomal doxorubicin in lieu of doxorubicin, have been adopted.[44]

• Severe mucositis is miserable. The dysphagia contributes to severe fluid and nutritional deficits. Mucositis is a severe problem for patients receiving "chemorads" treatment for head and neck cancers. It is sometimes not possible for patients to take oral nutrition, and they are temporarily tube fed. Although the treatment is debilitating and painful, the cure rate is high for those who can tolerate the toxicity. Palliative agents include oral anesthetics and coating agents, "magic mouth wash." A newer oral solution of glutamine (AES12) is a keratinocyte growth factor that reduces incidence and severity of mucositis from high-dose chemotherapy. The substitution of capecitabine, an oral prodrug activated into fluorouracil inside the neoplastic tissue for intravenous fluorinated pyrimidines (fluorouracil and floxuridine), minimizes the exposure of the normal mucosa to fluorouracil.[45]

• In addition to capecitabine and pegylated liposomal doxorubicin, a number of new drugs with favorable toxicity profiles are useful in older individuals. These include taxanes in low weekly doses, vinorelbine, and gemcitabine.

## Targeted Therapy

New insights in cancer cell biology have allowed the development of drugs that target specific components or specific metabolic processes of the tumor. Theoretically, targeted therapy would spare normal tissues that do not express the intracellular machinery or cell surface markers of the malignant cells.

Monoclonal antibodies may target either tumor surface antigens or intercept growth factors or growth factor receptors. They may destroy the tumor by an immune mechanism, by using cell surface receptors to carry the cytotoxic substance into the tumor, or by interfering with the vital processes of the tumor. Rituximab and alemtuzumab target respectively the CD 20 and the CD 52 antigens and are effective in lymphoid malignancies. Trastuzumab and cetuximab target different components of the epithelial growth factor receptors and are effective in cancer of the breast and of the large bowel, respectively. Bevacizumab is a monoclonal antibody directed to the vascular endothelial growth factor and is used in several solid tumor cancers.[42]

All monoclonal antibodies may cause anaphylactic reactions. Alemtuzumab may cause severe, prolonged myelosuppression and immune deficiency (neutropenia.) Trastuzumab may cause reversible heart failure by a different mechanism than the anthracyclines, which is irreversible. Cetuximab causes a severe acne-like reaction. Bevacizumab is used only with caution in older adults because of associated hypertension, bleeding, and visceral perforation.[42]

Rituximab and similar antibodies have been tagged with radioisotopes (radioimmunotherapy) to deliver high radiation doses to the tumor. Although highly effective, radioimmunotherapy may still be associated with severe myelosuppression. Thalidomide and recently developed congeners (lenalidamide) have substantial activity in multiple myeloma with relatively little toxicity. Side effects include somnolence, constipation, and thromboembolism.[42]

A relatively new group of drugs are the tyrosine kinase inhibitors (TKIs). Tyrosine kinase (TK) is a key enzyme of intracellular signal transduction. A number of small adenosine triphosphate-like molecules inhibit this enzyme and consequently tumor growth. Imatinib inhibits the soluble TK and is effective in chronic myelogenous leukemia (CML), in the acute lymphoblastic leukemias (ALL) with Ph chromosome, in stromal tumors of the stomach, and in hypereosinophilia. Gefitinib (unavailable in the United States) and erlotinib inhibit the TK associated with growth factor receptors and are sometimes effective with little toxicity in non—small cell lung cancer, particularly tumors with certain epidermal growth factor receptor mutations. In general, monoclonal antibodies and antiangiogenic factors represent an alternative to cytotoxic chemotherapy for older patients because they are less symptomatically toxic. Several are oral drugs so travel is reduced, and some patients experience strong tumor response.[42]

## CASE 1

### Jane Thompson (Part 2)

Mrs. Thompson's three children disagree on what they believe their mother would prefer. You review the options for therapy with the oncologist, and after 3 days, the family agrees to a trial of therapy. Mrs. Thompson, now fully awake and in agreement, will be treated with cyclophosphamide, vincristine, doxorubicin, and prednisone (CHOP regimen) with rituximab at reduced doses because of her recent kidney injury. She is given one round of reduced CHOP-R and discharged to an SNF on TPN. After 20 days Mrs. Thompson returns to the oncologist's office able to eat on her own. She has also regained her independence with ADLs. TPN is discontinued, and the patient receives five more courses of chemotherapy at full doses with G-CSF support (pegfilgrastim, a hemopoietic growth factor). After 4 years, she is still independent and in complete remission.

## CASE 1

### Discussion

The specific disease and Mrs. Thompson's health status are both important aspects of this case. This disease, DLBCL, is highly responsive to chemotherapy. Although age is a poor prognostic factor, more than 50% of persons older than 60 years will have a complete response to chemotherapy, and 30% are curable (defined as 5 years with no recurrence). Although Mrs. Thompson had a poor performance status when she was brought to the hospital, she had been totally independent 2 weeks before. Her poor condition was the result of an acute change that was reversed with fluid resuscitation and treatment of the gastric obstruction. Given their diminished organ reserve, older individuals' general condition may deteriorate more quickly in response to stress. To judge the fitness of older individuals for chemotherapy, their condition should be judged from the patient's functional status before the acute event and his or her response to treatment of the acute problem.

## CASE 2

### Mary Davis (Part 1)

A nursing aide finds a 1.5-cm nodule on the right breast of your patient, Mary Davis. She is a 90-year-old woman confined to a wheelchair by arthritis. She is quite conversational, and her last documented minimental state examination (MMSE) was 20/30. She has a history of congestive heart failure but has never been symptomatic over the 2 years you have cared for her. You are aware that independent of age, her ADL dependence and dementia are risk factors for toxicity of cytotoxic chemotherapy and for

postoperative delirium if surgery is attempted. Mrs. Davis defers decisions to her family.

After discussion with the patient's family and a medical oncologist, you recommend that a fine-needle aspiration biopsy be performed in radiology. Mrs. Davis becomes agitated, and the procedure is aborted. Her son refuses to consent to reattempting the procedure. The nodule is watched and does not seem to be changing over the next 6 months.
1. What is the natural history of untreated breast cancer in women age 70 years? 80 years? 90 years?
2. What diagnostic steps are appropriate for a woman with RLE less than 5 years, 5 to 9 years, more than 10 years? Mammography? Needle biopsy? Excisional biopsy? Observation?
3. Should you empirically treat with a SERM or AI? Or do nothing?

## Breast Cancer

### Carcinoma In Situ

Stage migration has affected the presentation of breast cancer in the older adult population. Approximately 20% of newly diagnosed breast cancers are in situ, found on mammograms and often not palpable. This is an increase from 1% in 1970. The most common form is ductal carcinoma in situ (DCIS), which is treated with simple or partial mastectomy. With a disease as heavily screened for as breast cancer, interpreting treatment results should take account of the so-called "Will Rogers effect." That is, with discovery and treatment of early stage disease that includes disease with both indolent and aggressive potential, treatment effectiveness will likely be overestimated. Because of this effect, treatment outcomes should be interpreted by both biological and stage criteria. Thus, the need for radiotherapy, especially in older women, is in doubt and is reserved for excisions with affected margins and higher-grade tumors. Taking tamoxifen for 5 years decreases the risk of local recurrence after partial mastectomy by 80%.[46,47]

◆◆ **Stage migration has affected the presentation of breast cancer in the older adult population; approximately 20% of newly diagnosed breast cancers are in situ, found on mammograms and often not palpable.**

### Localized Carcinoma of the Breast

Localized carcinoma of the breast (stages I—IIIA) is a surgically curable disease. The decision tree for management has grown more complex as less invasive treatments have been shown to be effective. Examples are simple or partial mastectomy (lumpectomy) alone or with radiotherapy for larger tumors, if the surgical pathology shows infiltrated margins or tumors have aggressive histology. Postoperative irradiation has no impact on freedom from distant metastases and overall survival. It only affects the likelihood of local recurrence. Irradiation of the breast has minimal complications in older women, but it is inconvenient and expensive. The risk of local recurrence after partial mastectomy declines with the age of the patient.[47] If the risk of local recurrence within 5 years is 10% or less and this risk is acceptable to the patient, postoperative radiation probably offers no advantages to an older woman.

Axillary lymph node dissection is a complicated subject. The options are sentinel node sampling, partial dissection, and complete dissection. Axillary lymph node dissection is associated with substantial morbidity, including chronic lymphedema and functional limitations of the upper extremity. Lymph node mapping may obviate the need of this procedure in the majority of patients. After the injection of a radioactive tracer, it is possible to identify the so-called sentinel lymph node. If this lymph node is clear of metastases, axillary dissection is unnecessary. Also, a localized stage I or small stage II tumor might not require axillary sampling at all in an older woman with good histology in the initial biopsy.[48]

Adjuvant chemotherapy should be reserved for women who are similar to the women who participated in the clinical trials and should be based on likelihood of recurrence during the woman's RLE. A node-negative simple mastectomy requires no radiation or adjuvant cytotoxic therapy. All mastectomy specimens should be tested for hormone receptors, proliferation rate, and HER2/neu antigens (the antigen for the epithelial growth factor receptor). This provides important prognostic information, as well as data for treatment. More centers are offering genomic profiling of other genetic markers of biological behavior and drug susceptibility to match tumor, drugs, and patients with the greatest chance of benefit. Oncotyping allows patients to think about the likelihood of recurrences for the type of breast cancer they have (or other cancers for which prognostic markers are available). They can decide how to balance their likelihood of recurrence with their willingness to take adjuvant chemotherapy. The benefits of adjuvant chemotherapy decline with age. In aggregated data, based on randomized controlled trials (RCTs) completed before the era of widely available oncotyping, there appears to be no benefit beyond the age of 70 years. Cytotoxic therapy is usually reserved for locally advanced stage II and III tumors with biologically aggressive histology and positive lymph nodes or for metastatic disease.

If it is the woman's choice, chemotherapy should be reserved for fit women with negative hormone receptors and overexpression of HER2neu. Anthracyclines are very effective against these tumors, doubling the cure rate.[8]

Adjuvant treatment with AIs delays the recurrence of breast cancer more effectively than do SERMs in hormone receptor–rich tumors and is preferred by the majority of practitioners.[49] Current practice suggests that SERMS and AIs be used for 5 years and then stopped.

## Metastatic Carcinoma of the Breast

All management of metastatic breast cancer is palliative. The goal of palliative chemotherapy is to reduce tumor burden and delay progression to symptomatic disease or to lessen symptoms that are caused by the cancer itself, such as bone pain. The choice depends on the patient's overall performance status, biology of the tumor, the specific symptoms to be palliated, and the woman's wishes with regard to quality of life. It is important to clarify advance directives if they have not yet been documented.

Cytotoxic chemotherapy is indicated for (apparently) hormone receptor–rich tumors that have failed at least two forms of hormonal treatment, or for tumors that lack hormone receptors. Isolated brain metastases may be managed with surgery or radiotherapy, but multiple brain metastases will require a decision about hospice or whole brain radiation therapy. Isolated bone metastases involving weight-bearing bones, such as the femur, the tibia, or the humerus, should undergo surgical fixation to prevent pathological fractures in otherwise functionally intact women. Such findings in a previously nonambulatory patient would suggest early referral for palliative care. It is important to remember that, in general, with symptomatic metastatic disease in a chronically ill, debilitated patient, treatment has little or no impact on survival. However, some women may live several years with stable metastatic disease,

| TABLE 46.4 | Median Survival in Months of Patients With Metastatic Breast Cancer by Location of Metastases | |
|---|---|
| **Location** | **Survival (Months)** |
| Liver ($>$ 30% replacement | 3 |
| Lung (lymphangitic) | 3 |
| Lung (nodular) | 22 |
| Skin | 27 |
| Bones | 36 + |

as shown in Table 46.4. The risks, costs, and benefits of tumor-directed palliation should be assessed and reassessed.[8]

Several forms of chemotherapy with limited toxicity are available. For patients with tumors that overexpress the HER2/neu antigen, a combination of trastuzumab and weekly taxane is the treatment of choice. For the other patients, weekly Taxol, Taxotere, or vinorelbine (Navelbine), oral capecitabine, or pegylated liposomal doxorubicin every 4 weeks are well tolerated and of similar efficacy.

## CASE 2

### Discussion

We do not know how long Mrs. Davis's tumor was there before it was discovered, so we do not know if it is growing rapidly or slowly. No change over 6 months, however, suggests slower growth. The recommendation of a biopsy for Mrs. Davis was reasonable because the procedure has negligible morbidity and might have provided prognostic information about the aggressiveness of the tumor, use of SERMs or AIs, and the value of simple excisional biopsy. If Mrs. Davis's fine needle aspiration revealed DCIS, observation alone would be acceptable in view of her estimated RLE; DCIS is unlikely to cause local symptoms or metastasize. The patient's reaction, however, and the denial of permission to try again prevented the biopsy.

The suspicion of metastatic disease was low, so further imaging with bone scans and CT did not appear necessary. A chest radiograph could show lung metastasis and possible humerus, rib, and thoracic spine lytic lesions. Basic blood work, including a complete blood count to exclude significant anemia and a metabolic blood panel, could show significant liver and bone metastasis by transaminases, albumin, alkaline phosphatase, and calcium levels.

In a 90-year-old woman, a breast nodule should be considered as cancer unless proved otherwise. There is an 80% chance the tumor was hormone receptor positive. A number of approaches were reasonable in this case. A local resection under local anesthesia would be diagnostic and curative and prevent local complications, such as fungating, painful, and ulcerating masses. However, Mrs. Davis's reaction to the biopsy precludes a local anesthesia approach. Empiric treatment with tamoxifen would have had a 60% to 80% chance of a measurable response. The chief disadvantage of tamoxifen is risk of deep vein thrombosis, which is increased for an older woman immobilized by arthritis. An AI could worsen her osteoporosis, and she would have to be treated with either oral or IV bisphosphonate. Close observation was reasonable because the average life expectancy of this woman with moderate dementia and functional impairment was probably less than 2 years. The median time for her tumor to metastasize or cause local problems, such as erosion through the skin, is more than 3 years based on observational studies of local breast cancer. Because breast masses are superficial, it is easy enough to follow with observation alone.

## CASE 3

### Zhao Min Xi (Part 1)

Zhao Min Xi comes to your office with his son as an interpreter. He is a 79-year-old man who has been losing weight and suffering from sweats at night since his arrival from China several months back. He is otherwise independent around the house. Mr. Zhao does little outside the home because he does not speak English, and the family operates a small factory in a small town with few other Chinese people. You discover that he has enlarged lymph nodes in both axillae. You exclude active tuberculosis infection. After referral for biopsy, the pathologist confirms peripheral T-cell lymphoma (PTCL). CT scans of the chest and abdomen and a bone marrow biopsy are negative for lymphoma. During the workup of the lymphoma, the patient went to a urologist because of difficulty urinating. As a result of this consultation, Mr. Zhao's prostate-specific antigen (PSA) was found to be 82 ng/mL. Transrectal prostatic biopsy reveals a Gleason 8 (aggressive) prostatic adenocarcinoma. The patient's hemoglobin is 10.2, serum creatinine is 1.7, and blood urea nitrogen is 26. Serum erythropoietin levels are 3 mg/mL (low). You are unable to formally assess cognition and depression, but he appears to be quite conversational with his son; he asks questions through his son and otherwise appears to be quite lively.

## Prostate Cancer

For American men, prostate cancer is the most common cancer and the second most common cause of cancer death. Incidence in Asian men is somewhat lower on a population level. The widespread use of PSA for screening asymptomatic men has led to a doubling of the reported incidence of prostate cancer in the last decade.[50] There is no conclusive evidence that screening has reduced the risk of death from prostate cancer, especially for men older than 65 years. Much of the current debate has to do with the contribution of radical prostatectomy and of radiation to survival of men after diagnosis.[51] The current staging and treatment of prostate cancer are summarized in Table 46.5.

Close observation (active surveillance) for patients with localized disease is a reasonable approach for men age 70 years or older with well-differentiated tumor (Gleason score $\leq 7$). In all other cases, some form of local treatment is appropriate. Brachytherapy (radiation by internal implant) may have fewer complications than external beam radiation therapy (EBRT). In younger men, there is increased risk for a second, radiation-induced cancer. Early symptoms of fatigue generally worsen over the course of radiotherapy but resolve when therapy is completed. Late complications of radiation include chronic cystitis and proctitis that can only be managed symptomatically.

Poor prognostic factors for localized disease (stages A, B, and C) include a poorly differentiated tumor Gleason grade 8 or higher, extracapsular involvement beyond the seminal vesicles, and a PSA level greater than 30 ng/mL.

The role of androgen ablation for asymptomatic lower Gleason-grade tumors is debatable because castration levels of testosterone induce secondary morbidities, including increased cardiovascular risk, osteoporosis, muscle wasting, weight gain, and subjective symptoms of hot flashes, loss of libido, and subsyndromal depression. Only one-third of these patients will develop clinical metastases within 10 years.[52]

Hormonal treatment is the mainstay of management of metastatic prostate disease. It has been demonstrated that hormonal treatment initiated immediately upon diagnosis of asymptomatic metastases is superior to delaying hormonal treatment until symptoms develop. It is unclear, however, whether hormonal treatment should be instituted for biochemical progression, that is, rising PSA after radical prostatectomy (stage D1.5 disease) without evidence of metastasis. The role of cytotoxic chemotherapy is limited to treating symptomatic metastatic disease that has become resistant to hormonal agents. Treatment is not curative. Spot radiation may help pain from bone metastasis; some centers use intravenous heavy particle isotopes, such as strontium 89, which produces more prolonged responses but also more severe myelosuppression. Most centers will use zoledronate prophylactically or symptomatically to prevent or treat the pain and delay the progression of bony metastases.

### TABLE 46.5  Clinical Staging of Prostate Cancer

| Stage | Clinical Description | Treatment |
|---|---|---|
| A | No palpable lesion, biopsy only | Observation |
| B1 | Palpable nodule 1 lobe | Radical prostatectomy, EBRT or brachytherapy |
| B2 | Palpable nodule both lobes or one dominant nodule >1.5 cm | Same |
| C | Locally advanced, invading the capsule | Radiation and hormonal therapy |
| D1 | Extracapsular involves pelvic lymph nodes | Lymph node dissection and hormonal therapy |
| D1.5 | Chemical recurrence, rising PSA after prostatectomy | Hormonal therapy if PSA doubling time is <10 months, occurs within 2 years of prostatectomy, or if the primary was Gleason 8 or higher |
| D2 | Extensive retroperitoneal lymph node involvement, distant metastasis | Hormonal therapy |
| D2.5 | Rising PSA after definitive treatment | Consider cytotoxic therapy if second- and third-line hormonal therapy fails, or treat only if symptomatic metastasis occurs. |

EBRT, External beam radiation therapy; PSA, prostate-specific antigen.

## CASE 3

### Zhao Min Xi (Part 2)

Mr. Zhao and both sons arrive for a family meeting in which the oncologist proposes CHOP (rituximab, cyclophosphamide, doxorubicin, vincristine, and prednisone) given every 3 weeks and G-CSF daily injections for a week following chemotherapy. If he becomes symptomatically anemic, transfusion would be considered. The prostate cancer will be treated simultaneously with goserelin, an LHRH analog, and anastrozole (Casodex), an antiandrogen. Any further treatment of the prostate cancer would be deferred until the lymphoma is addressed. In any case, the survival benefit of additional radiation to the prostate is debatable.

The more immediate problem is how to support Mr. Zhao through the next few months of chemotherapy for lymphoma. As an immigrant, Mr. Zhao did not have Medicare, nor did he have a privately paid major medical policy. His family had sufficient funds to cover his treatment and to house him in an SNF located on the campus of the hospital and cancer center. On admission to the SNF his weight was 92 lb, which declined to 89 lb. However, his son said Mr. Zhao never weighed as much as 100 lb. He refused restorative physical therapy largely because he did not speak English and found it tiring to try to comply with instructions he did not understand. He tended to stay in his room and sleep most of the day. You are concerned about his apparent decline in functional status. The evening nurse reported he got up in the early evening and walked independently in the hall while other residents were at dinner or asleep. A problem was that he missed scheduled meals. Once a month, his out-of-town daughter came for a week and he went home with her until his next cycle of chemotherapy. Mr. Zhao's standing orders in the nursing home covered follow-up labs, GI toxicity, fluids, and nutrition. Pegfilgrastim (G-CSF) was prescribed. He ultimately received six cycles of CHOP with complete remission. He was briefly hospitalized overnight for an episode of neutropenic fever. His PSA declined to 0.3 mg/mL, and further prostate cancer–directed therapy was deferred indefinitely.

## CASE 3

### Discussion

Mr. Zhao's case allows examination of common problems related to cancer and age. First, Mr. Zhao lives in a small town more than an hour away from the cancer center and is dependent on his son for transportation because neither he nor his wife can drive and his daughter-in-law does not feel safe with highway driving. Mr. Zhao is socially isolated by language even though he has no ambulatory problems.

Geriatric assessment for this older adult man with two cancers was limited by the language barrier; however, close observation of family interactions and gait assessment performed by the evening shift nurse indicated that although he was very thin by Western standards, Mr. Zhao was in good physical condition and his functional limitations were not caused by physical or cognitive impairments. Care planning was designed to minimize the stress on his support system. The nursing home relieved the patient and the family of tiring long-distance drives. Coordination of care between the physician at the SNF and the oncologist at the cancer center allowed standing orders to anticipate chemotoxicity in a safe environment where his nutrition, ambulation, and fluid status could be monitored.

Multiple neoplasms are common in older individuals. The management should start with the neoplasm that most immediately threatens the patient's life. Median survival of PTCL is approximately 18 months without treatment. Mr. Zhao's very high PSA suggests a more advanced cancer, but no metastatic disease was identified, so it is prostate cancer stage C, which has an approximately 5-year survival expectation. First attention should be directed to the lymphoma.

Mr. Zhao has an aggressive disease. The treatment of diffuse large B-cell non-Hodgkin lymphoma (the most common form of intermediate-grade lymphoma) involves a combination of an alkylating agent, an anthracycline,

a glucocorticoid, and rituximab. The most popular of these combinations is R-CHOP (rituximab, cyclophosphamide, doxorubicin, vincristine, and prednisone). In early disease (stages I and II), three courses of R-CHOP followed by radiation therapy produce a cure rate of 60% to 80%.[53,54] In more advanced disease, six cycles of chemotherapy are administered with a cure rate of 60% to 80%.[54]

Although he had a complete response to his treatment for non-Hodgkin lymphoma, Mr. Zhao has a high likelihood of recurrence within 5 years. Attention is turned to his prostate cancer. The survival advantage attributed to radical prostatectomy is experienced by men who have an RLE of more than 10 years. Mr. Zhao has a high likelihood of recurrent PTCL early in this period, so his estimated RLE is less than 10 years. Furthermore, the subjective harms of surgery include incontinence and impotence. Delayed risks from radiation include proctitis, cystitis, second cancers, and impotence. This should be balanced against the risk of accelerated frailty caused by androgen ablation in this small man.

## CASE 4

### Geraldine Brown (Part 1)

Geraldine Brown is a 72-year-old woman who came to your office for follow-up of a newly discovered microcytic anemia. You are following her for uncomplicated hypertension and mild hypothyroidism. You are concerned about her memory because her MMSE was recently 23/30. She had not finished high school and had been a domestic worker and hotel maid during her working years. Mrs. Brown lives alone, drives a car locally, and has a daughter nearby. You ordered a diagnostic colonoscopy, which reveals an apple core lesion of the ascending colon. She subsequently underwent surgical resection without incident. Surgical pathology revealed stage III disease. She was able to return home with home health care and help from her daughter a week after surgery. She did not experience hospital-acquired delirium.

Should Mrs. Brown receive adjuvant chemotherapy?

## Colon Cancer

Cancer of the large bowel is the second leading cause of cancer death in women and the third leading cause in men. Incidence of this neoplasm increases with age, at least until age 95 years. The staging of colon cancer follows the tumor size, nodes involved, metastasis present (TNM) system. TNM stage I, T1–T2, is limited to mucosa and submucosa. Stage IIA, invades muscularis propria, and stage IIB invades the outer layer of colon proper, the serosa. Stage III is any lymph node involvement. Stage IV involves distant metastases, typically the liver, regional abdominal lymph nodes, or lung because of the lymphatic drainage of the large bowel. The clinical workup of cancer of the large bowel includes a full colonoscopy and a CT scan of the chest, abdomen, and pelvis, or a positron emission tomography scan to evaluate for metastases. The serum carcinoembryonic antigen (CEA) should not be used as a diagnostic serum marker because a number of different conditions can cause false positives. It is useful to draw the CEA level before surgery because if it is elevated, return to low levels implies that the surgery was effective, and elevated levels suggest recurrence or incomplete resection.

Resection of stage I and IIA colorectal cancer results in a cure rate as high as 90%. Several studies have demonstrated the benefits of adjuvant treatment in stage III cancer and in some subsets of stage IIB cancer. Adjuvant treatment consists of a combination of fluorouracil and leucovorin administered over 6 months. The addition of oxaliplatin to a multiagent protocol improves the cure rate by 5%, but it is associated with significant toxicity, especially painful neuropathy and thrombocytopenia.[55] In metastatic disease, the combination of fluorouracil, leucovorin, and irinotecan or oxaliplatin produces a response rate of approximately 40% with a median duration response of 8 months.[55] The addition of bevacizumab (Avastin), cetuximab (Erbitux), and aflibercept (Zaltrap) further improve response and survival, but they have not been specifically studied in the older adult population.[55] Bevacizumab has been associated with adverse cardiovascular events and colonic perforation, especially in the older adult population.

◆◆ **Cancer of the large bowel is the second leading cause of cancer death in women and the third leading cause in men; incidence increases with age, at least until age 95 years**.

## CASE 4
### Geraldine Brown (Part 2)

Mrs. Brown has several comorbidities, including mild dementia, but none affecting her physical functional status. Her surgical risk for abdominal surgery was acceptable, and she did well after surgery. She and her daughter agreed to adjuvant therapy, which she tolerated very well, and she continued to drive her car. Her 1-year follow-up colonoscopy was clear.

About 3 years later, however, Mrs. Brown complained of feeling tired and had lost 10 pounds. Her MMSE was now 20/30. Abdominal CT revealed several small metastatic lesions. The oncologist recommended a second course of multiagent chemotherapy, which she and her daughter agreed to; however, this time the toxicities were severe enough that despite shrinkage of the tumors, they elected to stop multiagent therapy.

Mrs. Brown was continued on single-agent treatment, capecitabine, without apparent side effects. Follow-up imaging revealed stable liver disease. The situation remained as such for over a year and then Mrs. Jackson began to develop worsening cognitive performance. Her daughter took over transportation, medication, and money management, and reported that sometimes when she came over in the afternoon, Mrs. Brown had not yet been out of bed or eaten. Her weight began to decline again, and she looked gaunt. Imaging of her liver remained unchanged. Her MMSE was now 13/30. The oncologist wished to continue capecitabine, but the patient deferred to her daughter, who chose to stop active treatment. Hospice was initiated, and Mrs. Brown passed away without discomfort 8 months later in her own home.
1. What caused Mrs. Brown's weight loss?
2. Was her cognitive decline a result of cancer, cancer treatment, or progression of dementia unrelated to cancer?
3. Do you agree with Mrs. Brown's daughter's decision?

In approximately 50% of patients with colon cancer, the only site of metastatic disease is the liver. When feasible, local management of liver metastases may prolong survival and may even result in cure. Surgical resection of liver metastases followed by infusional chemotherapy with floxuridine in the hepatic artery results in prolonged remission in approximately 40% of patients.[43] Thermoablation of metastases with ultrasound is an alternative to surgery suitable for older individuals at poor surgical risk, but cure is rare.

All patients who have had a curative resection of cancer of the large bowel should undergo surveillance colonoscopy. The first examination is generally performed 1 year after surgery; the other examinations are performed at 3- to 5-year intervals. Yearly abdominal CT and periodic determinations of CEA for 5 years are also indicated.

## CASE 4
### Discussion

Mrs. Brown lived about 5 years after her first diagnosis, most of it with good quality of life. The single-agent therapy probably did effectively control her cancer, but the progression of her dementia was the chief threat to her quality of life. Although her daughter was able to provide some in-home care once Mrs. Brown's dementia had progressed, she was at high risk for nursing home placement. Her daughter made the substituted judgment that staying home was her mother's first priority. With hospice, her daughter, and her granddaughter, Mrs. Brown was able to stay home.

## Cancer Screening and Chemoprevention of Cancer

Cancer screening remains highly controversial and emotional in the public and in general. Medical specialties exhibit cultural differences in their acceptance of the US Preventive Services Task Force recommendations[56] (see Chapter 5).

Chemoprevention of cancer involves administration of substances that block or offset the late stages of carcinogenesis, where the gradual accumulation of transcriptional errors over time may impair naturally occurring apoptosis. Although chemoprevention of cancer is an enticing strategy of tumor control in the older person, the general use of drugs and dietary supplements cannot be recommended for the following reasons:
- No proof yet exists that chemoprevention reduces cancer-related morbidity and mortality. For example, finasteride reduced the total incidence of prostate cancer but appeared to increase the risk of the most aggressive forms of the disease.
- Medications used for chemoprevention may have serious complications. For example, tamoxifen has been associated with cerebrovascular accidents, deep vein thrombosis, and endometrial cancer. Cyclooxygenase 2 (COX-2) inhibitors may also be associated with cardiovascular and renal complications and for that reason alone are off many pharmacy formularies.

At least four groups of substances have demonstrated chemopreventive activity in humans.

### Hormonal Agents

SERMs, including tamoxifen and raloxifene, and AIs, including anastrozole, letrozole, and exemestane, may prevent breast cancer. The SERMs may also prevent osteoporosis but are associated with increased risk for venous thromboembolism. The AIs that are currently considered first line for adjuvant therapy of hormone-sensitive breast cancer also are known to cause osteoporosis and should not be given without bisphosphonate therapy. If there is a contraindication to bisphosphonates, other considerations should be taken on an individualized basis.

The 5-a reductase inhibitor finasteride, which is often used in conjunction with alpha-1 blockers for symptomatic management of benign prostatic hyperplasia (BPH) with lower urinary tract symptoms (LUTS), may prevent prostate cancer.[12] Other 5-a reductase inhibitors have been developed for BPH with LUTS but have not been studied for prostate cancer effect. Stronger androgen deprivation therapies are used for treatment of confirmed prostate cancer.

## Retinoids

Retinoids may prevent cancer of the upper airways in smokers. The current recommendation, however, is to avoid such use because of the apparent adverse effects found in the one clinical trial.

## Nonsteroidal Antiinflammatory Drugs

Specific nonsteroidal antiinflammatory drugs, the COX-2 inhibitors, and aspirin may prevent cancer of the large bowel and of the breast. Colon cancers in the older adult population more often express COX-2 receptors than those in younger patients. Aspirin use has been associated with better outcomes of diagnosed colon cancer, but a causal link is not established.

## HMG-CoA Reductase Inhibitors

Recent studies indicate that the cholesterol-lowering drugs HMG-CoA reductase inhibitors may prevent different cancers, including cancers of the large bowel and of the breast. There is no recommendation to prescribe statins for this indication.

## Summary

Cancer is the second leading cause of death and a major cause of morbidity for older adults. The biology of some cancers is age-associated. Specifically, some common cancers are more indolent, such as breast and prostate cancer, non–small cell lung cancer, and some subtypes of lymphoma and ovarian cancer. However, several are more aggressive in older patients, including several acute leukemias and lymphomas. Therefore, age alone should not determine the treatment of cancer. The cancer and the patient must be staged separately, and the treatment must be grounded in evidence-based expectations. Often there is limited evidence for cancer treatment in the older adult population. A geriatric assessment should be used to determine how well or poorly the evidence fits the patient. This calculation should take into account the patient's goals in terms of survival and quality of life, and the probability of achieving them. All geriatric cancer patients should be provided with best supportive and symptomatic care regardless of prognosis, good or bad. Continuous communication between the oncologist and the geriatrician should improve treatment tolerance and thus treatment effectiveness.

### Web Resources

American Cancer Society: www.cancer.org.
National Cancer Institute: www.nci.nih.gov.
Agency for Healthcare Research and Quality's National Guideline Clearinghouse: www.guidelines.gov.
U.S. Preventive Services Recommendations for Adults: www.uspreventiveservicestaskforce.org/adultrec.htm.
Decision-making tools for healthcare professionals: www.adjuvantonline.com.
National Comprehensive Cancer Network: www.nccn.org/professionals/physician_gls/f_guidelines.asp.
International Society of Geriatric Oncology: www.siog.org.

## Acknowledgments

The author and editors would like to acknowledge the authors of this chapter from the 6th edition of this book — Dr. Miriam Rodin, Dr. James Wallace, and Dr. Tanya Wildes. They contributed the majority of the outstanding content for that chapter, which has been carried forward to the 7th edition.

## Key References

**13.** Aapro M, Köhne C-HS, Cohen HJ, Extermann M. Never too old? Age should not be a barrier to enrollment in cancer clinical trials. *Oncologist* 2005;10(3):198–204.

**16.** Biganzoli L, Wildiers H, Oakman C, et al. Management of elderly patients with breast cancer: updated recommendations of the International Society of Geriatric Oncology (SIOG) and European Society of Breast Cancer Specialists (EUSOMA) [review]. *Lancet Oncol.* 2012;13(4):e148–160.

**19.** Rodin MB, Mohile SG. A practical approach to geriatric assessment in oncology [review]. *J Clin Oncol.* 2007;25(14):1936–1944.

**25.** Hurria A. Communicating treatment options to older patients: challenges and opportunities. *J Natl Compr Canc Netw* 2012;10(9):1174–1176.

**33.** Rodin M. Cancer patients in nursing homes: what do we know? *J Am Med Directors Assoc.* 2008;9(3):149–156.

**52.** Droz JP, Balducci L, Bolla M, et al. Background for the proposal of SIOG guidelines for the management of prostate cancer in senior adults. *Crit Rev in Oncol-Hem.* 2010;73:68–91.

**References available online at** expertconsult.com. ▶

# 47

# Anemia in Older Adults

MICAH T. PROCHASKA AND ANDREW ARTZ

## OBJECTIVES

*After completing the chapter readers should be able to:*

- Define hemoglobin thresholds for anemia in older adults.
- Understand the specific etiologies of anemia in older adults.
- Outline the workup of anemia in older adults and when to consider referral to a specialist.

- Understand principles of treatment in older adults with anemia.

## Introduction

Anemia is a common condition in older adults and is associated with adverse outcomes, making it a significant health problem. The pathophysiology of anemia in older adults differs from younger adults as a result of aging-related physiologic changes, and therefore there are special diagnostic and therapeutic considerations when evaluating and treating an older adult with anemia. As the population of the United States continues to age, primary care physicians will increasingly encounter anemia in older adults, and an understanding of the unique etiologies, pathophysiology, workup, and treatment of anemia in older adults will be an important part of primary care.

### CASE

#### Mrs. Johnson

Mrs. Johnson is a 74-year-old Caucasian female who has a past medical history of osteoarthritis. She presents to your office for a routine presurgical evaluation before hip replacement. In obtaining Mrs. Johnson's history you determine she has been feeling fatigued and having difficulty ambulating because of hip pain, but otherwise she has no complaints or notable symptoms. On routine laboratory tests you find her hemoglobin (Hb) level is 10.8 g/dL; hematocrit 32.3%, white blood count 6.4 × 10³ μL (normal differential), mean cell volume 95.6 fL; mean corpuscular hemoglobin concentration 35 g/dL (normal); platelet count 210,000 × 10³ μL. Her renal function is within normal limits (creatinine clearance 71 mL/min/1.73m²). In reviewing her medical record you note that 3 years prior, her Hb level was 11.2 g/dL, and 6 years prior her Hb was 11.4 g/dL.
1. What is the differential diagnosis for Mrs. Johnson's anemia?
2. What are your next steps in evaluating her anemia?

## Definition of Anemia in Older Age

Anemia in older and younger adults has been historically diagnosed using the World Health Organization (WHO) criteria of a hemoglobin (Hb) threshold < 13 g/dL for men and < 12 g/dL for women.[1] These Hb threshold criteria, established in 1968 by a WHO panel focused on nutritional anemias, were never intended to be universal standard criterion for defining anemia. Therefore more recently modified population-based Hb thresholds for

| TABLE 47.1 | Definition of Anemia in Adults Over 60 Years of Age | |
|---|---|---|
| | World Health Organization Hemoglobin (Hb) Definition | NHANES III Hb Definitions (age, race, gender adjusted) |
| **Females** | 12 g/dL | |
| Black | | 11.5 g/dL |
| White | | 12.2 g/dL |
| **Males** | 13 g/dL | |
| Black | | 12.7 g/dL |
| White | | 13.2 g/dL |

*NHANES III*, National Health and Nutrition Examination Survey III.

defining anemia have been proposed by Beutler and Waalen.[2] Using data from the large National Health and Nutrition Examination Survey III and Scripps Kaiser databases, their thresholds for anemia were determined by identifying the lower limit (fifth percentile) of normal Hb based on age, race, and gender, after excluding patients have inflammation, kidney disease, or iron deficiency.[2] These newer Hb thresholds define anemia in adults age ≥ 60 years as a Hb < 12.7 g/dL for Black men, 13.2 g/dL for White men, 11.5 g/dL for Black women, and 12.2 g/dL for White women (Table 47.1). Although these newer Hb thresholds are likely more valid than the WHO criteria, the clinical significance of the difference between the two criteria is unclear. Moreover, the use of either Hb threshold criteria should only be used for the general identification of anemia, with a subsequent workup to more specifically classify and define the etiology of anemia.

## Epidemiology of Anemia in Older Age

Anemia is common in older adults, and the prevalence of anemia increases with age.[2–6] In community-dwelling adults age ≥ 65 years, the estimated prevalence of anemia is 10% to 11%, but for those age ≥ 85 years the estimated prevalence increases to 20% to 25%.[3,4] In institutionalized older adults, the prevalence of anemia is even higher, estimated to be 40% in hospitalized patients and 50% in adults living in a nursing home.[4,7] The prevalence rate of anemia is also influenced by race and ethnicity, with the rate

of anemia among non-Hispanic Black adults (men and women) estimated to be three times that of non-Hispanic White adults.[3,4] Although there is variation between studies in the estimated prevalence of anemia in older adults, it is likely the result of study design, and there is a consistent agreement across studies that the prevalence of anemia increases with advancing age and varies by both race and sex. Therefore in the coming years, the number of anemic older adults will increase significantly given the aging population in the United States.

## Clinical Significance of Anemia

Anemia is a significant health problem in older adults given its high prevalence and because it is a risk factor that is associated with clinically important conditions and adverse outcomes. Anemia is associated with cardiovascular disease,[8,9] congestive heart failure,[10] dementia and cognitive impairment,[11–15] insomnia,[16] and depression.[17] In addition, anemia is associated with significant reductions in patient's quality of life (QOL)[18–20] and functional status,[18,19,21–24] and an increased risk of falls and hospitalization.[25]

In addition to increased morbidity, there is a significant body of literature demonstrating that anemia is an independent risk factor for mortality.[8,11,19,25–28] An important question is whether anemia itself is the causative pathologic process driving increases in patient mortality, or whether the presence of anemia is the byproduct of another underlying pathologic process (i.e., inflammation) driving an increased risk of mortality. Whereas the association between anemia and increased mortality has been demonstrated in large well-done epidemiologic studies, as observational studies they cannot answer this fundamental question of whether the association between anemia and mortality is indeed causal.

❖ **It is not uncommon for there to be more than one cause for anemia in an older person.**

## Causes of Anemia

Although there is a wide range of etiologies of chronic anemia in older adults, they are generally divided into four common categories based on the underlying pathophysiology of anemia: (1) anemia resulting from micronutrient deficiency (primarily iron deficiency), (2) anemia resulting from chronic inflammation, (3) anemia resulting from chronic kidney disease, and (4) unexplained anemia (Table 47.2). The etiologies of anemia in older adults and their epidemiologic distribution differ from the common

| TABLE 47.2 | Etiologies and Prevalence of Anemia in Older Adults From Different Databases | | |
|---|---|---|---|
| | NHANES III[3] | Chicago[6] | SHC/VAPAHCS[29] |
| Iron deficiency | 17% | 25% | 12% |
| B$_{12}$ and/or folate | 2% | <1% | <1% |
| Anemia of chronic inflammation | 20% | 10% | 6% |
| Anemia of chronic kidney disease | 8% | 3% | 4% |
| Unexplained anemia of the older adult population | 34% | 44% | 35% |
| Hematologic malignancy | NR | 7.5% | 6% |

*NHANES*, National Health and Nutrition Examination Survey III; *NR*, Not reported; *SHC*, Stanford Hospital and Clinics; *VAPAHCS*, the VA Palo Alto Health Care System.

etiologies of anemia in younger adults, and given the high burden of comorbid disease in older adults, it is not uncommon for there to be multiple etiologies contributing to anemia in an older adult. In addition, although these four categories capture the common causes of anemia in older adults, there are other less common etiologies of anemia in older adults that clinicians should remain aware of (hematologic malignancy, alcohol abuse, thalassemia, thyroid disorder, etc.).[6]

## Anemia Resulting From Micronutrient Deficiency

Anemia resulting from micronutrient deficiency is primarily the result of a deficiency of either iron, vitamin $B_{12}$, or folate, although other micronutrients have been implicated as well. Frequently termed "nutritional deficiency," micronutrient deficiency is preferred because such anemias frequently result from acquired pathology rather than poor oral intake alone, and dietary modification will rarely correct the deficiency. Iron deficiency anemia (IDA) is by far the most common micronutrient deficiency anemia in older adults, often the result of gastrointestinal (GI) tract bleeding.[30] Bleeding from the GI tract resulting in IDA is common in older adults given the high percentage of individuals using blood thinning antiplatelet and anticoagulant medications (i.e., aspirin, warfarin, direct oral anticoagulants). In addition, the prevalence of primary GI disease (i.e., cancer, diverticulitis, gastritis) increases with age and can result in GI bleeding and IDA. Even when upper and lower endoscopies are unrevealing in older patients, small bowel interrogation often implicates small bowel angiodysplasia as the source of bleeding and IDA.[31,32]

Although not typically caused by poor nutrition alone, low iron intake predisposes and exacerbates IDA. Dietary preferences influence iron stores: Heme from the diet (such as meat and fish), supplemental iron, and vitamin C all result in increased iron stores.[33] Poor nutrition and low iron intake may emerge as a result of decreases in functional capacity and increased social isolation that hinder preparing and consuming nutritious meals. Finally, GI pathology can further reduce iron absorption, compounding factors predisposing to iron deficiency. IDA should always be considered in the differential diagnosis of an older adult presenting with anemia given that it is relatively common, the underlying pathophysiologies can be catastrophic, and it is correctable with iron replacement and/or treatment of the underlying processes.

$B_{12}$ and folate deficiency, although less common than iron deficiency, can also result in anemia in older adults. $B_{12}$ deficiency may perhaps be rising in prevalence given the pervasive use of acid-reducing agents (i.e., proton-pump inhibitors) and because of *Helicobacter pylori* infections, resulting in the poor absorption of $B_{12}$.[34] Atrophic gastritis, resulting in the classic pernicious anemia caused by the loss of intrinsic factor and the ability to uptake $B_{12}$, is estimated to be a relatively rare cause of anemia in older adults. Folate deficiency can be the result of malnutrition associated with alcohol abuse, or the use of drugs, such as methotrexate or anticonvulsants. However, given the 1998 US Food and Drug Administration decision to fortify enriched grain products in the United States with folate, folate deficiency is rare in the United States. Given that they are relatively rare, the workup of $B_{12}$ and/or folate as a cause of anemia in an older adult should be guided by the presence of risk factors for these conditions (e.g., gastric surgeries) or in the presence of macrocytic anemia. However, early and correct diagnosis remains important because both $B_{12}$ and

folate deficiency are easily treatable with supplementation and/or medication. Last, it is worth noting that anemia develops from moderate to severe $B_{12}$ or folate deficiency, whereas the nonhematologic manifestations, such as cognitive/neurologic dysfunction, emerge with mild $B_{12}$ or folate deficiency.

## Anemia Resulting From Chronic Inflammation

Anemia resulting from chronic inflammation, or anemia of chronic inflammation (ACI), is the most common cause of anemia in chronically ill or hospitalized older adults.[35] There are numerous immune system activating chronic conditions that can drive three different pathophysiologic mechanisms, which contribute to and result in ACI. First, chronic inflammation results in reduced erythropoietin production in the kidneys and erythropoietin response of erythroid progenitor cells.[35,36] Secondly, chronic inflammation increases hepcidin, a liver-derived acute phase protein that reduces iron gut absorption, and reduces iron release from macrophages that have consumed senescent red blood cells (RBCs). The overall result of increased hepcidin is a relative-iron deficient erythropoiesis, often thought of as functional iron deficiency with low serum iron but adequate iron stores.[36,37] Third, chronic inflammation results in enhanced erythrophagocytosis by splenic and hepatic macrophages, decreasing erythrocyte survival time.[35,36] Classically, chronic inflammatory conditions, such as advanced cancer, infection, and autoimmune diseases, have given rise to the classic ACI phenotype. More common chronic conditions, such as diabetes, congestive heart failure, and obesity, may be implicated in less profound inflammation and also predispose patients to ACI. However, the severity of anemia (either in absolute Hb level or rate of Hb decline) because of chronic inflammation does not necessarily correlate with the severity or progression of the chronic underlying condition. Therefore although anemia in the presence of a chronic condition suggests ACI, providers should still pursue a directed anemia evaluation to ensure there are no other concomitant causes of anemia. For example, there is accumulating data suggesting that the coexistence of ACI and IDA is more prevalent than previously thought.[35] Lastly, although ACI is common in older adults, the clinical significance of ACI independent of the underlying chronic disease remains unknown. ACI may simply be a marker of the progression and severity of an underlying chronic disease, and/or it may contribute to the progression and severity of an underlying chronic condition.

**◆◆ The coexistence of ACI and IDA is fairly common; always check iron stores.**

## Anemia Resulting From Chronic Kidney Disease

Chronic kidney disease (CKD) is another important etiology of anemia in older adults. The pathophysiologic mechanisms of anemia caused by CKD overlap with ACI and include decreased renal erythropoietin production, uremic-induced inhibitors of erythropoietin, disordered iron hemostasis, and decreased erythrocyte survival time.[38] In patients with CKD, as the glomerular filtration rate (GFR) declines, there is also a gradual decline in patients' Hb level. The exact relationship between kidney disease progression and the development and progression of anemia is, however, not well characterized.[39] As a consequence, the optimal frequency of monitoring Hb levels in patients with CKD is unknown. Evidence for the association of anemia and CKD is strongest at a GFR $< 30$ mL/min, although data also suggest a hemoglobin decrement and/or reduced serum erythropoietin at a GFR in the range of 30 to 60 mL/min if not higher in older adults.[40–43] Similar to patients with ACI, patients with anemia caused by CKD also are at risk of anemia from other etiologies, most notably IDA. As such, in patients with stable CKD, the progression of anemia (included requiring higher doses of erythropoiesis stimulating agents to maintain hemoglobin) should be investigated and evaluated for other potential causes of anemia.

## Unexplained Anemia and Hematologic Malignancies

Approximately one-third of anemia in older adults will be categorized as unexplained anemia of the elderly (UAE), in which the etiology of their anemia is not attributable to micronutrient deficiencies, chronic inflammation, renal disease, or other established causes (hematologic malignancies, alcohol, medications, hemolysis, etc.), despite a thorough evaluation and workup. Typically UAE is mild (Hb 10–12 g/dL), normocytic, and hypoproliferative (low reticulocyte count). Several aging-related changes in physiology likely contribute to the development of UAE, including (1) declining testosterone levels,[44,45] (2) aging-related declines in renal function and serum erythropoietin in the absence of clinically recognized renal disease,[46–49] (3) occult chronic inflammation that is insufficient to meet the pathophysiologic criteria of ACI,[50] and (4) occult myelodysplasia.[51] It is likely that the pathophysiology of UAE is the multifactorial combination of several of these factors and perhaps others, such as shortened red cell survival.

A diagnosis of UAE can be challenging because UAE is typically a mild anemia that can be easily overlooked, and because UAE is a diagnosis of exclusion there is not a definitive test for UAE. Moreover, the pathophysiologic overlap of UAE with other etiologies of anemia can complicate the certainty a provider has in making the diagnosis. Although clinicians may struggle to categorize UAE, the diagnosis holds important value because it indicates a negative medical workup as opposed to a deferred workup. In addition, patients with UAE should be monitored for progression of their anemia because some of these patients may in fact have early or occult myelodysplasia or hematologic malignancy.[6]

❖ **After evaluation, about one-third of anemias in older people remain unexplained. This is called UAE.**

## Diagnostic Principles

A systematic evaluation in older adults presenting with anemia is recommended to exclude serious causes and detect treatable conditions and causes of anemia. Because multiple etiologies can be responsible for a patient's anemia, accurate classification of anemia can be a challenge, and a thorough history and a routine panel of anemia laboratory tests are justified (Box 47.1).

An anemia evaluation should be initiated when a patient's absolute Hb value falls below the Beutler and Waalen criteria (see earlier), but also based on the Hb trajectory over time when available. In older adults the average Hb declines about 1 g/dL over 15 years, so a consistent decline of 1 g/dL in <5 years or 2 g/dL over 10 years should be considered significant and warrant a complete evaluation.[52] Moreover, a stable Hb concentration over years is unlikely to be attributable to a sinister etiology.

❖ **Anemia evaluation is warranted when the Hb declines 1 g/dL in <5 years or 2 g/dL in <10 years.**

---

### • BOX 47.1 Routine Anemia Laboratory Evaluation

- Complete blood count, white blood cell differential, RBC indices
- Reticulocyte count
- Iron studies: serum ferritin, serum iron, TIBC, transferrin saturation
- Serum creatinine
- Thyroid stimulating hormone
- Vitamin B$_{12}$
- C-reactive protein
- RBC or serum folate (only when specific risk factors)

*RBC*, Red blood cell; *TIBC*, total iron binding capacity.

---

In obtaining a patient's history, the clinician should elicit the patient's fatigue level, especially in relation to Hb changes. An emphasis should be made to determine whether the patient has had signs or symptoms of bleeding or recent surgery, dietary preferences (including PICA, which strongly suggests IDA), alcohol abuse, or whether there are other risk factors that may portend anemia of a specific etiology. In addition, the history should elicit whether the patient has ever had a previous RBC transfusion (indicating prior severe anemia), prior chemotherapy or radiation (suggesting a therapy related myelodysplasia), or a family history of anemia (e.g., thalassemia). Patient report and the use of available past laboratory values should document a prior history of anemia, its duration, severity, prior evaluation, and treatment (including transfusion). Hb declines should be noted when coincident to major events, such as prolonged hospitalization or major surgery. Special attention to Hb values before a surgery or admission will alert the clinician to preexisting anemia.

Recognizing that anemia in older adults can be multifactorial, a routine laboratory workup in all patients with anemia should include a complete blood count, white blood cell differential, RBC indices, reticulocyte count, serum ferritin, serum iron, total-iron binding capacity (TIBC), transferrin saturation, serum creatinine (estimated GFR), vitamin B$_{12}$, C-reactive protein, and thyrotropin levels (see Table 47.2). These lab tests should be helpful in diagnosing micronutrient deficiencies, ACI, and anemia of CKD (Fig. 47.1). Low folate levels are rare in the United States given mandatory dietary fortification, and folate levels need not be drawn routinely nor repeatedly but only when there is a specific clinical risk factor (i.e., poor diet, intestinal malabsorption [gastric bypass], medication use [methotrexate, anticonvulsants]). In patients with unexplained IDA, subsequent testing should include both fecal guaiac tests for blood and an endoscopic GI evaluation. An additional workup should be done if after the aforementioned laboratory tests there remains diagnostic uncertainty. A review of the peripheral smear by the pathologist (routinely available by request) can be invaluable for abnormalities on the white blood cell differential or unexplained macrocytosis.

Diagnosing concomitant IDA and ACI is difficult because ferritin is an acute phase reactant that will be elevated in the context of ACI, and because chronic inflammation will drive serum iron and often mean cell volume (MCV) down mirroring mild iron deficiency. The value of novel markers to distinguish IDA in the presence of ACI, such as serum transferrin receptor or hepcidin, have yet to be clinically established nor are they routinely available.[35,53] Thus in the presence of significant inflammation known by medical history (e.g., advanced cancer, autoimmune disorders) or a high C-reactive protein (e.g., >10 mg/L), and a ferritin <30 to

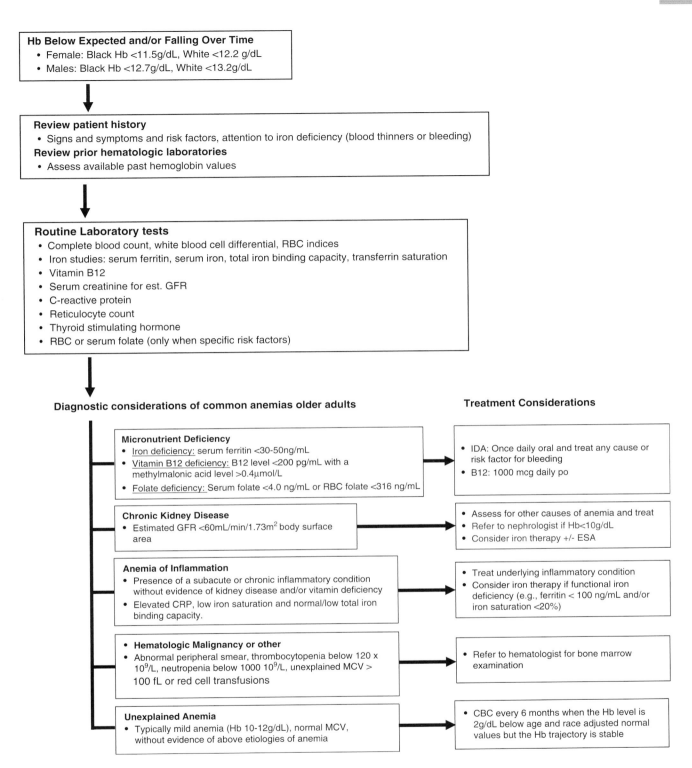

• **Figure 47.1** Workup of older adult presenting with anemia

50 ng/mL, it is reasonable to treat the patient for IDA. In contrast, in such a situation, a high ferritin ($>300$ ng/mL) would render iron deficiency unlikely. In patients with intermediate iron stores, a gray zone exists with respect to whether or not treat for IDA, but it is reasonable to treat empirically for IDA in the presence of significant ACI if the ferritin is below 100 ng/mL and/or a transferrin saturation of $<20\%$.

▸▸ **Because ACI and IDA often coexist, adjust ferritin thresholds for treatment with iron in ACI. Ferritin $<30$ to $50$ ng/mL is probable iron deficiency, and ferritin $<100$ ng/mL is possible iron deficiency. Treat and assess response.**

Referral to hematology/oncology to consider bone marrow examination is recommended should hematologic malignancy be a consideration. Specifically, patients with anemia and any of the following factors: thrombocytopenia $< 120 \times 10^9$/L, neutropenia $< 1000 \ 10^9$/L, an abnormal peripheral blood smear, unexplained macrocytosis, and/or unexplained requirement for RBC transfusions.

When the workup of anemia has revealed no clear etiology and the Hb level is 2 g/dL below age and race adjusted normal values but the Hb trajectory is stable, a complete blood count every 6 months is recommended to monitor for progression of anemia and any underlying pathophysiology, including occult myelodysplastic syndrome.

## Treatment of Anemia

Treatment of anemia and the intensity of treatment should be tailored to the symptoms of anemia, the underlying diagnosis, and the risks and benefits of the treatment. Treatment decisions should be influenced by the patient's symptoms because the relief of symptoms, such as fatigue, is often the most important consideration for patients with anemia.[54,55] In addition to the treatment of anemia, concurrently addressing the specific pathophysiology of the patient's anemia is critical.

Micronutrient anemias should almost always be treated given that there are readily available treatments, and treatment will result in resolution of the patient's anemia and confirm the deficiency as the etiology of their anemia. For patients with IDA, numerous oral and intravenous (IV) formulations are available. Oral iron therapy with around 50 mg of elemental iron daily (e.g., iron sulfate 325 mg has 65 mg of elemental iron) or every other day is recommended as first-line therapy for most patients. Paradoxically, less frequent dosing enhances iron absorption and improves tolerance relative to historical recommendations of three-times-daily dosing.[56-58] However, in older adults who may have severe anemia, reduced GI uptake, difficulty with compliance of oral medications, or are hospitalized, IV formulations of iron are also available and safe. Iron therapy should be continued until repletion of iron stores and the underlying pathophysiology has been resolved, and low-dose maintenance iron therapy may be used for intermittent bleeding or poor absorption. For patients with $B_{12}$ deficiency both oral and nonoral formulations (intranasal, intramuscular, subcutaneous) of vitamin $B_{12}$ (cobalamin) are also available and effective. Oral therapy at 1000 mcg daily is generally recommended. Regardless of the specific nutritional deficiency, iron or vitamin replacement used as both a diagnostic and therapeutic trial is appropriate for 3 months, with discontinuation of the treatment when ineffective with adequate adherence.

❖ **Oral iron replacement should be dosed once daily or every other day rather than three times daily.**

Anemia of CKD treatment involves ensuring that the patient has no other easily treatable concurrent conditions or micronutrient

deficiencies, and then if necessary using erythropoiesis stimulating agents (ESAs) for severe anemia. Typically the goal Hb in patients with CKD is $\geq 10$ g/dL, and patients with iron deficiency benefit from iron (oral or often intravenous) before giving an ESA because a significant portion of CKD patients have been shown to respond to iron with an increase in Hb.[39] In the presence of CKD, it is recommended that patients with a transferrin saturation $< 30\%$ and a serum ferritin $< 500$ ng/mL be treated with iron.[39] Ensuring that a patient is iron replete before starting ESAs is necessary to ensure that once an ESA is started there will be an appropriate bone marrow response. ESAs have been shown to increase Hb, thereby reducing the need for RBC transfusion and improve QOL in patients with anemia of CKD.[39]

In patients with either ACI or UAE, there are no definitive treatment options for anemia or increasing a patient's Hb. As discussed earlier, for ACI it is important to treat the underlying chronic condition and to test for and treat concomitant IDA when present.

RBC transfusion remains an effective and necessary therapy to avoid life-threatening consequences for severe symptomatic anemia. Recent guidelines in hospitalized patients with anemia have emphasized restrictive transfusion thresholds, or transfusion only when patient's Hb drops below 7 g/dL or 8 g/dL during hospitalization.[59] The studies informing these guidelines are randomized controlled trials that studied the effect of higher or lower Hb values on patient mortality, although there is a growing body of observational data suggesting that lower transfusion thresholds in hospitalized patients may have deleterious effects on patients' QOL.[60,61] In the outpatient setting, there are no formal guidelines or Hb criteria for RBC transfusion. However, in ambulatory oncology patients, there is good evidence to suggest that RBC transfusion to treat anemia improves patient's QOL.[62-65] It is therefore reasonable to assume that the use of RBC transfusion to treat symptomatic anemia will improve QOL in other patient populations as well, although further data are needed to better guide clinicians in this area.

### CASE

#### Discussion

Mrs. Johnson's presentation is notable for a chronic stable anemia in the context of fatigue. Although the stability of her Hb and her history are reassuring, you order follow-up laboratory values to identify any significant underlying pathology and determine if there is a treatable cause of her anemia. Follow-up laboratory values reveal a reticulocyte production index of 1.2% (underproduction), a ferritin level of 63 ng/mL, normal iron/TIBC, transferrin saturation, $B_{12}$, C-reactive protein, and thyrotropin levels. Given her mild stable anemia and unrevealing labs, you diagnose unexplained anemia and plan to monitor her Hb level over time. Although her Hb fell after surgery to 9 g/dL, it recovered after 3 months to her baseline of 11.2 g/dL and was unchanged after 6 months and 1 year.

## Summary

Anemia is a common condition among older adults and is associated with significant adverse consequences. Older adults also are at risk for anemia from different etiologies than are younger adults, and anemia in older adults is often caused by (1) micronutrient deficiencies, (2) anemia of chronic inflammation, (3) anemia of chronic kidney disease, and (4) unexplained anemia. It is also not uncommon for older adults to have anemia from multiple different

etiologies. Given the adverse consequences of anemia, all older adults presenting with anemia should receive a routine workup consisting of a thorough history and standard laboratory tests to identify the underlying pathophysiology of their anemia. Patients found to have either a micronutrient anemia and/or anemia of chronic kidney disease should receive standard treatment to resolve their anemia and/or improve their Hb level.

❖❖ Anemia is a common problem in older adults independently associated with worse outcomes and higher future mortality risk.

❖❖ The common causes of anemia in older adults are iron deficiency, anemia of chronic inflammation, anemia of chronic kidney disease, and unexplained anemia.

❖❖ An anemia evaluation should be triggered based on hemoglobin below expected normal levels, as well as based on hemoglobin change from prior values.

❖❖ Around one-third of older anemic adults will be categorized as unexplained; this is typically a mild normocytic anemia.

❖❖ Oral iron treatment may be initiated once a day or every other for most adults with iron deficiency anemia.

❖❖ Severe unexplained anemia, need for a transfusion, unexplained macrocytosis, or abnormalities of white cells or platelets should prompt hematology referral.

## Key References

2. Beutler E, Waalen J. The definition of anemia: what is the lower limit of normal of the blood hemoglobin concentration? *Blood.* 2006;107(5):1747–1750.
25. Penninx BWJH, Pahor M, Woodman RC, Guralnik JM. Anemia in old age is associated with increased mortality and hospitalization. *J Gerontol A Biol Sci Med Sci.* 2006;61(5): 474–479.
36. Stauder R, Valent P, Theurl I. Anemia at older age: etiologies, clinical implications, and management. *Blood.* 2018;131(5): 505–514.
49. Artz AS, Fergusson D, Drinka PJ, et al. Mechanisms of unexplained anemia in the nursing home. *J Am Geriatr Soc.* 2004;52(3):423–427.
59. Carson JL, Guyatt G, Heddle NM, et al. Clinical practice guidelines from the AABB: red blood cell transfusion thresholds and storage. *JAMA.* 2016;316(19):2025–2035.

**References available online at** expertconsult.com.

# 48

# Pulmonary Disease

KATHLEEN M. AKGÜN AND MARGARET A. PISANI

## OUTLINE

## OBJECTIVES

*Upon completion of this chapter the reader will be able to:*

- Recognize the changes in pulmonary physiology associated with aging.
- Identify the signs and symptoms associated with a variety of lung diseases in older adults with multiple comorbidities.
- Understand which diagnostic tests are indicated for the workup of dyspnea in older adults.

- Know when to refer for further evaluation of lung disease, including for pulmonary fibrosis, interstitial lung disease, and lung cancer screening.

## Changes in the Respiratory System With Aging

The respiratory system undergoes numerous changes as part of physiologic aging that contribute to pulmonary-related symptoms (Table 48.1).[1] Rhinitis, cough, and shortness of breath (dyspnea) are frequently reported by older persons and are common symptoms that bring patients to seek medical attention. Upper airway nasal passages become less cartilaginous and, as a consequence, less rigid, reducing nasal passage patency. Proximal and distal airways experience similar changes, resulting in air trapping in the smaller airways and less efficient ventilation and oxygenation. At the alveolar level, lung

## TABLE 48.1 Physiologic Changes in the Respiratory System Associated With Aging

| Anatomic Area | Change With Aging | Associated Symptoms/Signs |
|---|---|---|
| Nasal passages | Narrowed, decreased collagen | Chronic rhinosinus drainage<br>Postnasal drip |
| Sinuses | Decreased effective ciliary clearance<br>Change in microbiome | |
| Pharynx and larynx | Narrowed, thickened cartilage | Voice changes |
| Trachea | More collapsible, especially with expiration | Dyspnea, especially with hyperventilation<br>Tracheomalacia |
| Bronchioles | Decreased collagen and impaired airway clearance | Dyspnea on exertion<br>Positional dyspnea<br>Hypoventilation/chronic hypercapnic respiratory failure |
| Alveoli | Destruction, reduced numbers | |
| Diaphragm | Decreased contractility | |
| Skeletal muscle | Sarcopenia | |
| Rib cage and spine | Reduced expansion, kyphosis, disadvantaged mechanics of diaphragm | |

function begins to decline in the fourth decade at a rate of approximately 35 to 50 mL/year, leading to decreased alveolar surface for gas exchange to occur. Cigarette smoking accelerates this loss in effective alveoli.

Intercostal skeletal muscle atrophies and the diaphragm weakens, also contributing to inadequate ventilation by restricting vital capacity and further reducing lung compliance (Fig. 48.1).[2] These changes lead to reduced lung function down to the alveolar level, leading to decreased alveolar surface area and impaired gas exchange. The respiratory system begins to experience these declines in the fourth decade at a rate of approximately 35 to 50 mL/year. Cigarette smoking accelerates this loss in effective alveoli.

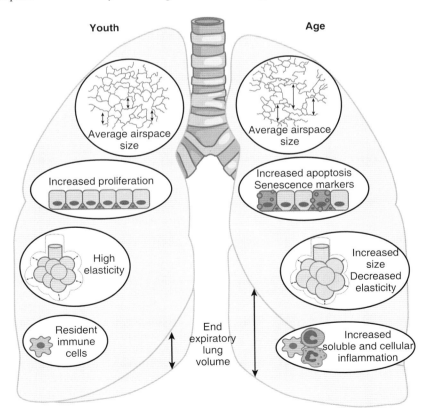

• **Figure 48.1** Representative changes to the lung observed with aging. (From Bowdish DME. The aging lung: is lung health good health for older adults? *Chest* 2019;155(2):391–400. Used with permission license number: 4678771389901.)

# Prevalence, Presentation, and Evaluation of Common Pulmonary Symptoms in Older Patients

Aging-related changes to the respiratory system lead to pulmonary-related symptoms in older persons. Patient-reported onset and patterns of symptoms can be helpful to narrow down the cause(s) of pulmonary symptoms. During a thorough evaluation of patients with pulmonary symptoms, it is also important to remember that other comorbid conditions may be present, and clinicians should continue to assess therapeutic success and consider additional diagnoses when needed.

The most common pulmonary-related symptoms include rhinitis, dyspnea, and cough (Table 48.2). The prevalence of these symptoms is either remaining stable or increasing because older persons are living longer with multiple chronic conditions.[3] Approximately one in four older adults report daytime and sleep-related rhinitis and shortness of breath. More than 30% of older adults report cough symptoms. Pulmonary-related diseases are common and increasing in older populations. The characteristics of pulmonary-related symptoms are nonspecific. Multimorbidity further complicates the identification of pulmonary disorders in older persons. Common pulmonary diseases in older adults along with common pulmonary function test findings are described in Table 48.3.

## TABLE 48.2 Pulmonary Symptom Prevalence and Differential

| Symptom | Prevalence | At-Risk Groups | Differential |
|---|---|---|---|
| Rhinitis | 24.7% | Women Younger age Snoring GERD | Allergy |
| Cough | 9.0% | Women Smoking status Obesity Snoring GERD | Asthma ILD Postnasal drip Cancer OSA GERD Chronic bronchitis Chronic aspiration Cancer Bronchiectasis (Non-CF and CF-related) |
| Dyspnea | 25.0% | Chronic lung disease Multimorbidity Current smokers Obesity | Asthma COPD Central airway obstruction/ cancer Cardiac etiologies Deconditioning |
| Wheezing/chest tightness | 12.0%–18.6% | Women Obesity Occupational exposures | Asthma COPD Cardiac etiologies |

CF, Cystic fibrosis; COPD, chronic obstructive pulmonary disease; GERD, gastrointestinal reflux disease; ILD, interstitial lung diseases; OSA, obstructive sleep apnea.

## TABLE 48.3 Differential Diagnosis for Common Pulmonary Diseases in Older Adults

| Condition | Pulmonary Evaluation Findings |
|---|---|
| Asthma | Obstruction on PFT with bronchodilator response |
| Chronic obstructive pulmonary disease (COPD) | Obstruction on PFT Diffusion impairment Hyperinflated |
| Mechanical obstruction by mass or lymph node in upper airways | Obstruction Blunted inspiratory limb of flow volume loop |
| Vocal cord dysfunction | Blunted inspiratory limb of flow volume loop |
| Interstitial lung diseases | Restriction on PFT Diffusion impairment |
| Lung cancer | Can be normal or have obstruction, restriction, or diffusion impairment |

PFT, Pulmonary function test.

## Pulmonary Function Testing

For patients with chronic dyspnea and/or sputum production, pulmonary function testing (PFTs) should be completed. PFTs require a patient who has the ability to create and hold a closed seal between the mouth and the PFT equipment mouthpiece. Patients also must be able to follow instructions to have valid PFT measurements. These requirements can make completion of PFTs challenging, especially for patients with neurocognitive disorders or skeletal muscle weakness. Because the results of PFTs are effort dependent, measurements may be of limited utility if patients have difficulty completing the maneuvers. Standard PFTs include three types of testing: spirometry, lung volume assessment, and diffusion capacity (Fig. 48.2). Spirometry is an effort-dependent test that evaluates airflow limitation because of obstructive diseases of the airways (e.g., chronic obstructive pulmonary disease [COPD], asthma). Key measurements from spirometry are the forced expiratory volume in the first second ($FEV_1$) of a forced expiratory maneuver and the forced vital capacity (FVC), the total volume a person can exhale during the forced maneuver. A valid study requires at least a 6-second exhalation. The $FEV_1$ and FVC are used to identify airflow limitations ($FEV_1$/FVC), to quantify the severity of airflow limitation ($FEV_1$), and may suggest if restrictive lung diseases are also present (proportional reduction in $FEV_1$ and FVC). With increased prevalence of asthma in older persons, overlap between asthma and COPD is common. For this reason, reversible airflow obstruction should be tested for a significant bronchodilator response, defined as a postbronchodilator improvement of $FEV_1$ or FVC by at least 200 mL and 12%. Lung volumes are determined by nitrogen dilution testing or a body box and are used to evaluate for restrictive lung diseases because of intrinsic (e.g., interstitial lung diseases [ILDs]) or extrinsic (e.g., obesity) causes. Diffusion capacity measures the ability of gas exchange to occur at the alveolar level and can be used to identify pulmonary vascular disorders, although it can also be used to further characterize obstructive and restrictive conditions (Fig. 48.3). Respiratory muscle weakness can also be studied by requesting maximal voluntary ventilation (MVV), maximal inspiratory pressures (MIPs), and maximal

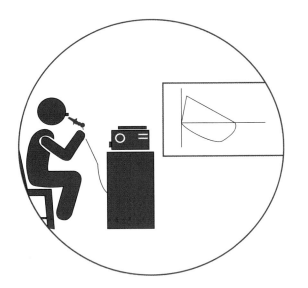

• **Figure 48.2** Cartoon representation of pulmonary function testing for patients.

expiratory pressures (MEPs). In most cases, PFTs take between 15 and 30 minutes to complete. It is recommended that PFTs are repeated at least annually for patients with chronic pulmonary conditions. However, comprehensive cost-effective analyses of PFTs in

improving chronic pulmonary disease management has not yet been reported.

The 6-minute walk test (6MWT) is used to evaluate the response to therapy for patients with cardiopulmonary conditions. The 6MWT may also assist in determining exertional supplemental oxygen needs. Key steps of performing the 6MWT include the following: use a measured straight corridor to estimate distance walked, have patient wear comfortable shoes, encourage patient to walk (not run) as far as possible in 6 minutes, measure heart rate and pulse oxygen saturation ($SpO_2$) continuously; at end of test assess pulse $SpO_2$, dyspnea, and fatigue levels, and measure distance walked.

## Imaging

Chest x-ray remains the most frequent radiologic lung study used in clinical practice. Chest x-rays can be used to identify acute changes, such as pneumonia, and can be used during initial evaluation for patients with more subacute or chronic pulmonary conditions, such as hyperinflation from COPD or interstitial markings associated with ILD. Chest computed tomography (CT) scans (including low-dose screening CT scans and high-resolution CT scans) have become increasingly common in clinical use for better sensitivity in detecting lung abnormalities, including lung nodules and cancers, airway abnormalities, pulmonary emboli, and pleural effusions. Ventilation/perfusion scans may be performed to assess surgical candidacy for potential lung resections or to evaluate for chronic thromboembolic disease.

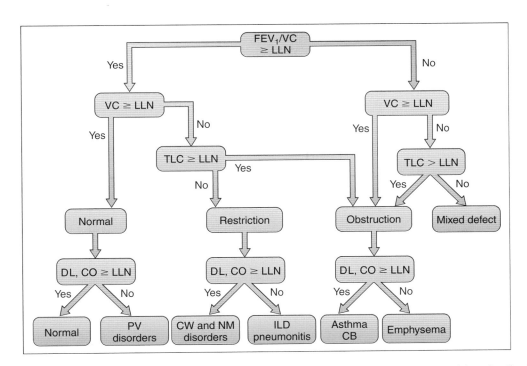

• **Figure 48.3** Patients may or may not present with the classic patterns, depending on their illnesses, severity, and lung function before the disease onset. The decisions about how far to follow this diagram are clinical and will vary depending on the questions being asked and the clinical information available at the time of testing. The forced expiratory volume in 1 second *(FEV₁)*/vital capacity *(VC)* ratio and VC should be considered first. Total lung capacity *(TLC)* is necessary to confirm or exclude the presence of a restrictive defect when VC is below the lower limit of normal *(LLN)*. The algorithm also includes diffusing capacity for carbon monoxide *(DL,CO)* measurement with the predicted value adjusted for hemoglobin. In the mixed defect group, the DL,CO patterns are the same as those for restriction and obstruction. *CB,* Chronic bronchitis; *CW,* chest wall; *ILD,* interstitial lung diseases; *NM,* neuromuscular; *PV,* pulmonary vascular. (From Pellegrino R, Viegi G, Brusasco V, et al., Interpretative strategies for lung function tests. *Eur Respir J.* 2005;26(5):948–968.)

## Rhinosinusitis

### Definition and Epidemiology

Rhinosinusitis is a heterogeneous syndrome resulting from interactions between host factors, microbial factors, and the environment. Age-related anatomic and functional factors, including decreased ciliary beat frequency, nasal mucosal atrophy, decreased nasal vasculature, and nasal mucous secretion likely all play a role in the development of rhinosinusitis. Changes in physiology of the nasal cartilage with aging contribute to a lengthening of the nose and drooping of the tip. These changes can restrict nasal airflow and cause narrowing of the nasal passages, which can lead to rhinitis, often termed geriatric rhinitis.

Rhinosinusitis is defined as acute (<4 weeks duration), subacute (4−12 weeks duration), and chronic (>12 weeks duration). Rhinosinusitis can be uncomplicated where signs and symptoms of inflammation are restricted to the nasal cavity and sinuses or complicated when inflammation extends to soft tissues or there is neurologic involvement.

Chronic rhinosinusitis (CRS) affects 10% of the general population. CRS is defined by the presence of two or more of the following symptoms for >12 weeks: nasal discharge, nasal congestion or obstruction, facial pain or pressure, and reduction or loss of smell. Increasing age is associated with increased incidence of chronic rhinosinusitis. In addition to age, smoking is also a major risk factor for CRS.[4]

Despite the highest prevalence of nasal polyps observed in persons age ≥60 years, older patients with CRS are more likely to report loss of smell and less rhinorrhea or nasal obstruction than young patients. Among patients with CRS with nasal polyps, 60% also have asthma, although the mechanisms underlying this association are not fully understood. In older patients with late-onset asthma, CRS with nasal polyps was closely related to severe eosinophilic asthma and elevated serum immunoglobulin (Ig)E levels. In addition to potential immune-mediating therapies for patients with CRS, polyps, and elevated IgE levels, identification and management of nasal polyps can be important to relieve CRS symptoms. The recurrence rate of nasal polyps following surgical resection during 2-year follow-up was lower in older patients compared to younger patients (11.6% vs. 28.2%; $P = .05$). Older patients with CRS more frequently have colonization of the nasal mucosa by *Staphylococcus aureus*, seen in up to 73.2%. Importantly, *S. aureus* colonization is associated with IgE levels and eosinophils within nasal polyps. Otitis media is also frequently seen in patients with CRS, and the association is significant in older adults (>50 years) but not in younger adults.

### Diagnosis

There is no data to support that rhinosinusitis manifests differently in older adults, and guidelines from the American Academy of Otolaryngology-Head and Neck Surgery do not recommend different approaches to diagnosis and treatment based on age. Diagnosis of rhinosinusitis is based on history, duration of symptoms as noted earlier, and clinical examination. Bacterial rhinosinusitis is often associated with purulent nasal discharge and facial pain or pressure.

### Treatment

In patients with clear nasal discharge the etiology of rhinosinusitis is usually viral, and treatment should focus on pain relief with analgesics and relief of nasal obstruction with saline irrigation. Topical treatment with α-adrenergic decongestants are effective, but they should be used with caution in older adults, especially those with hypertension or enlarged prostates. Antibiotics are usually only prescribed when symptoms are present for >7 days or if they continue to worsen. CRS can be treated with saline irrigation and topical steroids. A Cochrane review demonstrated that saline irrigation is more effective compared to placebo and is safe in older patients. Topical nasal steroids have been shown to be more effective than saline irrigation but can cause epistaxis. If the rhinosinusitis is secondary to allergens, there is a role for antihistamines, but these should be used judiciously because of the anticholinergic side effects.

---

### CASE 1

#### Mr. Walker

Mr. Walker, an 81-year-old man, is in your office today asking for symptom relief and to return to his prior activity level. Until a few months ago, he was an active swimmer, spending at least 1 hour in the pool four to five times per week. However, he has noticed increasing dyspnea on exertion, and now can barely complete 20 minutes in the pool once per week. He quit smoking 45 years ago, and before that had a 15 pack-year smoking history. He has no prior history of lung disease, and he has no associated rhinosinus symptoms, but does note an audible wheeze when he exerts himself. His PFTs show a ratio of FEV1/FVC = 55%, with an FEV1 of 1.67 L (67% predicted). After bronchodilator, his FEV1 = 2.50 L (93% predicted). What is his likely pulmonary-related diagnosis? How should it be managed?

---

## Asthma

### Definition and Epidemiology

Asthma is characterized by reversible airflow obstruction and is an inflammatory disorder characterized by variable and recurring symptoms of airway inflammation, hyperresponsiveness, and bronchoconstriction. The prevalence of self-reported asthma in patients >65 years is 6.8%, and the lifetime prevalence is estimated to be 13% in this population.[5,6] Asthma is particularly challenging in older persons because they have the highest rates of asthma-related deaths, perhaps owing to decreased patient recognition of symptoms as well as underdiagnosis and misdiagnosis.[7,8] A recent review on asthma in older adults provides an overview of the epidemiology, pathophysiology, clinical features, and treatment.[9]

There are two phenotypes of asthma in older persons. Longstanding asthma, which begins in childhood and is frequently associated with atopy, and late onset asthma, which typically begins after middle age and is less commonly associated with atopy.[10,11] Although there is often a link between atopy and asthma in younger patients, the role of atopy in older patients in unclear. Whereas asthma in older patients has been traditionally characterized as nonallergic, there is new, albeit conflicting evidence that atopy in not uncommon in older adults.[12] Studies of older, inner-city populations with asthma found that 60% had at least one detectable allergen-specific IgE antibody and that 41% were sensitized to at least one antigen.[13,14] Viral infections are frequently a precipitating factor for an asthma exacerbation in older patients. Data regarding specific pathogens are sparse, but respiratory syncytial virus and influenza virus strains have been frequently implicated.[15,16] Asthma in older adults often coexists with other diseases, such as COPD or pulmonary fibrosis and can result in a more severe phenotype that is often irreversible.

## Diagnosis

The diagnosis of asthma relies on assessment of clinical symptoms and the presence of reversible airway obstruction.[17] These symptoms include chest tightness, intermittent and nocturnal wheezing, and dyspnea. Oftentimes cough may be the only symptom. These symptoms of asthma overlap with COPD and heart disease, which can make the diagnosis challenging in older patients. Spirometry is an important tool for diagnosis of obstructive lung diseases, and improvement in FEV1 of at least 12% after inhalational treatment with a short-acting bronchodilator is key to the diagnosis, although patients with COPD can also have improvement confounding the picture. Between 10% and 20% of older patients are unable to appropriately perform spirometry because of poor physical or cognitive function.[18,19] As a result of accelerated decline in FEV1 with increasing age, it is important to use age-adjusted values when interpreting spirometry results in older patients to avoid overdiagnosis.[20] Fig. 48.4 lists criteria for asthma severity in adults.

Airways hyperresponsiveness (AHR) is an exaggerated bronchoconstrictor response to inhaled stimuli and correlates to the severity and frequency of asthma exacerbations. Assessment of AHR can be performed through a provocation test, such as a methacholine challenge.[21] Biomarkers that support a diagnosis of asthma include peripheral and/or sputum eosinophilia, elevated total serum IgE, and/or elevated fractional excretion of nitric oxide ($FE_{NO}$).[14]

$FE_{NO}$ can be measured easily in clinical practice and is increased in atopic asthma. $FE_{NO}$ can be used to monitor response to therapy as it is reduced with corticosteroid treatment but is unchanged with bronchodilator therapy.[22] In addition, $FE_{NO}$ has been found to correlate with AHR but there are no published data specifically examining levels in patients over age 65 years.[23,24]

◆◆ **Asthma in an older adult may be more severe and have an irreversible component as the result of airway remodeling, age of onset, and coexistence of COPD or pulmonary fibrosis.**

## Treatment

Treatment of asthma is similar regardless of age and is directed at controlling symptoms and eliminating or reducing exacerbating triggers. Table 48.4 lists common medication classes used to treat asthma. Older patients with asthma should be managed according to The National Institutes for Health and Global Initiative for Asthma.[17] Factors important to consider in older patients with asthma include presence of multiple chronic conditions, polypharmacy and potential drug interactions, and medication cost. Common cooccurring comorbidities with asthma include gastroesophageal reflux disease (GERD), chronic rhinosinusitis, congestive heart failure, diabetes mellitus, and obesity. Another consideration for older patients with asthma, especially with uncontrolled symptoms, includes inhaler technique. This can be compromised in older persons because of cognitive impairments and oropharyngeal and respiratory muscle strength.

| Components of severity | | Classification of asthma severity (youths ≥ 12 years of age and adults) | | | |
|---|---|---|---|---|---|
| | | Intermittent | Persistent | | |
| | | | Mild | Moderate | Severe |
| **Intermittent** Normal $FEV_1/FVC$: 8–19 yr 85% 20–39 yr 80% 40–59 yr 75% 60–80 yr 70% | Symptoms | ≤ 2 days/week | > 2 days/week but not daily | Daily | Throughout the day |
| | Nightime awakenings | ≤ 2x/month | 3–4x/month | > 1x/week but not nightly | Often 7x/week |
| | Short-acting beta$_2$-agonist use for symptom control (not prevention of EIB) | ≤ 2 days/week | > 2 days/week but not > 1x/day | Daily | Several times per day |
| | Interference with normal activity | None | Minor limitation | Some limitation | Extremely limited |
| | Lung function | • Normal $FEV_1$ between exacerbations • $FEV_1$ > 80% predicted • $FEV_1/FVC$ normal | • $FEV_1$ ≥ 80% predicted • $FEV_1/FVC$ normal | • $FEV_1$ > 60% but < 80% predicted • $FEV_1/FVC$ reduced 5% | • $FEV_1$ < 60% predicted • $FEV_1/FVC$ reduced > 5% |
| **Risk** | Exacerbations requiring oral systemic corticosteroids | 0–1/year | ≥ 2/year ─────────────────────────→ | | |
| | | Consider severity and interval since last exacerbation. ←── Frequency and severity may fluctuate over time for ──→ patients in any severity category. | | | |
| | | Relative annual risk of exacerbations may be related to $FEV_1$ | | | |

• **Figure 48.4** Classification of asthma severity. *EIB*, Exercise-induced bronchoconstriction. (From Expert Panel Report 3 [EPR-3]. Guidelines for the diagnosis and management of asthma-summary report 2007. *J Allergy Clin Immunol.* 2007;120[5 Suppl]:S94–138.)

## TABLE 48.4  Medications for Asthma Treatment

| Therapy | Use | Effectiveness | Side Effects | Examples |
|---|---|---|---|---|
| Short-acting β-adrenergic agonist (SABA) | Rescue medication | Bronchodilator Effect may be reduced in older adults | Tachycardia Hypokalemia | Albuterol |
| Inhaled corticosteroid (ICS) | Maintenance or controller therapy. Cornerstone of asthma treatment | Reduce hospitalizations and mortality. May not have effect in neutrophilic-driven asthma | Candidiasis, hoarseness Osteoporosis, cataracts after many years of use | Beclometasone Budesonide Ciclesonide Fluticosone Mometasone Triamcinolone |
| Long-acting β-adrenergic agonist (LABA) | Long-acting bronchodilator Should not be used alone without ICS | | Tachycardia Muscle tremors Usually well tolerated | Formoterol Olodaterol |
| Long-acting muscarinic antagonist (LAMA) | Add on therapy to ICS/LABA | Effective bronchodilator Useful in patients with asthma/COPD overlap syndrome | Well tolerated in older adult patients | Tiotropium |
| Leukotriene receptor agonist (LRA) | Controller medication. Not as effective as ICS | Improvement in symptoms although less than seen in younger patients | Safe agent | Montelukast |
| Anti-IgE | Atopic asthmatics not responding to ICS/LABA and/or LAMA | Reduced asthma exacerbations and ER visits. May be effective at advanced age | Adrenal insufficiency Increased risk of parasitic infections | Omalizumab |
| Immunotherapy Anti-IL 5/5R Anti-IL 4R | Use in specific patient with refractory asthma | May be effective in select older atopic patients | Need to weigh risks and benefits | Mepolizumab Dupilumab |
| Systemic corticosteroids | Acute exacerbations uncontrolled with ICS | | Diabetes, weight gain, osteoporosis, glaucoma, myopathy | |

*COPD*, Chronic obstructive pulmonary disease; *ER*, emergency room; *IgE*, immunoglobulin E; *IL*, interleukin.

---

### CASE 2

#### Mrs. Brown

Mrs. Brown, a 72-year-old woman who currently smokes half a pack of cigarettes per day (started when she was 14 years old, smoked approximated one pack per day for 40 years, then current level for the past 18 years) comes into your office to ask about dyspnea on exertion. She reports increased shortness of breath unloading and putting away her groceries from her car up to her four-step walk-up home. She completed PFTs that showed moderate airflow obstruction by FEV1/FVC < 0.7 and FEV1 of 62% of predicted. She was given a short-acting beta-agonist, which she uses three to four times per day every day. It helps relieve some dyspnea, but she still remains symptomatic.

What is her likely pulmonary-related diagnosis? How should it be managed?

## Chronic Obstructive Pulmonary Disease

### Definition and Epidemiology

COPD affects 15.7 million Americans and is the fourth leading cause of death in the United States. Worldwide COPD kills more than 3 million people.[25] COPD is defined as fixed airway obstruction and is identified by a reduction in the FEV1/FVC ratio on PFTs. In addition to decreases in lung function that inevitably occur with age, exposure to tobacco smoke and environmental factors, such as pollution and biomass exposure, accelerate the rate of decline in lung function. The majority of patients with COPD are affected by other comorbidities, including cardiovascular disease, lung cancer, muscle weakness, osteoporosis, anxiety, and depression. This likely relates to the shared risk factor of tobacco use among many of these diseases.

Like the majority of lung diseases, the symptoms of COPD are nonspecific and include dyspnea, cough, sputum production, wheezing, and chest pain. Beyond the pulmonary-related symptoms, COPD is also a systemic disease and is commonly associated with sarcopenia, increases in inflammatory biomarkers, and reduced exercise capacity. Acute exacerbations of COPD (AECOPD) are a common reason for hospitalization; further, AECOPD are associated with increased cardiovascular events up to 1 year following a hospitalization.

### Diagnosis

There are several key factors to evaluate when considering a diagnosis of COPD (Table 48.5). Confirmatory tests should include PFTs. Spirometry will exhibit irreversible airflow obstruction. If lung volumes are obtained there may be evidence of hyperinflation and/or air trapping indicated by an elevated residual volume (RV) or a residual volume to total lung capacity (TLC) ratio (RV/TLC). Diffusing capacity may also be reduced in patients with COPD. The spirometric classification for airflow obstruction for grading severity of COPD according to the Global Initiative for Chronic

## TABLE 48.5   Factors for Considering a Diagnosis of Chronic Obstructive Lung Disease

| Dyspnea | Progressive over time<br>Worse with exercise<br>Persistent (present daily)<br>Described as "increased effort to breathe," "heaviness," "air hunger," "gasping" |
|---|---|
| Chronic cough | May be intermittent and nonproductive |
| Sputum production | Any pattern of chronic sputum production can indicate chronic obstructive lung disease |
| Risk factors | Tobacco smoke<br>Occupational dusts and chemicals<br>Smoke from home cooking and heating fuel<br>Family history, genetic variant ($\alpha$-1 antitrypsin deficiency) |

## TABLE 48.6   Spirometric Classification of Airflow Obstruction in Chronic Obstructive Lung Disease

### FEV1/FVC  <70%[a] applies to each category

| Mild | FEV1 $\geq$ 80% predicted |
|---|---|
| Moderate | 50% $\leq$ FEV1 <80% predicted |
| Severe | 30% $\leq$ FEV1 <50% predicted |
| Very severe | FEV1 <30% predicted or FEV1 <50% predicted and chronic respiratory failure[b] |

*FEV1*, Forced expiratory volume in 1 sec; *FVC*, forced vital capacity.

[a]Using the criteria FEV1/FVC <70% may overdiagnose COPD in older, nonsmoking adults; some experts recommend using as the lower limit of normal the fifth percentile of the normal distribution of the FEV1/FVC ratio for the reference (older) population. The Global Lung Initiative recommends using this fifth percentile value as the cutoff. Most recent gold recommendations for COPD diagnosis and severity assessment are to use a combination of spirometric classification, symptoms, and exacerbation history.

[b]Chronic respiratory failure entails the need for chronic invasive or noninvasive ventilator support.

Obstructive Lung Disease (GOLD) guidelines defines four levels of severity (Table 48.6).

◆◆ **A diagnosis of COPD in a patient with dyspnea, a chronic cough with sputum production, and exposure to risk factors, including tobacco, needs to be confirmed by spirometry.**

## Treatment

Key aspects of COPD treatment include inhaler therapies, smoking cessation, supplemental oxygen, and pulmonary rehabilitation. Inhaled therapies include combinations of bronchodilators and inhaled corticosteroids, depending on symptoms and exacerbation history. Table 48.7 lists medications used to treat COPD. COPD exacerbations present with an acute increase in breathlessness, wheezing, cough, and increase in sputum production. Treatment may include increasing short-acting $\beta$-adrenergic agonist dose or frequency, use of nebulizers, short-course oral or intravenous (IV) steroids and antibiotics, and supplemental oxygen (target SpO$_2$

88%—92%). Patients not responding to outpatient treatment with an increase in respiratory rate ($\geq$25/min) and/or increased work of breath and fatigue will need additional monitoring and treatment in the emergency room or as an inpatient.

Smoking cessation is important to reducing AECOPD. Smoking cessation can also reduce lung cancer risk and slow the rate of decline in lung function over time. Supplemental oxygen should only be prescribed for patients with evidence of hypoxemia. Influenza and pneumococcal pneumonia vaccinations are also key aspects of health maintenance for older persons living with COPD.

### CASE 3

#### Mr. Thompson

Mr. Thompson, a 76-year-old man, is in your office today reporting symptoms of subacute dyspnea on exertion and dry cough. He smoked approximately 1 pack per day for 12 years but quit 38 years ago. He has no associated joint aches or pain and denies reflux symptoms. He worked as an accountant and has been retired for the past 6 years. He lives in the same home he purchased with his partner 20 years ago. They have had cats for much of their time in the home. Hobbies include bird watching, antique collecting, and domestic travel. His PFTs demonstrate moderate restriction and moderate diffusion impairment. His chest computed tomography (CT) image shows subpleural honeycombing in the bases and scattered areas of ground glass opacities.

What is the most likely pulmonary diagnosis? What diagnostic tests would you order? What are the potential treatment options available to him?

## Interstitial Lung Disease

### Definition and Epidemiology

ILD includes a spectrum of diffuse parenchymal and fibrotic lung injuries with interstitial pulmonary fibrosis (IPF) being the most closely related to aging. Symptoms of ILD include dyspnea and cough with crackles on lung examination, restrictive ventilatory impairment on PFTs, diffuse interstitial opacities on imaging, and alveolointerstitial inflammation with progression to fibrosis on histology. A recent study examined ILD in patients age $\geq$ 70 years and found that the majority of older subjects were White men. The most common diagnoses were unclassifiable ILD (45%), IPF (34%), connective-tissue disease ILD (11%), and hypersensitivity pneumonitis (8%).[26]

IPF is a chronic, progressive, fibrotic interstitial pneumonia of unknown cause limited to the lung, and its diagnosis is based on clinical, radiologic, and histopathologic examination. It is associated histopathologically with usual interstitial pneumonia (UIP) and a radiologic pattern of honeycombing. IPF disproportionally affects older adults with symptoms typically occurring between ages 50 and 70 years and the majority of patients > 60 years of age at the time of clinical presentation. The course of IPF is variable, with some patients experiencing rapid declines and others experiencing slow declines with acute exacerbations.

### Diagnosis

IPF presentation is normally one of insidious dyspnea and nonproductive cough, with dry inspiratory rales on examination. Clubbing is often a prominent finding on physical examination in IPF (40%—70%), as opposed to emphysema, which rarely causes

## TABLE 48.7   Medications Used in Patients With Chronic Obstructive Pulmonary Disease

| Medication | Inhaler Type | Duration of Action | Common Side Effects |
|---|---|---|---|
| **Short-acting β-2 agonist (SABA)** | | | |
| Fenoterol | MDI | 4–6 hours | Tremors, tachycardia, arrhythmia, hypokalemia |
| Levalbuterol | MDI | 6–8 hours | |
| Salbutamol (albuterol) | MDI/DPI | 4–6 hours | |
| | | 12 hours | |
| Terbutaline | DPI | 4–6 hours | |
| **Long-acting β-2 agonist (LABA)** | | | |
| Aformoterol | Nebulizer | 12 hours | Tremors, tachycardia, arrhythmia, hypokalemia |
| Formoterol | DPI | 12 hours | |
| Indacaterol | DPI | 24 hours | |
| Olodaterol | SMI | 24 hours | |
| Salmeterol | MDI/DPI | 12 hours | |
| **Short-acting muscarinic antagonistmus (SAMA)** | | | |
| Ipratropium bromide | MDI | 6–8 hours | Urinary retention, tachycardia, dry mouth, blurry vision, constipation |
| Oxitropium bromide | MDI | 7–9 hours | |
| **Long-acting muscarinic antagonist (LAMA)** | | | |
| Aclidinium bromide | DPI/MDI | 12 hours | Urinary retention, tachycardia, dry mouth, blurry vision, constipation |
| Glycopyrronium bromide | DPI | 12–24 hours | |
| Tiotropium | DPI/SMI | 24 hours | |
| Umeclidinium | DPI | 24 hours | |
| **Combination SABA/SAMA** | | | See earlier |
| Fenoterol/ipratropium | SMI | 6–8 hours | |
| Salbutamol/ipratropium | SMI/MDI | 6–8 hours | |
| **Combination LABA/LAMA** | | | See earlier |
| Formoterol/aclidinium | DPI | 12 hours | |
| Formoterol/glycopyrronium | MDI | 12 hours | |
| Indacaterol/ glycopyrronium | DPI | 12–24 hours | |
| Vilanterol/umeclidinium | DPI | 24 hours | |
| Olodaterol/tiotropium | SMI | 24 hours | |
| **Methylxanthines** | | | Multiple drug interactions |
| Aminophylline | Solution | 24 hours | Arrhythmias, seizure, hypercalcemia, headache, insomnia |
| Theophylline | Pill | 24 hours | |
| **Combination LABA/ICS** | | | See earlier |
| Formoterol/beclomethasone | MDI | | Pneumonia |
| Formoterol/budesonide | MDI/DPI | | |
| Formoterol/mometasone | MDI | | |
| Salmeterol/fluticasone | MDI/DPI | | |
| Vilanterol/fluticasone | DPI | | |
| **Triple combination (LABA/LAMA/ICS)** | | | See earlier |
| Fluticasone/umeclidinium/ vilanterol | DPI | | Pneumonia |
| Beclometasone/formoterol/ glycopyrronium | MDI | | |
| **Phosphodiesterase-4 inhibitor** | | | |
| Roflumilast | | Daily | Diarrhea, nausea, anorexia, weight loss, sleep disturbance, headache |
| **Mucolytics** | | | |
| Erdosteine | | | |
| Carbocysteine | | | |
| N-acetylcysteine | | | |

(From *Global Initiative for Chronic Obstructive Lung Disease (2020 Report).* 2019. Available at: https://goldcopd.org/wp-content/uploads/2018/11/GOLD-2019-v1.7-FINAL-14Nov2018-WMS.pdf.)
*DPI,* Dry powder inhaler; *MDI,* metered dose inhaler; *SMI,* soft mist inhaler.

clubbing. IPF should be considered in older adults with a restrictive ventilatory defect or a reduced diffusing capacity on PFT, or both. However, IPF and other ILDs can overlap with COPD, which can lead to pseudonormalization of the lung volumes on PFTs, where hyperinflation from obstructive lung disease masks the severity of restriction from ILD that is detected, warranting chest imaging to narrow in on the diagnosis. Chest radiographs often show reticular opacities in the mid and lower lung zones. High-resolution CT scans show characteristic areas of subpleural reticulation and honeycombing. A diagnosis of UIP can often be made based on clinical and radiographic factors. Compared with patients with a highly consistent chest CT for UIP, patients with probable or indeterminate UIP and/or patients for whom an alternative diagnosis is considered may warrant invasive testing with bronchoscopy or a surgical lung biopsy.

## Treatment

Treatment for IPF is largely supportive and once the diagnosis is made, early referral should be made to an experienced pulmonary physician for further assessment of etiology and discussions of treatment options. For patients who meet criteria and are willing to consider lung transplant, an early referral should be made to a transplant center. There are conditional recommendations for the use of nintedanib, pirfenidone, and antiacid medications in patients with IPF.[27] Data pooled from several studies suggest a reduction in mortality with pirfenidone and a reduced decline in FVC compared with placebo. Nintedanib has been shown to reduce acute exacerbations, FVC decline, and mortality compared with placebo in pooled trial data.

Acute exacerbations of IPF are defined as acute deterioration in pulmonary function associated with new findings on high-resolution CT and worsening dyspnea of unknown or known etiology. No treatments have been shown to be effective in the treatment of acute exacerbations. Most patients will be hospitalized and receive supportive care with oxygen, as well as antibiotics and steroids.

## Pulmonary Embolism

### Epidemiology

Older patients are at increased risk of developing venous thromboembolism (VTE) and pulmonary embolism (PE). In addition, they are at increased risk of adverse clinical outcomes, including recurrent VTE, bleeding related to anticoagulation, and death.[28] Hospitalization rates for pulmonary emboli in persons age $\geq 65$ years have remained essentially stable over the past decade at around 180 to 190 per 100,000 Medicare-beneficiary years.[29]

### Risk Factors

Cancer is the strongest risk factor for PEs. Surgery and traumatic fractures also increase risk for developing a PE. Prolonged bed rest or prolonged sedentary periods, such as long flights or train rides, are additional risk factors. However, a substantial proportion of PEs are unprovoked.

### Diagnosis

The first step in the diagnostic strategy of PE is assessing the pretest, presenting clinical probability of an embolus. Several different

---

> ● **BOX 48.1** Wells Clinical Prediction Score for Pulmonary Embolism

The Wells clinical prediction score for a PE is calculated using the following history and examination findings:
Clinically suspected DVT—3 points
Alternative diagnosis is less likely than PE—3 points
Tachycardia (heart rate >100 beats per minute)—1.5 points
Immobilization ($\geq$3 days)/surgery in previous 4 weeks—1.5 points
History of DVT or PE—1.5 points
Hemoptysis—1.0 point, malignancy treatment (within 6 months) or palliative—1.0 point
Score >6—High probability
Score 2 to 6—Moderate probability
Score <2—Low probability

*DVT*, Deep vein thrombosis; *PE*, pulmonary embolism.

---

clinical prediction rules have been developed to standardize the initial assessment of patients with suspected PE. The most frequently used decision tools are the Wells criteria and the Geneva score (Box 48.1).[30–33] D-dimer blood test (a fibrin degradation product, a small protein fragment present in the blood after a blood clot is degraded by fibrinolysis) can exclude VTE without need for further testing in patients with a low clinical probability of PE.[34] However, D-dimer increases with age so that older patients often have false-positive test results, with lower specificity of the test in older patients. Age-adjusted D-dimer testing can be useful if PE is suspected, although it is less helpful in hospitalized patients, or patients with cancer or prior VTE.[35] Ultrasonography can be performed to evaluate for deep venous thrombosis. CT pulmonary angiography (CTPA) has a good diagnostic accuracy for PE and in most situations has replaced ventilation/perfusion (V/Q) scintigraphy and pulmonary angiography as the imaging choice for suspected PE.[36] CTPA false positives may occur if performed in a patient with low pretest probability, and false negatives may occur in patients with high pretest probability for an embolus. Contraindications to CTPA include renal impairment and dye allergy, although appropriate premedication may permit safe, monitored administration of contrast dye.

### Treatment

Treatment of PEs has become increasingly simplified for the majority of patients who are identified as having PEs. Direct oral anticoagulants (apixaban, dabigatran, rivaroxaban) are recommended over warfarin for most patients with PEs, are usually prescribed as a fixed dose, and do not require routine laboratory monitoring.[37] Caution should be used when prescribing these medications in patients with renal insufficiency and in patients at the extremes of weight. Patients with PEs in the setting of cancer are recommended to receive low-molecular-weight heparin. A recent review discusses the advances in diagnosis and treatment of VTE.[38]

## Lung Cancer

### Epidemiology

Lung cancer is the leading cause of cancer deaths in men and women in the United States. Two-thirds of new lung cancer diagnoses are in patients over the age of 65 years. With the aging general population, this number is expected to continue to increase in the next 2 decades. Mortality from lung cancer exceeds that of other cancers, and 72% of deaths occur in those age $\geq 65$ years.[39] There are well described racial and socioeconomic disparities in lung cancer diagnosis and treatment, with Black and Hispanic patients having higher incidence and lower survival rates.[40] These disparities have been noted in older adults; among those age $\geq 86$ years, Black men had higher lung cancer incidence compared with White men.[41] In addition, White persons had more than three times the relative survival rate of Black persons for both local and regional disease. Several investigators have also found that older patients are less likely to be enrolled in clinical trials, referred to medical oncologists, receive chemotherapy or immunotherapy, or undergo surgery for lung cancer.[39]

## Treatment

Treatment strategies in older patients with lung cancer need to consider comorbidities, polypharmacy, frailty, and functional status. The traditional performance status measures used in oncology, such as the Eastern Cooperative Oncology Group performance status and Karnofsky Performance Scale, did not capture cognitive impairment or inability to perform instrumental activities of daily living.[42] For older patients with cancer, consensus guidelines from the National Comprehensive Cancer Network recommend the use of a Comprehensive Geriatric Assessment.[43]

For patients with early-stage non–small cell lung cancer, the treatment is surgical resection in those who are deemed surgical candidates. In patients who are at high risk for perioperative complications, local therapy may include both surgical resection and definitive radiation treatment. In deciding on treatment strategies, one must consider both patient and tumor-related factors, including patient preference. A recent review on lung cancer in the older patient discusses various treatment options.[39] Once the diagnosis is made, referral should be made to a thoracic oncology program for evaluation of treatment options.

## Tracheoesophageal Disorders, Chronic Aspiration, and Bronchiectasis

Oropharyngeal dysphagia increases in age, especially in the setting of underlying neurologic disorders, sedating medications, and/or requirements for feeding tubes for nutritional support. Chronic, repeated aspiration events can result in inflammation of the lung, airway remodeling, and pneumonia. Insufficient oral care also contributes to risk for aspiration pneumonia, especially from gram-negative organisms. Recurrent aspirations, with or without pneumonia, can cause airway changes, such as bronchiectasis, which results from repeated injury to the bronchiolar epithelium and alterations in the lung microbiome (see Chs. 28, 50, and 53).

## Management of Chronic Respiratory Failure

Oxygen supplementation is used by more than 1.5 million patients in the United States.[44] Home oxygen therapy is most frequently prescribed to manage chronic hypoxemia, defined as an oxygen saturation of 88% or less. The Nocturnal Oxygen Therapy Trial and the Long-term Oxygen Therapy Trial studies established that the benefits of supplemental oxygen use are only seen in patients with COPD and sustained, significant desaturations, and that benefits

were only achieved with at least 18-hour days of therapy.[45] Nocturnal supplemental oxygen may be indicated in patients with significant desaturations during sleep only; however, this is best determined with a polysomnogram. Portable oxygen concentrators (POCs) might be an option for patients but are often limited to patients who require lower liter flow of supplemental oxygen. POC prescription also requires counseling regarding insurance coverage and maintenance.

High-flow oxygen therapy (HFOT) is increasingly used for the care of patients with acute hypoxemic respiratory failure. HFOT has been especially beneficial for patients with cancer and may reduce the need for invasive mechanical ventilation and improve 90-day mortality.[46] The utility and efficacy in immunocompromised patients has not been demonstrated, and the therapy has not been shown to improve dyspnea and other related symptoms, calling into question the evidence to support the wide-spread support of the therapy.[47] Despite these concerns, patients in long-term care institutional settings with severe chronic hypoxemic respiratory failure can sometimes benefit from HFOT in terms of adequate oxygenation. HFOT is not routinely available for home use. Regardless of how supplemental oxygen is delivered, clinicians should identify these modes of oxygen delivery as life-sustaining treatments. It is important to determine the indications and limitations of these therapies and ensure that ongoing use is aligned with patients' preferences and values.

Noninvasive ventilation (NIV) is used to support patients with chronic hypercarbic respiratory failure from primary lung diseases, such as advanced COPD, or patients with neuromuscular disorders. In addition, NIV may be used for patients with complex sleep disordered breathing and/or those with obesity hypoventilation syndrome. NIV can also relieve dyspnea symptoms in both acute and chronic settings and can be prescribed for use in the home. Regardless of the indication, primary care clinicians should coordinate care with pulmonary and/or sleep experts. Palliative medicine consultation regarding ongoing use of NIV can be helpful, especially among patients with neuromuscular diseases.

---

**CASE 4**

**Mrs. Lewis**

Mrs. Lewis is a 72-year-old woman with moderate COPD who currently smokes half a pack of cigarettes per day (approximately 60 pack-year smoking history) and comes to see you to discuss smoking cessation. She reports improved shortness of breath since starting tiotropium and has not had any COPD exacerbations. In terms of smoking cessation, she has only tried to quit "cold turkey" in the past and is asking what she can do to improve her lung health.

What are some key components of counseling about smoking cessation?

In addition to smoking cessation, what other strategies would you recommend for her to optimize her lung health?

---

## Pulmonary Health Maintenance

### Smoking Cessation

Cigarette smoking is the leading cause of death from pulmonary disease between lung chronic pulmonary diseases, such as COPD, and cancer. Repeat quit attempts are needed for most smokers, and repeated assessments by clinicians are essential. The "5 As" provide a framework for clinicians to explore patients' readiness to quit smoking (Ask about tobacco use, Advise to quit, Assess willingness to attempt to quit, Assist in quit attempt, Arrange follow-up). Smoking cessation is the single most important treatment to improve and optimize lung health. Successful smoking cessation is individual for each patient but is highest when a commitment to a quit date is made and patients engage with various support networks and strategies to assist with smoking cessation. Nicotine is highly addictive, and "cold turkey" strategies for smoking cessation may be more efficacious than gradual reductions in nicotine use, but 6-month abstinence rate is still only 22%.[48]

Pharmacologic treatments for smoking cessation include nicotine replacement therapies (NRTs), bupropion, and varenicline and are recommended for all patients who are trying to quit smoking, as long as there are no contraindications to the medication.[49] Behavioral therapies and support groups are also helpful for patients age $\geq 50$ years.[50] Vaporized nicotine delivery systems (i.e., "vaping") are perceived by older adults to be safer and less stigmatizing than combustible cigarette use.[51] Indeed, public health leaders were receptive to rigorous testing of vaping as a potential harm reduction strategy to support smoking cessation. However, robust clinical trials to establish safety and efficacy of this in achieving smoking cessation are lacking. Furthermore, reports of acute lung injury associated with use of these devices raise additional concerns over safety of these devices and formulations and should not be recommended for clinical use.[52] Multimodal strategies for smoking cessation are most successful, but still are only successful for approximately one in every four patients who attempt to quit smoking (see Ch. 5).

⧫⧫ **Tobacco dependence is an addiction that is relapsing and remitting. Combinations of counseling, support groups, quit lines, and pharmacologic treatments are most effective in assisting patients to quit smoking.**

## Vaccinations

Prevention of pneumonia is a hallmark to caring for older patients and preventing morbidity and mortality, regardless of comorbidity burden. Annual influenza vaccinations are recommended for all persons. Annual influenza vaccination is associated with 50% reduction of influenza infection, which would likely also spare patients from developing pulmonary-related complications and other poor outcomes. Mutations to the virus prevent higher effectiveness of the vaccination, but vaccination remains beneficial. Progress toward a universal influenza vaccine, one that includes all virulent strains of the virus for each year, has been made. A universal vaccine would further increase the benefits of annual vaccination, but it is still in the development stage. Influenza vaccination is usually administered intramuscularly and does contain egg antigens. Patients with severe allergic reactions or a history of adverse effects from influenza vaccination may still be able to tolerate influenza vaccination in supervised settings but consultation with their healthcare provider is advised. Pneumococcal conjugate (PCV13; Prevnar) and pneumococcal polysaccharide (PPSV23) are also indicated for all persons age $\geq 65$ years. Ideally, PCV13 should be administered first, with PPSV23 administered 1 year later for immunocompetent patients and 8 weeks later for immunocompromised patients. If a patient has already received the PPSV23, PSV13 should be administered 1 year later. A second immunization of PPSV23 can be administered for patients age $\geq 65$ years at 5 years from the first vaccination, with at least 1 year from the PCV13 vaccination (see Ch. 5).

⧫⧫ **Vaccinations are recommended for older individuals, with annual influenza vaccinations and PCV13 administered 1 year before PPSV23 vaccinations.**

## Lung Cancer Screening

Until 2013 the evidence for lung cancer screening was discouragingly ineffective. However, the National Lung Cancer Screening Trial (NLST), published in 2011, was the first multicenter study to demonstrate an efficacious approach to reduce lung cancer mortality,[53] with relative mortality risk reduction of 20%. NLST enrolled approximately 50,000 relatively healthy, asymptomatic patients aged 55 to 74 years who were current or former (within the past 15 years) smokers with at least a 30 pack-year smoking history. Although the false-positive rate for detecting nonmalignant nodules was 96%, the study has impacted clinical care and prioritized lung cancer screening for patients at risk based on age and smoking history. The American Cancer Society based its recommendations for lung cancer screening on these data. Based on these results and subsequent real-world studies following implementation, the US Preventative Services Task Force recommends screening for patients age 55 to 80 years with a 30 pack-year smoking history within the past 15 years. Future work will be needed to address the role of screening for patients in their ninth decade and beyond. Table 48.8 lists current screening recommendations for lung cancer.

⧫⧫ **Low-dose lung cancer screening is indicated for asymptomatic patients with at least 30 pack-year smoking history who are current smokers or quit within the past 15 years and who have no known life-limiting condition.**

**TABLE 48.8  Lung Cancer Screening Recommendations**

| | | | |
|---|---|---|---|
| Asymptomatic patients age 55–77 years | > 30 pack-years | Current smoker or quit < 15 years | Annual screening with low-dose CT |
| Asymptomatic patients >77 years | < 30 pack-years | Quit smoking >15 years ago | Low-dose CT screening should not be performed |
| Patients with comorbidities that adversely influence their ability to tolerate treatment of early-stage screen-detected lung cancer, or that substantially limit their life expectancy | | | Low-dose CT screening should not be performed |

*CT,* Computed tomography.

## Summary

Lung diseases such as asthma and COPD are common with important health outcome and quality-of-life—related implications for older adults. In addition, older adults are more susceptible to chronic sinusitis, aspiration, and IPF. As the population ages, more research into the impact of age on the pathogenesis and outcomes of lung disease is occurring. Many pulmonary guidelines that address issues specific to older adults are being developed.[54]

## Key References

**9.** Braman SS. Asthma in the Elderly. *Clin Geriatr Med.* 2017;33(4):523—537.

**39.** Tritschler T, Kraaijpoel N, Le Gal G, Wells PS. Venous thromboembolism: advances in diagnosis and treatment. *JAMA.* 2018;320(15):1583—1594.

**40.** Barta JA, Zinner RG, Unger M. Lung cancer in the older patient. *Clin Geriatr Med.* 2017;33(4):563—577.

**45.** Jacobs SS, Lederer DJ, Garvey CM, et al. Optimizing home oxygen therapy. An official American Thoracic Society Workshop report. *Ann Am Thorac Soc.* 2018;15(12):1369—1381.

***References available online at** expertconsult.com.*

# 49
# Infectious Diseases

SUZANNE F. BRADLEY

## OUTLINE

*Additional online-only material indicated by icon.*

## OBJECTIVES

*Upon completion of this chapter, the reader will be able to:*

- Recognize the most common causes of infection in older adults.
- Understand how the causes of infections in older adults vary with the place of acquisition.
- Understand how the clinical presentation of infection differs with increasing age.
- Understand how to manage, treat, and prevent the most common infectious syndromes found in the older adult.

## General Prevalence and Impact

Despite medical advances, infection remains a major cause of morbidity and mortality in older adults. When considering causes of infection in older adults, it is important to know where the infection was acquired, what infections are most common in those settings, and what microorganisms cause those infections. Urinary tract infection (UTI), lower respiratory tract infection (LRTI), and skin and soft tissue infection (SSTI) are the most common infectious syndromes seen among older adults regardless of whether the infection was acquired in the community, in a nursing home, or in a hospital. Bloodstream infections (BSI) are reported more frequently among older adults who are in hospital, whereas a wider variety of gastrointestinal (GI) infections are found among community-dwelling older adults and nursing home residents. Overall rates of infection in nursing homes and hospitals are similar, but those in chronic care settings are generally thought to be less severe.[1-8]

Microorganisms vary with the setting in which the infection is acquired. Infections are generally defined to be nursing home acquired or hospital acquired if the patient has been in the facility for at least 72 hours. Older adults may also acquire healthcare-associated infections even if they have not been hospitalized recently through contact with outpatient clinical settings, such as a dialysis unit or outpatient intravenous (IV) therapy center.

Delayed recognition that an older patient is infected can result in delayed treatment. Consequently, older adults are more likely to die from their infections; their mortality is 2-fold to 20-fold higher than in young adults.[9-12]

## General Pathophysiology and Risk Factors

Why the older adult population are at increased risk of infection with poor outcome is a complex question. Predisposing risk factors for infection include immunosenescence, frailty with impaired functional status, increased prevalence of predisposing comorbid illnesses, exposure to pathogens within institutional settings, and complications of medical treatment.[13]

Changes in the immune system are found with normal aging. However, all aspects of the immune system of the older adult are not necessarily affected or depressed to the same degree. The most prominent impact of age is seen on the acquired or adaptive immune system. The adaptive immune system recognizes new infections through generation of specific T-lymphocytes and antibody-producing B-lymphocytes. Age-related defects have been described predominantly in T-cells. Other acquired conditions in the older adult population, such as malnutrition, can contribute to further decline in T-cell function. T-cells are important for host defenses against pathogens that can reside within cells. Antibody production is essential to facilitate uptake and killing of encapsulated bacteria by phagocytic cells. Neoplasms seen with increasing frequency in older adults can contribute to depressed antibody production and function. Defects in antibody response may explain why some responses to vaccinations and outcomes from infections are often poor in older adults.[14]

## General Principles of Diagnosis, Assessment, and Management

Recognition that the older patient has an infection may be delayed in part because his or her symptoms and signs of infection are atypical. Clinicians may also ascribe complaints or abnormal physical findings to preexisting illnesses and not consider infection as the cause. In addition, cognitively impaired older adults may not be able to perceive symptoms of infection or communicate them to their healthcare provider.[15]

⬥⬥ **Infections are not recognized in the older adult population because their clinical presentation may be atypical.**

The febrile response may be blunted or the onset delayed. Furthermore, appropriate increases in body temperature of 2° F (1° C) diagnostic of fever may not be recognized because the normal temperatures of older adults are lower at baseline. In addition, other markers of inflammation, such as leukocytosis, may be lacking. In one study, 48% of infected older adults were afebrile and 58% did not demonstrate significant leukocytosis. Because of a lack of an inflammatory response, more than half of older adults may not have localizing symptoms of infection, and focal findings for infection may be minimal or absent on physical examination.[15–21]

⬥⬥ **Approximately half of infected older adults will not have localizing symptoms or findings on physical examination. Approximately half of infected older adults will not have a fever or have inflammation on laboratory examination.**

Many older adults take medications with antiinflammatory effects, such as aspirin, acetaminophen, nonsteroidal antiinflammatory agents, corticosteroids, cytokine inhibitors, and antineoplastic agents that may further cloud the interpretation of the patient's history,

physical examination, and laboratory findings. Therefore it is not surprising that the diagnosis of infection is often missed or delayed in the older adult population. It is essential to consider infection in the older patient even if typical signs and symptoms are absent.

Diagnosis of infection in older adults is further compromised by limited access to laboratory and diagnostic procedures in some settings. There is also a lack of diagnostic algorithms that have been specifically validated for use in the older adult population. The McGeer Criteria were developed following a rigorous systematic review of the scientific literature related to the diagnosis of infectious syndromes in older adults.[22] Although these criteria are intended for the retrospective detection of infections acquired in nursing home residents, they may provide a useful evidence-based conceptual framework for the clinician who is trying to diagnose infections in the older adult population (Tables 49.1–49.4).

The following sections discuss a few aspects of the general diagnostic approach that have been shown to be of potential use in the assessment for infection in older adults.[15–27]

## General Symptoms

### Changes in Functional Status

An acute change in the ability to perform basic activities of daily living (ADLs) has been shown to be predictive of infection 77% of the time in nursing home residents. Acute change in functional status is a simple and potentially important clue that infection might be present.[15]

### Confusion

The symptom of confusion or altered mental status has traditionally been closely associated with presence of infection in older people. Unfortunately, this terminology is vague and does not differentiate between new symptoms (delirium) that might herald the presence of a new problem (such as infection) versus more chronic conditions that alter mental status (such as dementia, depression, and other psychiatric disorders). In addition, confusion and altered mental status do not provide any indication whether these chronic symptoms are stable or have acutely worsened.

## General Signs and Laboratory Findings

### Fever

A temperature of 101° F or higher is a highly specific indication of infection, but many older adults will not achieve this definition for fever. Alternative definitions for fever have been recommended as more sensitive means to detect infection in older adults. It has been shown that a fever threshold of 100° F or higher detects 70% of infections in nursing home residents with a specificity of 90%. Other definitions of fever in older adults include a 2.4° F increase over baseline temperature or higher than 99° F orally or 99.5° F rectally.[15,22]

### Dehydration

Dehydration may accompany fever and suggest possible infection in this population. Nonspecific findings of decreased oral intake, dry mucous membranes, or furrowed tongue could be important clues that fever and infection are present.[15,25–27]

### Delirium

The Confusion Assessment Method can be performed rapidly to differentiate delirium from other chronic psychiatric conditions

## TABLE 49.1  Criteria for Urinary Tract Infection

| Criteria | Comments |
|---|---|
| A. Without an indwelling catheter:<br>  Both criteria 1 and 2 present:<br>  1. At least one of the following signs/symptoms subcriteria (a–c) present:<br>    a. Acute dysuria or acute pain, swelling, or tenderness of the testes, epididymis, or prostate<br>    b. Fever or leukocytosis<br>      and<br>      At least one of the following localizing urinary tract subcriteria:<br>      i. Acute costovertebral angle pain or tenderness<br>      ii. Suprapubic pain<br>      iii. Gross hematuria<br>      iv. New or marked increase in incontinence<br>      v. New or marked increase in urgency<br>      vi. New or marked increase in frequency<br>    c. In the absence of fever or leukocytosis, then at least two or more of the following localizing urinary tract subcriteria:<br>      i. Suprapubic pain<br>      ii. Gross hematuria<br>      iii. New or marked increase in incontinence<br>      iv. New or marked increase in urgency<br>      v. New or marked increase in frequency | A urinary tract infection (UTI) should be diagnosed when there are localizing genitourinary signs and symptoms and a positive urine culture<br>A diagnosis of urinary infection can be made without localizing symptoms if a blood culture isolate is the same as the organism isolated from the urine, and there is no alternate site of infection<br>In the absence of a clear alternate source, fever or rigors with a positive urine culture in the noncatheterized resident or acute confusion in the catheterized resident will often be treated as urinary tract infection However, evidence suggests most of these episodes are likely not from a urinary source<br>Pyuria does not differentiate symptomatic UTI from asymptomatic bacteriuria<br>Absence of pyuria in diagnostic tests excludes symptomatic UTI in residents of long-term care facilities |
|   2. One of the following microbiologic subcriteria:<br>    a. $\geq 10^5$ cfu/mL of no more than two species of microorganisms in a voided urine<br>    b. $\geq 10^2$ cfu/mL of any number of organisms in a specimen collected by in-and-out catheter | Urine specimens for culture should be processed as soon as possible, preferably within 1 to 2 hours. If urine specimens cannot be processed within 30 minutes of collection, they should be refrigerated. Refrigerated specimens should be cultured within 24 hours |
| B. With an indwelling catheter:<br>  Both criteria 1 and 2 present:<br>  1. At least one of the following signs/symptoms subcriteria (a–d) present:<br>    a. Fever, rigors, or new onset hypotension, with no alternate site of infection<br>    b. Either acute change in mental status or acute functional decline with no alternate diagnosis and leukocytosis<br>    c. New onset suprapubic pain or costovertebral angle pain or tenderness<br>    d. Purulent discharge from around the catheter or acute pain, swelling, or tenderness of the testes, epididymis, or prostate | Recent catheter trauma, catheter obstruction, or new onset hematuria are useful localizing signs consistent with UTI, but not necessary for diagnosis |
|   2. Urinary catheter culture with $\geq 10^5$ cfu/mL of any organism(s) | Urinary catheter specimens for culture should be collected following replacement of the catheter (if current catheter has been in place > 14 days) |

(Modified from Stone ND, Ashraf MS, Calder J, et al. and the Society for Healthcare Epidemiology Long-Term Care Special Interest Group. Definitions of infection for surveillance in long-term care facilities: Revisiting the McGeer criteria. *Infect Control Hosp Epidemiol.* 2012;33:965–977.)
*cfu/mL,* Colony-forming units per milliliter.

with high interobserver reliability, high sensitivity (>94%), and high specificity (90%–100%) (see Ch. 17).[15,22,24]

### Complete Blood Count

A complete blood count is one laboratory test that has been shown to be highly predictive of infection in older adults. Presence of leukocytosis, neutrophilia, and left shift may be useful if present when evaluating the older adult patient with suspected infection (neutrophilia is present with >14,000 leukocytes/mm$^3$; left shift is present with >6% bands or $\geq$ 1500 bands/mm$^3$).[15,22,23]

## Management

### Empiric Therapy Versus Culture-Based Treatment

Although antibiotics can be beneficial, their unnecessary use can lead to toxic side effects and emergence of antibiotic resistance.

Strategies to help clinicians decide when or when not to use antibiotics has been termed *antibiotic stewardship*. The decision to start antibiotic therapy should be based on the patient's clinical condition. All patients with possible infection do not require urgent treatment. If urgent treatment is needed, then the choice of antibiotic should be based on the most likely clinical syndrome, the common organisms causing that condition, and knowledge of local antibiotic resistance patterns. Decision algorithms for when to begin treatment have been developed for nursing home residents (Table 49.5).[28–32] The optimum route of antibiotic administration may be influenced by the severity of the patient's clinical condition and access to healthcare resources.

Ideally treatment should be based on results of cultures and antimicrobial susceptibilities. Duration of therapy should be based on the presumed clinical syndrome to be treated and the organism isolated. Oral therapy can be considered for some severe infections if

TABLE
49.2 **Criteria for Lower Respiratory Tract Infection**

| Criteria | Comments |
|---|---|
| A. Influenza-like illness:<br>    Both criteria 1 and 2 present:<br>    1. Fever<br>    2. At least three of the following symptom subcriteria (a–f) present:<br>        a. Chills<br>        b. New headache or eye pain<br>        c. Myalgias or body aches<br>        d. Malaise or loss of appetite<br>        e. Sore throat<br>        f. New or increased dry cough | If criteria for influenza-like illness and another upper or lower respiratory tract infection (LRTI) are met at the same time, only the diagnosis of influenza-like illness should be recorded<br>Because of increasing uncertainty surrounding the timing of the start of influenza season, the peak of influenza activity, and the length of the season, "seasonality" is no longer a criterion to define influenza-like illness |
| B. Pneumonia:<br>    All criteria 1–3 present:<br>    1. Interpretation of a chest radiograph as demonstrating pneumonia or the presence of a new infiltrate<br>    2. At least **one** of the following respiratory subcriteria (a–f):<br>        a. New or increased cough<br>        b. New or increased sputum production<br>        c. $O_2$ saturation <94% on room air or a reduction in $O_2$ saturation of >3% from baseline<br>        d. New or changed lung examination abnormalities<br>        e. Pleuritic chest pain<br>        f. Respiratory rate of 25/min<br>    3. At least one constitutional criterion | For both pneumonia and LRTIs, presence of underlying conditions that could mimic a respiratory tract infection presentation (e.g., congestive heart failure or interstitial lung diseases) should be excluded by a review of clinical records and an assessment of presenting symptoms and signs |
| C. Lower respiratory tract (bronchitis or tracheobronchitis):<br>    All criteria 1–3 present:<br>    1. Chest radiograph not performed, or negative for pneumonia or new infiltrate<br>    2. At least **two** of the respiratory criteria (B. 2. a–f) listed earlier<br>    3. At least **one** constitutional criterion | |

(Modified from Stone ND, Ashraf MS, Calder J, et al., and the Society for Healthcare Epidemiology Long-Term Care Special Interest Group. Definitions of infection for surveillance in long-term care facilities: Revisiting the McGeer criteria. *Infect Control Hosp Epidemiol.* 2012;33:965–977.)

the medication is 100% bioavailable, the patient is clinically stable, and he or she has a functional GI tract. Other considerations when choosing an antibiotic include cost, drug interactions, and toxicity. Appropriate adjustments in dose and frequency of administration should also be made for renal and hepatic dysfunction if present.[33]

## Antibiotic Resistance

In the past, we could assume that antimicrobial-resistant bacteria were found primarily in healthcare settings where antibiotic use is most intense. Methicillin-resistant *Staphylococcus aureus* (MRSA), vancomycin-resistant enterococci (VRE), multidrug-resistant *Streptococcus pneumoniae* (DRSP), and multidrug-resistant gram-negative bacilli are still found primarily in hospitals, nursing homes, and in patients recently discharged from those facilities. However, emergence of community-acquired MRSA (CA-MRSA) and multidrug-resistant gram-negative infections in healthy older people has become an increasing problem. Some strains of gram-negative bacilli, particularly *Escherichia coli* and *Klebsiella pneumoniae*, have become increasingly resistant to β-lactam antibiotics. Dependence on the carbapenems (imipenem, meropenem, ertapenem) as the last resort to treat severe gram-negative infections is greatly threatened by the emergence of carbapenemase-producing strains.[34-36] Even strains of antifungal-resistant *Candida auris* have emerged in hospital and nursing homes, posing a threat to older adult patients.[36]

Because of increasing antibiotic-resistant strains in hospitals, nursing homes, and in the community, it is imperative that providers ask themselves if patients with positive cultures, particularly for MRSA, VRE, or extended spectrum β-lactamase-positive bacteria have significant symptoms and signs of infection that warrant antimicrobial therapy rather than observation. In general, treatment of asymptomatic colonization with these bacteria will not permanently eradicate the organism, prevent infections, or improve patient outcomes.

## CASE 1

### Florence Rowe

Florence Rowe is a 97-year-old woman who has resided in a skilled nursing facility for many years. She has had a chronic indwelling urethral catheter in place to manage urinary incontinence She develops fever and low blood pressure that improves after you order IV fluids. She is alert and tells you that her right side hurts. The presence of right-sided flank pain is confirmed by palpation. The rest of her examination is unremarkable. The catheter is changed, and a urinalysis is obtained that shows white blood cells in her urine too numerous to count. She previously had cultures of urine in the past that grew >100,000 colony-forming units of *Providencia stuartii*; urine cultures and susceptibilities were not done. Mrs. Rowe was treated with cephalexin for 3 days, but her fever and flank pain recur. New cultures of blood and urine grew *P. stuartii*.

1. Was initiation of empiric antibiotic therapy appropriate?
2. Was her management and treatment appropriate?

**TABLE 49.3 Criteria for Skin and Soft Tissue Infection**

| Criteria | Comments |
|---|---|
| A. Cellulitis/soft tissue/wound infection<br>At least **one** of the following criteria present:<br>1. Pus present at a wound, skin, or soft tissue site<br>2. New or increasing presence of at least four of the following signs/symptoms subcriteria:<br>  a. Heat at the affected site<br>  b. Redness at the affected site<br>  c. Swelling at the affected site<br>  d. Tenderness or pain at the affected site<br>  e. Serous drainage at the affected site<br>  f. One constitutional criterion | More than one patient with streptococcal skin infection from the same serogroup (e.g., A, B, C, G) in a healthcare institution may suggest an outbreak<br>For wound infections related to surgical procedures use the Centers for Disease Control and Prevention's National Healthcare Safety Network Surgical Site Infection criteria<br>Presence of organisms cultured from the surface (e.g., superficial swab culture) of a wound is not sufficient evidence that the wound is infected |
| B. Scabies<br>  Both criteria 1 and 2 present:<br>  1. A maculopapular and/or itching rash<br>  2. At least **one** of the following subcriteria:<br>    a. Physician diagnosis<br>    b. Laboratory confirmation (scraping or biopsy)<br>    c. Epidemiologic linkage to a case of scabies with laboratory confirmation | Care must be taken to rule out rashes related to skin irritation, allergic reactions, eczema, and other noninfectious skin conditions<br>An epidemiologic linkage to a case can be considered if there is evidence of geographic proximity, temporal relationship to the onset of symptoms, or evidence of common source of exposure (e.g., shared caregiver) |
| C. Fungal oral/perioral and skin infections<br>Oral candidiasis: Both criteria 1 and 2 present:<br>1. Presence of raised white patches on inflamed mucosa, or plaques on oral mucosa<br>2. A medical or dental provider diagnosis<br>Fungal skin infection: Both criteria 1 and 2 present:<br>1. Characteristic rash or lesions<br>2. Either a medical provider diagnosis or laboratory-confirmed fungal pathogen from scraping or biopsy medical | Mucocutaneous candida infections are usually caused by underlying clinical conditions, such as poorly controlled diabetes or severe immunosuppression. Although not transmissible infections in the healthcare setting, they can be a marker for increased antibiotic exposure<br>Dermatophytes have been known to cause occasional infections, and rare outbreaks, in the LTC setting |
| D. Herpes viral skin infections:<br>  Herpes simplex infection:<br>  Both criteria 1 and 2 present:<br>  1. A vesicular rash<br>  2. Either physician diagnosis or laboratory confirmation<br>  Herpes zoster infection: | Reactivation of herpes simplex ("cold sores") or herpes zoster ("shingles") is not considered a healthcare–associated infection<br>Primary herpes viral skin infections are very uncommon in an LTCF, except in pediatric populations where it should be considered healthcare associated |
| E. Conjunctivitis<br>  At least one of the following criteria present:<br>  1. Pus appearing from one or both eyes, present for at least 24 hours<br>  2. New or increased conjunctival erythema, with or without itching<br>  3. New or increased conjunctival pain, present for at least 24 hours | Conjunctivitis symptoms ("pink eye") should not be caused by allergic reaction or trauma |

(Modified from Stone ND, Ashraf MS, Calder J, et al., and the Society for Healthcare Epidemiology Long-Term Care Special Interest Group. Definitions of infection for surveillance in long-term care facilities: Revisiting the McGeer criteria. *Infect Control Hosp Epidemiol.* 2012;33:965–977.)
*LTC,* Long-term care; *LTCF,* long-term care facility.

## Urinary Tract Infection

**Prevalence and Impact.** UTI is the most common infection seen in older adults in the community, nursing home, or hospital. Overdiagnosis is common. Many clinicians erroneously assume that only a positive urinalysis and culture are required for diagnosis. It is well established that significant but asymptomatic bacteriuria ($\geq 10^5$ colony-forming units [cfu] per mL) increases with age and debility.[22,37–43]

**Pathophysiology and Risk Factors.** Why are bacteriuria and UTI so common in older adults? Conditions or diseases that lead to alterations in normal flora and urinary stasis and obstruction are associated with increased risk of bacteriuria. Shifts in normal perineal flora may occur because of estrogen deficiency with a shift in the normal acidic vaginal pH to a more alkaline environment. With the shift in the local vaginal environment, normal gram-positive vaginal flora may be

**TABLE 49.4  Criteria for Gastrointestinal Infection**

| Criteria | Comments |
|---|---|
| A. Gastroenteritis<br>At least one of the following criteria present:<br>1. Diarrhea, three or more liquid or watery stools above what is normal for the resident within a 24-hour period<br>2. Vomiting, two or more episodes in a 24-hour period<br>3. Both of the following signs/symptoms subcriteria present:<br>  a. A stool specimen positive for a pathogen (such as Salmonella, Shigella, *Escherichia coli* O157:H7, Campylobacter species, rotavirus)<br>  b. At least **one** of the following GI subcriteria present:<br>    i. Nausea<br>    ii. Vomiting<br>    iii. Abdominal pain or tenderness<br>    iv. Diarrhea | Care must be taken to exclude noninfectious causes of symptoms. For instance, new medications may cause diarrhea, nausea, or vomiting; initiation of new enteral feeding may be associated with diarrhea; nausea or vomiting may be associated with gallbladder disease<br>Presence of new gastrointestinal (GI) symptoms in a single resident may prompt enhanced surveillance for additional cases<br>In the presence of an outbreak, stool specimens should be sent to confirm the presence of norovirus, or other pathogens (such as rotavirus or *E. coli* O157:H7) |
| B. Norovirus gastroenteritis:<br>Both criteria 1 and 2 present:<br>1. At least one of the following GI subcriteria present:<br>  a. Diarrhea, three or more liquid or watery stools above what is normal for the resident within a 24-hour period<br>  b. Vomiting, two or more episodes in a 24-hour period<br>2. A stool specimen positive for detection of norovirus either by electron microscopy, enzyme immunoassay, or a molecular diagnostic test such as polymerase chain reaction (PCR) | In the presence of an outbreak, stool specimens should be sent to confirm the presence of norovirus, or other pathogens (such as rotavirus or *E. coli* O157:H7)<br>In the absence of laboratory confirmation, an outbreak (two or more cases occurring in the long-term care facility [LTCF]) of acute gastroenteritis because of norovirus infection in an LTCF may be assumed to be present if all of the following criteria are present ("Kaplan criteria"):<br>  a. Vomiting in more than half of affected persons<br>  b. A mean (or median) incubation period of 24–48 hours<br>  c. A mean (or median) duration of illness of 12–60 hours<br>  d. No bacterial pathogen is identified in stool culture |
| C. *Clostridium difficile* infection:<br>Both criteria 1 and 2 present:<br>1. One of the following GI subcriteria present:<br>  a. Diarrhea, three or more liquid or watery stools above what is normal for the resident within a 24-hour period<br>  b. The presence of toxic megacolon (abnormal dilatation of the large bowel documented radiologically)<br>2. One of the following diagnostic subcriteria present:<br>  a. The stool sample yields a positive laboratory test result for *C. difficile* toxin A or B, or a toxin-producing *C. difficile* organism is identified in a stool culture or by a molecular diagnostic test, such as PCR<br>  b. Pseudomembranous colitis is identified during endoscopic examination or surgery, or in histopathologic examination of a biopsy specimen | A "primary episode" of *C. difficile* infection is defined as one that has occurred without any previous history of *C. difficile* infection, or that has occurred more than 8 weeks after the onset of a previous episode of *C. difficile* infection<br>A "recurrent episode" of *C. difficile* infection is defined as an episode of *C. difficile* infection that occurs 8 weeks or less after the onset of a previous episode, provided that the symptoms from the earlier (previous) episode resolved<br>Individuals previously infected with *C. difficile* may continue to remain colonized even after symptoms resolve<br>In the setting of a GI outbreak, individuals could test positive for *C. difficile* toxin because of ongoing colonization and be coinfected with another pathogen. It is important that other surveillance criteria are used to differentiate infections in this situation |

(Modified from Stone ND, Ashraf MS, Calder J, et al. and the Society for Healthcare Epidemiology Long-Term Care Special Interest Group. Definitions of infection for surveillance in long-term care facilities: Revisiting the McGeer criteria. *Infect Control Hosp Epidemiol*, 2012;33:965–977.)

suppressed allowing potentially pathogenic enteric gram-negative bacilli to emerge. Functional dependency in toileting and need for assistance by healthcare personnel can lead to contamination of the urethral orifice with pathogenic bacteria. Bacteria can be introduced into the bladder with introduction of a urinary device.

Urinary obstruction and stasis can also occur because of normal aging and local or systemic comorbid disease. In males, prostatic hypertrophy that occurs with normal aging can lead to obstruction, urinary stasis, and increased frequency of UTI. Neoplasms and stones that occur with increasing age may lead to obstruction and infection throughout the urinary tract. Cystocele, cerebrovascular accident, and diabetic neuropathy may impair bladder emptying and encourage the development of urinary stasis and bacteriuria.[38,40,41]

## Differential Diagnosis, Assessment, and Management

### Asymptomatic Bacteriuria

A major dilemma for clinicians is differentiating UTI from asymptomatic bacteriuria. Presence of significant pyuria ($\geq 10$ white blood cells per low-power field) in older adults is not a useful indicator of UTI. A significant proportion of asymptomatic older adults (30%) will have significant and persistent pyuria. Pyuria can be found in conditions such as nephrolithiasis and primary diseases of bowel found adjacent to the urinary tract, such as diverticulitis, inflammatory bowel disease, and intraabdominal abscess. Absence of pyuria is useful, however. A negative urinalysis for pyuria is 99% predictive that bacteriuria, and hence UTI, is not present. Alternate diagnoses should be pursued.[38,40–43]

**TABLE 49.5  Minimum Criteria for the Initiation of Antibiotics in Residents of Long-Term Care Facilities**

| Urinary Tract Infection | Categories | Minimum Criteria |
|---|---|---|
| Fever[a] | No catheter | One or more of the following: new or worsening urgency, frequency, suprapubic pain, gross hematuria, CVA tenderness, urinary incontinence |
| Fever | Chronic indwelling catheter | New CVA tenderness *and* rigors without cause *or* new onset delirium[b] |

| Respiratory Tract Infection | Categories | Minimum Criteria |
|---|---|---|
| High fever | >102° F (>38.9° C) | Respiratory rate >25 breaths/minute *or* productive cough |
| Fever | ≤102° F (≤38.9° C) | Cough *plus one* of the following: tachycardia >100 beats/minute, delirium, rigors, respiratory rate >25 breaths/minute |
| Afebrile | COPD | New or increased cough and purulent sputum production |
| Afebrile | No COPD | New cough with purulent sputum and one of the following: respiratory rate >25 breaths/minute *or* delirium |

| Skin/Soft Tissue Infection | Categories | Minimum Criteria |
|---|---|---|
| Applies to intact skin, devices, or ulcers | | Fever or new or increasing redness, tenderness, warmth or swelling at the affected site[c] |

| Fever/Focus Unknown | | Minimum Criteria |
|---|---|---|
| | | Fever *and one* of the following: new onset delirium *or* rigors |

(Modified from Loeb M, Bentley DW, Bradley S, et al. Development of minimum criteria for the initiation of antibiotics in residents of long-term-care facilities: Results of a consensus conference. *Infect Control Hosp Epidemiol.* 2001;22:120–124.)

*COPD*, Chronic obstructive pulmonary disease; *CVA*, costovertebral angle.

[a]Fever is defined as a single temperature of >100° F (>37.9° C) or >2.4° F (>1.5° C) unless otherwise stated.

[b]Delirium is defined by the *Diagnostic and Statistical Manual of Mental Disorders,* 4th edition.

[c]Does not include nonbacterial infections (herpes), deep tissue, or bone infection; noninfectious causes, such as burns, thromboembolic disease, and gout can be mistaken for skin/soft tissue infection.

## Symptomatic UTI

The diagnosis of UTI rests principally on patient history of symptoms and physical signs referable to the urinary tract (see Table 49.1).[22,40–43] The symptoms and signs must be new or worsening of chronic symptoms. Symptoms of lower UTI or cystitis include suprapubic pain, dysuria, frequency, and urgency. Flank pain and fever are more typical of upper tract infection or pyelonephritis. Odiferous or cloudy urine indicate the presence of metabolites, urine concentration, crystals, and sediment and are not useful indicators for the presence of a UTI.[40,41]

Even in the cognitively impaired nursing home resident, physical signs referable to the urinary tract can be helpful especially if they resolve with treatment. Reproducible pain over the external genitalia (in a male), bladder, or flanks in the presence of significant bacteriuria and pyuria provides presumptive evidence that a UTI is present. In nursing homes, only 10% of fevers are caused by a urinary source. As a result, fever associated with change in mental status is rarely the result of a UTI and another cause should be sought. Special consideration should be given to patients with urinary catheters; 50% who have fever will have secondary bacteremia with the same organism present in urine.[22,40–43]

## Management and Treatment

**Asymptomatic Bacteriuria.** If an older adult has significant bacteriuria, pyuria, and symptoms, then treatment for UTI is appropriate. However, treatment of asymptomatic bacteriuria does not permanently eradicate the organism and, with rare exception, no benefit of treatment for the older adult has been demonstrated

in terms of improved wellbeing, relief of chronic symptoms, or survival. One exception is the treatment of patients with asymptomatic bacteriuria who undergo a prostatic resection; postoperative bacteremia is substantially reduced in that population. Otherwise, treatment of asymptomatic bacteriuria is a major cause of inappropriate antibiotic use and emergence of antibiotic resistance.[22,37,38,42,43]

⯀⯀ **Treatment of "dirty urine" in the older adult population with asymptomatic bacteriuria is not beneficial.**

**Uncomplicated UTI.** Predictability of the infecting organism and its response to treatment relates in part to gender, general health, and anatomy of the genitourinary tract. Many postmenopausal women have had a history of UTI throughout their lives that responds predictably to empiric treatment directed against *E. coli* (uncomplicated UTI). Uncomplicated UTI requires that the woman be healthy without diabetes and immunosuppression. In addition, there are not functional or anatomic abnormalities of the urinary tract or the need for catheter use. An uncomplicated UTI cannot be nosocomially acquired.[40,41,44]

Women with an uncomplicated cystitis do not necessarily require culture before initiation of treatment unless they have symptoms of pyelonephritis, they have recurrence of symptoms, or if local antibiotic resistance is a concern (Table 49.6). Otherwise, the optimum antibiotic treatment of urinary symptoms in older adults should be based on culture results and antimicrobial susceptibilities.

| TABLE 49.6 | Treatment of Woman With Uncomplicated Urinary Tract Infection |
|---|---|

| Cystitis | Pyelonephritis |
|---|---|
| Able to tolerate medication<br>Absence of:<br>• pyelonephritis symptoms<br>• fever, flank pain<br>• allergy history | Obtain a urine culture<br>Hospitalized—give IV dose initially<br>• ceftriaxone<br>• aminoglycoside<br>• quinolone (unless resistance >10%) |
| **First-Line Oral Treatment Options**<br><br>Nitrofurantoin 100 mg BID × 5 days[a]<br>TMP/SMZ DS BID × 3 days<br>(avoid if prior UTI in 3 months, or 20% resistance to sulfas in the community)<br>Fosfomycin 3 gm single dose[a]<br>(lower efficacy)<br>Pivmecillinam 400 mg BID × 5 days[a]<br>(lower efficacy) | **First-Line Oral Treatment Options**<br><br>Ciprofloxacin 500 mg BID × 7 days<br>Levofloxacin 750 mg QD × 7 days<br>TMP/SMZ DS BID × 14 days<br>β-lactam 10–14 days (less efficacious) |
| **Second-Line Treatment Oral Options**<br><br>Quinolones | |

(Modified from Gupta K, Hooton TM, Naber KG, et al. International clinical practice guidelines for the treatment of acute uncomplicated cystitis and pyelonephritis in women: A 2010 update by the Infectious Diseases Society of America and the European Society for Microbiology and Infectious Diseases. *Clin Infect Dis.* 2011;52:e103-120.)

*IV,* Intravenous; *TMP/SMZ DS,* trimethoprim-sulfamethoxazole double-strength.

[a]Avoid if early pyelonephritis suspect.

If symptoms are severe with impending sepsis, then empiric antibiotic choices can be initiated based on local epidemiology data and antimicrobial susceptibility patterns. Use of nitrofurantoin may be limited in older adults because of contraindications in patients with renal insufficiency (creatinine clearance <40 cc/min). Fosfomycin and nitrofurantoin are not indicated for pyelonephritis. The duration of treatment for cystitis and pyelonephritis is dependent on the antibiotic chosen (see Table 49.6).[44]

Topical estrogen use may reduce recurrent episodes of UTI in healthy older women by normalizing vaginal pH and restoring normal flora. Cranberry juice may reduce significant bacteriuria in older women by inhibiting binding of gram-negative bacilli to uroepithelial cells. Prophylaxis with postcoital or once-daily low doses of trimethoprim-sulfamethoxazole, quinolones, or nitrofurantoin may be considered on older women, as well as younger women with uncomplicated and recurrent UTI.[40,41]

**Complicated UTI.** For the remainder of older adults with UTI symptoms who have abnormal urinary tract anatomy, require a urinary device, or are exposed to antibiotic-resistant pathogens in hospitals and nursing homes (complicated UTI), appropriate management requires obtaining a urine sample for culture and antimicrobial susceptibilities because their infecting organisms and treatment responses are not predictable. Most of these patients have reinfection with a new organism rather than relapse with the same organism.[30,39–43]

◆◆ **The optimal treatment of complicated UTI in the older adult must be based on results of the urine culture; the organisms causing the infection and their resistance patterns are not predictable.**

When UTIs in men occur, they have a complicated UTI because urinary tract abnormalities or catheter use is invariably present. In contrast with uncomplicated UTI in healthy older women, bacteriuria in healthy men is most commonly the result of not only *E. coli,* but also of *Proteus mirabilis* and enterococci. In hospitalized older adult patients with complicated UTI, *E. coli* is still the predominant pathogen, but *Pseudomonas aeruginosa* occurs with increasing frequency, followed by *Candida albicans* and other antibiotic-resistant gram-negative bacilli. Chronic catheter-use has been associated with infections resulting from *P. stuartii* and coagulase-negative staphylococci. True polymicrobial infection can occur in institutionalized older adult patients even in the absence of an indwelling catheter.[39–41]

In the clinically stable patient, therapy can be withheld until culture results are known. When the diagnosis of UTI is uncertain, empiric antibiotic use may obscure the true diagnosis. Empiric treatment of complicated UTI should be based on the place of acquisition and primarily directed against gram-negative bacilli. For patients with complicated UTI, therapy must be reevaluated once culture and antimicrobial susceptibilities are available given the high prevalence of antibiotic resistance within and outside healthcare settings.[30,40,41]

Duration of treatment for complicated UTIs is based on response to symptoms and predisposing factors. For patients with short-term catheters in whom the catheter is removed and there are no upper tract symptoms, 3 days of antibiotic treatment may be sufficient. Some recommend 5 to 7 days if the patient is not severely ill and the clinical response is prompt. Longer therapy of 10 to 14 days is recommended for a delayed response (Box 49.1). If there is a relapse of symptomatic bacteriuria, a longer course of antibiotics may be needed to eradicate a chronic bacterial prostatic focus. Use of antimicrobial agents that penetrate prostatic tissue (quinolones, trimethoprim-sulfamethoxazole, cephalexin) is required for 6 to 12 weeks.[39–43]

Management of patients who do not have symptoms localized to the urinary tract or cannot report them present a problem,

## • BOX 49.1  Indwelling Urinary Catheters: Appropriate Care, Treatment, and Prevention of Urinary Tract Infection

Indwelling catheters should:
    Be used only for appropriate indications.
    Be removed immediately when they are no longer needed.
    Be inserted using aseptic technique and sterile equipment.
    Be used only in conjunction with a closed drainage system.
Indwelling urinary catheters should not be used for incontinence except when all other approaches have failed.
Catheter care *not* recommended:
    Enhanced meatal care
    Routine catheter changes
    Routine irrigation of catheters
    Routine use of antimicrobial prophylaxis
Urine cultures
    A urine culture should be obtained before initiating antimicrobial treatment.
    A urinary catheter should be changed or removed before obtaining a urine culture.
Duration of appropriate treatment
    Prompt resolution of symptoms: 7 days
Delayed resolution of symptoms: 10—14 days

(Modified from Hooton TM, Bradley SF, Cardenas DD, et al. International clinical practice guidelines for the diagnosis, prevention, and treatment of catheter-associated urinary tract infection. *Clin Infect Dis.* 2010;50:625—663.)

particularly in nursing homes. Febrile nursing home residents that meet criteria for fever and delirium could receive empiric therapy with close reevaluation. For a patient with frequent and transient episodes of mental status that do not meet criteria for delirium, a trial of IV fluids to treat dehydration and promote urinary tract flushing could be considered. Alternatively, a trial of empiric antibiotics could be started, but stopped at 72 hours if the evaluation is negative for urinary abnormalities, the patient does not improve on empiric therapy, or another diagnosis becomes evident. UTI can be excluded if improvement is seen but the bacterial isolates found are not susceptible to empiric antibiotic choices. Treatment of bacteriuria related to chronic indwelling urinary catheters should be considered only when typical symptoms or fever are present without another focus evident. A randomized trial found that nursing homes that used this algorithm had similar outcomes and reduced antibiotic use compared with nursing homes that were randomized to usual care.[30,42,43]

❖ **UTI in the patient with a chronic indwelling catheter is a diagnosis of exclusion.**

Follow-up samples of urine for culture should be obtained only if symptoms of infection persist or recur to verify if a secondary infection with a new organism resistant to therapy has emerged during treatment. In addition, ultrasound or computerized tomography (CT) should be considered if fever or bacteriuria fails to improve on appropriate therapy or if the patient has recurrent UTI to rule out the presence of obstruction or abscess. Surgical or pharmacologic relief of obstruction or stasis may be effective, particularly if the patient has relapsing episodes of UTI with the same organism.[40,41]

❖ **Recurrent UTI with the same organism should prompt a search for anatomic defects that can be remediated.**

Indications for urinary catheter use and alternative means of toileting should be reviewed, especially if incontinence and convenience are the only indications. Intermittent urethral catheterization may be associated with fewer infections. Routine catheter changes or irrigation with antimicrobial agents is not effective in preventing infection. Suppressive antibiotics can reduce the frequency of recurrent UTIs in spinal cord patients with chronic catheters, but resistance rapidly emerges.[39]

## CASE 1

### Discussion

Mrs. Rowe has fever and flank pain; the most likely diagnosis is pyelonephritis. Patients with chronic indwelling urinary catheters and fever are at increased risk of sepsis and bacteremia, so initiation of empiric antibiotic therapy is appropriate. However, several mistakes were made in her management.

Because Mrs. Rowe resides in a nursing home and has a urinary catheter, she has a complicated UTI. Therefore the etiology of her pyelonephritis is not predictable, and she is more likely to have an antibiotic-resistant bacterium as the cause of her UTI. Patients with complicated UTI must have a urine specimen sent for culture to confirm what the organism is, and if it is susceptible to the therapy chosen. Mrs. Rowe had a history of prior UTI with *P. stuartii*, which is a very resistant bacterium that commonly causes infections in patients with chronic urinary catheters; susceptibility to cephalexin is unlikely.

Finally, 3 days of antibiotic therapy for pyelonephritis, particularly in a patient with catheter-associated UTI, is not adequate. For residents who have not responded promptly to initial treatment, 10 to 14 days of therapy would be appropriate.

In summary, Mrs. Rowe's pyelonephritis symptoms recurred because the initial antibiotic chosen was not confirmed to be effective by urine culture and susceptibility, and the duration of therapy would have been inadequate.

## Lower Respiratory Tract Infection

### Prevalence and Impact

Pneumonia and bronchitis are common causes of hospitalization among older adults. They comprise the second most common cause of infection in nursing homes; rates of pneumonia range from 33 to 114 cases per 1000 residents per year or 0.3 to 2.5 episodes per 1000 days of resident care.[5–8,45–48] Despite advances in antibiotics, vaccines, and other treatments, LRTI remains one of the top 10 causes of death in older adults.[45–48]

Tuberculosis (TB) continues to be a problem in the United States but it has declined to approximately 9000 cases of illnesses diagnosed each year; approximately 2700 (30%) of cases occur in US-borne patients.[49] Most cases of TB disease occur in community-dwelling older adults, but nursing home residents are at greatest risk for poor outcomes.[50,51] Of those cases, 1.6% were diagnosed in nursing home residents and 57% were born in the United States.[49]

### Pathophysiology and Risk Factors

Risk factors for LRTIs are particularly common in older adults either because of the consequences of aging, acquired conditions, or treatment of those illnesses. Multiple host defenses reduce the likelihood that pneumonia will develop in the normal host.[45–48,52]

In older adults, microaspiration and inhalation of potential oral flora pathogens is an everyday occurrence. Handling respiratory secretions appropriately is a major barrier to the development of pneumonia. Common neurologic and psychiatric conditions or sedating medications can impair recognition that aspiration is occurring or result in a swallowing disorder.[45–48,52] Achlorhydria may result because of aging itself or from the use of medications that neutralize or block the production of stomach acid. Age-related declines in lung elasticity, respiratory musculature, and kyphosis contribute to diminished cough reflexes. Common conditions, such as obstructive airways disease, emphysema, bronchiectasis, and presence of neoplasms can also reduce mucociliary clearance.[45–48,52]

Normal aging, age-associated conditions, and their treatments also result in changes in oropharyngeal flora. Alterations in oropharyngeal environment allow the flora to change from predominantly gram-positive cocci to carriage with gram-negative bacilli.[45–48,52,53] Older adults also have more exposure to pathogens that cause respiratory disease through more frequent interactions with healthcare settings.[53]

Acquisition of respiratory pathogens via inhalation of droplets (influenza) or airborne pathogens (*Mycobacterium tuberculosis*) is less common. Older adults generally acquired asymptomatic latent TB infection (LTBI) when they were young and the infection was prevalent.[50,51] Aging and conditions that lead to waning cell-mediated immunity increase the likelihood that reactivation of symptomatic TB disease will occur.[50,51]

## Differential Diagnosis, Assessment, and Management

Although LRTI is common in older adults, making a definitive diagnosis can be difficult. The symptoms of cough and dyspnea are common among older adults with underlying cardiopulmonary disease and are not specific for LRTI. The diagnosis of LRTI is easily missed if one relies only on the presence of inflammatory signs, such as fever and leukocytosis; many frail older adults may lack a typical presentation. Only 56% of nursing home residents with pneumonia will have the symptom triad of cough, dyspnea, and fever; 60% will have isolated cough, and 40% will have dyspnea alone.[28,45–48,56] Presence of rales on physical examination is lacking in 45% of residents with pneumonia. It is therefore important that the clinician have a low threshold to evaluate older adult patients for pneumonia with careful attention to new or worsening symptoms and signs, both typical and atypical for pneumonia (see Table 49.2).[15,22,28,54]

New or worsening dyspnea seems to be a particularly important clue that LRTI is present. Tachypnea with tachycardia was noted in 66% of older adults with pneumonia and may be one of the earliest clues that LRTI is present. A strong association between respiratory rates of 25 breaths per minute or faster and the presence of pneumonia has been made in the older adult population. This elevated respiratory rate coupled with a pulse oximetry < 90% is an accurate predictor of impending respiratory failure.[15,22,28,54–56]

Chest radiographs, regardless of quality, technical difficulties, or lack of prior films for comparison, are helpful to confirm LRTI in > 90% of nursing residents. Chest radiographs can provide useful prognostic information (multilobar disease), as well as detect issues that might alter how the patient is evaluated and treated, such as empyema or possible neoplasms.[15,22,28,56]

### CASE 2

#### Evelyn Rafferty

Evelyn Rafferty is an 85-year-old woman who had a subdural hematoma following a fall several years ago with residual expressive aphasia. She requires assistance with many of her ADLs, but lives at home with assistance of a home health aide and a home-based primary care team. She was hospitalized 4 months ago with MRSA pneumonia. Today, her visiting nurse tells you that Mrs. Rafferty has a new cough and shortness of breath. She verifies that the patient's temperature is 100° F with a respiratory rate of 35 breaths per minute and a pulse oximetry of 90% on room air. You are also told that the patient appears to have an acute change in her mental status and has new crackles on lung examination.
1. What is Mrs. Rafferty's most likely diagnosis?
2. What are the next most appropriate steps in the management of her respiratory problem?

## Where Should the Patient With Pneumonia Be Treated?

Decisions about where and how to treat patients for community-acquired pneumonia (CAP) are based on several factors: (1) Does the patient require admission to hospital? The Pneumonia Severity Index (PSI) and CURB-65 (confusion, urea level, respiratory rate, blood pressure, and age > 65 years) have been used to determine if a patient can be treated safely in the outpatient setting.[57] Although there is more evidence to support the use of the PSI in terms of effectiveness and safety, it is recognized that the CURB-65 is a much simpler tool to remember and use (Table 49.7).[57] (2) How severe is the patient's pneumonia? Does the patient have three or more signs and symptoms of severe pneumonia (Box 49.2)? The presence of

**TABLE 49.7   Community-Acquired Pneumonia Severity of Illness Score (CURB-65 Criteria)**

| Factor | Criteria |
|---|---|
| **C**onfusion | Disoriented person, place, time |
| **U**remia | ≥ 20 mg/dL |
| **R**espiratory rate | > 30 breaths/minute |
| Low **B**lood pressure | Systolic/diastolic 90/60 mmHg |
| Age ≥ **65** years | Increased age |

| Number of Factors | 30-Day Mortality (%) | Recommended Treatment Site |
|---|---|---|
| 0 | 0.7 | Outpatient |
| 1 | 2.1 | Outpatient |
| 2 | 9.2 | Inpatient ward |
| 3 | 14.5 | ICU |
| 4 | 40.0 | ICU |
| 5 | 57.0 | ICU |

(Modified from Mandell LA, Wunderink RG, Anzueto A, et al. Infectious Diseases Society of America/American Thoracic Society consensus guidelines on the management of community-acquired pneumonia in adults. *Clin Infect Dis*. 2007;44:S27–72.)
*ICU*, Intensive care unit.

## • BOX 49.2  Defintions for Severe Pneumonia

Severe pneumonia = 3 or more minor criteria or 1 major criteria:

### Minor criteria

- Severe tachypnea ≥30 breaths per minute
- Hypoxemia $PaO_2/FIO_2$ ratio ≤250
- Multilobar infiltrates
- Confusion/disorientation
- Hypotension requiring aggressive fluid resuscitation
- Leukopenia <4
- 000 white blood cells/mL
- Thrombocytopenia <100,000 platelets/mL
- Uremia—blood urea nitrogen >20 mg/dL
- Hypothermia—temperature <36° C

### Major criteria

- Septic shock requiring vasopressors
- Respiratory failure requiring mechanical ventilation

    $FiO_2$, Fraction of inspired oxygen; $PaO_2$, partial pressure of oxygen.

(Modified from Metlay JP, Waterer GW, Long AC, et al. Diagnosis and treatment of adults with community-acquired pneumonia: an official clinical practice guideline of the American Thoracic Society and Infectious Diseases Society of America. *Am J Respir Crit Care Med.* 2019;200:e45—67.)

severe pneumonia would indicate the need for hospitalization and would change diagnostic and treatment recommendations.

Collection of clinical specimens from older patients who cannot cooperate or are too weak to cough, contamination with upper airway secretions is frequent, so routine collection of sputum in outpatients is not recommended. However, a sputum Gram stain and cultures of sputum and blood can be useful in establishing the cause of the pneumonia.[28,45–48,57] Specimens of sputum and blood are recommended for patients who require admission to hospital for pneumonia.[57]

Table 49.8 summarizes the common causes of CAP based on disease severity, comorbidity, and risk factors. For CAP, less emphasis is now placed on where the patient acquired the infection and more emphasis is based on patient comorbidities and risk factors when choosing therapy. For these reasons, the designation healthcare—associated pneumonia (HCAP), is no longer recommended.[57] Gram-negative bacillary LRTIs remain rare in outpatient settings and have tended to be less common in nursing homes when compared with hospitals; *Klebsiella* has been one of the most common organisms when they occur.[28,45–48,57]

In healthy community-dwelling older adults, LRTI resulting from *Streptococcus pneumoniae, Haemophilus influenzae,* and *Moraxella* have been described most commonly. In debilitated patients who have had hospital or ventilator-acquired pneumonia, resistant gram-negative bacilli, especially *P. aeruginosa* and *S. aureus,* are more likely. So, empiric treatment directed against MRSA and *Pseudomonas* infection may be warranted, if there is a history of prior treatment for MRSA or *Pseudomonas* respiratory tract infection, until results of sputum and blood cultures are known. If there is a known local risk of MRSA or *Pseudomonas* infection hospitalization and prior treatment with IV antibiotics within the past 90 days, awaiting results of diagnostic specimens is reasonable before initiating treatment if the patient is clinically stable.[57] MRSA infections are no longer confined to healthcare

## TABLE 49.8  Common Etiologies of Community-Acquired Pneumonia

| Patient Type | Etiology | Treatment |
|---|---|---|
| Outpatient | *Streptococcus pneumoniae* <br> *Mycoplasma pneumoniae* <br> *Haemophilus influenzae* | No comorbidities <br> Amoxicillin, doxycycline, or macrolides <br> (if local macrolide resistance <20%) |
|  | *Chlamydophila (Chlamydia)* <br> *pneumoniae* <br> Respiratory viruses | With comorbidities[a] <br> Combination therapy—amoxicillin/clavulanate or cephalosporin <br> AND macrolide or doxycycline <br> OR monotherapy with respiratory fluoroquinolone (levofloxacin or moxifloxacin) |
| Inpatient <br> (non-ICU) | *S. pneumoniae* <br> *M. pneumoniae* <br><br> *H. influenzae* <br> *Legionella* species <br> Aspiration <br> Respiratory viruses | Standard regimen <br> β-lactam + macrolide or respiratory fluoroquinolone <br> Prior respiratory isolate for methicillin-resistant *Staphylococcus aureus* (MRSA) or *Pseudomonas* <br> Obtain a nasal MRSA PCR and respiratory culture—add coverage until confirmed <br> Hospitalization and IV antibiotics within 90 days and local risk factors for MRSA or *Pseudomonas* <br> Obtain MRSA nasal PCR and cultures for MRSA or *Pseudomonas*, but do not treat until presence of <br> organisms confirmed |
| Inpatient (ICU) | *S. pneumoniae* <br> MRSA <br> *Legionella* species <br> Gram-negative bacilli – <br> *Pseudomonas* <br> *H. influenza* | Standard regimen <br> β-lactam + macrolide or β-lactam + fluoroquinolone <br> Prior respiratory isolate for MRSA or *Pseudomonas* <br> Obtain a nasal MRSA PCR and respiratory culture—add coverage until confirmed <br> Hospitalization and IV antibiotics within 90 days and local risk factors for MRSA or *Pseudomonas* <br> Add coverage—continue until results of a nasal MRSA PCR and respiratory culture confirm that the <br> organisms are present |

(Modified from Mandell LA, Wunderink RG, Anzueto A, et al. Infectious Diseases Society of America/American Thoracic Society consensus guidelines on the management of community-acquired pneumonia in adults. *Clin Infect Dis.* 2007;44:S27—72; Metlay JP, Waterer GW, Long AC, et al. Diagnosis and treatment of adults with community-acquired pneumonia: an official clinical practice guideline of the American Thoracic Society and Infectious Diseases Society of America. *Am J Respir Crit Care Med.* 2019;200:e45—67.)

Respiratory viruses = influenza A and B, adenovirus, respiratory syncytial virus, parainfluenza. *ICU,* Intensive care unit, *IV,* intravenous; *PCR,* polymerase chain reaction.

[a]Comorbidities include chronic heart, lung, liver, or renal disease; diabetes mellitus; alcoholism; malignancy; or asplenia.

settings and *Pseudomonas* may be found in patients with various comorbid illnesses, so empiric treatment directed against these organisms may be prudent.

**❖ For CAP, less emphasis is now placed on where the patient acquired the infection and more emphasis is based on patient comorbidities and risk factors when choosing therapy.**

### Atypical Pneumonia

*Legionella pneumophila*, other *Legionella* species, *Chlamydophila (Chlamydia) pneumoniae*, and *Mycoplasma pneumoniae* may cause atypical pneumonitis in older adults. *Legionella* occurs predominantly in older persons with underlying illness. Parainfluenza, respiratory syncytial virus (RSV), rhinovirus, metapneumovirus, coronaviruses, influenza, and adenovirus are increasingly recognized as causes of atypical pneumonia in older adults.[58,60–65] Identification of atypical causes of pneumonia is more difficult than identification of typical causes. Outbreaks of RTI, particularly during winter months, generally favor a viral etiology. Newer molecular diagnostic tests for multiple pathogens using nasopharyngeal specimens are increasingly available.

In healthcare facilities, the presence of influenza would prompt initiation of antiviral treatment, prophylaxis of exposed patients, and more intensive infection control measures. Diagnosis of influenza in individual outpatients still should rely on history and symptoms. Knowledge that influenza is in the community with fever and new respiratory symptoms of < 48-hour duration is just as sensitive as current diagnostic testing and at less expense.[57,58,60,64,65]

**❖ Consider atypical respiratory pathogens if a similar illness occurs in multiple patients, healthcare personnel, and visitors.**

### Management and Treatment

For older adults with CAP, empiric outpatient treatment should be based on the presence of comorbid illnesses and risks factors for antibiotic-resistant pathogens[57] (see Table 49.8). For inpatients without severe pneumonia or risk factors for MRSA or *Pseudomonas*, therapy should also target gram-negative bacilli using an IV penicillin/β-lactamase inhibitor combination (ampicillin plus sulbactam) or β-lactamase-resistant cephalosporins (ceftriaxone or cefotaxime) or a respiratory fluoroquinolone (levofloxacin or moxifloxacin). Therapy directed against atypical bacteria, such as macrolides and doxycycline, should also be given if the patient is not being treated with a fluroquinolone. Patients with severe pneumonia, but no risk factors for MRSA or *Pseudomonas*, should receive a β-lactam antibiotic in addition to therapy for atypical bacteria (macrolide or fluroquinolone). For severe pneumonia, a patient should also receive treatment for MRSA (vancomycin or linezolid) or *Pseudomonas* with an antipseudomonal penicillin (piperacillin-tazobactam), cephalosporin (cefepime or ceftazidime), or carbapenem (imipenem or meropenem) pending results of sputum, blood cultures, and nasal MRSA polymerase chain reaction (PCR, see Table 49.8).[57] If influenza is in the community, prompt initiation of neuraminidase inhibitors, such as oseltamivir, should be considered.[59]

### Mycobacterial Infection

Failure of an infiltrate to respond to reasonable antibiotic therapy for common pathogens suggests that other infectious and noninfectious etiologies should be considered. Tuberculosis should be considered particularly if there is a history of familial or occupational exposures or other risk factors, such as residence in

an endemic geographic area, prison, or a nursing home.[49–51] Pulmonary TB is found most commonly in the older adult population, whereas extrapulmonary disease may be seen more often in younger persons. Negative TB screening tests, such as the tuberculin skin test (TST) or interferon gamma-based assays (Quantiferon Gold in Tube or T-SPOT) do not exclude the diagnosis of TB disease. In older patients with active TB infection, 25% of TSTs will be negative.

Chest roentgenographic findings that are often seen with TB infection are frequently misinterpreted in older adults because of lack of clinical suspicion. Although reactivation disease seen in the upper lobes is most typical for TB, lower lobe infiltrates, adenopathy, and pleural effusions can occur. Evaluation for TB disease should be directed by abnormalities noted on physical and laboratory examinations; body fluids and tissues should be sent for culture and smear for acid-fast bacilli (AFB). Some specimens found to have AFB on smear may be probed directly to rapidly identify these organisms as related to TB.[49–51]

**❖ Negative screening tests for latent TB do not exclude the possibility of TB disease in the symptomatic patient with suspected infection.**

In the patient with positive TB smears or a clinically compatible illness, empiric four-drug RIPE (rifampin, isoniazid, pyrazinamide, and ethambutol) therapy is generally given until culture and susceptibility results are known. Experts in the management of TB disease should be consulted especially if the patient has a history of prior therapy for TB or has resided in a part of the world where multidrug-resistant or extremely resistant drug strains are found.[49–51]

Prevention of pneumonia in older adults should focus on reduction of individual risk factors and vaccination.[52,66,67] Vaccination of older adults has been effective in reducing the complications of influenza and the prevention of invasive pneumococcal disease.[58,59,68] Screening for LTBI and its treatment should be considered for all older adults.[50,51]

---

### CASE 2

#### Discussion

A temperature of 100° F is indicative of significant fever in older adults. Mrs. Rafferty also has symptoms of new or worsening cough and tachypnea with rales on examination that are commonly associated with LRTI. The respiratory rate of 25 breaths per minute is clearly abnormal; this degree of tachypnea has been strongly associated with the presence of pneumonia in older adults. Mrs. Rafferty's oxygen saturation of 90% in the face of a high respiratory rate and worsening lethargy are indicators that she has impending respiratory failure related to pneumonia.

Mrs. Rafferty's CURB-65 score of 3 (age, confusion, increased respiratory rate) indicates that she needs intensive care for severe pneumonia that would be appropriate given her advance directives. She has severe CAP given that her last hospitalization was > 90 days ago. However, because Mrs. Rafferty requires intensive care and had a prior history of respiratory MRSA infection, she is immediately started on an antipseudomonal β-lactam antibiotic, a macrolide, and vancomycin; sputum cultures and nasal swabs for MRSA are obtained. Sputum and blood cultures grow *Moraxella*; no *Pseudomonas* or MRSA is isolated from her respiratory tract. Her antipseudomonal β-lactam antibiotic is changed to ceftriaxone to treat her *Moraxella* pneumonia, and vancomycin is stopped. She slowly improves and eventually is discharged to a skilled nursing facility for rehabilitation.

## Skin and Soft Tissue Infection

### Prevalence and Impact

SSTIs are the third most common infection seen in older adults. In nursing homes, rates of 1% to 9% have been reported with a prevalence of 0.9 to 2.1 per 1000 patient days.[69-72] Primary infection of soft tissue and secondary infection of preexisting wounds are some of the most common manifestations of SSTI. Primary SSTIs range from common, superficial, and less severe pyodermas involving skin and mucous membranes to less common life-threatening infections extending to fascia (fasciitis), muscle (myositis), and bone (osteomyelitis).[73-76] Secondarily infected ulcers and postoperative wound infections are particularly common among nursing home residents and hospitalized older adults. Approximately 6% of pressure ulcers in nursing home residents will become infected at a rate of 1.4 infections per 1000 resident days.[77-81]

### Pathophysiology and Risk Factors

Intact skin and mucous membranes are major barriers to invasion by microorganisms. Even small breaks in mucocutaneous barriers can facilitate the introduction of many different pathogens, including bacteria, fungi, and viruses. Thinning of skin, decreased mobility, maceration related to incontinence, edema, reduced blood flow, medications, and devices are some of the many factors that alter the integrity of mucocutaneous barriers and contribute to the development of SSTIs in the older adult.[82] Other risk factors involved in the development of SSTIs include waning immunity, exposures to potential pathogens, and conditions that promote overgrowth of the patient's flora. Reactivation of latent viral mucocutaneous infections is common; 10,000 to 20,000 cases of herpes zoster occur annually in nursing home residents.[76,83]

Older adults who reside in shared living quarters are more likely to be exposed to potential pathogens that cause SSTIs. Ectoparasitic infections, such as scabies *(Sarcoptes scabiei),* lice *(Pediculus humanus capitis* [head lice], *P. humanus corporis* [body lice], and *Phthirus pubis* [pubic lice]), and bed bugs *(Cimex lectularius)* through direct exposure to another infected person or from contaminated fomites.[76,84-88]

Preexisting wounds can become secondarily infected by contamination from the hands of healthcare personnel and from contact with the environment (exogenous acquisition) or from the patient's own flora (endogenous acquisition). Other factors contribute to overgrowth of endogenous flora, such as fungi, including antibacterial drugs and corticosteroids.[89-91]

### Differential Diagnosis, Assessment, and Management

#### Primary Skin and Soft Tissue Infection

**Clinical Manifestations.** Primary bacterial SSTIs are most often caused by β-hemolytic streptococci *(S. pyogenes)* and *S. aureus,* and common and superficial manifestations of these infections include cellulitis, erysipelas, impetigo, paronychia, and conjunctivitis (see Table 49.3).[22,76,77] A cause of conjunctivitis may be established in fewer than 40% of cases; most are the result of *S. aureus, Moraxella catarrhalis,* and *Haemophilus* spp.

Primary infections of fascia and muscle do occur, but they are much less frequent; outbreaks of deep infection have been reported in the community and in healthcare settings. In older adults that have cellulitis, increasing pain and worsening symptoms out of proportion with physical findings should immediately raise suspicion for deeper infection and prompt emergent evaluation.[76]

❖❖ **Increasing pain and worsening symptoms out of proportion with findings on skin examination must prompt urgent evaluation for deeper soft tissue infection.**

Nonbacterial causes of primary SSTI also occur. *Candida* infections, primarily *C. albicans,* involve skin and mucosa resulting in many clinical manifestations, including thrush, denture stomatitis, chelitis, paronychia, and intertrigo. Dermatophyte infections involving various body sites include tinea corporis, tinea pedis, tinea cruris, and tinea unguium (onychomycosis) (see Table 49.3).[89-91]

Herpes infections are typically painful or pruritic. Mucocutaneous vesicles or ulcerations because of herpes simplex typically involve nasolabial, genital, or rectal skin and mucosa. A vesicular rash located in a dermatomal distribution is diagnostic for herpes zoster infection (see Table 49.3).[76,83]

❖❖ **Consider the diagnosis of herpes zoster infection if a rash does not cross the midline.**

Scabies infection can manifest atypically in the debilitated older nursing home resident or hospital patient where efficient person-to-person transmission occurs. The typical inflammatory response with resulting pruritus may be lacking in these patients. Burrows and rash in intertriginous areas are often absent and hyperkeratotic or crusting may be more typical (Norwegian scabies). The diagnosis is frequently made when pruritus and more typical rash are seen in family members, visitors, or healthcare workers (see Table 49.3).[76,84-87] Bed bugs are generally a community-associated infection. Acquisition of bed bugs in the healthcare setting is unusual because furniture must be easily cleaned. Red pruritic nodules are noted in a linear distribution.[88]

❖❖ **Consider the diagnosis of scabies if rashes occur in healthcare personnel and visitors.**

**Diagnosis.** The diagnosis of primary SSTIs is generally based on the clinical appearance and location of the lesion. When the presentation is atypical or the patient is not responding to treatment, appropriate samples of pus, blister fluid, or skin scrapings can be useful to verify the diagnosis.[28] Presence of giant cells on Tzanck smear is pathopneumonic for herpes infection. Speciation of herpes viruses as simplex or zoster can be confirmed by obtaining vesicle fluid for immunofluorescence antigen and culture. Differentiation between the two viral species is important because of infection control issues and the higher doses of antivirals required for herpes zoster.[28,76,83]

❖❖ **Swabs of superficial wounds do not predict what bacteria are invasive and causing infection; only send deep specimens, such as tissue and bone for culture.**

Frail older adults are often heavily infested with scabies; examination of deep skin scrapings under immersion oil readily detects mites, ova, and feces. Lice are typically found crawling at the base of hair follicles (nits), in the scalp (head lice), or in the seams of clothing (body lice). Adult bed bugs run rapidly; they are flat, red brown, and the size of an apple seed. Bed bugs are rarely found on the patient; they infest clothing and furniture. Remnants of bugs and blood are typically found along the seams of mattresses and overstuffed furniture.[76,84–88]

**Management and Treatment.** Treatment for primary SSTIs of presumed bacterial etiology may be started empirically if the patient has significant signs of systemic illness or deferred pending the results of cultures if the patient is clinically stable. Empiric treatment should be based on the place of acquisition and directed against the most likely causative organisms, generally *S. aureus* and β-hemolytic streptococci. For severe infection, empiric IV therapy would be appropriate. For less severe symptoms, oral antibacterial agents may be considered.[28,75]

Unfortunately, MRSA is no longer confined to hospitals and now accounts for >50% of primary bacterial SSTIs seen in the community, and decisions regarding empiric treatment of less severe infections with oral agents are no longer simple. Some experts recommend that all community-associated primary SSTIs be treated with clindamycin, a drug that treats many CA-MRSA strains, as well as β-hemolytic streptococci. Others note that the risk for CA-MRSA is increased if the primary SSTI has evidence for abscess formation or drainage when compared with cellulitis alone. In that instance, a β-lactam antibiotic is recommended for cellulitis alone and clindamycin or trimethoprim-sulfamethoxazole when abscesses or drainage are present. Still others note that the choice of antibiotic has little impact on CA-MRSA and surgical incision and drainage is most important.[28,92]

❖ **A scalpel is the best treatment for large MRSA skin abscesses.**

For treatment directed against methicillin-sensitive *S. aureus* and streptococci, oral treatments with first-generation cephalosporins (cephalexin) and antistaphylococcal penicillins (dicloxacillin, amoxicillin-clavulanate) are appropriate. For penicillin-allergic patients, clindamycin or a quinolone with activity against streptococci (moxifloxacin) can be used. For severe bacterial SSTIs, empiric treatment should be directed against MRSA until results of cultures are known; vancomycin, daptomycin, tigecycline, or oral linezolid could be considered.[28,75,92]

Oral acyclovir, famciclovir, or valacyclovir are effective for herpes simplex and localized herpes zoster infections; herpes zoster requires higher doses of these agents. Antiviral treatment is recommended for older adults to reduce postherpetic neuralgia and if they have ophthalmic involvement or disseminated disease. Disseminated herpes zoster should be treated intravenously.[76,83] Herpes zoster can be prevented and postherpetic neuralgia attenuated in older adults given a live virus vaccine.[93]

Topical treatments with nystatin or clotrimazole troches or systemic treatment with oral fluconazole are effective for oral candidosis. Topical clotrimazole or oral fluconazole is also effective for cutaneous candidosis. For dermatophyte infection, oral itraconazole or terbinafine is most beneficial. Drug interactions and hepatotoxicity are significant issues with systemic azoles and terbinafine; careful monitoring is essential during therapy. Onychomycosis typically requires months of therapy with an effective oral agent.[89–91]

Treatment of scabies can be difficult in the debilitated patient. To avoid lindane-associated central nervous system toxicity, permethrin 5% cream is preferred. The cream should be applied from the neck to toes and left in place for up to 12 hours, and nails should be trimmed. Oral ivermectin should be considered for patients with crusted scabies. For head and pubic lice, permethrin or lindane shampoo is applied to the affected area followed by frequent combing to remove nits. Patients should be reexamined weekly to ensure that the scabies and lice have been eradicated.[76,84–87]

Empiric treatment for conjunctivitis should be directed against *S. aureus* and β-hemolytic streptococci until results are known. Appropriate topical ophthalmic antibiotic drops or ointments are erythromycin, quinolones, sulfonamides, and tetracyclines. There are no specific treatments for viral conjunctivitis. Treatment should focus on symptomatic relief with the use of cool compresses, analgesia, and artificial tears. Patients should be monitored closely for bacterial superinfection.[77]

### Secondary Skin and Soft Tissue Infection

**Clinical Manifestations.** Secondary infections of wounds (e.g., pressure ulcers, diabetic ulcers) can range from localized involvement of skin to extension into subcutaneous tissue, muscle, and bone associated with bacteremia and severe systemic infection. Secondary infection of wounds is diagnosed primarily by the presence of localized clinical signs and symptoms; local findings may range from nonhealing to erythema, warmth, tenderness, and purulence to presence of necrotic tissue and crepitus. Systemic inflammatory signs of fever and leukocytosis may be absent (see Table 49.3).[22,28,75]

**Diagnosis.** Wound assessment should include its location and measurement of its circumference and depth using a probe or at the time of surgery. Involvement of underlying structures, such as bone, should be noted. Superficial bacterial colonization of wounds is universal. Superficial swab culture of the exposed surface of the wound does not reflect the cause of infection. Cultures of deep pus, tissue, and blood are required for accurate diagnosis and optimum treatment of infected open wounds. Debridement of superficial necrosis and fibrinous tissue should be performed before obtaining tissue for deep culture.[75,78–81,94]

Many secondary wound infections are polymicrobial. Aerobic gram-negative bacilli (*E. coli, Proteus, Pseudomonas*), gram-positive cocci (streptococci and staphylococci), and anaerobic flora (*Bacteroides, Peptostreptococci, Clostridium perfringens*) commonly infect perineal and lower extremity wounds. Culture of obligate anaerobes from tissue requires special handling by the microbiology laboratory.[75,78–81]

If the wound is contiguous with bone, osteomyelitis may be present. In the diabetic foot, palpable bone on the probe-to-bone test correlates well with the presence of bone infection.[94] In the pressure ulcer, confirmation of osteomyelitis by histopathology on bone biopsy is the gold standard, but sampling error is an issue. The most sensitive and specific imaging study for the diagnosis of osteomyelitis is magnetic resonance imaging (MRI). MRI is also useful to choose an optimal site for bone biopsy, histopathology, and culture. In the patient with a pressure ulcer, radiography and radionucleotide scintigraphy are not helpful because they cannot differentiate osteomyelitis from pressure-related heterotopic bone formation. In contrast, CT is relatively insensitive to detect osteomyelitis and its use should be limited to evaluation of the soft tissues.[75,78–81]

❖ **Proper evaluation of the diabetic foot requires debridement and exploration of all wounds with a probe; palpable bone is diagnostic for osteomyelitis.**

**Management and Treatment.** Initial treatment of secondary wound infection should focus on remediation of the underlying cause and local wound care in addition to antibiotic treatment. Improvement in mobility, relief of pressure, control of diabetes, incontinence, and edema, and improvement in arterial flow, are just a few of the issues that need to be addressed if successful wound healing is to occur. Use of negative pressure occlusive dressings has substantially shortened the time to healing for some patients with large wounds that are not located over major vessels[75,94] (see Ch. 30).

For severe systemic infection, empiric therapy should be given based on community or nosocomial acquisition and knowledge of local resistance patterns. Initial empiric treatment for serious infection is typically IV and directed against MRSA with antibiotics that treat aerobic and anaerobic pathogens. Single agents such as cefoxitin or cefotetan, broad-spectrum penicillin-β-lactamase combinations such as ticarcillin-clavulanate or piperacillin-tazobactam, or carbapenems are appropriate choices. Ciprofloxacin and levofloxacin do not have anaerobic activity, but they can be combined with clindamycin or metronidazole.[75,94]

Definitive therapy is based on the results of deep tissue and blood cultures. Acute wound infections that involve bone or bacteremia with *S. aureus* generally require prolonged IV therapy for 6 weeks or more. Otherwise, the duration of IV therapy is based on clinical experience. Serial measurement of a number of parameters may be helpful in making this decision, including the following: improvement in pain, resolution of fever, erythema, drainage, tissue necrosis, reduction in the size of the wound, clearance of bacteremia, and improvement in elevated inflammatory markers such as leukocytosis, neutrophilia, thrombocytosis, erythrocyte sedimentation rate, and C-reactive protein. Once the patient's clinical status and wound have substantially improved, transition from IV to oral therapy can be considered based on culture results.[75,94]

Prevention of secondary SSTI should focus on prevention of wounds and alleviation of the underlying cause.[78,95]

# Gastrointestinal Infection

## Prevalence and Impact

Manifestations of intraabdominal infection in older adults include infectious diarrhea, gastroenteritis, and intraabdominal abscesses. Infectious diarrhea with or without the nausea and vomiting of gastroenteritis is very common in older adults.[95,96] Although precise rates of GI infection are not known, approximately one-third of nursing home residents will have an episode of diarrhea each year. More than 50% of all deaths caused by diarrhea in the United States occur in adults age 75 years and older.[71,97–102] One-third of diarrheal deaths occur in nursing home residents. Infections with *Salmonella* may be particularly severe. Complications and fatality rates from enteric (typhoid) fever are greatest in persons age $\geq 50$ years. Salmonella gastroenteritis outbreaks in nursing homes have been associated with mortality rates of 10% or more.[103,104]

Intraabdominal abscesses, although less common, pose major problems for older adults.[98] Intraabdominal abscess is a leading consideration in the older adult with fever of unknown origin. Cholecystitis and diverticulitis are common; 10% to 20% of patients with diverticulitis will have the complication of diverticular abscess. Appendicitis is rare in older adults; only 5% to 10% of cases will be in this age group. A disproportionate number of older adult patients will die of appendicitis and diverticular abscess; mortality in this group exceeds 50% for both infections.[95,96,99,100]

## Pathophysiology and Risk Factors

For *C. difficile*, aging and debility have been associated with increased frequency of colonization and infection in older adults. Increased predisposition to *C. difficile* in older adults is also thought to be related in part to defects in the innate immune system, inadequate production of toxin A antibody, or inadequate neutralization of toxin A by antibody. Even so, most older adults who carry toxin-producing *C. difficile* strains will not develop symptomatic infection until they receive an antibiotic. It is thought that *C. difficile* emerges because it is resistant to the antibiotic prescribed and not because other bacteria are suppressed or killed by the drug.[102]

More than one-third of nursing home residents will acquire *C. difficile* within 2 weeks of receiving antibiotic therapy, illustrating how pathogens that cause diarrhea easily spread in closed environments of group homes and chronic healthcare facilities. Devices, such as feeding tubes and thermometers, have been shown to provide effective means of introducing *C. difficile* and other organisms into the GI tract. *C. difficile* spores readily survive in the healthcare environment and can contaminate devices and the hands of personnel.[102,105] Outbreaks of diarrhea have also occurred because of contaminated food or water, or by pets.[71,101]

## Differential Diagnosis, Assessment, and Management

### Classification and Clinical Manifestations

Inflammatory signs of pain, fever, and leukocytosis may be lacking in patients with intraabdominal abscess. Clinical suspicion and early imaging by CT scanning and radionucleotide scintigraphy are critical to diagnosing appendicitis and finding abscesses involving the liver, biliary tract, spleen, and gut.[95,96,106]

Diarrhea is typically defined as more than three watery, loose, or unformed stools per day for 48 hours or more. Symptoms can be mediated by direct invasion of the GI tract by the organism or by the elaboration of toxins. The causes of diarrhea are generally deduced by place of onset, exposure history, the presence or absence of inflammatory signs, and bloody stool, and if an outbreak is present (see Table 49.4).[22,102,105,107]

**Invasive Bacterial Diarrheas.** Invasive bacterial diarrheas, caused by *Salmonella*, *Shigella*, *Campylobacter*, and others, can be characterized by symptoms and signs of inflammation. Pain, fever, and leukocytosis, with blood found on occasion in stool, are prominent findings. Diagnosis of bacterial diarrhea may be suspected if fecal leukocytes are present. Elevated peripheral leukocyte counts may be seen with invasive diarrheas. Diagnosis of invasive bacterial diarrhea is made by culture of stool.[107]

**Toxin-Mediated Diarrheas.** Some bacterial diarrheal illnesses are mediated by the effects of toxin on the GI tract rather than by direct invasion. Shiga toxin—producing strains of enterohemorrhagic *E. coli* are associated with outbreaks of foodborne disease and hemolytic uremic syndrome. This noninvasive infection is not associated with inflammatory signs, but bloody diarrhea can be impressive because of the effects of the toxin on the GI tract. Shiga toxin—producing *E. coli* can be detected by stool culture using special media. Molecular assays are also available that detect specific Shiga toxin—producing strains of *E. coli*, such as 0157:H7.[107,108]

Clinical manifestations of another toxin-mediated bacterial diarrhea, *C. difficile*, range from asymptomatic to mild diarrhea, pseudomembranous colitis, and toxic megacolon. Symptoms can vary from fever with mild crampy abdominal pain to ileus and peritonitis. More recent *C. difficile* strains appear to cause more severe manifestations in older adults and immunosuppressed with increased risk of toxic megacolon and death. Very high peripheral leukocyte counts ($>30,000$ cells/mm$^3$) are suggestive, but not specific, for *C. difficile* infection.

The laboratory diagnosis of *C. difficile* now requires a multistep procedure. A stool assay for glutamine dehydrogenase (GDH) antigen is performed first as a marker that the *C. difficile* bacterium is present in stool and possible infection. Assays for the presence of toxin A and B are performed on GDH-positive specimens using an antigen-based method or by a less commonly available molecular method. Antigen-based tests for toxin A and toxin B are easily performed and rapid, but false-negative tests occur. The more sensitive molecular test for both toxins A and B is done on those GDH-positive/toxin-negative tests. This approach eliminates toxin testing of all stools that do not contain the *C. difficile* bacterium. Detection of toxins A and B is more sensitive, thus eliminating the need to send more than one stool specimen for diagnosis.[102,105]

❖ **Consider the diagnosis of *C. difficile* infection in any patient with a white blood cell count $>30,000$ cells/mm$^3$.**

Carriage of toxin-producing *C. difficile* in older adults without diarrhea is common, and treatment of this asymptomatic colonization does not alter outcome. Thus submission of nondiarrheal stools that do not conform to the shape of the container will not be tested. Endoscopy is not a substitute for stool toxin assays because few *C. difficile* infections are associated with presence of pseudomembranes, and isolated right-sided disease can be missed.[102,105]

❖ **Patients who no longer have diarrhea but had stools positive for *C. difficile* toxin do not benefit from treatment.**

**Noninvasive Diarrheas.** Acute gastroenteritis caused by noninvasive pathogens is characterized by nausea and vomiting associated with watery, nonbloody stools, with absence of fever and other signs of inflammation. Outbreaks of watery diarrhea are typically caused by viruses, such as norovirus, calciviruses, adenoviruses, enteroviruses, and rotavirus.[71,107,109–111] Food poisoning or intoxications caused by ingestion of preformed toxins made by *Bacillus cereus*, *C. perfringens*, and *S. aureus* may mimic outbreaks of viral gastroenteritis.[71,101,107] The onset of food poisoning occurs within hours of ingesting food. Outbreaks of giardiasis *or* cryptosporidiosis that cause chronic diarrhea has been reported in nursing homes related to contaminated water and food, and in childcare programs.[107,111–115] Specific diagnosis of noninvasive gastroenteritis is generally not warranted unless an outbreak is suspected. In healthcare facilities, infection control procedures for enteric precautions should be initiated and hand washing emphasized. Laboratories increasingly rely on antigenic detection for *Giardia lamblia* and *Cryptosporidium parvum* and molecular methods for the diagnosis of some viruses.[107]

### Management and Treatment of Diarrhea

Early identification and treatment of dehydration are important for treatment of all diarrheal illnesses.

**Management and Treatment of Invasive Diarrheas.** For invasive diarrheas, the decision to treat should be based on the patient's clinical condition and results of cultures and antibiotic susceptibilities. For empiric therapy of severe infection, most invasive pathogens remain susceptible to the quinolones. Older adults with *Shigella* infection are at greater risk of bacteremia and death. They should be treated given the potential severity of illness and to eradicate the organism and prevent transmission to others. Treatment of nontyphoidal *Salmonella* infections is generally not recommended in younger patients. However, metastatic seeding to extraintestinal sites, such as vascular and musculoskeletal systems, has been reported following gastroenteritis with *Salmonella* in the older adults; many experts recommend treatment for this age group.[107]

**Management and Treatment of Toxin-Mediated Diarrheas.** For Shiga toxin–producing strains of *E. coli*, antibiotic treatment is not recommended because of increased risk of development of hemolytic uremic syndrome. Avoid administering antimotility agents with bloody diarrhea and proven infection with Shiga toxin–producing *E. coli*.

For the treatment of *C. difficile* infection, all antibiotics that precipitated the episode should be stopped if possible.[105] Initial treatment for CDI with vancomycin or fidaxomicin is recommended over metronidazole; patients who meet criteria for severe infection may benefit from treatment with vancomycin. IV vancomycin solution has been given orally as a substitute for vancomycin capsules at significantly lower cost. Table 49.9 summarizes the approach to the treatment of initial and recurrent episodes of *C. difficile* infections.[105]

**Management and Treatment of Noninvasive Diarrheas.** For patients with noninvasive viral gastroenteritis, no specific treatment is available, and symptomatic treatment is sufficient. Chronic diarrheas caused by *Giardia* should be treated with metronidazole. There is no specific therapy for cryptosporidiosis; most patients improve with supportive therapy. Persistent infection tends to occur in the immunosuppressed and human immunodeficiency virus (HIV) patients; no effective therapy directed against the infection is available. These patients should be referred to a specialist.[107]

## Blood Stream Infection

### Prevalence and Impact

#### Primary Versus Secondary Blood Stream Infection

Most blood stream infection (BSI) occurs as a secondary consequence of infection at another site or source, such as the urinary or respiratory tracts (secondary BSI). Most are associated with the presence of a device, such as a urinary or IV catheter or a surgical procedure. *E. coli* and *Klebsiella* account for most secondary BSIs occurring in community-dwelling older adults and nursing home residents. In hospitalized older adults, *E. coli* and *S. aureus* are the most common causes of secondary BSI.[116–126]

There are some BSIs without an obvious source (primary BSI) that are found predominantly in older adults; these include *L. monocytogenes*, miliary TB, and extraintestinal nontyphoidal salmonellosis.[50,51,103,104,127] These uncommon disseminated infections have been associated with increasing debility, achlorhydria, and waning cell-mediated immunity and comorbid diseases. Extraintestinal salmonellosis has also been related to the presence of vascular disease, gallstones, malignancy, and cirrhosis.[103,104]

The source of BSI has important prognostic implications in older adults. The best survival rates occur following intravascular

**TABLE 49.9　Recommendations for the Treatment of *Clostridium difficile* Infection**

| Clinical Definition | Supportive Clinical Data | Recommended Treatment |
|---|---|---|
| Initial episode, mild or moderate | WBC <15,000 cells/mL<br>Cr <1.5 mg/dL | Vancomycin, 125 mg QID × 10 days<br>OR<br>Fidaxomicin 200 mg BID × 10 days |
| Initial episode, severe | WBC ≥ 15,000 cells/mL<br>OR<br>Cr >1.5 mg/dL | Vancomycin 125 mg QID × 10 days<br>OR<br>Fidaxomicin 200 mg BID × 10 days |
| Initial episode, severe, complicated | Hypotension, shock<br>Ileus, megacolon | Vancomycin 500 mg QID po<br>If ileus present, consider giving vancomycin enema and metronidazole 500 mg TID IV |
| First recurrence | | If metronidazole given first, then vancomycin 125 mg QID × 10 days<br>OR<br>Fidaxomicin 200 mg BID × 10 days |
| Second recurrence | | Vancomycin taper and/or pulsed regime<br>OR<br>Vancomycin 125 mg QID × 10 days followed by rifaximin 400 mg BID × 20 days<br>OR<br>Fidaxomicin 200 mg BID × 10 days<br>OR<br>Fecal transplantation |

(Modified from McDonald LC, Gerding DN, Johnson S, et al. Clinical practice guidelines for Clostridium difficile infection in adults and children: 2017 update by the Infectious Diseases Society of America (IDSA) and Society For Healthcare Epidemiology of America (SHEA). Clin Infect Dis. 2018:66:e1—48.)

*BID,* Two times a day; *Cr,* serum creatinine; *QID,* four times a day; *TID,* three times a day; *WBC,* white blood cells.

catheter-related, genitourinary, and GI tract infections. The poorest survival is found among older adult patients with pneumonia complicated by BSI. Poor outcome following bacteremia is particularly great in older adults who are afebrile, have few localizing symptoms, and have multiorgan system failure. Poor outcome is typically related to delayed or inappropriate treatment.[1,116–126]

### Complications of Blood Stream Infection

Unrecognized or inadequately treated BSI can also lead to complications and metastatic infection at other sites seeding native structures, such as heart valves (infective endocarditis) and vertebrae (vertebral osteomyelitis) and implanted devices. Infective endocarditis (IE) and vertebral osteomyelitis are uncommon but serious complications of BSI that are found with increasing frequency among older adults. Older adults are almost fivefold more likely to acquire IE than younger patients. Older adults are more likely to have IE associated with degenerative valvular disease and less commonly related to rheumatic or congenital valvular disease. IE caused by enterococci and *S. bovis* are also seen more often in the older adult population related to increased genitourinary and GI disorders, such as neoplasms. Older adults are twice as likely to die from their infection as younger persons, with an overall infection-related mortality rate in older adults of 25%.[128–130]

Infection infrequently complicates the placement of 1% to 2% of hip and knee arthroplasties caused by inoculation of the implantation site at the time of surgery or hematogenous seeding. Hematogenous seeding may occur at any time after implantation. In older adults, >60% of prosthetic hip infections are caused by staphylococci. It is estimated that 8% of older adults die because of this infection.[131–133]

**Differential Diagnosis, Assessment, and Management.** In the older adult patient with systemic illness, BSI must be suspected because the consequences of nontreatment are grave. A minimum of two blood samples should be obtained for culture at separate times before starting antibiotics to document that BSI is present. A secondary source of suspected BSI should be sought based on history of predisposing factors and presence of focal symptoms and signs. Appropriate cultures of those secondary sites and imaging should be obtained.

Recognition of the diagnosis of IE can be very difficult. Although older adults are at the greatest risk of acquiring IE, they are also the group most often misdiagnosed. Older adults are significantly less likely to have the diagnosis of IE made by physical examination alone. Fever (55%), leukocytosis (25%), and splenomegaly (20%) may be lacking. Embolic complications are found less often. Obtaining multiple sets of blood cultures before beginning antibiotics is essential to make the diagnosis of IE. In addition, transthoracic echocardiography may be more difficult to interpret in the patient with mitral annular disease or presence of prosthetic valve. Use of transesophageal echocardiography is recommended in those instances to confirm the presence of vegetations.[128–130]

Empiric therapy for BSI and its complications should be based on the place of acquisition, likelihood of antibiotic resistance, and the most likely source. Definitive therapy should be based on results of cultures obtained from blood and suspected secondary sources. Common bacterial causes of IE in adults age ≥ 65 years include MRSA (36%), *S. aureus* (28%), Enteroccoci (17%), coagulase-negative staphylococci (14%), *Viridans streptococci* (14%), and *Streptococcus bovis* (8%).[129] Isolation of the same organism and identical antimicrobial susceptibility patterns suggests that a secondary BSI is present.

Given the severity of BSIs, most treatment will be given intravenously, and the duration of treatment will depend on the source of the infection, the organism, the response of the patient to treatment, and the presence of devices. Abscesses should be drained, particularly if the patient remains symptomatic and particularly if BSI persists despite appropriate antibiotic treatment. Devices associated with the infection should be removed when feasible to facilitate clearance of the infection. Consultation for management of BSI is recommended.[128–133]

## Human Immunodeficiency Virus Infection

### Prevalence and Impact

Rates of HIV infection are rising most rapidly in older adults; 50% of persons living with HIV are age $\geq 50$ years.[134] Minority populations account for most of the new cases. Despite these findings, the diagnosis of HIV is made relatively late in older adults. Therefore more older adult patients progress to acquired immunodeficiency or death (53%) within 12 months of diagnosis compared with younger patients (39%).[134,135]

### Pathophysiology and Risk Factors

Many older adults are sexually active, but few patients used methods to protect themselves against sexually transmitted diseases in 2016. Thus the older patient is more likely to acquire HIV from sexual contact. A significant proportion of older men will have HIV risk factors, such as men having sex with men (67%) and injection drug use (9%).[134,135]

Delayed diagnosis in the older adult contributes to lower $CD_{4+}$ T-cell counts at baseline and more advanced HIV infection than in younger patients. Acquired immunodeficiency syndrome, defined in part by a $CD_{4+}$ T-cell count of 200 cells/mm$^3$, is associated with development of opportunistic infections, neoplasms, and increased risk of death.

In addition to the direct effects of HIV on the immune system, older adults with HIV frequently have a wasting syndrome suggestive of frailty. Cognitive dysfunction, bone loss, and vitamin D deficiency, commonly found in older HIV patients, are also associated with frailty, leading some to postulate that aging and HIV may have sarcopenia, inflammation with elevated cytokine levels, and insulin resistance as common pathways. It is known that untreated HIV also has a detrimental effect on commonly found comorbid conditions in the older adult population, such as cardiovascular disease, hepatitis, and metabolic syndrome.[136]

### Management and Treatment

Many clinicians never ask their older patients whether they have risk factors for HIV or counsel their patients about how to prevent the disease. Few older adults know how to protect themselves or ask to be tested. It is essential that geriatricians consider HIV infection in their patients because early diagnosis is essential to improve survival. HIV must be excluded in older adults with wasting syndrome or encephalopathy rather than assuming these are complications of aging.[135–137]

◆◆ **HIV should be considered in older adults who have dementia or wasting syndrome.**

Referral of HIV-positive patients to clinicians with expertise in administration of highly active antiretroviral therapy (HAART) and monitoring of HIV infection is also crucial. Older patients are just as likely to tolerate their medications, with better compliance than younger patients. However, because older patients are on many more medications than the young, the potential for serious drug interactions is great. Geriatricians should consult with the HIV expert whenever a change in medications is contemplated to ensure that drug interactions are minimized.[137]

HAART leads to increases in numbers of $CD_{4+}$ cells and suppression of viral replication with reduced risk of opportunistic infections. Once $CD_{4+}$ counts exceed 200 cells/mm$^3$ for approximately 12 months, the risk of opportunistic infections, such as *Pneumocystis jiroveci (carinii)* pneumonia, candidosis, *Mycobacterium avium* complex (MAC) infection, toxoplasmosis, and others, declines significantly, and preventative medications can be stopped.[137]

Older adults who adhere to an effective HAART can generally expect that they will not die as a direct consequence of their HIV infection, and prevention of disease becomes a major focus of their care. HAART benefits HIV patients in other ways; cardiovascular and metabolic disease remains a bigger threat to their survival. Suppression of viral replication improves control of hyperlipidemia and progression of coronary artery disease.[137]

In addition to routine screening for colon carcinoma and immunizations, other challenges ensue in the surviving HIV patient. Chronic hepatitis C and hepatitis B infection may require additional treatment and close monitoring for cirrhosis and hepatocellular carcinoma. Papillomavirus associated with the presence of condyloma has been associated with squamous cell carcinoma of the rectum. HAART has been associated with aseptic necrosis of the hip; routine screening for osteopenia is recommended.[135–137]

## Summary

Diagnosis and management of infectious diseases in older adults poses a significant challenge for healthcare providers. Attention to the history along with risk factors and exposures may yield important clues about the causes of infection in complicated patients. Individual physical findings can be subtle, and laboratory findings may be atypical. The astute clinician must make diagnostic and treatment decisions by focusing first on the most common infectious syndromes and the pathogens that cause them. Broad empiric treatment alone is not a substitute for a careful and thorough clinical assessment and systematic evaluation of the evidence for or against a diagnosis.

As one infectious diseases specialist once put it: "You just figure out what the problem is, what bug that is causing it, and treat it. Infectious disease really is that simple!"

### Web Resources

Infectious Diseases Society of America: www.idsociety.org.
Society for Healthcare Epidemiology of America: www.shea-online.org.
Association for Practitioners in Infection Control and Epidemiology: www.apic.org.
American Thoracic Society: www.thoracic.org.
Centers for Disease Control and Prevention: www.cdc.gov.

## Key References

**69.** Bradley SF. Infections and infection control in the long-term care setting. In: Yoshikawa TT, Norman DC, eds. *Infectious Diseases in the Aging. A Clinical Handbook.* Totowa, New Jersey: Humana Press; 2001: p. 245–256.

**28.** Jump RL, Crnich CJ, Mody L, Bradley SF, Nicolle LE, Yoshikawa TT. Infectious diseases in older adults of long-term care facilities: update on approach to diagnosis and management. *J Am Geriatr Soc.* 2018;66:789–803.

**15.** High KP, Bradley SF, Gravenstein S, et al. Clinical practice guideline for the evaluation of fever and infection in long-term care facilities 2008: update by the Infectious Diseases Society of America. *J Am Geriatr Soc.* 2009;57:375–394.

**22.** Stone ND, Ashraf MS, Calder J, et al. Definitions of infection for surveillance in long-term care facilities: revisiting the McGeer criteria. *Infect Control Hosp Epidemiol.* 2012;33:965–977.

**References available online at** expertconsult.com.

# 50

# Gastroenterology

AMIR E. SOUMEKH AND PHILIP O. KATZ

## OUTLINE

*Additional online-only material indicated by icon.*

## OBJECTIVES

*Upon completion of this chapter the reader will be able to:*

- Identify and differentiate the signs and symptoms of common gastroenterology diseases in the geriatric population.
- Demonstrate understanding of the diagnostic workup of dysphagia, gastroesophageal reflux disease, peptic ulcer disease, and NSAID-induced gastric complications.

- Recognize the basic medical, surgical, and endoscopic management of those diseases.

## Dysphagia

### CASE

#### Agnes B (Part 1)

Agnes B is a 74-year-old Caucasian woman who presents to your office with 6 months of difficulty swallowing food. She noted a gradual onset of symptoms with the food sticking in the middle of her chest. Her symptoms have progressed over the past 2 to 3 months and now she also has trouble with swallowing liquids. She denies nausea, vomiting, chest pain, or abdominal pain, and has no history of food regurgitation. She does note occasional heartburn—about three episodes per week for which she either uses over-the-counter (OTC) antacids or famotidine. She has lost over 15 lbs. in the past 3 months.

1. What diagnoses should be considered on the differential for this patient and what is the next appropriate step in Ms. B's workup?

## Epidemiology

Dysphagia refers to the sensation of difficulty swallowing and may be caused by any disruption in the swallowing process. The prevalence of dysphagia appears to increase with age and in patients age ≥65 years has been reported to be 15% to 40% in the outpatient setting. The prevalence can be even higher in institutionalized settings, with up to 50% in older adults living in nursing homes affected.[1]

◆◆ **Older adult patients experience esophageal motility changes as a normal part of aging; however, dysphagia is always considered an alarmsymptom and all patients should undergo evaluation.**

## Risk Factors and Pathophysiology

Dysphagia is typically classified as either oropharyngeal or esophageal. Anatomic or physiologic abnormalities along any portion of the oropharynx or the esophagus, including the upper and lower sphincters, may lead to the sensation of difficulty swallowing. There are physiologic changes associated with aging that may lead to dysphagia—these include fewer and less forceful primary peristaltic wave, decreased salivary production (which aids in food bolus clearance), and decreased ability to clear refluxed gastric material (via secondary persistalsis). Nonetheless, in all patients, dysphagia is considered an alarm symptom that must prompt evaluation and should never be attributed to normal aging without an appropriate evaluation.

◆◆ **Differentiating oropharyngeal dysphagia from esophageal dysphagia is critical to selecting appropriate further testing.**

Oropharyngeal dysphagia is characterized by the inability to initiate a swallow or transfer food from the mouth to the esophagus. In addition to the sensation of dysphagia, typical symptoms include coughing, choking, nasopharyngeal regurgitation, aspiration (with or without subsequent pneumonia), and retained food in the mouth after an attempted swallow. In patients with advanced dementia, oropharyngeal dysphagia may result from apraxia and be misinterpreted as a refusal to swallow. Multiple changes in the physiology of the aging gut, as well as specific disorders, may lead to oropharyngeal dysphagia.[2] Physiologic studies have shown reduced tongue strength, reduced pharyngeal wall contraction, decreased salivary flow, and impaired gag reflexes in healthy older adults, all of which likely contribute to dysphagia. Poor dentition may lead to inadequate mastication of food bolus and contribute as well. Neurologic disorders (such as stroke, Parkinson disease, Alzheimer dementia, myasthenia gravis) and malignancies of the oropharynx are common causes of oropharyngeal dysphagia. Structural abnormalities, such as a Zenker diverticulum or prominent cervical osteophytes, are also common in this age group.

In contrast, esophageal dysphagia typically presents as the sensation of food getting stuck in the esophagus (or chest) several seconds after initiating a swallow. Age-related physiologic changes such as decreased salivary flow and loss of neurons in the myenteric and submucosal plexus lead to altered motility of the esophagus and contribute to the high rates of dysphagia among older adults, especially those age ≥80 years. Further, medications can exacerbate these changes, often through anticholinergic effects.[3]

The etiology of esophageal dysphagia is usually subclassified into structural disorders, motility disorders, and infectious or inflammatory diseases (Box 50.1). Dysphagia for solids that progresses later to involve liquids suggests mechanical obstruction. In the older age group, multiple causes of mechanical obstruction are seen. Malignancy must be excluded in all patients. The most common cancers tend to be adenocarcinomas occurring in the distal esophagus as a complication of Barrett esophagus—a metaplastic change of esophageal mucosa from squamous to intestinal mucosa because of chronic

reflux. In the United States, squamous cell cancers are less common and are typically caused by toxic exposures, such as cigarette smoke, alcohol, or even food stasis because of severe motility disorders, such as achalasia.[4] Benign strictures may be caused by reflux, prior radiation, or pill-induced esophageal injury. Esophageal rings (concentric) and webs (eccentric) are benign, idiopathic, or reflux-induced, thin mucosal structures that partially occlude the esophageal lumen. A triad of webs, dysphagia, and iron deficiency anemia, typically seen in older Caucasian women, is known as Plummer-Vinson syndrome and is associated with an increased risk of future esophageal squamous cell cancers. Extrinsic compression may be caused by variant vasculature, a large aortic aneurysm, an enlarged left atrium, or extraesophageal malignancies, such as lymphoma.

In contrast with mechanical obstruction, dysphagia for both solids and liquids from the onset usually implies a motility disorder of the esophagus. Common primary motility disorders include achalasia, hypoperistaltic disorders (ineffective esophageal motility)—often associated with gastroesophageal reflux disease (GERD)—and hypertensive or spastic disorders (jackhammer esophagus, distal esophageal spasm). Although achalasia does not appear to be seen in greater frequency older adults it may present later in its course with greater esophageal dilation because of delay in presentation and diagnosis in the older adult population. Less is known about the epidemiology of the other motility disorders and aging.

Dysphagia accompanied by odynophagia (painful swallowing) is suspicious for an infectious etiology, such as a viral or fungal infection. Candidal infections are the most common and often seen in the setting of systemic immunosuppression or with use of inhaled steroids for asthma or chronic obstructive pulmonary disease. Common viruses are the herpes simplex virus, which can be seen in immunocompetent older adults, and cytomegalovirus, which is typically found only in immunosuppressed patients.

## Differential Diagnosis and Assessment

The differential diagnosis of dysphagia is broad, as noted earlier. Obstructive causes include malignancies of the esophagus (adenocarcinoma and squamous cell cancer being the most common), benign strictures (most commonly because of gastroesophageal reflux), diverticula (such as a Zenker diverticulum), or extrinsic compression (such as cardiac enlargement or osteophytes). Primary motility disorders (such as achalasia or esophageal spasms or hypoperistaltic disorders) should be considered after obstructive causes have been ruled out.

Systemic disorders—typically those with a neurologic component—tend to cause oropharyngeal dysphagia. However, some rheumatologic disorders (such as scleroderma or systemic sclerosis) can lead to an esophageal motility disorders. In older patients with dysphagia of any kind, systemic disorders should be considered.

In patients with dysphagia and pain (either chest pain or pain with swallowing), infectious etiologies, such as candida or herpes or cytomegalovirus, should be considered, especially in a patient who is immunosuppressed. Spastic esophageal disorders can be evaluated after infections are ruled out. Cardiac and pulmonary causes of chest pain must always be considered and sufficiently ruled out before a gastrointestinal (GI) evaluation.

## History and Physical Examination

Historical details to obtain from a patient who complains of swallowing difficulty help differentiate oropharyngeal from esophageal causes, structural from motility etiologies, and may raise the possibility of an underlying systemic disorder.

In all patients, a medication review should be done, particularly focusing on anticholinergic drugs that may worsen dysphagia of any etiology.

Patients whose symptoms include coughing, choking, nasopharyngeal regurgitation, aspiration, and retained food in the mouth after an attempted swallow should be evaluated for oropharyngeal dysphagia, as well as for systemic disorders with a neurologic or neuromuscular component.

Patients whose dysphagia is initially with solids and later progresses to involve liquids should be evaluated for mechanical obstruction. If the dysphagia occurs for both solids and liquids from the onset of symptoms, a motility disorder of the esophagus is more likely.

Rapidly progressive dysphagia of any kind is worrisome for malignancy. Although malignancy must be ruled out in all patients with dysphagia, rapidly progressive dysphagia requires more urgent and complete workup for an underlying cancer.

Physical examination is of limited utility in the workup of dysphagia. Supraclavicular lymph nodes may be palpated in metastatic cancer.

## Laboratory Testing

Laboratory testing is of limited utility in the workup of dysphagia. Anemia—particularly, iron deficiency anemia—is worrisome for an esophageal malignancy. In patients in whom dysphagia has caused weight loss, nutritional testing for vitamin or mineral deficiencies may be considered.

## Radiographic Imaging and Other Nonlaboratory Testing

Radiographic and endoscopic testing are the mainstay in the evaluation of dysphagia. All patients with dysphagia should undergo an upper endoscopy to evaluate for structural abnormalities, rule out malignancy, and allow for biopsy and histologic examination of the esophageal as needed.

◆◆ **All patients with esophageal dysphagia should undergo an upper endoscopy; preendoscopy imaging with a barium esophagram may provide additional information and help maximize the utility of the endoscopy by identifying diverticula (which can be missed or perforated during an endoscopy), strictures (which can be dilated, with planning, during an endoscopy), and motility abnormalities that suggest an esophageal manometry should be performed in addition to an endoscopy.**

In patients with oropharyngeal dysphagia, videofluoroscopy (often referred to as a modified barium swallow) can assess swallowing mechanics and detect aspiration. Patients can also be referred to otolaryngology and to speech/swallow therapy for a nasopharyngolaryngoscopy and a fiberoptic evaluation endoscopic of swallowing (FEES) study. During a FEES, a nasopharyngolaryngoscopy is performed while food and liquid boluses are given to the patient to assess oropharyngeal structure and function. There is good correlation between a modified barium swallow and a FEES and providers can choose either or both tests to obtain a complete assessment of pharyngeal swallowing. Access to FEES testing may be limited because it requires practitioners with specialized ear, nose, and throat (ENT) training. Together, these can assess for masses, pooled secretions, retained food, sensory abnormalities, and specific oropharyngeal movement abnormalities.[2]

In patients with esophageal dysphagia, a barium esophagram may be helpful by evaluating structural abnormalities (including diverticula, which can be missed on endoscopy) and by helping assess possible motor abnormalities and reflux.

Patients who appear to have a primary motility disorder should be referred to a GI motility center for esophageal manometry, the primary testing modality for esophageal motor abnormalities.

### CASE

#### Agnes B (Part 2)

Agnes B undergoes a barium esophagram (Fig. 50.1) and endoscopy (Fig. 50.2).
1. What are the findings noted on these studies? What is the patient's likely diagnosis? What is the primary risk factor for this diagnosis?

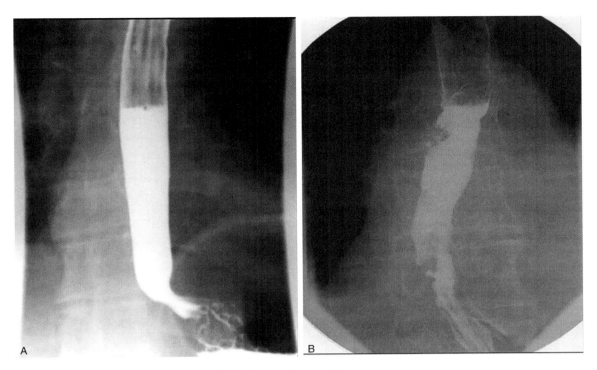

• **Figure 50.1** Normal barium esophagram (A) and Agnes B's barium esophagram (B).

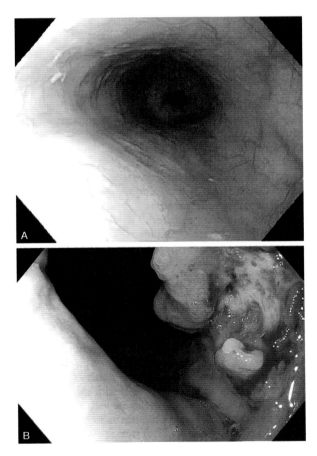

• **Figure 50.2** Normal endoscopy (A) and Agnes B's endoscopy (B).

## Management

Treatment of dysphagia depends on the underlying cause. Treatment of oropharyngeal dysphagia may require swallowing rehabilitation or dietary modifications, such as thickening liquids, or careful hand feeding with a spoon, cup, or straw. In cases in which dementia is the cause of dysphagia, the placement of a percutaneous gastrostomy with tube feeding has not demonstrated improvement in survival, function, or symptoms, and tube feeding is recognized as a risk factor for aspiration.

Multiple treatment options exist for achalasia, the most severe of the primary motility disorders. Injection of the lower esophageal sphincter with botulinum toxin may provide months of symptomatic relief in patients who are not surgical candidates or have a very limited life expectancy. In most patients, however, definitive treatment with surgical or endoscopic myotomy is indicated. Spastic motility disorder can often be treated medically. Calcium channel blockers or phosphodiesterase inhibitors (such as sildenafil) may provide relief by relaxing smooth muscle.[5]

Treatment of malignancy is primarily surgical, often with adjunct chemotherapy and/or radiation. However, in nonadvanced cancers or in patients who are not surgical candidates, endoscopic treatments may be available for curative or palliative intent.

Benign strictures are treated with endoscopic dilation, with a very high success rate, although they often require ongoing medical treatment of the underlying cause as well (e.g., reflux). The treatment of reflux is discussed separately.

Infectious causes require targeted antiviral or antifungal therapy.

## Summary

Dysphagia is a common complaint in the older adult population and can be caused by a variety of primary GI disorders or secondary to systemic disorders. Diagnosis requires careful history taking, but further testing, such as an upper endoscopy, barium esophagram, or motility testing is almost always required.

Therapy is tailored to the underlying disease. Treatment of oropharyngeal dysphagia is limited. For most causes of esophageal dysphagia, highly efficacious, minimally invasive treatment options exist.

## Gastroesophageal Reflux Disease

### CASE

#### Agnes B (Part 3)

Upon further history taking, Agnes B states that she has had "occasional heartburn" for decades. She used to "live on Tums" until she discovered cimetidine and, later, famotidine, which she has been using for over 10 years now. It mostly controlled her symptoms, so she never complained of reflux to her primary care doctor or sought further care. She admits, however, that she would be awakened one to two times per week with severe heartburn or regurgitation, particularly after eating late in the evening.

1. Had the patient sought care, what treatments options would have been available and appropriate for her reflux symptoms?

### Epidemiology

GERD is defined as symptoms or complications resulting from the reflux of gastric contents into the esophagus or beyond to the oropharynx, nasopharynx, larynx, or lung.[6] The typical symptoms of GERD are heartburn and regurgitation. Patients with heartburn will often describe a burning sensation in the chest, usually rising from the epigastric region. Regurgitation is the painless sensation of food or other gastric contents moving into the chest or mouth. Less typical symptoms of GERD include dyspepsia, epigastric pain, dysphagia, nausea, bloating, belching, asthma, chronic cough, globus, and laryngitis or voice changes. Patient with typical heartburn or regurgitation can often identify trigger foods, such as alcohol, acidic foods (e.g., citrus or tomatoes), or trigger lifestyle factors, such as symptoms brought on by stress or intake of larger meals or eating late in the evening.

**❖ GERD is a common GI symptom in the general population, as well as in the older adult population.**

GERD is the most commonly seen upper GI condition in primary care. Among adults age $\geq 65$ years, symptoms of heartburn or acid regurgitation occur at least weekly in 20% of the population and at least monthly in 59%.[7] Prolonged pH studies show that esophageal acid exposure frequency and duration increases with age, and endoscopic data suggest that esophagitis is more severe in older adults. However, likely because of decreased pain perception in this age group, the severity of symptoms often does not correlate with the severity of disease.

### Risk Factors and Pathophysiology

The underlying pathophysiology in GERD is a compromised lower esophageal sphincter (LES). The LES, located at the junction of the intraabdominal stomach and intrathoracic esophagus, is comprised of thickened esophageal and gastric muscle fibers that are tonically contracted and is augmented by the crural diaphragm.

Inappropriately frequent or prolonged relaxations of the LES is a primary cause of GERD. A hiatal hernia—a separation of the LES and the crural diaphragm—leads to a lower pressure at the esophagogastric junction and is another primary cause of GERD. Hiatal hernias are more common and larger in older adult patients and are associated with more severe symptoms.[8] Factors that increase intraabdominal pressure, such as obesity, pregnancy, or straining, can increase the pressure gradient between the stomach and esophagus and allow gastric contents to overcome the LES pressure leading to reflux.

Although often discussed, the role of specific foods and dietary choices is not well established in the pathophysiology of reflux.

Medications can play a role in reflux by reducing LES tone, acidifying gastric contents, or reducing salivary production. These include anticholinergics, benzodiazepines, opiates, nitrates, and calcium channel antagonists.

### Differential Diagnosis and Assessment

Symptoms of reflux can be extraesophageal, variable, and vague and therefore a large differential diagnosis should be considered. In patients with chest symptoms, cardiac disease should be ruled out. Patients who primarily complain of pulmonary symptoms (asthma, shortness of breath, cough) should be referred for pulmonary evaluation.

The differential for esophageal symptoms of GERD include infectious esophagitis, pill esophagitis, eosinophilic esophagitis, motility disorders, strictures, and malignancies.

### History and Physical Examination

The diagnosis of GERD can be difficult by history alone because older patients can present with more vague or atypical symptoms. Current guidelines allow for a presumptive diagnosis of GERD in patients with typical symptoms (heartburn and/or regurgitation), regardless of patient age. In these patients, an empiric trial of acid-suppression therapy with a proton-pump inhibitor (PPI) is warranted. As a test for GERD, an empirical PPI trial with improved symptoms has a sensitivity of 68% to 83%.[6]

History taking should be targeted to identify the specific symptoms of reflux to help determine if cardiology, pulmonology, and/or laryngology consults are needed. Alarm features, such as rapid-onset of symptoms, dysphagia, odynophagia, or weight loss should be elicited.

Patients with atypical symptoms, extraesophageal symptoms, or alarm symptoms need further testing. The physical examination is of limited utility in the patient complaining of typical reflux symptoms.

### Laboratory Testing

Laboratory testing is of limited utility in the patient complaining of typical reflux symptoms.

### Radiographic Imaging and Other Nonlaboratory Testing

Patients with alarm signs or symptoms, those with longstanding reflux, and who do not respond to a trial of PPI should undergo endoscopy to exclude severe esophagitis, strictures, Barrett esophagus, dysplasia, and malignancy. The threshold for endoscopic evaluation should be lower for older patients as age alone is a risk factor for esophageal malignancy.

◆◆ **Threshold for testing with upper endoscopy should be low as they may present with atypical symptoms and more severe disease.**

Patients who have persistent symptoms despite appropriate antisecretory therapy and in whom an upper endoscopy is unremarkable should be evaluated with formal reflux testing. A wireless pH capsule can measure acid reflux for up to 96 hours while a 24-hour catheter-based pH-impedance study can confirm or exclude both acid and nonacid reflux.

Motility testing with an esophageal manometry is used to exclude an underlying esophageal motility disorder, such as achalasia, as the cause of the symptoms, as well as to document the presence of effective esophageal peristalsis in patients in whom antireflux surgery is being considered.

## Management

Although data are limited, dietary and lifestyle modifications are an integral part of the initial management of reflux. Elevation of the head of the bed (> 30 degrees), fasting for 2 or more hours before bedtime, and sleeping in the left lateral position have been shown to reduce nocturnal reflux. Smoking and alcohol should be minimized or avoided. Weight loss, smaller meals, avoiding known dietary triggers, or avoiding common food triggers (such as high-fat foods, caffeine, peppermint, chocolate, carbonated beverages, and acidic foods) may be helpful, although data whether specific foods are refluxogenic are limited.[9] Medications that reduce LES pressure should be limited whenever possible. These include anticholinergics, benzodiazepines, opiates, nitrates, and calcium channel antagonists.

◆◆ **A variety of treatments are available, ranging from diet and lifestyle changes to medications to surgery, depending on disease severity and patient preference.**

Multiple classes of medications exist for the treatment of GERD. The choice of treatment depends primarily on the

frequency and severity of the patient's reflux symptoms, as well as payer coverage. An outline of the basic treatment options for GERD is provided in Table 50.1.

Short-acting antacids or alginic-acid containing medications (e.g., Gaviscon) may be helpful for patients with mild, transient reflux symptom, especially when heartburn is the primary symptom. The duration of action of these is limited and they have minimal to no ability to heal reflux inflammation.

OTC histamine-2 receptor antagonists (H2RAs) (e.g., ranitidine, famotidine, cimetidine) provide relatively rapid-onset relief of symptoms, with a duration of acid suppression of several hours. However, the level of acid suppression is limited, providing incomplete symptom relief in patients with moderate to severe symptoms and only moderate improvement of reflux esophagitis.[9] Of the H2RAs, cimetidine has been the least commonly used because of its side effect profile and possible drug interactions. Formulations of ranitidine have very recently been removed from the market because of possible carcinogenic impurities.[10]

◆◆ **PPIs are the most commonly used medication and are safe.**

PPIs provide the most effective acid suppression, the highest level of symptom reduction, and the highest rates of reflux esophagitis improvement—with healing of erosive esophagitis in more than 80% of patients, compared with 50% to 60% with H2RAs.[6] Multiple PPIs are available in the United States, including omeprazole, esomeprazole, lansoprazole, dexlansoprazole, pantoprazole, and rabeprazole. Esomeprazole is the isolated S-enantiomer of the racemic mixture of R- and S-enantiomers in omeprazole. Similarly, dexlansoprazole is the isolated R-enantiomer of the racemic mixture of R- and S-enantiomers in lansoprazole. Dexlansoprazole also has a dual-release mechanism, which allows it to achieve two peak concentrations at various times, within 2 and 5 hours of administration. There is some data showing various differences in acid suppression (based on pH testing) and symptom improvement between various PPIs—with marked intra- and intersubject variability. In practice,

**TABLE 50.1   Medical Management/Medication Treatment Options for Gastroesophageal Reflux Disease**

| Medication Class | Mechanism of Action | Specific Medications |
|---|---|---|
| Antacids | Alkaline ions that neutralize hydrochloric acid | Tums (calcium carbonate), Rolaids (calcium carbonate, magnesium hydroxide), Milk of Magnesium (magnesium hydroxide), Maalox or Mylanta (aluminum hydroxide, magnesium hydroxide) |
| Alginic acid | An additive to antacids that precipitates to form a gel-foam substance that floats to the gastroesophageal junction to provide a physical barrier to refluxate entering the esophagus | Gaviscon |
| Histamine 2 receptor antagonist (H2RAs) | Competitive antagonists of the H2 receptors. Meal-induced gastrin secretion leads to histamine release, which stimulates H2 receptors, which trigger HCl release. Blocking H2 receptors stops this pathway for gastric acid release/production | Famotidine, ranitidine, cimetidine, nizatidine |
| Proton-pump inhibitors (PPIs) | Permanently inactivates the active form of the proton pump (H + -K + -ATPase), completely blocking H + secretion from a given pump. A new pump must be created to restart acid secretion. Typically requires 3 days of consistent PPI use to inhibit gastric proton pumps | Prilosec (omeprazole), Nexium (esomeprazole), Protonix (pantoprazole), Aciphex (rabeprazole), Prevacid (lansoprazole), Dexilant (dexlansoprazole) |

the first choice of PPI is based on cost considerations. In patients who do not respond to an initial PPI choice, a dose increase or switching to a different PPI is recommended. Patients who do not respond to a dose increase or a brand switch should be referred to a dedicated reflux center for further testing.

There have been concerns over the long-term safety of PPIs. A large number of observational studies and several metaanalysis have investigated a possible link between long-term PPI use and potential adverse effects. These include increased risk of *Clostridium difficile* and other infections, osteopenia/osteoporosis, micronutrient deficiency, kidney disease, and dementia. Data on these side effects are limited and inconsistent.[11]

Of particular concern to the older adult community are the potential adverse effects of osteoporosis and dementia. Purported mechanisms by which PPIs may cause osteoporosis are decreased calcium absorption and augmented osteoclastic activity caused by PPI-induced hypochlorhydria; however, neither of these effects have been proven. The data on the effects of PPIs have been conflicting, with some studies showing worsening bone mineral density whereas others showed no association. Overall, studies do suggest a modest increase of fracture risk, although again, this is not a consistent finding and no causal link has been proven. The research has been limited and inconsistent enough for the US Food and Drug Administration to retract a warning it had placed on PPIs and increased fracture risk in 2011, just 1 year after placing the initial warning.[12] In addition, guidelines on GERD management recommend the use of PPIs in patients with osteoporosis if other medications are insufficient to control symptoms. Regardless, it is reasonable to adjust the regimen in patients with known osteoporosis risk factors, such as smoking. For PPI users who require calcium supplementation, a soluble form such as calcium citrate is preferred.

As with osteoporosis, the link between PPIs and dementia is unclear. Purported mechanisms by which PPIs may affect dementia risk include the following: by interfering with clearance of amyloid-beta and tau proteins in the central nervous system, through drug-drug interactions, and interference with B12 and other micronutrient absorption.[13] The data on whether PPIs actually increase dementia risk are conflicting with several observational studies suggesting an increased rate of dementia in long-term PPI users and others showing no such risk.[14]

Overall, PPIs are safe. However, patients should use the lowest doses necessary for the shortest period of time. Patients on PPIs should routinely be reevaluated and attempt to taper off PPIs or transition to H2RAs if possible.

Patients who cannot tolerate PPIs because of a class allergy or adverse effects and patients whose symptoms cannot be controlled with medications may be candidates for antireflux surgery, such as a hiatal hernia repair and fundoplication (GERD guidelines). Age alone is not a contraindication to surgical treatment and older adult patients may benefit more from surgical referral because of higher rates of hiatal hernias and severe disease, including pulmonary disease because of GERD.[15] Laparoscopic fundoplication appears to be as safe and efficacious in older patients as it is in younger ones.[16]

## Summary

GERD is a common disease in the general population and its prevalence and severity appear to increase in the older population. This is likely caused by inherent age-related physiologic changes, as well as increased use of medications that can cause or exacerbate GERD. Cardiac and pulmonary diseases should be ruled out in patients who present with atypical GERD symptoms. Treatment options include diet and lifestyle changes, antacids, H2RAs, PPIs, and antireflux surgery.

# Peptic Ulcer Disease and Nonsteroidal Antiinflammatory Drug-Induced Gastric Complications

## Epidemiology

The term *peptic ulcer* refers to acid-induced injury of the digestive tract, typically in the stomach or duodenum, resulting in loss of the mucosal layer. The incidence and prevalence of peptic ulcer diseases (PUD) vary greatly depending on geography and socioeconomic status but have been falling sharply over the past several decades.[17] Lifetime prevalence of PUD in the general population has been estimated to be about 5% to 10%, and incidence 0.1% to 0.3% per year, and does appear to increase with age.[18] The declining rates of PUD are likely caused by decreased prevalence of *Helicobacter pylori* (with decreased transmission rates as a result of improved hygiene and higher rates of *H. pylori* testing and treatment), as well as higher rates of PPI use.[19]

❖❖ **High rates of NSAID use, including low-dose cardioprotective aspirin, place geriatric patients at risk for PUD.**

Nonsteroidal antiinflammatory drug (NSAID)—induced injury to the GI tract range from mild mucosal changes (edema and erythema) to mucosal loss (erosions and ulcers), possibly complicated by pain, GI bleeding, and/or perforation. As the rates of *H. pylori*—induced disease declines, the proportion of NSAID-induced gastric complications has been rising.[20] The growth of NSAID-induced gastric diseases parallels the rise of NSAID use, including low-dose aspirin, as cardiovascular diseases become more prevalent in an aging population.[21]

## Risk Factors and Pathophysiology

Most *H. pylori* infections are acquired during childhood in both developed and developing countries.[22] Most infections appear to occur by the age of 5 years, from infected family members or chronic exposure to others living in close quarters. The risk of acquiring *H. pylori* increases with overcrowding, the number of siblings or household family members, inadequate hygiene practices, or poor access to running water. Countries with rising economic status and improvement in household sanitation typically see a decline in infection rates.[23]

The pathophysiology of *H. pylori*—induced gastric disease is caused by the bacteria's exclusive affinity for the gastric mucosa and its unique adaptions to the caustic gastric environment. *H. pylori* is not an invasive bacteria—instead, it uses adhesins and other membrane proteins to attach to gastric mucosal cells and then cause tissue damage through a variety of direct and indirect mechanisms.[24] Urease allows the bacteria to alkalinize its surrounding environment whereas phospholipases, catalases, and other proteolytic enzymes break down the protective mucous barriers of the stomach. This allows stomach acid to directly contact gastric cells causing tissue damage that is then exacerbated by the inflammatory response to the *H. pylori*'s enzymatic products.[24] Chronic inflammation and cellular damage can then progress to superficial mucosal loss (erosions) and then to complete mucosal loss (ulcers) causing pain, bleeding, or even perforation. In a small subset of patients, the chronic inflammation induced by the bacteria can ultimately lead to gastric malignancies.[25]

NSAID-induced gastric injury appears to occur primarily as a consequence of inhibition of cyclooxygenase (COX)-1 in the upper GI tract. COX is the key enzyme in prostaglandin synthesis. The two functional forms of the enzyme—COX-1 and COX-2—play different roles in the human body. COX-1 is a "housekeeping" constitutive enzyme; it is chronically expressed in healthy gastric and duodenal mucosa (as well as several other tissues throughout the body), leading to continuous production of local prostaglandins. Prostaglandins in turn exert several mucosal protective effects, including stimulation of mucin secretion, bicarbonate secretion, and phospholipid secretion by the gastric epithelial cells, increased epithelial cell proliferation, and improved vascular flow.[26] The COX-2 enzyme is inducible and produced in response to infection or inflammation and it is responsible in triggering a further inflammatory cascade.

Most NSAIDs, including low-dose aspirin, nonselectively inhibit both COX-1 and COX-2, thereby reducing pain and inflammation (the intended goal) and incidentally inhibiting several gastric mucosal protective mechanisms. Without COX-1 induced gastric protection, local tissue ischemia, as well as unbuffered exposure to luminal acid, leads to inflammation, mucosal breakdown, and ultimately ulceration.

In addition to advanced age, risk factors for NSAID-induced disease include high-dose NSAID use, a prior history of PUD, and concurrent use of two NSAIDs (typically, low-dose aspirin in addition to another NSAID). Patients also taking anticoagulants, glucocorticoids, antiplatelet medications (such as clopidogrel), or selective serotonin reuptake inhibitors (which exhibit antiplatelet activity) appear to have an increased risk of bleeding with NSAIDs. Several studies have shown that *H. pylori* and NSAIDs are independent and synergistic risk factors for ulcer development and that eradication of *H. pylori* can reduce the risk of PUD in patients who require chronic NSAID use.[27,28]

## Differential Diagnosis and Assessment

The differential diagnosis of PUD (or gastritis) consists of other diseases that cause epigastric discomfort or pain, such as gastric malignancy, gallstone disease, celiac disease, inflammatory bowel disease (Crohn disease, in particular), gastroparesis, and chronic pancreatitis. For patients presenting with bleeding, the differential diagnosis is larger and includes all potential causes of GI bleeding, including any GI malignancy, angioectasias, severe erosive esophagitis, proximal colonic diverticulosis, and Meckel diverticulum.

## History and Physical Examination

Patient's with symptomatic gastritis or PUD typically present with dyspepsia, defined as predominant epigastric pain lasting at least 1 month, possibly associated with any other upper GI symptom, such as epigastric fullness, nausea, vomiting, or heartburn.[29] A detailed history is necessary to determine the underlying cause and to identify patients with alarm features. Weight loss, anorexia, vomiting, dysphagia, odynophagia, and a family history of GI cancers suggest the presence of an underlying gastroesophageal malignancy.

More urgently, as the mucosal damage progresses, and the ulcer depends, patients will present with upper GI bleeding (typically melena) or even frank perforation (with severe abdominal pain, fever, or distension).

◆◆ **Bleeding is the most common worrisome complication and thus early diagnosis with endoscopy and treatment are critical.**

The physical examination in patients with dyspepsia is typically unrevealing except for epigastric tenderness (which is a nonspecific finding). The examination should note any palpable masses, jaundice or ascites (because of liver disease) or pallor (because of anemia) and signs of potential malignancy, such as muscle wasting. In patients with possible perforation, signs of peritonitis (such as rigidity or rebound tenderness) should be noted.

## Laboratory Testing

Like history, laboratory testing should be geared toward identifying alarm signs, as well as to rule out potentially nongastric causes of dyspepsia. Routine blood counts and iron studies should be performed to identify patients with iron deficiency anemia, suggestive of GI bleeding from a potential malignancy. Liver function tests, amylase/lipase, and bloody chemistries (including a hemoglobin A1C) can identify hepatobiliary causes of dyspepsia, as well as metabolic disorder such as diabetes, which can mimic PUD.

◆◆ **All patients should be tested for *H. pylori* infection with biopsy, breath test, or stool test and then retested after completing treatment to confirm eradication.**

In all patients with suspected or confirmed PUD, *H. pylori* testing should be performed. Noninvasive testing options include serology (serum *H. pylori* immunoglobulin G antibody testing), urea breath testing, and a stool antigen assay.[29] In most cases, serology is not recommended because antibody testing does not reliably distinguish between active and past infection. The urea breath test (UBT) is based upon the hydrolysis of urea by *H. pylori* to produce $CO_2$ and ammonia. Carbon-labeled urea is given orally and then a breath sample is taken and analyzed for labeled $CO_2$ (which is released only if *H. pylori* and its urease enzyme are presents in the patient's stomach). The sensitivity and specificity of the UBT both approach 100%, but can be lowered in patients who have recently taken PPIs or antibiotics.[30] Stool sample testing to identify *H. pylori* bacterial antigen using a monoclonal enzyme immunoassay has a sensitivity and specificity similar to UBT. And like the UBT, its accuracy is reduced by PPI or antibiotic exposure. It is recommended, to reduce false-negative results, that patients should be off antibiotics for 4 weeks, and PPIs for 1 to 2 weeks, before testing.[29]

## Radiographic Imaging and Other Nonlaboratory Testing

Peptic ulcers are diagnosed via upper endoscopy, which has a sensitivity of more than 90% and also allows for treatment of bleeding lesions (and lesions at high risk of bleeding). Endoscopy also allows for biopsies to differentiate benign ulcers from gastric cancers, as well as to exclude an underlying *H. pylori* infection.

Although an empiric trial with antisecretory therapies is often used, prompt endoscopy should be performed in older adults because of the increased rate of organic disease (including malignancy) in this age group.[29] Endoscopy for evaluation of dyspepsia in older adults has been shown to obtain diagnostic information in more than 90% of patients and is associated with a significant reduction in PPI use and an improvement in quality-of-life measures. Endoscopy has been shown to be safe in older adults who are

| TABLE 50.2 | Common First-Line Treatment Regimens for *Helicobacter Pylori* Infection | | |
|---|---|---|---|
| **Regimen Name** | **Drug and Dose** | **Frequency** | **Duration** |
| Clarithromycin triple therapy | Clarithromycin 500 mg | BID | 14 |
| | Amoxicillin 1 g | BID | 14 |
| | ªMetronidazole 500 mg TID can be used in place of amoxicillin in cases of penicillin allergy | | |
| Bismuth quadruple therapy | Bismuth subcitrate 120–300 mg or subsalicylate 300 mg | QID | 10–14 |
| | Tetracycline 500 mg | QID | 10–14 |
| | Metronidazole 500 mg | TID | 10–14 |
| Concomitant therapy | Clarithromycin 500 mg | BID | 10–14 |
| | Amoxicillin 1 g | BID | 10–14 |
| | Nitroimidazole 500 mg | BID | 10–14 |
| Levofloxacin triple therapy | Levofloxacin 500 mg | QD | 10–14 |
| | Amoxicillin 1 g | BID | |

Adapted from Chey WD, Leontiadis GI, Howden C, et al. ACG clinical guideline: treatment of *Helicobacter pylori* infection. *Am J Gastroenterol*. 2017;112:212–238.

ªAll regimens must include a PPI (either once or twice daily)

otherwise healthy. The risk of endoscopy in older adult patients with cardiac, pulmonary, or other systemic disease depends on disease severity. The decision to perform endoscopy should be made on a case-by-case basis.

Clinicians should have a low threshold for repeat endoscopy in older patients with gastric ulcers to confirm ulcer healing and to exclude malignancy, because initial biopsies for gastric cancer can have a sensitivity as low as 70%.

## Management

The management of PUD will depend partially on the presenting symptom, stability of the patient, and the underlying etiology.

Patients who present with bleeding or whose history and examination are at all suggestive of peritonitis should be referred to the emergency department for urgent medical, endoscopic, and possibly surgical treatment.

❖ **PPIs are the standard of care for the treatment of PUD.**

Once a presumptive (or definitive) diagnosis of PUD is made, PPI therapy should be instituted in all patients. In the emergent setting, intravenous PPIs should be used. In patients who are bleeding, PPIs neutralize the gastric pH, thereby allowing platelet aggregation and clot formation over the ulcer. In all patients, the removal of chronic acid exposure allows for ulcer healing. Multiple studies and metaanalysis show that PPIs markedly increase the rates of ulcer healing, are more effective than any other class of

gastroprotective medications, and prevent recurrent PUD or PUD-induced bleeding.[31] The duration of PPI use as well as the possibility of a repeat upper endoscopy to confirm ulcer healing depends on the severity of the presentation. Patients should be reassessed for resolution of symptoms or endoscopic proof of healing between 4 to 8 weeks and, if possible, the PPI should be tapered off.[32]

In all patients, the underlying cause of the peptic ulcer should be identified to prevent ulcer recurrence. *H. pylori* testing should be performed in all patients. Multiple treatment options exist and the choice of the antibiotic regimen will depend on the patient allergies, prior antibiotic exposure, and local resistance patterns (Table 50.2).[33] Approximately 20% of patients fail first-line treatment regimens.[34] Therefore all patients should be tested to confirm eradication after treatment with stool or breath testing. Patients with persistent infection should receive an alternative medication regimen and then undergo repeat testing. Culture and sensitivity of biopsy samples are difficult to perform and are of limited utility; empiric treatment with standard regimens is recommended.

Patients in whom NSAIDs are the presumed cause of ulcer formation should reduce or eliminate their NSAID exposure if possible. If NSAID avoidance is not possible, COX-2 selective inhibitors should be considered. Multiple trials have shown that COX-2 inhibitors reduce the risk of gastroduodenal toxicity when compared to nonselective NSAIDs (23726390). Patients who cannot avoid chronic NSAID use should be placed on prophylactic acid suppression with a PPI as this appears to reduce the risk of PUD and bleeding recurrence. The optimal dosing of PPIs for chemoprevention has not been clarified and low doses are often used.

## Summary

PUD is defined by acid peptic injury of the digestive tract, resulting in loss of the mucosal layer. Although common, the causes of PUD are changing in incidence as the primary cause worldwide, *H. pylori* infection, becomes less prevalent and NSAID use, the second major cause of PUD, increases, especially in the older adult population. The range of presenting symptoms varies greatly, from the asymptomatic patient with incidentally found iron deficiency from occult bleeding, to pain, to overt bleeding and even perforation. Treatment includes medical management with PPIs, endoscopic treatment of bleeding lesions, testing and treatment of *H. pylori*, and avoidance of NSAIDs when possible.

## Key References

2. Christmas C, Rogus-Pulia N. Swallowing disorders in the older population. *J Am Geriatr Soc.* 2019;67:2643–2649.

6. Katz PO, Gerson LB, Vela MF. Guidelines for the diagnosis and management of gastroesophageal reflux disease. *Am J Gastroenterol.* 2013;108(3):308–328.

7. Pilotto A, Maggi S, Noale M, et al. Association of upper gastrointestinal symptoms with functional and clinical characteristics in elderly. *World J Gastroenterol.* 2011;17 (25):3020–3026.

11. Haastrup PF, Thompson W, Søndergaard J, et al. Side Effects of long-term proton pump inhibitor use: a review. *Basic Clin Pharmacol Toxicol.* 2018;123(2):114–121.

21. Sung JJ, Kuipers EJ, El-Serag HB. Systematic review: the global incidence and prevalence of peptic ulcer disease. *Aliment Pharmacol Ther.* 2009;29(9):938–946.

32. Chey WD, Leontiadis GI, Howden CW, et al. ACG Clinical guideline: treatment of helicobacter pylori Infection. *Am J Gastroenterol.* 2017;112(2):212–239.

**References available online at** expertconsult.com.

# 51

# Benign Prostate Disease

LISA J. GRANVILLE AND NIHARIKA SUCHAK

## OBJECTIVES

*Upon completion of this chapter, the reader will be able to:*

- Describe the clinical anatomy, physiology, and age-related changes of the prostate.
- Describe common lower urinary tract symptoms (LUTS) in an aging male.
- Know how to diagnose benign prostatic hyperplasia (BPH).

- Delineate the treatment options for BPH.
- Understand the framework for the diagnosis and treatment of prostatitis.

## Incidence and Prevalence

This chapter reviews the two common benign conditions of the prostate gland: benign prostatic hyperplasia (BPH) and prostatitis. With advancing age, the prevalence of prostate diseases increases dramatically. Self-reported prostate disease affects about 3 million American men. BPH develops in more than half of men age $\geq 65$ years and affects the overwhelming majority of men older than age 85 years. The prevalence of prostatitis is similar to that of ischemic heart disease or diabetes mellitus.

### CASE 1

**Ben Proctor (Part 1)**

Ben Proctor is a 68-year-old man who comes to your office asking for "something to stop me from going so often." He notes being unable to hold his urine for very long once he has an urge to void and arising three to four times each night to urinate. He is often tired in the morning because the frequent nighttime voiding interferes with his sleep. He is concerned that his urinary symptoms cause interruptions in his daily golf game. He drinks an energy drink about three times a day and has an evening cocktail four or five times a week.

His past medical history is remarkable for occasional constipation (he uses a stool softener two to three times a month), osteoarthritis of the knee which he manages with Tylenol extra strength two to three times a week, and bilateral cataracts for which he limits night driving. He takes a daily multivitamin and uses Stay Awake alertness pills about four times a month when his sleep has been significantly interrupted.

1. What initial evaluation and management would you recommend for Mr. Proctor's lower urinary tract symptoms?

## Risk Factors and Pathophysiology

### Overview of Anatomy and Physiology, Including Age-Related Changes

The male lower urinary tract is composed of the urinary bladder, prostate, and urethra. The prostate gland is an accessory gland of the male reproductive system. The retroperitoneal organ is located anterior to the rectum and encircles the neck of the urinary bladder and part of the urethra. Its main function is to produce fluid for semen, which transports sperm. A healthy adult prostate is walnut shaped with an average size of 20 g.

Upon gross appearance, the prostate includes a base and an apex. The base of the prostate is near the inferior surface of the bladder, and a large part of the base is continuous with the bladder wall. The apex or lower end of the prostate is adjacent to the external urethral sphincter.

The prostate is a collection of 30 to 50 irregularly shaped tubuloalveolar glands that open into the prostatic urethra via separate branching ducts. These glands are embedded in fibromuscular stroma, dense with collagen, and irregularly arranged smooth muscle. The outer layer of the prostate is a thin, indistinct fibroelastic capsule mixed with smooth muscle. Age-related changes in the prostate, such as glandular enlargement, increased smooth muscle tone, and decreased compliance secondary to altered collagen deposition, can lead to urinary symptoms.

The prostate is divided into four lobes. The anterior lobe lies in front of the urethra and consists of fibromuscular tissue. The median lobe is situated between the two ejaculatory ducts and the urethra. The right and left lateral lobes make up the bulk of the prostate and are separated by the prostatic urethra. The posterior lobe is the medial part of the lateral lobes and can be palpated through the rectum during digital rectal examination (DRE).

The prostate can be divided histologically into three concentric zones: the peripheral zone (the outermost area of the prostate that constitutes 70% of the glandular tissue), the central zone (which represents 25% of the glandular tissue), and the transitional zone (the innermost area that rests next to the urethra and constitutes 5% of the glandular tissue). This distribution of zones has clinical significance. The peripheral zone is the area that is palpated on DRE, is most commonly affected by chronic prostatitis, and is where 70% of adenocarcinomas are found. BPH commonly arises in the transitional zone.

The white serous prostatic fluid contains acid phosphatase, citric acid, zinc, prostate-specific antigen (PSA), and other protease and fibrolytic enzymes involved in liquefaction of semen. With aging, there is an increase in the number and calcification of prostatic concretions (mixture of prostatic secretions and debris from degenerated epithelial cells). It is postulated that prostatic concretions serve as a nidus for development of chronic bacterial prostatitis.

The prostate is under neurohormonal influence; alpha-1 adrenergic receptors are the predominant type of adrenergic receptors present in the smooth muscle of the prostate and help maintain urethral tone and intraurethral pressure. Testosterone is converted to dihydrotestosterone (DHT) by 5-alpha-reductase in prostatic stromal cells. Androgen stimulation of glandular tissue via DHT contributes to the development and growth of the prostate gland and may lead to BPH. The prostate gland enlarges during a man's life via multiple growth spurts, with the last growth phase starting when a man is in his 50s. Problems with urinary flow usually appear only after the age of 50 years as a consequence of the final growth phase. There is some evidence to suggest that the relative increase in circulating estrogen associated with aging may strengthen the effect of DHT on the prostate with promotion of cellular growth and glandular enlargement.

The pathophysiology of urinary symptoms associated with BPH can be attributed to both static and dynamic factors. The static component is a result of the enlargement of the prostate impinging upon the prostatic urethra and bladder outlet, whereas the dynamic component is related to the tension of prostatic smooth muscle. The static component may cause urinary symptoms because of excessive growth of the glandular tissue in the periurethral zone or stromal tissue in the transition zone. The direction of growth of glandular tissue can affect urinary flow. Growth toward the inside will probably cause direct urinary flow obstruction. The beginning phase of an outward growth of glandular tissue is less likely to cause urinary flow obstruction. The prostatic capsule may prevent progressive outward expansion of the prostate. Therefore ongoing outward growth may ultimately result in compressive forces on the prostatic urethra. If the prostate can be thought of as a donut, then the hole in the middle of the doughnut becomes smaller by inward growth of tissue and/or inward compression when the capsule restricts outward expansion. Thus the size of the prostate as detected by a DRE, which correlates with outward growth, may not correlate with urinary flow symptoms. In addition, an increase in the tone of prostatic smooth muscle may lead to obstructive urinary symptoms without any prostate enlargement.

Voiding of urine is a synchronized action between the bladder and urethra. The bladder is innervated by parasympathetic nerves and their stimulation causes bladder muscle contraction leading to voiding of urine. Stimulation of sympathetic nerves that innervate the bladder neck and prostate causes closure of the bladder outlet. A voluntary sphincter in the bladder neck, supplied by the pudendal nerve and controlled by the higher cortical centers and diencephalons, enables conscious control of urine voiding. Multiple factors, including changes in the bladder, prostate, and/or urethra, can lead to voiding dysfunction in an aging male.

◆◆ **LUTS can occur from a variety of conditions within and outside of the urinary tract; a diagnostic evaluation is necessary to determine etiology.**

## Clinical Manifestations

Historically, prostatism and symptoms of BPH have been used to describe LUTS in men. Although the term *prostatism* implies a prostatic cause for urinary symptoms, frequently no evidence exists for such an implication. LUTS are very common both in older adult men and women. BPH is a precise histologic term, yet many older men with LUTS are described as suffering from the symptoms of BPH or from clinical BPH without this level of diagnostic evaluation. The use of the specific histologic term is confusing in routine clinical practice.

The preferred term, *LUTS*, describes patients' complaints without implying their cause. This is important because the symptoms are not gender, age, or disease specific. Transient causes of LUTS include drugs, dietary factors, restricted mobility, constipation, infection, inflammation, polyuria, and psychological causes. Stimulation of the alpha-1 adrenergic receptors in the smooth muscle of the stroma and capsule of the prostate, as well as in the bladder neck, can cause an increase in smooth muscle tone, which can worsen LUTS.

Diseases that originate from the lower urinary tract (prostatic and nonprostatic diseases) and diseases that do not originate from the lower urinary tract (such as those that can affect the neural control of voiding mechanisms [e.g., diabetes mellitus, cerebrovascular accident, Parkinson disease, multiple sclerosis, and spinal cord injury]) can affect the primary structures and systems involved with voiding and lead to LUTS.

Histologically, BPH is categorized as a hyperplastic process that results in enlargement of the prostate that may cause restriction in the flow of urine from the bladder. Subsequently obstruction induces bladder wall changes, such as thickening, increase in trabeculations, and irritability, that contribute to LUTS. Increased bladder sensitivity (detrusor overactivity [DO]) occurs even with small volumes of urine in the bladder. The bladder may gradually weaken and lose the ability to empty completely, leading to increased residual urine volume and, possibly, acute or chronic urinary retention.

The International Continence Society has published standard terminology to define symptoms, signs, urodynamic observations, and conditions associated with lower urinary tract dysfunction.[1] LUTS are divided into three groups: storage, voiding, and postmicturition symptoms. Storage (irritative) symptoms include increased daytime frequency (voiding too often during the day), nocturia (to wake at night one or more times to void), urgency (sudden urge to urinate that is difficult to defer), incontinence (complaint of any involuntary leakage of urine), and bladder sensation (defined by five categories: normal, increased, reduced, absent, and nonspecific). Voiding (obstructive) symptoms are experienced during the voiding phase and include a slow stream (perception of reduced urine flow), splitting or spraying (character of stream), intermittent stream (urine flow that starts and stops), hesitancy (difficulty in initiating micturition), straining (muscular effort used to initiate, maintain, or improve the urinary stream), and terminal dribble (prolonged final part of micturition, when flow has slowed to a trickle/dribble). Postmicturition symptoms are experienced immediately after micturition and include a feeling of incomplete emptying (sensation of not emptying the bladder completely after finishing urinating) and postmicturition dribble (involuntary loss of urine immediately after completion of urination, usually after leaving the toilet in men, or after rising from the toilet in women).

---

### CASE 1

#### Ben Proctor (Part 2)

Mr. Proctor's initial assessment reveals urinary frequency, urgency, nocturia, and straining with an International Prostate Symptom Score (IPSS) of 12. DRE reveals normal sphincter tone, prostate about 20 g with no asymmetry or nodules. Urinalysis is unremarkable. You educate Mr. Proctor about LUTS, discuss transient causes, including caffeine and alcohol, and recommend discontinuation of Stay Awake alertness pills, avoidance of fluids 2 hours before bedtime, and dietary modifications with use of a bladder diary to help him identify triggers.

---

Two months later at a follow-up visit Mr. Proctor reports his frequency, urgency, and nocturia are much improved, with an IPSS of 5. He notes, "Now I can spend time with my friends and play a round of golf without worrying."

1. How frequently will Mr. Proctor need to be monitored for BPH? When would it be appropriate to initiate BPH medication?
2. Medications should always be considered in the differential diagnosis as a cause of LUTS or worsening BPH symptoms.

---

## Benign Prostatic Hyperplasia: Differential Diagnosis and Assessment

The diagnosis of BPH in men is typically clinical, and one of exclusion. When a urinary symptom is noted, a standardized questionnaire, such as the IPSS, is used to quantify the severity of LUTS (Fig. 51.1). The IPSS assesses seven symptoms during the past month. The questions address the following factors: feeling of incomplete bladder emptying, frequency, intermittency, urgency, weak stream, straining, and nocturia; each is rated on the scale where 0 = none and 5 = almost always. The symptom categories are based on the summative score: 0–7 mild, 8–19 moderate, and 20–35 severe.

Other possible contributors are queried, such as endocrine (e.g., poorly controlled diabetes), neurologic (e.g., neurogenic bladder), symptoms of urinary tract infection, and previous urologic conditions (e.g., urethral stricture, bladder neck contracture, interstitial cystitis). Although nonspecific for BPH, DRE is performed to rule out other conditions. The prostate size, tenderness, and presence of nodules are noted. Because hyperplasia may only involve the transitional zone, the DRE can be unremarkable, or it may reveal an enlarged, smooth, rubbery, symmetric gland. Lower abdominal/suprapubic palpation may identify a distended bladder. Urinalysis is routinely performed to evaluate for urinary tract infection, hematuria, and glycosuria; BPH is associated with an unremarkable urinalysis.

❖ **Lifestyle modifications can be effective in reducing urinary symptoms, and bladder diaries often assist a person in making these changes.**

Additional tests are considered optional and are based on clinical indications. If urinary retention is suspected, postvoid residual urine volume (often done by office or bedside bladder scan) is performed. Serum creatinine measurement may be used to assess kidney function and the possibility of obstructive uropathy and/or intrinsic renal disease. Pressure-flow urodynamic studies are commonly performed before surgical interventions. These tests can also be considered when the diagnosis is uncertain.

## Benign Prostatic Hyperplasia: Management

The initiation of BPH therapy depends on the patient and is driven by the effect of the symptoms on the patient's quality of life (Table 51.1 and Fig. 51.2). All patients should be educated regarding lifestyle modification. Men with mild to moderate symptoms may be satisfied with lifestyle modification only. Both medical and surgical treatments are also available, with medication the usual first approach. Indications for surgical treatment include patient preference, dissatisfaction with medication, and refractory urinary retention. Complications from prostatic obstruction, including

## INTERNATIONAL PROSTATE SYMPTOM SCORE (I-PSS)

Patient name: _____ Date of birth: _____ Date completed: _____

| In the past month: | Not at all | Less than 1 in 5 times | Less than half the time | About half the time | More than half the time | Almost always | Your score |
|---|---|---|---|---|---|---|---|
| **1. Incomplete emptying** How often have you had the sensation of not emptying your bladder? | 0 | 1 | 2 | 3 | 4 | 5 | |
| **2. Frequency** How often have you had to urinate less than every two hours? | 0 | 1 | 2 | 3 | 4 | 5 | |
| **3. Intermittency** How often have you found you stopped and started again several times when you urinated? | 0 | 1 | 2 | 3 | 4 | 5 | |
| **4. Urgency** How often have you found it difficult to postpone urination? | 0 | 1 | 2 | 3 | 4 | 5 | |
| **5. Weak stream** How often have you had a weak urinary stream? | 0 | 1 | 2 | 3 | 4 | 5 | |
| **6. Straining** How often have you had to strain to start urination? | 0 | 1 | 2 | 3 | 4 | 5 | |
| | **None** | **1 Time** | **2 Times** | **3 Times** | **4 Times** | **5 Times** | |
| **7. Nocturia** How many times did you typically get up at night to urinate? | 0 | 1 | 2 | 3 | 4 | 5 | |
| **Total IPSS score** | | | | | | | |

Score: 1–7: *Mild*    8–19: *Moderate*    20–35: *Severe*

| Quality of life due to urinary symptoms | Delighted | Pleased | Mostly satisfied | Mixed | Mostly dissatisfied | Unhappy | Terrible |
|---|---|---|---|---|---|---|---|
| If you were to spend the rest of your life with your urinary condition just the way it is now, how would you feel about that? | 0 | 1 | 2 | 3 | 4 | 5 | 6 |

• **Figure 51.1** The International Prostate Symptom Score (IPSS) is based on the answers to seven questions related to lower urinary tract symptoms. Each symptom is scored 0 to 5 for a possible total score between 0 and 35. Question 8 refers to the patient's perceived quality of life but is not included in the scoring of the IPSS. The IPSS is similar to the American Urological Association's Symptom Index. (From Barry M, Fowler FJ, O'Leary MP, et al. The American Urological Association Symptom index for benign prostatic hyperplasia. *J Urol.* 1992;148:1549–1557.)

renal dysfunction, bladder stones, recurrent urinary tract infections, and hematuria, are also managed surgically. The selection of surgical approach is dependent on patient anatomy and the surgeon's experience, as well as the potential benefits and risks for complications.

## Lifestyle Interventions and Self-Management

BPH is a chronic condition with symptoms that impact men's quality of life. As with other chronic conditions, patients benefit from self-management interventions (SMIs) that empower the individual's involvement and control of treatment. SMI helps patients learn what to do and develops their belief in their own ability to use knowledge and skills toward achieving realistic, desired outcomes. SMI has been shown to be effective in men with BPH LUTS as an alternative to initial pharmacologic management and as adjuvant therapy for men who are using alpha-blockers.[2,3] Three major categories for LUTS SMI are (1) education and reassurance, (2) lifestyle modification, and (3) behavioral interventions.

| TABLE 51.1 | Management Options for Benign Prostatic Hyperplasia | | | |
|---|---|---|---|---|

| Category | Interventions | Rationale | Comments | Level of Evidence for Effectiveness[a] |
|---|---|---|---|---|
| Self-management interventions | Education and reassurance, lifestyle modification (reduce nighttime fluids to manage nocturia; eliminate dietary diuretics, such as caffeine, alcohol), behavioral interventions (e.g., bladder retraining) | Empowers individuals to comanage chronic condition; factors outside the urinary tract contribute to urinary symptoms | Often sufficient management for mild symptoms; complements management for moderate to severe symptoms | A |
| Pharmacologic management | Alpha-blockers: terazosin, doxazosin, tamsulosin, silodosin, alfuzosin | Works on dynamic component: relaxation of smooth muscle in prostate and bladder neck decreases resistance to urinary flow | Considered to have equal clinical effectiveness | A |
| | 5-alpha-reductase inhibitors: finasteride, dutasteride | Works on static component: reduced tissue levels of dihydrotestosterone result in prostate gland size reduction | Most effective for men with large prostates ($> 40$ g); results may not be evident for up to 6 months | A |
| | Combination therapy: alpha-blockers and 5-alpha-reductase inhibitors | Over several years of combined treatment slower progression of BPH than when each used alone | Most effective for men with large prostates ($> 40$ g) | A |
| | Combination therapy: alpha-blockers and anticholinergics | Combined with alpha-blockers, inhibition of muscarinic receptors in the bladder relieves irritative voiding symptoms (frequency, urgency, nocturia) | Low risk of urinary retention in men with a postvoid residual volume $<250$ mL | A |
| | Phosphodiesterase-5 inhibitors | Sexual dysfunction is prevalent in aging men with LUTS associated with BPH; underlying mechanisms have not been determined | Tadalafil is the only FDA-approved agent; combination with alpha-blockers has not been studied and may trigger hypotension | B |
| Phytotherapy | Variety of agents available: *Urticae radix, Secale cereale, Serenoa repens, Pygeum africanum* | Complementary and alternative medicine use is common practice | These agents are well tolerated but appear comparable to placebo | *Serenoa repens*: X Others: C |
| Surgery | Transurethral resection of the prostate; transurethral incision of the prostate; open prostatectomy; transurethral microwave thermotherapy or laser | Removal or expansion of periurethral prostate tissue reduces obstruction to urinary flow | Considered to have equal clinical effectiveness; indicated for complications of prostate obstruction: recurrent urinary tract infections, hematuria, bladder stones, renal insufficiency | A |

*BPH,* Benign prostatic hyperplasia; *FDA,* US Food and Drug Administration.

[a]*A,* Supported by one or more high-quality randomized clinical trials (RCTs); *B,* supported by one or more high-quality nonrandomized cohort studies or low-quality RCTs; *C,* supported by one or more case series and/or poor-quality cohort and/or case-control studies; *D,* supported by expert opinion and/or extrapolation from studies in other populations or settings; *X,* evidence supports the treatment being ineffective or harmful.

Education and reassurance provides knowledge about male anatomy and the relationship of the bladder and enlarged prostate to voiding symptoms. Patients are reassured that LUTS commonly occur in the absence of cancer. Illustrations and written information facilitate understanding and retention of information. Group settings can also be used for providing education and sharing effective strategies.

Lifestyle modifications address avoiding caffeine and alcohol and the timing of fluid intake, such as avoiding fluids 2 hours before bedtime if bothersome nocturia is present. Dietary factors

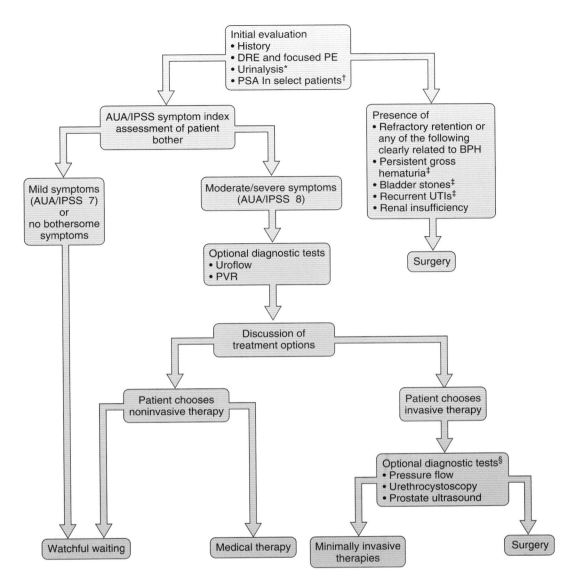

• **Figure 51.2** Algorithm for evaluation and treatment of BPH. *AUA*, American Urological Association; *BPH*, benign prostatic hyperplasia; *DRE*, digital rectal exam; *IPSS*, International Prostate Symptom Score; *PE*, physical exam; *PSA*, prostate-specific antigen; *PVR*, postvoid residual urine; *UTI*, urinary tract infection. *In patients with clinically significant prostatic bleeding, a course of a 5-alpha-reductase inhibitor may be used. If bleeding persists, tissue ablative surgery is indicated. [†]Patients with at least a 10-year life expectancy for whom knowledge of the presence of prostate cancer would change management or patients for whom the PSA measurement may change the management of voiding symptoms. [‡]After exhausting other therapeutic options as discussed in detail in the text. [§]Some diagnostic tests are used in predicting response to therapy. Pressure-flow studies are most useful in men before surgery. (Modified from American Urological Association. © 2003 American Urological Association Education and Research, Inc.)

may also include avoiding bladder irritants, such as carbonated beverages and artificial sweeteners.[4] Bladder diaries document urinary frequency, volume, and circumstances surrounding urinary symptoms and can assist individuals in identifying lifestyle contributors. Education regarding medications is also provided. Medication review may lead to adjustment of existing therapy, such as timing of diuretics to reduce nocturia. Patients are informed about BPH medical therapy and how to adjust medication dosing to improve LUTS at times of greatest inconvenience, such as when traveling.

Behavioral interventions address voiding habits, replacing maladaptive behaviors with more healthful approaches. For example, patients with urgency may void at inappropriately short intervals to stay ahead of the urge and as a result diminish bladder capacity.

Bladder retraining is used to appropriately lengthen the time between voids.

## CASE 1

### Ben Proctor (Part 3)

It is 7 years later, and Mr. Proctor is in your office for an annual visit. Over the past year he has noticed progressive slowing of his urinary stream, difficulty initiating urination, a sense of incomplete emptying, increased frequency of urination, and awakening to void three to four times per night; his IPSS score is 16. Mr. Proctor used a bladder diary and was unable to identify any triggers. He started using saw palmetto herbal therapy 3 months ago but is unsure if his urinary symptoms are improved. He reports his cataracts are

worse and his blurry vision now also interferes with golfing. On physical examination, there is no suprapubic fullness or tenderness, and the prostate is about 25 g without discrete nodules or tenderness.
1. Before initiating medication, what further evaluation would you recommend for Mr. Proctor?

## Medical Therapy

### Alpha-Blockers

When patients do not wish to pursue lifestyle modifications, or have an insufficient response, medical therapies are available for BPH. Medications have become the first-line treatment for most patients with BPH. The two main pharmacologic approaches are alpha-adrenergic antagonist and 5-alpha-reductase inhibitor therapy. Anticholinergic agents may be used when irritative symptoms of LUTS predominate.

Alpha-adrenergic antagonists, or alpha-blockers, are directed at the dynamic component of urethral obstruction. Smooth muscle of the prostate and bladder neck has a resting tone mediated by alpha-adrenergic innervation. Alpha-blockers relax the smooth muscle in the hyperplastic prostate tissue, prostate capsule, and bladder neck, thus decreasing resistance to urinary flow. Of the two major alpha-adrenergic receptors, alpha-1 receptors predominate in the prostate. Alpha-blockade development for BPH therapy progressed from a selective alpha-1 agent (e.g., prazosin) to long-acting selective alpha-1 agents (terazosin, doxazosin) that allowed once-a-day dosing but still required blood pressure monitoring and dose titration to reduce orthostatic hypotension. Initially it was thought that the effects on blood pressure would allow treatment of two common conditions, hypertension and BPH, with one drug. Subsequently, the Antihypertensive and Lipid-Lowering Treatment to Prevent Heart Attack Trial (ALLHAT) demonstrated that alpha-blockers were inferior to other classes of antihypertensive agents as first-line therapy.[5] Therefore these two common conditions tend to be treated independently.

With the understanding that the alpha-1A subtype comprises 70% of the prostate receptors, the development of more targeted therapy was attempted.[6] Tamsulosin, the first alpha-1A subtype selective agent released, has the advantage of minimal effects on blood pressure thus avoiding the need for dose titration, but it has a side effect of ejaculatory dysfunction.[7] Alfuzosin, originally thought to be alpha-1A subtype selective, with additional testing was found to lack this selectivity. However, like tamsulosin, it offers once daily dosing without affecting blood pressure. In addition, alfuzosin appears to have no effect on ejaculation.[8] Silodosin is highly selective of the alpha-1A receptor. Compared with tamsulosin's 9.55 times selectivity for alpha-1A versus alpha-1B, silodosin is 162 times more alpha-1A selective.[9] Silodosin has an excellent cardiovascular safety profile but causes ejaculatory dysfunction in almost one-third of patients.[10]

Evidence has shown that alpha-blockers relieve LUTS via mechanisms in addition to prostate smooth muscle relaxation. As a result, the effectiveness and adverse effects of these medications cannot be predicted solely by how well they target alpha-1A subtype receptors. The most common adverse events of alpha-1 agents are dizziness, mild asthenia (fatigue or weakness), and abnormal ejaculation. For patients undergoing cataract surgery, intraoperative floppy iris syndrome (IFIS) is a potential risk of all alpha-blockers. IFIS is characterized by sudden intraoperative iris prolapse and pupil constriction and may result in surgical complications, such as iris damage, torn lens capsules, and vitreous prolapse. The greatest frequency and severity of IFIS has been reported among those using tamsulosin.[11] Moreover it has been shown that IFIS can occur more than 1 year after tamsulosin has been discontinued.[12] It is suggested that men with plans for cataract surgery delay initiation of alpha-blockers until surgery is completed. Alternatively, men who have already used alpha-blockers should advise their ophthalmologists, so this can be factored into planning for cataract surgery.

The five long-acting alpha-1 selective blockers, namely terazosin, doxazosin, tamsulosin, alfuzosin, and silodosin, are approved by the US Food and Drug Administration (FDA) for the treatment of symptomatic LUTS arising from BPH and are considered to have equal clinical effectiveness.[13] All five of these medications have the convenience of once-daily dosing. Side effect profiles are generally similar except that alfuzosin appears less likely to cause ejaculatory dysfunction. Terazosin and doxazosin are less costly, older, generic options but require dose titration and blood pressure monitoring.

### 5-Alpha-Reductase Inhibitors

The enzyme 5-alpha-reductase is required for the conversion of testosterone to the more active dihydrotestosterone. Finasteride and dutasteride are inhibitors of 5-alpha-reductase and reduce tissue levels of dihydrotestosterone, thus reducing prostate gland size, the static component of urethral obstruction. Improvements in LUTS scores and urine flow rates may not be evident for up to 6 months. The 5-alpha-reductase inhibitors are most effective in men with larger prostates (> 40 g, about the size of a plum).[14] The reduction in prostate size results in decreased risk of acute urinary retention and delay of BPH-related surgery.[15,16] Finasteride has been shown to suppress prostatic vascular endothelial growth factor and reduce or cease recurrent hematuria related to BPH.[17] Dutasteride is thought to function in a similar fashion.[13]

Finasteride and dutasteride have similar clinical efficacy and side effects.[18] Side effects are primarily sexual and include decreased libido, erectile dysfunction, and ejaculation dysfunction. Less often, gynecomastia and breast tenderness occur. Sexual side effects may persist after discontinuation of the medication. These medications are not to be handled by pregnant women because of the possibility of absorption and subsequent risk to a male fetus.[19]

Because 5-alpha-reductase inhibitors reduce serum PSA levels by an average of 50%, after 6 months of therapy, men receiving prostate cancer surveillance will need a new baseline serum PSA determination.[14] The primary prevention of prostate cancer with 5-alpha-reductase inhibitors showed unexpected results; while less cases of prostate cancer occurred, there was a higher unexplained incidence of more aggressive cancers.[20]

❖ **Patients determine the level of bother from lower urinary symptoms and guide treatment initiation and selection between medications and surgery.**

### Combination Therapy: Alpha-Blockers and 5-Alpha-Reductase Inhibitors

Combinations of doxazosin and finasteride, as well as tamsulosin and dutasteride, have been studied.[21,22] When used together over several years, the combination of alpha-adrenergic antagonists with 5-alpha-reductase inhibitors has been shown to be safe and to reduce clinical progression of BPH better than either agent alone. In particular, a lower risk of urinary retention, urinary incontinence, renal insufficiency, and recurrent bladder infections is associated with combination therapy. Higher rates of side effects occur with combination therapy compared with either agent used alone. As with 5-alpha-reductase inhibitors, the benefits of combination therapy are best realized by men with large prostates.

### Combination Therapy: Alpha-Blockers and Anticholinergic Medications

Anticholinergic agents (e.g., oxybutynin, tolterodine) inhibit muscarinic receptors in the detrusor muscle and relieve irritative voiding symptoms. Commonly used for overactive bladder, the use of anticholinergics was discouraged in patients with BPH because of concerns of causing urinary retention. Several randomized controlled trials have now shown that anticholinergics can be safely used in combination with alpha-blockers.[23,24] These trials demonstrated a low risk (about 3%) of urinary retention in men who had a postvoid residual volume of < 250 mL. The use of anticholinergics as monotherapy for BPH LUTS has not shown clinical benefit. Common side effects of anticholinergics include dry mouth, dry eyes, and constipation.

### Phosphodiesterase-5 Inhibitors

Phosphodiesterase-5 inhibitors, initially approved for the treatment of erectile dysfunction, have been studied for the treatment of LUTS. Compared with placebo, the daily use of sildenafil, tadalafil, or vardenafil demonstrated improvement in both erectile function and IPSS scores.[25] Although relief of urinary symptoms was reported, no improvement in peak urinary flow rate was demonstrated. When phosphodiesterase-5 inhibitors were used in combination with alpha-blockers, peak urinary flow rate increased beyond that achieved with alpha-blockers alone. Side effects from phosphodiesterase-5 inhibitors include headache, dyspepsia, and back pain. Presently only tadalafil is FDA approved for the treatment of BPH-associated urinary symptoms in men with or without erectile dysfunction.

## Phytotherapy

The use of plants and herbs for the treatment of BPH is common although there are limited data to support this practice. Most clinical trials indicate that these agents are well tolerated and comparable to placebo. However, common methodologic concerns among studies of phytotherapy include small numbers of participants, short study duration, varied doses and preparations, and lack of or inconsistent use of standardized, validated measures of efficacy.[26–28] Some examples of phytotherapy for BPH-associated LUTS include *Urticae radix* (stinging nettle root), *Secale cereale* (rye grass pollen), *Serenoa repens* (saw palmetto), and *Pygeum africanum* (African plum tree). *Serenoa repens* has been well studied and serves as an example of the type of data available for phytotherapies. Limited data from smaller studies suggested that *Serenoa repens* improves urinary symptoms and flow measures in men with BPH. However, a 2012 Cochrane review that included 32 randomized controlled studies involving 5666 men found that compared with placebo, *Serenoa repens* monotherapy does not improve urinary symptoms or maximum urinary flow rate even at double and triple the usual dose.[29]

## Surgical Therapy

The surgical approaches for managing LUTS of BPH are constantly evolving. Surgical approaches offer the best chance for symptom improvement but also have the highest rates of complications. The benefits of various surgical treatments are generally considered equivalent, but complication rates and retreatment rates differ. Because medications have evolved as first-line therapy, the indications for surgery have shifted toward moderate to severe LUTS refractory to medical therapy, coupled with abnormal objective parameters, such as impaired flow rate and increased residual volume.[30]

Transurethral resection of the prostate (TURP), in use for over 90 years, is the standard of care to which other BPH surgical treatments are compared. TURP has a high success rate for improving symptoms, urinary flow, and postvoid residual with low retreatment rates.[31] Usually performed under spinal anesthesia, TURP involves passage of an endoscope through the urethra to surgically remove the inner portion of the prostate. Long-term complications can include retrograde ejaculation, bladder neck contracture, and erectile dysfunction. One unique complication of TURP is TUR syndrome, a dilutional hyponatremia resulting from systemic absorption of irrigant solution. The development of a bipolar generator (bipolar TURP) to replace the conventional monopolar TURP allows the use of isotonic irrigating fluids and eliminates the risk of electrolyte disturbance.[32]

Transurethral incision of the prostate (TUIP) is an endoscopic procedure via the urethra to make one or two cuts in the prostate and prostate capsule, relieving urethral constriction. Limited to use in small prostate glands (<30 g), TUIP results in lower rates of retrograde ejaculation but higher rates of requiring secondary procedures.[13]

Open prostatectomy involves removal of the inner portion of the prostate, while leaving the outer capsule, through a retropubic or suprapubic incision. Currently, open prostatectomy is reserved for patients with larger prostates (> 80 g) or with complicating conditions, such as bladder stones or diverticula.[13,33] Open prostatectomy is associated with incisional morbidity, longer hospitalization, and greater risk of erectile dysfunction. These risks can be reduced by using less invasive robot-assisted techniques for simple prostatectomy, but high costs of this technology may limit its application.[34]

With advancing technologies, a variety of surgical approaches have evolved in an effort to maintain the efficacy of TURP while reducing the associated risks. Current modalities include transurethral microwave thermotherapy (TUMT), laser vaporization, laser enucleation, and aquablation. These modalities appear to have similar short-term efficacy compared with TURP in improving symptoms and urinary flow rate.[13] There is insufficient evidence to state that any one procedure is superior to the others. National trends in surgical therapy support the growing interest in using minimally invasive therapies and providing care in an outpatient setting. Since the 1990s, the number of TURPs has been steadily declining whereas laser vaporization is the fastest growing modality, with 70% performed as an outpatient procedure.[35]

Three emerging minimally invasive modalities are the prostatic urethral lift (PUL), convective water vapor energy (WAVE) ablation, and prostatic artery embolization (PAE). PUL involves the placement of tissue retracting implants into the lateral lobes of the prostate to open an anterior channel. Predictors of success include prostate gland volume 20 to 70 cm$^3$ and typical lateral lobe obstruction. Relative contraindications include prostate size > 100 cm$^3$, high bladder neck, and protruding middle lobe. PUL has been shown to decrease LUTS, enhance quality of life, and improve urine flow rate with sustained results for up to 5 years. PUL has no negative effects on erectile or ejaculatory function and does not limit any future surgical approaches, such as TURP. WAVE therapy delivers small amounts of steam that damages prostate cells and reduces overall size. Usually one to three injections are given to each lateral lobe. This therapy can be used on the median lobe. WAVE therapy has been shown to decrease LUTS, enhance quality of life, and improve urine flow rate with sustained results for up to 3 years.[36] PAE, used for years as a treatment for prostate-related hematuria, has more recently been used for LUTS caused by BPH. PAE induces ischemia of prostatic tissue with an initial swelling followed by reorganization to a smaller, less dense gland. An advantage of PAE is that it can be used in large glands ($> 80$ cm$^3$). PAE has been shown to decrease LUTS, enhance quality of life, and improve urine flow rate with sustained results for up to 2 years.[37] The American Urological Association recommends that PAE treatment of BPH-related LUTS remain within the context of clinical trials until further data are available.[38]

## Indications for Referral to Specialist

Referral to a urologist is recommended for patients with clinically significant LUTS who fail to adequately respond to medical therapy. Men with complications from BPH, including bladder stones, urinary retention, recurrent urinary tract infections, or renal dysfunction, should also be referred.

---

### CASE 2

#### Blake Lutz (Part 1)

Blake Lutz, a 66-year-old man, comes to your office with persistent LUTS over the past week and a concern about recurrent "bladder infections." His past medical history includes hypertension and BPH with no history of sexually transmitted diseases and no new sexual partners. During the past year, he visited an urgent care center three times for bothersome urinary symptoms (increased urinary urgency, frequency, and sensation of incomplete emptying). Each time a urine specimen was obtained, a 10- to 14-day course of antibiotics was prescribed, and his urinary symptoms resolved.

Physical examination reveals no fever, no abdominal tenderness, and a diffusely enlarged, nontender prostate with no asymmetry or nodules. A recent ultrasound of the bladder at the urgent care center showed postvoid residual volume as 50 mL and no bladder stones. Today his urinalysis reveals 4 red blood cells, 10 white blood cells, and is Gram stain negative. Your review of urine culture reports from the urgent care visits show *Escherichia coli* bacteria grew each time.

1. What would be the next step in the evaluation and management of Mr. Lutz's symptomatology?
2. Are there any additional tests that should be performed?

---

## Prostatitis: Differential Diagnosis and Assessment

Prostatitis is an infection or inflammation of the prostate gland that can present as one of numerous syndromes with variable and nonspecific clinical features. The term *prostatitis* denotes microscopic inflammation of the tissue of the prostate gland and is a diagnosis that covers a wide range of clinical conditions. The differential diagnosis of prostatitis includes acute cystitis, BPH, urinary tract stones, bladder cancer, prostatic abscess, enterovesical fistula, and foreign body within the urinary tract.

The prevalence of prostatitis is estimated at 9% with prostatitis-like symptoms reported from as low as 3% to as high as 16%. Approximately 1% of visits to primary care physicians are related to prostatitis, whereas 8% of all visits to urologists are for prostatitis.[39–41]

The National Institutes of Health's consensus classification of prostatitis includes four categories.[42]
- Category I: Acute bacterial prostatitis
- Category II: Chronic bacterial prostatitis
- Category III: Chronic prostatitis / chronic pelvic pain syndrome (CP/CPPS)
  - Inflammatory
  - Noninflammatory
- Category IV: Asymptomatic inflammatory prostatitis

Bacterial prostatitis is described as either acute or chronic based on the duration of symptoms, with chronic reflecting duration of at least 3 months. Acute and chronic bacterial prostatitis are the most easily recognized but the least common of the prostatitis syndromes. Clinical presentation of acute bacterial prostatitis includes acute symptoms suggestive of a urinary tract infection, such as urinary frequency and dysuria. Symptoms suggestive of a systemic infection such as malaise, fever, and myalgias may also occur.

Patients with chronic bacterial prostatitis have recurring episodes of bacterial urinary tract infection caused by the same organism, usually *E. coli*, another gram-negative organism, or enterococcus. Lower urinary tract cultures performed between symptomatic episodes can be useful in confirming an infected prostate gland as the nidus of these recurrent infections.

An overwhelming majority ($> 90\%$) of symptomatic patients have CP/CPPS. This term acknowledges the partial comprehension of the basis of this syndrome and the possibility that organs other than the prostate gland may have a significant role in its origin.[43,44] The definition of CP/CPPS recognizes urologic pain as a primary symptom component of this syndrome, in the absence of other diagnoses, such as urethritis, urogenital cancer, urinary tract disease, functionally significant urethral stricture, or neurologic disease affecting the bladder. Leukocytes are found in the expressed prostatic secretions, postprostatic massage urine, or semen of patients with the inflammatory subtype of CP/CPPS, whereas patients with the noninflammatory subtype have no evidence of inflammation. CP/CPPS may be the most prevalent of all prostate diseases and it is the most common symptomatic type of prostatitis. The European Association of Urology defines the duration of CP/CPPS as 6 months or longer.[44]

High concentrations of leukocytes in the prostate tissue or seminal fluid are a common incidental finding in patients who undergo evaluation for other genitourinary tract concerns (e.g., during prostate biopsy for evaluation of possible prostate cancer or during evaluation of infertility). Such patients with no corresponding urinary symptoms and no lower urinary tract pain are believed to have asymptomatic inflammatory prostatitis.

## Diagnosis: Initial Evaluation, Physical Examination, Diagnostic Studies

When prostatitis is considered in the differential diagnosis, history should include sexual activity, previous episodes of prostatitis, duration and nature of symptoms and any association with voiding of urine and ejaculation, and impact on function and quality of life.

The typical physical examination will include the abdomen, pelvis, genitalia, including the perineal area, and a DRE of the prostate in addition to other targeted examinations based on the history. Evaluation of the pelvic floor musculature may be completed as part of the clinical examination. A postvoid residual urine volume should be measured if urinary retention is suspected.

Laboratory tests include urinalysis for evidence of inflammation, including blood, leukocytes and leukocyte esterase, and urine culture. Bacteriuria and pyuria indicate infection of the prostate and/or bladder, usually caused by common uropathogenic bacteria, especially *E. coli*. A complete blood count will assist in determining any peripheral leukocytosis, and a blood culture may be performed, if indicated. The four-glass test includes culture and microscopic examination of (1) initial stream urine representing the urethra, (2) midstream urine representing the bladder, (3) expressed prostatic secretion (EPS), and (4) postprostatic massage urine. The preprostatic and postprostatic massage urine evaluation test, a simpler screen of the lower urinary tract, became more popular in the 1990s and is considered a reasonable alternative to the four-glass test for diagnosing prostatitis.[45,46]

Patients with acute bacterial prostatitis have acute onset of symptoms. Clinical presentation may include fever, chills, dysuria, low back pain, or urinary obstruction and a swollen and tender prostate on physical examination. Prostatic massage is contraindicated.

The National Institutes of Health chronic prostatitis symptom index is one of the symptom questionnaires used for the quantification of symptoms in CP/CPPS.[47] The questionnaire contains four questions regarding localization of pain or discomfort, two regarding urination (incomplete emptying, frequency), and three related to quality of life.

### CASE 2

#### Blake Lutz (Part 2)

Mr. Lutz returns for renewal of primary care services 5 years after last being seen. His interval history is remarkable for recurrent urinary tract infections, low back pain, and depression managed by urgent care and a local urologist with several "long courses of antibiotics" without adequate relief. He describes persistent and bothersome symptoms for 2 years: aching pain between his rectal and testicular area, significant pain upon ejaculation, and persistent urinary symptoms (urgency, frequency, and sensation of incomplete emptying). He states "I've had it" with urologists and does not want a referral. Review of systems reveals chronic fatigue, insomnia, poor appetite, and intermittent depressed mood without suicidal ideation.

On physical examination, he is afebrile and appears frustrated and slightly angry at times. He has a normal musculoskeletal and neurosensory examination of his back and legs. Genitourinary examination shows normal nontender testicles and a normal phallus. He has moderate tenderness to palpation of the perineum and a diffusely enlarged, nontender prostate with no asymmetry or nodules. Urinalysis shows no white blood cells or red blood cells, and a bladder scan shows a negligible postvoid residual.

1. How would you treat Mr. Lutz?
2. Would you prescribe antibiotics?

## Prostatitis: Management

### Acute Bacterial Prostatitis

Antimicrobial therapy is essential in the patient with acute bacterial prostatitis. The type and route of antibiotic treatment are determined by the acuity and severity of the symptoms, as well as the other components of the clinical presentation. Acute bacterial prostatitis, when presenting as a serious infection, may require parenteral administration of high doses of a bactericidal antibiotic, which may include a broad-spectrum penicillin, a third-generation cephalosporin, or a fluoroquinolone. An aminoglycoside may be added to the initial therapy. Duration of treatment is based on timing of systemic symptom relief and normalization of infection parameters. In less severe cases, a fluoroquinolone may be given orally for 10 days.

### Chronic Bacterial Prostatitis

Chronic bacterial prostatitis is the most frequent cause of recurrent urinary tract infections in men. A 4- to 6-week course of oral fluoroquinolones may be prescribed after the initial diagnosis in chronic bacterial prostatitis if infection is strongly suspected. Herbal extracts or phosphodiesterase-5 inhibitors when combined with antibiotics may improve symptoms and quality of life. When chronic bacterial prostatitis is caused by *Trichomonas vaginalis*, a 14-day course of metronidazole has been shown effective.[48]

### Chronic Prostatitis/Chronic Pelvic Pain Syndrome

Patients with chronic prostatitis/chronic pelvic pain syndrome (CP/CPPS) are treated empirically with numerous pharmacologic approaches such as analgesics, antiinflammatory agents, antibiotics, and alpha-blockers, and nonpharmacologic approaches such as neural blockade and neural stimulation.[44] Despite numerous studies related to diagnosis and management of CP/CPPS, there is lack of consensus on specific recommendations. An initial approach to a patient with suspected CP/CPPS could be to consider their clinical phenotype in which the symptoms appear to be primarily perceived, and then treat with a multimodal approach. The UPOINT system classifies patients into urinary, psychosocial, organ-specific, infection, neurologic/systemic, and tenderness of muscles domains.[49] A "urinary" patient presenting with urgency, frequency, nocturia, and intermittency may be treated with diet modification, alpha-blockers, and anticholinergics. A "psychosocial" patient with depressive symptoms, stress, and poor coping mechanisms may be treated with cognitive behavioral therapy, meditation, and antidepressants. An "organ specific" patient in whom the prostate has been implicated with prostate tenderness, leukocytosis in the prostatic fluid, and blood in ejaculate could be treated with antiinflammatory medication, acupuncture, or extracorporeal shockwave therapy.[50,51] CP/CPPS represents a diverse group of diseases and therefore the use of many approaches, both pharmacologic and nonpharmacologic, offers the best approach.

⯮⯮ **CP/CPPS is the most common type of prostatitis with long-lasting, difficult-to-resolve symptoms for which patients will access multiple providers. Nonmedication approaches, alpha-blockers, anticholinergics, antibiotics, and combinations of these therapies improve symptoms.**

## Summary

The prevalence of LUTS increases with age. Symptoms in men with an enlarged prostate can be attributed to BPH and managed accordingly after an initial evaluation reveals an absence of other common etiologies, such as medication side effects, urinary tract infection, or diabetes mellitus. The level of bother from LUTS guides initiation and selection of therapy. Evidence of obstruction, such as decreased force of stream, supports the likelihood of benefit from a surgical approach to BPH. Prostatitis symptoms are common in men, chronic symptoms become more prevalent with age, and in > 90% of cases no infectious agent is identified.

National Institute on Aging Health Information Center: www.nia.nih.gov/health.

National Kidney and Urologic Diseases Information Clearinghouse: www.kidney.niddk.nih.gov.

## Web Resources

American Geriatrics Society: www.americangeriatrics.org.

AGS Foundation for Health in Aging: www.healthinaging.org.

## Key References

4. Bradley CS, Erickson BA, Messersmith EE, et al. Evidence of the impact of diet, fluid intake, caffeine, alcohol and tobacco on lower urinary tract symptoms: a systematic review. *J Urol.* 2017;198(5):1010−1020.

14. Alawamlh OAH, Goueli R, Lee R. Lower urinary tract symptoms, benign prostatic hyperplasia, and urinary retention. *Med Clin North Am.* 2018;102:301−311.

36. Magistro G, Weinhold P, Stief G, et al. The new kids on the block: prostatic urethral lift (Urolift) and convective water vapor energy ablation (Rezūm). *Curr Opin Urol.* 2018;28:294−300.

37. Young S, Golzarian J. Prostatic artery embolization for benign prostatic hyperplasia: a review. *Curr Opin Urol.* 2018;28:284−287.

38. Foster HE, Barry MJ, Gandhi M, et al. *Benign Prostatic Hyperplasia: Surgical Management of Benign Prostatic Hyperplasia/Lower Urinary Symptoms (2018, amended 2019).* American Urological Association. Available at: https://www.auanet.org/guidelines/benign-prostatic-hyperplasia-(bph)-guideline. Accessed 02.09.19.

48. Bonkat G, Bartoletti RR, Bryere F, et al. *2018 EAU Guidelines on Urological Infections.* Available at: https://uroweb.org/guideline/urological-infections/. Accessed 02.09.19.

50. DeWitt-Foy ME, Nickel JC, Shoskes DA. Management of chronic prostatitis/chronic pelvic pain syndrome. *Eur Urol Focus.* 2019;5(1):2−4.

51. Franco JVA, Turk T, Jung JH, et al. Non-pharmacological interventions for treating chronic prostatitis/chronic pelvic pain syndrome. *Cochrane Database Syt Rev.* 2018;5: CD012551.

**References available online at** expertconsult.com.

# 52

# Parkinson Disease

MONICA STALLWORTH

## OBJECTIVES

*Upon completion of this chapter, the reader will be able to:*

- Define and recognize the clinical features that justify a clinical diagnosis of Parkinson disease (PD).
- Describe the differences in clinical features and medication responsiveness of the illnesses from which PD must be differentiated, including other Lewy body dementias.

- Understand the role of levodopa in diagnosis and treatment and the indications for the use of adjunctive medications in PD in older persons.
- Recognize and optimally manage the motor and nonmotor complications of PD.

## Prevalence and Impact

Parkinson disease (PD) is a progressive disorder that results in severe disability 10 to 15 years after its onset. It is the second most common neurodegenerative disorder after Alzheimer disease (AD). PD is characterized by rigidity, tremor, and bradykinesia; it is usually asymmetric and is usually responsive to dopaminergic treatment. Parkinson-plus syndromes refer to disorders that include parkinsonism with other clinical signs: they include Lewy body dementia (LBD), multiple system atrophy (MSA), progressive supranuclear palsy (PSP), and corticobasal degeneration (CBD). As in other industrialized countries, the prevalence is approximately 1% in persons age >65 years in the United States, and rises to 3% in those age >85 years. PD is twice as common in men.[1,2]

## Risk Factors and Pathophysiology

Although its incidence increases with age, PD is generally not considered a normal part of aging. Most people with PD do not have a family history, but 15% do have a first-degree relative with PD, often without a clear mode of inheritance.[3] Several genetic loci for PD are identified, although a common environmental etiology could explain familial patterns. Pesticides, rural environments, and well water have all been associated with PD. In the early 1980s, a perthine analog was reported: it is the only environmental agent directly linked to levodopa-responsive parkinsonism.[4,5] Parkinsonian features are seen in head injury, including boxers and football players, and also in cerebrovascular disease, both presumably because of traumatic injury to the basal ganglia. PD in any one individual is likely to represent several factors acting together.

## Pathology

The underlying pathologic change in PD is injury to the dopaminergic projections from the substantia nigra pars compacta to the caudate nucleus and putamen. Intraneuronal Lewy bodies and Lewy neurites are other pathologic features of PD. Lewy neurites are often observed in the cortex, amygdala, locus coeruleus, vagal nucleus, and peripheral autonomic nervous system; this could explain some of the nonmotor features of PD. Pathologic changes may be detected up to 20 years before the onset of motor symptoms and are accompanied by a clinical prodrome of nonspecific symptoms, such as hyposmia, constipation, and fatigue.[6]

### CASE

#### Robert Wilmington (Part 1)

Mr. Wilmington is a 65-year-old right-handed building contractor who has been healthy and active most of his life. Over the past 3 years his work has become more supervisory by necessity, with ongoing complaints for several years of shoulder and limb joint discomfort followed by increased difficulty manipulating hand tools. He started hiding his dominant hand under his desk or sitting on it when in public after embarrassing questions about what he was rolling between his thumb and index finger. Six months later, he noted his newspaper shaking in both hands when held in his lap. Subsequently, he blamed his joint pains and stiffness for difficulties standing up and not walking at the pace to which he was accustomed.

His family noticed at the dinner table that he was now the last one to finish eating. He also made sure a handkerchief was handy to wipe unexpected drool from his lower lip. Most recently, it startled him that when standing and shaving in front of a mirror he lost his balance. He has had a few stumbles without falls when his body seemed to get ahead of his feet. He was prompted to seek medical attention after his first fall; it occurred when attempting to turn suddenly when called from behind.

1. Name the cardinal features of PD found in this case. What is the order these features present in this patient? Which symptoms may be attributable to bradykinesia?
2. What examination signs could be related to his rigidity and postural instability?
3. What cardinal feature is most helpful in distinguishing PD from other causes of parkinsonism?

❖ **A clinical diagnosis of PD requires the presence of bradykinesia with at least one the following cardinal signs: resting tremor, rigidity, and asymmetric onset.**

## Differential Diagnosis and Assessment

### Is It Parkinson Disease?

Although only autopsy makes the definitive diagnosis of PD, an accurate clinical diagnosis is based on the classic features that Parkinson originally described, plus other features recognized to be associated with PD since that time. Box 52.1 lists four cardinal features. Because some of these features are signs or symptoms seen with aging, the diagnosis of PD should be considered when at least two of the four are present. Box 52.2 lists significant supportive motor features.[7,8]

### Levodopa Responsiveness

Treatment with levodopa or a dopamine agonist (DA) usually provides improvement in the motor manifestations, therefore a

---

### • BOX 52.1 Primary Features of Parkinson Disease

- Resting tremor
- Bradykinesia
- Rigidity
- Asymmetric onset
- *Plus* responsiveness to levodopa

---

### • BOX 52.2 Some Supportive Features of Parkinson Disease

- Sustained response to levodopa (i.e., more than transient)
- Expressionless face (hypomimia)
- Sialorrhea (producing drooling)
- Speech and swallowing problems (hypophonia, dysarthria, dysphagia)
- Loss of fine motor skills (such as writing, producing micrographia)
- Abnormal gait (shuffling, reduced arm swing, flexed posture, freezing, and festination)
- Reduced upward gaze, positive glabellar tap, and decreased blinking)

---

definite response to levodopa is regarded as a confirmatory test and is required for a diagnosis of probable (i.e., clinically definite) PD. Although levodopa responsiveness can help differentiate classic PD, in most instances initial response can occur in Parkinson-plus syndromes, such as LBD and MSA. However, the sustained response to levodopa is confirmatory of PD, and it is the motor features that are most improved.

❖ **Slow and rigid with a resting asymmetric tremor: think Parkinson disease, consider a trial of levodopa.**

The National Institute of Neurologic Disorders and Stroke (NINDS) provides criteria that guide the diagnosis of PD and its differentiation from other related conditions. Criteria provide for definite, probable, or possible PD. In the NINDS Diagnostic Criteria for PD, the features summarized in Box 52.3 are considered suggestive of diagnoses other than PD. The presence of these features makes a diagnosis of PD less likely and should prompt a neurology referral. The NINDS criteria require a confirmatory autopsy for PD to be described as **"definite."** The presence of three of the four clinical features (see Box 52.1) present for at least 3 years yields a **"probable"** diagnosis in the presence of a

---

### • BOX 52.3 Findings in Potential Parkinson Disease That Suggest Other Diagnoses

Any of these three occurring in the **first 3 years**:
1. Nonmedication-related **hallucinations**
2. **"Freezing"** phenomenon
3. Prominent **postural instability**
4. **Dementia** occurring before Parkinson disease (PD) motor symptoms or in the first year of illness
5. Certain **eye movement** abnormalities other than limited upward gaze
6. Nonmedication-related, severe symptoms of **autonomic dysfunction**
7. Conditions present, which are themselves likely causes of PD symptoms (e.g., **neuroleptic use** in prior 6 months)

sustained, definite response to L-dopa (or a DA) and in the absence of symptoms found in Box 52.3. A diagnosis of **"possible"** PD requires only two of the four primary features (see Box 52.1) (provided one of the two were bradykinesia or tremor), does not require medication responsiveness if an adequate trial had not yet taken place, and—if symptoms had been present for 3 years—one or more of the findings that suggest other diagnoses (see Box 52.3) could be present.[8]

## Motor Features

**Resting tremor**, pronation-supination, or pill-rolling with a frequency of 4 to 6 Hz[9] is the **presenting symptom in 70%** of PD patients. Tremor is characteristically asymmetric at onset and worsens with anxiety, contralateral motor action, and ambulation.

**Muscular rigidity is resistance noted during passive joint movement** in the normal range of motion of that joint and is often termed cogwheeling. It is often more prominent in the most tremulous extremity. Rigidity is increased by contralateral motor movement or a mental task.

**Bradykinesia** causes the **most dysfunction in the initial stages** of the illness. The patient is unable to perform fine-motor tasks effectively. Recognition of this feature requires observation of a patient suspected of having PD walking, tying shoelaces, or writing a sentence. Other manifestations can include softening of the voice (hypophonia) or loss of amplitude and legibility of handwriting (micrographia).

**Postural instability** presents more insidiously with progressively **poor balance**. It leads to increased **fall risk**. Testing for postural reflexes includes pushing the patient forward (propulsion) or backward (retropulsion) to check for balance recovery.

**Gait dysfunction** or changes include shuffling, slowness of walking, and turning "enbloc." Further, a person with PD can accelerate while walking and have difficulty moderating speed or slowing appropriately. This is termed festination.

**Freezing** is shown by difficulty initiating walking or by a striking gait hesitation (transient loss of movement). This often occurs on turning or on arriving at a real or perceived obstacle.

## Nonmotor Features

Autonomic dysfunction is common and causes bowel and bladder dysfunction, excessive sweating, and orthostatic hypotension. However, dysautonomia as an early and particularly severe feature suggests a diagnosis other than PD.[9]

Dementia develops in an estimated 40% of PD patients, although in a study that followed patients until death, significant cognitive impairment was present in over 80% in the end stage of the illness. Thus the primary care provider (PCP) must monitor for cognitive decline and other characteristic symptoms of dementia in patients with a diagnosis of PD. Differentiating PD dementia (PDD) from other causes of cognitive decline presents challenges. This is particularly true for **LBD** as this dementia is much more common than has been historically taught. Convention holds that if PD symptoms and/or signs have existed for at least 1 year before signs of dementia, the diagnosis is PDD, whereas if dementia occurs first or concurrent with PD symptoms, a diagnosis of LBD should be considered (see later). Importantly, any diagnosis of dementia predisposes patients treated with antiparkinsonian drugs to hallucinations and other psychotic symptoms.[10]

Depression is common in PD, affecting nearly half of patients. Serotonin reuptake inhibitors (SSRIs) can be effective, and the dopaminergic qualities of sertraline can be therapeutic but can also complicate levodopa dosing.

Sensory symptoms in PD are quite varied and include anosmia, paresthesia, and pain.

Sleep disorders are common. Causes include nocturnal stiffness, nocturia, depression, restless legs syndrome, and rapid eye movement (REM) sleep behavior disorder (RSBD).

## Differential Diagnosis

**Essential tremor** is the most common tremor and tends to be familial. It occurs with voluntary movement and is often first noted when it interferes with eating or other activities of daily living. It can usually be detected in the finger to nose test. It is also absent at rest and tends to be bilateral. It has a higher frequency range (5–10 Hz) than the typical tremor in PD; although in older patients, the frequency is in the lower range. In advanced cases, essential tremor can be present at rest and thus confused with PD; and a patient with PD can have both! If rigidity and bradykinesia are present, a trial of levodopa may be appropriate.

The following differential diagnoses are summarized in Table 52.1.

**Drug-induced parkinsonism** occurs after exposure to neuroleptics, antiemetics, promotility agents, and some calcium channel blockers. Symptoms are symmetric. It characteristically resolves when the drug is stopped, although resolution can take weeks or months.

**PSP** is a rare disorder with typical onset in the 50s. Approximately 4% of parkinsonian patients have PSP. It progresses rapidly and is characterized by oculomotor disturbance, speech and swallowing difficulties, imbalance with falls, and frontal dementia. It is symmetric. Postural instability occurs early. Additional clinical manifestations include severe axial rigidity, absence of tremor, and a poor response to dopaminergic treatment. The defining characteristic is supranuclear gaze palsy, especially of downward gaze. Marked incapacity occurs within 3 to 5 years of onset, with death typically within 10 years. Compared with PD, the rigidity in PSP tends to be more severe and axial and postural instability is an early feature.

**MSA** involves the central, autonomic, and peripheral nervous systems. The prominence and severity of autonomic dysfunction differentiates it from PD. The term MSA includes a cluster of diseases previously regarded as separate entities, including Shy-Drager syndrome, olivopontocerebellar atrophy, and striatonigral degeneration. There is little or no response to levodopa. Presentation typically includes parkinsonism, cerebellar and autonomic dysfunction (orthostatic hypotension, bladder and bowel dysfunction, temperature dysregulation), and pyramidal dysfunction in various combinations. MSA-P (formerly called striatonigral degeneration) is characterized by symmetric parkinsonism without tremor and early, pronounced postural instability. MSA-C (formerly called olivopontocerebellar atrophy) manifests with cerebellar signs and parkinsonism. Corticospinal tract signs and respiratory stridor occur in all categories of MSA.

**CBD** is a progressive movement disorder that has a range of manifestations, including rigidity and akinesia, dystonias, and focal myoclonus. Motor symptoms often start in a single limb and spread to other areas as the disease progresses. In

| TABLE 52.1 Distinguishing Parkinson Disease From Its Differential Diagnosis | | | | | | |
|---|---|---|---|---|---|---|
| Disease | Bradykinesia and Rigidity | Tremor | Dementia | Other Features | L-dopa Responsiveness | Antipsychotic Sensitivity |
| Parkinson disease | Yes Limb | Yes | | More common in late onset | Yes | + |
| Drug-induced | Yes Limb | No | | | No | + + |
| Progressive supranuclear palsy | Yes Axial | No | Yes, early | Loss of conjugate gaze (especially downward) | No | |
| Lewy body dementia | Yes Axial | No | Yes, early | Hallucinations | Yes, initially | + + + |
| Vascular parkinsonism | Yes Limb | No | Yes, in some | Pyramidal signs | No | + |
| Multisystem atrophy | Yes | No | Yes, in some | Pyramidal and cerebellar signs Dysautonomia | | |

(Reproduced with permission from The Royal Australian College of General Practitioners from Chan DK. The art of treating Parkinson's disease in the older patient. *Aust Fam Physician* 2003;32:927–931. Available at www.racgp.org.au/afpbackissues/2003/200311/20031101chan.pdf)

addition, affected patients develop distressing and functionally disruptive signs related to motor planning (ideomotor apraxia) and self-awareness (alien limb phenomenon). Unlike MSA, patients with CBD develop a progressive cognitive disorder characterized by a frontal pattern of impairment, including executive dysfunction, aphasia, apraxia, and behavioral changes. Like other parkinsonian syndromes, CBD inexorably progresses over years and motor symptoms are not responsive to levodopa.

**LBD** is a progressive dementia in which cognitive decline is often the primary, initial clinical feature, but occasionally the earliest symptoms suggest a more atypical depressive disorder. As the dementia progresses, parkinsonian features may develop, and in most cases there are complex visual hallucinations, considered the "psychiatric" hallmarks of this disease. Unfortunately, there is also marked sensitivity to parkinsonian (extrapyramidal) side effects of neuroleptics (both the traditional and the "atypical" antipsychotics). Typical antipsychotics (those with high affinity for D2 receptors) should especially be avoided. Judicious use of low doses of atypical antipsychotics (especially quetiapine) by experienced specialists may be indicated with refractory hallucinations leading to harmful behaviors, but clear guidelines are lacking. Resting tremor is rare. Frontal lobe disinhibited behaviors are often present. Sleep disorders can occur, including REM sleep behavior disorder, which is characteristic and may precede cognitive symptoms by several years. Dopaminergics usually produce no improvement in motor manifestations. Cognitive symptoms can respond to cholinesterase inhibitors (ChEI), perhaps more so than in patients with AD.

**Normal pressure hydrocephalus (NPH)** is another progressive primary dementia, unrelated to PD pathologically, which classically presents with gait dysfunction, plus urinary incontinence and progressive dementia. The typical wide-based shuffling gait is often the initial presentation. Tremor is usually absent. Imaging may help when the clinical presentation makes it difficult to differentiate PD from another disorder with similar characteristics. The radiographic hallmark is ventricular dilatation. There should be no therapeutic response to dopaminergic treatment. When diagnosed early, NPH can improve or even reverse with placement of a ventriculoperitoneal shunt.

**Vascular parkinsonism** has a similar etiology to vascular dementia (VaD); that is, multiple infarcts occur. The infarcts in vascular parkinsonism are in the basal ganglia and the subcortical white matter. Tremor is usually absent, and there is no therapeutic response to dopaminergic treatment. Vascular parkinsonism tends to be accompanied by dementia, pseudobulbar affect, urinary symptoms, and pyramidal signs. Brain imaging showing extensive small vessel disease is supportive, and treatment is mostly the management of the vascular risk factors.

◆ **The diagnosis of parkinsonism can be difficult to make particularly in early stages as the differential diagnosis of tremor and gait changes is broad; a neurology referral for initial diagnosis is usually required.**

## Management

Management of individual patients requires careful consideration of multiple factors but with a primary emphasis on patient preferences and goals of care. The others include age, stage of disease, degree of functional disability, and level of physical activity and productivity. Treatment modalities include pharmacologic, non-pharmacologic, and surgical therapy. Most available treatments target symptom relief and do not appear to slow or reverse the natural course of the disease.

The key therapeutic strategies for PD (Box 52.4) include:
1. Increased dopaminergic stimulation
2. Decreased cholinergic stimulation
3. Decreased glutamatergic stimulation

In most cases, anticholinergics should be avoided in older patients as detailed in many other places in this text!

The American Academy of Neurology has published evidence-based reviews of several aspects of the management of PD. The review of initiation of treatment is especially of interest to the

## • BOX 52.4   Ablative and Stimulation Procedures for Parkinson Disease

Ablative procedures
Thalamotomy
Pallidotomy
Subthalamotomy
Deep brain stimulation procedures (DBS) procedures
Thalamus (Vim nucleus)
Globus pallidus pars interna (Gpi)
Subthalamic nucleus (STN)
Restorative procedures
Fetal cell transplantation
Stem cell transplantation

primary care clinician, who will frequently be the first prescriber when the diagnosis is made in the primary care setting. An algorithmic (decision tree) approach to PD management has also been published.[15–18]

## CASE

### Robert Wilmington (Part 2)

He starts a therapeutic trail of levodopa/carbidopa (LD/CD) gradually increased to 25/100 three times a day. His tremor improves and he declines addition of anticholinergic medication because of concerns about side effects. His bradykinesia partially improves resulting in fewer problems with feeding and walking. He requires increased frequency of dosing eventually to every 4 hours while awake to prevent end-of-dose return of motor symptoms. Initially, he feels there is improvement in his postural instability, but this is not confirmed on examination. His imbalance is still present. His reduced falling is a result of cautious gait, gait training, and—later—the use of assistive devices. With time, his maximum benefit from each dose of LD/CD, as well as its duration of benefit, diminishes. His dose is gradually doubled with some further improvement. This is accompanied by minimal dyskinesias at peak dose, which are not noticeable until the dose is increased to 25/250.

1. What are the benefits and risks of starting levodopa versus a DA in this patient?
2. What are the options when side effects develop from levodopa?
3. At what point would you refer him to a neurologist?
4. How should his nonmotor symptoms be treated?

## When to Start Medications

Clinicians should always try to find the lowest dose of dopaminergic medication, either singly or in combination, that adequately manages the patient's symptoms according to his or her individual needs. In addition, patients should be reassured that the onset of motor fluctuations likely depends on the rate of progression of underlying disease, rather than choice of initial therapy, and that any delay in onset of motor fluctuations using DAs occurs at the expense of reduced efficacy when compared with levodopa.

The decision to begin symptomatic therapy in PD is determined by the patient's choice and by the degree of functional impairment.[11] For example, a mild resting tremor that does not impact function does not warrant treatment. When the tremor is severe or affecting function, **levodopa** is the first-line treatment in the older adult population. The progression of PD over the years is not uniform. If gait or other aspects of functional independence

become affected, treatment should be considered at that time, even if the tremor is tolerable.[12]

Because many patients have motor complications from long-term levodopa, considerable work in recent years has led to the emergence of other antiparkinsonian therapies, especially for younger patients. **DAs** include ropinirole or pramipexole. These agents are less effective, but the incidence of motor side effects is much lower; however, they have other side effects (edema of the legs, sleepiness, impulsive behaviors, and confusion) and are more expensive.[13,14] They are best used in younger patients, who are better able to tolerate the side effects. In fact, treatment for early PD in younger, healthy patients generally begins with DA monotherapy.

## How to Choose Initial Therapy?

The decision to start pharmacotherapy in patients with PD is based on assessment of both motor and nonmotor symptoms, side effects, and patient choice (Table 52.2). There is no single preferred therapy, and trade-offs are common. Optimal care requires a flexible trial-and-error approach. The four main drugs or classes of drugs that have antiparkinson activity are monamine oxidase type B (MAO B) inhibitors, amantadine, DAs, and levodopa. They differ with respect to potency, dosing frequency, and side effects. All primarily target symptom relief, and none have been firmly established as disease modifying or neuroprotective. Ultimately, the goal of treatment is to increase the amount of available dopamine to decrease PD symptomatology. Most patients require some kind of symptom management 2 to 5 years after onset.[15–18]

The most important patient-related factor is age. Age has important implications for tolerability of certain drug classes and severity of side effects depending on the antiparkinson potency of different classes. Anticholinergics must generally be avoided in older adults.

## Levodopa

Levodopa is the preferred initial drug in older, frail patients (and is less expensive!). It remains the most potent antiparkinson drug. Like any symptomatic medication in PD, treatment starts when symptoms become bothersome or cause functional disability.

### Lack of Levodopa Responsiveness May Mean Inaccurate Diagnosis

Levodopa is also the most effective drug for the symptomatic treatment of idiopathic PD, especially for **bradykinesia and rigidity.** It is generally combined with a peripheral decarboxylase inhibitor—**carbidopa** in the United States—to block its conversion to dopamine in the systemic circulation; this reduces the peripheral effects of nausea, vomiting, and orthostatic hypotension. The carbidopa/levodopa combination in the immediate release form is available in 10/100, 25/100, and 25/250 mg.

### "Start Low and Go Slow" With Levodopa and Most Neurologic Drugs

The starting dose is generally one-half tablet of 25/100 mg three times daily, titrated upward over several weeks to a whole 25/100 mg tablet three times daily, as tolerated and according to the response. "Start low and go slow" is the rule, owing to adverse reactions, especially if dementia is present. There is a wide range of dose response in the older adult population. The majority of those with idiopathic PD have a significant therapeutic response to moderate doses (400–600 mg/day of levodopa). No response to 1000 to 1500 mg/day strongly implies that the diagnosis should be reviewed.

Controlled-release carbidopa-levodopa is less well absorbed, requiring doses up to 30% higher than the immediate-release form; each tablet typically results in a less dramatic symptom benefit than the immediate-release preparation, as the controlled-release form penetrates more slowly to the brain. Thus therapy should start with an immediate-release preparation, switching to controlled-release when the dose is stable.

Carbidopa-levodopa should be taken on an empty stomach, 30 to 60 minutes before or 45 to 60 minutes after meals because of competitive absorption of other amino acids. This also increases the duration of response to each dose. This is more crucial in advanced disease with motor fluctuations. Unfortunately, initial nausea from levodopa is more likely on an empty stomach, so such patients may take it with a snack or after meals. However, nausea often occurs because of insufficient carbidopa; manage this with supplemental carbidopa or with antiemetics, such as trimethobenzamide or ondansetron given beforehand. Phenothiazine antiemetics and metoclopramide must be avoided; they can themselves cause drug-induced parkinsonism.

Increasing the levodopa dosage should be tried if responsiveness drops. If that fails or side effects become unacceptable, an adjunctive therapy (next section) should be tried. Nausea on levodopa? Try more carbidopa.

### Withdrawal Syndrome

The DA withdrawal syndrome is described in some patients with PD who abruptly stop taking a DA. In retrospective studies, the frequency of the syndrome among patients who withdraw from DAs ranged from 8% to 19%. Symptoms resemble those of cocaine withdrawal and include anxiety, panic attacks, depression, sweating, nausea, pain, fatigue, dizziness, and drug craving. These symptoms were refractory to other antiparkinson medications, including levodopa, and only responded to resuming the DA.

## Motor Fluctuations

The primary cause of motor fluctuations is the short half-life of levodopa (90–120 minutes). After years on the medication, as the disease progresses, the duration of responsiveness to levodopa becomes shorter and the patient experiences a "wearing off" reaction.[19,20] Some patients react to "off" states with panic attacks, screaming, or even drenching sweats. With disease progression, there is a tendency for the fluctuations to become increasingly less predictable. The "on-off" effect is the most unpredictable of these states. "Delayed-on" and "no-on" as well as dyskinesias, occur. Motor complications are a major cause of disability in advanced PD patients. Treatment for these fluctuations focuses on trying to improve absorption, altering the timing of doses, and prolonging the effect of every dose. As noted earlier, a high protein meal can reduce levodopa absorption; so spreading protein intake throughout the day can help reduce motor fluctuations.

Controlled-release levodopa unfortunately only slightly lengthens the duration of action of levodopa. The therapeutic effects are more unpredictable than those of immediate-release levodopa, which is especially important in older patients. Controlled-release levodopa reduces "off" time by 20% to 70%, increases the total daily dose of levodopa by about 20%, yet decreases the number of doses by 30%. Catechol-o-methyl transferase (COMT) inhibitors, which relieve end-of-dose wearing off by lengthening the half-life

of circulating levodopa, and DAs, which enhance effectiveness of levodopa and help to reduce off time, are options detailed in "Adjunctive Therapy" later. Surgery can also reduce "off" time. Both pallidotomy and deep brain stimulation (DBS) of the globus pallidus or the subthalamic nucleus can be highly effective in this regard. However, surgery may be contraindicated in frail older patients who could potentially most benefit from this effect (see later).

## Dyskinesias

Chorea or choreodystonia, usually accompanying the "on" state, is most commonly induced by levodopa at the peak of its clinical effect ("peak-dose" dyskinesias). The movements are typically choreiform or dystonic, and range from mild to severe and disabling. Most medical strategies for reducing "off" states can cause increased dyskinesias as a side effect, so a therapeutic balance must be sought.

DAs sometimes help by allowing a reduction of levodopa dosage. However, note that COMT inhibitors tend to worsen dyskinesias. Amantadine, 100 to 300 mg per day, may reduce dyskinesia through the inhibition of glutamate-mediated neurotransmissions, but anticholinergic side effects can be problematic. Propranolol (up to 20 mg three times per day) has some potential benefit. For pure dystonia that does not respond to levodopa adjustment, anticholinergics may be helpful, but again, side effects need to be balanced against benefits. Also again, surgery (pallidotomy or DBS) may be considered, but is used in frail older adults with caution.

## Adjunctive Medications

Adjuncts to levodopa (amantadine and a number of dopaminergic medications) reduce the overall quantity of "off" time in patients with motor fluctuations. The dopaminergics have either longer half-lives or an ability to extend the half-life of levodopa, thus leading to more continuous dopaminergic stimulation. None of them completely relieve the "off" time problems.

**Amantadine:** This drug has been used for years as a treatment for early PD. More recently, it has been studied for its effects in fluctuating disease. Its most impressive effect in advanced PD is its efficacy against dyskinesias; one report showed a reduction in the severity of dyskinesias by 50%. Problems that limit the wider use of amantadine in older adults include edema of the legs, with a characteristic rash (livido reticularis), plus hallucinations and anticholinergic effects.

**DAs: Bromocriptine** was the first of these to be used clinically. Others now available include **pramipexole, ropinirole, rotigotine (patch), and apomorphine** (injection). They reduce "off" time as their half-lives are longer than that of levodopa. Extended-release formulas offer more continuous dopaminergic stimulation and improved compliance. They should be used cautiously.[21–23] The dose is increased gradually over 4 to 8 weeks to an optimal level. If dyskinesia occurs, reduction of levodopa may be required. Motor score improvement is seen in around 20% to 35% of patients. Their antiparkinsonian efficacy is significantly less than that of levodopa. They work primarily by improving "off" episode disability and can be used as the sole therapy in mild to moderate disease, as well as an adjunct in severe PD conditions. Adverse effects often limit their use, including orthostatic hypotension, delirium, nausea, and vomiting.

**MAO-B inhibitors: Selegiline, rasagiline, and safinamide** are inhibitors available in the United States. These medications decrease the central catabolism of dopamine by blocking MAO-B but are generally less effective. They may be used as sole therapy from mild to moderate disease or adjuncts in severe disease. They have a long half-life, so once daily dosing is possible with minimal side effects.

**COMT inhibitors:** The enzyme COMT is key to peripheral catabolism of levodopa. Blocking it with COMT inhibitors (entacapone or tolcapone) lengthens the plasma half-life of levodopa by 40% to 80%. Adverse effects are diarrhea and dyskinesia. Tolcapone has liver toxicity, so monitoring of liver function is recommended. This class tends to worsen dyskinesias.

**Neuroprotective agents:** Several substances have been studied as potential neuroprotective agents to slow disease progression. **Vitamin E** was not beneficial in a large, multicenter trial of patients with early PD. The effectiveness of **coenzyme Q** is not yet certain. At this time for PD there are no proven neuroprotective agents.

## Nonpharmacologic Strategies

Emerging evidence supports a variety of nonpharmacologic activity-based interventions for patients with PD.[24] In general, regular aerobic exercise appears to help with motor symptoms in mild PD, particularly high-intensity exercise. In addition, tai chi, a martial art focused on movement and balance, improved postural stability, stride length, and functional reach. In addition, participants reported fewer falls and had small but discernible improvements in objective measures of movement, including timed up and go and 6-minute walk. A wide range of interventions has focused on improving balance, flexibility, and strength with a focus on improving functional outcomes. This includes modalities such as dance, boxing, treadmill training, and bicycling. External cues also seem to improve pace and maintenance of mobility, including music, metronome, lasers, and mirrors. Not surprisingly, many participants also experience improvements in confidence, mood, and other nonmotor symptoms. An early referral to a physical therapist and an occupation therapist with specific experience in the treatment of patients with PD is strongly recommended.[25]

## Management of Nonmotor Symptoms

**Autonomic dysfunction** in patients with PD manifests as orthostatic hypotension, constipation, urinary symptoms, and sexual dysfunction. Symptomatic orthostatic hypotension occurs in 15% to 20% of PD patients, with potentially devastating results, including falls. Droxidopa is a synthetic amino acid precursor that acts as a prodrug for norepinephrine but is capable of crossing the blood-brain barrier. Post hoc analysis of randomized controlled trials with droxidopa has shown efficacy and tolerability with Parkinson patient with neurogenic orthostatic hypertension.[26,27] Neurogenic orthostatic hypertension may be from PD-related autonomic dysfunction but is also a side effect of many PD treatments. Reduction of the dose of antiparkinson drugs, enhancement of salt and fluid intake, and addition of fludrocortisone or midodrine are treatment options for hypotension. If systolic hypertension coexists, pindolol may be useful. Aggressive management of constipation entails escalation of water and fiber intake, addition of fiber supplements (e.g., psyllium),

and use of stool softeners, suppositories, and enemas. Urinary urgency can be treated with peripheral anticholinergic drugs (oxybutynin and tolterodine) but is limited because of the side effects; adrenergic-blocking agents (prazosin and terazosin) unfortunately exacerbate hypotension.

**Depression** affects about 40% of PD patients.[28] Coexistent depression may significantly affect both the symptoms and rehabilitation efforts. Affective symptoms can be difficult to differentiate from PD symptoms, so regular screening with the Patient Health Questionnaire will allow the PCP to identify it. An unblinded study has SSRIs to be useful. Of the antidepressants shown in small controlled studies, citalopram and venlafaxine are among those most useful in older adults. Although SSRIs are associated with extrapyramidal symptoms, sertraline has a greater effect on dopamine reuptake inhibition making it also a rational choice as an SSRI for use in persons with PD. No head-to-head studies exist to provide evidence if one antidepressant is superior to another in PD. Tricyclics can exacerbate orthostatic hypotension. In hypotensive patients, venlafaxine may be the drug of choice because it increases blood pressure. In bipolar patients, note that lithium may worsen parkinsonism.

**Sleep disorders** in PD include daytime somnolence and sleep attacks, nighttime awakenings attributable to overnight rigidity and bradykinesia, RSBD, restless legs, or periodic limb movements of sleep. Daytime somnolence and sleep attacks have been linked to DAs, and patients should be warned of these adverse effects. The prevalence has been estimated to be as high as 50%. Elimination of the agonist or even use of a stimulant might be necessary. Patients and families should be warned about safety issues, such as driving. Nighttime awakenings and restless legs can be alleviated with a bedtime dose of long-acting levodopa or the addition of entacapone. Melatonin is the safest and most effective treatment for RSBD.

**Psychosis** occurs rarely in untreated PD and is thought to be mostly drug induced.[28] DAs are more likely to cause hallucinations than is levodopa. The first step in management is to discontinue the agonist or any anticholinergic drugs and to use the lowest levodopa dose possible.[29,30] However, addition of an atypical neuroleptic is sometimes necessary. Two randomized controlled trials have shown that clozapine is useful for symptoms, such as visual hallucinations. However, because of potentially fatal agranulocytosis, blood counts must be measured every week or biweekly. Therefore quetiapine has become the most popular atypical neuroleptic in PD because of the absence of agranulocytosis and fewer extrapyramidal adverse effects than other atypical antipsychotics.[31] Several open-label studies have suggested that dementia and psychosis in PD respond to ChEIs—consistent with the efficacy of ChEIs in LBD.

**Dementia** is common but has limited evidence for specific treatments.[28] There is no evidence that one ChEI is superior to another in PD patients with dementia. A small, randomized controlled trial has shown that donepezil is useful in improving cognition in demented parkinsonian patients. Another randomized trial has shown that rivastigmine is useful in LBD.[32] Cholinergic stimulation theoretically would be counterproductive in parkinsonism. Both anticholinergics and DAs should be used with caution in patients with dementia because of the risk of increasing confusion, hallucinations, and other psychotic symptoms.

**Bladder impairment**: The most common and earliest bladder abnormality in patients with PD is nocturia. Urgency and frequency may also occur because of detrusor hyperreflexia. In some people with PD, detrusor hyporeflexia and urinary sphincter problems occur. Because bladder disturbance in patients with PD can be complex, urodynamic studies may be required to make the correct diagnosis to the nature of the problem. Management includes timed voiding, intermittent catheterization, and pharmacologic agents to avoid nocturia.

**Thermoregulation and sweating:** Individuals with PD may complain of impaired sweating and cold/heat intolerance. The exact mechanisms are not known, thermoregulatory and vasomotor tone problems may result from dopamine system abnormalities. Dopaminergic agents may help alleviate these symptoms.

**Gastrointestinal (GI) impairment**: GI motility disorders are believed to be the most common autonomic dysfunction in persons with PD, manifesting as dysphagia, constipation, and problems with gastric emptying. The problem may result from pathologic changes in the myenteric plexus from the esophagus to the rectum. Neurohistochemical studies have demonstrated the presence of Lewy bodies in the myenteric plexus of persons with Parkinson.

## Management of the Secondary Effects of Parkinson Disease

Primary care clinicians often take the lead in addressing the functional, social, emotional, economic, sexual, and nutritional (and other) effects of this progressive and disabling condition. The PCP often assumes the active care of these effects of PD on daily life.

**Swallowing impairment and nutrition:** Up to 75% of people with PD complain of dysphagia. The problem is related to abnormalities in striated muscles under dopaminergic control and smooth muscles under autonomic influence. **Dysphagia and aspiration** risk should be approached proactively, and the input and expertise of speech therapists (who are really "speech and swallowing therapists"—patients and families still often do not realize this) should be ordered when either symptom presents. A speech pathologist may help by teaching oral-motor exercises and providing education on compensatory strategies to prevent penetration and aspiration. **Undernutrition** (often presenting as weight loss) and poor fluid intake with dehydration (frequently overlooked as contributory factor to hypotension and orthostasis) are common risks in the PD patient; problems with swallowing and choking/aspiration further compromise both food and fluid intake. **Hypophonia** is another important symptom that leads to difficulty with communication and social isolation. Engagement with speech therapy on exercise to improve voice volume and projection have proven helpful as long as patients continue exercises.

❖ **PD requires a multidisciplinary, interprofessional team for optimal patient-centered outcomes. Team members includes occupational, physical, and speech therapy.**

## Parkinsonism-Hyperpyrexia Syndrome

There have been reports of patients with PD who developed neuroleptic malignant syndrome in the context of sudden withdrawal or dose reductions of levodopa or DAs, and rarely, as well as with switching from one agent to another. In this context, the condition has been termed the "parkinsonism-hyperpyrexia syndrome." Prompt recognition and treatment are important, as severe cases

and even fatalities have been reported.[33,34] Management of parkinsonism-hyperpyrexia syndrome involves replacing antiparkinson medications at the dose used before the onset of the syndrome. Levodopa and DAs can be given orally or via nasogastric tube. Nonoral options for DAs include transdermal and by injection of continuous infusion. The use of injectable apomorphine requires a test dose before ongoing treatment. In addition to replacing antiparkinson medications, patients with significant hyperthermia and rigidity should be admitted to an intensive care unit setting and undergo aggressive supportive care, as well as monitoring for potential dysautonomia and other complications.

## Surgical Treatment for Parkinson Disease

Interest in surgical intervention in PD has reemerged in the past few years, especially in patients who do not achieve adequate symptom control with medication (see Box 52.4). Surgical intervention should be considered when medical therapy is no longer effective.

**Ablative therapy** (pallidotomy) consists of surgical destruction of part of the brain (usually the globus pallidus). The patient is usually awake during the procedure to monitor movement in real time, so that surgeons can ablate the appropriate location and amount of tissue to restore the balance between excitation and inhibition of movement. Pallidotomy is effective at reducing contralateral dyskinesias, as well as reducing symptoms, such as bradykinesia. However, patients who have even a minor degree of cognitive impairment or who are age >70 years seem to tolerate the procedure poorly.

**DBS** is the placement of a stimulator in the globus pallidus, the subthalamic nucleus, or the thalamus. DBS placement has the advantage of being adjustable as opposed to the permanence of ablation. The amount of energy sent through the device, as well as the rate at which the device operates, can be adjusted as the patient's symptoms progress. The procedure has similar benefits to ablative surgery in terms of reducing dyskinesia and bradykinesia but also may benefit tremor (depending on where the device is placed). Complications include bleeding and infection, hardware problems (such as dislocation of electrodes), or battery failure. The unit is expensive and requires considerable time to adjust for optimal response. Older adults with PD appear to derive similar benefits to younger patients.[35]

❖ **DBS should be offered to patients with significant symptoms and functional impairment despite an adequate trial of optimal medication.**

Inpatient considerations—Given the high prevalence of motor fluctuations in PD, and the disabling nature of both "off" periods and severe dyskinesias, care should be taken in the inpatient setting to administer all PD medications at the appropriate dose and the correct time. Patients should be advised to bring a medication list (including when doses are taken) and the medications themselves, in case some are not available on the hospital formulary. Failure to conform to the patient's individualized regimen can result in either complications of untreated parkinsonism, such as falls, aspiration, or rigidity, or adverse effects of medications, including orthostasis, confusion, and hallucinations. Dopamine-blocking agents, including antipsychotics and antiemetics, must be avoided.

Swallowing restrictions—Most patients with PD can go without antiparkinson medications for a brief period (i.e., <24 hours) when oral intake is temporarily restricted (e.g., perioperative or periprocedural) or when seriously ill. In patients who are critically ill and bedbound, the parkinsonian symptoms are typically over-shadowed by the burden of other medical problems, and antiparkinson medications may not provide any clear benefit. However, sudden withdrawal or dose reduction of antiparkinson medications can rarely precipitate the parkinsonism-hyperpyrexia syndrome.

When treatment is still desired for patients who are restricted to take nothing by mouth, options include transdermal rotigotine and apomorphine by injection or continuous infusion. The use of apomorphine requires a test dose before ongoing treatment. Initiation of rotigotine or apomorphine in the inpatient setting requires a thorough review of historical reactions to DAs, and careful consideration of benefits versus risks, which include orthostasis, confusion, and hallucinations. For patients with a nasogastric feeding tube, levodopa tablets can be crushed and given through the tube.

## CASE

### Robert Wilmington (Part 3)

Other symptoms were present but not volunteered by the patient. Specific inquiry by the examiner revealed constipation and nocturia, depression and inattentiveness, and sleep disturbances, including apparent acting out during vivid dreams.

1. Which of these could be nonmotor symptoms related to PD?
2. Name another category of nonmotor symptoms that can be recognized in his case?
3. Among the causes for disturbed sleep, which specific disorder is likely being described here?

## TABLE 52.2  Pharmacotherapy of Parkinson's Disease

| Drug | Mechanisms of Action | Usual Dosing | Side Effects | Comments |
|---|---|---|---|---|
| Levodopa + Carbidopa | Levodopa activates D1 and D2 dopamine receptors in the brain. Carbidopa is a peripheral dopa-decarboxylase inhibitor. It increases therapeutic potency and decreases gastrointestinal side effects of levodopa | Levodopa/carbidopa 25/100 titrated upward to achieve desired clinical effects (Brands/dosage strengths available: Sinemet, 10/100, 25/100, 25/250; Sinemet-CR 25/100, 50/200) | Nausea, vomiting, hypotension (usually due to inadequate doses of carbidopa); dyskinesias; motor fluctuations; neuropsychiatric problems (e.g., confusion) | Most potent antiparkinsonian drug; may improve mortality rate; levodopa forms free radicals, which may cause progress of IPD. |
| Dopamine agonists: Bromocriptine Pergolide Cabergoline Pramipexole Ropinirole | Stimulate dopamine receptors | 2.5–40 mg/day 0.1–5 mg/day 0.5–1 mg/day 1.5–4.5 mg/day 0.75–24 mg/day | Similar to levodopa; Bromocriptine may cause red, inflamed skin (St. Anthony's fire), which is reversible on drug discontinuation | Reduced incidence or levodopa-related side effects; selective stimulation of dopamine receptor subtypes; potential neuroprotection; limited antiparkinsonian effect |
| Amantadine | Promotes synthesis and prevents reuptake of dopamine; increases dopamine release; stimulates dopamine receptors | 100 mg every other day for 1 week, with subsequent dose increase to up to 100 mg t.i.d. | Insomnia, confusion, hallucination, ankle edema, livido reticularis | Limited clinical efficacy |
| Anticholinergics: Trihexyphenidyl | Restore imbalance between dopaminergic and cholinergic neurotransmitters | 0.5–1 mg b.i.d. and gradually increased to 2 mg t.i.d. | Significant cognitive (e.g.; confusion, hallucination, memory impairment) and peripheral antimuscarinic side effects (e.g.; dry mouth, blurred vision, constipation) | Limited clinical efficacy |
| Benztropine | | 0.5–2 mg b.i.d. | | |
| COMT inhibitors: Entacapone | Considered neuroprotective. Rescues dopaminergic neurons by inducing changes in transcription with new protein synthesis and alteration in gene expression | 200 mg per dose (up to 1,600 mg/day) | Dyskinesia Diarrhea Liver toxicity/(tolcapone) | Increases levodopa availability; smother levodopa plasma levels, thus, reducing levodopa related side effects |
| Tolcapone Selegiline hydrochloride (Deprenyl or Eldepryl) | | 100–200 mg t.i.d. 5 mg at breakfast and 5 mg at noon | Fulminant liver failure Hypertensive reactions may occur if taken with theophylline, ephedrine, carbidopa/levodopa and foods containing tyramine | May potentiate levodopa; some clinicians use it as monotherapy in early IPD. May delay the need for levodopa for about 9 months. Used with levodopa to potentiate its effects and reduce the dose of levodopa |

(From Francisco GE. et al. Rehabilitation of person with Parkinson's disease and other movement disorders 4th edition physical medicine and rehabilitation principles and practice p. 817.)

*bid,* Twice a day; *COMT,* catechol-o-methyl transferase; *IPD,* idiopathic Parkinson's disease; *tid,* three times a day.

## Discussion

Mr. Robinson demonstrates a frequently seen initial presentation of PD.

PD is characterized by the motor symptoms of bradykinesia, rigidity, and hypokinesia. Mr. Robinson observed a decrease in manipulation of hand tools demonstrating the bradykinesia and hypokinesia seen in PD. Asymmetric reduced or absent arm swing of his dominant hand with associated public embarrassment is a characteristic presentation. Rigidity of PD typically results in complaints of joint pain, which is later demonstrated as disease progresses to difficulties standing up with stooped posture and shuffling gait. Six months later, the tremor becomes evident while reading the newspaper.

In Mr. Wilmington's case, although resting tremor appeared to be the most obvious initial symptom, the rigidity and bradykinesia actually began earlier. The rigidity caused the pains that he assumed were from his joints—an often unrecognized symptom of rigidity. The rigidity could have also contributed to his ambulation problems. Bradykinesia was the second of his PD-associated features—with impaired fine motor control of hand tools and the later difficulties with standing, with the speed of ambulation and eating, as well as the drooling and festination. His falling was mainly because of the onset of postural instability and the gait dysfunction. Mr. Wilmington also has RSBD, a nonmotor symptom.

In regard to treatment there are no disease-modifying medications or any proven efficacy to slow disease progression of PD. There have been randomized controlled trials, as well as observation studies that demonstrate the benefits of daily exercise, which improves gait and motor function.

Pharmacologic therapy should be initiated with clear endpoints regarding functionality. Because the PD population is heterogeneous, functional impairment must be addressed in a multidisciplinary framework accounting for personal factors and an environmental context.

## Summary

The incidence of PD increases with age. Diagnosis requires a careful symptom history and physical examination focused on cardinal features, including bradykinesia, tremor, cogwheeling, and asymmetric onset. PD must also be differentiated from a variety of other conditions causing parkinsonian symptoms. The decision to initiate symptomatic medical therapy in patients with PD is influenced by the degree to which symptoms interfere with functionality and quality of life and patient preferences regarding use of medications. The four main drugs or classes of drugs that can be used as monotherapy are MAO B inhibitors, amantadine, DAs, and levodopa. The choice of which pharmacotherapy to use ultimately requires trial and error. The most important patient-related factors are age, tolerability, and a given patient's perceived degree of functional impairment. MAO B inhibitors have relatively modest antiparkinson effects, whereas levodopa is the most potent antiparkinson therapy. When motor symptoms of PD begin to interfere with daily function and quality of life, symptomatic therapy with a DA or levodopa is indicated. For the geriatric population with symptoms of PD that affect daily life, levodopa is the treatment of choice. Doses should be started low and slowly titrated. If symptoms continue with no response to levodopa, it may mean PD is not the correct diagnosis. DAs are less well tolerated in older adults and those with cognitive dysfunction.

## Key References

11. Miyasaki JM, Martin W, Suchowersky O, et al. Practice parameter: initiation of treatment for Parkinson's disease: an evidence-based review: report of the Quality Standards Sub-committee of the American Academy of Neurology. *Neurology*. 2002;54:2292.
15. Spindler, Meredith A, et al. Internal pharmacological treatment. Nov 20, 2019. Available at: https://www.uptodate.com/contents/initial-pharmacologic-treatment-of-parkinson-disease. Accessed June 4, 2020.
20. Fox SH, Katzenschlager R, Lim SY, et al. International Parkinson and movement disorder society evidence based medicine review: update on treatments for the motor symptoms of Parkinson's disease. *Mov Disord*. 2018;33:1248.
28. Miyasaki JM, Shannon K, Voon V, et al. Practice parameter: evaluation and treatment of depression, psychosis, and dementia in Parkinson disease (an evidence-based review): Report of the Quality Standards Subcommittee of the American Academy of Neurology. *Neurology*. 2006;66:996.

**References available online at** expertconsult.com.

# 53

# Oral Disorders and Systemic Diseases

**JULIE ZACHARIAS SIMPSON, AURELIO MUYOT, KIKI DOUNIS, DONG-HUN HAN, SOO KIM, AND GEORGIA DOUNIS**

## OBJECTIVES

*Upon completion of this chapter, the reader will be able to:*

- Relate the risk of poor oral health to systemic health.
- Explain the increased susceptibility of older adults to dental caries and periodontal disease.
- Discuss the clinical significance of mouth dryness and its causes.
- Name the indications for referral to a dentist.

- Describe the guidelines for antibiotic prophylaxis in cardiac patients at risk for infective endocarditis and in patients with total joint replacement.
- List the major risk factors for oral cancer, its sites, and its public health significance.

## Oral Health and the Primary Care of Older Adults

An examination of the mouth and teeth is a vital part of even a brief encounter with an older patient who is coming under your care. It is comparable in importance to observing and examining for gait and balance (also often omitted!). The oral examination can provide insight about your patient's state of health, nutrition, and hydration, whether the mouth is dry (often from medication) and/or the teeth and gums are diseased. One can assess whether there is a commitment to self-care or whether there is self-neglect. If poor dental hygiene is found, the patient can be instructed about the importance of improving oral care and to follow up long term with a dental professional. Family and patient often fail to realize the effect of poor dental hygiene on their future health and quality of life in the years ahead.

❖ **Always look carefully into the mouth, especially of your older patients. There is a lot to learn during a brief examination.**

## Oral Health—Systemic Health Interactions

Health and wellbeing is determined by the interactions of environmental, lifestyle, behavioral, social, economic, and educational factors. Most chronic systemic conditions and oral disease share common modifiable lifestyle risk factors mediated by the same range of genetic, environmental, behavioral, and socioeconomic factors. These chronic diseases can result in oral manifestations, thus impacting the individual's oral health (Table 53.1). Oral health affects general health and emotional, psychosocial, and functional wellbeing. The specific diseases of oral and craniofacial tissues are chronic inflammatory conditions, affecting the majority of older Americans. Chronic, noncommunicable bacterial infections

| TABLE 53.1 | Oral Manifestations of Systemic Disease | |
|---|---|
| **Chronic Systemic Condition** | **Oral Manifestation** |
| Diabetes | Advanced periodontal disease, polydipsia, xerostomia, periodontal abscesses, loss of sensation |
| Cardiovascular disease Stroke | Tooth loss, advanced periodontal disease, injured tongue, or cheek biting |
| Alzheimer disease/ cognitive decline | Advanced periodontal disease, dental caries |
| Osteoarthritis | Dental caries, periodontal disease, and decrease range of motion open/close |
| Cancer | Dental caries/root caries, candidiasis, difficulty with speech and swallowing |

resulting in disorders of the oral soft and hard tissue are often preventable, reversible, and linked to social and behavioral lifestyle practices. Unmanaged infection of the periodontal tissue (periodontitis) and dentition (caries) can result in cumulative irreversible disease progression over the course of life, which impacts the chronic systemic conditions common in old age.

❖❖ **Poor oral health affects the impact of the chronic systemic conditions common in old age.**

**CASE**

**Wilma Dean (Part 1)**

Wilma Dean is an 80-year-old Hispanic-American female with a sixth-grade education who makes a routine visit to your primary care clinic. She has multiple systemic conditions, including hypertension, lower extremity edema, type 2 diabetes, degenerative joint disease, benign paroxysmal positional vertigo, depression, and urinary incontinence. She is prescribed several appropriate medications to manage these conditions. She smokes about 10 cigarettes per day while gambling. She is experiencing bleeding gums and found droplets of blood on her pillow. She changed her diet to softer foods thinking her gums were getting softer because of her age.
1. What do you emphasize regarding her oral health during a short appointment time?
2. Can the medications she is prescribed be contributing to her problems?
3. What might be causing her bleeding gums?
4. Does she need to be referred to a dentist?

## Oral Cavity

Oral health affects and is affected by nutrition, deglutition, digestion, speech, social mobility, employment, self-esteem, and quality of life. The oral cavity is one of the microhabitats of the human body that contains its exclusive microbiome and metagenome. Over 1 billion dynamic biodiverse microflorae (balanced prohealthy and prodisease bacterial species) contribute to the oral microbiome (microbial communities) that occupy the various oral cavity niches, such as the dorsum of the tongue, buccal mucosa, teeth, periodontal tissues, soft palate, and tonsils. These microflorae

contribute to maintaining a healthy and balanced physiologic oral ecosystem. The oral mucosa and gingival tissue function as defense barriers to continual exposure to harmful agents, foreign substances, and diverse oral microbiome. The immune system is key to the defense against disease at these barrier sites while maintaining homeostasis with the communal microbiome. Saliva is essential to maintaining homeostasis and defending against disease. A shift in the oral ecosystem may occur and may disrupt the once commensal relationship among microbes to pathologic acidogenic (acid forming) and aciduric (tolerate acidic habitat) microbes associated with oral disease development in the older adults. Oral health deterioration will limit nutritional intake options, reduce chewing efficiency, affect body mass index (weight loss and/or obesity), increase frailty risk, contribute to systemic conditions (e.g., diabetes, heart disease) and associated comorbidities, compromise communication, contribute to social isolation, and exacerbate depression.

## Assessment of Oral Health

The Oral Health Assessment Tool (OHAT) is a validated and reliable instrument (Table 53.2) used to assess oral health and to facilitate oral hygiene. It is comprised of eight assessment components with maximum of 2 points, with 0 = healthy, 1 = oral changes, and 2 = unhealthy with maximum score of 16 and lowest score of 0. The eight assessment categories include lips, tongue, gums, tissues, saliva, natural teeth/dentures, oral cleanliness, and dental pain. The OHAT was originally designed for institutionalized settings, including cognitively compromised residents; however, more recently it has been adapted to community and primary care settings. The application of the OHAT will help the primary care provider to determine the severity of oral disease and select the appropriate intervention.[1]

## Dental (Coronal and Root) Caries

The majority of independent older adults retain their natural dentition. Dental caries development is a multifactorial shift within the complex dental biofilm impacted by salivary composition and flow.[2] Dental caries initiation requires four elements: host, bacteria, time, and fermentable carbohydrates.[3] Dental biofilm is a nonmineralized/soft, sticky coating that entraps food particles, human proteins, oral bacteria, and viruses and preserves their deoxyribonucleic acid. Biofilm attaches to teeth, dental restorations, and fixed and removable prostheses.[4] Dental calculus development entails metabolic activities to strengthen the bacterial colony attachment on tooth surfaces, dental restorations, and dental prostheses. Early stages of the disease are reversible; however, unmanaged dental caries results in a chronic slow developing infection. Disease progression modulating factors comprise host, biophysiologic, sociobehavioral, and socioenvironmental factors that result in disease expression. Ninety-three percent of dentate older adults suffer from transmissible bacterial (*Streptococci mutans* and related acidogenic species) infections of the hard tissues (tooth) dental caries, whereas 18% have unrestored/untreated dental caries (Fig. 53.1).[5]

Older adults are four times more likely to have unrestored dental caries than schoolchildren because of social-behavioral risk factors such as smoking, limited financial resources, and access to care barriers that can result in pain, infection, reduced quality of life, and increased risk of morbidity and mortality. Unrestored dental caries account for over 50% of tooth losses. Over 32% of older adults are missing at least six permanent teeth, compromising nutritional intake and contributing to social isolation.[3] Visible dental calculus always harbors nonmineralized biofilm that

## TABLE 53.2   Oral Health Assessment Tool for Dental Screening

Client:__ Completed by:__                                                                          Date: / /

Scores — *You can circle individual words as well as giving a score in each category and can write notes in the category scores column also*

| Category | 0 = healthy | 1 = changes[a] | 2 = unhealthy[a] | Category scores |
|---|---|---|---|---|
| Lips | smooth, pink, moist | dry, chapped, or red at corners | swelling or lump, white/red/ulcerated patch; bleeding/ulcerated at corners | |
| Tongue | normal, moist roughness, pink, | patchy, fissured, red, coated | patch that is red and/or white, ulcerated, swollen | |
| Gums and tissues | pink, moist, smooth, no bleeding | dry, shiny, rough, red, swollen, one ulcer/sore spot under dentures | swollen, bleeding, ulcers, white/red patches, generalized redness under dentures | |
| Saliva | moist tissues, watery and free flowing saliva | dry, sticky tissues, little saliva present, resident thinks they have a dry mouth | tissues parched and red, very little/no saliva present, saliva is thick, resident thinks they have a dry mouth | |
| Natural teeth Yes/No | no decayed or broken teeth/roots | 1 to 3 decayed or broken teeth/ roots or very worn down teeth | ≥ 4 decayed or broken teeth/roots, or very worn down teeth, or <4 teeth | |
| Dentures Yes/No | no broken areas or teeth, dentures regularly worn, and named | 1 broken area/tooth or dentures only worn for 1 to 2 h daily, or dentures not named, or loose | >1 broken area/tooth, denture missing or not worn, loose and needs denture adhesive, or not named | |
| Oral cleanliness | clean and no food particles or tartar in mouth or dentures | food particles/tartar/plaque in 1–2 areas of the mouth or on small area of dentures or halitosis (bad breath) | food particles/tartar/plaque in most areas of the mouth or on most of dentures or severe halitosis (bad breath) | |
| Dental pain | no behavioral, verbal, or physical signs of dental pain | are verbal &/or behavioral signs of pain, such as pulling at face, chewing lips, not eating, aggression | are physical pain signs (swelling of cheek or gum, broken teeth, ulcers), as well as verbal &/or behavioral signs (pulling at face, not eating, aggression) | |
| | | | TOTAL____ SCORE: 16 | |

[a]Refer person to have a dental examination by a dentist unless person and/or family/guardian refuses dental treatment
Complete oral hygiene care plan and start oral hygiene care interventions for person
Review this person's oral health again on   Date: / /

(a) referenced within the table. a). Chalmers J, Johnson V, Tang JH, Titler MG. Evidence-based protocol: oral hygiene care for functionally dependent and cognitively impaired older adults. *J Gerontol Nurs.* 2004;30(11):5−12. doi:10.3928/0098-9134-20041101-06 Citation (b) illustrates the validity and reliability of the instrument. b). Chalmers JM, King PL, Spencer AJ, Wright FA, Carter KD. The oral health assessment tool—validity and reliability. *Aust Dent J.* 2005;50(3):191−199. doi:10.1111/j.1834-7819.2005.tb00360.x

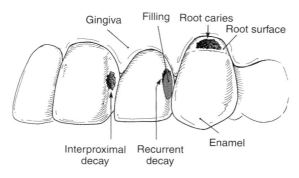

• **Figure 53.1** The most common form of dental caries in older adults is root caries: decay that attacks the portion of the tooth not protected by enamel, that is, the root. Root caries may appear as a tan, brown, or black discoloration in this area or as frank cavitation. Recurrent caries develop adjacent to a filling at its margin. Interproximal caries occur between teeth and may not be observed clinically.

compromises the dental-gingival and implant-mucosal apparatus. Clinical attachment loss of the periodontal tissues, compromising social habits and insufficient or aggressive oral hygiene practices, increases the risk for root caries development in older adults.[6] With advanced age, compromised manual dexterity and health-destructive social habits cause an increased risk of coronal and root caries, as well as tooth fracture and increase risk of tooth loss.[7] Past caries experience is the single most robust predictor of future caries development. Moreover, recurrent caries occurring between the interface of the existing restoration and natural tooth structure are more prevalent in older adults. The rate of recurrent caries may be caused by restorative material's susceptibility to degradation of the surrounding tooth structure encircling the restoration.[8] Enamel requires a pH of 5.5 to demineralize, whereas dentin/cementum will demineralize at a pH of 6.5; however, carcinogenic bacterial survive at a pH of 4.5.[9,10] Dental coronal, recurrent, and root caries share the same etiology; however, the rate of disease expression is dependent on the host. Past caries experience along with sociodemographic factors, salivary flow, buffering capacity, noncompliance to good oral hygiene practices, and dietary selection accelerate disease expression and do not always directly correlate with a fermentable carbohydrate diet.[11]

The majority of older adults have high dental plaque scores, multiple restored tooth surfaces, high caries risk profile, fractured teeth, and premature tooth loss often related to physical limitations, as well as systemic conditions. Topical and systemic exposure to fluoride, good oral hygiene practices, and access to oral healthcare will reduce the risk for dental caries progression. Dental caries assessment and disease prevention options are illustrated in Table 53.3 based on key (intraoral/systemic/psychosocial/behavioral) risk factors and rated as low, moderate, high risk, as well as recommended over-the-counter supplements that may be used for disease prevention.[12,13]

## Periodontal Disease

Both dental caries and periodontal diseases are common nonage-related, often silent conditions that contribute to tooth loss. Both diseases can impact self-esteem, social isolation, and depression and can lead to compromise in nutritional intake and frailty. The etiology of periodontal disease is dental plaque-initiated and multifactorial with typically gram-negative anaerobes with bacterial

virulence factors to trigger systemic inflammation upon entry into the circulation. This chronic infectious disorder affects the gingiva, the connective tissue supporting the teeth and alveolar bone (Fig. 53.2). Dietary accumulation of subgingival plaque biofilm on the retentive surfaces of the natural dentition, lack of oral hygiene practices, and social habits elicit an irreversible gingival inflammatory response that affects at least 70% of older adults.[14] The host response to the bacterial challenge and byproducts triggers a complex inflammatory cascade that results in soft tissue damage and alveolar bone loss.

There are two types of periodontal diseases: gingivitis and periodontitis. Gingivitis can occur in systemically healthy individuals and is the more common multifactorial, plaque induced, reversible, less-severe form of periodontal disease. It is clinically described as inflammation that will spread over the periodontal supporting structures of the gingiva with lack of periodontal (bone and connective tissue) breakdown. Symptoms may include minor swelling, redness, halitosis, blood in the saliva, and bleeding with tooth brushing.[6]

Unmanaged gingivitis progresses to advanced stages of periodontal disease, which affects 10% to 20% of the population. Prevalence varies with sociobehavioral factors. Compromised host and local and chronic systemic conditions have been identified as precursors of disease progression and tooth loss.[15] Periodontal disease is described as gingival inflammation with irreversible breakdown of the root attached connective tissue, as well as the dentoalveolar structures.[16] Advanced stages of disease progression result in breakdown of connective tissue attachment, alveolar bone resorption, and thus apical relocation of the epithelial (junctional) attachment to result in periodontal pocket formation. The outcome of unmanaged chronic periodontal disease is increase in tooth hypermobility, tooth loss, and edentulousness.[17]

The American Academy of Periodontology with the European Federation of Periodontology in a joint effort conducted an evidence-based review of the literature to reach an agreement on periodontal disease classification and staging.[18] Social habit of smoking and type 2 diabetes synergistic affect the subgingival microbiome. Other rare systemic (genetic, autoimmune, endocrine/metabolic, physiologic) conditions affect the periodontium independent of dental biofilm/plaque accumulation.[18]

Oral bacteria toxins are able to penetrate blood vessels and connective tissue, and progress to invade tissues, organs, and systemic pathways that contribute to other systemic disease processes.[19] Other studies have found individuals with advanced periodontal disease that includes alveolar bone loss suggesting the individual had a higher risk of mortality. Patient-tailored oral hygiene instructions, as well as oral health destructive behavior modification and access to oral cleaning aids designed to meet the physical limitations of older adults, are warranted to promote disease prevention.

Common types of periodontal diseases in older adults are illustrated in Table 53.4, which offers description (cause, timeline, concise clinical presentation, and management options) of periodontal disease stages and management options.

## Edentulism

The erroneous perception that increases in chronologic age coincide with increases in the prevalence of edentulousness is waning. The current findings show that only 25% to 30% of older adults have lost all of their natural dentition, primarily because of lack of access to oral healthcare services postretirement.[20,21] Most epidemiologic studies have indicated that the incidence of edentulism is

## TABLE 53.3   Dental Caries Assessment and Disease Prevention for Older Adults

| Risk | Risk Factors | Over-the-Counter Supplements or Prescription |
|---|---|---|
| **Low risk**<br>• No decay or broken teeth/roots<br>• Moist tissues and free flowing saliva<br>• Clean and no food particles/tartar on teeth<br>• No signs or verbal dental pain | • Normal salivary flow<br>• Good oral hygiene (clean and no food particles, tartar on teeth or dentures)<br>• Regular dental visits (once/year)<br>• No new lesions in the last 3 years | Daily oral (tooth-brushing, flossing) care, community water fluoridation, avoid acidic and or sugary foods and drinks, Dentifrice ($\sim$1100 ppm) |
| **Moderate risk**<br>• 1–3 decayed/broken teeth/roots<br>• Dry, sticky tissues, little saliva present<br>• Moderate –high consumption of dietary sugar<br>• Moderate to high consumption of carbonated beverages<br>• Food particles/tartar in 1–2 areas of the mouth or denture<br>• Tobacco and alcohol use<br>• 1–3 prescription medications<br>• Verbal or signs of pain | • Frequent intake of carbohydrates or sugars (mints, lozenges, candy, sweet baked goods etc.)<br>• Brushes teeth >2 times per day and no other source of fluoride<br>• Uses multiple medications that may reduce quality and quantity of saliva<br>• Multiple broken/missing teeth<br>• Teeth with carious root surfaces<br>• Occasional visits to the dentist or NO visits to dentist<br>• Use of removable dental prosthesis<br>• 1–2 new visible carious lesions | Daily oral (tooth-brushing, flossing) care, avoid acidic and or sugary foods and drinks<br>0.05% NaF (sodium fluoride) rinse 1–2 times daily OR<br>Prescribe 1.1% NaF (5000 ppm) paste/gel brushed on the teeth at bedtime after flossing and brushing with regular strength toothpaste 1–2 times per day<br>Prescribe casein phosphopeptide-amorphous calcium phosphate (CPP-ACP) *MI Paste Plus* applied in morning and night to teeth after flossing and brushing with regular strength toothpaste<br>Refer to dentist |
| **High risk**<br>• ≥4 decayed/broken teeth<br>• Very little to no saliva<br>• Food particles and tartar in most areas of the mouth<br>• Physical signs of pain, such as aggression or including not eating | • Low salivary flow<br>• Poor quality of daily oral care brushing less than 2x per day<br>• Chronic systemic conditions that contribute to caries susceptibility (mental health issues, minimal manual dexterity, drug abuse, etc.)<br>• Frequent intake of carbohydrates or sugars (mints, lozenges, candy, sweet baked goods)<br>• Multiple teeth with carious root surfaces<br>• Multiple medications and over-the-counter supplements<br>• Use of ill-fitting removable dental prosthesis<br>• NO visit to dentist<br>• Prosthetic retainer teeth | Daily oral (tooth-brushing, flossing) care, avoid acidic and or sugary foods and drinks<br>Prescribe 1.1% NaF paste used 1–2 times per day OR<br>Prescribe 1.1% NaF gel brushed on the teeth after flossing and brushing with regular strength toothpaste applied on teeth 1–2 times per day<br>CPP-ACP *MI Paste Plus* applied in morning and night to teeth after flossing and brushing with regular strength toothpaste<br>Refer to dentist |

(From Slayton RL, Urquhart O, Araujo MWB, et al. Evidence-based clinical practice guideline on nonrestorative treatments for carious lesions: a report from the American Dental Association. *J Am Dent Assoc.* 2018;149(10):837–849. e19.; McReynolds D, Duane B. Systematic review finds that silver diamine fluoride is effective for both root caries prevention and arrest in older adults. *Evid Based Dent.* 2018;19(2):46–47.; Patel J, Anthonappa RP, King NM. Evaluation of the staining potential of silver diamine fluoride: in vitro. *Int J Paediatr Dent.* 2018. [Epub ahead of print].)

dependent upon sociodemographic variables that include race, education, geographic location, dental service utilization, economic status, and damaging oral health habits.[22,23] Other studies indicate edentulism is more prevalent among women with socioeconomic disparities, lack of dental insurance coverage, inability to access oral care, and lower level of education that will affect quality of life, self-rated wellbeing, and self-esteem. Artificial prostheses will impair chewing efficiency by 30% to 40% in comparison with natural teeth, as well as impair the swallowing threshold requiring seven times more chewing strokes to mill the bolus of food before swallowing, therefore food selection is compromised and less enjoyable.[24,25] Impaired chewing efficiency results in consumption of low fiber,

high saturated fat, less carotene, and fewer fruits/vegetables and demonstrated to increase levels of C-reactive protein, interleukin-6, and fibrinogen that increase risk of coronary heart disease. Some studies have indicated that many older adults perceive that it is unnecessary to visit a dentist postdental extractions. The primary cause of partial or total edentulism is caused by chronic oral infection of the teeth and/or of the supporting structures leading to tooth mortality.

Edentulous older adults with compromised social habits are at risk for oral cancer, and an annual oral cancer screening is recommended. Early diagnosis and treatment is recommended particularly for patients that have chronic behavioral risks, including

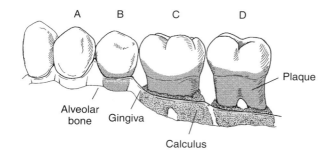

• **Figure 53.2** The periodontium consists of alveolar bone and gingiva, the anatomic foundation for sound teeth (*tooth A*). Healthy periodontium is maintained by thorough oral hygiene practices. When plaque remains on teeth, gingivitis develops (*tooth B*). The accumulation of plaque and calculus on teeth results in destruction of the periodontium known as *periodontitis* (*tooth C*). Periodontitis is considered severe when more than 50% of supporting bone has been lost (*tooth D*).

tobacco and alcohol consumption. Lesions that do not heal shortly after denture adjustments should be addressed as potential malignancies.[26]

Complications of edentulism can be prevented. They include denture stomatitis and angular cheilitis. Denture stomatitis is also known as denture-induced stomatitis, denture sore mouth, inflammatory papillary hyperplasia, and chronic atrophic candidiasis. This is a candida-induced inflammation of the edentulous mucosal tissues causing infection, irritation, and lesions. Some 65% of the partially and totally edentulous individuals and many institutionalized edentulous older adults experience this condition. Transmissible opportunistic pathogens live as nonpathogenic members of the normal microflora. They grow and proliferate in response to alterations of the host's immunologic and physiologic responses. Behavioral habits, including tobacco and alcohol use, promote the pathogenicity of these organisms in combination with the inability to cleanse the oral prosthesis.[21] These habits enable these pathogens to proliferate on the tissue surface of the acrylic resin of the denture. These organisms proliferate in hospitalized older adults (88%) or among those who reside in long-term care facilities and who are unable to manage their oral hygiene needs. Patients who are immunocompromised, suffer from malnutrition (i.e., iron, folate, or vitamin $B_{12}$ deficiency) or have uncontrolled type 2 diabetes are prone to this condition. Those with cancer (acute leukemia, agranulocytosis), or

**TABLE 53.4  Common Types of Periodontal Diseases in Older Adults**

| Stages | Cause | Time Interval | Concise Clinical Description | Management options for primary care clinician |
|---|---|---|---|---|
| Gingivitis Reversible Mild form of periodontal disease Grade A | Systemic factors: medication-induced xerostomia, gingival enlargement (calcium channel blockers, phenytoin), immune status, genetics, mouth breathing, social habits (smoking/alcohol), poor nutrition conditions that depress immunity (i.e., leukemia, HIV/AIDS, or cancer) Local factors: biofilm, plaque (gram-positive cocci and filaments), calculus deposits induced inflammation | 4–7 days initial lesion >14 days chronic lesion Local host response | Erythema, minor tissue edema, halitosis, bleeding on probing/tooth-brushing tenderness | • Disease is reversible • Patient motivation and oral hygiene instruction • Use plaque-reducing dentifrice such as stannous fluoride/sodium fluoride dentifrice • Professional mechanical plaque removal by an oral healthcare professional |
| Advanced lesion transition to periodontitis Grade B and C | Systemic factors: medications, xerostomia, physical/cognitive impairment, chronic illness (i.e., diabetes, obesity), social habits (smoking/alcohol), financial constraints, oral health literacy, poor nutrition, conditions that depress immunity (i.e., leukemia, HIV/AIDS, or cancer treatment) Local factors: biofilm (gram-negative bacteria and spirochetes) expands into the subgingival space, calculus deposits, occlusion, tooth morphology/proximal contact, defective restorations, chronic advanced endodontic lesions | Local host response, >14 days Distant host dependent response | Inflammation has extended to clinical loss of adjacent attachment, pocket depth 4–5 mm in moderate disease, advanced disease pocket depth >5 mm, evidence of alveolar bone loss Tooth mobility is associated with chronic inflammation Bad taste | • Disease is irreversible • Use plaque-reducing dentifrice such as stannous fluoride/sodium fluoride dentifrice • Nonalcohol-based fluoridated mouth rinse • Antiseptic oral mouth rinse • Chlorhexidine gluconate 0.12% alcohol-free mouth rinse • At least quarterly professional mechanical plaque/calculus removal by the oral healthcare professional team as well as oral hygiene instruction to facilitate patient motivated self-care oral hygiene practices |

(From Tonetti MS, Eickholz P, Loos BG, et al. Principles in prevention of periodontal diseases: consensus report of group 1 of the 11th European workshop on periodontology on effective prevention of periodontal and peri-implant diseases. *J Clin Periodontal.* 2015;42(16):5; James P, Worthington HV, Parnell C, et al. Chlorhexidine mouthrinse as an adjunctive treatment for gingival health. *Cochrane Database Syst Rev.* 2017;3:CD008676.)

receiving antibiotic therapy, corticosteroids, radiation therapy, and/or chemotherapy, are also susceptible.

◆◆ **Oral lesions that do not heal shortly after denture adjustments should be addressed as potential malignancies.**

Continuous swallowing or possible aspiration of these pathogens from denture plaque is a risk for pleuropulmonary and gastrointestinal infections. Denture plaque naturally adheres and accumulates on the dental prosthesis forming a dense microbial layer. Intraoral fungal microbe is primarily located on the tongue and tonsillar areas of the oral cavity. Candida biofilm along with bacteria adherence in microcracks, voids on the intaglio/unpolished side of the denture, may compromise the denture stability and support.

Continuous wearing of the denture can result in traumatic ulceration. Salivary proteins, mainly histatins, inhibit the pathogenicity of Candida and can control drug-resistant antifungal infections. Histatins are synthesized in the parotid and submandibular glands and provide fungicidal and bactericidal activity. Good oral hygiene of the edentulous mucosa and of the prosthesis, as well as limiting use of the prosthesis while resting, is recommended to prevent traumatic ulceration. This practice is advised to reduce the possibility of candidiasis.

◆◆ **Continuous wearing of the denture can result in traumatic ulceration.**

Angular cheilitis (cracking of the lips) is often associated with *Candida albicans* or *Staphylococcus aureus*, as well as nutritional deficiencies. Excessive use of antibiotics and immunosuppressive therapies contribute to this condition. Oftentimes the lesion will spontaneously resolve. Recurrence is not uncommon and may require use of topical antifungals (nystatin oral suspension 100,000 U/mL, chlorhexidine gluconate 0.12% nonalcohol-based rinse), nutritional intervention, evaluation of the dental prosthesis, or treatment of lesions with a soft tissue laser to prevent future recurrence.[26,27]

## Oral Cancer

Oral cancer is the eighth most common cancer in the United States with the average age of diagnosis at 62 years and a 65% overall 5-year survival rate. Most common sites are lips, tongue, salivary glands, floor of the mouth, gums, oropharynx, and tonsillar areas. Oral pharyngeal cancer is more visible and deforming than other cancers, and it is unfortunately detected and diagnosed at advanced stages. Lack of implementation of the national oral cancer screening standard recommendations, public awareness, and limited health literacy regarding risk factors, signs, and symptoms contribute to the morbidity and mortality rates.[28] Risk factors for oral cancer are a complex interaction of behavioral, social, hereditary, systemic, economic, and environmental conditions. Pathogenesis includes social habits, such as poor oral hygiene, history of tobacco, alcohol use, unprotected exposure to ultraviolet radiation, and exposure to sexually acquired human papillomavirus (HPV), especially HPV-16, as well as inadequate consumption of grains, fruits, and vegetables. Recent studies have shown HPV contributes to 70% of oropharyngeal cancer. HPV vaccination early in life may prevent HPV-mediated oropharyngeal cancer.[29–31]

Early signs and symptoms of oropharyngeal cancer are asymptomatic with minimal discomfort and indiscernible tissue changes.

Early signs may include recurring mouth sore and persistent white or red patches on the tongue, mucosa, gums, and tonsillar area. Leukoplakia (white patch) is a frequent finding in individuals with history of tobacco, alcohol use, cheek biters/bruxism, and denture wearers that have the potential to progress to oral cancer. Intraoral red patches (erythroplakia) are rarer lesions with a greater potential to become malignant. Clinical signs and symptoms of advanced stages of oral cancer include chronic mouth pain, sore throat, voice alteration, difficulty swallowing, chewing, moving tongue, and jaw, swelling of the edentulous areas with chief complaint "dentures do not fit." Numbness in the mouth, teeth with hypermobility, loss of weight, lumps in the neck, and persistent bad breath are additional indicators of possible advanced oral cancer.

Risk reduction, early detection, diagnosis, staging of oral cancer, and follow-up will result in a better prognosis. Preventive strategies for oral cancer should include community-based education and interprofessional training/practice of oral and primary healthcare providers to manage the oral-systemic healthcare needs of at-risk patients.[30,31]

## Xerostomia

Over 400 medications prescribed to older adults are associated with dry mouth that affect over 30% of hexagenerians ($\geq$65 years) and 40% of the octogenarians ($\geq$80 years). Medication affects functional or organic disturbances of the salivary gland, leading to lack of normal salivary secretion.[32,33]

Saliva inhibits demineralization of the tooth surface and enhances remineralization. It has both buffering and lubricating capability. Furthermore, saliva is part of a natural defense system with antifungal, antiviral, and antibacterial properties.[34] It enhances taste, bolus formation, and digestion of food. As salivary flow decreases, Candida count increases, thus patients that suffer from xerostomia have a higher prevalence of Candida infection. Salivary substitute options (Table 53.5) for older adults suffering from xerostomia at high risk of dental erosion suggest the use of salivary supplements with high viscosity and neutral pH to minimize enamel erosion.

**TABLE 53.5   Salivary Substitutes**

| Brand Name | Manufacturer | pH |
| --- | --- | --- |
| **Mouth Sprays** | | |
| Biotene | SmithKline Beechman Ltd. | 6.18 |
| Emofluor | Dr. Wild & Co | 7.42 |
| Oasis | Oasis Consumer Healthcare | 6.28 |
| **Gels** | | |
| Biotene *oral balance* | GlaxoSmithKline, Brentford Middlesex | 5.49 |
| GC Dry Mouth Gel | GC Corp. | 7.38 |

(From Aykut-Yetkiner A, Wiegand A, Attin T. The effect of saliva substitutes on enamel erosion in vitro. *J Dent*. 2014;42(6):720–725.)

Helpful hint: Patients suffering from xerostomia and at high risk for dental erosion should use high viscous saliva substitutes, but should avoid saliva substitutes with low pH or containing citric acid.

## Systemic Diseases and Oral Disorders

### Diabetes Mellitus

Periodontal disease, periapical lesions, xerostomia, and taste disturbances are more prevalent in diabetics. Other associated conditions include dental caries and oral mucosal lesions.[35]

The risk of periodontal disease is increased twofold in diabetics and could be the initial presentation of the disorder. Progressive disease worsens glycemic control, and an updated systematic review reported that treatment of periodontal disease resulted in a 0.29% reduction in hemoglobin (Hb) $A_{1C}$ at 3 to 4 months, but the effect after 4 months was unclear.[36] The Federation of Periodontology suggests that medical health professionals recommend initial and periodic thorough oral examinations, including comprehensive periodontal examinations, for patients with diabetes.[37]

Oral mucosal disorders are common with diabetes, and xerostomia is one of the more frequent oral complaints. Poor glycemic control has been associated with xerostomia and lower salivary flow rates, as well as polyuria and osmotic diuresis. Medications often are contributory. Sodium-glucose cotransporter 2 inhibitors increase glucose excretion and can lead to dehydration and increased thirst. Tricyclic antidepressants (for neuropathy) and some antihypertensives are xerogenic. Hence the evaluation of a diabetic patient presenting with the complaint of a dry mouth should include a thorough medication review and assessment of blood sugar control. Other oral mucosal disorders frequently encountered in diabetics include fungal infection related to dentures (denture stomatitis) and tongue alterations such as migratory glossitis, coated tongue, and fissured tongue.[38] Diabetic patients with dental prosthesis should undergo frequent dental checkups to prevent denture stomatitis.

### Cardiovascular Disorders

Periodontal disease is also associated with an increased risk of developing a stroke or coronary artery disease, with inflammation thought to be the pathophysiologic link. In a large cohort study, periodontal disease was shown to be a risk factor for ischemic stroke (adjusted hazard ratio [HR], 1.89 with mild disease; HR, 2.20 with severe disease), and those who received routine dental care reduced their risk (HR, 0.77).[39] Stroke patients are more likely to have poorer oral health (dental caries, periodontal disease, and tooth loss) and less frequently receive dental care.[40] Aspiration pneumonia, a significant cause of mortality poststroke, may be associated with oral health. A review concluded that evidence was weak on whether improving oral care reduces the risk of pneumonia or mortality after a stroke and that guidelines on the subject acknowledged the lack of supporting evidence.[41] In patients with cardiovascular disease and chronic periodontitis, a review found only one study of low quality and concluded that there was insufficient evidence to support or refute whether periodontal therapy can prevent recurrence of cardiovascular events.

Patients with cardiac disease or symptoms are often encountered in dental practices. When surgery is planned, primary care clinicians are consulted to assess their risk of a major adverse cardiovascular event perioperatively. Similar to recommendations for patients undergoing other surgeries, elective procedures should be deferred for any unstable cardiac conditions, such as unstable angina, acute heart failure, significant arrhythmias, symptomatic valvular heart disease, and a recent myocardial infarction (within 60 days). A blood pressure reading of 180/110 mmHg or higher is also considered as an absolute cutoff for procedures. Additional factors that increase major adverse cardiac event risk are poorly controlled cardiac risk factors (ischemic heart disease, chronic heart failure, stroke, chronic kidney disease, and diabetes), related comorbidities, $O_2$ saturation of $\leq 94\%$, body mass index $> 35$ m$^2$/kg, sleep apnea, low functional capacity, significant anxiety, and more invasive procedures.[42]

Antihypertensive medications can also have a negative impact on oral health. Dry mouth (xerostomia) has been associated with thiazide diuretics, loop diuretics, clonidine, and angiotensin-converting enzyme (ACE) inhibitors. Gingival hyperplasia has been reported as a side effect of calcium channel blockers. Dysgeusia (altered taste) has been associated with beta-blockers, diltiazem, and ACE inhibitors. Lichenoid reactions have been reported in patients taking captopril, methyldopa, furosemide, thiazide diuretics, or beta-blockers. The recommended approach to patients presenting with medication-related symptoms or conditions is to change the offending drug(s).[43]

### Thrombolytic Therapy

A 2013 review indicated a trend toward increased occurrence of immediate postoperative bleeding for patients on dual antiplatelet therapy compared with single therapy or controls, but there was no increase in the occurrence of intraprocedure or late postoperative bleeding complications.[44] Given the importance of antiplatelet therapy in reducing the risk of poststent thrombosis, a consensus opinion from the American Heart Association (AHA), the American College of Cardiology, the Society for Cardiovascular Angiography and Interventions, the American College of Surgeons, and the American Dental Association (ADA) recommended that dentists concerned about periprocedural and postprocedural bleeding should contact the patient's cardiologist regarding the patient's antiplatelet regimen to discuss optimal patient management before discontinuation.

For warfarin, a 2015 systematic review concluded that patients with an international normalized ratio within the therapeutic range can safely continue taking their regular dose of warfarin before dental extractions.[45] More recently, a systematic review that included novel oral anticoagulants found that continuing anticoagulation during dental procedures did not increase the risk of bleeding in most trials, and that heparin bridging was associated with an increase in bleeding incidence.[46] The ADA does not deem it necessary to alter anticoagulation or antiplatelet therapy before dental intervention, and a monograph is available on their website.

### Prevention of Infective Endocarditis

The mouth has been recognized as a portal of entry for bacteremia more than 100 years ago, and initial recommendations in 1955 for antibiotic prophylaxis against Streptococcus from the AHA were for individuals with rheumatic heart disease and congenital heart disease. Since then, the guideline has been revised several times because of a shift in prevailing cardiac conditions, concerns about efficacy, antibiotic resistance, lack of randomized clinical trials, and questions about the contribution of dental procedures to infective endocarditis (IE). Transient bacteremia can result from activities such as chewing food, tooth brushing, flossing, and using toothpicks, but these usually do not result in IE. The increasing number of cardiovascular electronic cardiovascular devices, prosthetic valve implants, transcatheter aortic valve implantations, along with frequent invasive procedures, are thought to contribute to the rise of IE in older adult patients. The rate of bacterial-IE related hospitalizations in the United States rose from 11.4 per

100,000 population-years to 16.6 per 100,000 population-years from 1999 to 2008, driven primarily by an increase in *S. aureus* IE. Staphylococci were isolated in 57.5% of cases, followed by strepto-cocci/enterococci (33%).[47] The most common portal of entry (POE) identified was the cutaneous route (40%), and associated with intravenous drug use and healthcare. The second most common POE was oral or dental (29%), and more commonly associated with a dental infection (59%) rather than a dental procedure (12%).[48] This suggests that maintenance of good oral health may be another strategy to reduce the risk of IE.

The 2007 guidelines from the AHA on antibiotic prophylaxis (AP) on prevention of viridians group streptococcus IE for individuals undergoing dental procedures are directed at high-risk individuals, based on the cardiac condition and the type of procedure.[49] AP is recommended for cardiac disorders listed in Table 53.6, and only for procedures involving manipulation of gingival tissue or the periapical region of teeth, or perforation of the oral mucosa (Table 53.7). The antibiotic regimens are outlined in Table 53.8. A metaanalysis of the impact of AP guidelines showed a reduction in bacteremia, but case-control studies suggest it did not translate to a significant protective effect against IE in low-risk patients.[50] After publication of the guidelines, an analysis of US healthcare data from 2003 to 2015 showed a fall in AP prescribing and a rise in the incidence of IE in high-risk individuals, but it did not establish a cause-and-effect relationship.[51]

In summary, the role of the primary care clinician in the prevention of IE with dental procedures is to identify at-risk patients based on their cardiac condition and type of procedure planned, educate patients at high risk on the benefits and risks of AP, recommend which agent to use based on the AHA guidelines, and encourage them to maintain good oral health.

## Dementia

Dementia is considered a risk factor for poor oral health, and older patients with dementia have higher levels of plaque, periodontal disease, and dental caries. They are more likely to need help with tooth brushing and tend to wear their dentures less as cognitive impairment progresses.[52] Oral hygiene deficiencies, plaque, and gingival inflammation worsen with increasing severity of cognitive impairment.[53] A review of studies investigating the impact of strategies to improve oral health in cognitively impaired individuals suggests improvement can be achieved in some respects, with more pronounced benefits in patients who need assistance with oral hygiene tasks or had poorer oral health at baseline (Level of evidence [LOE] = C).[54]

⇥ **To improve the oral health in cognitively impaired individuals, the interprofessional healthcare team is crucial in the development and implementation of a treatment plan that incorporates the patient's goals, level of functioning, and comorbidities.**

Individuals with dementia and psychological symptoms and/or who have difficulty cooperating with more invasive procedures pose another treatment dilemma. Intravenous sedation (IVS) is an available option to reduce dental accidents and allow for the

**TABLE 53.7  Dental Procedures for Which Endocarditis Prophylaxis Is Recommended for Patients With Conditions Listed in Table 53.6**

- All dental procedures that involve manipulation of gingival tissue or the periapical region of teeth, or perforation of the oral mucosa
- This includes all dental procedures except the following procedures and events:
  - Routine anesthetic injections through noninfected tissue
  - Taking of dental radiographs
  - Placement of removable prosthodontic or orthodontic appliances
  - Adjustment of orthodontic appliances
  - Shedding of deciduous teeth and bleeding from trauma to the lips or oral mucosa

(From Wilson W, Taubert KA, Gewitz M, et al. American Heart Association Guideline: Prevention of Infective Endocarditis. *Circulation.* 2007;116(15):1736–1754.)

**TABLE 53.6  Cardiac Conditions Associated With the Highest Risk of Adverse Outcome From Endocarditis for Which Prophylaxis With Dental Procedures Is Recommended**

- Prosthetic cardiac valve
- Previous infective endocarditis
- Congenital heart disease (CHD) only in the following categories:
  1. Unrepaired cyanotic CHD, including those with palliative shunts and conduits
  2. Completely repaired CHD with prosthetic material or device by surgery or catheter
     Intervention during the first 6 months after the procedure
     Prophylaxis is recommended because endothelialization of prosthetic material occurs within 6 months after the procedure
  3. Repaired CHD with residual defects at the site or adjacent to the site of a prosthetic patch or prosthetic device, which inhibits endothelialization
- Cardiac transplantation recipients who develop cardiac valvulopathy

(From Wilson W, Taubert KA, Gewitz M, et al. American Heart Association Guideline: Prevention of Infective Endocarditis. *Circulation.* 2007;116(15):1736–1754.)

**TABLE 53.8  Regimens for Dental Procedures**

| Regimens for Dental Procedures | Agent (Single Dose 30–60 Minutes Before Procedure) |
| --- | --- |
| Oral | Amoxicillin 2 g |
| Allergic to oral penicillin or amoxicillin | Cephalexin 2 g, or clindamycin 600 mg, or azithromycin or clarithromycin 500 mg |
| Unable to take oral medication | Ampicillin 2 g IM or IV, or cefazolin or ceftriaxone 1 g IM or IV |
| Allergic to penicillins or ampicillin and unable to take oral medication | Cefazolin or ceftriaxone[a] 1 g IM or IV, orc Clindamycin 600 mg IM or IV |

(From Wilson W, Taubert KA, Gewitz M, et al. American Heart Association Guideline: Prevention of Infective Endocarditis. *Circulation.* 2007;116(15):1736–1754.)
*IM,* Intramuscular; *IV,* intravenous.
[a]Cephalosporins should not be used in a person with a history of anaphylaxis, angioedema, or urticaria with penicillins or ampicillin

performance of such procedures. A retrospective study on outpatients reported completion of almost all dental treatments with IVS but recommended stringent attention to circulatory (46% of all cases) and respiratory changes (52% of all cases) especially with tooth extractions.[55] Postoperative delirium (POD) is another concern in patients with dementia. A retrospective study on outpatient anesthesia management for dental treatment in patients with severe Alzheimer disease, none of the patients exhibited POD in the recovery period. These patients underwent a preanesthetic evaluation, received smaller drug doses, and the facility had an aggressive nondrug prevention strategy, suggesting the importance of appropriate anesthesia management.[56] Given the various aspects and challenges in oral health in cognitively impaired individuals, the interprofessional healthcare team is crucial in the development and implementation of a treatment plan that incorporates the patient's goals, level of functioning, and comorbidities.

## Joint Replacement

Total hip and total knee replacements are cost-effective procedures for end-stage arthritis. Postoperative, periprosthetic joint infections have always been a concern, and in 2014 the rate of periprosthetic joint infection in the first year ranged from 0.58% to 1.6% after knee arthroplasty and 0.67% to 2.4% after hip arthroplasty.[57] Historically, prophylactic treatment with antibiotics for any dental procedure was given to all patients who had a prosthetic joint. The hypothesized mechanism was that transient bacteria from manipulation of the gums could lead to seeding the prosthetic joint, which would lead to infection. This hypothesis has never been proven. Berbari et al. found that antibiotic prophylaxis in high-risk or low-risk dental procedures did not decrease the risk of subsequent hip or knee infection (adjusted odds ratio [OR], 0.9; 95% confidence interval [CI], 0.5−1.6; and 1.2; 95% CI, 0.7−2.2).[58]

In 2012 a panel of experts representing the American Academy of Orthopedic Surgeons (AAOS) and the ADA published a systematic review and clinical practice guidelines, entitled "Prevention of Orthopedic Implant Infection in Patients Undergoing Dental Procedures: Evidence-based Guidelines and Evidence Report." In 2014 the ADA panel convened to update and clarify the 2012 clinical practice guidelines.[59] The panel identified four case-controlled studies to review and used these studies to construct their recommendations.[58,60−62] Fig. 53.3 reviews the clinical recommendations published by the 2014 ADA expert panel (LOE = D).

In summary, most patients with prosthetic joint implants do not need prophylactic antibiotics before dental procedures. The ADA panel found no association between dental procedures and prosthetic joint infections.[63] In one case-control study, three major risk factors were identified that placed patients at higher risk for prosthetic joint infection and therefore should be considered for prophylactic antibiotics.[58] These risk factors were postoperative complications, including postoperative wound drainage (OR, 18.7; 95% CI, 7.4−47.2), postoperative hematoma (OR, 2.5; 95% CI, 1.3−9.5), and postoperative urinary tract infection (OR, 2.7; 95% CI, 1.04−7.1).[58,63] There was also a strong association

# Management of patients with prosthetic joints undergoing dental procedures

## Clinical Recommendation:

In general, for patients with prosthetic joint implants, prophylactic antibiotics are *not* recommended prior to dental procedures to prevent prosthetic joint infection.

For patients with a history of complications associated with their joint replacement surgery who are undergoing dental procedures that include gingival manipulation or mucosal incision, prophylactic antibiotics should only be considered after consultation with the patient and orthopedic surgeon.* To assess a patient's medical status, a complete health history is always recommended when making final decisions regarding the need for antibiotic prophylaxis.

## Clinical Reasoning for the Recommendation:

- There is evidence that dental procedures are not associated with prosthetic joint implant infections.

- There is evidence that antibiotics provided before oral care do not prevent prosthetic joint implant infections.

- There are potential harms of antibiotics including risk for anaphylaxis, antibiotic resistance, and opportunistic infections like *Clostridium difficile*.

- The benefits of antibiotic prophylaxis may not exceed the harms for most patients.

- The individual patient's circumstances and preferences should be considered when deciding whether to prescribe prophylactic antibiotics prior to dental procedures.

ADA. Center for Evidence-Based Dentistry™

* In cases where antibiotics are deemed necessary, it is most appropriate that the orthopedic surgeon recommend the appropriate antibiotic regimen and when reasonable write the prescription.

Sollecito T, Abt E, Lockhart P, et al. The use of prophylactic antibiotics prior to dental procedures in patients with prosthetic joints: Evidence-based clinical practice guideline for dental practitioners — a report of the American Dental Association Council on Scientific Affairs. JADA. 2015;146(1):11-16.

• **Figure 53.3** Management of patients with prosthetic joints undergoing dental procedures.

with patients who are immunocompromised or have a medical condition, such as diabetes, that may increase the risk of prosthetic joint infection. Despite these associations there was a lack of clinical relevance seen in the observational studies, and further studies are needed.[58] Ultimately, the decision to use prophylactic antibiotics during invasive dental procedure for prevention of periprosthetic joint infection should be a shared decision between orthopedic surgeons, the primary care physician, and subspecialists.

## Chemotherapy and Radiation

### Mucositis

In addition to multiple systemic side effects patients experience from chemotherapy, oral complications are a common complaint. Oftentimes patients fail to discuss or report disruption in their oral health during follow-up with their primary care physician or oncologist. Oral complications are broken down into acute or chronic. Acute complications include mucositis, infection, and saliva and neurosensory changes. Chronic complications in survivors include neurosensory changes; saliva, taste, and functional changes; oral and dental infections; and risk of dental disease and necrosis of the jaw.[64]

Mucositis is mucosal damage secondary to chemotherapy and radiation therapy. It occurs in approximately 20% to 40% of patients receiving conventional chemotherapy and 80% of patients receiving high-dose chemotherapy as seen in hematopoietic stem cell transplantation. In those patients receiving head and neck radiation therapy, 80% to 100% will experience mucositis and is a major dose limiting toxicity.[65]

Oral mucositis can present as erythema of the mucosa and can progress to full ulcerations of the mucosa. This can span into the pharyngeal, laryngeal, and esophageal mucosa. Patients typically have pain with mucositis leading to decrease in nutritional intake and quality of life.[65] Clinically, mucositis starts shortly after therapy has begun, typically around 7 to 10 days of treatment. It is often a self-limiting disease and resolves within 1 to 2 weeks. Some patients who have severe disease might endure a longer course.[66] There are different grading scales when evaluating mucositis. The World Health Organization Scale is shown in Fig. 53.4, and the National Cancer Institute Common Terminology Criteria for Adverse Events is described in Table 53.9.

Although acute mucositis is typically self-limiting and resolves within 2 to 4 weeks after stopping treatment, there are clinical guidelines published for prevention and treatment for oral mucositis. In general, patients undergoing chemotherapy and radiation should be urged to get a comprehensive dental examination and maintain good oral hygiene. This includes brushing regularly with a soft toothbrush, eating a soft diet low in sugar and acid, flossing unless patients have low platelets, rinsing with a nonirritating solution like saline, avoid smoking and alcohol, and minimizing denture use.[67]

In 2004 the Mucositis Study Group of the Multinational Association of Supportive Care in Cancer and International Society of Oral Oncology (MASCC/ISOO) published evidence-based clinical practice guidelines for mucositis. These have been revised and updated by other organizations. The most revised edition of the MASCC/ISOO Clinical Practice Guidelines will be available in 2020.

## Osteonecrosis of the Jaw

The diagnostic criteria prescribed by The International Task Force on Osteonecrosis of the Jaw defines it as exposed bone in the maxillofacial region that does not heal within 8 weeks after identification by healthcare provider, exposure to an antiresorptive agent, and no history of radiation therapy to craniofacial region.[68] The bare bone could lead to infection, pain, swelling, and potentially a break.

Oncology patients receiving bisphosphonates or denosumab have an estimated risk of 1% to 15% of developing osteonecrosis of the jaw. The higher incidence in this population is caused by the higher doses and longer duration used in these patients compared with patients receiving antiresorptive therapy for osteoporosis. Typically, the doses are 12 to 15 times higher for oncology patients. In patients receiving high-dose intravenous bisphosphonate or denosumab therapy, who are at high risk of developing osteonecrosis of the jaw, early and accurate detection of dental disease is imperative.

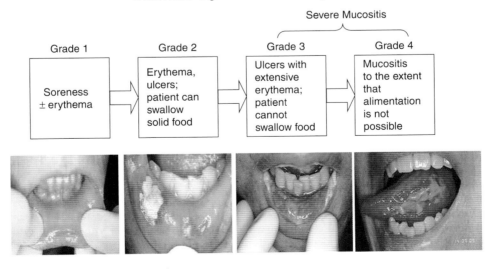

World Health Organization's Oral Toxicity Scale

Severe Mucositis

| Grade 1 | Grade 2 | Grade 3 | Grade 4 |
|---------|---------|---------|---------|
| Soreness ± erythema | Erythema, ulcers; patient can swallow solid food | Ulcers with extensive erythema; patient cannot swallow food | Mucositis to the extent that alimentation is not possible |

• **Figure 53.4** World Health Organization's oral toxicity scale.

| TABLE 53.9 | National Cancer Institute Common Toxicity Criteria | |
|---|---|---|
| Grade | Clinical Examination | Function/Symptoms |
| Grade 1 (mild) | Erythema of the mucosa | Minimal symptoms, normal diet |
| Grade 2 (moderate) | Patchy ulcerations of pseudomembranes | Symptomatic but can eat and swallow modified diet |
| Grade 3 (severe) | Confluent ulcerations or pseudomembranes, bleeding with minor trauma | Symptomatic and unable to adequately aliment or hydrate orally |
| Grade 4 (life threatening) | Tissue necrosis, significant spontaneous bleeding, life-threatening consequences | Symptoms associated with life-threatening consequences |

Major and necessary dental surgeries in oncology patients should be performed before the start of high-dose bisphosphonate or denosumab.[70] There are several imaging modalities that are used for periodic evaluation in patients that are high risk of developing osteonecrosis of the jaw. Plain films are typically used first because they are readily available. If there is concern for progression or further evaluation is warranted, a cone beam computed tomography imaging can be used in diagnosing periapical and periodontal disease. Other imaging modalities that are used include magnetic resonance imaging, bone scans, and positron emission tomography.

In individuals taking high doses of antiresorptive medications, there may be a benefit in withholding them following oral surgery until the soft tissue heals. Bisphosphonates are known to have a high affinity to bone and have a half-life of > 10 years even after cessation.[70] However, bisphosphonates have increased skeletal uptake at the site of local bone injury; therefore withholding the bisphosphonate following surgery may allow the mandible and maxilla to remodel at a faster rate.[71]

## Osteoporosis

In patients receiving bisphosphonates or denosumab for osteoporosis, the incidence for developing osteonecrosis of the jaw is estimated to be 0.001% to 0.01%.[72] This is only a slight increase compared with the general population not taking these medications. Although the incidence is low in patients receiving osteoporosis therapy doses, there are key risk factors that increase the risk for developing osteonecrosis of the jaw (Box 53.1). If the risk of osteonecrosis of the jaw is increased and the risk of fracture is low (fracture risk assessment tool [FRAX] score <10% over the next 10 years) or moderate (FRAX score 10%–20% over the next 10 years), then stop

### • BOX 53.1  Risk Factors for Osteonecrosis of the Jaw

Invasive dental procedure
Diabetes
Glucocorticoid therapy
Periodontal disease
Denture use
Smoking
Antiangiogenic agents

antiresorptive therapy. If risk of fracture is high (FRAX score of ≥ 20% over the next 10 years) and major invasive oral surgery is planned, consider stopping antiresorptive therapy. Consider the use of teriparatide during the time off antiresorptive therapy if no contraindications. If contraindications to teriparatide (hypercalcemia, high parathyroid hormone levels, prior skeletal radiation, malignancy, elevated alkaline phosphatase) are present, stop antiresorptive therapy after dental procedure until surgical site heals. In all patients with increased risk of osteonecrosis of jaw, consider antimicrobial mouth rinse, antibiotics, and always good oral hygiene.

If a patient is at low risk for osteonecrosis of jaw, there is no need to stop antiresorptive medication for dental procedures. The treatment plan must be individualized for each patient in regard to comorbidities, risk of osteonecrosis of jaw, and extent of planned surgery.[71] Conservative therapy of osteonecrosis of jaw focuses on improving oral hygiene, treating active dental and periodontal disease, topical antibiotic mouth rinses, and systemic antibiotic therapy. A referral to a dentist or oral surgeon for possible debridement is required for advanced disease.

### CASE

#### Wilma Dean (Part 2)

Wilma Dean will benefit from an interprofessional team approach to manage her oral systemic conditions. During her visit to your primary care office you assessed her blood glucose level, as well as HbA$_{1C}$ level. The HbA$_{1C}$ result was 8.5%, and her fasting blood glucose was 170 mmol/L. Her cognitive status tested normal, and she denied alcohol consumption. Ms. Dean's OHAT score was 12 and required referral to an oral healthcare provider. The oral healthcare team's findings included advanced chronic periodontal disease, several dental carious lesions, and xerostomia. Ms. Dean's teeth were restored, she received professional mechanical plaque and calculus removal by the oral healthcare professional team, as well as oral hygiene instruction to facilitate patient-driven self-care oral hygiene practices. She was advised to use a nonalcohol antiseptic oral rinse, prescribed salivary (normal pH and high viscosity), and placed on quarterly dental visits. Ms. Dean postintervention follow-up to primary care clinic reports she has not experienced bleeding gums or blood on her pillow, her HbA$_{1C}$ is 6.8%, and her fasting blood glucose is 120 mmol/L.

## Summary

Management of chronic oral systemic conditions requires coordination of services from multiple healthcare professionals at various sites and settings. Patient-centered interprofessional collaborative health promotion strategies in formulating a patient-centered action plan that includes family/caregiver and community resources are critical in managing oral systemic chronic conditions of older adults. The older adult's self-motivation to daily self-manage the oral-systemic condition or to adopt health promoting lifestyle choices will have greater impaction in mitigating chronic disease progression. This approach will lead to positive patient-provider relationships, enhanced patient satisfaction, and improved emotional wellbeing.

### Web Resources

The American Dental Association (ADA) monograph on managing anticoagulants and antiplatelet medications: https://www.ada.org/en/member-center/oral-health-topics/anticoagulant-antiplatelet-medications-and-dental-.

Mucositis Study Group of the Multinational Association of Supportive Care in Cancer and International Society of Oral Oncology (MASCC/ISOO) evidence-based clinical practice guidelines for mucositis: www.mascc.org/mucositis-guidelides.

## Key References

1. Chalmers JM, Pearson A. A systematic review of oral health assessment by nurses and carers for residents with dementia in residential care facilities. *Spec Care Dent.* 2005;25(5):227–233.

35. Mauri-Obradors E, Estrugo-Devesa A, Jané-Salas E, Viñas M, López-López J. Oral manifestations of diabetes mellitus. A systematic review. *Med Oral Patol Oral Cir Bucal.* 2017;22(5):e586–e594.

50. Cahill TJ, Harrison JL, Jewell P, et al. Antibiotic prophylaxis for infective endocarditis: a systematic review and meta-analysis. *Heart.* 2017;103(12):937–944.

54. Rozas NS, Sadowsky JM, Jeter CB. Strategies to improve dental health in elderly patients with cognitive impairment: a systematic review. *J Am Dent Assoc.* 2017;148(4):236–245. e3.

63. Sollecito TP, Abt E, Lockhart PB, et al. The use of prophylactic antibiotics prior to dental procedures in patients with prosthetic joints: Evidence-based clinical practice guideline for dental practitioners--a report of the American Dental Association council on scientific affairs. *J Am Dent Assoc.* 2015;146(1):1–16. e8.

**References available online at** expertconsult.com.

# 54

# Skin Problems

**JUSTIN ENDO**

## OUTLINE

*Additional online-only material indicated by icon.*

## OBJECTIVES

*Upon completion of this chapter, the reader will be able to:*

- Describe lesions and rashes using a four-point process to facilitate differential diagnosis formulation, triage, and communication of dermatologic problems.
- Diagnose and manage common, benign neoplastic skin growths in older patients.
- Diagnose and discuss evidence-based management options for actinic keratosis and common skin cancers in the geriatric population.

- Discuss the differential diagnoses and approach to older patients presenting with itch but without intact primary lesions.
- Discuss the diagnosis and management of common rashes associated with aging, including how to estimate appropriate potency and quantity of topical steroids.
- Discuss evidence-based prevention and treatment of acute herpes zoster and management options for postherpetic neuralgia.

---

### CASE 1

#### Cándido Aguado (Part 1)

You are in the middle of a busy clinic. The next patient is an 84-year-old otherwise healthy Hispanic man, Cándido Aguado, who is in for an annual physical. He immediately hands you a meticulously written list of medical questions. He shakes his head as he explains his friend had a fourth skin cancer removed. The patient has two changing spots (Figs. 54.1 and 54.2) and a request for a general skin check. Because your clinic is running behind, you have only 20 minutes to do his usual healthcare maintenance and also answer his questions.

1. What strategies can you use to balance the needs of addressing healthcare maintenance during his visit while also efficiently examining Mr. Aguado's skin?
2. If you had to succinctly communicate the skin findings to a dermatologist to ask for help, how would you describe what you see?

---

## Dermatologic Examination: Challenges and Practical Approaches

The skin examination is a common and important part of primary care. More than one-third of patients presenting to primary care providers have at least one skin complaint.[1] Ironically, older adults tend to underestimate their risk of skin cancer. Because skin cancers are the most common malignancy,[2] the primary care provider can play an important role in patient education and skin cancer screening.[3] Total body skin cancer screening might be associated with decreased melanoma mortality.[4,5] One study showed cost effectiveness of skin cancer screening at least once in individuals over 50 years of age.[6]

Many challenges exist in the dermatology examination for the nondermatologist. First, many of us had very limited exposures during medical school or residency training.[7] This barrier creates difficulty in approaching the skin from a systematic approach and

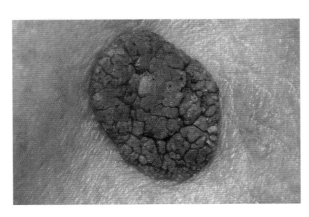

• **Figure 54.1** See Case 1: A lesion of concern. (From Nooshin Brinster, Vincent Liu, Hafeez Diwan, Phillip McKee. *Dermatopathology*. St Louis: Elsevier; 2011: p. 365–366. [Chapter 216: Seborrheic Keratosis, Fig. 2].)

recognizing dermatologic conditions.[8] Second, many primary care providers have time constraints and medically complex patients with a multitude of nondermatologic comorbidities.[9] Third, there might be access limitations to dermatologic specialists, particularly in rural or inner-city areas.[10]

Triaging patients with skin problems and communicating the urgency to the specialist can seem daunting. The purpose of this section is to facilitate the dermatologic examination and to address these barriers. Proposed approaches to general skin cancer screening will be outlined first, followed by a framework for describing skin findings. The remainder of the chapter will focus on common dermatologic problems in primary care of geriatrics rather than providing an exhaustive litany of diagnoses. The primary care provider will be empowered to describe lesions and rashes to a dermatologist or to use clinical decision making tools (see Web Resources section) to facilitate referral, when needed.

## Total Body Skin Examination

❖❖ **The total body skin examination (TBSE) is important for identifying premalignant and malignant skin disorders as part of the routine complete physical, but also should be considered for new rashes or to look for cutaneous clues of underlying systemic diseases.**

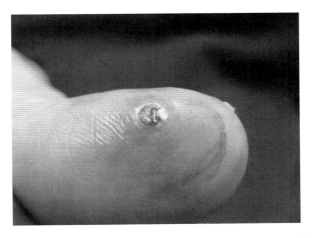

• **Figure 54.2** See Case 1: Another lesion of concern. Used with permission, University of Utah Department of Dermatology.

The TBSE is important for identifying premalignant and malignant skin disorders as part of the routine complete physical, but also should be considered for new rashes or to look for cutaneous clues of underlying systemic diseases.[11] It should be especially encouraged in patients with a personal history of skin cancers or precancers, history of transplantation or immunosuppressant use, chronic antitumor necrosis factor use, exposure to known cutaneous carcinogens (e.g., tanning bed use, arsenic), multiple moles (> 12), or family history of skin cancer.[12,13] Although fair-skinned patients are known to be at highest risk for skin cancer, a recent study highlighted the increasing incidence of melanoma among Hispanic persons and suggested a potential practice gap in preventive education and screening for minority ethnic groups.[14]

Several practical considerations can improve the efficiency and thoroughness of TBSE. During the routine primary care examination that includes palpation and auscultation, the overlying skin can be visually inspected. The patient should ideally disrobe and remove anything that might obscure skin findings, such as accessories (e.g., watches, glasses, hearing aids, toupees, bracelets) and makeup.[11,15] The mucous membranes, anogenital regions, interdigital spaces of fingers and toes, scalp and hair, nails, and retroauricular neck are ideally inspected. Although skin cancers are less common in these areas that are not as sun exposed, delayed diagnosis can lead to potentially devastating outcomes—particularly in non-White patients.[16] Furthermore, some inflammatory conditions of the anogenital region, such as lichen sclerosus, are more common in postmenopausal women and clinically diagnosed with visualization rather than symptomology; when undiagnosed and untreated, they can lead to morbidity, reduced quality of life, and sometimes malignant transformation.[17] Adequate lighting is required to visualize the skin, especially for subtle lesions or areas that cast shadows. Natural sunlight is ideal, otherwise bright lamps can be used with the patient positioned underneath.[11] A portable light, such as penlight or otoscope, held in front of or tangentially to lesions can be helpful to detect subtle changes, such as wrinkling, fluid within lesions, and lesion margins.[11]

The ABCDE (asymmetry, irregular border, color variation, diameter >6 mm, evolving characteristic over months) rule is a simple and popular screening method for melanoma (Fig. 54.3).[18,19] However, by itself, there are limitations in missing the rare amelanotic variant of melanoma or misdiagnosing seborrheic keratosis (see Fig. 54.1) as melanoma.[13] Furthermore, this heuristic does not apply to nonpigmented skin cancers (see later section). For routine skin cancer screening, especially in patients with many skin lesions, a practical, rapid, gestalt approach is the "ugly duckling" detection method.[20] A lesion that does not resemble the overall color, shape, texture of other pigmented lesions on a given patient is considered suspect. Dermoscopy (using a special magnifying lens with polarized light) can be a helpful extension of the unaided eye, but is operator dependent and requires training.[21] Promising noninvasive tools, such as confocal microscopy technology, might facilitate the skin examination in the future. However, cost and technological limitations are current barriers to their routine implementation.[22]

## Four-Point Dermatologic Description

❖❖ **In patients with a specific lesion or rash complaint, the most succinct approach is a systematic four-point method that describes (1) anatomic distribution, (2) configuration, (3) primary lesion and color, and (4) secondary change, if present.**

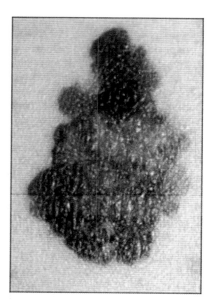

• **Figure 54.3** Melanoma violating the ABCDE rule. (From *The Lancet*, 2015; 385(9985):2323–2323. © 2015. Original figure legend: Melanoma research gathers momentum)

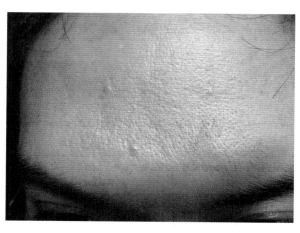

• **Figure 54.4** Small, yellow to flesh-colored papules with central dells on the forehead. Sometimes sebaceous hyperplasias have a pink color and mimic basal cell carcinoma (From Dr. Endo.)

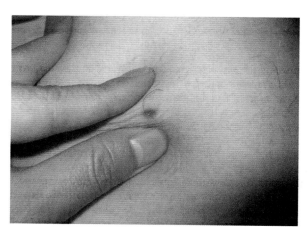

• **Figure 54.5** Brown papule with a "dimple" upon squeezing. Dermatofibromas are often mistaken for other pigmented lesions.

In patients with a specific lesion or rash complaint, the most succinct approach is a systematic four-point method that describes (1) anatomic distribution, (2) lesion configuration, (3) primary lesion and color, and (4) secondary change.[11] History and medications can sometimes be important, but these four descriptors are quintessential for efficiently framing the skin examination and formulating a differential diagnosis. No singular component of this four-point system is necessarily weighted more than the others. It is important to accurately describe skin findings to facilitate patient triage but also to be able to take advantage of Internet and smart-device clinical decision making aids that are currently available (see Web Resources later).[23]

Anatomic distribution of the dermatologic finding, and areas that are relatively spared, can sometimes provide rapid clues about a rash. Configuration (Table 54.1) refers to how the lesion or rash is patterned. Sometimes lesions can be solitary or scattered without any particular pattern (e.g., seborrheic keratoses). Distribution and configuration are sometimes interrelated. For example, a photosensitizing drug eruption might be on the arms and legs in sun-exposed areas while sparing the palms and soles.

| TABLE 54.1 | Examples of Configurations | |
|---|---|---|
| | **Description** | **Example** |
| Annular | Ringlike | Tinea corporis (ringworm), granuloma annulare (Fig. 54.4), porokeratosis (Fig. 54.5) |
| Dermatomal (zosteriform) | Confined to a dermatome and abruptly stops at midline | Herpes zoster (Fig. 54.6) |
| Grouped (herpetiform) | Clustered lesions | Herpes simplex (Fig. 54.7) |
| Linear | Lesions arranged in a line, suggestive of an external cause | Contact dermatitis (Figs. 54.8 and 54.9), scabies burrows (Fig. 54.10) |
| Reticular (retiform) | Netlike or meshlike, suggesting a process affecting the cutaneous vascular network | Livedo reticularis (Fig. 54.11), erythema ab igne (red-brown patch in area of heating pad use) |

(From Bolognia J, Jorizzo JL, Rapini RP. Dermatology. 2nd ed. St. Louis, MO: Mosby/Elsevier; 2008.)

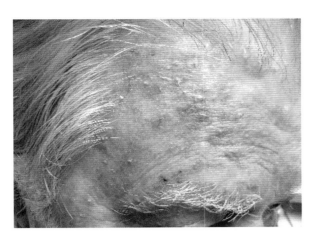

• **Figure 54.6** Actinic keratoses are pink, gritty, scaly papules on sun-exposed skin. (From Dr. Robert Norman.)

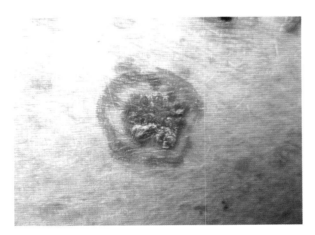

• **Figure 54.7** Squamous cell carcinoma. (From University of Utah Department of Dermatology. With permission.)

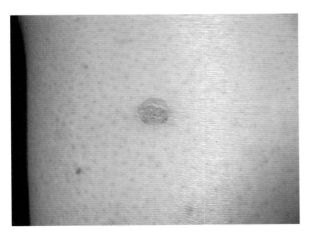

• **Figure 54.8** Nummular eczema consists of scaly, red, coin-shaped patches and plaques that often favors the lower extremities. Unlike psoriasis, it lacks the distinct silvery scale and well-demarcated borders and does not favor extensor surfaces. (From University of Utah Department of Dermatology. With permission.)

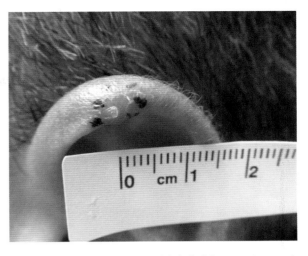

• **Figure 54.9** Chondrodermatitis nodularis helicis presents as a tender nodule or ulcer on the helical (or antihelical) rim of the ear. It is generally considered to be a pressure sore on sun-damaged skin. Clinically, it can be difficult to distinguish from a squamous cell carcinoma, especially if inflamed. (From University of Utah Department of Dermatology. With permission.)

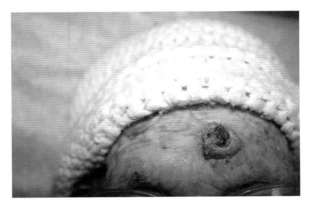

• **Figure 54.10** Keratoacanthoma is an exophytic tumor with central keratotic plugging. It is controversial whether these truly self-resolve. (From Dr. Robert Norman.)

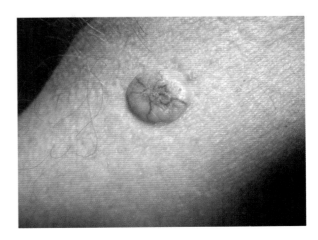

• **Figure 54.11** Basal cell carcinoma showing a pearly nodule with prominently dilated vessels. (From University of Utah Department of Dermatology. With permission.)

| TABLE 54.2 | Examples of Primary Lesions | |
|---|---|---|
| | Description | Examples |
| Macule or patch | Flat without induration or significant elevation | Idiopathic guttate hypomelanosis (Fig. 54.12), lentigo |
| Nodule/tumor | Deep-seated, indurated lesion, often fixed | Squamous cell carcinoma, basal cell carcinoma (Fig. 54.13) |
| Papule or plaque | Elevated lesion confined to upper dermis ± epidermis | Nevus (mole), seborrheic keratosis (see Fig. 54.1), lichen planus (Fig. 54.14), psoriasis |
| Purpura, petechiae or ecchymosis | Nonblanching dark red-purple lesion, suggesting extravasated erythrocytes in skin (in contrast, "violaceous" means a purple color that blanches) | Vasculitis (inflammation and destruction of vascular walls), solar purpura from chronic sun damage, hypercoagulable state (see Fig. 54.11) |
| Pustules | Yellow, pus-filled | Folliculitis, rosacea (Fig. 54.15) |
| Telangiectasia | Prominent blood vessel, blanches easily | Spider telangiectasia, rosacea (see Fig. 54.15), basal cell carcinoma (see Fig. 54.13) |
| Vesicle/bulla | Blister filled with nonpurulent material (e.g., serum, blood). If deeply seated in dermis, it is a cyst (e.g., sebaceous cyst) | Bullous pemphigoid (Fig. 54.16), bullous tinea pedis, acute allergic contact dermatitis (see Figs. 54.8, 54.9), insect bite, herpes (see Fig. 54.7) |
| Wheal/urticaria | Pink-white, blanchable, edematous, pruritic lesions | Hives, serum sickness (Fig. 54.17) |

(From Bolognia J, Jorizzo JL, Rapini RP. Dermatology. 2nd ed. St. Louis, Mo.: Mosby/Elsevier; 2008.)

The primary lesion (Table 54.2) refers to an intact, unmanipulated representation of the process and includes color description. Sometimes it can be difficult to identify a primary lesion if the patient has already self-medicated or excoriated the lesions, or if the lesion is short-lived (e.g., urticaria) or friable. In general, if there is not an intact primary lesion, biopsy tends to be of low diagnostic value. Secondary change (Table 54.3) refers to the findings caused either by the evolution of a primary lesion or an external factor modifying the lesion. In some cases, secondary changes are absent.

**CASE 1**

**Cándido Aguado (Part 2)**

You successfully incorporate a general skin examination of Mr. Aguado while you do your usual healthcare maintenance examination, which is otherwise unremarkable. Fig. 54.1 is a brown, stuck-on, waxy, scaly plaque on the back that he admits to picking. You reassure the patient it is an irritated seborrheic keratosis. The lesion in Fig. 54.2 concerns you, and the patient relays change over a few months following trauma. It is tender and frequently bleeds. You call a dermatologist: "On the left thumb is a solitary red, bleeding, tender nodule that is eroded, rapidly growing, and painful."

## Benign Cutaneous Processes

Recognizing common benign conditions can minimize unnecessary referrals and provide patient reassurance.

Seborrheic keratoses (SKs) are ubiquitous, benign epidermal hyperplasia that often have a yellow, brown, and/or black, waxy, stuck-on appearance (see Fig. 54.1). They sometimes have a

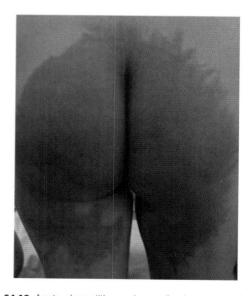

• **Figure 54.12** Acute dermatitis, such as allergic contact dermatitis to povidone iodine, can cause oozing papules and vesicles that might be confused for infection. (From de la Cuadra-Oyanguren J, Zaragozá-Ninet, Sierra-Talamantes, C, et al. Postsurgical contact dermatitis due to povidone iodine: a diagnostic dilemma. *Case Rep.* 2014;105(3):300–304. © 2012. Fig. 2.)

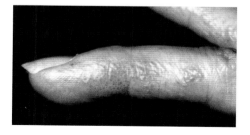

• **Figure 54.13** Eczema on the hands can present with vesicles, particularly along the lateral fingers. This appearance can be mistaken for infection or warts. (From McIntee TJ. *Eczematous Dermatitis, Dermatology Secrets Plus.* 2016:70-81. © 2016. Fig. 8.4 Pompholyx. Characteristic "tapioca" vesicles on the sides of the fingers.)

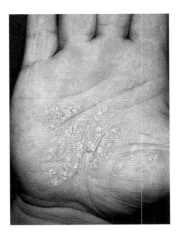

• **Figure 54.14** Chronic eczema consists of dry, scaly patches that sometimes can evolve into thickened plaques with accentuated skin lines (lichenification). (From Zug KA. Eczema. In: Habif, Thomas P. (ed.). *Skin Disease: Diagnosis and Treatment*, 4th ed. Elsevier; 2018: p. 12–84. © 2018. Fig. 2.54.)

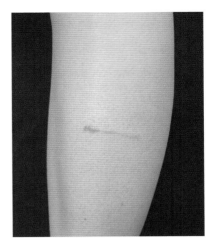

• **Figure 54.16** Contact dermatitis from poison oak with linearly arranged, succulent papules and vesicles. (From University of Utah Department of Dermatology. With permission.)

wartlike texture. They might be caused by mutations in fibroblast growth factor receptor 3 and sun exposure, although they are not considered potentially premalignant.[24,25] A distinctive variant consisting of smaller papules that are reminiscent of flat warts on the bilateral cheeks of ethnic skin is known as *dermatosis papulosa nigra*. Another variant, stucco keratoses, appear as white, warty, scaly papules on the ankles and legs. The sign of Lesar-Trelat, or eruptive appearance of multiple SKs as a paraneoplastic phenomenon, is a rare and controversial entity.[26] Three case-controlled studies[27–29] suggest most eruptive SKs are not associated with underlying malignancy and probably do not justify aggressive testing in the absence of other concerning review of systems. SKs can

become symptomatic when they become irritated, such as catching on clothing, although sometimes they spontaneously become inflamed with a pink or purple hue. Anecdotally, many patients report the lesions disappearing (probably excoriated or coincidentally traumatized) but only to return. The differential diagnosis might include melanoma, verruca, or lentigines (sunspots).[12] There are no preventive measures. Reassurance is all that is generally required. If lesions are symptomatic, they can be treated (Level of Evidence [LOE] = D) with liquid nitrogen (cryotherapy) or shave removal; the US Food and Drug Administration (FDA) recently approved a topical formulation of hydrogen peroxide 40% (LOE = A).[25] See Box 54.1 for pearls about effectively applying liquid nitrogen.

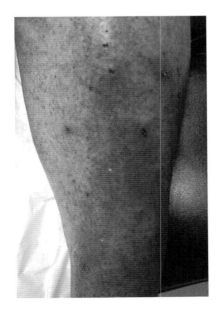

• **Figure 54.15** Stasis dermatitis mimics "bilateral leg cellulitis." (From Stasis dermatitis with ill-defined erythema. Ill-defined erythema with relative loss of hair on the lower extremity. From Brinster NK et al. Stasis dermatitis. In: Brinster NK et al, eds. *Dermatopathology: High-Yield Pathology*. Philadelphia, PA: Saunders)

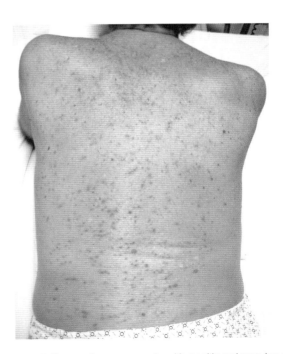

• **Figure 54.17** Grover disease presents with pruritic red papules on the chest, abdomen, or back that are often worse with heat. (From University of Utah Department of Dermatology. With permission.)

| TABLE 54.3 | Examples of Secondary Changes | |
|---|---|---|
| | Description | Example |
| Atrophy | Thinning of skin. When epidermis is involved, fine wrinkling, transparency of skin, stretch marks, or visualization of underlying dermal vessels might be present. When dermis or fat is involved, there is often skin depression | Lichen sclerosus, steroid-induced atrophy (Fig. 54.19) |
| Crust | Dried blood, honey-colored, or serum (clear/straw-colored) | Impetigo (Fig. 54.20), scab (Fig. 54.21) |
| Erosion or avulsion | Partial thickness epidermal loss. In contrast, ulceration means full thickness loss of epidermis with exposure of at least dermis | Excoriated skin (see Fig. 54.6) |
| Necrosis | Dead cutaneous tissue | Eschar (Fig. 54.22), wet gangrene |
| Scale | Desiccated, flaky keratinocytes | Psoriasis, eczema (Fig. 54.23), porokeratosis (see Fig. 54.5), seborrhea (Fig. 54.18) |

(From Bolognia J, Jorizzo JL, Rapini RP. Dermatology. 2nd ed. St. Louis, MO: Mosby/Elsevier; 2008.)

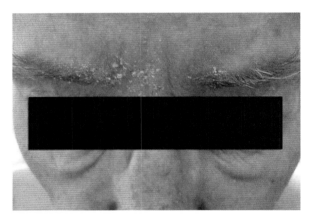

• **Figure 54.18** Seborrheic dermatitis often involves the glabella, eyebrows, nasolabial folds. (From Dr. Robert Norman.)

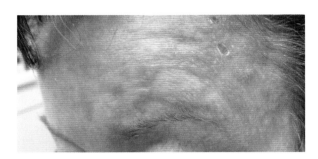

• **Figure 54.20** Herpes zoster involves a dermatome, as demonstrated by papules and vesicles that abruptly stop at the facial midline. Erosions are also present in the upper right hand corner of the figure. (From Dr. Robert Norman.)

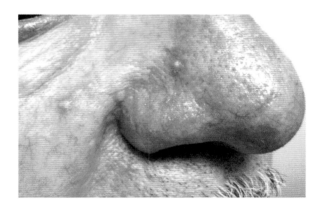

• **Figure 54.19** Rosacea commonly manifests with pustules and telangiectasias. (From Dr. Robert Norman.)

Sebaceous hyperplasias (Fig. 54.24) are benign overgrowths of normal sebaceous oil glands that are usually found on the face. They can be seen commonly on the face, vermilion lips and buccal mucosa (Fordyce spots), eyelids (meibomian glands), areola (Montgomery tubercles), and glans penis or clitoris (Tyson glands). There is a yellow to flesh-colored appearance and often

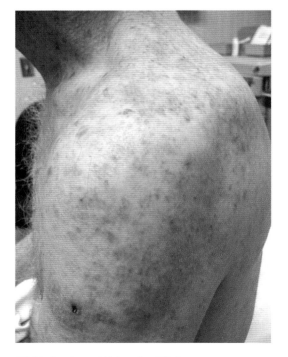

• **Figure 54.21** Courtesy of University of Utah.

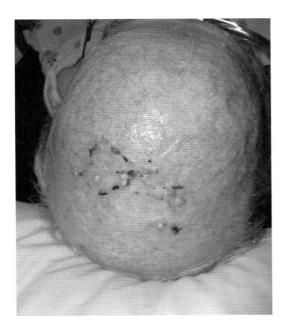

• **Figure 54.22** See Test question 3.

associated central umbilication. The condition is usually idiopathic, although cyclosporine has been reported to cause diffuse lesions.[30] The major differentials include basal cell carcinoma (which has a more pearly and pink appearance), fibrous papule/angiofibroma (flesh colored and firm), sebaceous adenoma or carcinoma (usually much larger), and milium (more white and dome-shaped). Treatment is usually not required because they are typically asymptomatic, but removal options include electrodesiccation, serial topical liquid nitrogen, or topical retinoids (LOE = C).[30–32]

Dermatofibromas (benign fibrohistiocytomas) often appear on the lower extremities (or sometimes on the torso or upper extremities) as pink-brown dome-shaped firm papules. There will often be a characteristic "dimple sign" when squeezed (Fig. 54.25). The lesions are usually asymptomatic, although sometimes can be pruritic or

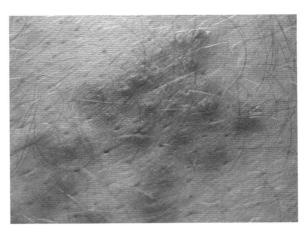

• **Figure 54.24** Herpes simplex, showing grouped papules and vesicles. (From University of Utah Department of Dermatology. With permission.)

### • BOX 54.1  Pearls on Liquid Nitrogen (Cryotherapy)

Topical liquid nitrogen treatment is a versatile technique for removing a variety of benign irritated lesions, as well as potentially premalignant, nonpigmented ones. First, it is important to counsel patients about expectations. There will be stinging, redness, swelling that typically begins shortly after treatment. The lesion might take several days to weeks to scab or form a sore before eventually coming off. The lesion might not completely go away with just one treatment. To optimize healing, counsel patients to apply unscented petrolatum jelly until sores heal; and to avoid traumatizing the area (e.g., scratching, shaving, scrubbing). Second, it is important to adequately freeze. A general rule-of-thumb is to freeze until there is a 1- to 2-mm white rim around the lesion; the time to achieve this will vary depending on lesion thickness, size, and anatomic location. Be sure to shield surrounding critical structures (e.g., eyes). After the white discoloration fades, a second application is generally performed to increase the likelihood of removal. The liquid nitrogen may be safely applied using a cannister gun or cotton-tipped applicator. Two cycles are typically used to reduce lesion recurrence.

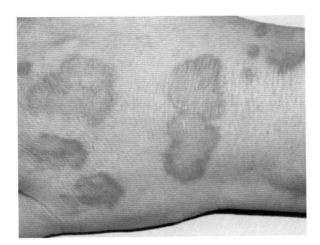

• **Figure 54.23** Granuloma annulare, with a ring-like plaque. (From Andrew I, Bardhan A. Granuloma annulare. In: Lebwohl, M., ed. *Treatment of Skin Disease: Comprehensive Therapeutic Strategies*, 5th ed. Elsevier; 2018: p. 302–306. © 2018.)

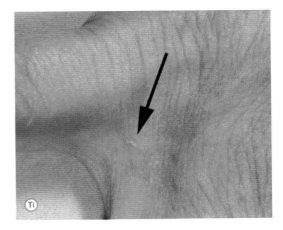

• **Figure 54.25** Scabies infestations can present with burrows: intensely pruritic and linear scaly papules. (From Marks JG, Miller JJ. *Principles of Diagnosis. Lookingbill and Marks' Principles of Dermatology*. Elsevier; 2019: p. 11–28. © 2019.)

painful. They are thought to be caused by trauma, because the histologic appearance is similar to scar. The primary differential includes irritated nevus (when more brown in color or raised), melanoma, or dermatofibromosarcoma protuberans. When symptomatic, they can be excised, treated with intralesional triamcinolone acetate or topical ultrapotent steroids (LOE = D), or frozen with liquid nitrogen (LOE = C).[33] Recurrences can occur, because the process can often spread laterally and into the deep dermis.

## Precancerous and Malignant Cutaneous Diseases

### Actinic Keratosis

Actinic keratoses (AKs, solar keratoses) are potentially precancerous lesions that are thought to be in the middle of the spectrum between photo-aged skin and squamous cell carcinoma (SCC).[34] The prevalence in fair-skinned adults is at least 25%, with a somewhat higher prevalence among men.[35,36] The dogma had been that the risk of progression of AK to SCC was 0.03% to 20% per lesion year,[37] but several experts suggest that AKs are more of a general marker of sun damage and overall skin cancer risk rather than individual lesions that are destined to transform into cancers.[34,38] Clinically, AKs are usually pink- to brown-colored papules or patches with scale on sun-exposed areas (Fig. 54.26). The gritty texture on palpation is a helpful diagnostic clue. For small lesions, the tactile presence of rough scale is sometimes easier to detect than relying only on visual appearance.[12]

Several variants based on clinical appearance or anatomic location have been described.[12] Pigmented AKs can sometimes resemble small SKs. Actinic cheilitis (solar cheilosis) is clinically characterized as grayish-white rough patches on sun-exposed portions of the vermilion lip.[39] Hypertrophic AKs (i.e., thickened, conical) can be difficult to differentiate from SCC, verruca, or irritated SKs. Certain high-risk features that favor SCC over AK have been proposed, including "IDRBEU: Inflammation or Induration, Diameter over 1 cm, Rapidly Enlarging, Bleeding,

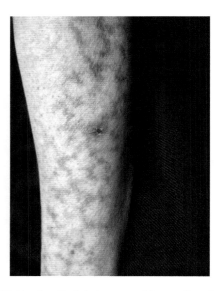

• **Figure 54.26** Livedo reticularis has a meshlike configuration of purpura that overlies the cutaneous vascular network. (From University of Utah Department of Dermatology. With permission.)

Erythema, Ulceration."[37] Sometimes AK can be partially treated and recur, but consider biopsy when the same lesion has been treated more than once or twice (LOE = D).[38]

◆◆ **Traditionally, liquid nitrogen has been the preferred treatment modality when there are a relatively small number of AKs. For patients who have diffuse disease, a recent randomized trial found that 5-fluorouracil appears to be superior to other topical modalities. Combination of liquid nitrogen and topical prescriptions can be more effective than monotherapy, particularly for hypertrophic lesions. Ultimately, the patient's care goals and overall state of health should be considered.**

A plethora of treatment options exist to reduce or prevent AKs, although the data for long-term skin cancer prevention are somewhat limited.[34,40] Treatment is traditionally with cryotherapy (LOE = D) when lesions are discrete and few.[38] See Box 54.1 for pearls about liquid nitrogen cryotherapy. However, cryotherapy directed at individual lesions does not address the surrounding sun-damaged areas where subclinical precancerous lesions likely exist.[8] Some advocate that thin AKs need be treated with only consistent sun protection because approximately 25% of lesions may spontaneously regress—although recurrences are not uncommon.[34,41–44] Field therapy to eradicate subclinical photodamaged skin is increasingly recommended (LOE = B).[40,45] Currently, FDA-approved topical therapies include photodynamic therapy with amino-levulinic acid or methyl-5-aminolevulinate (LOE = A), 5-fluorouracil (LOE = A), imiquimod (LOE = A), and diclofenac (LOE = A).[34] A recent randomized controlled trial found 5-fluorouracil 5% to be superior at reducing the number of AKs compared with imiquimod, methyl-5-aminolevulinate photodynamic therapy, and ingenol mebutate.[46] Topical tretinoin monotherapy is generally not recommended (LOE = X), because a randomized controlled trial failed to show chemopreventive effect and treatment was associated with an inexplicably increased risk of all-cause mortality.[47,48] Combination therapy (e.g., cryotherapy with topical field therapy) can be effective for hypertrophic lesions (LOE = B).[49] It is the author's opinion that the decision to treat or closely monitor AKs should also consider the patient's overall life expectancy and care goals, given the natural history of lesions. For instance, a relatively healthy patient with history of skin cancers might derive more benefit for AK treatment compared with one with relatively limited life expectancy or few AKs and no history of skin cancer.

### Cutaneous Malignancies

◆◆ **Skin cancers are prevalent in the geriatric population, and the incidence has been on the rise. Primary care providers have continuity of care of their patients and are uniquely positioned to identify suspicious lesions that the patient might not even notice.**

Skin cancers are prevalent in the geriatric population, and the incidence has been on the rise.[2,50] Primary care providers have continuity of care of their patients and are uniquely positioned to identify suspicious lesions that the patient might not even notice.[51] This section will review the more common skin cancers in geriatric patients to empower the primary care provider to recognize and triage appropriately. See Box 54.2 for information about nonmelanoma skin cancer chemoprevention.

For all patients as primary and secondary prevention of skin cancers, sun protection is advised using either clothing and hats and/or broad-spectrum sunscreen with sun protection factor (SPF) of at least 30 (LOE = D). In some travel destinations, only zinc or titanium ingredients are allowed because of possible concerns of the impact of chemical-based sunscreens on coral reefs.[52]

It is generally recommended that patients with nonmelanoma skin cancers should have ongoing examinations, although there is considerable variability and lack of evidence base for the ideal frequency or duration (LOE = D).[53,85] The majority of recurrences or new skin cancers occur within the first few years from the time of initial skin cancer diagnosis (LOE = D).[54]

For patients with a history of two or more basal or squamous cell carcinomas, niacinamide (nicotinamide) 500 mg orally twice daily has been shown to reduce the risk of additional nonmelanoma skin cancers (LOE = B).[55] Note: It is not the same as niacin. Another study of patients with a history of actinic keratoses and nonmelanoma skin cancers demonstrated topical 5-fluorouracil reduced the risk of subsequent nonmelanoma skin cancers.[46]

## Squamous Cell Carcinoma

Cutaneous SCC is full thickness epidermal atypia and subcategorized as in situ (Bowen disease) or invasive (extending into or below the dermis). Major risk factors include sun exposure, fair skin, radiation exposure (e.g., cancer survivors, historical acne treatments), and immunosuppression (e.g., solid organ transplant patients).[12] Occasionally, patients with chronic inflammatory skin conditions (e.g., lichen planus, lichen sclerosus) can develop SCC.[12] There are also associations with long-term voriconazole in transplant patients, vemurafenib, tumor necrosis factor antagonists, and hydrochlorothiazide.[56–60] Damaged deoxyribonucleic acid repair and tumor suppression pathways seem to be the underlying pathophysiology, and certain human papillomavirus strains have been implicated in some cases.[61] The clinical appearance is usually an indurated, pink-red, scaly plaque or tumor (Fig. 54.27) that is sometimes symptomatic. It can also manifest as a nonhealing ulcer that does not respond to wound care.

According to the eighth edition of the American Joint Commission on Cancer guidelines, staging depends on the histologic features, depth, anatomic site, and presence of perineural invasion or nodal involvement.[62] The recommendation of complete excisional biopsy and histologic staging reporting tumor invasion depth have not been widely accepted and implemented yet. The National Comprehensive Cancer Network 2019 guidelines describe lesions in the H-zone of the face (ears, temples, jawline, nose) or head and neck, mucosal sites, immunosuppressed patients, and tumor size > 2 cm as high risk for recurrence or poor prognosis.[54]

Differential diagnoses of SCC include hypertrophic actinic keratosis, nummular eczema (see Fig. 54.23), lichen planus, benign lichenoid keratosis, superficial basal cell carcinoma (simulates SCC in situ), and chondrodermatitis nodularis helicis when present on the ear (Fig. 54.28). However, irregular borders or ulceration is concerning for SCC.

Treatment options for SCC depend on anatomic site, histologic features, and patient preference. Expert consensus guidelines (LOE = D) have recommended electrodesiccation and curettage for nonhair-bearing, low-risk in situ tumors that do not extend too deeply into the dermis in noncosmetically sensitive areas. Excision with histologic confirmation should be at least 4-mm margins for low-risk and 6-mm margins for high-risk cases (LOE = C).[54,63]

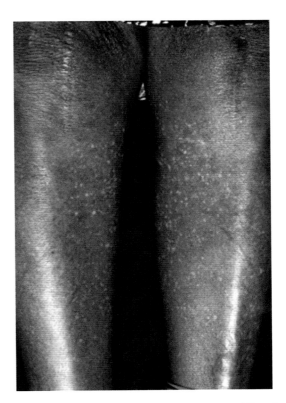

• **Figure 54.27** Idiopathic guttate hypomelanosis. Unlike vitiligo, there are multiple, small, white, monomorphous, circular macules that appear symmetrically on sun-exposed limbs. (From James WD, Elston DM, Treat JR, et al. Disturbances of pigmentation. In: *Andrews' Diseases of the Skin*, 13th ed. Elsevier; 2020: p. 862–880.e2. © 2020. eFig. 36.10 Idiopathic guttate hypomelanosis)

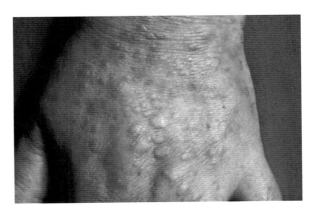

• **Figure 54.28** Lichen planus with violaceous-purple polygonal papules. (From Brinster NK, Diwan AH, Liu V. *Dermatopathology*. St Louis: Elsevier; 2010: p. 48–49. © 2011. [Fig 1]); (From the collection of the late NP Smith, MD; the Institute of Pathology, London.) Lichen planus. Polygonal, violaceous flat-topped papules on the dorsal hand.)

Mohs micrographic surgery (Box 54.3) should be considered for high-risk tumors, those with poorly demarcated clinical edges, recurrent lesions, and those involving critical anatomic sites to spare normal tissue (LOE = D).[12]

Second-line nonsurgical therapy for thin and low-risk tumors, which should be discussed with a dermatologist, might include

**• BOX 54.3** Mohs Micrographic Surgery

Mohs surgery, named after Dr. Frederick Mohs, is an in-office surgical method that removes tumors with a low recurrence rate while sparing normal tissue.[64] The surgeon removes discs of tissue, prepares frozen histologic sections using a special technique to allow complete margin examination, and repeats the process until the tumor is completely removed. Wound closure is obtained through many techniques, including but not limited to secondary intent, intermediate closure, skin flap, or graft. Appropriate Use Criteria for Mohs Micrographic Surgery are available here: https://www.aad.org/member/clinical-quality/clinical-care/au/mohs-surgery

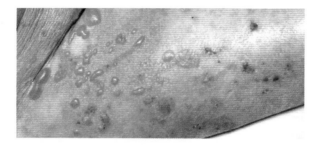

**• Figure 54.29** Bullous pemphigoid. Pruritic tense bullae on the torso and extremities. (From University of Utah Department of Dermatology. With permission.)

aggressive cryotherapy (LOE = C), topical imiquimod (SCC in situ; LOE = C), or topical 5-fluorouracil (LOE = C)—although these are off-label uses.[65-67] For advanced or inoperable cutaneous SCC, comanagement with an oncologist to discuss radiation therapy or systemic chemotherapeutics is appropriate.[12,68,69]

One variant worth mentioning is keratoacanthoma. This controversial entity is a firm nodule with central hyperkeratotic plug (Fig. 54.29). Some characterize these as a form of well-differentiated SCC that should be treated as such, although others believe them to be generally benign, self-limited processes.[70-72] It is the author's opinion that in cases of patients being reasonable surgical candidates, especially in those with high-risk features, surgical management should be discussed.

## Basal Cell Carcinoma

Basal cell carcinoma (BCC) (see Fig. 54.13) is a malignant growth of the basal layer keratinocytes and the most common human skin cancer.[73] The major risk factors include sun exposure and fair-colored skin.[73] The tumor is generally slow growing and often has excellent prognosis with appropriate treatment.[74] BCC rarely metastasizes, although it can be locally invasive, painful, and disfiguring.[73] The pathophysiology of most BCCs is related to tumor suppression mutations in either p53 or patched-sonic hedgehog (PTCH-SHH) pathways.[75] The differential includes scar (morpheic BCC variant), melanoma (pigmented BCC variant), fibrous papule, intradermal nevus, sebaceous hyperplasia, eczema (superficial BCC), or nonhealing ulcer ("rodent ulcer" BCC). Sometimes it can be confused with rosacea because of the telangiectasias overlying papules.

As with SCC, treatment of BCC depends on factors, such as histologic features, size, depth, anatomic site, and patient's immune status. Therapeutic approaches are similar to that outlined for SCC, with the notable exception that BCC might behave less aggressively and is not as strongly associated with mortality.[76] Historically, the standard of care is generally surgical with either simple excision or Mohs micrographic surgery (LOE = B; see Box 54.3). For nonsurgical candidates, especially for superficial or nodular (not micronodular) histology in low-risk and cosmetically insensitive areas, second-line therapies that should be discussed with a dermatologist might include electrodesiccation and curettage (LOE = D)[77]; aggressive cryotherapy with or without curettage (LOE = B)[73]; topical imiquimod 5% qHS 5 times per week for 6 weeks (LOE = A; FDA-approved for superficial BCC); photodynamic therapy (LOE = B); vismodegib (FDA-approved SHH inhibitor) (LOE = B) or intralesional chemotherapeutics (LOE = C).[78-81] Radiation therapy can also be used (LOE = C).[82] Ultimately, the patient's care goals and anticipated life expectancy should be considered in the treatment decision (LOE = D)—particularly if the risks and morbidity of treatment might outweigh potential benefit for these generally slow-growing tumors.[83]

## Melanoma

Melanoma (see Fig. 54.3) is a dreaded melanocytic cancer that can affect the skin or, less commonly, the retina. Several risk factors exist, including genetics, skin and eye color (fair skin, blue eyes, red or blond hair), and total number of atypical-appearing nevi.[12] The incidence of melanoma has unfortunately been increasing in the United States over the past few decades and is suspected to be related to tanning practices.[84] Diagnosis is discussed under "Total Body Skin Examination" earlier in this chapter. The differential diagnosis of melanoma includes atypical nevus, seborrheic keratosis, pigmented BCC, dermatofibromas, and very dark benign vascular growths that usually can be discerned with adequate lightning (e.g., cherry angiomas, venous lakes, angiokeratomas). It should be noted that current evidence does not support the notion that mildly and moderately dysplastic nevi transform into melanoma (LOE = C).[85] There is controversy and limited data as to whether such lesions need to be reexcised (especially if initial biopsy margins are positive), but it is the author's opinion that it is unnecessary in the majority of cases (LOE = D).

Staging, treatment, and follow-up are beyond the scope of this text. Prognosis depends on several factors—including advanced age, male gender, tumor site, Breslow depth (which has supplanted Clark level), ulceration, and presence of nodal or distant metastasis. Subtypes (e.g., nodular, superficial spreading) are not directly pertinent to staging.[12,86] Close clinical follow-up of the patient and first-degree relatives is recommended (LOE = D). It is the author's opinion that an interspecialty care approach is ideal, which might include dermatologists, radiation oncologists (where appropriate), medical oncologists (for advanced disease), Mohs surgeons (for earlier stage disease), and surgical oncologists (if sentinel node is offered). Depending on cancer staging, patients can be educated about sentinel node biopsy, the role of targeted therapy in advanced-stage disease, or possibly be enrolled in clinical trials.

## CASE 2

### Sally Maloney (Part 1)

Sally Maloney, a 72-year-old frail female, visits your clinic with an approximately 6-month history of progressively worsening pruritus that is "head to toe." She denies any new personal products or medications. Upon examination, Ms. Maloney's skin is somewhat dry and scaly and there are many linearly configured erosions and hemorrhagic crusts but not intact primary lesions.

1. What other focused pertinent history and examination will help you understand possible causes of Ms. Maloney's pruritus?
2. What features of pruritus might warrant further investigation?

# Pruritus

Pruritus is often caused by dry skin in older patients. However, the clinician should be astutely aware of other etiologies of intractable itch, including occult malignancy or serious metabolic derangement. A practical framework to consider is itch with rash and itch without rash.

Pruritus, or itch, is one of the most common problems of older patients and is often multifactorial from age-related changes of skin barrier function and immunology.[87–89] One framework is to consider itch with versus without rash.[89] Itch with rash (not just scabs or dry skin) can be caused by inflammatory skin conditions, such as hives, dermatitis, folliculitis, immunoblistering conditions, and infectious diseases. Itch without rash is often caused by xerosis (asteatosis, dry skin). It can also be idiopathic, but underlying systemic causes, such as neuropathy or a systemic cause, should be considered. See Table 54.4 for the differential diagnosis and suggested history and workup. Subacute to chronic generalized and severe pruritus without rash that awakens the patient should alert the practitioner to search for secondary causes (especially lymphoma or hematologic conditions).[12,90]

If no underlying treatable cause of pruritus is found, symptomatic treatment can be challenging and must be individualized to the patient. Of note, antihistamines are generally not helpful for pruritus, unless hives are present (LOE = D).[90] Mirtazapine up to 15 mg by mouth at night (LOE = C) can help mitigate pruritus along with providing a sedating effect to provide additional relief.[87] It is the author's opinion that it should be started at 7.5 mg in older adults and gradually uptitrated to effect. Topical 5% doxepin cream can be cost prohibitive; it frequently causes contact dermatitis; and it can lead to systemic side effects, if applied to large body surfaces.[12] Topical steroids are generally not recommended if there is not visible inflammatory rash (LOE = D).[90] In select severe and intractable cases, phototherapy, antiepileptics, antidepressants, neurokinin inhibitors, or opioid receptor modulators such as naltrexone might be helpful (LOE = C).[90] The side effects of oral medications must be weighed and discussed with the patient, and the patient should be counseled not to discontinue many of these medications abruptly (e.g., gabapentin, opioid receptor modulators) because of withdrawal potential.[90]

---

**CASE 2**

**Sally Maloney (Part 2)**

You gather additional history, and Ms. Maloney has been feeling somewhat fatigued recently and has noticed cold intolerance. Her thyroid-stimulating hormone is markedly elevated and you diagnose her as having hypothyroidism. You know thyroid replacement should be started at a low dose and slowly titrated; thus general dry skin recommendations and topical emollients are also recommended.

---

# Common Rashes of Aging

## Eczematous Dermatoses

Eczema (dermatitis) is a common clinical sign that refers to a group of conditions that share histologic features but have differing etiologies and clinical appearances. *Dermatitis* is a misnomer, because the inflammation and edema (spongiosis) is at the level of the epidermis, not the dermis. In the acute phase, it is often confused as being infected because of the oozing papulovesicles (see Fig. 54.8) or vesicular appearance on acral surfaces (Fig. 54.30). Chronic eczema usually appears as dry, scaly patches or sometimes lichenified (thickened) plaques with fissures (cracks) (Fig. 54.31).[12]

▸▸ **Stasis dermatitis, caused by underlying venous insufficiency, is commonplace in older patients from acquired venous incompetence, saphenous vein grafting, or prior thromboembolism. The patient is often misdiagnosed as having bilateral leg cellulitis and has partial or no response to antibiotic therapy, which leads to unnecessary cost, hospitalization, and interventions.**

Several etiologies can lead to the final common pathway of eczema.[12] Stasis dermatitis (Fig. 54.32), caused by underlying venous insufficiency, is common in older patients from acquired venous incompetence, saphenous vein grafting, or prior thromboembolism. The patient is often misdiagnosed as having bilateral leg cellulitis and has partial or no response to antibiotic therapy, which leads to unnecessary hospitalization, interventions, and cost.[94] Sometimes amlodipine can exacerbate the peripheral edema and rash. Nummular (discoid) eczema is an idiopathic variant with solitary or multiple coin-shaped plaques, typically on the extremities (see Fig. 54.23). It is often mistaken for "refractory" tinea corporis, although a skin scraping mounted in potassium hydroxide (KOH) can differentiate the two.[12]

Contact dermatitis is another common cause of eczema. It is typically well demarcated and geometrically (see Fig. 54.8) or linearly configured (see Fig. 54.9). It can be caused by a nonimmunologic response to a chemical irritant, such as soap residue.[95] Allergic sensitization (i.e., type IV delayed hypersensitivity cell-mediated reaction), which is exemplified by poison ivy or nickel allergy, is probably as common in older patients as irritant dermatitis.[95,96] Ask about all personal products and topical medicaments, because geriatric patients and those with stasis dermatitis who are self-medicating have a high prevalence of allergic contact dermatitis, particularly to neomycin and fragrance mixes.[95,97] Eyelid dermatitis can result from eyedrops or from nail cosmetic products.[98] Airborne allergens (e.g., pollens) can mimic photodistributed rashes on exposed areas.

Autoeczematization ("id" reaction, autosensitization) is a symmetric eruption of eczematous papules and plaques that occur distant to the primary sites of chronic skin inflammation. The classic example is symmetrically distributed eczematous papules on the upper extremities or torso in the context of chronic tinea pedis.[12] It can also be seen with severe contact or stasis dermatitis.[99] The presumed pathophysiology is lymphocytes at the site of chronic inflammation circulate peripherally and deposit at other anatomic sites.[100]

The differential diagnosis of eczema includes cutaneous T-cell lymphoma (particularly if confined to sunprotected areas), scabies, early SCC or BCC (if irregularly shaped), mammary or extramammary Paget disease, and dermatophytosis (tinea).[95] Eczematous drug reactions have been described with calcium channel blockers and thiazides.[101] Consider skin biopsy or skin scraping if lesions are not responding or worsening with topical corticosteroids or if it is predominantly on the areas that are not sun-exposed (particularly the buttocks and torso in the setting of negative KOH test).

Treatment regimens generally include dry skin care instructions (Box 54.4), brief courses of topical corticosteroids (LOE = D), or calcineurin inhibitors (e.g., tacrolimus or pimecrolimus) (LOE = D) for symptomatic relief.[12] Tips for how to choose the steroid molecule

**TABLE 54.4  Causes of Pruritus in Older Patients and Possible Treatment Options**

| Causative Factor | Rash Usually present | Comments and Suggested Management Approach |
|---|---|---|
| Chronic kidney disease | No | • Check renal function<br>• Does not always respond to dialysis and can be challenging to treat<br>• Emollients are first line (LOE = C)[91]<br>• Gabapentin 100–300 mg after dialysis (LOE = B)[91]<br>• Naltrexone (LOE = C, mixed results)[91]<br>• Transplantation is generally considered to be the more successful treatment, if the patient is a candidate (LOE = D) |
| Dermatitis (e.g., nummular eczema, stasis dermatitis, contact dermatitis from an allergen or irritant) | Yes | • Avoid sensitizing agents (e.g., Balsam of Peru, lanolin, vitamin E, topical antibiotics)<br>• Compression garments if leg swelling<br>• Topical corticosteroids<br>• Consider dermatology referral for skin patch testing, if sharply demarcated areas (type IV hypersensitivity reaction). This is different from scratch or prick testing (type I hypersensitivity). |
| Dry skin (xerosis) | No | • See Dry Skin Care Recommendations in Box 54.4<br>• Senescent changes in epidermal lipid production and skin barrier function[92] |
| Folliculitis | Yes | • Scraping of pustule to look for yeast (potassium hydroxide mounting) and/or bacterial culture<br>• Counsel patient about frequency of relapses<br>• Treat underlying cause |
| Immunoblistering conditions (e.g., bullous pemphigoid [see Fig. 54.16], dermatitis herpetiformis) | Yes | • Requires high index of suspicion because pruritus may present before blisters<br>• Dermatologic referral for immunofluorescence studies of skin and possibly serum<br>• Systemic immunosuppression or topical steroids, when appropriate |
| Infestation or infection (e.g., bed bugs, scabies, tinea corporis, parasites) | Yes | • Skin scraping in potassium hydroxide (tinea) or mineral oil (scabies) or other parasite screening tests<br>• Treat underlying cause<br>• Treat close contacts, when appropriate (e.g., scabies) |
| Medications (e.g., statins, calcium channel blockers, hydrochlorothiazide, angiotensin-converting enzyme inhibitors, opioids) | Yes | • Discontinue offending agent<br>• Allow for 1–2 month drug holiday before judging improvement<br>• Do not exclude the possibility that a chronically prescribed antihypertensive medication might be the cause of unexplained widespread pruritus with eczematous changes[93] |
| Metabolic or endocrine derangements (e.g., anemia, cholestasis, hypercalcemia, nutritional deficiency, thyroid disease) | No | • Complete blood count with differential<br>• Complete metabolic panel<br>• Electrolyte panels<br>• Iron studies<br>• Nutritional studies<br>• Thyroid studies<br>• Correcting underlying cause<br>• Note: Cholestatic itch can be notoriously refractory |
| Neuropathy (e.g., diabetic, degenerative spinal disease) | No | • Tends to be localized rather than generalized<br>• Treat underlying condition<br>• Brachioradial pruritus presents as itching of the arms (particularly dorsolateral) that is only alleviated by ice<br>• Notalgia paresthetica manifests as chronically rubbed, thickened, brown skin near the shoulder blades<br>• Consider symptomatic treatment with judicious prescription of psychoactive medications (e.g., selective serotonin reuptake inhibitor, selective serotonin-norepinephrine reuptake inhibitor, tricyclic antidepressant) or antiepileptic agent |
| Paraneoplastic (especially lymphoma, leukemia, myeloma) | ± | • History, physical examination, review of systems to identify possible source<br>• Unexplained pruritus has been described to precede lymphoma by several years<br>• Lactate dehydrogenase (LDH)<br>• Erythrocyte sedimentation rate (ESR)<br>• Imaging, as appropriate<br>• Cancer screening tests, as appropriate |
| Psychogenic (diagnosis of exclusion) | No | • Referral for cognitive-behavioral techniques or medication, when appropriate |

(From Bolognia J, Jorizzo JL, Rapini RP. *Dermatology.* 2nd ed. St. Louis, MO: Mosby/Elsevier; 2008; Patel T, Yosipovitch G. The management of chronic pruritus in the elderly. *Skin Therapy Lett.* 2010;15 (8):5–9.)
*LOE,* Level of Evidence.

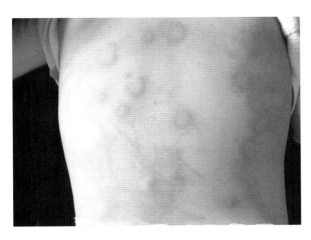

• **Figure 54.30** Serum sickness. Multiple, annular, edematous coalescing urticarial plaques.

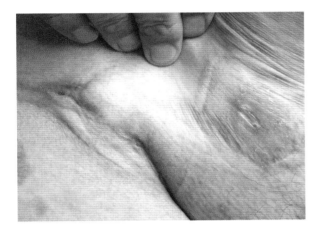

• **Figure 54.31** Topical steroid-induced atrophy and associated ulceration caused by a commonly prescribed antifungal/steroid combination. (From University of Utah Department of Dermatology. With permission.)

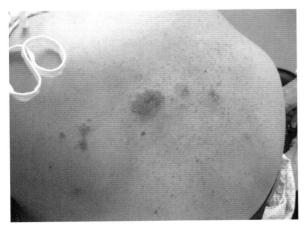

• **Figure 54.32** Honey-crusted impetiginized eczema. (From University of Utah Department of Dermatology. With permission.)

---

**• BOX 54.4  Pearls: Dry Skin Care Recommendations (LOE = D)**

Avoid soaps that are not sensitive-skin products, bubble baths. Note: Unscented products often contain neutralizing fragrances, which can cause contact dermatitis. Unfragranced products are therefore preferable.

Minimize exposure to chemical irritants by wearing gloves when doing chores.

Apply cream or ointment emollients before the skin dries (within 3 minutes). Lotions are less effective.

Avoid abrasive scrubbing.

Avoid hot water or long baths.

Focus cleansing areas that are hair-bearing or visibly soiled rather than lathering the entire body indiscriminately; avoid excessing bathing.

Consider a humidifier (adjust to about 50% humidity) in dry climates.

(From Bolognia J, Jorizzo JL, Rapini RP. *Dermatology*. 2nd ed. St. Louis, MO: Mosby/Elsevier; 2008; White-Chu EF, Reddy M. Dry skin in the elderly: complexities of a common problem. *Clin Dermatol*. 2011;29(1):37–42.)

---

**TABLE 54.5  Pearls for Choosing Potency or Vehicle of Topical Antiinflammatory Medications**

| Characteristic | Comments |
|---|---|
| Anatomic site[104] | Acral sites absorb medications the least and can withstand a mid- to high-potency steroid molecule[a]<br>Facial and intertriginous areas require a weaker steroid molecule[a]<br>Hair-bearing skin is easier to treat with gels, lotion, shampoo, oil, or foam (rather than ointments and creams) |
| Patient preference[12] | Patient adherence often dictates vehicle (e.g., avoid ointment if patient is unwilling to apply something that feels greasy) |
| Rash attributes[12] | Thickened, scaly skin difficult to penetrate and requires a high-potency steroid molecule.<br>For severely inflamed, lichenified or eroded skin, consider occluding the steroid with moistened dressings or plastic food wrap to help penetration. Ideally leave in place for as long as the patient can tolerate, up to several hours |
| Vehicle attribute[12] | Alcohol-based (e.g., solution), especially on open or inflamed skin, tends to be irritating<br>Ointment are more potent compared with other vehicles<br>Propylene glycol, which is found in many topical medicaments, can sometimes cause an irritant contact dermatitis |

[a]High-potency steroids include clobetasol 0.05%, halobetasol 0.05%, betamethasone diproprionate 0.05%, fluocinonide 0.05%; midpotency steroids include triamcinolone 0.1%, betamethasone valerate 0.1%, fluocinolone propionate 0.05%; and low-potency steroids include hydrocortisone butyrate 0.1%, hydrocortisone 2.5% and desonide 0.05%.[12]

potency, vehicle, and dispensed quantity are described in Tables 54.5 and 54.6. When dermatitis is acute, severe, and widespread, systemic steroids (0.5–1 mg/kg per day for 3–4 weeks) can be considered if the benefits outweigh potential risks and side effects (LOE = D).[12] However, systemic steroids are not considered sustainable long-term

| TABLE 54.6 | **Pearls on Quantity of Topical Medication** | |
|---|---|---|
| Body Site | Fingertip Units[a] | Grams Required for Twice Daily Application over 2 Weeks |
| Entire hand | 1 | 14 |
| One foot | 2 | 28 |
| Neck and face | 2.5 | 35 |
| One arm | 3 | 42 |
| One leg | 6 | 84 |
| Torso (only anterior *or* posterior) | 7 | 98 |

(From Bolognia J, Jorizzo JL, Rapini RP. *Dermatology.* 2nd ed. St. Louis, MO: Mosby/Elsevier; 2008; Long CC, Finlay AY. The finger-tip unit--a new practical measure. *Clin Exp Dermatol.* 1991;16(6):444–447.)

[a]Based on the assumption that approximately 0.1-mm layer of medication should be applied, one fingertip unit is a strip of medication dispensed to cover the volar index finger between the distal interphalangeal joint to the fingertip.

treatments for chronic eczema. If allergic contact dermatitis is suspected, the allergen should be avoided completely because even one exposure can cause a skin reaction to last for over 1 month.[12] Referral to dermatology for skin patch testing (rather than scratch or prick allergy testing) should be considered. Dietary restrictions (except in cases of test-proven allergens or additives) and water softeners are of uncertain value.[12,102,103]

## Grover Disease (Transient Acantholytic Dermatosis)

Grover disease has been classically described as a recrudescent, pruritic, pink-brown, papulovesicular eruption on the torso of middle-aged to older men that is worse with warmth (see Fig. 17). However, it can occur in females or during cooler conditions. Grover disease is an idiopathic condition, but those afflicted with cancer or taking certain chemotherapeutics, febrile illness, or prolonged bed rest seem to be particularly predisposed.[95,105,106] The differential can include folliculitis and seborrheic dermatitis of the chest. Usually the diagnosis is made clinically, and patients are advised to avoid excessive heat or sweating (LOE = D).[105] There are weak data supporting multiple treatment options, but it is the author's opinion that topical nonprescription menthol-containing lotions are the safest first-line therapy. Consider a topical medium-potency steroid for more severe symptoms. In rare instances, systemic therapies, such as acitretin or methotrexate, might be considered.[107]

### Seborrheic Dermatitis (Dandruff, Cradle Cap, Seborrhea)

Seborrheic dermatitis is relapsing, pruritic, greasy, scaly, poorly demarcated patches (see Fig. 54.18). It is frequently found on the scalp, eyebrows, forehead, nasolabial folds, external meati, retro-auricular neck; and sometimes on the central chest and axilla. It affects about 10% of the population. Patients with neurologic conditions seem to be at risk for unclear reasons.[108] Particularly severe inflammatory eruptions are sometimes associated with human

immunodeficiency virus. The pathophysiology has been attributed to an exuberant inflammatory response to *Malassezia* (formerly *Pityrosporum*), although this yeast exists as flora in people without seborrheic dermatitis and treatment responses occur even if the organism is not eradicated.[109,110] Another hypothesis is alteration of skin surface lipid composition, which might be altered by bacteria and yeast flora composition.[109] This condition is chronic, thus treatment is directed toward symptom management (Table 54.7). In general, topical antifungals are first-line therapy, followed by either calcineurin inhibitors or short courses of low-potency topical steroids.

The differential diagnosis includes psoriasis (which can often overlap with or closely mimic seborrheic dermatitis), eczema, and dermatophyte infection (*Tinea capitis* or *T. faceii*).[108] Seborrheic dermatitis can involve the cheeks and be mistaken for the malar rash of systemic lupus erythematosus. Psoriasis is the most difficult differential to distinguish from seborrheic dermatitis, but a family history, nail abnormalities (e.g., pits, oil spots), and psoriasiform lesions on extensor surfaces of extremities or in the umbilicus or buttocks can be helpful clues. Usually seborrheic dermatitis is more diffuse, whereas psoriasis tends to be well demarcated. Eczema typically has a drier scaly appearance and does not tend to favor the glabella, nasolabial folds, and central chest to the same extent as seborrhea. Dermatophytosis is excluded by KOH skin scraping or fungal culture.

### Rosacea

Rosacea, also known as adult acne, is common among adults.[122] It is a chronic condition of unclear etiology, although it may be triggered by an inflammatory response to Demodex mite overabundance in hair follicles.[123] The inflammation is exacerbated by vasodilatory responses to triggers, such as ultraviolet light, exercise, heat, embarrassment, spicy foods, and chocolate.[12] The role of caffeine has recently been called into question.[124] Clinical presentations include the classic papulopustular eruption of the nose and cheeks, erythematotelangiectatic variant consisting of ruddy cheeks and nose (see Fig. 54.15), and rhinophymatous changes with a bulbous nose (akin to that of WC Fields). Patients commonly report "sensitivity" such as stinging or burning.

One noteworthy variant, ocular rosacea, is thought to occur in up to 50% of rosacea cases.[125] The presentation is variable, ranging from sicca to blepharitis (scale and inflammation of the eyelid margin and eyelashes) to pruritus and, rarely, visual impairment.[12]

The differential diagnosis varies with the most prominent rosacea feature.[12] For the papulopustular variant, the main differentials are acne vulgaris or folliculitis. Rosacea notably lacks the comedones (whiteheads, blackheads) of acne vulgaris. In erythematotelangiectatic rosacea, the primary differential is the malar rash of acute systemic lupus erythematosus or a sun-induced or exacerbated dermatosis. Individual blanching telangiectasias, presence of pustules or inflammatory papules, and absence of systemic symptoms militate against systemic lupus rash. Both rosacea and systemic lupus rash can be exacerbated by sunlight, but the lupus malar rash generally spares the nasolabial folds. Ocular rosacea sometimes mimics other causes of blepharitis or conjunctivitis, including allergic and infectious etiologies, in addition to seborrheic dermatitis (which also commonly causes blepharitis).

Management is tailored to the most prominent clinical features, disease severity, and patient preference (Table 54.8). In patients with eye symptoms, consider eyelid hygiene scrubs and warm compresses and referral to an eye provider. Patients should be counseled about the chronicity of the condition and avoidance of aforementioned triggers (LOE = D).

## TABLE 54.7 Treatment Options for Seborrheic Dermatitis

| Regimen | Level of Evidence | Comment |
|---|---|---|
| **TOPICAL THERAPIES** | | |
| Antifungals | B | Ketoconazole 2% and ciclopirox 1% have relatively more supporting data compared with miconazole, clotrimazole[111] |
| Topical calcineurin inhibitors | A (tacrolimus),[112] B (pimecrolimus)[112] | Advantageous for the face, because it does not cause atrophy<br>Counsel patients about black box warning; topical use has not been shown to increase risk of cancers[113] |
| Metronidazole | B[114] | |
| Promiseb | B | Proprietary nonsteroidal FDA-cleared medical device |
| Selenium sulfide 2.5% | B | Comes as shampoo for scalp or lotion for other sites<br>Ketoconazole might be somewhat better tolerated[115] |
| Zinc pyrithione 1% | B | Shampoo is available without a prescription, but might not be quite as efficacious as ketoconazole[116] |
| Corticosteroids | B[a], D | [a]For the scalp, clobetasol 0.05% shampoo twice weekly for 4 weeks with at least 10 minutes of dwell time before rinsing<br>It is also available in leave-on lotion, solution or foam formulations<br>Patients must be counseled about side effects of long-term use and should be encouraged to have drug holidays<br>One survey found a high proportion of nondermatologists prescribed high-potency topical steroids for the face, which can cause significant adverse effects[117] |
| Salicylic acid | D[118] | |
| **ALTERNATIVE MEDICINES (TOPICAL)** | | |
| Aloe vera | B | Reduction in pruritus and scale but not erythema[119] |
| Tea tree oil 5% (melaleuca) | B[120] | |
| **ORAL THERAPIES** | | |
| Antifungals | B (terbinafine, fluconazole)<br>C (itraconazole)[121] | In general reserved for more widespread or refractory disease because of theoretical side effects and interactions of oral medications |
| Vitamins and minerals | C | Weak or conflicting data |

(From Naldi L. Seborrhoeic dermatitis. *Clin Evid.* 2010;2010; Borda LJ, Perper M, Keri JE. Treatment of seborrheic dermatitis: a comprehensive review. *J Dermatolog Treat.* 2019;30(2):158–169, unless otherwise noted.)

*FDA,* US Food and Drug Administration.

## Herpes Zoster (Shingles) and Postherpetic Neuralgia

Zoster refers to reactivation of the varicella virus (chickenpox), to which most of the general population has been exposed in childhood. It occurs in almost one-quarter of people exposed to chickenpox, but further zoster recurrence in otherwise immunocompetent hosts is low irrespective of zoster vaccination status.[12,127,128] Immunosuppression (e.g., iatrogenic, immunosenescence), often in conjunction with an acute physical or emotional stressor, leads to unchecked viral replication in the dorsal root ganglion.[129] The classic presentation is a prodrome of unilateral pain or pruritus followed by corresponding dermatomal vesiculopustular eruption within days to a week (see Fig. 54.6). Disseminated zoster is an uncommon presentation when 20 or more vesicles appear outside of a single dermatome.[12] The host is contagious during the prodrome (via respiratory route) and through direct contact until the lesions become dried and crusted.[12,130,131]

The diagnosis is usually made clinically, although several laboratory tests can be performed when the vesicles are carefully unroofed and the fluid collected. Polymerase chain reaction (PCR) is a rapid, sensitive, and specific assay that is generally preferable over direct fluorescent antibody assay and viral culture.[132] The Tzanck smear is a rapid diagnostic tool but is operator-dependent. The clinical differential diagnosis is sometimes challenging. The prodrome of pain can sometimes mimic cardiac angina if on the chest. Zoster might be confused for impetigo, herpes simplex, or bacterial folliculitis, but the dermatomal band configuration and viral PCR are often helpful. Currently, FDA-approved vaccines for patients over 50 years old include Zostavax (attenuated live virus) and Shingrix (recombinant, 2-doses). The former should not be given to immunosuppressed individuals.

First-line treatment of acute varicella zoster virus is systemic antiviral therapy (see Table 54.9 for uncomplicated zoster treatment options), preferably within 72 hours of rash onset with the goals of faster resolution of the rash and decreasing the severity and duration of acute pain.[133,134] However, dose-adjustments and

**TABLE 54.8  Treatment Options for Cutaneous Rosacea**

| Regimen | Rosacea Variant | Level of Evidence | Comments |
|---|---|---|---|
| **ORAL THERAPIES** | | | |
| Doxycycline | Erythema, ocular [a] | A[b] | FDA approved as 40-mg daily (immediate + delayed release), which was as efficacious, had fewer side effects, and has no antimicrobial resistance compared with higher doses for cutaneous disease<br>[a]Modest improvement in ocular disease in one trial (LOE = B)<br>Avoid in liver disease<br>[b]The immediate release form is generic and often used off-label when the FDA-formulation is cost prohibitive (LOE = D) |
| Tetracycline 250 mg TID | Erythema, papulopustular | B | Mixed study results regarding efficacy<br>Modest improvement in ocular disease that might best doxycycline<br>Consider renal dose adjustment<br>Frequency of dosing might limit adherence |
| Zinc sulfate | Papulopustular, erythemato-telangiectatic | B | Inconclusive if effective because of limited data |
| **Topical Therapies** | | | |
| Azelaic acid 15%–20% | Erythema, papulopustular | A | FDA-approved (available as generic)<br>More effective for papulopustular variant than topical metronidazole but can be more irritating and cause stinging<br>Daily dosing as effective as BID<br>Sometimes cost prohibitive, even though available as generic<br>Can be purchased in lower strengths OTC from online vendors |
| Brimonidine 0.5% gel once daily | Erythema | A | FDA-approved (currently no generic) |
| Ivermectin | Papulopustular | A | FDA-approved (currently no generic). Demodex mites appear to contribute to rosacea pathogenesis. Ivermectin might have other mechanisms of action other than anti-Demodex mite effect |
| Metronidazole BID | Erythema, papulopustular | A | FDA-approved (available as generic). Effective in treatment of active disease and maintenance therapy to reduce flares<br>No difference between 0.75% and 1% formulations (generic versus trade)<br>Available as generic |
| Oxymetazoline | Erythemato-telangiectatic | A | FDA-approved in 1% cream form (currently no generic). Note: this is the same ingredient but much higher strength than the OTC nasal decongestant spray (which has mixed anecdotal response) |
| Clindamycin 1% BID | Papulopustular and erythemato-telangiectatic rosacea | B | Unclear if effective even if combined with benzoyl peroxide; very limited data |
| Erythromycin 2% BID | Erythemato-telangiectatic | B | Very limited and weak data, patient-reported measures |
| Permethrin 5% BID | Papulopustular | B | Inconclusive if effective; perhaps if Demodex mites found in abundance on skin scraping |
| Sodium sulfacetamide | Erythema | B | Also helps seborrhea<br>± sulfur formulations, which theoretically might have additional benefit |
| Pimecrolimus 1% BID | Papulopustular | C | Very limited and weak data; rare case reports of rosacea exacerbation |
| Retinoids | Anecdotal reports of papulopustular or erythemato-telangiectatic | C[126] | Can be very irritating to rosacea skin |

(From van Zuuren EJ, Kramer SF, Carter BR, et al. Effective and evidence-based management strategies for rosacea: Summary of a Cochrane systematic review. *Brit J Dermatol.* 2011;165(4):760–781; Del Rosso JQ, Tanghetti E, Webster G, Stein Gold L, Thiboutot D, Gallo RL. Update on the management of rosacea from the American Acne & Rosacea Society (AARS). *J Clin Aesthet Dermatol.* 2019;12 (6):17–24, unless otherwise noted.)

*BID,* Twice a day; *FDA,* US Food and Drug Administration; *LOE,* Level of Evidence; *OTC,* over the counter; *PO,* by mouth; *TID,* three times a day.

caution are advised in patients with chronic kidney disease. Treatment might be considered beyond 72 hours, if additional lesions appear (LOE = D).[135] Treatment with IV antivirals should be considered for all patients with ocular involvement, immunosuppression, suspected meningitis, or sepsis (LOE = D).[12,133] The patient should have contact and respiratory droplet

## TABLE 54.9  Antiviral Treatment Options for Acute Uncomplicated Zoster in Otherwise Immunocompetent Patients

| Regimen | Level of Evidence | Comments |
|---|---|---|
| Acyclovir 800 mg PO five times daily for 1 week[a] | A | It is relatively inexpensive in generic form, but the dosing frequency can be cumbersome<br>Some evidence suggests famciclovir and valacyclovir might be superior[136] |
| Famciclovir 500 mg PO TID for 1 week[a] | A | Prodrug of penciclovir<br>Available as generic |
| Valacyclovir 1000 mg PO TID for 1 week[a] | A | Prodrug of acyclovir<br>Available as generic |

*PO*, By mouth; *TID*, three times a day.

[a]Dose adjustment for renal insufficiency is required.

precautions, particularly around unvaccinated, pregnant, or immunosuppressed individuals (LOE = D).[133]

Acute zoster pain management can be challenging, and there are limited data. Some experts recommend nonsteroids or acetaminophen for milder pain; and careful consideration of opioids for more severe pain.[137] There is limited evidence that systemic steroids might reduce acute pain, but it does not prevent subsequent postherpetic neuralgia (PHN, see later section).[138] It is the author's opinion that the potential risks of systemic steroids in older adults probably do not justify routinely prescribing in acute pain (LOE = D). Current data do not support the use of gabapentin for acute pain management or for preventing PHN.[139,140] There are insufficient data to routinely recommend tricyclic antidepressants or other antiepileptics.

For postexposure prophylaxis in certain high-risk patients (e.g., immunosuppressed, not vaccinated), passive immunization with FDA-approved varicella immunoglobulin (VARIZIG) can be considered 96 hours (possibly up to 10 days) after exposure to provide passive immunity (LOE = D). This form replaces VZIG and is much more widely available than its predecessor.

Several complications of zoster are worth noting to ensure antiviral therapy without delay and specialty consultation when appropriate, regardless of duration of rash (LOE = D).[141] These include neurologic impairment (e.g., Ramsay Hunt syndrome, meningoencephalitis) or viral hepatitis.[12] Hutchinson sign, or zoster rash affecting the nasal tip or sidewall, and eye redness are highly suggestive of ophthalmic involvement (LOE = C).[141,142]

## TABLE 54.10  Selected Treatment Options for Postherpetic Neuralgia

| Regimen | Level of Evidence | Comments |
|---|---|---|
| Gabapentin, pregabalin | A | FDA-approved<br>Sedation can be limiting side effect<br>Caution with renal insufficiency<br>Response may take up to 2 weeks |
| Topical capsaicin | A[a] | [a]FDA-approved capsaicin 8% patch; potential challenges of in-clinic application[144]<br>For lower concentration creams (not FDA-approved), a systematic review found no statistically significant pain reduction percentage but almost one-quarter withdrawal because of adverse effect[149] |
| Topical lidocaine | A[150] | FDA-approved in patch form |
| Tricyclic antidepressants (amitriptyline, desipramine, nortriptyline) | A[151] | Pain reduced, but potential side effects must be considered, especially with tertiary amines (amitriptyline, doxepin) |
| Opiates | C | Controversial, mixed evidence; difficult to determine if benefits outweigh risks, particularly for long-term use[144,152] |
| Acetaminophen | X[144] | |
| Acupuncture | X | |
| Antiviral therapy | X[144] | |
| Nonsteroidal antiinflammatory drugs | X[144] | |

*FDA*, US Food and Drug Administration.

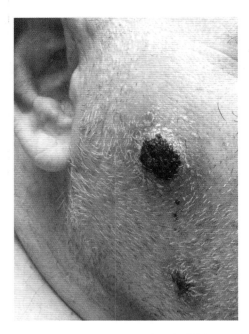

• **Figure 54.33** Hemorrhagic crusting (scab). (With permission from University of Utah Department of Dermatology). See Test question 1: What is the primary lesion?

◆◆ **PHN is a debilitating chronic neuropathic pain condition that can persist for months to years after zoster rash resolution. PHN occurs most commonly in older patients with zoster, probably as a function of immunosenescence.**

PHN is a dreaded, debilitating chronic neuropathic pain condition that persists for at least 3 months after zoster rash resolution. PHN risk factors include the initial severity of the zoster acute pain and rash, chronic conditions, or immunosuppressed states, such as diabetes or pulmonary disease, and advanced age.[143,144] Zoster vaccination is considered the first-line prevention of PHN. In the minority of vaccinated patients who still develop zoster, some data suggest subsequent PHN might be associated with less severe pain in women.[145] A Cochrane review did not support the following practices in preventing PHN after zoster rash resolution: antivirals, systemic steroids, and vaccination.[131,138,146,147]

PHN medical treatment options are listed in Table 54.10. In severe, refractory cases, consider referral to a pain or neurosurgery clinic to discuss sympathetic block, spinal cord stimulators, or other procedures (LOE = C).[148]

## Summary

◆◆ **Dermatologic problems are common chief complaints in the primary care of older patients. Incorporating a skin examination during the primary care provider's routine examination is important for formulating a differential diagnosis.**

Dermatologic problems are common chief complaints in the primary care of older patients.[153] Tips for incorporating a skin examination during the primary care provider's routine physical examination were discussed, in addition to a simple and systematic method of succinctly describing dermatologic findings. These skills are important to help formulate a differential diagnosis and triage patients appropriately. Several common, benign

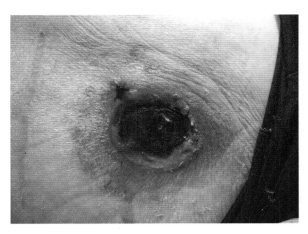

• **Figure 54.34** Eschar. (From University of Utah Department of Dermatology. With permission.)

### CASE 1

#### Discussion

Primary care providers see the bulk of dermatologic problems and are well equipped to manage the majority. When a lesion or rash is unknown or not responding as expected to treatment, accurately and succinctly describing the cutaneous examination findings to the specialist is paramount to triage the patient. For the lesion that was in question (see Fig. 54.2), the patient was urgently seen and diagnosed as having a pyogenic granuloma (benign vascular lesion) that was surgically removed.

### CASE 2

#### Discussion

Although most cases of pruritus in older patients are caused by xerosis and correcting this is a reasonable step, new onset pruritus in geriatric patients should not be ignored. When abrupt in onset, the practitioner should inquire about new medications, personal products, or infestations. However, when an obvious trigger is not elicited or the process is more subacute, focused history and examination can help identify secondary causes. It can be helpful to categorize itch as being associated with or without rash. Generalized pruritus that is intractable and awakens the patient at night should push the clinician to search for an occult metabolic, endocrine, or malignant process.

lesions associated with aging were reviewed; proper diagnosis can spare patients from unnecessary referrals, delay in care, and anxiety. Eczematous skin conditions are common in geriatric patients, and practical recommendations for treatment, including choosing appropriate steroid potency, vehicle, and size, can be helpful to improve patient outcome and minimize preventable side effects. Skin premalignancies and malignancies tend to increase with age, and management options for the more common conditions were summarized. Although pruritus can be caused by simply dry skin, other not-to-miss differential diagnoses were discussed. Common inflammatory skin conditions of aging were reviewed. Lastly, the impact and evidence-based prevention and management of herpes zoster and PHN were discussed.

## Web Resources

American Academy of Dermatology core curriculum. Useful for review of general dermatology topics; good resource for students or non-dermatologists: https://www.aad.org/education/basic-derm-curriculum.

DermNet NZ. New Zealand Dermatological Society online reference of clinical photos; includes diagnostic and management synopses: http://dermnetnz.org.

VisualDX. Web or smartphone-based application to create dermatologic differential diagnoses. Available for free at many institutions, including Veterans Affairs hospitals (under clinical tools): www.visualdx.com.

## Key Reference

12. Bolognia J, Jorizzo JL, Rapini RP. Dermatology. 2nd ed. St. Louis, Mo.: Mosby/Elsevier; 2008.

*References available online at* expertconsult.com.

# Index

Page numbers followed by *f* indicate figures; *t*, tables; *b*, boxes.